ACSM's
Clinical Exercise Physiology

Second Edition

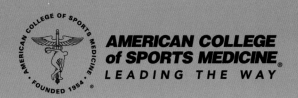

AMERICAN COLLEGE
of SPORTS MEDICINE®
LEADING THE WAY

ACSM's
Clinical Exercise
Physiology

Second Edition

EDITORS

Walter R. Thompson, PhD, FACSM, ACSM-CEP, RCEP, PD

Regents' Professor Emeritus and
 Associate Dean
College of Education & Human Development
Georgia State University
Atlanta, Georgia

Cemal Ozemek, PhD, FACSM, ACSM-CEP

Clinical Associate Professor, Director — Doctor
 of Clinical Exercise Physiology Program
Department of Physical Therapy
University of Illinois at Chicago
Chicago, Illinois

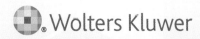
®. Wolters Kluwer

Philadelphia • Baltimore • New York • London
Buenos Aires • Hong Kong • Sydney • Tokyo

Acquisitions Editor: Lindsey Porambo
Senior Development Editor: Amy Millholen
Editorial Coordinator: Nancy Dickson
Marketing Manager: Danielle Klahr
Production Project Manager: Nancy Devaux
Design Coordinator: Stephen Druding
Manufacturing Coordinator: Margie Orzech
Compositor: S4Carlisle Publishing Services

ACSM Publications Committee Chair: Karyn L. Hamilton, PhD, RD, FACSM
ACSM Certification-Related Content Advisory Committee Chair: Daniel L. Carl, PhD, FACSM
ACSM Chief Operating Officer: Katie Feltman
ACSM Assistant Director of Publishing: Angie Chastain

Second Edition

Library of Congress Cataloging-in-Publication Data

ISBN-13: 978-1-9751-9679-0
ISBN-10: 1-975196-79-1

Library of Congress Control Number: 2023915107

DISCLAIMER

Care has been taken to confirm the accuracy of the information present and to describe generally accepted practices. However, the authors, editors, and publisher are not responsible for errors or omissions or for any consequences from application of the information in this publication and make no warranty, expressed or implied, with respect to the currency, completeness, or accuracy of the contents of the publication. Application of this information in a particular situation remains the professional responsibility of the practitioner; the clinical treatments described and recommended may not be considered absolute and universal recommendations.

The authors, editors, and publisher have exerted every effort to ensure that drug selection and dosage set forth in this text are in accordance with the current recommendations and practice at the time of publication. However, in view of ongoing research, changes in government regulations, and the constant flow of information relating to drug therapy and drug reactions, the reader is urged to check the package insert for each drug for any change in indications and dosage and for added warnings and precautions. This is particularly important when the recommended agent is a new or infrequently employed drug.

Some drugs and medical devices presented in this publication have Food and Drug Administration (FDA) clearance for limited use in restricted research settings. It is the responsibility of the health care provider to ascertain the FDA status of each drug or device planned for use in their clinical practice.

To purchase additional copies of this book, call our customer service department at (800) 638-3030 or fax orders to (301) 223-2320. International customers should call (301) 223-2300.

For more information concerning the American College of Sports Medicine certification and suggested preparatory materials, call (800) 486-5643 or visit the American College of Sports Medicine Website at www.acsm.org.

shop.lww.com

QUADM1023

Dedication

This book is first dedicated to the pioneers in clinical exercise physiology, several of whom were my teachers and mentors, all of them lifelong friends.

To Paul Ribisl who, when recruiting for the first graduate exercise science class at Wake Forest University in 1978, took a big chance on a not-so-good student.

To Henry Miller who taught me (among many other things) venipuncture techniques and when I finally was successful gave me a high five. Both of us forgot the needle was still in the arm of my volunteer. She didn't bleed to death, but it was close. She married me anyway.

To the late Ed Fox, my major professor and dissertation advisor at The Ohio State University, who passed away — far too young.

To Noel Nequin, who in 1979 was searching for a director for his program and, after calling Phil Wilson at the University of Wisconsin — LaCrosse (who had no candidates), called Paul Ribisl at Wake Forest (who had one student graduating that semester). Luckily that person was me, and we remain great friends to this day.

To Dan Benardot who recruited me to Georgia State University and taught me how to work with and assess elite athletes including gold medal–winning Olympic teams. He also became one of my closest friends. We traveled the world together both professionally and with our families. It was an honor to have served as Best Man at his wedding to Robin.

To Yves Vanlandewijck of Leuven, Belgium, who introduced me in 1995 to his work with athletes who had physical or intellectual impairments. Since that time, we have served together on the Sports Science Committee of the International Paralympic Committee (IPC), traveled around the world, coordinating research projects at IPC-sanctioned events, including Paralympic Games, and edited two books together that are part of the IOC series. He also skillfully extracted me from a ravine after a very bad snowmobile accident in Whistler, Canada, on March 19, 2010.

Finally, this book is dedicated to my family: to Deon, my wife of 45 years; my daughter Jessica and her husband Daniel; my son Aaron and his wife Joellyn; and to the four most amazing grandchildren in the world, Alison, Annalee, Kinsley, and Andy. All of you inspire me every day to be the greatest husband, father, and Papaw. I love all of you more than you can imagine.

Walter R. Thompson, PhD, FACSM, ACSM-CEP, RCEP, PD

To my mentors, Pete Brubaker, Lenny Kaminsky, Kerrie Moreau, and Ross Arena. Each of these incredible individuals has had a profound impact on not only my growth as a professional but most importantly as a person. Despite their renowned professional achievements and international recognition, each is as humble as the next and has always made time for me regardless of their inconceivable workloads. They serve as my North Star and I am honored to be able to refer to them as close colleagues and lifelong friends.

Most of all, this book is for my parents, Sera and Haluk, and sister, Hale, for being a strong and supportive presence throughout my life; to my dear wife and colleague, Hannah, for showing limitless patience (…can't express that enough) and unwavering support through my academic and life pursuits; and to my daughter Lillian, who is a constant reminder of what is truly important in life and has the ability to dissolve any work-related stress as soon as I see her bright smile. My accomplishments to date would not have been possible without the love and guidance they provided in every stage of my life.

Cemal Ozemek, PhD, FACSM, ACSM-CEP

Contributors

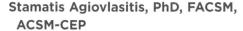

Stamatis Agiovlasitis, PhD, FACSM, ACSM-CEP
Mississippi State University
Mississippi State, Mississippi
Chapter 12

Kevin D. Ballard, PhD, FACSM
Miami University
Oxford, Ohio
Chapter 17

J.P. Barfield, FACSM
University of North Carolina Charlotte
Charlotte, North Carolina
Chapter 12

Melissa J. Benton, PhD, RN, FACSM
University of Colorado — Colorado Springs
Colorado Springs, Colorado
Chapter 2

Barry Braun, PhD, FACSM
Colorado State University
Fort Collins, Colorado
Chapter 10

Natasha T. Brison, JD, PhD
Texas A&M University
College Station, Texas
Chapter 19

Katie M. Brown, PhD
Texas Tech University
Lubbock, Texas
Chapter 19

Peter H. Brubaker, PhD, FACSM
Wake Forest University
Winston-Salem, North Carolina
Chapter 5

Kristin L. Campbell, BSc, PT, PhD, FACSM
University of British Columbia
Vancouver, British Columbia, Canada
Chapter 13

Heather Chambliss, PhD, FACSM
St. Jude Children's Research Hospital
Memphis, Tennessee
Chapter 15

Brian Coyne, MEd, ACSM-CEP, ACSM/NCHPAD-CIFT, RCEP
Duke University Health System
Durham, North Carolina
Chapter 7

Melanie Cree, MD, PhD
University of Colorado Anschutz
Aurora, Colorado
Chapter 10

Bhibha M. Das, PhD, MPH, FACSM
East Carolina University
Greenville, North Carolina
Chapter 4

Sonja de Groot, PhD
Reade & Vrije Universiteit
Amsterdam, the Netherlands
Chapter 12

Gregory B. Dwyer, PhD, FACSM, ACSM-CEP, EIM, RCEP, ETT
East Stroudsburg University
East Stroudsburg, Pennsylvania
Chapter 1

Tim Edwards, MS, ACSM-CEP, EIM
Arkansas Children's Nutrition Center
Little Rock, Arkansas
Chapter 6

Ellen M. Evans, PhD, FACSM
Indiana University
Bloomington, Indiana
Chapter 4

Bradley S. Fleenor, PhD
Ball State University
Muncie, Indiana
Chapter 5

Judy Foxworth, PT, PhD, OCS
Winston-Salem State University
Winston-Salem, North Carolina
Chapter 11

Ginny M. Frederick, PhD
University of Georgia
Athens, Georgia
Chapter 4

Matthew S. Ganio, PhD, FACSM
University of Arkansas
Fayetteville, Arkansas
Chapter 17

Carol Ewing Garber, PhD, FACSM, ACSM-CEP, ACSM-EP, ETT, PD, RCEP, EIM
Teachers College, Columbia University
New York, New York
Chapter 3

Matthew P. Harber, PhD, FACSM
Ball State University
Muncie, Indiana
Chapter 5

Sandra K. Knecht, MS, ACSM-CEP, RCEP
Cincinnati Children's Hospital, Ohio
Cincinnati, Ohio
Chapter 9

Shel Levine, MS, ACSM-CEP
Eastern Michigan University
Ypsilanti, Michigan
Chapter 7

J. Timothy Lightfoot, PhD, FACSM, ACSM-CEP, RCEP
Texas A&M University
College Station, Texas
Chapter 18

Laurie A. Malone, PhD, MPH, FACSM
University of Alabama at Birmingham
Birmingham, Alabama
Chapter 12

Carrie McLean, PhD
MGH Institute of Health Professions
Boston, Massachusetts
Chapter 10

Monique Middlekauff, PhD, ACSMCEP, RCEP, EIM
St. Luke's Health System
Twin Falls, Idaho
Chapter 16

A. Lynn Millar, PT, PhD, FACSM
Winston-Salem State University
Winston-Salem, North Carolina
Chapter 11

Jaime M. Moore, MD, MPH
University of Colorado School of Medicine
Aurora, Colorado
Chapter 10

David C. Nieman, DrPH, FACSM
Appalachian State University
Kannapolis, North Carolina
Chapter 14

Stacey A. Reading, PhD
University of Auckland
Auckland, New Zealand
Chapter 8

Laura A. Richardson, PhD, FACSM, ACSM-CEP, RCEP
University of Michigan
Ann Arbor, Michigan
Chapter 9

Deborah Riebe, PhD, FACSM, ACSM-EP
University of Rhode Island
Kingston, Rhode Island
Chapter 3

Kathryn H. Schmitz, PhD, MPH, FACSM
University of Pittsburgh
Pittsburgh, Pennsylvania
Chapter 13

Kevin R. Short, PhD, FACSM
University of Oklahoma Health Sciences Center
Oklahoma City, Oklahoma
Chapter 2

Erica M. Taylor, PhD, FACSM
Columbus State University
Columbus, Georgia
Chapter 15

Sean Walsh, PhD, FACSM
Central Connecticut State University
New Britain, Connecticut
Chapter 1

Christie L. Ward-Ritacco, PhD, FACSM, ACSM-EP
University of Rhode Island
Kingston, Rhode Island
Chapter 3

Emma W. White, PT, DPT, OCS
Winston-Salem State University
Winston-Salem, North Carolina
Chapter 11

Kerri Winters-Stone, PhD, FACSM
Oregon Health & Science University
Portland, Oregon
Chapter 13

Reviewers

Eddie Davila, MS, ACSM-CEP, ACSM-EP
Urban Fitness
Bozeman, Montana

Glen Davison, PhD
University of Kent
Canterbury, United Kingdom

Kurt A. Escobar, PhD
California State University, Long Beach
Long Beach, California

Bo Fernhall, PhD, FACSM
University of Massachusetts Boston
Boston, Massachusetts

Ron Hager, PhD
Brigham Young University
Provo, Utah

**Trent A. Hargens, PhD, FACSM,
  ACSM-CEP, EIM**
James Madison University
Harrisonburg, Virginia

Brian P. Heermance, Esq.
Morrison Mahoney, LLP
New York, New York

Ira Jacobs, DrMedSc, FACSM
University of Toronto
Toronto, Ontario, Canada

Gary W. Mack, PhD, FACSM
Brigham Young University
Provo, Utah

Steven K. Malin, PhD, FACSM
Rutgers University
New Brunswick, New Jersey

Mindy M. Mayol, PhD, ACSM-EP
University of Indianapolis
Indianapolis, Indiana

Laurie A. Milliken, PhD, FACSM
University of Massachusetts Boston
Boston, Massachusetts

R. Andrew Shanely, PhD
Appalachian State University
Boone, North Carolina

**Pat R. Vehrs, PhD, FACSM, ACSM-CEP,
  ACSM-EP, ETT, PD**
Brigham Young University
Provo, Utah

Joseph R. Visker, PhD, ACSM-CEP
The University of Utah
Salt Lake City, Utah

Ashley Wishman, ACSM-CEP, ACSM-EP, EIM
Bozeman Health
Bozeman, Montana

Foreword to the First Edition

For many years, the American College of Sports Medicine (ACSM) has been a leader in the training and certification of clinical exercise physiologists (CEPs). The history is impressive and has led to the publication of this landmark book, the first edition of *ACSM's Clinical Exercise Physiology*. On May 2, 1972, at the annual meeting of ACSM in Philadelphia, a special interest group was convened, and it recommended that ACSM initiate definitive guidelines for the conduct of exercise testing and prescription; in December 1972 at a workshop in Aspen, Colorado, a subcommittee presented their first thoughts. Physicians, physiologists, and physical educators, representing 32 laboratories from 19 states and 3 Canadian provinces, reviewed the proposed guidelines, and in 1975, the first edition of *ACSM's Guidelines for Exercise Testing and Exercise Prescription* was published. Dr. John Faulkner, the 15th president of the ACSM (1971–1972), and Dr. Karl Stoedefalke are credited as chairs of that publication, which numbered 48 pages. The Behavioral Objectives appearing in that first edition were an initial attempt to define the role of what would become the CEP. *Guidelines*, now in its 10th edition at 472 pages, no longer contains the Behavioral Objectives. Now known as Performance Domains and Associated Job Tasks, they are so comprehensive that they are accessed as an online adjunct of *Guidelines* (https://www.acsm.org/get-stay-certified).

We have come a long way from that first edition. The role of the CEP in medical practices; in commercial, community, and medical fitness centers; and in corporate wellness programs has now been well defined. Today the CEP is an integral member of the team, providing continuous care to patients and the apparently healthy. They work side by side with physicians, nurses, physical therapists, occupational therapists, nutritionists, and other members of the health care team. ACSM's support certifications to prepare and accredit the CEP include the Exercise Physiologist, CEP, and Registered CEP. This book, *ACSM's Clinical Exercise Physiology*, will help build the foundation of knowledge necessary to be successful in clinical exercise physiology courses and to sit for these certification examinations.

Dr. Walt Thompson, the 61st president of the ACSM (2017–2018), has assembled a remarkable team of scientists and clinicians to write this first edition. Within these 19 chapters are the foundations for the science of clinical exercise physiology. The book should be used in advanced undergraduate and graduate exercise science curricula in colleges and universities. It should also be found on the bookshelves of every clinician and exercise professional around the world. It is, clearly, the most comprehensive clinical exercise physiology book in print. Having served as presidents of ACSM, we congratulate Dr. Thompson and his writing team for assembling this impressive, inspiring, and remarkable resource for exercise physiology and its clinical applications.

Howard G. Knuttgen	1973–1974
Charles M. Tipton	1974–1975
Roy J. Shephard	1975–1976
David L. Costill	1976–1977
James S. Skinner	1979–1980
David R. Lamb	1980–1981
Henry S. Miller, Jr.	1981–1982
William L. Haskell	1983–1984
Peter B. Raven	1987–1988
Barbara L. Drinkwater	1988–1989
Lyle J. Micheli	1989–1990
Neil B. Oldridge	1990–1991
Brian J. Sharkey	1991–1992
Robert C. Cantu	1992–1993
Russell R. Pate	1993–1994
Timothy P. White	1994–1995
Steven N. Blair	1996–1997
Charlotte A. Tate	1997–1998
Paul D. Thompson	1998–1999
Barry A. Franklin	1999–2000
Angela D. Smith	2001–2002
Edward T. Howley	2002–2003

W. Larry Kenney	2003–2004	William W. Dexter	2013–2014
William O. Roberts	2004–2005	Carol Ewing Garber	2014–2015
Carl Foster	2005–2006	Lawrence E. Armstrong	2015–2016
J. Larry Durstine	2006–2007	Elizabeth Joy	2016–2017
Robert E. Sallis	2007–2008	Kathryn H. Schmitz	2018–2019
Melinda Millard-Stafford	2008–2009	William E. Kraus	2019–2020
James M. Pivarnik	2009–2010	NiCole R. Keith	2020–2021
Thomas M. Best	2010–2011	L. Bruce Gladden	2021–2022
Barbara E. Ainsworth	2011–2012	Anastasia Fischer	2022–2023
Janet Walberg Rankin	2012–2013	Irene Davis	2023–2024

Foreword to the Second Edition

As international organization presidents dedicated to the advancement of clinical exercise physiology, we are pleased to write this Foreword to the second edition of *ACSM's Clinical Exercise Physiology*. Echoing the words of the former ACSM presidents who authored the Foreword to the first edition, we believe that the role of the clinical exercise physiologist (CEP) is well defined all over the world. They are now a recognized part of the health care team taking care of patients with a variety of both acute and chronic illnesses. Although the history of clinical exercise physiology may be in cardiac rehabilitation and pulmonary rehabilitation, today's CEP helps in the treatment plan of patients with diabetes, metabolic syndrome, peripheral arterial disease, and many other disease states that can benefit from therapeutic exercise programs. Outside of rehabilitation, the CEP also plays a vital role in the prevention of chronic disease and disability. Contemporary CEPs can be found in hospitals and medical centers, physician's office and clinics, as well as in commercial, community, corporate, and medical fitness centers.

Dr. Walt Thompson and Dr. Cemal Ozemek have recruited the world's experts to contribute to this second edition. All 19 chapters are relevant to the practice of clinical exercise physiology and can be applied immediately to CEP practice. We encourage anyone who teaches advanced undergraduate and graduate classes in CEP to consider using this extraordinary text in their classrooms. The text and ancillaries (question bank, videos, journal activities, slide decks, test bank and image bank) are simply extraordinary. We are pleased to add our names in the support of this second edition of *ACSM's Clinical Exercise Physiology*.

Ash Walker, DHSc, MA, ACSM-CEP, EIM, FAACVPR
President, American Association of Cardiovascular and
 Pulmonary Rehabilitation (AACVPR)

Professor Zoe Knowles, PhD, FBASES
Chair, British Association of Sport and Exercise Sciences
 (BASES)

Guoping Li, MD
President, Chinese Association of Sports Medicine
 (CASM)

Laura J. Newsome, PhD, ACSM-CEP, EIM
President, Clinical Exercise Physiology Association
 (CEPA)

Helen Jones, BSc, PhD
Chair, Clinical Exercise Physiology UK (CEP-UK)

Eleanor Nattrass, MSc, ACSM-CEP, CEPNZ-RCEP
Chair, Clinical Exercise Physiology
New Zealand (CEPNZ)

A. William Sheel, PhD, FACSM
Chair, Canadian Society for Exercise Physiology (CSEP)

Brendan Joss, BSc (Hons), PhD, AEP, ESSAF
President, Exercise & Sports Science Australia (ESSA)

Preface

The concept for *ACSM's Clinical Exercise Physiology* was launched in December 2015 with the approval of the American College of Sports Medicine (ACSM) Publications Committee, Committee on Certification and Registry Boards, Administrative Council, and the Board of Trustees. It had been determined that there was a need to re-envision the existing *ACSM's Resource Manual for Guidelines for Exercise Testing and Prescription* to meet the evolving needs of the field. The *Resource Manual* was originally developed as a comprehensive, explanatory companion text to *ACSM's Guidelines for Exercise Testing and Prescription*. As an outcome of this strategy, two additional resources to be paired with *Guidelines* were recommended for development and were to be called: *ACSM's Exercise Testing and Prescription* and *ACSM's Clinical Exercise Physiology*. Authors of the current book have provided thorough updates within each chapter to reflect advancements and current best practice recommendations in the respective topic areas.

This book, *ACSM's Clinical Exercise Physiology, 2nd edition*, fulfills a vision to create an advanced undergraduate and graduate textbook that could be used worldwide. International experts were selected to write key chapters, reflecting the work CEPs do every day in hospitals and medical centers; in neighborhood programs like commercial health clubs, corporate wellness programs, university recreation centers; and in not-for-profit family-oriented community fitness centers. Although the book is primarily intended to be used in college and university classrooms, it can also be of benefit to anyone studying for the ACSM Clinical Exercise Physiologist certification.

ORGANIZATION

The logical presentation of material provides a format that can be used over the course of one to two semesters in any college or university offering advanced undergraduate or graduate classes in clinical exercise physiology. Organized in a semisequential manner, the first chapter details the history of clinical exercise physiology. The second chapter provides an overview of the life cycle from birth to death with a special focus on women and children. After these two introductory chapters, the book builds sequentially, each chapter increasingly becoming more independent. Chapters 3 and 4 review the benefits and risks associated with exercise and physical activity and introduce preparticipation health screening, followed by a detailed description of how to develop exercise programs for the apparently healthy client. These chapters provide the foundation for subsequent topics that are more specific, such as cardiovascular disease, respiratory disease, diabetes, physical and intellectual impairments, cancer, diseases and conditions of the bones and joints, immunological disorders, and behavior and mental health as they relate to exercise. Chapter 16 focuses on multiple disorders (co- or multimorbidities), followed by environmental and genetic impacts. The final chapter describes and outlines potential legal issues facing the CEP.

FEATURES

Several features of this book distinguish it from other clinical exercise physiology books available today. First, there is **a single chapter dedicated to electrocardiography** written specifically for the CEP. Many electrocardiography books are written by and for clinicians, but seldom are there any directed to what the CEP might encounter during exercise testing or in a rehabilitation program. The electrocardiography chapter focuses primarily on those conditions typically seen by the CEP and does not include obscure, confusing, or abstruse conditions. Included also are many examples that can be used for review purposes. A second unique feature is **chapter review questions** (with answers) and **case studies**. Most of the chapters have multiple case studies, but what makes this unique is that each has accompanying **review questions** and short answers.

ADDITIONAL RESOURCES

Additional resources are available with purchase of Lippincott Connect.

Student Resources:

- Question Bank
- Videos
- ECG Animations

Instructor Resources:

- PowerPoints
- Test Bank
- Image Bank
- Answers to Text Questions

See inside the front cover of this text for more details.

Updates for the book can be found at https://www.acsm.org/education-resources/books/acsm-book-updates.

Acknowledgments to the Second Edition

Much appreciation should be noted to many groups and individuals for the concept, development, writing, and future success of the first and second editions of this book. Any omission of appreciation is entirely our fault. First, thanks to the ACSM Publications Committee, Committee on Certification and Registry Boards, Administrative Council, and the Board of Trustees for having the vision to recognize the potential significance of this book to ACSM and to college classrooms worldwide. Second, thanks to our publisher, Wolters Kluwer, who took a chance on this book and then put every available resource into making it the very best it could be. The superior quality of this book and its ancillary materials are attributable to our publisher, who believed in the project even more than we did, and for that we are grateful. ACSM is thankful and appreciates that each author worked hard with considerable investment of their personal resources and time — time they could have spent with family and friends. This book is an example of the collective efforts of an incredibly talented and dedicated writing team. We have tested the patience, benevolence, generosity, and goodwill of many people during the course of this project. For that, we would like to personally thank each author, ACSM Chief Operating Officer Katie Feltman, ACSM Assistant Director of Publishing Angie Chastain, Wolters Kluwer Senior Development Editor Amy Millholen, and our development editor Laura Bonazzoli, the incredibly talented word magician for the first edition who crafted the language and phrasing just right. This book could not have been possible without the four of them. We would also like to thank the present and past presidents of ACSM who agreed to author the Foreword for the first edition and to the president of all the major clinical exercise physiology professional societies around the world who agreed to author the Foreword for this second edition. They are all heroes of ours. Finally, we would like to thank our families, who often wondered why husband, Dad, Papaw would suddenly disappear, later to be found pounding at the keyboard during brief moments of inspiration. Walt thanks Deon, Jessica, Aaron, Daniel, Joellyn, Alison, Annalee, Kinsley, Andy, and Molly (the Thompson dog who probably showed the greatest patience). Cemal firstly thanks Walt for inviting and trusting him to serve as an editor. It was a career high point to work with you and it was truly impressive watching you conduct this massive undertaking while making it look seemingly effortless. And thank you to Hannah and Lily for their infinite support throughout this process.

Walter R. Thompson, PhD, FACSM, ACSM-CEP, RCEP, PD

Cemal Ozemek, PhD, FACSM, ACSM-CEP

Contents

Clinical Exercise Physiology Roots: Evolution, Professional Practice, and Future

"Lack of activity destroys the good condition of every human being, while movement and methodical physical exercise save it and preserve it." (Plato, a philosopher from ancient Greece, circa 428–347 BCE; note: the years of his birth and death are debated)

"Leave all the afternoon for exercise and recreation, which are as necessary as reading. I will rather say more necessary because health is worth more than learning." (Thomas Jefferson, former U.S. president, 1743–1826)

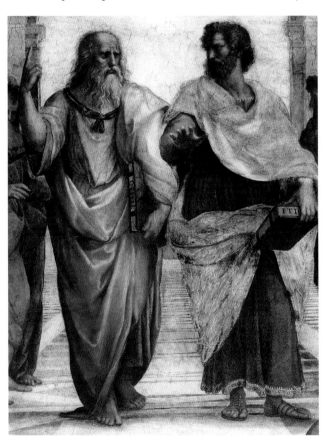

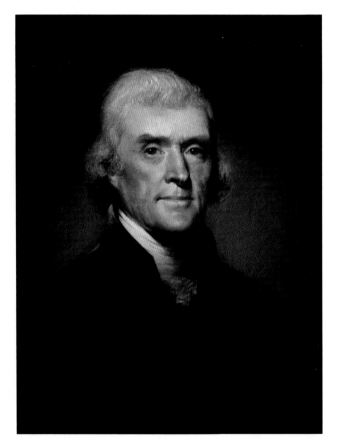

INTRODUCTION

Although no well-documented history has been published to date in peer-reviewed sources, it is clear that clinical exercise physiology evolved from and is a subspecialty of exercise physiology, the roots of which go back to ancient times. This first chapter begins, therefore, by providing a brief glimpse at this extraordinary evolution. It then explores the emergence of clinical exercise physiology in the U.S. and globally around the middle of the 20th century.

In the field's infancy, clinical exercise physiology services were largely provided for patients in hospital-based cardiac rehabilitation programs. Toward the end of the 20th century, health care providers began to recognize the value of clinical exercise physiology services for patients with significant lung disease in pulmonary rehabilitation programs. However, despite a great deal of research and discussion on the application of clinical exercise physiology services to other medical populations (including, but not limited to, patients with diabetes, cancer, and various musculoskeletal diseases and disorders), relatively few reimbursable clinical exercise physiology services are currently recognized. In fact, one goal of this textbook is to demonstrate the breadth of research and education efforts over the years involving the use of clinical exercise physiology with special populations, and thereby to promote its expanded scope of practice, in the hope that one day clinical exercise physiologists (CEPs) become recognized as qualified health care professionals. An important example of this is the ongoing efforts by the American College of Sports Medicine (ACSM; 1), along with other organizations, such as the Physical Activity Alliance, to advance policies leading to the recognition and reimbursement of CEPs and exercise physiologists within health care. In addition, one of ACSM's signature initiatives, Exercise is Medicine (EIM), seeks to make physical activity (PA) assessment and promotion a standard in clinical care, connecting health care with evidence-based PA resources, including professionals, programs, and facilities. Discussed in detail later in this chapter, EIM has attempted to place PA and exercise programming at the forefront of clinical services offered to patients with a variety of chronic diseases and even to apparently healthy patients. As it stands today, EIM offers a professional credentialing program that recognizes exercise professionals who possess the education and skills to work closely with the health care community, which will be seen later in this chapter.

Today, the practicing CEP in the U.S. has an almost unlimited, continuously growing collection of resources available from professional organizations, including textbooks, position stands, and professional certifications (2).

This chapter provides a brief overview of these resources, as well as CEP academic program accreditation and the potential for recognition as qualified health care professionals. The chapter concludes with a look at the future of clinical exercise physiology.

BRIEF HISTORY OF EXERCISE PHYSIOLOGY

To better appreciate the field of clinical exercise physiology, it is important to understand its roots in the broader discipline of exercise physiology. The human body was designed for movement; and a careful analysis of the etiology and pathophysiology of many chronic disease processes reveals an established hypokinetic (*lack of movement*) lifestyle. The primary focus of the clinical exercise physiology profession is the relationship between PA and/or exercise and disease prevention and rehabilitation. As evidenced by the quotations that opened this chapter, this profound relationship was understood and elucidated centuries ago.

Early History

Perhaps the history of exercise and/or PA *began* with the earliest humans on the plains of Africa. As they spread into Asia and Europe, humans tended to aggregate and establish the earliest civilizations near the banks of major rivers. There, these communities transitioned from hunter-gatherer to largely agricultural societies. Unfortunately, a constant threat to early humans was acute infectious and chronic diseases. The ravages of these diseases prompted the earliest attempts at prevention and treatment and a concern for health and hygiene, as well as an ever-changing template for the understanding of disease (3).

In the ancient world, many Indian, Chinese, Arabic, and Greek physicians and scholars were leaders in thinking about the importance of PA and/or exercise. Of these, a few stand out.

The much respected and influential Herodicus (circa 5th century BCE) was a Greek physician and athlete who used exercise in the treatment of disease (Figure 1.1). He is thought to have been a teacher of Hippocrates (circa 460–370 BCE), who is one of the key figures in the history of medicine. Hippocrates is strongly associated with a collection of more than 60 texts related to Greek medicine that are known as the *Corpus Hippocraticum* (Figure 1.2). He was responsible for separating medicine from superstition, religion, and magic and for the emergence of a more rational medicine. For this, he is often known as the father

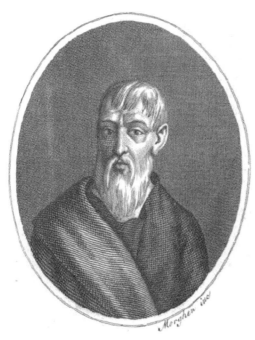

FIGURE 1.1 Herodicus (a Roman copy [2nd century CE] of a Greek bust of Herodicus from the first half of the 4th century BCE). (Available from: https://en.wikipedia.org/wiki/Herodotus#/media/File:Herodotos_Met_91.8.jpg)

of scientific medicine. He felt that PA and/or exercise was necessary in the prevention, treatment, and management of many diseases. Concerning the need for proper food and exercise to maintain a healthy state, he advised, "Food alone will not keep a man well. He must also take exercise.

For food and exercise, while possessing opposite qualities, work together to produce health." He also stated that excesses of either activity or inactivity could cause diseases, and that "those due to exercise are cured by rest, and those due to idleness are cured by exercise." Although these statements are centuries old, they clearly can be argued as the basis for clinical exercise physiology. To Hippocrates, exercise meant walking, running, wrestling, swinging the arms, push-ups, shadow boxing, and ball punching at a moderate intensity. Hippocrates was also one of the first to prescribe an amount of exercise for good health (3).

Galen (131–201 CE), a Greek physician, prolific researcher, and writer, lived several centuries after the time of Hippocrates (Figure 1.3). In addition to conducting several scientific experiments to learn more about the human body, he wrote a variety of medical treatises, including one on exercise that clearly hints at a continuum of exercise from light to moderate to vigorous. Interestingly, this concept of the continuum of exercise and the benefits of vigorous exercise are still being explored today.

Another influential figure in the ancient history of exercise and medicine is Sushruta from India (circa 6th century BCE), who recognized the prevention of diseases with physical exercise. In the Middle Ages, Avicenna from Persia (980–1037) wrote 40 texts on medicine and is considered by some to be the father of modern medicine. Many scientists from the Renaissance contributed to the evolution of exercise physiology, including the artist and

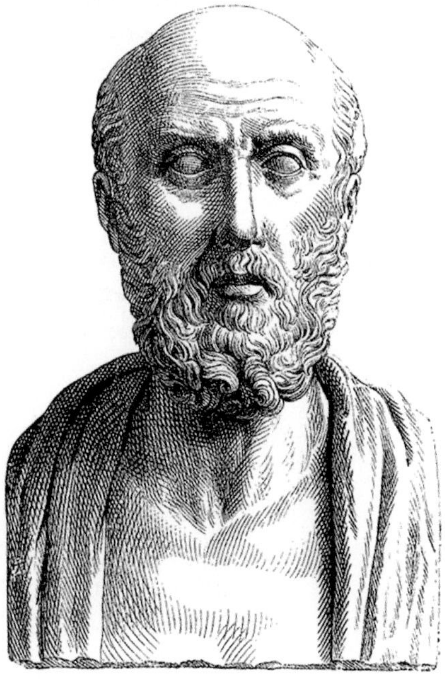

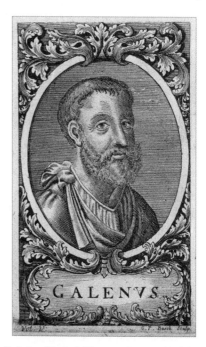

FIGURE 1.2 Hippocrates (From Young Persons' Cyclopedia of Persons and Places. Available from: https://commons.wikimedia.org/wiki/File:Hippocrates.jpg).

FIGURE 1.3 Galen (From 18th-century portrait of Galen by Georg Paul. Busch. Available from: http://www.wikiwand.com/en/Galen).

citizen scientist Leonardo Di Vinci (1452–1519), who explored human anatomy and movement through his art (3).

Development in the 19th and 20th Centuries

In the 19th century, several colleges and universities established academic programs in exercise physiology. One of the first began at Amherst College in Massachusetts in the 1860s. There, Edward Hitchcock and his son, Edward Hitchcock, Jr., developed a rudimentary exercise physiology program that included anthropometric studies and required exercises for all Amherst undergraduates. Edward Hitchcock, Jr. (Figure 1.4) continued the efforts of his father by having Amherst serve as a model for college physical education programs in the U.S. and globally. The initiatives at Amherst College also included the development of a formalized curriculum and a textbook in exercise physiology. Other colleges and universities around the U.S. and world would soon follow suit.

In 1927, David Bruce Dill (Figure 1.5) helped establish a research agenda in applied physiology at the Harvard Fatigue Laboratory located at Harvard University (Figure 1.6). This laboratory was active through 1946 and, during its two decades, produced close to 500 research

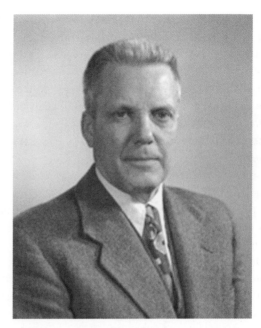

FIGURE 1.5 David Bruce Dill. (Used with permission from the American Physiological Society. Available from: http://www.the-aps.org/fm/About/presidents/introdbd.html)

publications establishing the early roots of exercise physiology. In fact, many of the early researchers in exercise physiology could trace their roots back to the Harvard Fatigue Laboratory (3).

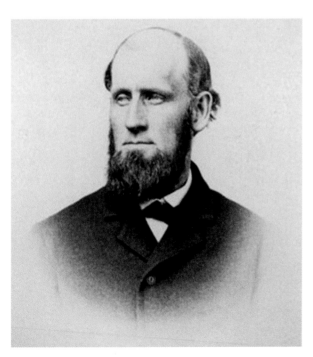

FIGURE 1.4 Dr. Edward Hitchcock, Jr. (Used with permission from Amherst College. Available from: https://www.amherst.edu/news/news_releases/2011/08/node/337711/.)

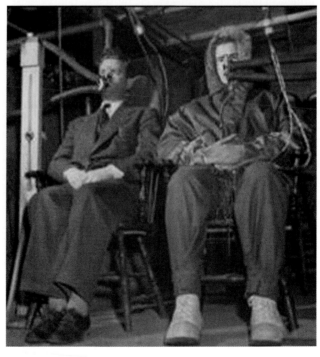

FIGURE 1.6 Fatigue Lab testing clothing. (From HBS Archives Photograph Collection, Baker Library, Harvard Business School [olvwork375058].)

Two decades later, in Europe, Per-Olof Åstrand (Figure 1.7) came into prominence in this early field of exercise physiology. Åstrand earned his PhD at the medical school at the Karolinska Institute in Sweden in 1952. From 1977 to 1988, he served as professor of physiology at the Karolinska Institute. His seminal *Textbook of Work Physiology* has been translated into eight languages and has been revised several times, and he and his many colleagues are credited with hundreds of research publications in the areas of work physiology, the human oxygen transport system, physical performance, health and fitness, preventive medicine, and rehabilitation. Åstrand is often considered one of the founding fathers of modern exercise physiology (3).

During the 20th century, departments of physical education became established in U.S. and international universities and provided leadership for exercise physiology instruction and research. By 1960, exercise physiology was entrenched in departments of physical education, and courses in biomechanics, motor learning, exercise physiology, and therapeutic exercise were being offered on a regular basis. Over the next two decades, graduate programs in physical education at many major institutions in the U.S. and around the world had a marked effect on the emergence and acceptance of exercise physiology as an academic discipline (4). As specialization increased, many departments of physical education split into departments of exercise science, kinesiology, movement sciences, or a combination thereof. This enhanced the scientific image, acceptance, and identity of this area of specialization without changing its character.

Development of Contemporary Clinical Exercise Physiology

Contemporary clinical exercise physiology began to enter the mainstream when the term *aerobics* was popularized by the flight physician and author Kenneth Cooper (Figure 1.8).

Dr. Cooper wrote an important series of books directed at the layperson, including the popular 1968 book titled *Aerobics* (3). In his 1970 text, *The New Aerobics*, Dr. Cooper stated that "countless people in every walk of life have found aerobics a workable way to achieve new levels of physical competence and personal wellbeing." This statement is almost a foreshadowing of what experts in this field would later state, particularly as it related to clinical exercise physiology. Dr. Cooper also went on to establish the world-renowned Cooper Aerobics Center in Dallas, Texas (3). Around this time, regular exercise was shown to be important to maintaining optimal health, whereas prolonged bed rest was found to be associated with marked loss of exercise capacity. Many clinical pioneers in this early discipline, such as Herman Hellerstein (Figure 1.9), demonstrated that

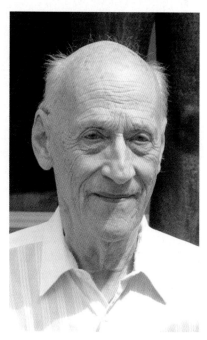

FIGURE 1.7 Per-Olof Åstrand. (Used with permission of The Swedish School of Sport and Health Sciences. Available from: http://www.gih.se/Nyheter/2015/Minnesstund-for-Per-Olof-Astrand/.)

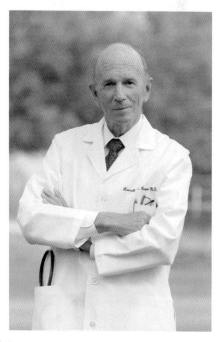

FIGURE 1.8 Dr. Kenneth H. Cooper, MD, MPH. (Used with permission of The Cooper Institute. Available from: http://www.cooperinstitute.org/research/.)

bed rest was detrimental to people with heart disease who were recovering from a myocardial infarction. Dr. Hellerstein and Dr. James Naughton and Irving Mohler published a new textbook in 1973, titled *Exercise Testing and Exercise Training in Coronary Heart Disease* (5). These early findings and work in the field gave way to the development and subsequent proliferation of cardiac rehabilitation programs throughout the 1970s and into the 1990s. Although there were several pioneers in this effort, many historians credit Dr. Hellerstein with the development of the first structured exercise rehabilitation program for cardiac patients (3).

Although exercise physiology had been an academic discipline from the time of the 1960s, it was not yet recognized as a profession (6). During these early years, exercise physiologists were either physicians or scientists with PhD degrees or some other form of advanced training. Several of these pioneers of the 1960s can trace their roots to the academic training and research studies conducted in the laboratory of T. K. Cureton at the University of Illinois (Figure 1.10). In the early 1970s, the question of "What is an exercise physiologist?" began to be discussed. The consensus of ACSM members at that time defined the exercise physiologist as a "doctoral-level

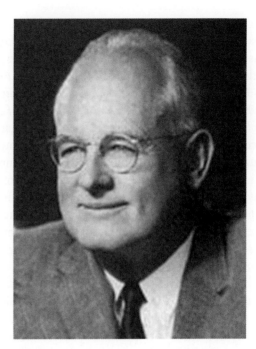

FIGURE 1.10 Dr. T. K. Cureton. (© 2018 University of Illinois Board of Trustees. Available from: http://lifetimefitnessprogram.kch. illinois.edu/about-us/sample-page/.)

research scientist" who studied mechanisms of biological function in relation to the exercise state (4, 7). At this same point in history, the first master's degree–prepared students began emerging from exercise physiology and cardiac rehabilitation preparatory programs. The question of whether these master's degree–prepared individuals were exercise physiologists began to be debated. A core group of exercise scientists recognized that appropriately trained "physical educators" could assimilate a multitude of information from the academic discipline of exercise physiology to create what began to be called the CEP. Collectively, they integrated this body of knowledge into the *Guidelines for Exercise Testing and Prescription*, first published by ACSM in 1975 (8). This arose from a special interest group meeting on Cardiac Rehabilitation at the Annual Meeting of ACSM held in Philadelphia in 1972 where a subcommittee was formed to develop guidelines for graded exercise testing and exercise prescription for both the healthy and the unhealthy. Many feel that with this publication, the field of clinical exercise physiology was born. This text has undergone regular revisions (the 11th edition was copyrighted in 2022) and serves as the foundation of much of clinical exercise physiology and continues to be the most widely circulated set of guidelines for exercise professionals, including CEPs.

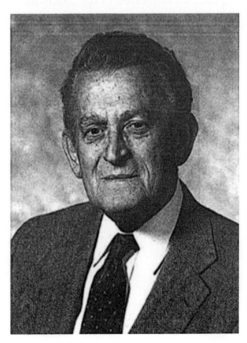

FIGURE 1.9 Dr. Herman Hellerstein. (Used with permission from Franklin BA. Dr. Herman K. Hellerstein world-renowned cardiologist. *J Cardiopulmonary Rehabil.* 1993;13(6):379–80. Available from: http://journals.lww.com/jcrjournal/Citation/1993/11000/Dr__Herman_K__Hellerstein_World_Renowned.1.aspx.)

Published in 1996, *Physical Activity and Health: A Report of the Surgeon General* remains a landmark report for the field of clinical exercise physiology (9). Using an evidence-based approach, it identified numerous chronic diseases and conditions whose risk increases among people lacking in exercise or PA. In 2008, ACSM and the American Heart Association (AHA) jointly published PA guidelines for healthy and older adults (10). These were updates to an earlier version published jointly by the U.S. Centers for Disease Control and Prevention (CDC) and ACSM (11). Also in 2008, the U.S. Department of Health and Human Services published its first Physical Activity Guidelines for Americans (12). And most recently, in 2018, *Physical Activity Guidelines for Americans*, 2nd edition was released (14; Figure 1.11).

With these publications, recognition grew that exercise limits disability and improves outcomes for many diseases and conditions, including chronic cardiovascular, skeletal muscle, metabolic, and pulmonary diseases. For these conditions, exercise training was increasingly incorporated into a comprehensive treatment plan. Additionally, research revealed that some population groups are at increased risk for developing a chronic disease or disability because of physical inactivity, including women, children, and people of certain races and ethnicities (9). More than ever before, clinical exercise physiology had moved to the forefront of advances in clinical care and public policy directed at improving health and attenuating future disease risk.

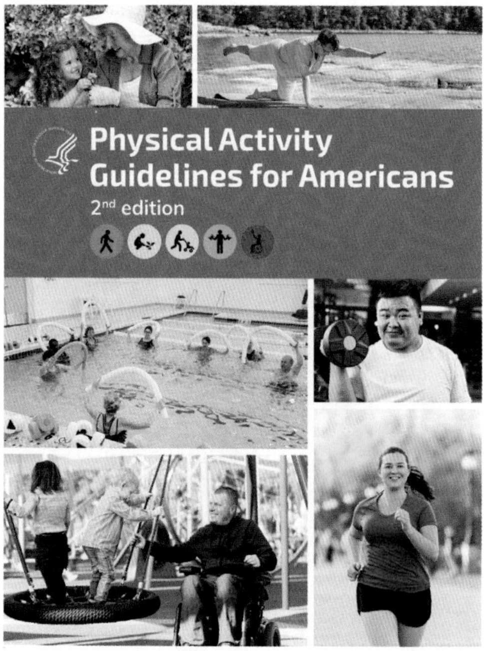

The 1996 Surgeon General's Report *Physical Activity and Health* spawned published practice guidelines, position statements, and ongoing research. Cardiac rehabilitation programs evolved into the sophisticated programs present today. Interdisciplinary teams of allied health professionals that include CEPs began to administer exercise training and behavioral management programs. Pulmonary rehabilitation, bariatric surgery, weight management, exercise oncology, neuromuscular, prenatal and postnatal exercise, and diabetes management programs have also developed from the research and clinical contributions of CEPs.

The body of knowledge underpinning the clinical exercise physiology profession is primarily contained in ACSM's *Guidelines for Exercise Testing and Prescription* published by Wolters Kluwer Health/Lippincott Williams & Wilkins. The first edition of this text was published in 1975 and was coedited by Karl G. Stoedefalke and John A. Faulkner (8). It is shown in Figure 1.12. Updated editions of this vital resource are published every 4 years. The 11th edition, copyright 2022, is the most recent (12). It contains over 460 pages of text as well as five appendices and is supported by more than 1,500 scientific references. The text is fittingly dedicated to the hundreds of volunteer professionals who since 1975 have contributed their

FIGURE 1.11 2018 Physical Activity Guidelines for Americans. (U.S. Department of Health and Human Services. 2008 Physical Activity Guidelines for Americans. Washington (DC): U.S. Department of Health and Human Services; 2008.)

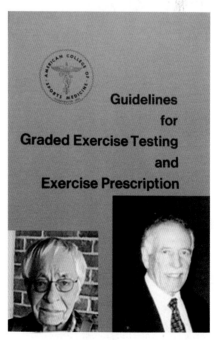

FIGURE 1.12 *Guidelines for Graded Exercise Testing and Exercise Prescription.* 1st ed. Cochairs: Karl Stoedefalke, John Faulkner (1975).

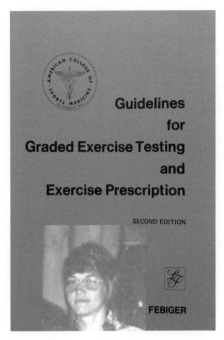

FIGURE 1.13 *Guidelines for Graded Exercise Testing and Exercise Prescription.* 2nd ed. Chair: R. Anne Abbott (1980).

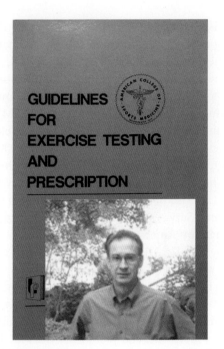

FIGURE 1.15 *Guidelines for Exercise Testing and Prescription.* 4th ed. Chair: Russ Pate (1991).

valuable time and expertise to develop and update the guidelines (see Figures 1.13–1.22).

ACSM's *Guidelines for Exercise Testing and Prescription* constitutes the most widely circulated set of guidelines used by professionals performing exercise testing or

designing science or evidence-based exercise programs. Notice, however, that the information it contains constitutes guidelines as opposed to standards of practice. The distinction is important because specific legal connotations may be attached to standards of practice that are not

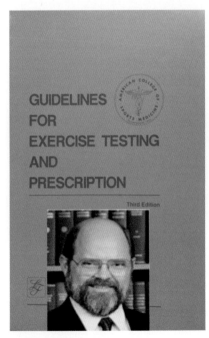

FIGURE 1.14 *Guidelines for Exercise Testing and Prescription.* 3rd ed. Chair: Steve Blair (1986).

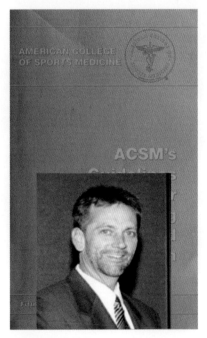

FIGURE 1.16 *ACSM's Guidelines for Exercise Testing and Prescription.* 5th ed. Senior Editor: Larry Kenney (1995).

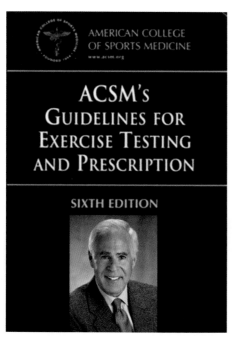

FIGURE 1.17 *ACSM's Guidelines for Exercise Testing and Prescription.* 6th ed. Senior Editor: Barry Franklin (2000).

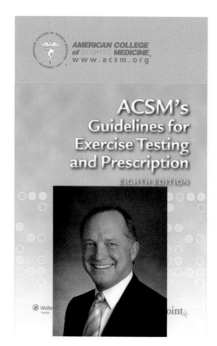

FIGURE 1.19 *ACSM's Guidelines for Exercise Testing and Prescription.* 8th ed. Senior Editor: Walt Thompson (2009).

ascribed to guidelines. The distinction acknowledges the CEP's freedom to deviate from these guidelines when necessary and appropriate while using independent and prudent judgment. The publication does, however, provide a

framework whereby the CEP may certainly, and in some cases has the obligation to, modify the program to the individual client's or patient's needs while balancing institutional and legal requirements (13).

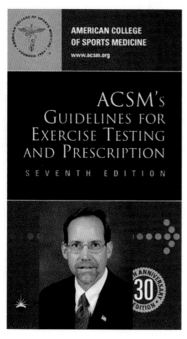

FIGURE 1.18 *ACSM's Guidelines for Exercise Testing and Prescription.* 7th ed. Senior Editor: Mitch Whaley (2005).

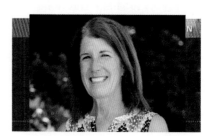

FIGURE 1.20 *ACSM's Guidelines for Exercise Testing and Prescription.* 9th ed. Senior Editor: Linda Pescatello (2013).

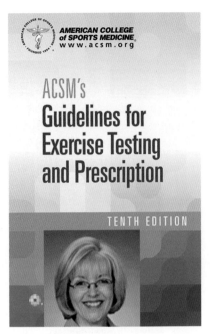

FIGURE 1.21 *ACSM's Guidelines for Exercise Testing and Prescription.* 10th ed. Senior Editor: Deb Riebe (2017).

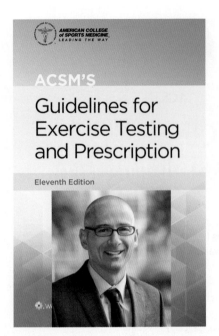

FIGURE 1.22 *ACSM's Guidelines for Exercise Testing and Prescription.* 11th ed. Senior Editor: Gary Liguori (2021).

PROFESSIONAL SOCIETIES FOR CLINICAL EXERCISE PHYSIOLOGY

Two professional societies with international standing in the field of clinical exercise physiology are ACSM and its affiliate, the Clinical Exercise Physiology Association (CEPA). It is incumbent upon CEPs to join at least one of these professional organizations, or perhaps one of the other global societies mentioned in the following subsections, to benefit the future of clinical exercise physiology. All the websites of these organizations are listed in the references to help with membership decisions.

American College of Sports Medicine

ACSM was established in 1954 in order to have like-minded individuals gather to celebrate the burgeoning fields of sports medicine and exercise science. The modest group of individuals credited with the founding of ACSM included Louis Bishop, Clifford Brownell, Albert Hyman, Peter Karpovich, Leonard Larson, Grover Mueller, Neils Neilson, Josephine Rathbone, Arthur Steinhaus, and Joseph Wolffe who would go on to become ACSM's first president.

From the beginning, the many scholars who helped found and form ACSM stressed the importance of research with application and collaboration. In fact, ACSM has a rich history of collaborating with other prominent allied health organizations around the globe. For example, as mentioned earlier, in 2008, ACSM and the AHA jointly published PA guidelines for healthy Americans (14). These were updates to the 1995 joint CDC and ACSM PA guidelines. Also in 2007, the American Medical Association (AMA) and ACSM colaunched EIM, a global health initiative that has been coordinated by ACSM (15).

With over 50,000 members and certified professionals, ACSM has contributed greatly to the clinical exercise physiology profession. The CEP has benefited greatly from ACSM's many efforts, from producing the periodically updated *Guidelines for Exercise Testing and Prescription*, and other certification and exercise publications (this text is one example), to offering a variety of certifications for exercise professionals. Indeed, its affiliate society, the CEPA, was formed inside the structure of ACSM to serve the needs of the expanding number of CEPs.

Clinical Exercise Physiology Association

As an affiliate society of ACSM, the CEPA is autonomous, but operates with administrative support from its parent organization (Figure 1.23). Established in 2008 as an independent, self-sufficient professional organization, its founding members include Dino G. Costanzo, Brian Coyne, Carol Harnett, Sam A. E. Headley, Steven J. Keteyian, Randi Lite, and Murray Low (16) and has become a critical professional organization for the field.

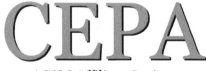

FIGURE 1.23 Clinical Exercise Physiology Association (CEPA) logo. (Clinical Exercise Physiology Association Web site [Internet]. Indianapolis (IN): American College of Sports Medicine; [cited 2021 Dec 10]. Available from: http://www.acsm-cepa.org.)

The primary purpose of CEPA is to advance the scientific and practical application of clinical exercise physiology for the betterment of the health, fitness, and quality of life for patients at high risk of living with a chronic disease. The focus of CEPA is to advance the profession of clinical exercise physiology through advocacy, education, and career development. As a professional network, CEPA is dedicated to the following:

- Enhancing the communication between CEPs by fostering and promoting the interchange of ideas, offering mutual support, and encouraging professional development
- Improving clinical practice by promoting established standards for programs, personnel, and facilities
- Working with employers and the public to promote the knowledge base and skill set of the CEP
- Promoting scientific inquiry and advancement of education for CEPs and for the public related to exercise and its application in the prevention and treatment of chronic diseases and special medical conditions
- Cooperating with other professional organizations, health care providers, insurers, legislators, scientists, and educators with the same or related concerns
- Supporting the development and maintenance of quality care
- Supporting the efforts of ACSM

The CEPA has defined the CEP as follows:

"A CEP is a certified health professional that utilizes scientific rationale to design, implement and supervise exercise programming for those with chronic diseases, conditions and/or physical shortcomings. They also assess the results of outcomes related to exercise services provided to those individuals. Clinical Exercise Physiology services focus on the improvement of physical capabilities for the purpose of: (a) chronic disease management; (b) reducing risks for early development or recurrence of chronic

diseases; (c) creating lifestyle habits that promote enhancement of health; (d) facilitating the elimination of barriers to habitual lifestyle changes through goal setting and prioritizing; (e) improving the ease of daily living activities; and (f) increasing the likelihood of long-term physical, social and economic independence." An individual with a bachelor's degree in exercise physiology, exercise or movement science, or kinesiology and certified as an ACSM-CEP are considered the minimum requirements to be a CEP (1, 16).

Notice that the CEPA defines a CEP as an individual who holds a bachelor's degree or higher in an exercise science–related field and/or is licensed or holds a clinical exercise certification such as ACSM-CEP. Because many CEPs currently work in cardiac rehabilitation, they may also be active members in other organizations such as the AHA and the American Association of Cardiovascular and Pulmonary Rehabilitation (AACVPR). Others are members of organizations that reflect the main patient group with whom they work (*e.g.*, American Diabetes Association, the American Lung Association). Still others are members of the Medical Fitness Association (MFA), whose interests may be aligned with those of the CEPA. Although expired, MFA and CEPA have had a more formal relationship in the past designed to strengthen both organizations. Nevertheless, the CEPA is the only organization that specifically serves the needs and interests of the CEP in the U.S. (16). It is worth highlighting the ever important role for the CEPA flagship journal, *Journal of Clinical Exercise Physiology*.

It should be noted that the CEPA's definition may not reflect the full scope of practice of the CEP in the U.S. or globally. The scope of practice is largely determined by local and institutional (workplace) policies and procedures.

Other Global Professional Societies

Other professional societies of interest to the CEP include the AACVPR, mentioned earlier, Exercise & Sports Science Australia (ESSA), and the Canadian Society for Exercise Physiology (CSEP).

American Association of Cardiovascular and Pulmonary Rehabilitation

Founded in 1985, AACVPR is dedicated to the mission of reducing morbidity, mortality, and disability from cardiovascular and pulmonary disease through education, prevention, rehabilitation, and research and disease management. Central to the core mission is improvement in quality of life for patients and their families (17).

AACVPR (Figure 1.24) is a multidisciplinary professional organization with a membership of health professionals who serve in the field of cardiac and pulmonary

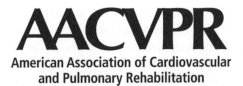

FIGURE 1.24 American Association of Cardiovascular and Pulmonary Rehabilitation (AACVPR) logo. (American Association for Cardiovascular and Pulmonary Rehabilitation Web site [Internet]. Indianapolis (IN): American Association for Cardiovascular and Pulmonary Rehabilitation; [cited 2021 Dec 10]. Available from: http://www.aacvpr.org; © American Association of Cardiovascular and Pulmonary Rehabilitation [AACVPR].)

rehabilitation. Members include cardiovascular and pulmonary physicians, registered nurses (RNs), exercise physiologists, physical therapists (PTs), behavioral scientists, respiratory therapists, dietitians, and registered nutritionists. CEPA has maintained a close relationship with AACVPR, which includes a professional liaison between the two organizations. Many CEPA members also hold a membership in AACVPR.

Exercise & Sports Science Australia

Founded in 1991, ESSA, formerly known as the Australian Association for Exercise and Sports Science (Figure 1.25), is a professional organization that is committed to establishing, promoting, and defending the career paths of exercise and sports science practitioners in Australia (18). ESSA has 11,000 members, of whom 7,600 are accredited exercise physiologists. ESSA and CEPA signed a strategic partnership agreement in 2016 designed to strengthen both organizations.

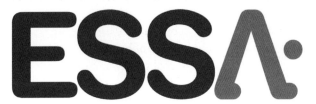

FIGURE 1.25 Exercise & Sports Science Australia (ESSA) logo. (Exercise and Sports Science Australia Web site [Internet]. Queensland (Australia): Exercise and Sports Science Australia; [cited 2021 Dec 10]. Available from: http://www.essa.org.au; © Exercise & Sports Science Australia.)

Canadian Society for Exercise Physiology

The CSEP is a voluntary organization composed of professionals involved in the scientific study of exercise physiology, exercise biochemistry, fitness, and health (Figure 1.26). CSEP (initially known as the Canadian Association of Sport Sciences) was founded at the Pan American Games, Winnipeg, Manitoba, in 1967, the result of 4 years of cooperative efforts by the Canadian Medical Association and the Canadian Association for Health, Physical Education, Recreation and Dance. CSEP celebrated its 50th-year anniversary in 2017 and has over 5,000 members. CSEP also has a robust certification program similar to that of ACSM in clinical exercise physiology. CSEP certification is titled the CSEP Certified Exercise Physiologist. This level of certification is targeted toward undergraduates in the Canadian education system (19). Recently, the CSEP and CEPA have become strategic partners that may help flourish clinical exercise physiology across a large part of North America.

British Association of Sport and Exercise Sciences and the Clinical Exercise Physiology UK

The British Association of Sport and Exercise Sciences (BASES) is the professional body for sport and exercise sciences in the UK whose vision is to deliver excellence in the sport and exercise sciences (Figure 1.27). Its mission is to lead the advancement of knowledge and evidence-based practice within the UK's sport and exercise sciences for the benefit of human performance, health, and education. BASES objectives are to develop and enhance professional and ethical standards in the sport and exercise sciences through its key strategic objectives including the promotion of research in sport and exercise sciences, encouragement of evidence-based practice in sport and exercise sciences, distribution of knowledge in sport and exercise sciences, development and maintenance of high professional standards for those involved in sport and exercise sciences, and representation of the interests of sport and exercise sciences nationally and internationally.

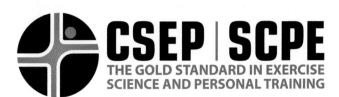

FIGURE 1.26 Canadian Society for Exercise Physiology (CSEP/SCPE) logo. (Canadian Society for Exercise Physiology Web site [Internet]. Ottawa, Ontario (Canada): Canadian Society for Exercise Physiology; [cited 2021 Dec 10]. Available from: http://www.csep.ca; © Canadian Society for Exercise Physiology.)

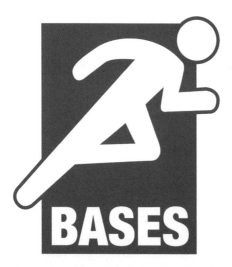

FIGURE 1.27 British Association of Sport and Exercise Sciences (BASES) logo. (British Association of Sport and Exercise Science Web site [Internet]. Headingley, Leeds, United Kingdom: British Association of Sport and Exercise Science; [cited 2022 Sept 1]. Available from: https://www.bases.org.uk/.)

Clinical Exercise Physiology UK (CEP-UK) was established in September 2021 and is the group setting the standards for UK CEPs (Figure 1.28). They have learned from international models and collaborations to shape the UK exercise health care and workforce provision. An agreement was signed in October 2021 whereby BASES would house CEP-UK within its organizational structure. CEP-UK has enabled registration and accreditation of a new health professional in the UK now known as CEPs.

Other CEP Societies

There are many other organizations across the globe that have a relationship to clinical exercise physiology. These organizations generally promote the role of the CEP in

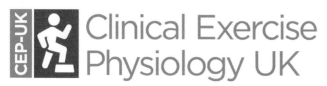

FIGURE 1.28 Clinical Exercise Physiology UK (CEP-UK) logo. (Clinical Exercise Physiology Web site [Internet]. Headingley, Leeds, United Kingdom: Clinical Exercise Physiology UK; [cited 2022 Sept 1]. Available from: https://www.clinicalexercisephysiology.org.uk/.)

their respective countries or regions. Several of these organizations have partnerships with ACSM. These include, but are not limited to, the:

- European College of Sport Science
- Chinese Association of Sports Medicine
- Sport and Exercise Science New Zealand
- National Strength and Conditioning Association
- American Council on Exercise
- National Academy of Sports Medicine
- International Confederation of Sport and Exercise Science Practice

This area is expected to grow at an exponential rate as the CEP's role is more clearly defined around the globe.

CURRENT STANDING OF THE CEP IN THE U.S.

The health care system in the U.S. is in flux, quite dynamic, and perhaps politically unstable. It is a system dominated by crisis medicine with relatively meager resources allocated toward disease prevention. Licensed allied health professions dominate the system; however, among allied health professionals working with high-risk patients with multiple comorbidities, only CEPs are unlicensed, with the state of Louisiana being the only exception (16).

A CEP is a certified health care professional who utilizes scientific evidence to design, implement, and supervise exercise testing and programming for people with chronic diseases, conditions, and/or physical shortcomings. The CEP also assesses the results of outcomes related to exercise services provided to those individuals. Clinical exercise physiology services focus on the improvement of physical capabilities for the following purposes:

- Chronic disease management
- Reducing risks for early development or recurrence of chronic diseases
- Promoting lifestyle habits that enhance health
- Facilitating the elimination of barriers to habitual lifestyle changes through goal setting and prioritizing
- Improving the ease of daily living activities
- Increasing the likelihood of long-term physical, social, and economic independence (16)

A CEP typically obtains a medical history and engages in risk stratification of a patient/client prior to administering exercise-related tests. From the test results, the CEP can design an individualized exercise prescription that meets the specific needs of each client. Many factors enter into risk reduction, and the CEP creatively counsels clients to set goals necessary to meet risk reduction objectives. In consultation with the patient/client, the CEP establishes achievable short-term and long-term goals. CEPs work with clients to prioritize PA and exercise as an enjoyable habitual lifestyle practice (16).

CEPs work in a variety of settings including hospitals, outpatient clinics, physician offices, university laboratories, or hospital-based research facilities. CEPs may work independently or as a member of a multidisciplinary team with other health professionals including PTs, occupational therapists, dietitians, social workers, physicians, and nurses (16).

CEPs also lead clients through a comprehensive program of health education and exercise as a means of managing risk factors for chronic disease. The CEP encourages and supports clients, helping them adhere to recommended lifestyle changes. The result is risk factor modification, greater ease in performing activities of daily living, and the incorporation of exercise as an enjoyable and permanent practice in the individual's lifestyle. Ultimately, the goal is to help clients effectively manage any chronic disease and improve their health-related quality of life (16).

In contrast, a PT treats patients who have acute or chronic pain because of injury and disability (an example is rehabilitation after knee or shoulder surgery). The PT uses exercise and other therapeutic modalities (ultrasound, traction, and electrical stimulation) to improve function relative to the area of concern (16).

Personal trainers generally work with clients who are healthy and, like CEPs, use different types of exercise to assist their clients in reaching their physical potential. Personal trainers are not required to have any formal training in exercise science, although it is helpful if they do have a degree in exercise science. The minimum educational level for the many certifications available to the personal trainer is a high school diploma (16).

CLINICAL EXERCISE PHYSIOLOGY CERTIFICATIONS, ACADEMIC PROGRAM ACCREDITATION, AND STATE LICENSURE

As noted earlier, the primary certifications for CEPs practicing in the U.S. are offered through ACSM. Other specialty certifications are also available.

Certifications From ACSM

The certification programs of ACSM originated in a meeting held in December 1974 in Aspen, Colorado. Conducted by John Faulkner and Karl Stoedefalke, this formative meeting led to one of the first certification levels, the Preventive and Rehabilitation Exercise Program Director, which is no longer actively offered (20). ACSM currently offers one health fitness certification and one clinical certification (Figure 1.29). Both the health fitness certification and clinical certification contain the term "exercise physiologist" in their title and have relevancy to the practicing CEP (21).

ACSM Certified Exercise Physiologist

ACSM Certified Exercise Physiologist (ACSM-EP) is a bachelor's level trained health professional who practices in the exercise field working with mostly apparently healthy and/or stable disease clients. ACSM-EP falls under the health fitness certification track. There are approximately 11,800 ACSM-EPs worldwide. Because this certification typically targets healthy and/or stable clients, it may not be completely appropriate to the CEP (21).

ACSM Certified CEP

ACSM-CEP works with patients challenged with cardiovascular, pulmonary, and/or metabolic diseases and disorders, as well as with apparently healthy populations in cooperation with other health care professionals (19). ACSM-CEPs have a minimum of a bachelor's degree in exercise science and hands-on practical experience (for the most current requirements, visit ACSM certification Web site). In addition to prescribing exercise and lifestyle management, ACSM-CEPs demonstrate knowledge in cardiovascular, pulmonary, metabolic, orthopedic/musculoskeletal, neuromuscular, neoplastic, immunologic, and hematologic disorders. Although working primarily

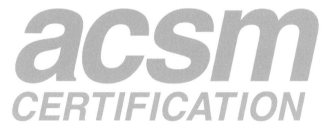

FIGURE 1.29 American College of Sports Medicine (ACSM) Certification logo. (American College of Sports Medicine Web site [Internet]. Get & Stay Certified; [cited 2021 Dec 10]. Available from: https://www.acsm.org/get-stay-certified.)

with individuals facing health challenges, ACSM-CEP builds better health outcomes through a combination of assessing risk, managing exercise implementation, and helping individuals attain positive health outcomes while recovering and rehabilitating from disease, injury, or other limiting factors. ACSM-CEPs turn disease challenges into healthier results. They also provide exercise-related consulting for research, public health, and other clinical and nonclinical services and programs. There are approximately 4,000 ACSM-CEPs worldwide today (21).

Cardiovascular Rehabilitation Certifications

In addition to the clinical exercise certification available from ACSM (ACSM-CEP) in the U.S., several other exercise-based clinical certifications are offered by other organizations, including the American Council on Exercise, National Academy of Sports Medicine, and the National Strength and Conditioning Association. The AACVPR has a newer certification titled the Certified Cardiac Rehabilitation Professional (CCRP).

The AACVPR CCRP has been developed over the past decade and is only recently available. Provided exclusively to cardiac rehabilitation professionals, the CCRP is the only certification aligned specifically with published program competencies. To sit for the exam, 1,200 clinical hours in cardiac rehabilitation and/or secondary prevention, and a minimum of a bachelor's degree or higher in a health-related field from an accredited college or university, *or* current RN licensure is required.

AACVPR's CCRP exam evaluates the knowledge and processes required to complete tasks in the following areas:

- Patient assessment
- Nutrition management
- Weight management
- Blood pressure management
- Blood lipid management
- Diabetes management
- Tobacco cessation
- Psychosocial management
- PA counseling
- Exercise training

The exam is based on AACVPR national standards. The CCRP certification is awarded by the AACVPR Professional Certification Commission solely upon achievement of a passing score on the exam. At this time, there is no requirement for any class, course, or other education or training programs provided by AACVPR or any other provider as a prerequisite for the CCRP examination (17).

The Coalition for the Registration of Exercise Professionals

An exciting development in the field for the certified exercise professional is the recent founding of the Coalition for the Registration of Exercise Professionals (CREP; Figure 1.30). CREP is a not-for-profit 501(c)(6) corporation composed of organizations that offer National Commission for Certifying Agencies (NCCA)-accredited certifications. Five member organizations, including ACSM, founded the CREP. Coalition members are committed to providing individuals of all ages and abilities with resources and leadership to assist in safely and effectively reaching their goals of achieving more active, healthy lifestyles through movement, PA, or exercise for recreation or performance. They also work to advance the fitness profession and earn recognition as a health care provider for individuals who have passed a competency-based certification exam that has been accredited by the NCCA.

The mission of CREP is to secure recognition of registered exercise professionals for their distinct roles in medical, health, fitness, and sports performance fields. CREP's vision is for consumers and other allied health professionals and policy makers to recognize registered exercise professionals for their leadership and expertise in the design and delivery of PA and exercise programs that improve the health, fitness, and athletic performance of the public. An initial effort to this end has been the development of a national and international registry for certified exercise professionals: CREP has a global reach in the International Confederation of Registers for Exercise Professionals (iCREPS; Figure 1.31) and a national effort in the U.S. Registry of Exercise Professionals (US-REPS; Figure 1.32), an internationally recognized registry of exercise professionals in the U.S. Current exercise

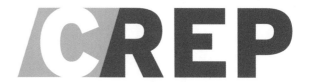

FIGURE 1.30 Coalition for the Registration of Exercise Professionals (CREP) logo. (U.S. Registry of Exercise Professionals Web site [Internet]. Available from: http://www.usreps.org/Pages/aboutus.aspx.)

iCREPS
INTERNATIONAL CONFEDERATION OF REGISTERS FOR EXERCISE PROFESSIONALS

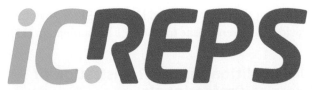

FIGURE 1.31 International Confederation of Registers for Exercise Professionals (iCREPS) logo. (The International Confederation of Registers for Exercise Professionals Web site [Internet]. Available from: https://icreps.org/.)

USREPS
US Registry of Exercise Professionals®

FIGURE 1.32 U.S. Registry of Exercise Professionals (USREPS) logo. (U.S. Registry of Exercise Professionals Web site [Internet]. Available from: http://www.usreps.org/Pages/default.aspx.)

certifications of member organizations listed in USREPS include ACSM-CEP (22).

ACSM Specialty Certifications

ACSM specialty certifications are designed to credential those who may already have an NCCA-accredited certification to work with clients with special needs. These ACSM specialty certifications are themselves NCCA accredited. They certify the CEP's ability to work with clients of different fitness levels, to address a variety of diseases and disabilities, and to promote PA in public health at national, state, and local levels. Currently, there are four relevant specialty certifications or certificates from ACSM. These are discussed briefly in the following subsections (21).

ACSM EIM Credential

ACSM EIM (Figure 1.33) credential recognizes exercise professionals who possess the education and training to collaborate with the health care community to provide PA guidance to referred patients, specifically those with common chronic medical conditions. EIM provides an opportunity for professional development to certified professionals through an interactive online course and the ability to be a part of EIM programs. The EIM Credential highlights how an exercise professional's services could extend a provider's reach of care and is a valuable conversation starter with providers who are curious about how an exercise professional could assist their patients within or outside the health care setting. The EIM program is discussed in more detail later in this chapter.

ExeRcise is Medicine®

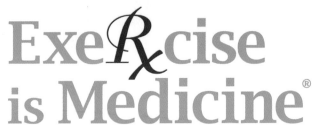

FIGURE 1.33 Exercise is Medicine logo. (Exercise is Medicine Web site [Internet]. Indianapolis (IN): Exercise is Medicine; [cited 2021 Dec 10]. Available from: http://www.exerciseismedicine.org.)

ACSM/American Cancer Society Certified Cancer Exercise Trainer

ACSM has collaborated with the American Cancer Society to develop a specialty certification allowing exercise professionals to work with clients who have a diagnosis of cancer and who have been cleared by their physician for independent exercise and PA. ACSM/American Cancer Society Certified Cancer Exercise Trainer (CET) credential may help with the demonstration of knowledge relating to the development of exercise programs for clients making lifestyle changes caused by cancer and related treatments.

ACSM/NCHPAD Certified Inclusive Fitness Trainer

In collaboration with the National Center on Health, Physical Activity and Disability (NCHPAD), ACSM has developed a specialty certification for exercise professionals to empower those who are challenged by physical, sensory, or cognitive disabilities. ACSM/NCHPAD Certified Inclusive Fitness Trainers (CIFT) give clients the knowledge and support to lead a healthy and comfortable lifestyle.

ACSM/NPAS Physical Activity in Public Health Specialist

ACSM, in collaboration with the National Physical Activity Society (NPAS), has developed a certification for exercise professionals who want to promote PA with focus on the public health setting. ACSM/NPAS Physical Activity in Public Health Specialist (PAPHS) develops key partnerships to establish legislation, policies, and programs that promote PA for people all over the country.

Academic Program Accreditation

In the U.S., educational programs to train the practicing CEP have been in existence since before the 1980s. These programs generally had their origins at the graduate level; however, in the recent past, there has been a competition for these educational programs at the baccalaureate level as well. Academic program accreditation is an effort to assess the quality of academic institutions and their programs and services, measuring them against agreed-upon standards and thereby ensuring that they meet those standards.

In the case of postsecondary education and training, there are two types of accreditations: institutional and programmatic (or specialized). Institutional accreditation helps to assure potential students that a school is a sound institution and has met certain minimum standards in terms of administration, resources, faculty, and facilities. Programmatic (or specialized) accreditation examines specific schools or programs within an educational institution (*e.g.*, the law school, the medical school, the nursing program).

The standards by which these programs are measured have generally been developed by the professionals involved in each discipline and are intended to reflect what a person needs to know and be able to do to function successfully within that profession. Accreditation in the health-related disciplines also serves a very important public interest. Along with certification and licensure, accreditation is a tool intended to help ensure a well-prepared and qualified workforce providing health care services.

ACSM has led the way toward the standardization of curriculum in the training of future CEPs. In fact, a program initiated by ACSM in the 1990s termed the University Connection was an attempt to standardize the educational program components springing forth from many universities. This University Connection program enjoyed a certain level of success before morphing into a program under the auspices of the Committee on Accreditation for the Exercise Sciences (CoAES) (22). The CoAES was formed initially by a handful of professional societies affiliated with the exercise sciences, including ACSM. The CoAES offers exercise science curriculum accreditation at both the baccalaureate and graduate degree levels. The CoAES accreditation entitled "Clinical Exercise Physiology" generally matches the job-task analyses done by ACSM. New standards for undergraduate programs were published effective January 1, 2022, with a strength and conditioning knowledge base needed for the first time as the field continues to evolve. Graduates from a CAAHEP-accredited Clinical Exercise Physiology graduate program at a university may enjoy greater marketability in today's health care job market (Figure 1.34).

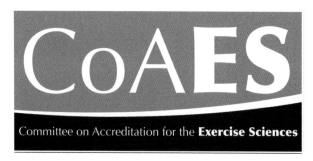

FIGURE 1.34 Committee on Accreditation for the Exercise Sciences (CoAES) logo. (Commission of the Accreditation for the Exercise Sciences Web site [Internet]. Indianapolis (IN): Commission of the Accreditation for the Exercise Sciences; [cited 2021 Dec 10]. Available from: http://coaes.org; © Commission on Accreditation of Allied Health Education Programs.)

The CoAES offers exercise science curriculum accreditation under the auspices of the Commission on Accreditation of Allied Health Education Programs (CAAHEP; Figure 1.35), a postsecondary accrediting agency recognized by the Council for Higher Education Accreditation. CAAHEP carries out its accrediting activities in cooperation with 25 review committees (committees on accreditation). Formed in 1994, CAAHEP currently accredits nearly 2,200 educational programs in 32 different health science professions (24).

CAAHEP is composed of both a commission and a Board of Directors. The commission includes representatives of the member organizations as well as certain other "communities of interest." These commissioners are responsible for determining which health sciences professions are to be recognized by CAAHEP (23). The

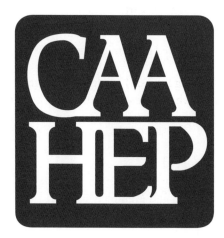

FIGURE 1.35 Commission on Accreditation of Allied Health Education Programs (CAAHEP) logo. (Commission on Accreditation of Allied Health Education Programs. Web site [Internet]. Seminole, FL: Commission on Accreditation of Allied Health Education Programs; [cited 2022 Aug 24]. Available from: https://www.caahep.org/.)

CAAHEP Board of Directors is the accrediting body of CAAHEP that awards or denies accreditation after reviewing the recommendations of the committees on accreditation. It is also the primary governing body that oversees the business of CAAHEP (24).

In April 2004, CAAHEP recognized the CoAES with Walt Thompson (2017–2018 ACSM president) as the founding chairman. The primary role of the CoAES is to establish standards and guidelines for academic programs in exercise science or related departments (kinesiology, human performance, etc.) that facilitate the preparation of students seeking employment in the health, fitness, and exercise industry. The secondary role of the CoAES is to establish and implement a process of self-study, review, and recommendation for all programs seeking CAAHEP accreditation (23).

Presently, CoAES participating organizations include the following:

- American College of Sports Medicine
- American Council on Exercise
- American Kinesiotherapy Association
- American Red Cross
- National Academy of Sports Medicine
- National Council on Strength and Fitness

Currently, there are only 11 Clinical Exercise Physiology programs and 77 undergraduate Exercise Science programs fully accredited by CAAHEP, and that number is growing yearly including Master of Science and Bachelor of Science programs (22). Ultimately, the goal is for most, if not all, academic programs related to exercise science to become accredited. This then fulfills one of the major requirements for recognition as a qualified health provider and is significant progress toward licensure. Recently, ACSM has announced that in order to sit for their certifications one will have to have graduated from a CAAHEP-accredited academic program (21).

Licensure

A natural progression for a health care profession is to evolve from

1. Certification, to
2. Registration, to
3. Accreditation, and eventually to
4. State licensure (24)

With the primary goal of protecting and best serving the U.S. population, the health care profession strives to be an integral component of a "continuity of care" model. CEPs wish to collaborate with and work beside colleagues in other allied health professions in a truly interdisciplinary

environment that is patient centered. This collaboration is currently occurring on a grassroots level, in real-world practice. It is the hope of ACSM, CEPA, and others that eventually this continued collaboration will dissolve some of the conflicts between professional organizations and health care providers. One current movement for the CEP profession to monitor may be the efforts toward individual reimbursement for CEP services.

Through the efforts of the many volunteers and staff of ACSM over the past 30 years, the first three steps of this process have been officially formulated. However, with the current confusion over which certifications should be pursued by the CEP (e.g., ACSM-EP or ACSM-CEP), a corresponding confusion remains among hospital administrators, physicians, clinic managers, and others with the authority to hire CEPs over the precise competencies of those in the profession (24). The fourth step toward fully becoming a health care profession, state-by-state licensure of the CEP, could help eliminate this confusion.

Although licensure has been widely contemplated and discussed within the profession over a significant number of years, there remain disparate views on this course of action. A point/counterpoint piece published in the inaugural issue of CEPA's *Journal of Clinical Exercise Physiology* provides a careful analysis of the advantages and disadvantages of CEP licensure (24, 25).

If a decision were made to pursue licensure, certain obstacles would need to be overcome. First, licensure is a regulatory process implemented by individual state legislatures. Hence it must be pursued on a state-by-state rather than a national basis. One licensure bill for each state requires 50 licensure bills. There is little doubt that all state licensures of CEPs would be identical.

Second, legislative consultants identify several "pillars" in the evolution of the licensure process. These "pillars" include a professional organization, certification or examination, accredited academic programs, and development of a defined evidence-based body of knowledge for a profession. In the field of clinical exercise physiology, although the skeletal outline of each pillar is in place, there is significant expert agreement that more work needs to be done to strengthen these pillars.

CEPs currently have the potential to be licensed only in the state of Louisiana (24). In 1995, a small group of CEPs, working primarily in cardiac rehabilitation, formed the Louisiana Association of Exercise Physiologists (LAEP). A 2012 analysis of the profession since the bill was enacted reveals that the benefits envisioned with state licensure (e.g., higher salaries, better professional recognition) have not yet been realized in Louisiana (26). Louisiana CEPs have not observed significant improvements in practice patterns or employment opportunities, and not all employers in Louisiana require licensed CEPs; thus, Louisiana CEPs continue to explore ways to increase opportunities and demand for their services.

There have been numerous state-by-state efforts led by CEPs to promote licensure for the profession in several states. None of these efforts have succeeded to date, except for Louisiana, for a multitude of reasons including lobbying against these efforts by other professional groups. Perhaps the future will hold more state-by-state licensure opportunities for CEPs. Perhaps a more national effort to recognize the CEP as a Qualified HealthCare Provider (QHP) may be the path forward toward greater acceptance in the health care field. More will be discussed about this effort, as well as the National Provider Identifier (NPI) program, later in the chapter.

EXERCISE IS MEDICINE

"The greatest medicine of all is teaching people how not to need it." (Hippocrates)

In 2007, the AMA and ACSM colaunched EIM, a U.S.-based health initiative that has since been coordinated by ACSM and has a strong global identification. The initial purpose of EIM was to publicize the scientifically proven benefits of PA and make them the standard in the U.S. health care system. Within 2 years of its launch, representatives from international public health, medical, and scientific associations asked ACSM to expand its initial scope beyond the U.S. and begin a multinational collaboration to make EIM a global effort. These requests led to the establishment of the EIM Global Headquarters in Indianapolis, Indiana. Currently, in the EIM Global Network there are 3 regional centers, 37 national centers (including the U.S.), and 1 affiliate partner.

The broad vision of EIM is to have health care providers assess every patient's level of PA at every clinic visit, determine if the patient is meeting the 2018 Physical Activity Guidelines for Americans, and provide patients with brief counseling to help them meet the guidelines and/or refer the patient to either health care or community-based resources for further PA counseling and guidance (14).

PA and exercise are powerful complements to traditional medical intervention and, in many instances, may allow a physician to reduce a patient's drug dosage or eliminate the need for medication altogether. CEPs can play an integral role in educating clients/patients, including those who require medical monitoring, about the benefits of becoming more active and teaching them how to converse

with their provider about ways to increase their PA and exercise. However, doing so requires a paradigm shift and systems approach, as health care policy decision-makers, CEPs, and health care providers must learn to see CEPs as extensions of the health care team (14).

As part of this transformation, EIM exercise professionals, both within and outside of the health care system, must possess the knowledge and skills to successfully integrate themselves as part of the health care continuum. For example, in this ever-changing health care environment, exercise professionals must be able to develop and implement exercise training programs for a variety of chronic medical conditions; utilize behavioral support techniques and technology to help clients to adopt and maintain a regular program of PA; facilitate small group fitness programs for clients with similar diagnoses; and communicate information about the patient back to the health care provider. To assist exercise professionals in this role, EIM has developed the interactive EIM online course, designed to prepare exercise professionals to successfully receive referrals from health care providers and have a positive impact on the health and well-being of those with common chronic diseases.

The EIM Credential is earned by exercise professionals with a qualifying degree, an NCCA-accredited fitness certification, and successful completion of the EIM online course. The EIM course provides continuing education to help exercise professionals work safely and effectively with many of the clients/patients and older adults who walk through their doors every day, regardless of whether they have been referred by a health care provider. Having the EIM Credential signifies that an exercise professional is an integral part of the EIM movement and is qualified to staff EIM community fitness programs.

Practicing CEPs "do EIM" every day. The EIM Credential provides additional recognition and continuing education. It sends a powerful message that exercise should be highly recommended as the drug of choice, positively impacting mental and physical health.

THE FUTURE OF CLINICAL EXERCISE PHYSIOLOGY

Through a comprehensive strategic planning process, CEPA is sharing in its charting of the way forward for the profession with many other professional societies. CEPA has identified several specific strategic priorities within the areas of research, education, advocacy, career, and health care. For instance, in the U.S., CEPA's strategic priority in health care is to document, promote, and firmly establish in the minds of physicians, hospital administrators, insurance companies, legislative bodies, and fellow health care professionals the significant role that CEPs can play in improving patient care and health care outcomes.

The CEPA is working for the recognition of PA and exercise as a treatment option that is equally or perhaps even more effective than other treatments that have benefited from better marketing, funding, and support. The EIM international movement briefly outlined in this chapter is a strong starting point. In addition, the CEPA is working toward an increased recognition of the benefits of PA and exercise that will be reflected at the federal level by reimbursement for CEPs. Early in 2021, ACSM formalized support for this effort by creating a task force to support the CEP as a QHP and to promote all CEPs obtaining their NPI to ultimately pursue insurance reimbursement (27). As the levels of chronic disease increase worldwide and one-third of the world's population remains physically inactive (15), it is reasonable to expect that a formalized, reimbursed exercise intervention to increase PA levels will become the standard in health care.

The CEP, because of education, training, and experience, is the allied health professional most uniquely qualified to provide exercise prescription to patients with chronic disease. The CEP has spent far more time and effort being educated specifically to perform these duties than any other allied health professional.

CEPA supports increased student enrollment in accredited, rigorous university-level clinical exercise programs and that graduates of these programs may earn a livable salary commensurate with colleagues in other licensed allied health professions. A new advancement in this field is the recent addition of a Professional Doctorate in Clinical Exercise Physiology at the University of Illinois at Chicago, the first of its kind. This is an important step, as we move toward the future, that CEPs are not confused with less educated personal trainers or a multitude of different questionably certified exercise "professionals."

In short, CEPs are allied health professionals, who as members of an interdisciplinary team provide individualized PA and exercise services and education to select populations who are either at risk for or have chronic diseases or other conditions warranting specific modifications. CEPs extend the continuum of care for patients who participate in or have been discharged from physical rehabilitation or chronic disease management programs. CEPs apply clinically accepted outcome measurements and evidence-based strategies to enhance their patients' physical function and health-related quality of life.

DISCLAIMER

The field of clinical exercise physiology is relatively new and is continuing to evolve and thus most of the data presented in this chapter must be referenced to the time of writing of the chapter — January 2022 — and are subject to change on a regular basis. The authors fully expect further advances in the exercise science accreditation movement and also in obtaining QHP status.

SUMMARY

Although both medicine and exercise physiology can trace their roots back for thousands of years, clinical exercise physiology is a relative newcomer in today's health care environment. During the last 50 plus years, efforts by ACSM and CEPA have helped the profession evolve. These efforts include establishment of exercise certifications and the publication of the first and subsequent editions of the *Guidelines for Exercise Testing and Prescription*. Countless volunteer time and effort from ACSM professional members and staff have been devoted to the development of the profession of the CEP. In short, the CEP has one single voice in the U.S., and that is the CEPA through the efforts of ACSM, but also has many voices throughout the world. Nevertheless, the CEP profession is fraught with challenges from academic program accreditation to professional certification to insurance billing. These challenges are discussed in this book with solutions offered for each.

The field of CEP grew out of the efforts of countless researchers and clinicians whose work has elucidated the important role of PA and exercise in attenuating the many chronic diseases and disabilities afflicting contemporary society. These findings are discussed in the numerous chapters that follow in this second edition of this landmark book. The monumental efforts of ACSM and the EIM movement have great potential for continued impact. It is truly an exciting time to practice the art and science of clinical exercise physiology.

CHAPTER REVIEW QUESTIONS

1. What is the leading international professional organization specializing in the study of the exercise sciences and sports medicine, and in what year was it founded?
2. What academic institution is credited with initiating the study of exercise physiology in the U.S.?
3. The first application of clinical exercise physiology is generally agreed to be cardiac rehabilitation programming. Who is credited with starting cardiac rehabilitation in the U.S.?
4. Which professional certification is most in line with the tasks and responsibilities of a CEP, and what is the minimal educational requirement for this certification?
5. Identify the professional organization in the world dedicated to the CEP and state their purpose and focus.
6. What are two professional organizations that you feel you are most aligned with to become a member and which certification do you feel is most aligned with your career goals?
7. Name the educational program launched by ACSM and AMA that is global in nature, attempts to place PA and exercise programming at the forefront of clinical services, and has as its goal the advancement of exercise and/or PA services for all.
8. Standardization of academic curriculum in the exercise sciences has been a recent move by the CAAHEP and CoAES. What do these initials stand for?
9. Many organizations around the world are attempting to register qualified exercise professionals. What is the name of the organization that is responsible for this effort?
10. What is the name of the school and the program that will now be offering a doctoral degree in clinical exercise physiology?

REFERENCES

1. American College of Sports Medicine Web site [Internet]. Indianapolis (IN): American College of Sports Medicine; [cited 2017 Mar 1]. Available from: https://www.acsm.org.
2. American College of Sports Medicine. Evolution of the clinical exercise physiologist. In: Farrell PA, Joyner MJ, Caiozzo VJ, editors. ACSM's Resources for Clinical Exercise Physiology. 2nd ed. Baltimore (MD): Wolters Kluwer/Lippincott Williams & Wilkins; 2009. p. 280-7.
3. Tipton CM. History of Exercise Physiology. Champaign (IL): Human Kinetics Publishers; 2014.
4. Foster C. ACSM and the emergence of the profession of exercise physiologist. *Med Sci Sports Exerc.* 2003;35(8):1247.
5. Naughton J, Hellerstein H. Exercise Testing and Exercise Training in Coronary Heart Disease. New York (NY): Academic Press; 1973.
6. Brown SP. Profession or discipline: the role of exercise physiology in allied health. *J Clin Exerc Physiol.* 2000;2:168.
7. Foster C, Roitman J, Harnett C. Profession or discipline: asking the right questions or turf protection? *J Clin Exerc Physiol.* 2000;2:168.
8. American College of Sports Medicine. Guidelines for Exercise Testing and Prescription. 1st ed. Philadelphia (PA): Lippincott, Williams & Wilkins; 1975.
9. U.S. Department of Health and Human Services. Physical Activity and Health: A Report of the Surgeon General. Atlanta (GA): U.S. Department of Health and Human Services, Centers for Disease Control and Prevention, National Center for Chronic Disease Prevention and Health Promotion; 1996.
10. Haskell WL, Lee IM, Pate RR, et al. Physical activity and public health: updated recommendation for adults from the American College of Sports Medicine and the American Heart Association. *Med Sci Sports Exerc.* 2007;39(8):1423-34.
11. Pate RR, Pratt M, Blair SN, et al. Physical activity and public health. A recommendation from the Centers for Disease Control and Prevention and the American College of Sports Medicine. *JAMA.* 1995;273(5):402-7.
12. U.S. Department of Health and Human Services. 2008 Physical Activity Guidelines for Americans. Washington (DC): U.S. Department of Health and Human Services; 2008.
13. American College of Sports Medicine. Guidelines for Exercise Testing and Prescription. 11th ed. Baltimore (MD): Wolters Kluwer Health; 2022.
14. U.S. Department of Health and Human Services. 2018 Physical Activity Guidelines for Americans. Washington (DC): U.S. Department of Health and Human Services; 2018.
15. Exercise is Medicine Web site [Internet]. Indianapolis (IN): Exercise is Medicine; [cited 2021 Dec 10]. Available from: http://www.exerciseismedicine.org.
16. Clinical Exercise Physiology Association Web site [Internet]. Indianapolis (IN): American College of Sports Medicine; [cited 2021 Dec 10]. Available from: http://www.acsm-cepa.org.
17. American Association for Cardiovascular and Pulmonary Rehabilitation Web site [Internet]. Indianapolis (IN): American Association for Cardiovascular and Pulmonary Rehabilitation; [cited 2021 Dec 10]. Available from: http://www.aacvpr.org.
18. Exercise & Sports Science Australia Web site [Internet]. Hamilton, QLD (Australia): Exercise & Sports Science Australia; [cited 2021 Dec 10]. Available from: http://www.essa.org.au.
19. Canadian Society for Exercise Physiology Web site [Internet]. Ottawa, ON (Canada): Canadian Society for Exercise Physiology; [cited 2021 Dec 10]. Available from: http://www.csep.ca.
20. Berryman J. Out of Many, One. A History of the American College of Sports Medicine. 1st ed. Champaign (IL): Human Kinetics; 1995.
21. American College of Sports Medicine Web site [Internet]. Get & Stay Certified; [cited 2021 Dec 10]. Available from: https://www.acsm.org/certification.

22. U.S. Registry of Exercise Professionals [Internet]. Kansas City (KA): United States Registry of Exercise Professionals; [cited 2021 Dec 10]. Available from: http://www.usreps.org.

23. Commission of the Accreditation for the Exercise Sciences Web site [Internet]. Indianapolis (IN): Commission of the Accreditation for the Exercise Sciences; [cited 2021 Dec 10]. Available from: http://coaes.org.

24. Berry R, Verrill D. Licensure for clinical exercise physiologists — an argument in favor of this proposal. *J Clin Exerc Physiol.* 2012;1:35–8.

25. Foster C, Procari, J. Licensure for clinical exercise physiologists — a desirable goal with an elusive outcome. *J Clin Exerc Physiol.* 2012;1:38–40.

26. Clinical Exercise Physiology Association Web site; Legislation Resources section [Internet]. Indianapolis (IN): American College of Sports Medicine; [cited 2021 Dec 10]. Available from: https://www.acsm-cepa.org/content.aspx?page_id=22&club_id=324409&module_id=291082.

27. Overstreet, B, Ward-Ritacco, C, Neric, F et al. Technical requirements for clinical exercise physiologists as qualified health providers. *ACSMs Health Fit J.* 2023;27(2):20–6.

CHAPTER 2

Transformations Across the Lifespan

INTRODUCTION

The human lifespan is typically separated into stages based on age that include childhood, adolescence, young adulthood, midlife, and old age. The first half of the lifespan is characterized by rapid growth and development, whereas the second half is characterized by gradual loss and deterioration. Although the rate of change varies greatly between individuals based on genetics and lifestyle choices, current evidence indicates that change is ultimately unavoidable. This chapter discusses normal age-related changes in body composition, muscle strength, cardiorespiratory fitness, and bone density that clinicians and clinical exercise physiologists (CEPs) should know to provide the best quality care for people at all stages of life.

Because behavior influences aging, normal aging is not necessarily optimal or healthy aging. An inactive lifestyle and poor diet contribute directly to the aging process and to premature morbidity and mortality. This "normal" premature aging does not reflect the true potential of the human body, which can achieve a projected lifespan of 120 years (1). To further confound the issue, many research studies screen out participants with disease and dysfunction, and thus, current research evidence may be skewed in favor of describing growth and aging that reflect either optimal lifestyle behaviors or protective genetics in those who practice suboptimal behaviors. The results of such studies may not be generalizable to adults who have accrued comorbidities with age. Moreover, the declines in health and functioning observed with age in adulthood are likely greater in our current population than what is commonly reported.

Finally, a word of caution is needed regarding the types of evidence available in studies of development and aging. Much of what is understood regarding change across the lifespan is derived from cross-sectional, rather than longitudinal, data. This allows comparisons between age groups but does not allow investigators to observe individuals as they age over time. Therefore, be cautious in the interpretation of some of those data. Longitudinal studies can provide stronger evidence about the magnitude of change in physiological characteristics over time but are harder to conduct because they can be very expensive and require many years to complete. This chapter presents a summary of our current understanding based on a mix of cross-sectional and longitudinal study results. When possible, data from meta-analysis of multiple studies have been used to provide the strongest available evidence.

CHILDREN

Childhood covers the period from infancy (2 years old) up to about 10–12 years old and is characterized by growth and development. During this time, sex differences in strength and body size are less profound than in later life.

Body Size and Composition

Pediatricians, clinicians, and scientists who work with children use growth charts to track growth rate against normative data. The World Health Organization (WHO) developed charts in 2006 that describe the growth of children from infancy up to 5 years based on patterns in six countries with environments believed to support optimal growth, including the U.S. (2). In the U.S., the Centers for Disease Control and Prevention (CDC) recommends using the WHO standards up to age 2 and then switching to growth curves developed specifically for the U.S. population. The CDC's standards were developed in the 1980s and revised in 2000 (3). As shown in Figure 2.1, body mass index (BMI) varies widely in boys and girls from 2 to 20 years. From approximately age 2 to 6, BMI declines because the annual rate of gain in height is faster than

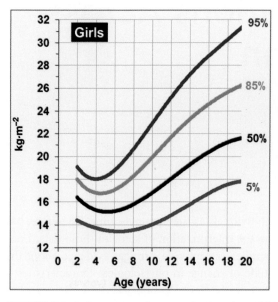
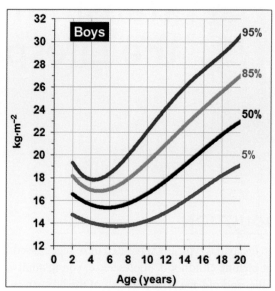

FIGURE 2.1 Reference growth curves for American children and adolescents. From the Centers for Disease Control and Prevention, revised in 2000. Values are shown as percentiles of body mass index (calculated as weight relative to height, $kg \cdot m^{-2}$). Underweight <5th percentile. Normal weight = 5th–84th percentile. Overweight = 85th–94th percentile. Obese ≥95th percentile. (Data from Kuczmarski RJ, Ogden CL, Guo SS, et al. 2000 CDC growth charts for the United States: methods and development. *Vital Health Stat.* 2002;11(246):1–190.)

the increase in body mass. From about age 7 through 20, however, the accrual of body mass is faster than the increase in height, and BMI increases steadily toward adult values. Many other countries and regions have growth curves for their populations that vary slightly from those for the U.S.

Figure 2.1 also shows BMI curves that define the normal-weight range (5th–84th percentile) and ranges that classify cut points for underweight (<5th percentile), overweight (85th–94th percentile), and obesity (≥95th percentile). These curves were developed from data acquired from large national surveys of children in the 1970s and early 1980s. At that time, approximately 5% of children and adolescents were considered obese and another 10% were in the overweight range (3). Over the past 40 years, however, the prevalence of overweight and obesity has risen markedly. Data from the U.S. collected in 2017–2018 showed that 15% children are overweight and another 19% are obese (4). Obesity rates are lower in children ages 2–5 (13%) than in children ages 6–11 (20%) or adolescents ages 12–19 (21%), and about 2% higher in boys than in girls in each of those age groups. Those estimates are derived by expressing the BMI of contemporary children relative to the growth curves in Figure 2.1. Thus, there are now nearly four times as many children and adolescents in the U.S. who exceed the 95th percentile (obesity range) as there were in 1980 (3, 4). There are two potential limitations for using standard BMI growth

curves to determine whether a child is overweight or obese. First, the use of chronological age does not account for variation in development. Children who enter puberty early may grow more rapidly than their peers and may be inappropriately classified as overweight if they exceed reference values for their age (5, 6). Second, BMI does not account for body composition. As a result, BMI reference curves tend to overestimate the presence of excess adiposity in African American children compared to measures of body fat obtained with dual-energy x-ray absorptiometry (7). Despite these caveats, BMI-based estimates of obesity prevalence are consistent with data showing that body fat in U.S. children is increasing. A comparison of body composition data using dual-energy x-ray absorptiometry performed on children during 1999–2006 and 2011–2018 showed that the average values for body fat (as percent body mass) rose from 25.6% to 26.3% in boys and 33.0% to 33.7% in girls (8).

During the age span from 6 to 12 years, total body muscle mass approximately doubled in size in healthy children, based on data from the U.S. and the United Kingdom (9, 10). Those surveys also revealed that from 6 to 12 years, skeletal muscle accounts for almost half of total body lean tissue. Figure 2.2 shows the rapid growth of total body lean mass and the lean mass in the legs during childhood. The data were acquired from a large ethnically diverse sample of U.S. children from 1999 to 2004 as part of the National Health and Nutrition Examination Survey

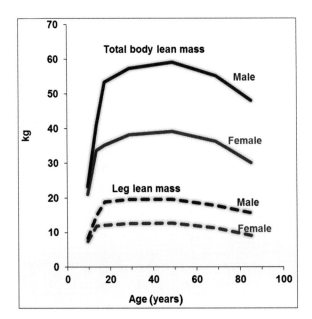

FIGURE 2.2 Reference values for total body lean mass and leg lean mass in American children and adults. Data from the National Health and Nutrition Examination Survey (NHANES) 1999–2004, using dual-energy x-ray absorptiometry (DEXA). Values shown are for the 50th percentile for females (~3,000 participants) and males (~11,000 participants) ages 8–80+. Total body lean mass is shown in solid lines, leg lean mass in dotted lines. (Data from Borrud LG, Flegal KM, Looker AC, Everhart JE, Harris TB, Shepherd JA. Body composition data for individuals 8 years of age and older: U.S. population, 1999–2004. National Center for Health Statistics. *Vital Health Stat.* 2010;11(250):1–87.)

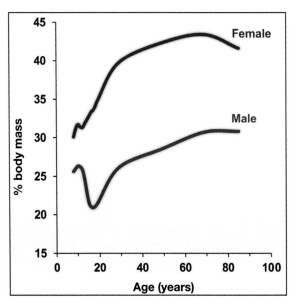

FIGURE 2.3 Reference values for body fat percentage in American children and adults. Data from the National Health and Nutrition Examination Survey (NHANES) 1999–2004, using dual-energy x-ray absorptiometry (DEXA). Values shown are for the 50th percentile for females (~3,000 participants) and males (~11,000 participants) ages 8–80+. (Data from Borrud LG, Flegal KM, Looker AC, Everhart JE, Harris TB, Shepherd JA. Body composition data for individuals 8 years of age and older: U.S. population, 1999–2004. National Center for Health Statistics. *Vital Health Stat.* 2010;11(250):1–87.)

(NHANES) (11). The developmental pattern of lean mass in the legs is presented because it is predominantly skeletal muscle, and the legs are so important for mobility, exercise performance, and metabolic health throughout life. Leg lean mass accounts for about 36% of the total body lean mass in the 6- to 11-year-old age range and does not markedly differ between girls and boys. In contrast, by age 6–11, body fat content, when expressed as a percentage of total body mass, is already significantly higher in girls than in boys (Figure 2.3). This difference in body fat between the sexes grows larger during childhood and is maintained during adolescence and adulthood.

Although developmental patterns in body mass and composition during childhood may be similar among countries, absolute values can differ. For example, compared to children from the U.S., children from both Austria and South Korea have lower lean mass and fat mass relative to their height (12, 13). These differences are likely due in part to the trends toward larger body sizes in the U.S. over the past 40 years. It also means that clinicians and scientists need to consider regional differences in body composition reference values when

evaluating patients or comparing research results across populations.

Physical Activity Patterns

The American Academy of Pediatrics, CDC, American Heart Association, and American College of Sports Medicine (ACSM) recommend that children and adolescents accumulate at least 60 minutes per day of moderate-to-vigorous physical activity (MVPA) on at least 5 days per week (*i.e.*, 300 min per wk). This is double the volume of physical activity recommended by ACSM for adults (14). The most recent ACSM guidelines, which specify exercise frequency, intensity, time, and type (FITT) for children and adults, recommend that children and adolescents spend most of their daily physical activity in moderate-to-vigorous aerobic-type activities, with vigorous aerobic activity, specifically, included on at least 3 days per week. Muscle strengthening and bone strengthening activities should also be included on at least 3 days per week, and these activities count toward the goal of 60 minutes of activity per day. Weight-bearing, vigorous activities like running and jump roping are ideal for meeting two or more of these specific recommendations.

To meet the activity guidelines through ambulatory activities, children require about 11,000–15,000 steps per day. Tudor-Locke et al. (15) conducted a review of studies, performed up to 2010, in which children and adolescents wore a pedometer for at least 3 days. They found that children 4–6 years old needed to complete 10,000–14,000 steps per day to achieve 60 minutes per day of MVPA, whereas elementary school–aged children required 13,000–15,000 steps for boys and 11,000–12,000 steps for girls. Another large study of children and adolescents found that boys and girls 6–10 years old need to complete approximately 12,000 steps per day to meet the recommended 60 minutes of MVPA (16).

In their review, Tudor-Locke et al. (15) also found that physical activity patterns were similar in preschool-aged boys and girls and that sex differences began to appear after age 6–7, with boys being more active. This pattern is commonly observed during childhood, although the reason for the sex difference is not understood.

In 2015, a group of investigators from 10 countries published results from the International Children's Accelerometry Database (ICAD), a pooled set of physical activity measurements from studies using similar methodology with more than 27,000 children ages 2–18 (17). In the summary analysis, a common finding across data sets was that boys 5–6 years old had the highest rates of daily physical activity relative to other age and sex groups. In reference to 5- to 6-year-old boys, as shown in Figure 2.4, daily physical activity declined during childhood and adolescence by about 1% every 5 years. Girls performed about 2% less physical activity per day than boys, and this difference was consistent during childhood. In contrast to physical activity, the time spent being sedentary (no physical activity) steadily increased from age 5 to 6, with girls spending slightly more time being sedentary than boys. The report also showed that U.S. children ages 9–10 met the 60-minutes-per-day level of MVPA on 40% of days for boys and 20% of days for girls, which were among the lowest levels in the database. In contrast, the highest values for MVPA were recorded in Norway, with boys reaching 60 minutes per day on 60% of days and girls meeting that standard on 45% of days. Another consistent finding was that children who were overweight or obese had lower levels of physical activity from age 6 onward, compared to their normal-weight peers. Collectively, the available data suggest that most children in the U.S. and Europe are not meeting current recommended levels of physical activity.

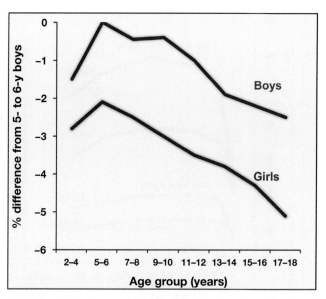

FIGURE 2.4 Daily time spent in moderate-to-vigorous physical activity (MVPA) during childhood and adolescence. Results are from the International Children's Accelerometry Database (ICAD), a compilation of data from studies performed in 10 countries. Because there was considerable variation in daily MVPA among countries and study groups, the results were presented as relative values, referenced to the percent difference from 5- to 6-year-old boys, who had the highest MVPA in several studies. (Data from Cooper AR, Goodman A, Page AS, et al. Objectively measured physical activity and sedentary time in youth: the International Children's Accelerometry Database (ICAD). *Int J Behav Nutr Phys Act.* 2015;12:113.)

Large, randomized controlled trials conducted in schools to increase physical activity in children have had some success, though results have been varied and the programs require considerable time and resources. A study in Australian children in grades 3–6 reported that MVPA measured with accelerometers was approximately 21 minutes per week higher in schools assigned to a 6-month intervention program to promote physical activity, compared to control schools that maintained their standard activity programs (18). A 1-year program for students ages 9–12 in China resulted in an increase in 33 minutes per week in MVPA (assessed with questionnaires) and was associated with slower rise in BMI and fewer children reaching thresholds for overweight or obesity compared to a control group (19). A large program in Canada to promote physical activity and healthy eating for children in grades 4–6 was notable for the efforts to tailor the intervention to accommodate the complex time, space, and resource differences among schools (20). They found that some intervention components like incorporation of physical activity in the classroom were associated with improvements in measured physical activity, running performance, and bone health in initial efficacy trials. However, as the program was scaled up, there was a modest decrease in the number of schools meeting the intervention goals, highlighting the challenges of these types of programs.

Metabolic Changes

Resting metabolic rate (RMR) is the amount of energy consumed by cellular activity while a person is awake and lying quietly. RMR is also referred to as resting energy expenditure (REE). Because RMR is the sum of energy-consuming processes (*e.g.*, maintenance, transport, and repair activities), as children grow, their total RMR (reported in units of either kilocalories or kilojoules) increases in proportion to the change in the body size. To assess the relative metabolic activity among people of different size, the RMR value is typically adjusted for either total body mass or lean body mass (because lean mass accounts for most of the metabolic activity). When expressed in kilocalories per kilogram body mass or kilocalories per kilogram fat-free mass, RMR declines throughout childhood and adolescence as shown in Figure 2.5 (21–35). The decline in RMR continues during adulthood, although at a much slower rate, as described later in this chapter.

Muscle

Normal Changes

Muscle strength increases during childhood, but differences between boys and girls do not emerge until adolescence. This is demonstrated in Figure 2.6, which shows values for knee extensor strength that were collected in NHANES and the NHANES National Youth Fitness Survey (NNYFS). In children 6–11 years old, boys and girls had similar values for knee extension strength, hand grip strength, the number of modified pull-ups performed, and the duration of time they could maintain a plank position (36). Boys and girls 12–15 years old performed significantly better than their younger counterparts, but in the older group boys were stronger than girls on all four tests. There is good agreement with findings from surveys of children in other countries. Figure 2.7 shows average values for handgrip strength across the lifespan, measured in participants in the U.S. and South Korea (37, 38). Although the absolute values differ between the two countries, both data sets show that strength differences between boys and girls are evident after age 10–12 and

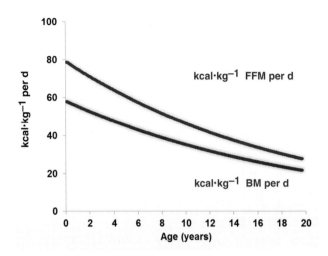

FIGURE 2.5 Decline in resting energy expenditure during childhood and adolescence. As body mass increases during youth, the absolute value for resting energy expenditure increases but the normalized value relative to either body mass (BM, blue line) or fat-free mass (FFM, red line) declines. Even when more complex modeling adjustments are used to account for changes in body size and composition, there is a decline in resting energy expenditure in response to the inherent slowing of cellular metabolism. Curves are drawn from a compilation of several studies of infants, children, and adolescents. (Data from references 21–34, 488.)

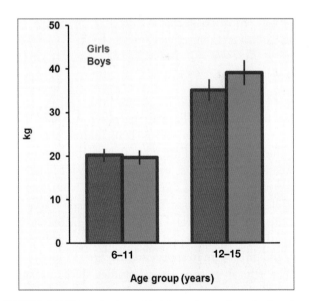

FIGURE 2.6 Values for isometric knee extensor force in American children and adolescents. Data collected in healthy children (ages 6–11) and adolescents (ages 12–15) in the National Health and Nutrition Examination Survey (NHANES) and the NHANES National Youth Fitness Survey (NNYFS) in 2012. Force was measured while seated in 600 girls and 600 boys, using a handheld dynamometer on the right leg. Boys were stronger than girls in the older but not the younger age range. (Data from Ervin RB, Wang CY, Fryar CD. Measures of muscular strength in U.S. children and adolescents, 2012. National Center for Health Statistics. *NCHS Data Brief*. 2013;139:1–8.)

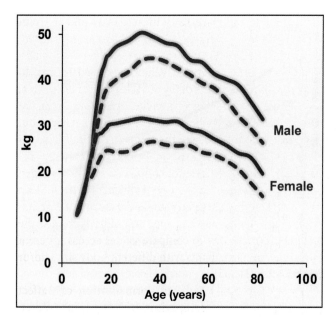

FIGURE 2.7 Reference values for handgrip strength in children and adults. Solid lines show data from more than 13,000 people tested in the U.S. National Health and Nutrition Examination Survey (NHANES) from 2011 to 2014. Dotted lines show results from nearly 8,000 people tested in the Korean NHANES from 2014 to 2016. Values shown are for the 50th percentile for females and males in each study. (Data from Wang YC, Bohannon RW, Li X, et al. Summary of grip strength measurements obtained in the 2011–2012 and 2013–2014 National Health and Nutrition Examination Surveys. *J Hand Ther.* 2019;32(4):489–96; Kim CR, Jeon YJ, Kim MC, et al. Reference values for hand grip strength in the South Korean population. *PLoS One.* 2018;13(4):e0195485.)

persist throughout the lifespan thereafter. A pooled analysis of multiple studies with 50,000 children and adults combined in the United Kingdom showed the same developmental patterns and same average values for hand grip strength as the U.S. data shown in Figure 2.7 (39). Reports on children from Europe, Chili, and Canada also agree that the strength of several muscle groups increases continuously during childhood and that differences between boys and girls begin to appear around age 11 (40–42).

For ethical reasons, fewer studies have measured the histochemical or biochemical properties of skeletal muscle tissue in children than in adults. Acquiring small amounts of tissue for such analyses using the muscle biopsy technique is relatively simple and painless and does not result in residual scarring or muscle damage. However, the procedure is still considered to involve more than minimal risk, so it is seldom approved for research studies in healthy children who are not already undergoing another medical procedure or surgery. Nevertheless, data from a small number of children have shown

that the proportion of type I (slow twitch) fibers in the quadriceps muscle by age 6 is similar to, or slightly higher than, what is reported for untrained adults (43). Muscles of children may be better prepared for endurance exercise than activity that relies on anaerobic metabolism, such as repeated sprinting. This is due in part to the finding that the amount of muscle glycogen and enzymes in the glycolytic pathway in children is lower than that typically measured in adults (44). These differences begin to disappear during adolescence.

Role of Physical Activity and Exercise

Despite lower muscle mass and strength than adults, children demonstrate improved muscle strength and motor- and sport-specific performance in response to structured exercise programs. The conclusion of a 2014 position paper published by a group of British and American sport medicine experts was that resistance training is safe and effective for improving the health and function of children and adolescents (45). The panel found no evidence for increased risk of injury or growth impairment in children who performed resistance training if the exercises were designed and supervised by qualified professionals and the activities were tailored for the developmental and motor skill level of the children. The most recent *ACSM's Guidelines for Exercise Testing and Prescription* also recommend that children engage in strengthening activities on at least 3 days per week (14).

A systematic review from 2016 examined the results of resistance training studies conducted with athletes 6–18 years old to determine the effect of age, sex, and training program design on the development of muscle strength and physical performance (46). A key feature of the review was that it was limited to interventions with children who were already involved in team or individual sports, and studies that included a recreationally active control group. A control group that maintains normal physical activity is an important study design feature as children are expected to gain strength over time because of normal growth and maturation. Fewer studies performed with children ($n = 10$) than adolescents ($n = 22$) were available, but the data showed that children can improve performance on tests of muscle strength, vertical jump, running sprints, agility tasks, and sport-specific skills in response to resistance training. Furthermore, the magnitude of those changes in children was similar to that observed in adolescents. Girls and boys had similar relative gains in strength and performance. The authors of this review concluded that strength training programs can be safe and effective for child athletes.

For children not already involved in competitive sports, more generalized physical activity programs can also improve strength. A group of Swedish investigators conducted a school-based intervention to increase physical activity time in children starting at ages 6–9 (47, 48). Children at the intervention schools increased physical education time to 200 minutes per week (40 min per d, 5 d per wk), whereas control schools remained at 60 minutes per week. The types of games and sports activities at the intervention schools remained the same and no special effort was made to specifically target muscle strength or endurance, or to provide additional physical activity on weekends or school holidays. After 3 and 5 years, both boys and girls in the intervention group demonstrated greater gains in muscle strength than children in the control group. As discussed later in this chapter, increasing muscle strength during youth is associated with better health in adulthood.

Cardiorespiratory

Normal Changes

Cardiorespiratory, or aerobic, fitness is defined as the highest rate of oxygen consumption achieved during exercise ($\dot{V}O_{2max}$). It is typically measured in laboratory settings during a graded exercise test in which the participant completes increasing levels of work on a treadmill or bicycle ergometer, and expired air is directed to a metabolic measurement instrument to quantify the rate of oxygen consumption. Performing such standard laboratory-based graded exercise tests with children can be challenging. Special accommodations may be needed to ensure that the exercise and measurement equipment is appropriately sized for children. Young children may not be able to follow safety precautions on a treadmill, may not be able to maintain a steady walking gait or cycling cadence, or may lack the necessary focus or motivation to provide a true maximal effort. For these and other reasons, aerobic fitness has often been estimated in young children using field tests such as timed runs, shuttle runs, or step tests or extrapolated from submaximal tests (41, 49–51). When standard graded exercise tests are performed with children, the resulting values are frequently described as $\dot{V}O_{2peak}$, because it is acknowledged that the highest rate of oxygen consumption may approach but not quite reach a true physiological maximum according to classic definitions from studies of adults.

Despite the potential challenges, many aerobic fitness data on children ages 8 and up show that absolute values (in liters per minute, $L \cdot min^{-1}$) for $\dot{V}O_{2peak}$ increase during childhood (52–54). The age-related increase becomes most evident around 10 years old and is mostly attributable to the increase in muscle mass and strength in both sexes. On average, values for $\dot{V}O_{2peak}$ in children, like adults, are 5%–20% lower when tested on a stationary bicycle than on a treadmill. When expressed relative to body mass (in milliliters of O_2 per kilogram of body mass per minute, $mL \cdot kg^{-1} \cdot min^{-1}$), values for $\dot{V}O_{2peak}$ tend to stay the same in prepubescent boys as they get older but values for girls tend to stay the same or decline. This has been attributed, in part, to higher body fat in girls. Because adipose tissue does not contribute much to oxygen use during exercise and because children increase lean mass as they grow, there is ongoing debate about whether expressing values for $\dot{V}O_{2peak}$ per unit of body mass is the most appropriate way to compare values across different age groups or participants with different body size and/or composition (54, 55).

An example of how data normalization can affect interpretation is in a comparison of $\dot{V}O_{2peak}$ in children classified as normal weight or obese. Children who are overweight or obese tend to score lower on most fitness tests than their normal-weight counterparts. However, Goran et al. (56) showed that normalization for body weight versus lean mass can affect interpretations. They compared $\dot{V}O_{2peak}$ measured during a treadmill test performed by 39 children who were normal weight and 39 children who were obese, who were about 9 years old. The group with obesity had 5 kg (11 lb) more lean mass and 15 kg (33 lb) more fat mass than the normal-weight group. The children who were obese had a shorter time to exhaustion (11 vs. 15 min for the normal-weight group) but reached a higher absolute value for $\dot{V}O_{2peak}$ than the normal-weight group (1.56 vs. 1.24 $L \cdot min^{-1}$). When expressed relative to total body weight, $\dot{V}O_{2peak}$ was 27% lower in the obese group (44 vs. 32 $mL \cdot kg^{-1} \cdot min^{-1}$), but when expressed relative to lean body mass $\dot{V}O_{2peak}$ did not differ between groups (59 vs. 58 $mL \cdot kg^{-1} \cdot min^{-1}$). Thus, this study demonstrated that the absolute capacity of the cardiorespiratory system may not be limited in children who were obese, especially those who are physically active, but the extra body mass imposes a limitation on submaximal exercise ability and time to fatigue, especially during a weight-bearing activity. In children who were obese who have habitually low physical activity, however, both the absolute and normalized $\dot{V}O_{2peak}$ may be low.

Role of Physical Activity and Exercise

Like adolescents and adults, prepubescent children who are active in sports and exercise typically have higher values for $\dot{V}O_{2peak}$ than untrained children (52, 53). This difference is maintained in physically active children over 2–3 years of follow-up. McNarry et al. (52) followed a group of children annually for 3 years, from age 10 to 12, and showed that swimmers who trained 8–12 hours per week had higher absolute $\dot{V}O_{2peak}$ and peak cardiac output each year than an age-matched group of recreationally active healthy peers. Furthermore, the authors showed that expressing $\dot{V}O_{2peak}$ or cardiac output relative to body mass masked differences between the trained and untrained groups, as well as the increase in both variables over the course of the observation period. Instead, they recommended that a statistical modeling approach, called allometric scaling, is better for adjusting $\dot{V}O_{2peak}$ than dividing the absolute $\dot{V}O_{2peak}$ value by either body mass or lean body mass, and should be used to control for the growth in body size in children and adolescents. Using that scaling method allowed for the detection of the effects of training and maturation on $\dot{V}O_{2peak}$ over time. Similar approaches have been used for regression-based or allometric scaling of values for $\dot{V}O_{2peak}$, daily energy expenditure, physical activity, and other metabolic variables that vary with age, body size, and body composition (54, 55, 57–61). Such approaches can be useful in research studies that include participants with widely varying age, body size, or body composition. However, in most clinical settings, the convention of expression of $\dot{V}O_{2peak}$ as milliliters per kilogram body mass per minute remains widely used because of the simpler application and because measures of lean mass are often not available. CEPs should be aware of the potential pitfalls of using simple ratio scaling to express commonly measured variables per unit body mass and when it may be appropriate to apply alternate approaches.

There is a long-standing debate about the "trainability" of prepubescent children. When comparing children who are very active in sports to boys and girls who are only recreationally active or predominantly sedentary, it is unclear how much of the difference between groups is attributable to the effects of extra physical activity versus inherent factors such as genetics. When prepubertal children undertake an exercise program, there is often little or no change in $\dot{V}O_{2peak}$ reported (62). It is unclear whether physiological changes that accompany puberty, such as androgens or other factors, are required for improvement in aerobic fitness (62). However, there are many challenges to conducting training studies with children, which may contribute to the inconclusive results in some studies. The length of training programs and individual training sessions may be shorter than those performed by adults, the number of participants may be small and limited by high attrition rates, the background level of physical activity may not be well characterized, and exercise programs must be designed to keep the children interested and engaged. Despite those challenges, plus those described

earlier for obtaining accurate and reliable measures of aerobic fitness, when children complete at least 8 weeks of structured exercise with sufficient duration and intensity, the median increase in cardiorespiratory fitness is about 5%–10% (63–65). That level of improvement may be smaller than in adults but is consistent with the hypothesis that trainability of children is somehow impaired.

Even under controlled conditions, improvement in aerobic fitness in children can be variable. For example, McManus et al. (66) had 9- to 10-year-old girls complete 3 days of training per week for 8 weeks, performing either 20 minutes of cycling at 85% of peak heart rate or a series of 10- and 30-second sprints. The two programs resulted in an increase in $\dot{V}O_{2peak}$ of 10% and 8%, respectively. However, when the same investigators performed a similar training program with boys, there was no significant improvement in $\dot{V}O_{2peak}$ (67). Likewise, another study from the same research group reported that 8 weeks of cycling performed for 20 minutes on 3 days per week by 10-year-old girls did not result in an increase in $\dot{V}O_{2peak}$ (68).

Exercise programs that are longer than 8 weeks and/or have a higher volume of exercise per week may be more likely to promote improvement in aerobic fitness in children. For example, 8- to 12-year-old boys who completed 14 weeks of running training demonstrated a 13% improvement in $\dot{V}O_{2peak}$ (69). Another study showed improved fitness in 10- to 11-year-old boys and girls after they trained for 60 minutes on 3 days per week for 13 weeks (70). Each week, the children performed one session of continuous moderate-intensity running, one session with higher-intensity interval running, and one session of other sports such as swimming, soccer, or basketball. There was improvement in $\dot{V}O_{2peak}$ in both boys (+5%) and girls (+9%) at the end of the program. The greater magnitude of change in girls could be explained by their lower initial aerobic fitness. When the same investigators conducted a follow-up study with a similar population of children and a similar training program, the improvement in $\dot{V}O_{2peak}$ was higher in boys (15%) than in girls (8%), once again revealing the variability in training responses in young participants (71). In the latter study, the authors also showed that the training resulted in an increase in peak cardiac output. Because peak heart rate was unchanged, the improvement in cardiac output was due to an 11% increase in cardiac stroke volume in girls and 15% in boys. Thus, the change in cardiac function occurred in both boys and girls and paralleled the change in aerobic capacity.

The studies described earlier examined trainability in healthy children who were normal weight. Many studies are being conducted in children who were overweight and obese to determine whether exercise is effective at improving aerobic fitness and metabolic health, and if so, how much exercise is needed to produce clinically meaningful changes. For example, Davis et al. (72) conducted an after-school intervention for children ages 7–11 who were overweight and obese. Participants were assigned to either 20 or 40 minutes of structured exercise on 5 days per week for 13 weeks or a control condition in which they maintained their current level of physical activity. At the end of the intervention, both training groups improved $\dot{V}O_{2peak}$ on a treadmill by about 8%–9%, whereas the control group was unchanged. There were no differences in the magnitude of improvement in aerobic fitness between the 20- and 40-minute exercise groups. Likewise, both exercise groups had improvements in risk factors for diabetes and metabolic disease, including reduced total body fat and visceral fat, and improved insulin sensitivity. The study showed that daily exercise can improve metabolic health in children who were overweight/obese and that significant clinical benefits can be achieved at exercise volumes well below the current recommendation of 60 minutes per day.

Collectively, the available evidence shows that prepubertal children can improve aerobic capacity, but the likelihood of observing improvement is enhanced if the training program is at least 8 weeks in duration and includes at least 100 minutes per week of moderate-to-vigorous exercise.

Bone

Normal Changes

Like lean body mass, bone mineral density (BMD) increases rapidly during childhood and does not differ much between boys and girls until adolescence, as shown for U.S. children in Figure 2.8 (73). Similar reference data for BMD are available for children in other countries, including Mexico, South Korea, and the United Kingdom (74–76). Total bone size also increases during childhood. The long bones of the arms and legs have epiphyseal plates at each end where active growth of new bone occurs during childhood and adolescence. These growth plates, which are visible on x-rays, are weaker than the developed bone areas and can be vulnerable to fracture. However, as described in the following section, typical physical activity and sport participation pose low risk of bone fracture in children.

Role of Physical Activity and Exercise

Weight-bearing exercise is safe for the bone health of children and can increase bone strength, and this is reflected

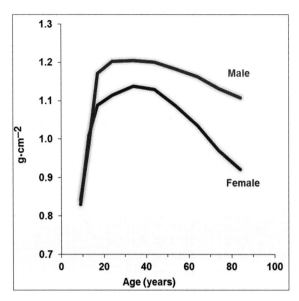

FIGURE 2.8 Reference values for total body bone mineral density in American children and adults. Data from the National Health and Nutrition Examination Survey (NHANES) 1999–2006, using dual-energy x-ray absorptiometry (DEXA). Values shown are for the 50th percentile for females (~14,000 participants) and males (~14,000 participants) ages 8–80+. (Data from Looker AC, Borrud LG, Hughes JP, Fan B, Shepherd JA, Sherman M. Total body bone area, bone mineral content, and bone mineral density for individuals aged 8 years and over: United States, 1999–2006. *Vital Health Stat 11*. 2013;11(253):1–78.)

in the most recent ACSM guidelines (14). In 2004, ACSM released a position stand on "Physical Activity and Bone Health" in which the expert committee recommended that children perform 10–20 minutes of bone-loading activities, such as running and jumping, on at least 3 days per week (77).

A 2014 review of 37 studies conducted with children and adolescents examined the effect of physical activity on bone strength, either through observation of children with different activity levels or in response to specific exercise interventions (78). Bone strength was measured with a variety of methods that provide values for mineral density, size, or structure. The majority of studies agreed that exercise has a positive effect, by promoting increased bone strength in children. The strongest effects were achieved with weight-bearing activities like running or jumping. The authors speculated that exercise may have the biggest impact on bone strength during childhood and early adolescence, because increases in bone strength in response to exercise appear to be smaller in later adolescence and young adulthood. A more recent review that focused specifically on school-based physical education interventions also confirmed that children who increase their exercise activity have greater accrual of bone mineral in the lumbar spine and femoral neck (79).

The loading forces on bone imposed by normal exercise do not appear to increase the risk of bone fracture in children. As described in the section on muscle, a Swedish study with more than 700 children 6–9 years old tested the effects of having schools increase their weekly physical activity time from a starting level of 60 minutes per week to 200 minutes per week for up to 7 years (47). In addition to showing gains in muscle strength, after 3 and 5 years of the intervention, there was no evidence for increased risk of bone fractures in the intervention group when compared to 1,500 age-matched control children who maintained the standard 60 minutes per week of physical education instruction at school (48). More importantly, a subset of participants completed annual bone density tests (using dual-energy x-ray absorptiometry) and after 2 and 3 years of the intervention, BMD, particularly in the spine, had increased more than what was observed in the control group. In another subset of children who were retested 4 years after the intervention was over, the magnitude of increase in bone mass and knee extensor strength remained higher than that of the control group, demonstrating the lasting benefits of physical activity on childhood bone development (80).

ADOLESCENTS

Adolescence is the period of physical and cognitive development between the onset of puberty and the attainment of adulthood, generally beginning at ages 10–12. Puberty, which is the development of sexual maturity, is typically complete by age 17. The end of adolescence, however, is often described as extending to 18–21 years of age, varying based on the components of physical and cognitive development under consideration, as well as legal definitions, and cultural norms.

The onset of puberty is marked by an increased production in the pituitary of the gonadotropin hormones, luteinizing hormone (LH) and follicle-stimulating hormone (FSH). LH and FSH act on the testes and ovaries to increase production of testosterone and estrogen, respectively, which promotes sexual maturation and affects growth, body composition, metabolism, and physical and cognitive function.

Because the age of puberty onset and rate of development are variable, pediatricians often classify

developmental stages in adolescents using an anatomic scoring system developed by James Tanner (81, 82). There are five Tanner stages, defined by the degree of pubic hair growth in both sexes, plus breast development in girls and testicular growth in boys. Tanner stage I is prepubertal, whereas Tanner stage V is completion of puberty, with stages II–IV defining intermediate development. In research studies with adolescents, outcomes are often considered in relation to chronological age and/or anatomical maturational level (Tanner score). There is also increasing recognition for the value of using hormone measurements like LH and FSH to classify the stage of development.

Body Size and Composition

As shown in Figures 2.1 and 2.2, growth continues rapidly from childhood through adolescence, particularly the accrual of lean mass. After puberty, differences between boys and girls become larger, with boys adding muscle mass and total lean mass at a higher rate than girls. Figure 2.3 shows that the onset of puberty in girls results in greater deposition of body fat and a steeper annual increase in body fat percentage than during childhood. By comparison, boys experience, on average, a decrease in body fat percentage during adolescence, which widens the difference between the sexes.

Physical Activity Patterns

To meet the daily recommendation of 60 minutes of MVPA, adolescents need to complete about 11,000–12,000 steps per day. Colley et al. (16) estimated that adolescent boys and girls need to complete close to 12,000 steps per day, similar to daily step rate for children in their study. That value is only slightly higher than the 11,000–11,700 steps per day for adolescents calculated in the review by Tudor-Locke et al. (15). However, more than half of adolescents do not reach these recommendations.

As mentioned in the previous section on children, Figure 2.4 displays values for daily physical activity in children and adolescents (17). The ICAD data set, which was compiled from more than 27,000 participants from 10 different countries, shows that daily MVPA declines from childhood to adolescence. Among the groups contributing data to the ICAD were investigators from the Iowa Bone Development Study (83). In that study, a cohort of nearly 600 children born between 1993 and 1997 underwent repeated assessments of growth and health. Starting when the children were 5 years old, physical activity was measured every 2–3 years until the children reached 19 years. The average level of MVPA declined as the children grew older, and girls had lower values than boys. However, more complex patterns of change occurred, depicted in Figure 2.9. Participants were subdivided into four different MVPA pattern groups. Group 1, comprising 15% of the cohort, had consistently low MVPA throughout childhood and adolescence. Group 2 (18% of participants) had a consistently moderate level of MVPA. Group 3 (53% of participants) had a decline in MVPA from moderate to low. Group 4 (14% of participants) had a decline from high to moderate MVPA. Girls made up 85% of group 1, 29% of group 2, 58% of group 3, and 12% of group 4.

The Iowa group found that involvement in organized sports also declined over time. However, there were three patterns of sport participation:

- Consistently little or no sports activity,
- Initially high sports activity but falling consistently over time, and
- Initially high activity that was maintained through age 17 before declining moderately.

Participation in organized sports, even at a declining level, was important for avoiding a consistently inactive lifestyle in those adolescents. Thus, a decline in physical activity during childhood and adolescence is a common and apparently normal development. However, opportunities and encouragement for physical activity are critical to avoid long-term sedentary lifestyle.

Metabolic Changes

As described in the section on children, the absolute value for RMR increases with growth, especially in lean mass. As shown in Figure 2.5, RMR declines throughout childhood and adolescence, though this trend is not linked to specific events or hormonal changes during adolescence.

The cellular response to insulin is clearly affected by the hormonal changes accompanying puberty (84–86). Insulin is the pancreatic hormone released when blood glucose rises, as occurs following a meal. One of the roles of insulin is to promote glucose uptake from the blood into tissues like skeletal muscle and adipose cells. Insulin resistance describes a condition in which muscle and adipose cells become less responsive to the insulin signal. The result is that blood glucose concentration may increase; moreover, the pancreas releases more insulin in an attempt to overcome the resistance. Type 2 diabetes develops when insulin resistance becomes prolonged and severe, and the pancreas does not produce enough insulin to keep glucose within the normal range. Insulin resistance is exacerbated by obesity and sedentary lifestyle, and the rise of both is a key reason that diabetes prevalence has increased so dramatically over the past 30 years.

FIGURE 2.9 Patterns of change in the daily time spent in moderate-to-vigorous physical activity (MVPA) during childhood and adolescence. Values shown for MVPA were measured in 573 children who completed follow-up measurements every 2–3 years starting at 6 years. Overall level of MVPA in the whole group declined over time, but there were four subgroups of behavior patterns evident. Groups 1 and 2 maintained their level of MVPA at low or moderate values, respectively. Groups 3 and 4 both declined, though group 4 was higher initially. (Data from Kwon S, Janz KF, Letuchy EM, Burns TL, Levy SM. Developmental trajectories of physical activity, sports, and television viewing during childhood to young adulthood: Iowa Bone Development Study. *JAMA Pediatr.* 2015;169(7):666–72.)

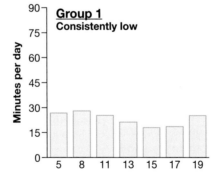

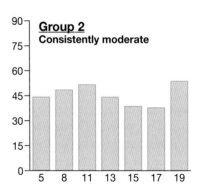

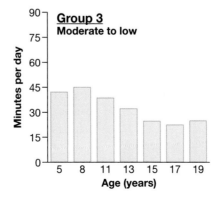

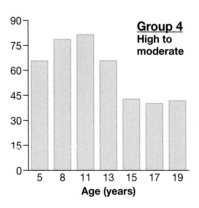

During puberty, a transient increase in insulin resistance is considered normal. Among the studies that have been performed on this topic, there is some variability in the reported magnitude of the change in insulin resistance. This may be due to the use of different measurement approaches, study populations, and study designs. However, the main finding is that, compared to Tanner stage I (prepubertal), insulin resistance is increased by 10%–20% during Tanner stages II–IV and then declines during Tanner stage V. This pattern was demonstrated in a cross-sectional study of 357 boys and girls ages 11–15 (84) and a longitudinal study in which insulin resistance was measured annually in a group of 60 boys and girls (85). In both of those adolescent cohorts, the change in insulin resistance could not be fully explained by changes in body fat, muscle mass, sex, or race, implying that endocrine changes may be responsible.

Extending those findings, more recent work showed that the rise in insulin resistance may begin even before the hormonal and anatomic changes of puberty. In the EarlyBird study, annual assessments were conducted on 307 children from Plymouth, United Kingdom, starting from when the participants were 5 years old (86, 87). Based on the age at which LH began to increase, the onset of puberty occurred at ages 9–10 in about 20% of boys and girls, and as late as age 14 in some children. Girls had higher LH values and advanced through puberty faster, based on Tanner staging, than did boys. Insulin resistance was calculated from values for fasting blood glucose and insulin. As shown in Figure 2.10, the average value for insulin resistance was lowest at 7 years, rose annually until age 13, and then declined in later adolescence. The rise in insulin resistance was evident before either the hormonal or anatomic signs of puberty, so the cause of that early change remains to be determined. The EarlyBird study also showed that insulin resistance was higher in girls than in boys throughout most of the observation period, a finding that agrees with prior investigations (84). Average blood glucose rose about 17% from ages 7 to 16, consistent with historical changes observed during puberty. The large change in insulin resistance was driven primarily by a large change in fasting insulin, which increased from ages 5 to 13 by about 60% in boys and 100% in girls, before declining thereafter.

Muscle

Normal Changes

Figure 2.2 shows that leg lean mass, which is predominantly comprised of muscle, increases rapidly during adolescence. In the NHANES sample, both boys and girls

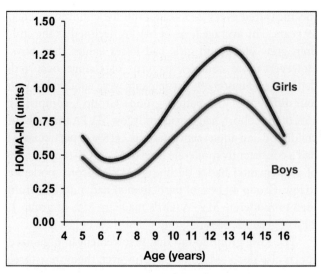

FIGURE 2.10 Changes in insulin resistance during childhood and adolescence. Values shown are for the homeostatic model of assessment — insulin resistance (HOMA-IR), a value calculated from the concentrations of fasting blood glucose and insulin. A higher value for HOMA-IR indicates higher insulin resistance. A cohort of 307 children was tested annually from age 5 to 16. Insulin resistance was higher in girls than in boys, increased during late childhood and early adolescence, and then declined in later adolescence. (Data from Mostazir M, Jeffery A, Voss L, et al. Generational change in fasting glucose and insulin among children at ages 5–16y: modelled on the EarlyBird study (2015) and UK growth standards (1990) (EarlyBird 69). *Diabetes Res Clin Pract.* 2017;123:18–23.)

demonstrated a near-doubling of leg lean mass from childhood (8–11 years) to early adolescence (12–15 years). However, boys continue to gain lean mass into late adolescence at a higher rate than girls, resulting in a higher final leg muscle mass upon reaching adulthood. Similar results were obtained in a study of boys and girls aged 6–18, in which detailed assessments of total body muscle mass were made using magnetic resonance imaging (9).

Role of Physical Activity and Exercise

As described in the section on children, expert consensus panels have concluded that resistance training is a safe and effective means to increase muscle strength in children and adolescents (45). Resistance exercise can also be used to improve speed, agility, and sport-specific tasks in adolescents who are already active in individual or team sports (46). Within the adolescent age range, girls and boys can achieve similar relative improvements in strength and performance in response to resistance training.

The high prevalence of childhood overweight and obesity, and the decline in physical activity during adolescence, may promote the development of cardiovascular and metabolic diseases earlier in adulthood. For that reason, resistance training has been tested as a means to improve both muscle mass and strength, and clinically relevant health outcomes in adolescents. Shaibi et al. (88) had overweight boys who were about 15 years old and Tanner stage III or above complete supervised resistance training for 60 minutes per session, twice per week, for 16 weeks. That program resulted in a 7% increase in lean body mass, a 26% increase in bench press and leg press strength, and a 45% reduction in insulin resistance. There was also a trend for a reduction in body fat. The same group conducted similar resistance training studies with overweight girls and boys that included a nutrition program to target weight loss (89, 90). Muscle strength was improved by about 30% but significant changes in body composition or insulin resistance were not observed. The authors speculated that the resistance training program may need to be more frequent than twice per week to promote body composition and metabolic benefits in adolescents.

Subsequent work by Sigal et al. (91) demonstrated the value of a higher volume and longer program of resistance exercise for adolescents. In their study, 300 boys and girls 14–18 years old who were overweight or obese were randomly assigned to aerobic training, resistance training, combined aerobic plus resistance training, or a no-training control group. The exercise programs were performed 4 days per week for 6 months. All participants received nutritional counseling to reduce energy intake. All three of the exercise groups showed improvement in leg press strength, but the difference was larger in the resistance training group (73%) than either the combined (58%) or aerobic training (44%) groups. All three exercise groups had a similar reduction in body fat (about 1.5 kg or 3 lb) and waist circumference (2.5–4.1 cm, or 1–1.6 inch). Though there were small changes in measures of insulin resistance and blood lipids, none were significantly altered during the intervention. The authors pointed out that the lack of change in those variables may have been because the participants were already within the normal ranges, and therefore had less margin for improvement than a cohort with, for example, diabetes or dyslipidemia. One of the challenges acknowledged in this study, which is common with exercise interventions, especially in overweight youth, was that adherence to the planned exercise program was only 60%, and about 25% of participants withdrew from the study before they finished. Thus, the exercise program may have produced larger changes if followed as prescribed, but a major obstacle is to promote behavior changes and reduce barriers to becoming physically active.

Together, the available evidence shows that strength training is effective for improving muscle size and strength in adolescents who are already active in sports as well as those who are inactive and overweight. In some adolescents, resistance training may have benefits on metabolic risk factors, such as insulin resistance or lipids, but those effects have been small and inconsistent.

Cardiorespiratory

Normal Changes

During adolescence, muscle mass and strength increase, permitting boys and girls to perform at higher workloads and achieve higher values for absolute $\dot{V}O_{2peak}$ ($L \cdot min^{-1}$) (52, 53, 92). For boys, the increase in absolute $\dot{V}O_{2peak}$ continues into late adolescence, whereas girls show signs of reaching a plateau by mid-adolescence (53, 92). Differences between boys and girls are attributed to boys having higher muscle mass and strength, higher cardiac output, and a higher concentration of hemoglobin than girls. In both boys and girls, exercise economy improves from childhood into adolescence, which means that exercise at submaximal workloads requires less energy, especially for weight-bearing activities like walking or running (93, 94). The improvement in exercise economy allows adolescents, as compared to children, to perform at a higher fraction of their aerobic capacity during continuous work such as a 1-mile run, thus achieving better performance without an increase in $\dot{V}O_{2peak}$. This gain in exercise economy is the result of increased motor unit coordination and/or motor unit activation, increased muscle perfusion, increased muscle mitochondrial content leading to higher lactate threshold, and longer stride length.

As noted earlier, values for $\dot{V}O_{2peak}$ have been historically expressed relative to body mass to normalize for the age-associated body size differences. $\dot{V}O_{2peak}$ is closely associated with lean mass, because active muscle mass is required for movement, but those data are not always available (54, 55). Values for $\dot{V}O_2$ in $mL \cdot kg$ body $mass^{-1} \cdot min^{-1}$ are either stable or increase in boys from ages 12 to 18, and stable or decline in girls (53, 95, 96). There is variation among studies about whether aerobic fitness relative to body mass increases, decreases, or stays the same as adolescents mature, but that can be explained by the inclusion of participants with different levels of physical activity and body fatness. Methods for measuring aerobic fitness can also vary among laboratories, with some using measurements of expired gases to determine $\dot{V}O_{2peak}$ and others predicting $\dot{V}O_{2peak}$ from submaximal workloads or heart rates during treadmill or cycle ergometry testing.

Because measurement of $\dot{V}O_{2peak}$ typically occurs under controlled laboratory settings and requires expensive equipment and skilled operators, alternate methods are often used in field studies or community- or school-based fitness screenings. For example, Lang et al. (51) compiled data for the 20-m shuttle run (also known as a PACER test or "beep" test) from 177 studies, with more than 1.1 million children and adolescents ages 9–17. Some caution should be used when interpreting results from field tests because they are indirect measures of $\dot{V}O_{2peak}$. For example, estimates of $\dot{V}O_{2peak}$ derived from a 20-m shuttle run performed with adolescent boys were not well matched with $\dot{V}O_{2peak}$ measured during treadmill test with expired gas measurements, and the estimated values were both higher and lower than measured values among individual participants (97).

The NHANES data set has assessments of cardiorespiratory fitness for participants aged 12–49, displayed by the dotted lines in Figure 2.11. For the 3,000 adolescents 12–18 years old tested in the years 1999–2002, $\dot{V}O_{2peak}$ on the treadmill increased with advancing age in boys and decreased in girls (95). A strength of the NHANES study is that it is a large, nationally representative data set that includes participants from several racial–ethnic groups, geographic areas, and socioeconomic classes. A limitation of that data set, however, is that the tests were not continued to maximal effort and expired gases were not measured, so $\dot{V}O_{2peak}$ was estimated from submaximal heart rate values. Eisenmann et al. (95) presented normative data for adolescents who were tested in NHANES, including percentile data for high and low fitness, but acknowledged that predicting $\dot{V}O_{2peak}$ from heart rate and workload in adolescents has not been extensively validated.

A comparison of large data sets from several countries published over the past 50 years suggests that average cardiorespiratory fitness in children and adolescents has declined over time (98). Data from NHANES show that aerobic fitness in adolescents tested in 2012 was significantly lower than in the adolescents tested from 1999 to 2002, and fewer reached the "healthy fitness zone" (99). The Cooper Aerobics Institute (Dallas, TX) defined healthy fitness zone based on the association of aerobic fitness with risk factors for cardiometabolic diseases like diabetes and cardiovascular disease (CVD). To reach the healthy fitness zone, boys need to achieve a $\dot{V}O_{2peak}$ between 40.2 mL·kg^{-1}·min^{-1} (10 years old) and 44.3 mL·kg^{-1}·min^{-1} (18 years old). Girls need a $\dot{V}O_{2peak}$ between 40.2 mL·kg^{-1}·min^{-1} (10 years old) and 38.6 mL·kg^{-1}·min^{-1} (18 years old). Over the two measurement periods, the percentage of boys 12–15 years old who reached the healthy fitness zone fell from 65% to 50% (99). The number of girls in the healthy fitness zone fell from 41%

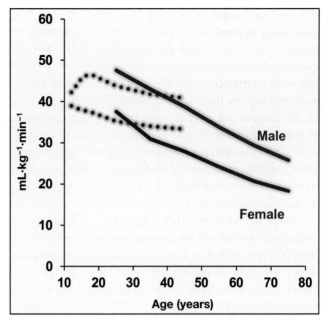

FIGURE 2.11 Reference values for cardiorespiratory fitness ($\dot{V}O_{2peak}$) in American children, adolescents, and adults. Dotted lines are for the 50th percentile for females (~3,000 participants) and males (~3,200 participants) tested in the National Health and Nutrition Examination Survey (NHANES) 1999–2004. In NHANES, children and adults aged 12–49 walked or ran on a treadmill until achieving at least 75% of the age-expected maximal treadmill stage and peak oxygen uptake ($\dot{V}O_{2peak}$) was estimated using heart rate. The solid lines show $\dot{V}O_{2peak}$ measured in the FRIEND study using expired breath analysis during a treadmill test to volitional fatigue. Values plotted are means for each decade from 20 to 79 years in ~3,200 women and ~4,600 men who did not have cardiovascular disease. (Data from Eisenmann JC, Laurson KR, Welk GJ. Aerobic fitness percentiles for U.S. adolescents. *Am J Prev Med.* 2011;41(4 Suppl 2):S106–10; Kaminsky LA, Arena R, Myers J. Reference standards for cardiorespiratory fitness measured with cardiopulmonary exercise testing: data from the fitness registry and the importance of exercise national database. *Mayo Clin Proc.* 2015;90(11):1515–23.)

to 34%. Similar trends were observed in both younger and older adolescents, across racial–ethnic groups, and across socioeconomic levels. A likely contributor to the reduced aerobic fitness is the increase in average body mass over time, because $\dot{V}O_{2peak}$ was presented as mL·kg^{-1}·min^{-1}.

Role of Physical Activity and Exercise

Tests performed on adolescent endurance athletes in the U.S. and Europe, primarily middle- and long-distance runners, showed that $\dot{V}O_{2peak}$ can reach 60–70 mL·kg^{-1}·min^{-1} in boys and 50–60 mL·kg^{-1}·min^{-1} in girls (100). Boys who consistently trained demonstrated minor increases in $\dot{V}O_{2peak}$ over 3–6 years of follow-up, whereas girls had a minor decline. Among the highest values for $\dot{V}O_{2peak}$ reported for adolescents were mean values of 74 mL·kg^{-1}·min^{-1} for boys and 62 mL·kg^{-1}·min^{-1} for girls living in rural Kenya (101). Kenyan runners are renowned for their success in middle- and long-distance events, so several studies have been conducted to determine the relative contributions of genetics, environment, and training on their athletic ability. The high $\dot{V}O_{2peak}$ of the Kenyan adolescents could be attributed, at least in part, to low body mass and habitually high volumes of MVPA (156 min per d). Even though the participants were not engaged in structured sports or training, they traveled on foot an average of 7.5 km (4.7 miles) per day to attend school.

There is a lot of evidence that $\dot{V}O_{2peak}$ can increase in response to training in adolescence (96, 102). The magnitude of improvement is likely to be higher if participants start with a habitually low level of physical activity. For example, van der Heijden et al. (103) enrolled sedentary boys and girls who were about 15 years old for a 12-week exercise program in which they performed 30 minutes of aerobic training twice per week. Starting values for $\dot{V}O_{2peak}$ were 38 mL·kg^{-1}·min^{-1} for normal-weight participants and 27 mL·kg^{-1}·min^{-1} for participants with obesity. In response to the training program $\dot{V}O_{2peak}$ improved by about 15% in both groups. In the study by Sigal et al. (91) described earlier, in which adolescents with excess body weight completed 6 months of aerobic exercise 3−4 days per week, $\dot{V}O_{2peak}$ increased by about 9% from a starting value of 30 mL·kg^{-1}·min^{-1}. Across studies, the range of improvement in $\dot{V}O_{2peak}$ in adolescents in response to training is similar to that reported in adults.

$\dot{V}O_{2peak}$ responses to training can be quite variable. Sénéchal et al. (104) found that following 6 months of aerobic training on 3 days per week, adolescents who were overweight/obese had a wide range of individual changes in $\dot{V}O_{2peak}$, demonstrating that "trainability" is an inherent trait that differs among individuals. That finding is consistent with prior work in adults, which also showed that the magnitude of improvement in $\dot{V}O_{2peak}$ is variable but clusters within families, revealing an underlying genetic regulation (105).

In addition to improving cardiorespiratory fitness, aerobic training has been shown to reduce body fat (particularly abdominal fat), lower insulin resistance, reduce blood pressure, and reduce triglycerides in adolescents (91, 103, 104, 106, 107). Those effects are usually more pronounced in participants who were initially overweight or obese compared to peers who were normal weight. For example, after 12 weeks of aerobic exercise on 3 days per week, teenagers who were obese had a 10% reduction in abdominal fat and a 25% reduction in liver fat content (103). Peers who were normal weight who completed the same exercise program had low values of abdominal and liver fat at the start of the program, so the exercise training did not have a measurable effect on those outcomes. However, the groups that were normal weight and obese each had a reduction in insulin resistance, with a trend for greater improvement in the obese group (59%) than the group that was normal weight (35%) (108). The obese group had greater insulin resistance at the beginning of the study and, despite the large reduction during the exercise program, remained higher than the starting level of the group that was normal weight.

There is growing evidence that exercise quality is important for achieving improvements in several health metrics in adolescents who are sedentary and/or overweight/obese. A focus on using high-intensity interval training (HIIT; alternating intervals of high-intensity exercise and low- to moderate-intensity recovery activity) has become popular. HIIT has been shown to induce larger improvement in $\dot{V}O_{2peak}$ and blood pressure in adolescents who were obese than a comparable volume of continuous moderate-intensity exercise (65, 106). When used in a school setting for brief periods on 3 days per week for 10 weeks, HIIT resulted in lower serum triglyceride concentration in 13- to 14-year-old boys and girls (107). The potential value of HIIT is that it imposes elevated levels of exertion on the cardiovascular and metabolic systems than moderate-intensity training, but the short segments of activity are manageable because they are typically 1−4 minutes in duration. The additional stress from higher-intensity work may provoke greater adaptive responses. If conducted with supervision, HIIT may be particularly useful for sedentary adolescents, for whom 60 minutes per day of MVPA is an unlikely goal. HIIT sessions can be completed in 20−30 minutes per session, including the warm-up.

Bone

Normal Changes

Attainment of peak height occurs in adolescence when the long bones, particularly the legs, stop growing. The epiphyseal growth plates of the legs typically fuse between age 12 and 16 in girls and between age 14 and 19 in boys (109). Fusion of the epiphyses is regulated by the actions of estrogen and testosterone. Although linear growth ends, bone architecture and remodeling remain active, and deposition of bone mineral continues to increase into young adulthood. As shown in Figure 2.8, boys reach a higher level of BMD by age 17 than girls and the difference is maintained throughout adulthood. In addition to sex differences, non-modifiable factors that regulate development of bone mass during adolescence and young adulthood include genetics, race/ethnicity, and age of pubertal onset (109). Studies of families show that peak bone mass is highly heritable, accounting for about 60%–80% of the variability. Young African Americans have higher bone density than all other racial/ethnic groups in the U.S., so the International Society for Clinical Densitometry recommends using reference tables with race-specific values when calculating bone development potential in children (110). The rate of accrual of bone mineral accelerates during puberty, but earlier onset of puberty is associated with higher peak bone mass development, especially in girls (109).

Role of Physical Activity and Exercise

As described in the section on children, weight-bearing exercise has been shown to increase bone strength in children and adolescents. ACSM recommends that adolescents perform weight-bearing exercise or resistance exercise for 10–20 minutes on at least 3 days per week to promote the development of strong bones (14, 77).

The amount of skeletal muscle mass is positively related to bone mineral content in children and adolescents (9). Thus, physical activity that promotes muscle development is also likely to support bone strength. However, there are fewer well-controlled studies on the effect of exercise on bone strength in adolescents than in children, so additional work is needed to determine how much exercise is required to produce a clinically significant change in bone strength (78).

Foundations for Adult Health and Disease Evident in Adolescence

Although overt cardiovascular or metabolic diseases are rare during adolescence, health-related behaviors practiced during this life stage can either promote or help prevent the development of these diseases in adulthood. Because few adolescents experience conditions like heart attacks, stroke, kidney failure, pulmonary disease, or Type 2 diabetes (which is increasing in adolescents but is still uncommon), studies monitoring predictors of those conditions rely on several other clinical and blood-based biomarkers. In the NHANES from 1999 to 2004, the panel of cardiovascular and metabolic risk factors measured in children and adolescents included blood pressure and blood concentrations of lipids, glucose, insulin, and C-reactive protein (an inflammatory marker produced by the liver). Children and adolescents with the lowest proportion of body mass as skeletal muscle were most likely

to have the highest values for those risk factors (111). Similarly, adolescents with the highest relative body fat were most likely to have the highest values for cholesterol and triglycerides (112). Thus, associations between body composition and known risk markers for cardiovascular and metabolic disease follow generally similar patterns in adolescents as in adults.

Cardiorespiratory fitness is also associated with metabolic health in youth. As described previously, the thresholds for the healthy fitness zone for $\dot{V}O_{2peak}$ were set based on associations with risk factors for the clustering of risk factors for CVD and diabetes known as the metabolic syndrome. The presence of metabolic syndrome is defined as having at least three of the following: high blood pressure, high fasting glucose, high triglycerides, high waist circumference, and low concentration of high-density lipoprotein (HDL) cholesterol. A large European study of 9- and 15-year-olds measured aerobic fitness on a bicycle and the components of metabolic syndrome to determine how closely they were related (113). About 15% of the children were at risk for metabolic syndrome, defined as having a composite metabolic risk score that was 1 standard deviation above the mean. Aerobic fitness was negatively correlated with metabolic risk, meaning that children with the highest fitness were at the lowest metabolic risk. Optimal fitness was defined as $\dot{V}O_{2peak}$ greater than 37 and 33 mL·kg^{-1}·min^{-1} in 9- and 15-year-old girls, respectively, and 44 and 46 mL·kg^{-1}·min^{-1} in 9- and 15-year-old boys, respectively.

Longitudinal studies showed that characteristics such as obesity, low fitness, and dyslipidemia tend to persist from adolescence into adulthood (114). Such findings have been used as the rationale for greater health and fitness promotion to establish healthy lifestyles during childhood and adolescence.

Several longitudinal studies of adolescents have identified variables that predict adult health and disease outcomes. For example, a study of Swedish men showed that both $\dot{V}O_{2peak}$ and muscle strength at age 18 were inversely related to the development of CVD and death by middle age in men (115). The authors of that study were able to use fitness assessments performed on 1.1 million men who completed mandatory military service screening when they were about 18 years old. Using public health databases, they could also track health events in those men over a median follow-up time of 26 years. Men with low aerobic fitness and/or handgrip strength when they were young were the most likely to develop arrhythmias, heart failure, stroke, and related diseases or to die of CVD during the follow-up period.

Similar types of observations have been made in European and U.S. populations. The Young Finns Study is an ongoing longitudinal study of more than 4,000 men and women in Finland. Among their many observations, the investigators found that high blood pressure and lipids (specifically, a high ratio of low-density lipoprotein [LDL] to HDL cholesterol and the apolipoproteins associated with those molecules) during childhood and adolescence were associated with greater thickening of the carotid artery and lower function of the vascular endothelium 21 years later in young adulthood (116, 117). Both of those vascular changes are risk factors for CVD. In the U.S., longitudinal studies involving children from Muscatine, Iowa, and Bogalusa, Louisiana, had findings like those of the European studies, showing that cardiometabolic disease risks that develop during childhood and adolescence carry forward into early adulthood (118–122).

Together, these longitudinal studies provide much of what we know today about markers for adult disease risk that are detectable in childhood and adolescence. The available evidence shows that a combination of low aerobic fitness and muscle strength, high blood pressure and blood lipids, and/or obesity during childhood and adolescence is associated with elevated cardiovascular and metabolic disease risk in adulthood.

YOUNG ADULTS

Young adulthood covers the period from approximately 20 to 39 years old. During this period, most people achieve their highest values for muscle mass and strength, and athletic performance. The differences in body composition and physical performance between boys and girls established in adolescence persist into young adulthood.

Unlike childhood and adolescence, which are marked by growth and development, young adulthood is predominantly characterized by maintenance of physical function.

Muscle

Normal Changes

As shown in Figure 2.2, leg lean mass is maintained throughout young adulthood. Those results agree with the findings of several other studies, including classic work by Lexell et al. (123–125). Lexell et al. (124) examined the size and contractile phenotype of the vastus lateralis muscle in healthy adults from 15 to 83 years old. Unlike studies that measured muscle fibers from small biopsy samples, a novel feature of Lexell et al.'s studies was that measurements were made on a cross-section of the entire muscle, obtained during autopsy from people who had died in accidents. Figure 2.12 shows a summary of the findings. As described in more detail in following sections, whole muscle size and the size and number of muscle fibers were reduced in middle-aged and older people compared to young adults. From 20 to 40 years old, however, muscle size and the proportion of fiber types were largely stable.

The strength of some muscle groups can continue to increase up to age 30 as shown for handgrip in Figure 2.7. For most other muscle groups, the level of muscle strength achieved in late adolescence or early adulthood is maintained through approximately 40 years old and declines thereafter. That pattern is shown for knee extensor strength in Figure 2.13, using data acquired from 654 healthy men and women in the Baltimore Longitudinal Study of Aging (126). Another report on the same cohort showed that arm strength (elbow flexors) followed

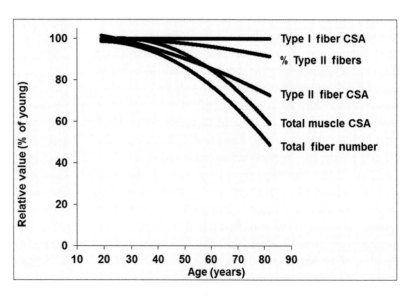

FIGURE 2.12 Age-related changes in quadriceps muscle size, and the proportion and cross-sectional area (CSA) of type I and type II muscle fibers. Values are shown as relative changes in the vastus lateralis muscle from young adults (~20 years), using samples from 83 people. The main finding was that the decline in muscle size could be attributed to a decline in the number of muscle fibers and a selective reduction in the area occupied by type II muscle fibers. (Data from Lexell J, Taylor CC, Sjostrom M. What is the cause of the ageing atrophy? Total number, size and proportion of different fiber types studied in whole vastus lateralis muscle from 15- to 83-year-old men. *J Neurol Sci.* 1988;84(2–3):275–94.)

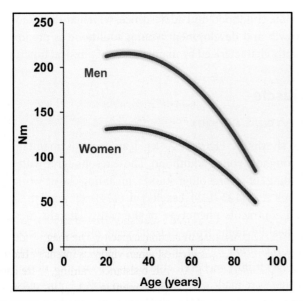

FIGURE 2.13 Values for isokinetic knee extensor torque in adults. Data collected in healthy adults 20–93 years old enrolled in the Baltimore Longitudinal Aging Study. Values shown are for the line of best fit for age vs. strength (torque at 30 degrees·s^{-1} [0.52 rad·s^{-1}], measured in Newton meters) for 308 females and 346 males. (Adapted with permission of American Physiological Society, from Lindle RS, Metter EJ, Lynch NA, et al. Age and gender comparisons of muscle strength in 654 women and men aged 20–93 yr. *J Appl Physiol (1985)*. 1997;83(5):1581–7.)

a similar pattern as the legs, with peak values maintained from 20 to 40 years old, before declining during middle age and beyond (127).

Role of Physical Activity and Exercise

It is well established that resistance training results in increased muscle strength in young adults, because of increases in muscle size (hypertrophy) and neuromotor activation (128). Classic studies performed with young adults showed that these changes occur in both arm and leg muscles. For example, Narici et al. (129) conducted a small but detailed examination of the quadriceps muscle in young men who completed knee extensor resistance exercise on 4 days per week for 9 weeks. As a result of training, muscle strength increased by 21%. The cross-sectional area (CSA) of the quadriceps increased 8.5% and electromyographic (EMG) activity during contractions increased 42%.

The hypertrophy response to resistance exercise is due to a net increase in muscle protein synthesis relative to protein breakdown. In response to an acute bout of resistance exercise, both muscle protein breakdown and synthesis are elevated for several hours (130, 131). This process of synthesis and breakdown is called protein turnover. With repeated training sessions, the elevation in protein synthesis outpaces breakdown, leading to a net gain of protein deposition, particularly the myofibril proteins responsible for contraction. This results in hypertrophy of individual muscle fibers. The process of protein breakdown allows for removal of older, damaged proteins, with many of the liberated amino acids available for synthesis of new proteins. Recycling of amino acids within the muscle alone is not sufficient to support muscle growth. Optimal enhancement of muscle protein synthesis occurs when a protein-containing meal or amino acid supplement is consumed within about 3 hours after resistance exercise (132–134). In this way, muscle contraction and the amino acids from the meal act synergistically to activate the protein synthesis pathways. However, attaining improvements in muscle size and strength in response to a resistance training program appears to be less dependent on meal timing than once assumed, and is more closely dependent on consuming a consistent diet with adequate daily protein (135–138).

An important characteristic of exercise adaptation that is only partly understood is the individual variability in physiological responses. A good example for resistance training was a study performed by a team of investigators from 10 academic centers called the Exercise and Genetics Collaborative Research Group (139). They had 585 young men and women, 18–39 years old, perform unilateral resistance training with only their nondominant arm. The exercise consisted of bicep curls and triceps extensions and was performed 2 days per week for 12 weeks. The strength of the biceps muscle was measured during dynamic (one-repetition maximum) and isometric (maximal voluntary contraction at a fixed elbow angle) contractions, and muscle size was measured with magnetic resonance imaging. The training program produced significant improvements in biceps muscle CSA (19%) and isometric (20%) and dynamic (54%) strength. Men had 2.5% greater hypertrophy than women and greater absolute gains in strength. Women had a greater relative change in strength than men: 22% versus 16% for isometric, 64% versus 40% for dynamic. However, a striking finding was that the responses were highly variable among both men and women. The range in relative change in muscle CSA from pre- to posttraining was −2% to +59%. For isometric strength, the range was −32% to +149%, and for dynamic strength, the range was 0% to +250%. A goal of the study was to explore potential genetic explanations for those variations. At least 17 genetic differences, known as single nucleotide polymorphisms (SNPs), were found to be related to either baseline strength or response to strength training (140). The best-studied of the gene candidates was α-actinin 3 (ACTN3). That gene accounted for about 2% of the baseline variability in strength and 2% of the change in strength, though these relationships were only evident in women. Thus, even the strongest SNP accounted for only a small fraction of the total variation in muscle strength. It is possible that further studies will reveal that muscle strength is regulated by clusters of multiple SNPs along with other types of regulatory factors affecting muscle contractile proteins. SNPs and other genetic mechanisms are discussed in detail in Chapter 18.

Cardiorespiratory

Normal Changes

Cardiorespiratory fitness and sport performance can continue to increase in young adults who maintain a high level of training, as demonstrated in competitive endurance athletes. For the average recreationally active person, $\dot{V}O_{2max}$ reaches the highest level in late adolescence, may be maintained into early adulthood (20–29 years old), and then begins to decline. Several studies have reported that $\dot{V}O_{2max}$ decreases about 1% per year on average, starting around age 30. That change in adults is shown in Figure 2.11, which depicts representative values for children and adults 12–49 years old in NHANES, and in adults 20–79 years old in the Fitness Registry and the Importance of Exercise National Database (FRIEND) study (141). The FRIEND study compiled values from treadmill tests for about 7,800 adults without CVD, performed at eight laboratories in the U.S. For young adults $\dot{V}O_{2max}$ acquired in NHANES (dotted lines in Figure 2.11) and FRIEND (solid lines in Figure 2.11) were similar, although they did not fully overlap. An important distinction between the two studies is the way that $\dot{V}O_{2max}$ was determined. In NHANES, $\dot{V}O_{2max}$ for each person was estimated based on submaximal values for heart rate, whereas in the FRIEND study, $\dot{V}O_{2max}$ was measured using expired gas analysis while the participant exercised to volitional exhaustion. Despite numerous attempts to create accurate and reliable prediction equations for $\dot{V}O_{2max}$, there are always potential errors because of the variability in heart rate during submaximal exercise; each person's maximal heart rate (HR_{max}); speed or grade of treadmill stages used in the prediction equations; and exercise economy. The FRIEND team published a separate set of reference values for $\dot{V}O_{2max}$ during a cycling ergometry test (142). Data were obtained from almost 5,000 adults tested at 10 laboratories. $\dot{V}O_{2max}$ values for cycling were, on average, 23% lower than the reference values attained during treadmill testing, but the age-related decline was about the same with both exercise modes.

Role of Physical Activity and Exercise

In young, highly competitive endurance athletes (*i.e.*, runners and cyclists), values for $\dot{V}O_{2max}$ can reach 75–85 $mL \cdot kg^{-1} \cdot min^{-1}$ in men and 65–78 $mL \cdot kg^{-1} \cdot min^{-1}$ in women (143–145). Some world-class cross-country skiers have even been reported to exceed 90 $mL \cdot kg^{-1} \cdot min^{-1}$ at their peak training (146). Achieving such high values requires the right genetics, low body mass, and heavy training. Even in nonathletes, however, it is well established that exercise training results in an increase in aerobic capacity. The magnitude of increase in $\dot{V}O_{2max}$ is greatest when vigorous intensity training is included (147). As with resistance training, there can be high variability in the improvement in $\dot{V}O_{2max}$ in response to aerobic training (105). This key concept was clearly shown in the HERITAGE study, in which 742 adults completed the same program of stationary bicycle exercise on 3 days per week for 20 weeks. Participants were clustered in family units that had two middle-aged or older parents and at least two of their young adult offspring. At the end of the program, the average improvement in $\dot{V}O_{2max}$ was 19%. However, there was a continuum of individual responses, with 5% of participants experiencing little or no change and another 5% experiencing a $\dot{V}O_{2max}$ improvement of at least 40% above baseline. The results showed that relative improvement was similar among the younger and older participants, and that genetics and shared family environment accounted for nearly half of the variability in $\dot{V}O_{2max}$ response to the training. Several other clinical and functional variables measured in the study (blood lipids, insulin resistance, blood pressure, body composition) also showed variable responses to the exercise training and evidence of genetic influences on those responses. Thus, a useful lesson for the CEP is to expect potentially high variability in client responses to exercise training programs. If initial responses in $\dot{V}O_{2max}$ to a training program are less than expected, adjusting the frequency, intensity, time, or type of exercise may be effective.

Bone

Normal Changes

In young adults, the long bones are no longer growing but the turnover of protein and bone mineralization remains active. In the cross-sectional comparison of people in NHANES, total body BMD increased between age 20 and 30 in both men and women (Figure 2.8). As in adolescents, bone strength during young adulthood is positively related to muscle mass. There is also evidence that exercise causes bone remodeling in young adults and that weight-bearing and higher impact activities can promote increases in bone strength. Because women have lower average BMD than men and because women are at higher lifetime risk of osteoporosis, more attention has been given to exploring the role of exercise on bone health in women.

Role of Physical Activity and Exercise

Load-bearing exercise is beneficial for increasing the BMD of the hip and spine in young adults. Several approaches have been used to test the hypothesis that weight-bearing activities can promote the accrual of bone mass after puberty, with the expectation that such efforts would offer protective benefit later in life. For example, a study of Korean women aged 19–26 collected their history of physical activity, including running, weightlifting, jumping, and other impact exercises (148). The volume of loading-type activities was positively correlated to BMD of the total hip and the femoral neck, a frequent site of osteoporotic fracture in old age. In those women, fat-free mass was also positively correlated to BMD. Similarly, a study of more than 1,000 young women from Sweden showed that those who regularly performed high-impact exercise had bone density values that were 4.7% higher in the femoral neck and 3.1% higher in the lumbar spine than women of the same age who were sedentary or performed only low-impact activities (149). Intervention studies showed that bone density in young women can be increased in response to at least 6 months of jumping exercise and/or resistance training of the legs and hips (150–152).

MIDDLE-AGED ADULTS

With the onset of midlife, at approximately 40–45 years of age, physiological changes are no longer characterized by growth and development. Peak gains in major systems have occurred among both men and women, and a pattern of loss becomes apparent in muscle, bone, and cardiorespiratory function that continues through the onset of old age at approximately 65 years. Although loss can be minimized and to a certain extent reversed by exercise and diet, age-related changes are inevitable and continue into senescence.

Muscle

Normal Changes

Loss of muscle mass is progressive with age, although during middle age, absolute and relative muscle mass vary by race and ethnicity (153). Men achieve greater absolute skeletal muscle mass than do women and generally retain more throughout the lifespan, but by the fifth decade loss is apparent in both sexes and comes primarily from the larger muscles of the lower body (154). Loss is gradual, with reductions of 3%–8% observed each decade after the age of 30 (155). Generally, the rate of change remains constant for both men and women (156), and by middle age, an average of 10% of peak muscle mass is lost (124). This loss of skeletal muscle with age is termed *sarcopenia*. Although often associated with old age, a 10% prevalence of sarcopenia has been reported in adults as early as 45 years of age (157).

Both the quantity and quality of muscle are diminished with age. Muscle quantity is the overall muscle mass or volume. It is determined by the total number of fibers and the CSA of those fibers (Figure 2.12), with the total number of muscle fibers having the greatest influence (124). In middle-aged adults, skeletal muscle is chiefly composed of slow twitch type I and fast twitch type II fibers, and there is little reduction in the total number of fibers compared to younger adults (125). However, a shift in fibers begins to occur during midlife associated with denervation and reinnervation of individual fibers and loss of motor units (123). Consequently, there is a reduction in type II fiber size (Figure 2.12), and as a result, type I fibers make up a greater proportion of the CSA (158). Muscle strength is influenced primarily by type II fibers, which may place women at greater risk for loss of strength than men. Hakkinen et al. (159) evaluated muscle fiber CSA in middle-aged men and women, finding that in men type II fibers made up 45% more of the CSA of the vastus lateralis, although the CSA of type I fibers was equal between sexes.

Muscle quality is the ability of muscle to generate force. It describes the physiological function of muscle. Changes in muscle quality reflect changes associated with performance or functional ability. Although muscle quality is not solely dependent on muscle mass, strength relative to muscle mass is the defining characteristic of muscle quality (160). With age, there is a loss of contractility in both type I and type II fibers that impairs the muscle's ability to generate force independent of the CSA (161). Compared to younger adults, Jozsi et al. (162) reported average losses in force production of 14% in midlife adults.

Fat deposition, both within and outside the muscle, is associated with loss of strength and, hence, loss of muscle quality with age. During middle age, adults experience weight gain accompanied by intra- and intermuscular fat deposition, and loss of muscle strength and quality (163,

164). Overend et al. (165) evaluated differences in fat deposition between young and elderly men, finding 35% or more increases in intra- and intermuscular fat, which would have accrued during middle age.

Loss of muscle is accompanied by a decreased RMR. In midlife, there is a positive relationship between lean mass and 24-hour energy expenditure (166). Through the fifth decade of life, skeletal muscle accounts for approximately 22% of RMR (167). A study of 700 healthy adults across the lifespan found that the relationship between muscle mass and RMR remained the same between young (18–39 years), middle-aged (40–59 years), and older (≥60 years) adults (168). However, after reaching a peak in young adults, RMR declines by 1%–2% per decade through midlife into old age (169). In a cohort of approximately 200 adults from the Quebec Family Study, RMR declined by 7% over 30 years between the ages of 24 and 54 (170). This decline mirrors age-related changes in lean mass.

Postexercise metabolism is characterized by a transient increase in energy expenditure known as the excess postexercise oxygen consumption (EPOC). Lean mass is a determinant of the extent and duration of EPOC (171), so as muscle is lost over the lifespan, there may be effects on EPOC as well. Gender differences in EPOC have been reported in men and women during middle age, but when normalized for lean mass, these differences are no longer apparent (172). Although evidence regarding age-related changes in EPOC is limited, EPOC remains intact or slightly blunted during midlife. In men between the ages of 59 and 77, a 3% increase in energy expenditure over a 48-hour period has been observed after an acute bout of resistance exercise (173). By comparison, a study using a similar bout of resistance exercise in young men elicited a 9% increase over 24 hours of recovery (174). Differences are less clear in women. After comparable bouts of resistance exercise, both young and middle-aged women experienced similar 2-hour increases in EPOC of 23% and 22%, respectively (175, 176).

Nutritional and Biochemical Influences

Changes in endogenous hormone production, metabolism, and physical activity during midlife contribute to loss of muscle. Beginning in middle age, total and bioavailable testosterone levels have been observed to decline in men by as much as 3% annually (177), although there is some evidence that total testosterone is relatively stable until the eighth decade, at which time it begins to decline (178). In women, evidence indicates a progressive decline in both

total and bioavailable testosterone with age (178). Total testosterone has been observed to increase slightly after menopause, but it does not achieve levels found during young adulthood (178). In men, the Leydig cells of the testes produce approximately 95% of total testosterone. In women, testosterone production is divided equally between the ovaries and the adrenal glands (179). Midlife is characterized by a decline in ovarian activity in women, and hence, testosterone production is limited to the adrenal glands, resulting in a 50% reduction in total testosterone (180).

The decline in testosterone contributes to a reduction in the rate of muscle protein synthesis and the ability to synthesize lean mass (181). By midlife, whole-body muscle protein synthesis diminishes by approximately 40% in both men and women compared to young adults (182). Amino acid metabolism is blunted secondary to insulin resistance, and as a result muscle protein synthesis is reduced following a meal (183). Consistent with other changes in the hormonal milieu, the prevalence of insulin resistance increases with age (184). In a cohort of over 2,500 adults with an average age of 54 from the Framingham Offspring Study, insulin resistance increased with age and the overall prevalence of prediabetes in middle age was approximately 30% (185).

Chronic inflammation with elevated levels of interleukin-6 (IL-6), IL-1, and tumor necrosis factor alpha (TNF-α) contributes to the catabolism of lean mass (186). Over the adult lifespan, cytokine levels increase and have been shown to trigger atrophic changes within skeletal muscle (187, 188). As levels of inflammatory markers increase with age, skeletal muscle protein synthesis decreases (189). There is evidence for differences in the production of inflammatory markers within different muscle fiber types, with IL-6 expressed predominantly in type I fibers and TNF-α expressed primarily in type II fibers (190). Furthermore, type II fibers appear to be more vulnerable to atrophy induced by chronic inflammation than type I fibers (191), a factor which may explain in part the selective atrophy of type II fibers with age.

Role of Physical Activity and Exercise

During midlife, physical activity declines by as much as 20% compared to young adulthood (192). This is unfortunate as research evidence consistently demonstrates the beneficial effects of exercise at recommended levels (14) to prevent and reverse age-related loss of muscle mass during midlife. In middle-aged men, an acute bout of resistance exercise increases muscle protein synthesis by 80% over a 4-hour recovery period (193). Furthermore, an acute bout of resistance exercise stimulates transient increases in total and free testosterone in middle-aged men, although not middle-aged women (194). Finally, in men and women approximately 40 years of age, resistance training stimulates hypertrophy of both type I and type II fibers (Figure 2.14) that is accompanied by average increases in muscle fiber force production of 30% (159) and increases in muscle CSA of 5%–10% (194). Overall, resistance training programs of two, three, or four times per week over a 6- to 8-week period elicit increases in lean mass of approximately 3% in middle-aged men and women (195, 196).

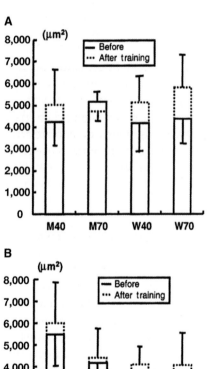

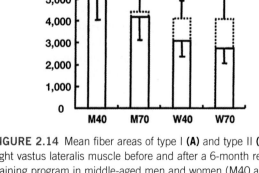

FIGURE 2.14 Mean fiber areas of type I **(A)** and type II **(B)** of the right vastus lateralis muscle before and after a 6-month resistance training program in middle-aged men and women (M40 and W40) and older men and women (M70 and W70). (Taken from Häkkinen K, Kraemer WJ, Newton RU, Alen M. Changes in electromyographic activity, muscle fibre and force production characteristics during heavy resistance/power strength training in middle-aged and older men and women. *Acta Physiol Scand.* 2001;171(1):51–62.)

Aerobic exercise also stimulates muscle protein synthesis in middle-aged adults. Chronic training can improve but does not eliminate age differences. Doering et al. (197) studied highly trained middle-aged triathletes, finding that muscle protein synthesis increased after an acute bout of exercise, but rates were reduced by 12% compared to young triathletes. In response to a 4-month cycling program, middle-aged adults demonstrated a 22% increase in muscle protein synthesis, which is comparable to increases observed in both younger and older adults (58). Cycling training can also increase CSA of the quadriceps muscle by 10% in middle-aged men (198). Both slow and fast twitch muscle fibers are affected by endurance training. Twelve weeks of high-intensity interval cycling stimulate an average increase of 10% in CSA of both type I and type II muscle fibers in middle-aged men (199).

Cardiorespiratory

Normal Changes

During midlife, cardiorespiratory fitness has long-term health implications. In a seminal study of more than 13,000 men and women, Blair et al. (200) found that low fitness increased all-cause mortality risk by more than 50%, and that achieving a fitness level equivalent to a brisk walk for at least 30 minutes per day alleviated this risk. Unfortunately, middle-aged men and women are 50% more likely to be sedentary than younger adults (201). Furthermore, $\dot{V}O_{2max}$ begins to decline during middle age, although there are apparent sex differences. Peak $\dot{V}O_2$ values have been found to be approximately 17% lower among middle-aged women compared to men of the same age, but when normalized for lean mass, differences are reduced to less than 4% (202). Cross-sectional data from more than 3,400 men and women (Figure 2.15) reflect a nonlinear rate of decline in cardiorespiratory fitness that accelerates after the age of 45, and is greater for men than for women (203). Data from meta-analyses provide overall estimates of 10-year changes in $\dot{V}O_{2max}$ for both men and women. Among sedentary men, the rate of decline is approximately 9% per decade, although regular endurance training can blunt declines to approximately 7% per decade (204). In contrast, both sedentary and endurance-trained women demonstrate similar rates of decline in $\dot{V}O_{2max}$ of approximately 10% per decade (205).

Declines in HR_{max} accompany loss of aerobic capacity with age. Cross-sectional data from approximately 5,000 healthy men and women demonstrate decreases of 3%–4% per decade during middle age (206, 207). Cardiac output and stroke volume also decline with age in both

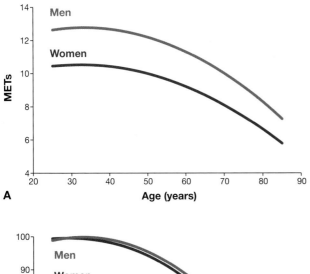

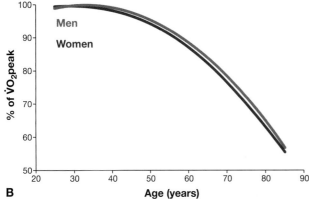

FIGURE 2.15 Age-related cardiorespiratory fitness (CRF) changes in women and men. Changes are expressed in metabolic equivalents (METs) (**A**) and as a percentage of peak CRF (**B**). (Taken from Jackson AS, Sui X, Hebert JR, Church TS, Blair SN. Role of lifestyle and aging on the longitudinal change in cardiorespiratory fitness. *Arch Intern Med.* 2009;169(19):1781–7.)

men and women (208). However, cardiac response to prolonged aerobic exercise in middle-aged adults is like that of young adults (209).

Influence of Age, Genetics, and Inactivity on Aerobic Capacity

The age-related decline in aerobic capacity appears to be constant, despite genetic and lifestyle factors. Individuals with a genetic predisposition for high peak $\dot{V}O_{2max}$, those who increase their $\dot{V}O_{2max}$ through high-intensity endurance training, and those who are habitually sedentary demonstrate a similar rate of decline with age despite initial differences, although those who achieve higher aerobic capacity at a younger age retain that advantage over the lifetime (204). However, younger men are more physically active than younger women and more likely to engage in vigorous activities that promote greater aerobic capacity (192). Hence, with age and inactivity, losses

among men are more dramatic than those observed among women (210).

Lean mass also influences aerobic capacity. In sedentary middle-aged adults, there is a strong relationship between $\dot{V}O_{2max}$ and muscle mass that attenuates the amount of decline normally attributed to age (211). Although regular exercise during young adulthood can promote greater peak aerobic capacity and lean mass, during middle age, $\dot{V}O_{2max}$ declines similarly in both athletic and sedentary adults, and these changes are attributable to loss of muscle (212). The relationship between lean mass and aerobic capacity may be explained by the oxidative capacity of skeletal muscle. Specifically, the mitochondrial respiratory capacity of skeletal muscle diminishes with age in healthy adults (213, 214), and this decline has been attributed to a decreased rate of mitochondrial protein synthesis (215). These reductions are accompanied by decreases in aerobic capacity (216). Middle-aged men with greater muscle oxidative capacity have also been observed to have greater $\dot{V}O_{2max}$ (217). Generally, in sedentary middle-aged and older adults, mitochondrial respiration is positively related to cardiorespiratory fitness and negatively related to BMI, and together, fitness and BMI explain as much as 45% of mitochondrial respiratory capacity (218). Furthermore, despite apparent loss with age, the capacity for mitochondrial biogenesis is retained in the aging muscle (219).

Role of Physical Activity and Exercise

Improvements in aerobic capacity secondary to exercise training are accompanied by improvements in skeletal muscle oxidative capacity. In middle-aged men between age 40 and 59, 6 months of running or jogging exercise increases mitochondrial density in type II muscle fibers by as much as 20% (220), whereas in men with an average age of 52, only 3 months of walking or jogging improves aerobic capacity by as much as 5% (221). Furthermore, long-term training ameliorates the expected age-related loss of aerobic capacity, and endurance-trained adults demonstrate superior aerobic capacity at any age compared to untrained adults of the same age (Figure 2.16) (222). Middle-aged Masters endurance athletes (runners, cyclists) demonstrate $\dot{V}O_{2max}$ levels that are 60%–90% greater than levels in untrained sedentary adults of the same age and that are comparable to levels in young athletes (223–227). Benefits of regular exercise during middle age are retained over time. Women who regularly exercised during middle age have been found to have a 15% greater aerobic capacity two decades later compared to women who were sedentary (228). Resistance training can also produce cardiorespiratory improvements in previously untrained

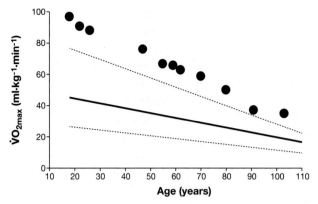

FIGURE 2.16 Highest maximum oxygen consumption ($\dot{V}O_{2max}$) values reported in the scientific literature for athletes of different ages (black circles). The solid line represents the 50th percentile of $\dot{V}O_{2max}$ according to the normative values provided by the American College of Sports Medicine (498), and the dotted lines represent the 5th and 95th percentiles. As reference values were only available up to the age of 65–75, references values from that age were estimated through linear extrapolation. ($\dot{V}O_{2max}$ individual data were taken from Valenzuela PL, Maffiuletti NA, Joyner MJ, Lucia A, Lepers R. Lifelong endurance exercise as a countermeasure against age-related $\dot{V}O_{2max}$ decline: physiological overview and Insights from masters athletes. Sports Med. 2020;50(4):703–16.)

adults. In middle-aged men and women, a brief 2-week resistance training program improved peak aerobic capacity by 3%–5%, compared to an 8% increase from 2 weeks of cycling (229). Finally, longitudinal data from large cohort studies demonstrate that the protective health benefits of cardiorespiratory fitness achieved during middle age can be retained for up to two decades (230, 231).

Bone

Normal Changes

Bone is not a static organ. In homeostasis, bone resorption (removal of old bone by osteoclasts) and formation (replacement with new mineralized bone by osteoblasts) should be balanced. With aging, bone remodeling is altered. There is a reduction in the volume of bone resorbed, accompanied by an even greater reduction in the volume of bone formed (232). As a result, bone mass decreases from young peak values. In an early study of postmortem skeletal weight, middle-aged adults were observed to have reductions of up to 35% of total bone mass compared to young adults, although middle-aged men retained as much as 50% more mass than women (233).

Loss of bone mass involves both the organic matrix that consists primarily of collagen and provides flexibility, and the inorganic mineral crystals that consist primarily of calcium and phosphorus and provide strength. Demineralization and loss of BMD occur in both trabecular

and cortical bone, although there is variability. Cross-sectional data from the Rochester Epidemiology Project demonstrate that loss of trabecular bone begins earlier than loss of cortical bone (234). Longitudinal data from the same study group demonstrate that 35%–40% of total trabecular bone loss occurs in women and men before the age of 50, whereas only 5%–15% of cortical bone is lost during the same time period (235). NHANES data reflect an overall 4% loss of BMD between young and middle adulthood (236). Sex differences have also been observed. For example, loss of spinal BMD during midlife can be 30%–40% greater among women, because of smaller declines in trabecular bone among men combined with little or no loss of cortical bone (237).

Changes in *morphology* or bone geometry also occur. Cortical bone thins and becomes more porous, whereas trabecular bone thins and loses connectivity (232, 238). Over time, bone CSA decreases, stiffness increases, and bones become fragile, with increased risk of stress-related fracture (238). Retrospective data from more than 1,200 women demonstrate that the occurrence of one or more fractures before age 50 increases risk for a second fracture after age 50 by approximately 75% (239). It is estimated that approximately 45% of women with osteoporosis at the age of 50 will experience a fracture in the following decade, compared to 30% of men with the same level of risk based on BMD (240). However, between the ages of 50 and 60, data from meta-analysis demonstrate that men and women with similar BMD have similar risks for osteoporotic fracture (241).

Influence of Genetics, Hormones, and Diet

Loss of BMD with age is influenced by genetics and hormonal changes that occur during middle age. As much as 40% of the lifetime variability in loss of BMD has been attributed to genetics (242). Furthermore, decreases in estrogen and testosterone during midlife contribute to bone loss in both men and women (243). Among women in their fifth decade, profound bone loss begins in the year prior to menopause and continues for at least 2 years subsequent to cessation of menses (244).

Diet may influence BMD. Higher protein intake, especially a high-dairy diet, may have a protective effect on BMD, particularly during periods of weight loss (245). In a cohort of approximately 3,000 men and women with an average age of 61, protein intake was found to be positively related to BMD only in women with low calcium intake (246). Subsequent analysis of this same cohort demonstrated a positive relationship between BMD and consumption of low-fat milk, which was contrasted by a negative relationship with consumption of red meat and processed foods (247). However, when data from intervention studies were pooled for meta-analysis, protein supplementation, either from plant or from animal sources, had no significant effect on BMD (248). The apparent discrepancy in findings may lie in the positive relationship found between lean mass and BMD (236). When regular protein intake is adequate to support maintenance of lean mass and subsequently BMD, a ceiling effect may exist in which supplemental protein may not have an additive effect on BMD.

Role of Physical Activity and Exercise

There is evidence that physical activity and exercise can be both detrimental and beneficial to BMD during middle age. In a cohort of 3,000 men and women from NHANES with an average age of 51, those who engaged in high levels of physical activity had higher BMD and were less likely to meet the diagnostic criteria for osteoporosis than those who engaged in low or moderate physical activity (249). Consistent with this finding, lower body muscular strength and power have been found to be positively related to hip BMD in men and women with an average age of 57 (250), and among competitive Masters athletes in their sixth decade, BMD is highest in strength athletes with greater lean mass (251).

In postmenopausal women with an average age of 61, prolonged moderate-intensity activity (60 min of brisk walking) decreases serum calcium and elicits an increase in bone resorption (252). Hence, short bouts of high-intensity exercise may be more beneficial. In women with an average age of 45, acute bouts of soccer training elicit immediate increases in bone turnover, and 15 weeks of training three times a week can increase hip and leg BMD (253). In middle-aged men with an average age of 44, 6 months of either jump or resistance training can increase spine and whole-body BMD, and improvements are maintained at 12 months with continued training (254). Finally, among middle-aged men and women with normal BMD, pooled analysis of randomized trials demonstrates that 6 months of high-load resistance training can significantly improve lumbar BMD (255).

Evidence regarding the long-term effects of regular exercise on BMD is mixed, although there is support for short, higher-intensity exercise from three cross-sectional studies. Data from male Masters track and field athletes with an average age of 50 demonstrate no effect of long-distance running on BMD, although sprinters and jumpers have been observed to have approximately 10% greater

total body BMD than either endurance runners or recreationally active controls (256). Furthermore, short-distance male and female athletes (sprinters and jumpers) with an average age of 54 have been found to have greater spine, hip, and leg BMD than long-distance runners of similar age (257). Finally, data from female Masters track and field athletes with an average age of 57 demonstrate calcaneal BMD equivalent to young adult women and 20% higher than nonactive middle-aged women, with runners, sprinters, and jumpers having higher BMD than racewalkers (258). In contrast, longitudinal data from a 12-year supervised resistance exercise and jumping program for women with an average age of 55 demonstrate progressive loss of lumbar and total spine BMD among all women (259). Nevertheless, loss was greatest among women who did not exercise and those who exercised less than twice a week, whereas loss was blunted and BMD preserved among those who exercised two or more times per week.

OLDER ADULTS

The onset of old age begins in the seventh decade, at approximately 65 years of age. Systemic losses continue in both men and women, although women are often considered at greater risk because they typically achieve lower peak lifetime values of muscle, bone, and cardiorespiratory capacity than men. Exercise and physical activity retain their effectiveness into the ninth and tenth decades, although response is generally blunted compared to young and middle-aged adults. Therefore, it is likely more prudent to prevent losses during middle age than try to reverse them in old age.

Muscle

Normal Changes

In old age, sex differences in body composition are clearly apparent, with older women having greater fat mass and lower lean mass compared to older men (260). Visser et al. (261) observed a decrease in lean mass of approximately 1%–2% per year among men and women in their eighth decade, with the rate of loss slightly greater in men. However, because of higher peak muscle mass achieved during young adulthood, older men retain significantly more lean mass in old age. Cross-sectional data from approximately 1,000 older adults from the Health, Aging, and Body Composition Study demonstrated 28% higher lean mass in men compared to women (262). Risk of sarcopenia, or loss of muscle, increases with advancing age. Using population-level data from NHANES, prevalence has been calculated to be as high as 20%–30% in community-dwelling older adults in general (263), whereas among centenarians, prevalence has been found to exceed 65% (264). However, older adults who maintain normal muscle mass during midlife are less likely to develop sarcopenia and more likely to remain functionally independent during old age (265).

Sarcopenia increases the risk for *frailty* that in turn increases the risk for morbidity and mortality in the elderly (266). Fried et al. (267) identified five criteria to define frailty that include weight loss, fatigue, weakness, slow walking speed, and low physical activity. All these criteria are influenced by or have an influence on muscle. Among most older adults, loss of both quantity and quality of muscle continues with age. Compared to peak muscle achieved in early adulthood, muscle mass declines by approximately 20% in men and women over the age of 70 (168), although the rate of decline varies by race and ethnicity (268). Furthermore, muscle CSA in the elderly can be reduced by as much as 40% compared to young adults (124), although among both men and women this loss is primarily observed in type II fibers (159) (Figure 2.12). In older men, the CSA of type II fibers has been reported to be 20% smaller than the CSA of type I fibers, despite an overall 5% greater number of type II fibers (269). Loss of contractile force in both type I and type II fibers accompanies loss of CSA. Compared to young men in their third or fourth decade, older men in their seventh or eighth decade exhibit loss of force production by as much as 25% in type I fibers and 33% in type II fibers (161). Loss of muscle strength in the elderly that is not related to neurological or muscular disease (270), referred to as "dynapenia," occurs at a faster rate than loss of muscle mass. Longitudinal data from more than 1,600 older adults in the Health, Aging, and Body Composition Study over a 5-year period demonstrate losses of 13%–16% in quadriceps strength compared to losses of only 3%–5% in thigh muscle mass (271). Although weight gain tends to stabilize in older adults, body composition changes continue. Visser et al. (261) followed 2,000 older men and women over a 2-year period, finding a 1% loss of lean mass that was balanced by a 2% gain in fat mass. Gains in intermuscular fat are accompanied by similar gains in intramuscular fat. In this same cohort of older adults, fatty infiltration within lower extremity muscles was observed in both sexes. Women were more affected than men, having more than 10% greater intramuscular thigh fat despite 40% less thigh muscle area, and at the same time greater intramuscular fat deposition effectively doubled the risk for mobility impairment in both men and women (272).

Commensurate with loss of muscle, RMR also continues to decline through the ninth decade (169). Data from more than 850 men and women in the Louisiana Healthy Aging Study demonstrate that, compared to young adults, RMR declines by an overall average of 8% in the seventh decade and by an additional 20% in the tenth decade (273). However, sex differences have been observed. Women, who on average achieve lower peak muscle mass in early adulthood compared to men, experience more profound decreases in RMR, and by the seventh decade demonstrate more than a 20% loss of 24-hour RMR compared to only a 13% loss among men (274). Generally, lean mass that primarily consists of muscle accounts for more than 60% of RMR (275). However, in elderly individuals, loss of muscle does not fully account for decreases in RMR. Atrophy of major organs also influences declines. Studies of measured versus predicted RMR in men and women over the age of 60 demonstrate differences of approximately 10% that reflect loss of metabolic activity from major organs (170, 276).

The acute effect of exercise on EPOC is retained in old age, although evidence is limited. Melanson et al. (277) compared 24-hour energy expenditure in old versus young men after an acute bout of stationary cycling, finding that both age groups increased similarly even though older men had 6% less lean mass. After an acute bout of resistance exercise, increases in RMR up to 72 hours have been observed among old men (278). Similar increases in RMR up to 72 hours have also been observed in young men after resistance exercise (279, 280), although a direct comparison of EPOC response is stymied by differences in exercise protocols.

Nutritional and Biochemical Influences

Periods of inadequate energy intake contribute to progressive loss of muscle with age. Longitudinal data from more than 2,000 older men and women in the Health, Aging, and Body Composition Study demonstrate that with weight loss, lean mass represents more than 50% of the weight lost, and when re-gain occurs, lean mass represents only 20% of the weight gained (260). The hormonal changes observed during midlife also continue into old age. Cross-sectional data from more than 1,600 older men and women in the Toledo Study of Healthy Aging reflect similar decreases in both sexes of 14% in free testosterone and more than 40% in total testosterone during the eighth decade (281). However, there are sex differences. Testosterone levels are more than 90% greater in older men than in older women; and compared to middle-aged adults, free testosterone is reduced by 40%

in older women and only 30% in older men (282). Loss of free testosterone may contribute to sex differences in lean mass. Yuki et al. (283) studied more than 500 women over an average period of 8 years, finding that the prevalence of low free testosterone ranged from 38% to 42% in the seventh and eighth decades, and the prevalence of sarcopenia among those with low free testosterone was more than three times that of women with high levels.

Muscle protein synthesis is also diminished. Compared to young adults, older adults in their seventh and eighth decades exhibit decreases in skeletal muscle protein synthesis of 20%–50% (189, 284). Specifically, quadriceps muscle protein synthesis in 65-year-old men has been found to be 25% lower than in 24-year-old men (285). By comparison, myosin heavy chain synthesis in older adulthood is reduced by 13% compared to midlife and by 44% compared to young adulthood, with no differences between sexes (182). Protein synthesis is further impaired during old age by inadequate availability of amino acids. Specifically, in older men and women in their seventh decade, blood levels of total amino acids, essential amino acids, and branched-chain amino acids are reduced by as much as 13% compared to young men and women (286). Diminished protein intake may contribute to reductions in muscle protein synthesis. More than one-third of older adults do not consume adequate protein to meet recommendations (287).

Insulin resistance appears to stabilize or even decrease during old age. Longitudinal data from 386 men in their seventh decade in the Cohort on Diabetes and Atherosclerosis Maastricht Study demonstrate this stability over a 7-year period (288). By comparison, data from a combined cohort of 5,000 men and women in the cross-sectional Di@bet.es and prospective Pizarra studies reflect a late-life decrease in insulin resistance where men and women in their seventh and eighth decades show a trend for increased insulin resistance consistent with that observed during middle age, but by the ninth decade insulin resistance decreases to approximately that of younger adults (289).

Inflammation also contributes to loss of muscle quantity and quality during old age. Increased fat mass promotes inflammation in older adults (290), so progressive fat deposition with age promotes chronic increases in cytokine production. During the eighth decade, increases in IL-6 and TNF-α are associated with decreased overall muscle mass, decreased appendicular skeletal muscle mass, and loss of upper and lower body strength (291). Furthermore, over a period of 5 years, older men and women with higher levels of IL-6 and TNF-α have been observed to lose 3%–5% of mid-thigh CSA, 7%–9% of upper body strength, and 16%–18% of lower body strength (292).

Role of Physical Activity and Exercise

Resistance training can increase both muscle quantity and quality in older adults, although less than 15% of older adults meet ACSM (14, 293) recommendations for resistance exercise (192). A 6-month program of resistance training increases muscle CSA in older adults, with greater gains observed in older women compared to older men (see Figure 2.14; (159)). A selective influence on type II fibers has been observed, with increases of up to 25% in quadriceps type II fiber size after 6 months of resistance training in older men (294). Furthermore, although force production increases in both older men and women after resistance training, their response is blunted and over a 6-month period the quality of older muscle remains diminished in relation to that of middle-aged adults participating in the same training program (159). Results from meta-analyses demonstrate average increases with resistance training of 1.1 kg in lean mass and 24%–33% in upper and lower body strength (295, 296). Nevertheless, losses cannot be entirely prevented or re-gained, so chronic exercise may provide greater protection against loss than what can be accrued from an acute exercise program. Aagaard et al. (297) compared older men with greater than 50 years of strength or aerobic training experience to older men with no training experience, finding that strength was 30% greater in the chronically trained, although type II CSA was greater only in those who engaged in strength training.

Although less effective in stimulating acute increases in muscle mass, aerobic exercise can be beneficial. Muscle protein synthesis in untrained older men and women has been found to be 19% lower than in untrained young adults, but a 16-week cycling program increases synthesis rates equally with those of trained young adults (58). Chronic aerobic training lowers insulin resistance among old men to levels below those observed in young inactive men (298). Furthermore, in elderly men and women who report lifelong regular exercise, overall lean mass remains similar to young and middle-aged adults. Wroblewski et al. (298a) compared male and female Masters athletes in their seventh and eighth decades to middle-aged athletes in their fifth and sixth decades, finding decreases in lean mass of only 9% in men and 16% in women.

Cardiorespiratory

Normal Changes

By old age, $\dot{V}O_{2max}$ declines from young peak capacity by approximately 35%–40% in sedentary men and women (204, 205), whereas female centenarians demonstrate a greater than 50% decrease in lung function and aerobic capacity compared to women eight decades younger (299). Among older adults, aerobic capacity is positively related to lean mass, and when age-related declines in $\dot{V}O_{2max}$ are adjusted for loss of lean mass, an average loss of 5% per decade is observed (214).

Declines in cardiac function are also observed. Compared to young adults, sedentary adults in their seventh decade experience a decrease of as much as 20% in cardiac output, primarily because of decreased stroke volume, and regular exercise training does not appear to attenuate loss (208). Furthermore, by the eighth decade, HR_{max} declines by as much as 16% compared to young adults in their third decade (206).

Influence of Inactivity on Cardiorespiratory Change

By the seventh decade, the predominant influence on cardiorespiratory change appears to be inactivity compounded by a blunted response to exercise training. Less than 25% of adults over 65 years of age participate in regular aerobic exercise (192). Among older adults, loss of aerobic capacity is accompanied by decreased skeletal muscle mitochondrial content (300) and energy production (214). Regular activity attenuates the decreases in mitochondrial biogenesis and oxidative capacity that are observed in sedentary older adults (301). Moreover, compared to older adults who are sedentary, those who are active demonstrate greater aerobic capacity and cardiac function (208, 302). However, the magnitude of improvements that can be achieved is diminished with age. In both young men (20–27 years) and old men (60–75 years), a 2-week period of inactivity decreases $\dot{V}O_{2max}$ by approximately 5%, whereas retraining improves aerobic capacity by only 12% in older men compared to 20% in young men (303).

Role of Physical Activity and Exercise

Improvements in cardiorespiratory capacity are observed in older adults as a result of exercise training. Masters athletes in their seventh decade demonstrate a $\dot{V}O_{2max}$ approximately 65% greater and a resting heart rate approximately 15% lower than sedentary adults of the same age (302). In older men and women in their seventh and eighth decades, 4 months of endurance exercise (cycling) improves aerobic capacity by approximately 10% (58), while extending training to 6 months increases $\dot{V}O_{2max}$ by approximately 20% (304). Six months of resistance training can also improve peak aerobic capacity by 15%–20% and time to exhaustion on a graded treadmill test by 20%–25% in 60- to 70-year-old men and women (305).

Nonetheless, loss over time is inevitable. Maintaining training intensity and volume can attenuate this loss to some extent (306), although Masters athletes pair matched with younger athletes based on performance ability still demonstrate a 10% lower $\dot{V}O_{2max}$ (307). Furthermore, a comparable rate of decline in aerobic capacity has been observed between older endurance athletes and sedentary men, although older athletes maintain a consistently higher $\dot{V}O_{2max}$ than their sedentary counterparts (308). However, the rate of decline accelerates when training intensity is not maintained over time (Figure 2.17). Similarly, chronic endurance training maintains a higher $\dot{V}O_{2max}$ in older women but the rate of decline has been observed to be greater despite training, such that absolute differences in aerobic capacity between trained and untrained women decrease with age (Figure 2.18) (309).

There is increasing interest in the effect of aerobic exercise on cognitive function for prevention or treatment of dementia. Cognitive decline in the eighth or ninth decade increases mortality by approximately 30% (310). Worldwide, the prevalence of dementia is approximately 5%, representing more than 35 million older adults (311).

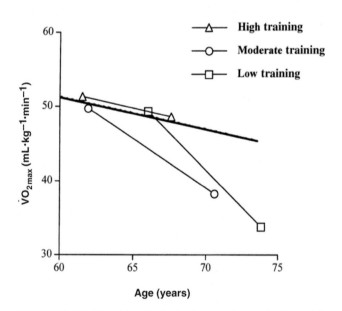

FIGURE 2.17 Mean longitudinal changes in maximal aerobic capacity ($\dot{V}O_{2max}$) with athletes categorized by training status at follow-up as "high training," "moderate training," and "low training" groups. Note the progressive reduction in $\dot{V}O_{2max}$ in the "moderate training" and "low training" groups compared with the "high training" group and the divergence from the regression line showing the baseline cross-sectional change in $\dot{V}O_{2max}$ with age. (With permission from Katzel LI, Sorkin JD, Fleg JL. A comparison of longitudinal changes in aerobic fitness in older endurance athletes and sedentary men. *J Am Geriatr Soc.* 2001;49(12):1657–64.)

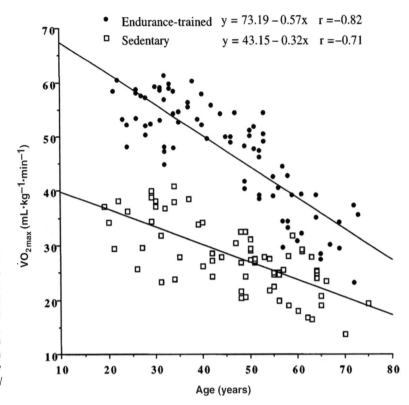

FIGURE 2.18 Relationship between maximal oxygen uptake ($\dot{V}O_{2max}$) and age in endurance-trained and sedentary women. Rate of decline in $\dot{V}O_{2max}$ with age is greater in endurance-trained women than in sedentary women. (Republished with permission of American Physiological Society, from Tanaka H, DeSouza CA, Jones PP, Stevenson ET, Davy KP, Seals DR. Greater rate of decline in maximal aerobic capacity with age in physically active vs. sedentary healthy women. *J Appl Physiol (1985)*. 1997;83(6):1947–53.)

The cardiovascular benefits of aerobic exercise suggest a biological mechanism for additional benefits on cognitive function (312). Cross-sectional data indicate a negative relationship between aerobic capacity and cerebral pathologies related to cognitive decline, and in Masters athletes, chronic endurance training decreases the occurrence of these pathologies by 80% (313). Longitudinal data from more than 21,000 participants in the Finnish Twin Cohort study demonstrate a 35% reduction in risk for onset of dementia with participation in vigorous aerobic exercise compared to sedentary behavior (314). Furthermore, longitudinal data from more than 1,700 adults over the age of 65 demonstrate a 30% overall reduction in risk for dementia among those who exercise at least three times per week (315).

However, data from meta-analyses do not support the effectiveness of acute aerobic exercise interventions for either prevention or treatment of dementia. In older adults without cognitive impairment, aerobic exercise programs of up to 6 months have not been shown to improve cognitive function despite improvements in cardiorespiratory fitness (316). Among older adults diagnosed with dementia, there is limited evidence that aerobic exercise may improve their ability to perform activities of daily living, but no evidence that it improves cognitive function (317).

Bone

Normal Changes

Bone strength is maintained by continual remodeling. Osteoclasts remove old, damaged bone to allow replacement with healthy bone by osteoblasts. However, as previously discussed, the remodeling process becomes imbalanced as individuals age. A greater volume of bone is resorbed and at the same time there is a decrease in the volume of bone formed. By old age, the rate of remodeling slows, so bone loss decreases, and results primarily from reduced formation rather than increased resorption (318). There are health implications related to bone loss. Longitudinal data from more than 700 older men demonstrate that greater bone resorption and lower BMD increase risk for all-cause mortality by 50% and double the risk for myocardial infarction (319, 320).

Postmortem measurement of skeletal mass demonstrates reductions of up to 30%–40% in older men and women compared to young adults (233). During the seventh and eighth decades, dramatic site-specific declines in BMD occur in both trabecular and cortical bones. Vertebral bone mass that is more than 80% trabecular and radial bone mass that is more than 95% cortical demonstrate a sharp increase in rate of decline in both men and women at approximately 65 years of age (234). Furthermore, on a population level, these two sites show unique patterns of

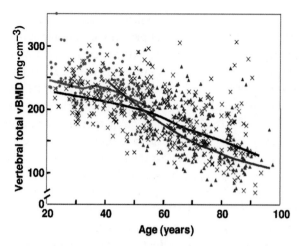

FIGURE 2.19 Values for BMD (milligrams per cubic centimeter) of the total vertebral body (>80% trabecular bone) of a population sample of adults from 20 to 97 years of age. Individual values and smoother lines are given for premenopausal women in orange, for postmenopausal women in blue, and for men in black. vBMD, volumetric bone mineral density. (Taken from Riggs BL, Melton LJ III, Robb RA, et al. Population-based study of age and sex differences in bone volumetric density, size, geometry, and structure at different skeletal sites. *J Bone Miner Res.* 2004;19(12):1945–54.)

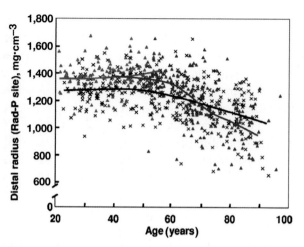

FIGURE 2.20 Values for total bone mineral density (BMD) of the distal radius (>95% cortical bone) at Rad-P scanning site in a population sample of adults from 20 to 97 years of age. Individual values and smoother lines are given for premenopausal women in orange, for postmenopausal women in blue, and for men in black. (Taken from Riggs BL, Melton LJ III, Robb RA, et al. Population-based study of age and sex differences in bone volumetric density, size, geometry, and structure at different skeletal sites. *J Bone Miner Res.* 2004;19(12):1945–54.)

change in which women have slightly greater BMD than men in young adulthood but experience greater rates of loss than men during midlife, resulting in lower BMD than men in old age. Adult changes in BMD of the vertebrae and distal radius are shown in Figures 2.19 and 2.20. In addition to gender differences, there are also racial and ethnic differences in bone density among older adults that are not explained by differences in BMI and body composition (321).

Influence of Diet on Aging Bone

Diet may influence BMD, possibly through its interaction with muscle. Cross-sectional data from more than 17,000 older adults analyzed by quartiles demonstrate that men and women in the highest quartile for dietary calcium intake and quadriceps strength had 11% and 15% higher BMD, respectively, than those in the lowest quartile (322). Nonetheless, evidence is not conclusive. Meta-analysis of five randomized controlled trials with more than 1,100 men and women in their seventh and eighth decades provides moderate-level evidence that higher protein intake has a protective effect on the lumbar spine, but not total hip, femoral neck, or total BMD (323).

Role of Physical Activity and Exercise

There is an increasing awareness of the interrelationship of bone and muscle. Stress applied to bone during muscle

activity stimulates bone remodeling, and as muscle is lost with age, mechanical stimuli are reduced (324). Elderly men with sarcopenia have lower femoral neck BMD than those with normal muscle mass (325). This is likely because of loss of the stimulus provided by the large muscles of the leg. Cross-sectional data from the Korean NHANES demonstrate an 87% prevalence of low BMD (osteopenia and osteoporosis) in older men with sarcopenia, compared to only 48% in those with normal muscle mass (326). By comparison, cross-sectional data from the Osteoporosis Fracture Prevention Study demonstrate more than a 12-fold increase in risk for low BMD (osteoporosis) among older women with sarcopenia compared to those with normal muscle mass (327).

Regular exercise throughout adolescence and young adulthood does not protect against loss of BMD during subsequent inactivity in midlife; however, a lifetime history of exercise does appear to have a protective effect. Masters athletes in their eighth decade with an average of 45–56 years of endurance or speed training have been found to have calcaneal BMD 11%–16% higher than nonathletes of the same age (328). Long-term losses can be blunted but not prevented altogether. Competitive Master sprinters in their seventh and eighth decades have tibial BMD more than 10% greater than younger recreationally active controls, but still demonstrate reductions in tibial BMD of 12% compared to younger competitive sprinters (329).

Improvements in BMD may be accrued in old age with participation in regular exercise, although evidence is inconsistent. A meta-analysis of randomized controlled trials of exercise alone (without hormone therapy) in adults 60 years of age and older calculated a weighted mean difference in BMD of 0.016 g·cm^{-2} at the femoral neck and 0.011 g·cm^{-2} at the lumbar spine as a result of resistance or odd-impact exercises (330). However, in a meta-analysis of randomized controlled trials for men between 41 and 79 years of age (average age 62), no effect of resistance training, jumping, or calisthenics was observed (331). By comparison, meta-analysis of studies with postmenopausal women provides support for resistance training to improve lumbar spine and total hip BMD when training frequency is less than two sessions per week (332). Furthermore, when different types of exercise are compared in postmenopausal women, resistance training appears to selectively promote lumbar spine and total hip BMD, whereas general weight-bearing exercises such as brisk walking, running, jumping, or rope skipping have superior effects on femoral neck BMD (333).

WOMEN

The vast majority of physiological changes that occur among women over the lifespan mirror those that are observed among men and have been covered as part of the other lifespan stages in this chapter. However, three physiological events over the lifespan are unique to women: menarche, pregnancy, and menopause. Here, we discuss both the advantageous and deleterious effects of exercise on women experiencing these events and provide current clinical recommendations.

Menarche

On average, girls experience menarche (onset of menses) at 12.4 years of age, approximately 1 year earlier than the average a century ago (334). This trend toward earlier puberty is associated with an increased BMI that has been attributed to improved nutrition, but may also reflect the increase in overweight and obesity observed in this age group (335). Observational data from more than 1,100 girls and women in the Bogalusa Heart Study demonstrate significantly higher BMI in girls who report onset of menses before age 12 compared to those who report menses after age 13.5 (336).

With onset of regular menses, normal menstruation occurs approximately every 28 days. One menstrual cycle

is calculated as the number of days between the first day of bleeding in one menstrual period and the first day of bleeding in the following menstrual period. Each menstrual cycle includes two phases, the follicular or proliferative phase, and the luteal or secretory phase. The follicular phase begins with the first day of bleeding and continues until ovulation. This phase is characterized by decreasing levels of FSH and concomitant increases in LH, estrogen, and testosterone, which peak prior to ovulation. The luteal phase begins with ovulation and lasts approximately 14 days. Levels of FSH and progesterone rise, whereas LH and testosterone levels fall. Estrogen levels initially decrease in the early luteal phase, followed by a secondary increase that mirrors the increase in progesterone.

Influence of the Menstrual Cycle on Metabolism and Exercise Performance

Data regarding the influence of the menstrual cycle on metabolism in "eumenorrheic" women are inconsistent. Earlier research measuring RMR every other day throughout the menstrual cycle demonstrated a distinct pattern of change in which metabolic rate decreased steadily over the follicular phase, reaching its lowest point prior to ovulation, and then increased throughout the luteal phase (337). Subsequent data obtained only at single time points in both the follicular and luteal phases demonstrated an elevated fasting metabolic rate during the luteal phase compared to the follicular phase (338, 339). By comparison, a study measuring RMR three or more times per week over one or more complete menstrual cycles found considerable day-to-day variability with no consistent pattern among women (340). Overall, research regarding the influence of menstrual cycle on RMR has been characterized by relatively small sample sizes, which may have influenced findings. However, meta-analysis of 26 studies with over 300 participants found a small but significant increase in RMR during the luteal phase compared to the follicular phase (341).

The effect of the menstrual cycle on energy and substrate response to consumption of a standardized meal has been evaluated in two studies. No differences were observed in postprandial energy expenditure or oxidation of fat and carbohydrate (338, 342). In one of the studies, protein oxidation was blunted during the luteal phase (342), whereas in the other, it was not (338).

Research into the effect of the menstrual phase on exercise-related metabolism in eumenorrheic women is also somewhat inconsistent. Initial research during continuous endurance exercise reported greater carbohydrate oxidation in the follicular phase (343). Subsequent studies are not in agreement, and during prolonged endurance exercise, no differences were observed in energy expenditure or substrate utilization between the follicular and luteal phases (344–346). Finally, although data are limited to two studies, menstrual cycle appears to have little or no influence on recovery energy expenditure. In eumenorrheic women who completed 60 minutes of continuous cycling, no differences in total EPOC were observed between the follicular and luteal phases (339, 347), although in one study during the luteal phase, there was a greater reliance on fat as a fuel source immediately postexercise (339).

The effect of the menstrual cycle on exercise performance has been studied in eumenorrheic women by measuring differences between the follicular and luteal phases. Anaerobic power was measured in untrained women using a force–velocity cycling test, multijump test, and squat jump test, with no differences in maximal power or jump height found (348). In studies of trained women, no differences in maximal oxygen consumption ($\dot{V}O_{2max}$) or peak running velocity were observed during a maximal treadmill test to exhaustion (349), nor were differences in maximal aerobic performance (maximal oxygen consumption) or the anaerobic threshold observed during an incremental rowing ergometer test (350). Furthermore, in a resistance training study comparing unilateral upper extremity exercise (arm curls) over 12 weeks (three menstrual cycles), the menstrual cycle had no effect on gains in either force production or muscle CSA (351). Finally, a meta-analysis of 51 studies found what the authors described as a trivial reduction in exercise performance during the early follicular phase, but when lower quality studies were excluded from the analysis, the effect was nullified (352).

Despite limited and somewhat inconsistent evidence regarding the effect of the menstrual cycle on exercise metabolism and performance, there is consistent and compelling evidence regarding the effect of exercise on the menstrual cycle. The female reproductive system is sensitive to a variety of stressors. Physical stress from excessive exercise, often combined with inadequate diet and weight loss, can result in menstrual abnormalities, including *amenorrhea.*

Primary Amenorrhea

More than 95% of girls begin menstruating by 15 years of age (353). If no menstrual period has occurred by 16 years, this is considered primary amenorrhea (354). Primary amenorrhea can be caused by genetic, hormonal, or physical factors. Genetic anomalies such as Turner syndrome are characterized by inadequate production of estrogen because of failure of the ovaries to develop normally (355). Polycystic ovary syndrome with elevated levels of testosterone can also result in primary amenorrhea (356). Finally, physical abnormalities linked to eating disorders, malnutrition, excessive exercise, or stress can impair hypothalamic function, causing primary amenorrhea by inhibiting release of LH and FSH (354).

Secondary Amenorrhea

After normal onset of menses, cessation of menstruation for three consecutive cycles is considered secondary amenorrhea (357). The majority of cases of secondary amenorrhea are linked to hypothalamic irregularity complicated by weight loss or low body weight (358). This condition, called functional hypothalamic amenorrhea, can result from emotional or physical stress, inadequate nutrition, or excessive exercise (357). Secondary amenorrhea is characterized by hormonal imbalances that include decreased LH and FSH (359) and increased cortisol that directly inhibits estrogen activity in the uterus (360).

Female Athlete Triad/Relative Energy Deficiency in Sport

The female athlete triad has been identified in women who participate in exercise and sports and is characterized by three interrelated conditions: menstrual dysfunction, low energy availability, and low BMD (361, 362). Among female athletes, the prevalence of menstrual disturbances in general is as high as 60%, especially in lean sports that emphasize endurance training, low body weight, lean physique, and aestheticism (363). Amenorrhea has the most serious long-term implications for bone and cardiovascular health (364, 365). Estrogen has a protective role through promotion of bone mineralization and endothelial function (366, 367), so estrogen-deplete, amenorrheic women are at risk for osteoporosis (see Chapter 11) and atherosclerosis (see Chapter 5).

Energy imbalance is a key factor in the female athlete triad. The low energy intake observed in female athletes is often the result of disordered eating, although common dieting behaviors without adequate knowledge or understanding of energy requirements can also result in low energy availability. Excessive exercise or sports activities compound energy deficits by increasing energy requirements. The proposed relationship between low energy availability and amenorrhea is based on the need for a critical minimum amount of body fat relative to body weight, with a threshold of 17% body fat needed to achieve menarche or for resolution of primary amenorrhea, and 22% body fat needed for restoration of menses

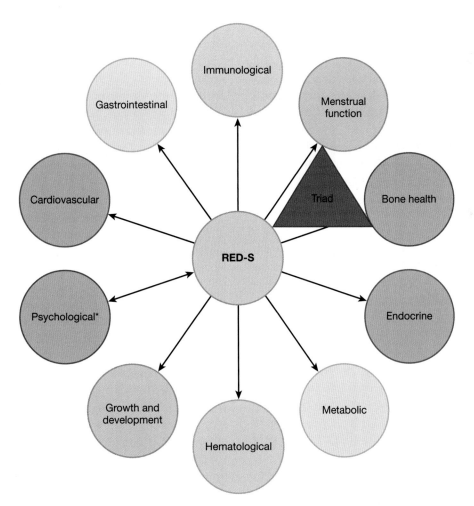

after cessation with secondary amenorrhea (368). There is also a relationship between inadequate energy intake and low BMD. Women diagnosed with anorexia nervosa have low relative weight for height that meets the criteria for underweight BMI and low femoral neck, hip, and whole-body BMD compared to women who were normal weight with no disordered eating (369). ACSM treatment recommendations for the female athlete triad focus on resolving energy imbalances by increasing energy intake or decreasing energy expenditure in order to promote weight gain and resumption of menses (361). With return of regular menstrual cycles, BMD will improve, although some loss may be irreversible (370).

Energy imbalance is also the defining characteristic of *relative energy deficiency in sport* (RED-S), an expansion of the female athlete triad (371, 372). This syndrome

of negative health and performance outcomes related to inadequate energy intake affects both female and male athletes. A detailed discussion is beyond the scope of this chapter, but a key feature of RED-S is the emphasis on individual variability between athletes in which energy deficiency is relative to individual athletes and their specific needs (373). Hormonal imbalances and low BMD remain principal health outcomes of RED-S (Figure 2.21), although both gender and race may influence etiology (371).

Pregnancy

Pregnancy is accompanied by profound physiological changes. Menstrual cycles cease for the duration of the pregnancy, which is approximately 40 weeks or 9 months.

FIGURE 2.21 Health consequences of Relative Energy Deficiency in Sport (RED-S) showing an expanded concept of the Female Athlete Triad to acknowledge a wider range of outcomes and the application to male athletes (*Psychological consequences can either precede RED-S or be the result of RED-S) (372, 497). (Taken from Mountjoy M, Sundgot-Borgen JK, Burke LM, et al. IOC consensus statement on relative energy deficiency in sport (RED-S): 2018 update. *Br J Sports Med.* 2018;52(11):687–97.)

During that time, estrogen and progesterone, which are at their nadir immediately following conception, rise continually. *Gestation* is traditionally divided into three phases — or trimesters — each lasting about 3 months. During this time, maternal health and behaviors can affect both fetal and maternal outcomes.

First Trimester

The first trimester is primarily dedicated to development of the *embryo*. By 8 weeks, embryonic development is complete, and major organs and body systems are differentiated (374). The embryo is now a *fetus*. Facial features are evident, and external genitalia can be observed. Most importantly, the placenta is mature, the umbilical cord is functioning, and the circulatory system is well established. In addition to its role in delivery of oxygen and nutrients to the fetus, the placenta at 8 weeks becomes the dominant source of estrogen and progesterone to sustain the pregnancy (375). By 12 weeks, at the end of the first trimester, the cardiovascular system is functioning, the liver is producing red blood cells, and the musculoskeletal and gastrointestinal systems are developing. In response to increased fetal circulation, maternal blood volume and cardiac output begin to increase (376). However, maternal weight gain should be minimal during the first trimester. Fetal development is emphasized over growth, and at 12 weeks, the fetus weighs an average of 28 g (1 oz) and is approximately 7.6 cm (3 inches) long (374).

Second and Third Trimesters

During the second and third trimesters, emphasis is on final development of major body systems and relatively rapid growth of the fetus. By the end of the second trimester at approximately 24 weeks, fetal movements are evident, heart rate can be auscultated, and the gastrointestinal system is intact with peristalsis. However, oxygen and all nutrients are obtained through the placenta, which increasingly stresses maternal reserves. Insulin resistance increases continuously beginning in the second trimester, allowing available glucose and amino acids to preferentially be used to support fetal growth (377). The fetus now weighs approximately 665 g (23.5 oz or 1.5 lb) and is 30.5 cm (12 inches) long (374, 378). As the pregnancy progresses, up to 75% of women report dyspnea (379). Growth of the fetus and increased size of the uterus displace the diaphragm upward by as much as 4 cm (1.57 inch), limiting diaphragmatic movement and reducing functional residual capacity by approximately 18% (376). Maternal lung volume decreases by approximately 5%,

while at the same time oxygen consumption increases by as much as 15% (380).

The third trimester is marked by gains in fat and lean mass. Fetal adipose tissue increases subcutaneously, and at birth, normal weight should average 3,300–3,500 g (116–123.5 oz or 7.3–7.7 lb), and length should average 48.3–53.3 cm (19–21 inches) (374, 378). These rapid gains in size increase maternal stress and by 40 weeks RMR has increased by approximately 15%, oxygen consumption has increased by 30%, and blood volume has increased by up to 50% (376). Maternal heart rate and systolic and diastolic blood pressure also increase, most likely because of increased blood volume (381). Both respiratory rate and tidal volume are increased, and dyspnea on exertion becomes more common (376).

Effect of Pregnancy on Musculoskeletal Health

Pregnancy is accompanied by musculoskeletal problems that impact maternal health. The abdominal muscles are stretched severely and there is a shift in the center of gravity that further decreases the support the abdominal muscles provide (382). Low back pain is common and reported by more than 60% of pregnant women (383, 384). In addition, gestational weight gain can contribute to discomfort. An increase in maternal body weight of only 20% can increase force on knee or hip joints by as much as 100% (385). Weight gain is impacted by fluid retention. During a normal pregnancy, women retain an additional 6,500 mL (219.79 oz) of fluid; this amount can further increase by 1,000 mL (33.81 oz) over a single day because of gravity and movement of fluids into the interstitial space (386).

Although weight gain and increased joint impact should mechanistically promote bone mineralization, this has not been the case. In response to fetal demands, maternal intestinal calcium absorption doubles beginning in the first trimester, but by the third trimester, bone resorption has also doubled, whereas the rate of bone formation is unchanged or decreased (387). Apparently, the increased demand for calcium by the fetus negates the effect of increased loading on weight-bearing joints, resulting in bone loss, especially during the third trimester (388). For each pregnancy, overall losses in maternal BMD range from 1% to 2% at the femoral neck (389, 390) to more than 3% at the spine (390, 391).

Gestational Weight Gain

Energy requirements increase during pregnancy, especially during the second and third trimesters when the rate

Table 2.1	2009 IOM/NRC (National Research Council) Guidelines for Weight Gain During Pregnancy		
Prepregnancy BMI (kg·m⁻²)	Mothers of Singletons		Mothers of Twins (Provisional)
	Total Weight Gain (lb)	Rate of Weight Gain in the Second and Third Trimesters (lb per wk)	Total Weight Gain at Term (lb)
Underweight (<18.5)	28–40	1.0 (1.0–1.3)	No guideline available
Normal-weight (18.5–24.9)	25–35	1.0 (0.8–1.0)	37–54
Overweight (25.0–29.9)	15–25	0.6 (0.5–0.7)	31–50
Obese (≥30.0)	11–20	0.5 (0.4–0.6)	25–42

BMI, body mass index; IOM, Institute of Medicine.

Source: Rasmussen KM, Catalano PM, Yaktine AL. New guidelines for weight gain during pregnancy: what obstetrician/gynecologists should know. *Curr Opin Obstet Gynecol.* 2009;21(6):521–6.

of fetal growth is increasing. However, increased maternal energy needs are estimated as only 89 kcal per day during the first trimester, 286 kcal per day during the second trimester, and 466 kcal per day during the third trimester (392). In 2009, the Institute of Medicine (IOM) published revised guidelines for weight gain during pregnancy based on prenatal weight (Table 2.1). Women who were normal weight should gain no more than 16 kg (35.27 lb), whereas women who were overweight and obese should limit weight gain to no more than 11.5 kg (25.35 lb) and 9 kg (19.84 lb), respectively (393).

Unfortunately, weight gain often exceeds recommendations. In a meta-analysis of studies including approximately 1.5 million women from 29 countries, the global prevalence of excessive weight gain above the 2009 IOM recommendations was 27.8%, with the highest rates in North America and the lowest in Asia (394). Although older maternal age increases the risk for prepregnancy overweight and obesity (395), it does not appear to influence gestational weight gain. In an analysis of 326,368 women, of whom 44% were overweight or obese, average gestational weight gain differed by less than 0.5 kg (1.1 lb) between 15- to 17-year-olds, 18- to 19-year-olds, and 20- to 34-year-olds (396). However, race and ethnicity may influence maternal weight gain, although evidence is conflicting. Kinnunen et al. studied more than 600 women from six racial and ethnic groups, finding that average gestational weight gain ranged from 12.0 to 13.1 kg (26.46–28.88 lb) in African and South Asian women, up to 17.6 kg (38.80 lb) in Eastern European women (397). Meta-analysis of studies with more than 1.3 million women provides initial support for these differences, but when

recommendations for weight gain are adjusted for regional BMI criteria, racial differences in excessive weight gain are eliminated (398). Finally, there is some evidence that prepregnancy weight offsets racial and ethnic influences. In a study of more than 3,000 women from eight countries in Europe, Asia, Africa, and North and South America who were normal weight, average gestational weight gain was only 13.7 kg (30.20 lb), which does not exceed recommendations (399).

Excess gestational weight gain is becoming an increasingly serious problem. When weight gain exceeds recommendations, excess weight is primarily fat rather than lean mass (400). Maternal health can be negatively affected. In both women who were normal weight and overweight/obese, excess weight gain during pregnancy is associated with maternal hypertension (401) and gestational diabetes mellitus (402, 403) and increases the risk for preeclampsia, preterm birth, and cesarean delivery (404, 405). Fetal outcomes are also affected. Excessive gestational weight gain is associated with "macrosomia" and cephalopelvic disproportion, which contribute to the risk for cesarean section (405–407). In contrast, when women who were obese gain less weight than recommended, the risk for preeclampsia, postpartum hemorrhage, and cesarean delivery decreases (408).

Exercise During Pregnancy

There is strong evidence from meta-analyses regarding the benefits of exercise during pregnancy. Exercise of any type can prevent excessive gestational weight gain (409–411), reduce the risk for cesarean delivery (412, 413), prevent maternal hypertension (410, 413), and also prevent gestational diabetes mellitus (411, 413). Regular maternal exercise can also reduce fetal birth weight and decrease the risk of macrosomia (411, 414). Furthermore, although evidence regarding higher-intensity exercise is limited, moderate-to-vigorous exercise before pregnancy and through the first and second trimesters appears to be safe and can improve glucose tolerance (415). Elite female athletes report continuing endurance and strength training throughout pregnancy, although with decreased volume (416) and approximately 50% of their prepregnancy training intensity (417). When compared to physically active controls, elite athletes that continue training during pregnancy demonstrate no differences in adverse outcomes including miscarriages, preterm births, cesarean sections, or low birth weight babies (416). Meta-analysis of elite female athletes who were training competitively immediately prior to pregnancy demonstrates improvements in complaints of low back pain and no negative effects on risk of preterm birth, low birth weight, macrosomia, or cesarean section (418).

Despite the evident advantages of regular exercise, general physical activity, particularly exercise, decreases during pregnancy (419), especially among overweight and obese women (420). Current guidelines from the American College of Obstetricians and Gynecologists (421) recommend a minimum of 20–30 minutes of moderate-intensity exercise on all or most days of the week, with intensity measured as a perceived exertion of "somewhat hard" (13–14 on the 6–20 Borg scale) or through the "talk test" (to avoid overexertion, women should be able to carry on a conversation while exercising) (422). These recommendations are consistent with the 2018 Physical Activity Guidelines for Americans (14, 423), discussed in Chapter 4. Recommended exercises include walking, swimming, stationary cycling, aerobics, and resistance training with weights and elastic bands. Education is needed to ensure safety and promote adherence. Maternal barriers to exercise during pregnancy include lack of advice and information, safety concerns, and lack of resources (424), all of which can be overcome with appropriate counseling. Women can be educated regarding warning signs to discontinue exercise, including vaginal bleeding, abdominal pain or regular contractions, leaking of amniotic fluid, chest pain, calf pain or swelling, or muscle weakness affecting balance (14, 421). Furthermore, although physiologic responses to exercise include increased maternal heart rate, cardiac output, and hyperventilation (425), fetal health is not impaired even with strenuous exercise, and with regular training maternal cardiorespiratory responses are attenuated (426).

Menopause

Cessation of menses at the time of menopause marks the end of reproductive function among women. The average age at natural menopause is approximately 50 (427), with the majority of women reporting cessation of menses by age 55 (428). Age at menopause has long-term health implications. Results from meta-analysis demonstrate that cessation of menses prior to age 45 increases risk for all-cause and heart disease–specific mortality by 10%–20%, and menopause prior to age 50 increases risk for coronary heart disease by 13% (429). Furthermore, longitudinal data from more than 68,000 women reflect a 20% increase in mortality because of gastrointestinal disease and a 40% increase in mortality because of genitourinary disease when menopause occurs prior to 45 years of age (430).

Age at menopause is influenced by genetic, lifestyle, and environmental factors. Genetic influences are manifested as familial similarities in menopausal age (i.e., if a woman's mother experienced menopause at an early age, then the likelihood of early menopause is greater for that woman). Studies of heritability estimate a genetic contribution to age at menopause of 40%–50% (431, 432), so it seems clear that lifestyle choices can have a significant impact. Behaviors such as breastfeeding, use of oral contraceptives, regular exercise, higher protein consumption, and avoiding underweight are protective and increase women's age at menopause (433, 434). In contrast, current smoking lowers menopausal age by approximately 1 year (435). There is also growing awareness of environmental influences on menopausal age. In addition to chemical compounds in cigarette smoke, higher lifetime lead exposure can decrease age at menopause by as much as 1.2 years (436).

Menopause results from decreases in bioavailable estrogen. Whether menopause occurs naturally because of ovarian aging or surgically because of removal of the ovaries, estrogen levels are diminished. In postmenopausal women, estrogen levels are 50%–90% lower than in premenopausal women (437). Estrogen has multiple roles in the body. In addition to its role in reproduction, estrogen influences body composition and BMD (438).

Body Composition

Menopause is associated with gains in fat mass. Cross-sectional data demonstrate that prior to menopause, overall women have more fat mass than men (439), although they tend to gain body fat at a similar rate until after the age of menopause, when women continue to gain fat while men remain stable or lose fat mass (440). Furthermore, after menopause, fat mass is preferentially deposited centrally in the abdominal area, and compared to premenopausal women, postmenopausal women have as much as 30% greater abdominal fat deposition (441). These gains in central body fat substantially increase the risk for insulin resistance (442), metabolic syndrome (443), CVD, and all-cause mortality (444). Data from meta-analysis of 11 longitudinal studies, including more than 650,000 participants, demonstrate that abdominal fat deposition with a high waist circumference decreases life expectancy among women by as much as 5 years (445).

In postmenopausal women, loss of lean mass accompanies gains in fat mass. Cross-sectional data from more than 550 women demonstrate an average difference in total body lean mass of 6% between pre- and postmenopausal women (446). Among postmenopausal women, muscle mass is estrogen dependent (447). Estrogen receptors are present on cell membranes of skeletal muscle, with a high proportion found on type II fibers (448). This may explain the decrease in size and CSA of type II fibers compared to type I fibers that has been observed in postmenopausal women (449). Type II fibers are critical for strength and force production, and in postmenopausal women, muscle strength is approximately 5% greater among those who receive estrogen replacement compared to those who do not, and when muscle force is calculated as strength normalized to size, the difference increases to approximately 10% (450, 451). Decreased muscle quality is also reflected in metabolic changes. Compared to premenopausal women, postmenopausal women exhibit an overall lower RMR per unit of lean mass (452). Finally, insulin resistance accompanies central body fat deposition (443) and may contribute to loss of lean mass after menopause. In obese and normal-weight women between the ages of 40 and 70, whole-body protein synthesis is blunted by insulin resistance (453, 454).

Bone Mineral Density

Menopause is associated with loss of BMD and is considered a risk factor for osteoporosis (see Chapter 11) in women. Longitudinal data from a cohort of approximately 2,000 women demonstrate average annual bone mineral losses of 0.018 g·cm^{-2} from the spine and 0.010 g·cm^{-2} from the hip during the menopausal transition (perimenopause; (455)). After completion of menopause, the rate of demineralization increases, with annual losses approximating 0.022 g·cm^{-2} from the spine and 0.013 g·cm^{-2} from the hip. Greater body weight slows the rate of loss by as much as 55% (455). With advancing age, the rate of loss appears to diminish. In a longitudinal study of postmenopausal women, the rate of bone loss was greatest in the decade immediately following menopause, and subsequently decreased by 50% in the second and third decades after menopause (456). In contrast, BMD increases by 2%–3% for every decade in which menopause is delayed (457).

In postmenopausal women, estrogen levels correlate with BMD (447). Estrogen directly promotes bone health through inhibition of bone breakdown by osteoclasts and stimulation of bone formation by osteoblasts (448). With estrogen deficiency, bone turnover accelerates because of increased remodeling and resorption (458). Approximately 2 years prior to completion of menopause, bone resorption increases significantly. After cessation of menses, resorption begins to decline, but remains approximately 20% higher than before menopause (459). Furthermore, although BMI appears to be protective and is inversely related to bone resorption among postmenopausal women, abdominal obesity and insulin resistance apparently promote bone loss, as they are negatively associated with serum osteocalcin, a bone protein and biochemical marker of bone formation (460).

Loss of BMD increases the risk of fracture (457). Longitudinal data from more than 11,000 postmenopausal women enrolled in the Women's Health Initiative study demonstrate a 50% increase in the risk of fracture for each standard deviation reduction in femoral neck and lumbar spine BMD (461). Early menopause increases fracture risk even more. In a longitudinal study of approximately 300 women over three decades, those who experienced early menopause at an average age of 42 had an 80% increase in risk for osteoporosis, a 70% increase in risk for fracture, and a 60% increase in mortality risk (456). Furthermore, in a larger cohort of more than 21,500 postmenopausal women from the Women's Health Initiative study, BMD (total body, hip, and spine) was 0.05–0.11 g·cm^{-2} less and risk of fracture was 20% more in women who experienced menopause before age 40 compared to those who experienced menopause at 50 years or older (462).

Role of Physical Activity and Exercise

Although estrogen replacement therapy can effectively reverse the negative effects of menopause including body composition, BMD, and insulin resistance (463), risks for adverse health outcomes including breast cancer, heart disease, thromboembolism, and stroke outweigh the benefits (464). Exercise provides an effective alternative. Regular moderate activity reduces the weight gain commonly observed among women in the first decade following menopause (465). Furthermore, at least 30 minutes a day of moderate-to-vigorous activity is associated with greater lower extremity strength (466).

Endurance exercise has multiple health benefits in postmenopausal women. Brisk walking at moderate to high intensity at least 3 days per week can reduce body weight by approximately 1.0 kg (2.2 lb) and relative body fat by more than 2.0% (467). Stationary cycling at least 3 days per week improves insulin sensitivity and selectively decreases abdominal fat (468, 469). Combined training with exercises such as cycling, treadmill walking, and rowing at least 3 days per week can maintain lean mass while decreasing fat mass (470), most likely by shifting substrate oxidation during exercise from carbohydrates to lipids (471). Finally, daily high-impact jumping exercises can decrease fat mass while increasing lean mass by as much as 1.0 kg (2.2 lb) over a 12-month period (472).

Resistance training also improves body composition after menopause. Over a 6-year period, postmenopausal women who reported resistance training as part of a regular exercise program gained less body weight, less body fat, and greater lean mass than sedentary women (473). In women between 60 and 70 years of age, resistance training 2–3 days per week can increase overall lean mass by 1.5 kg (3.31 lb) and selectively increase type II fiber area (474, 475). Meta-analysis of resistance training studies for postmenopausal and elderly women over a 20-year period reflects a somewhat reduced effect on gains in lean mass of approximately 0.5 kg (1.1 lb) and no effect on fat mass (476). However, when resistance training is combined with endurance training, lean mass is retained, whereas body weight, body fat, waist circumference, and insulin resistance are reduced (477, 478).

Evidence regarding the effects of exercise on BMD is inconsistent, and caution is needed because researchers have not consistently controlled for estrogen replacement therapy. Hence, only results from meta-analyses will be discussed here. As discussed previously, a meta-analysis that evaluated the effect of exercise on prevention of bone loss in postmenopausal women concluded that resistance training appeared to be the most effective exercise for total hip BMD, whereas combined resistance and weight-bearing endurance training such as walking or running appeared most effective for lumbar spine BMD (333). By comparison, both resistance training and ground-impact activities such as walking and jumping were found to improve both femoral neck and lumbar spine BMD (479, 480), although resistance training may be more effective for improvements in the lumbar spine at higher intensities (481) and when free weights are used instead of machines (332). Furthermore, improvements in BMD were estimated to reduce the 20-year relative risk of femoral neck fracture by 11% and lumbar spine fracture by 10% (480). Finally, in a meta-analysis of walking programs for women during and after menopause, there was no effect on lumbar spine BMD, although improvements in femoral neck BMD were found with programs lasting at least 6 months (482).

Current treatment guidelines from the International Menopause Society recommend at least 150 minutes of moderate-intensity aerobic exercise per week in addition to resistance exercise on 2 days per week (483), which is consistent with recommendations by ACSM (14) and the U.S. Physical Activity Guidelines (423). Unfortunately, both moderate and vigorous physical activity decline each decade following menopause, with an 18% decrease in moderate activity alone between 50 and 60 years of age (484). Clinical interventions for postmenopausal women are effective. Individual counseling regarding the perceived risks and benefits of exercise can increase participation in a regular exercise program by 50% (485), whereas use of technology such as activity trackers can double MVPA (486). Finally, if postmenopausal women are engaged in a regular exercise program for a sufficient period of time to promote self-efficacy, then they are three times more likely to continue exercise participation over time (487).

SUMMARY

Significant changes in body composition, muscle strength, cardiorespiratory fitness, and bone density occur across the lifespan in normal healthy people. A common pattern among these variables is that they steadily increase during childhood, until puberty, which marks the transition into adolescence. During adolescence, they increase rapidly for several years until the transition into young adulthood. Muscle size and strength, peak aerobic capacity ($\dot{V}O_{2peak}$), and bone density are similar in boys and girls through childhood, but during adolescence sex differences emerge (boys experience greater increases in muscle mass, muscle strength, bone density, $\dot{V}O_{2peak}$, and strength than do girls, whereas girls accrue more body fat), and those differences are maintained throughout adulthood. During young adulthood, muscle size and strength, $\dot{V}O_{2peak}$, and bone density are maintained or increase slightly, but middle age marks another major life transition point, when all these physiological systems begin to decline in the average person. Those declines continue into older adulthood when the loss of skeletal muscle mass and strength becomes more evident. This is described as the sarcopenia of aging. For women, the transition to menopause can result in a faster rate of decline in muscle mass, and particularly in bone density, increasing the risk for frailty, falls, and bone fractures.

Physical activity and purposeful exercise training have important, beneficial effects on multiple body systems throughout the lifespan. For children and adolescents, the current ACSM guidelines call for 60 minutes per day of MVPA with most of the time spent in endurance-type activities that support cardiorespiratory fitness, with muscle and bone strengthening activities on at least 3 days per week. For adults, ACSM guideline is for 30 minutes of MVPA on 5 or more days per week with 2 days of muscle and bone strengthening activities. Throughout the lifespan, resistance exercises have been shown to be safe and effective at increasing muscle size and strength and aiding the development and maintenance of bone density. Likewise, performing endurance activities has been shown to increase $\dot{V}O_{2peak}$ in children and adults of all ages. The relative change in aerobic capacity to endurance training or muscle strength response to resistance training is often greater in previously untrained people than in trained people but is remarkably similar in magnitude among studies of adolescents and adults, and in males and females, across the lifespan. Training-induced changes in aerobic capacity and muscle strength tend to be of smaller magnitude in children than in other age groups, but this may be attributed to the difficulty in keeping younger children engaged in exercise programs for long durations.

A challenge for CEPs and other health care providers that has emerged over the past 20–30 years is the elevated prevalence of obesity and a sedentary lifestyle. It is increasingly clear from longitudinal studies that attributes such as obesity, elevated lipids, and low aerobic fitness are becoming more common in adolescents and young adults and, when present, are predictive of increased risk for developing CVD and metabolic diseases like diabetes during young adulthood and middle age. Because the lifetime socioeconomic costs of managing cardiometabolic diseases are so high, promoting physical activity in children and adolescents, as well as adults, could have a major impact on this challenge.

Although men and women demonstrate similar changes over the lifespan, there are three physiological events unique to women: menarche (onset of menses), pregnancy, and menopause (cessation of menses). As previously discussed, regular exercise during adolescence is recommended. However, excessive exercise can either delay onset of menses (primary amenorrhea) or impair regular menstrual function after menarche occurs (secondary amenorrhea). During pregnancy, regular moderate-intensity exercise is recommended to decrease risk for excessive weight gain, which can have deleterious effects on both mother and child. Unfortunately, physical activity during pregnancy tends to decrease, especially among women who are already overweight or obese. Finally, menopause, which typically occurs naturally at approximately 50 years of age, is associated with gains in fat mass and loss of lean mass and BMD. Regular moderate-intensity exercise can improve body composition, but high-intensity, high-impact activities may be needed to maintain or improve BMD. Women should be encouraged to exercise regularly at all stages of life to promote healthy body composition and BMD as they age.

CHAPTER REVIEW QUESTIONS

1. In adult men and women, there are differences in body composition, with men having more muscle mass and women having more body fat (on average). Describe the differences that occur during childhood or adolescence.
2. What sex differences in muscle strength, if any, are present in childhood or adolescence?
3. Insulin resistance and diabetes are increasing clinical concerns for adults and children. What happens to insulin resistance during adolescence? Does insulin resistance in adolescence lead to diabetes in adulthood?
4. How does aerobic capacity ($\dot{V}O_{2peak}$) in adolescence compare to aerobic capacity in other phases of life? Describe any differences between boys and girls.
5. Respiratory capacity changes during adulthood. What genetic and lifestyle factors have the greatest influence on these changes?
6. What factors influence the development of sarcopenia?
7. Behaviors during pregnancy can influence both maternal and fetal health. How does exercise during pregnancy improve health for mothers and babies? What

recommendations would you make for a 24-year-old pregnant woman with a BMI of 23 kg·m^{-2} in her first trimester?

8. What are the three main concerns associated with the female athlete triad? What influence does exercise have?

9. What factors influence development of osteoporosis?

10. Long-term exercise has recognized health benefits. Describe the differences in body composition, muscle strength, cardiorespiratory fitness, and bone density observed in Masters athletes compared to sedentary adults of similar age.

Case Study 2.1

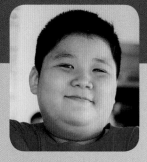

David is a 14-year-old boy who was given a referral by his health care provider to a wellness center for guidance in increasing his physical activity and physical fitness. As part of the assessment, his height is measured as 170.18 cm (67 inches) and his weight as 78.47 kg (173 lb). David performs a graded exercise test to volitional fatigue on a stationary bicycle. His final workload is 145 W and his $\dot{V}O_{2peak}$ is 2.020 L·min^{-1}. For a week, he wears a pedometer, which records an average of 7,000 steps per day. He currently attends physical education class at school once per week for 50 minutes but does not do any other structured exercise or sports activities. At the follow-up meeting with David and his parents, describe the findings and make recommendations for areas of improvement based on current guidelines.

Case Study 2.1 Questions

1. What is David's BMI and where does that place him relative to normative values?

2. How does David's aerobic fitness compare to average values for boys his age? Is he at a healthy level of fitness?

3. What is David's current level of physical activity relative to current recommendations?

4. What should be the exercise recommendation for David? What, if any, health concerns are there about his current fitness and physical activity level?

Case Study 2.2

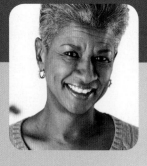

Clarice is 73 years old, with a height of 155 cm (61 inches) and body weight of 79 kg (156.53 lb). Her BMI is 32.9 kg·m^{-2}. She has lived alone in a two-story home since her husband died 6 years ago. She does not drive and once a week her daughter, who lives approximately 20 miles away, takes her grocery shopping. She reports falling twice last year — once when walking downstairs in her home and once when she tripped on a curb outside her home. She now uses a cane at home and a walker outside of home. When questioned, she reports feeling weaker than she did a year ago and having more difficulty climbing the stairs (13 steps) at home to get to her bedroom and bathroom. She says she feels out of breath and has to stop and rest midway. She denies smoking or regular alcohol consumption. Her blood pressure is 131/69 mm Hg and her heart rate is 88 beats per minute. She reports taking medication for her blood pressure but does not remember the name of the medication. When asked what her goal is, she responds that she wants to get stronger and would like to be able to climb the stairs at home without needing to rest.

Case Study 2.2 Questions

1. What recommendations would you make to help Clarice achieve her goal? Specifically address both weakness and feeling out of breath.

2. Download the current *ACSM Recommendations for Exercise Preparticipation Health Screening* from https://journals.lww.com/acsm-msse/Fulltext/2015/11000/Updating_ACSM_s_Recommendations_for_ Exercise.28.aspx. Does Clarice need physician clearance before beginning a regular exercise program? What factors influence your decision-making?

3. Clarice may be at risk for fracture if she falls again. What factors influence Clarice's risk?

4. What recommendations would you make specifically to address fracture risk?

Case Study 2.3

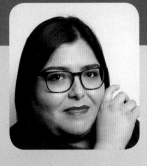

Phoebe is a 36-year-old woman, with a height of 173 cm (68 inches) and body weight of 88 kg (194 lb). Her BMI is 29.5 kg·m^{-2}. She is 5 weeks pregnant. This is her first pregnancy. Phoebe is married, lives with her spouse, and does not work. Prior to pregnancy she was diagnosed with insulin resistance and high blood pressure (135/90 mm Hg). She reports anxiety regarding potential weight gain and problems with pregnancy. Phoebe does not engage in regular physical activity or exercise and describes them as "too hard" and "too uncomfortable." She also believes that strenuous activity could hurt her baby. Her physician referred her to you to provide advice on maintaining appropriate weight gain during pregnancy.

Case Study 2.3 Questions

1. Phoebe is currently in what trimester? What changes in her body weight and physical function should she anticipate as part of the normal changes that are likely to occur during pregnancy?

2. Based on IOM guidelines for weight gain during pregnancy, how much total weight should Phoebe gain during pregnancy? What additional information do you need to make appropriate recommendations?

3. Describe the appropriate recommendations for exercise for Phoebe throughout her pregnancy. What warning signs should she be aware of that would indicate that she should discontinue exercise? What two strategies can she use to ensure that she does not exercise too vigorously?

4. What benefits can Phoebe anticipate for herself and her infant if she adheres to an appropriate exercise program throughout her pregnancy?

Case Study 2.4

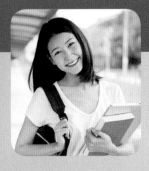

Louise is a 16-year-old female who was referred by her school nurse for menstrual irregularities. Louise is 160 cm (63 inches) tall, weighs 47.2 kg (104 lb), and has a BMI of 18.4 kg·m^{-2}, which places her at the 22nd percentile for 16-year-old girls. She recently lost 9.1 kg (20 lb) and reports having no regular menstrual cycles for 2 months. Louise plays competitive soccer on her high school team and 4 months ago her coach recommended that she lose weight to improve her performance. To achieve weight loss, she doubled her weekly running time and stopped eating breakfast, so that she eats only two meals per day. To help with weight loss, she stopped drinking milk and only drinks water and diet soda.

Case Study 2.4 Questions

1. What risks are associated with menstrual irregularities in adolescent female athletes and what is the underlying cause?

2. For what condition or syndrome is Louise at risk? What behaviors are placing Louise at risk?

3. What treatment recommendations are appropriate to promote Louise's health and prevent long-term health problems?

REFERENCES

1. Finch CE, Pike MC. Maximum life span predictions from the Gompertz mortality model. *J Gerontol A Biol Sci Med Sci.* 1996;51(3):B183–94.

2. World Health Organization. Child growth standards. 2006. Available from: https://www.who.int/toolkits/child-growth -standards.

3. Kuczmarski RJ, Ogden CL, Guo SS, et al. 2000 CDC growth charts for the United States: methods and development. *Vital Health Stat 11.* 2002;11(246):1–190.

4. Fryar CD, Carroll MD, Afful J. Prevalence of overweight, obesity, and severe obesity among children and adolescents aged 2–19 years: United States, 1963–1965 through 2017–2018. *NCHS Health E-Stats* [Internet]. 2020 [updated 2022 Jan 8]. Available from: https://www.cdc.gov/nchs/data/hestat/obesity -child-17-18/overweight-obesity-child-H.pdf.

5. Gillison FB, Grey EB, Cumming SP, Sherar LB. Does adjusting for biological maturity when calculating child weight status improve the accuracy of predicting future health risk? *BMC Public Health.* 2021;21(1):1979.

6. Bomberg EM, Addo OY, Sarafoglou K, Miller BS. Adjusting for pubertal status reduces overweight and obesity prevalence in the United States. *J Pediatr.* 2021;231:200–6.e1.

7. Weber DR, Moore RH, Leonard MB, Zemel BS. Fat and lean BMI reference curves in children and adolescents and their utility in identifying excess adiposity compared with BMI and percentage body fat. *Am J Clin Nutr.* 2013;98(1):49–56.

8. Stierman B, Ogden CL, Yanovski JA, Martin CB, Sarafrazi N, Hales CM. Changes in adiposity among children and adolescents in the United States, 1999–2006 to 2011–2018. *Am J Clin Nutr.* 2021;114(4):1495–504.

9. Dorsey KB, Thornton JC, Heymsfield SB, Gallagher D. Greater lean tissue and skeletal muscle mass are associated with higher bone mineral content in children. *Nutr Metab (Lond).* 2010;7:41.

10. McCarthy HD, Samani-Radia D, Jebb SA, Prentice AM. Skeletal muscle mass reference curves for children and adolescents. *Pediatr Obes.* 2014;9(4):249–59.

11. Borrud LG, Flegal KM, Looker AC, Everhart JE, Harris TB, Shepherd JA. Body composition data for individuals 8 years of age and older: U.S. population, 1999–2004. *Vital Health Stat 11.* 2010;(250):1–87.

12. Ofenheimer A, Breyer-Kohansal R, Hartl S, et al. Reference charts for body composition parameters by dual-energy X-ray absorptiometry in European children and adolescents aged 6 to 18 years—results from the Austrian LEAD (Lung, hEart, sociAl, boDy) cohort. *Pediatr Obes.* 2021;16(1): e12695.

13. Kang MJ, Hong HS, Chung SJ, Lee YA, Shin CH, Yang SW. Body composition and bone density reference data for Korean children, adolescents, and young adults according to age and sex: results of the 2009–2010 Korean National Health and Nutrition Examination Survey (KNHANES). *J Bone Miner Metab.* 2016;34(4):429–39.

14. American College of Sports Medicine. *Guidelines for Exercise Testing and Prescription.* 11th ed. Philadelphia (PA): Wolters Kluwer; 2022.

15. Tudor-Locke C, Craig CL, Beets MW, et al. How many steps/ day are enough? for children and adolescents. *Int J Behav Nutr Phys Act.* 2011;8(1):78.

16. Colley RC, Janssen I, Tremblay MS. Daily step target to measure adherence to physical activity guidelines in children. *Med Sci Sports Exerc.* 2012;44(5):977–82.

17. Cooper AR, Goodman A, Page AS, et al. Objectively measured physical activity and sedentary time in youth: the International Children's Accelerometry Database (ICAD). *Int J Behav Nutr Phys Act.* 2015;12:113.

18. Sutherland RL, Nathan NK, Lubans DR, et al. An RCT to facilitate implementation of school practices known to increase physical activity. *Am J Prev Med.* 2017;53(6):818–28.

19. Wang Z, Xu F, Ye Q, et al. Childhood obesity prevention through a community-based cluster randomized controlled physical activity intervention among schools in China: the health legacy project of the 2nd World Summer Youth Olympic Games (YOG-Obesity study). *Int J Obes (Lond).* 2018;42(4):625–33.

20. McKay HA, Macdonald HM, Nettlefold L, Masse LC, Day M, Naylor PJ. Action Schools! BC implementation: from efficacy to effectiveness to scale-up. *Br J Sports Med.* 2015;49(4):210–8.

21. Butte NF, Wong WW, Hopkinson JM, Heinz CJ, Mehta NR, Smith EOB. Energy requirements derived from total energy expenditure and energy deposition during the first 2 y of life. *Am J Clin Nutr.* 2000;72(6):1558–69.

22. Ekelund U, Aman J, Yngve A, Renman C, Westerterp K, Sjostrom M. Physical activity but not energy expenditure is reduced in obese adolescents: a case-control study. *Am J Clin Nutr.* 2002;76(5):935–41.

23. Jackson DM, Pace L, Speakman JR. The measurement of resting metabolic rate in preschool children. *Obesity*. 2007;15(8):1930–2.
24. Reichman CA, Davies PS, Wells JC, Atkin LM, Cleghorn G, Shepherd RW. Centile reference charts for total energy expenditure in infants from 1 to 12 months. *Eur J Clin Nutr*. 2003;57(9):1060–7.
25. Rising R, Duro D, Cedillo M, Valois S, Lifshitz F. Daily metabolic rate in healthy infants. *J Pediatr*. 2003;143(2):180–5.
26. Rising R, Lifshitz F. Lower energy expenditures in infants from obese biological mothers. *Nutr J*. 2008;7:15.
27. Salbe AD, Fontvielle AM, Pettitt DJ, Ravussin E. Maternal diabetes status does not influence energy expenditure or physical activity in 5-year-old Pima Indian children. *Diabetologia*. 1998;41(10):1157–62.
28. Short KR, Teague AM, Fields DA, Lyons TJ, Chernausek SD. Lower resting energy expenditure and fat oxidation in Native American and Hispanic infants born to mothers with diabetes. *J Pediatr*. 2015;166(4):884–9.
29. Spadano JL, Bandini LG, Must A, Dallal GE, Dietz WH. Longitudinal changes in energy expenditure in girls from late childhood through midadolescence. *Am J Clin Nutr*. 2005;81(5):1102–9.
30. Wang Z. High ratio of resting energy expenditure to body mass in childhood and adolescence: a mechanistic model. *Am J Hum Biol*. 2012;24:460–7.
31. Lee SJ, Arslanian SA. Fat oxidation in black and white youth: a metabolic phenotype potentially predisposing black girls to obesity. *J Clin Endocrinol Metab*. 2008;93:4547–51.
32. Bandini LG, Must A, Spadano JL, Dietz WH. Relation of body composition, parental overweight, pubertal stage, and race-ethnicity to energy expenditure among premenarcheal girls. *Am J Clin Nutr*. 2002;76(5):1040–7.
33. Ansell SKD, Jester M, Tryggestad JB, Short KR. A pilot study of the effects of a high-intensity aerobic exercise session on heart rate variability and arterial compliance in adolescents with or without type 1 diabetes. *Pediatr Diabetes*. 2020;21(3):486–95.
34. Short KR, Pratt LV, Teague AM. A single exercise session increases insulin sensitivity in normal weight and overweight/obese adolescents. *Pediatr Diabetes*. 2018. doi:10.1111/pedi.12684.
35. Treuth MS, Butte NF, Wong WW. Effects of familial predisposition to obesity on energy expenditure in multiethnic prepubertal girls. *Am J Clin Nutr*. 2000;71(4):893–900.
36. Ervin RB, Wang C-Y, Fryar CD, et al. *Measures of Muscular Strength in U.S. Children and Adolescents, 2012*. Hyattsville (MD): National Center for Health Statistics; 2013.
37. Wang YC, Bohannon RW, Li X, Yen SC, Sindhu B, Kapellusch J. Summary of grip strength measurements obtained in the 2011–2012 and 2013–2014 National Health and Nutrition Examination Surveys. *J Hand Ther*. 2019;32(4):489–96.
38. Kim CR, Jeon YJ, Kim MC, Jeong T, Koo WR. Reference values for hand grip strength in the South Korean population. *PLoS One*. 2018;13(4):e0195485.
39. Dodds RM, Syddall HE, Cooper R, et al. Grip Strength across the life course: normative data from twelve British Studies. *PLoS One*. 2014;9(12):e113637.
40. Hébert LJ, Maltais DB, Lepage C, Saulnier J, Crête M. Hand-held dynamometry isometric torque reference values for children and adolescents. *Pediatr Phys Ther*. 2015;27(4):414–23.
41. De Miguel-Etayo P, Gracia-Marco L, Ortega FB, et al. Physical fitness reference standards in European children: the IDEFICS study. *Int J Obes*. 2014;38(S2):S57–66.
42. Escobar RG, Munoz KT, Dominguez A, Banados P, Bravo MJ. Maximal isometric muscle strength values obtained by hand-held dynamometry in children between 6 and 15 years of age. *Muscle Nerve*. 2017;55(1):16–22.
43. Bell RD, MacDougall JD, Billeter R, Howald H. Muscle fiber types and morphometric analysis of skeletal muscle in six-year-old children. *Med Sci Sports Exerc*. 1980;12(1):28–31.
44. Boisseau N, Delamarche P. Metabolic and hormonal responses to exercise in children and adolescents. *Sports Med*. 2000;30(6):405–22.
45. Lloyd RS, Faigenbaum AD, Stone MH, et al. Position statement on youth resistance training: the 2014 International Consensus. *Br J Sports Med*. 2014;48(7):498–505.
46. Lesinski M, Prieske O, Granacher U. Effects and dose-response relationships of resistance training on physical performance in youth athletes: a systematic review and meta-analysis. *Br J Sports Med*. 2016;50(13):781–95.
47. Detter F, Nilsson J-Å, Karlsson C, Dencker M, Rosengren BE, Karlsson MK. A 3-year school-based exercise intervention improves muscle strength—a prospective controlled population-based study in 223 children. *BMC Musculoskeletal Disorders*. 2014;15:353.
48. Fritz J, Coster ME, Stenevi-Lundgren S, et al. A 5-year exercise program in children improves muscle strength without affecting fracture risk. *Eur J Appl Physiol*. 2016;116(4):707–15.
49. Institute of Medicine. *Fitness Measures and Health Outcomes in Youth*. Washington (DC): The National Academies Press; 2012.
50. Raghuveer G, Hartz J, Lubans DR, et al. Cardiorespiratory fitness in youth: an important marker of health: a scientific statement from the American Heart Association. *Circulation*. 2020;142(7):e101–18.
51. Lang JJ, Tremblay MS, Ortega FB, Ruiz JR, Tomkinson GR. Review of criterion-referenced standards for cardiorespiratory fitness: what percentage of 1 142 026 international children and youth are apparently healthy? *Br J Sports Med*. 2019;53(15):953–8.
52. McNarry MA, Mackintosh KA, Stoedefalke K. Longitudinal investigation of training status and cardiopulmonary responses in pre- and early-pubertal children. *Eur J Appl Physiol*. 2014;114(8):1573–80.
53. Armstrong N, Welsman JR. Assessment and interpretation of aerobic fitness in children and adolescents. *Exerc Sport Sci Rev*. 1994;22:435–76.
54. Armstrong N, Welsman J. Sex-specific longitudinal modeling of youth peak oxygen uptake. *Pediatr Exerc Sci*. 2019;31(2):204–12.
55. Welsman JR, Armstrong N. Interpreting cardiorespiratory fitness in young clinical populations-folklore and fallacy. *JAMA Pediatr*. 2019;173(8):713–4.
56. Goran M, Fields DA, Hunter GR, Herd SL, Weinsier RL. Total body fat does not influence maximal aerobic capacity. *Int J Obes Relat Metab Disord*. 2000;24(7):841–8.
57. Toth MJ, Goran MI, Ades PA, Howard DB, Poehlman ET. Examination of data normalization procedures for expressing peak VO_2 data. *J Appl Physiol*. 1993;75:2288–92.
58. Short KR, Vittone JL, Bigelow ML, Proctor DN, Nair KS. Age and aerobic exercise training effects on whole body and

muscle protein metabolism. *Am J Physiol Endocrinol Metab.* 2004;286(1):E92–101.

59. Müller MJ, Geisler C, Hübers M, Pourhassan M, Braun W, Bosy-Westphal A. Normalizing resting energy expenditure across the life course in humans: challenges and hopes. *Eur J Clin Nutr.* 2018;72(5):628–37.

60. McMurray RG, Butte NF, Crouter SE, et al. Exploring metrics to express energy expenditure of physical activity in youth. *PLoS One.* 2015;10(6):e0130869.

61. Pontzer H, Yamada Y, Sagayama H, et al. Daily energy expenditure through the human life course. *Science.* 2021;373(6556):808–12.

62. Rowland TW, Boyajian A. Aerobic response to endurance exercise training in children. *Pediatrics.* 1995;96:654–8.

63. Payne VG, Morrow JR Jr. Exercise and VO₂ max in children: a meta-analysis. *Res Q Exerc Sport.* 1993;64(3):305–13.

64. Baquet G, van Praagh E, Berthoin S. Endurance training and aerobic fitness in young people. *Sports Med.* 2003;33(15):1127–43.

65. Eddolls WTB, McNarry MA, Stratton G, Winn CON, Mackintosh KA. High-intensity interval training interventions in children and adolescents: a systematic review. *Sports Med.* 2017;47(11):2363–74.

66. McManus AM, Armstrong N, Williams CA. Effect of training on the aerobic power and anaerobic performance of prepubertal girls. *Acta Paediatr.* 1997;86:456–9.

67. Williams CA, Armstrong N, Powell J. Aerobic responses of prepubertal boys to two modes of training. *Br J Sports Med.* 2000;34(3):168–73.

68. Welsman JR, Armstrong N, Withers S. Responses of young girls to two modes of aerobic training. *Br J Sports Med.* 1997;31(2):139–42.

69. Mahon AD, Vaccaro P. Cardiovascular adaptations in 8- to 12-year-old boys following a 14-week running program. *Can J Appl Physiol.* 1994;19(2):139–50.

70. Mandigout S, Lecoq AM, Courteix D, Guenon P, Obert P. Effect of gender in response to an aerobic training programme in prepubertal children. *Acta Paediatr.* 2001;90(1):9–15.

71. Obert P, Mandigouts S, Nottin S, Vinet A, N'Guyen LD, Lecoq AM. Cardiovascular responses to endurance training in children: effect of gender. *Eur J Clin Invest.* 2003;33(3):199–208.

72. Davis CL, Pollock NK, Waller JL, et al. Exercise dose and diabetes risk in overweight and obese children: a randomized controlled trial. *JAMA.* 2012;308:1103–12.

73. Looker AC, Borrud LG, Hughes JP. Total body bone area, bone mineral content, and bone mineral density for individuals aged 8 years and over: United States, 1999–2006. *Vital Health Stat 11.* 2013;11(253):1–78.

74. Lee EY, Kim D, Kim KM, et al. Age-related bone mineral density patterns in Koreans (KNHANES IV). *J Clin Endocrinol Metab.* 2012;97(9):3310–8.

75. Crabtree NJ, Shaw NJ, Bishop NJ, et al. Amalgamated reference data for size-adjusted bone densitometry measurements in 3598 children and young adults-the ALPHABET study. *J Bone Miner Res.* 2017;32(1):172–80.

76. Lopez-Gonzalez D, Wells JC, Cortina-Borja M, Fewtrell M, Partida-Gaytán A, Clark P. Reference values for bone mineral density in healthy Mexican children and adolescents. *Bone.* 2021;142:115734.

77. Kohrt WM, Bloomfield SA, Little KD, Nelson ME, Yingling VR; American College of Sports Medicine. American College of Sports Medicine Position Stand: physical activity and bone health. *Med Sci Sports Exerc.* 2004;36(11):1985–96.

78. Tan VPS, Macdonald HM, Kim S, et al. Influence of physical activity on bone strength in children and adolescents: a systematic review and narrative synthesis. *J Bone Miner Res.* 2014;29(10):2161–81.

79. Mello JB, Pedretti A, Garcia-Hermoso A, et al. Exercise in school Physical Education increase bone mineral content and density: systematic review and meta-analysis. *Eur J Sport Sci.* 2022;22(10):1618–29.

80. Rosengren BE, Lindgren E, Jehpsson L, Dencker M, Karlsson MK. Musculoskeletal benefits from a physical activity program in primary school are retained 4 years after the program is terminated. *Calcif Tissue Int.* 2021;109(4):405–14.

81. Marshall WA, Tanner JM. Variations in the pattern of pubertal changes in boys. *Arch Dis Child.* 1970;45(239):13–23.

82. Marshall WA, Tanner JM. Variations in the pattern of pubertal changes in girls. *Arch Dis Child.* 1969;44(235):291–303.

83. Kwon S, Janz KF, Letuchy EM, Burns TL, Levy SM. Developmental trajectories of physical activity, sports, and television viewing during childhood to young adulthood: Iowa Bone Development Study. *JAMA Pediatr.* 2015;169(7):666–72.

84. Moran A, Jacobs DR, Steinberger J, et al. Insulin resistance during puberty: results from clamp studies in 357 children. *Diabetes.* 1999;48:2039–44.

85. Ball GD, Huang TT, Gower BA, et al. Longitudinal changes in insulin sensitivity, insulin secretion, and beta-cell function during puberty. *J Pediatr.* 2006;148(1):16–22.

86. Jeffery AN, Metcalfe BS, Hosking J, Streeter AJ, Voss LD, Wilkin TJ. Age before stage: insulin resistance rises before the onset of puberty. A 9-year longitudinal study (EarlyBird 26). *Diabetes Care.* 2012;35:536–41.

87. Mostazir M, Jeffery A, Voss L, Wilkin T. Generational change in fasting glucose and insulin among children at ages 5–16y: Modelled on the EarlyBird study (2015) and UK growth standards (1990) (EarlyBird 69). *Diabetes Res Clin Pract.* 2017;123:18–23.

88. Shaibi GQ, Cruz ML, Ball GD, et al. Effects of resistance training on insulin sensitivity in overweight Latino adolescent males. *Med Sci Sports Exerc.* 2006;38(7):1208–15.

89. Davis JN, Tung AMY, Chak SS, et al. Aerobic and strength training reduces adiposity in overweight Latina adolescents. *Med Sci Sports Exerc.* 2009;41(7):1494–503. doi:10.249/MSS.0b013e31819b6aea.

90. Davis JN, Kelly LA, Lane CJ, et al. Randomized control trial to improve adiposity and insulin resistance in overweight Latino adolescents. *Obesity.* 2009;17(8):1542–8.

91. Sigal RJ, Alberga AS, Goldfield GS, et al. Effects of aerobic training, resistance training, or both on percentage body fat and cardiometabolic risk markers in obese adolescents: the healthy eating aerobic and resistance training in youth randomized clinical trial. *JAMA Pediatr.* 2014;168(11):1006–14.

92. Armstrong N, Welsman J. Development of peak oxygen uptake from 11–16 years determined using both treadmill and cycle ergometry. *Eur J Appl Physiol.* 2019;119(3):801–12.

93. Walker JL, Murray TD, Jackson AS, Morrow JR Jr, Michaud TJ. The energy cost of horizontal walking and running in adolescents. *Med Sci Sports Exerc.* 1999;31(2):311–22.

94. Cureton KJ, Sloniger MA, Black DM, McCormack WP, Rowe DA. Metabolic determinants of the age-related improvement in one-mile run/walk performance in youth. *Med Sci Sports Exerc.* 1997;29(2):259–67.

95. Eisenmann JC, Laurson KR, Welk GJ. Aerobic fitness percentiles for U.S. adolescents. *Am J Prev Med.* 2011;41(4 Suppl 2):S106–10.

96. Krahenbuhl GS, Skinner JS, Kohrt WM. Developmental aspects of maximal aerobic power in children. *Exerc Sport Sci Rev.* 1985;13:503–38.

97. Welsman J, Armstrong N. The 20 m shuttle run is not a valid test of cardiorespiratory fitness in boys aged 11–14 years. *BMJ Open Sport Exerc Med.* 2019;5(1):e000627.

98. Fuhner T, Kliegl R, Arntz F, Kriemler S, Granacher U. An update on secular trends in physical fitness of children and adolescents from 1972 to 2015: a systematic review. *Sports Med.* 2021;51(2):303–20.

99. Gahche J, Fakhouri T, Carroll DD, Burt VL, Wang CY, Fulton JE. Cardiorespiratory fitness levels among U.S. youth aged 12–15 years: United States, 1999–2004 and 2012. *NCHS Data Brief.* 2014;153:1–8.

100. Eisenmann JC, Pivarnik JM, Malina RM. Scaling peak VO$_2$ to body mass in young male and female distance runners. *J Appl Physiol (1985).* 2001;90(6):2172–80.

101. Gibson AR, Ojiambo R, Konstabel K, et al. Aerobic capacity, activity levels and daily energy expenditure in male and female adolescents of the Kenyan Nandi Sub-Group. *PLoS One.* 2013;8(6):e66552.

102. Costigan SA, Eather N, Plotnikoff RC, Taaffe DR, Lubans DR. High-intensity interval training for improving health-related fitness in adolescents: a systematic review and meta-analysis. *Br J Sports Med.* 2015;49:1253–61.

103. van der Heijden G-J, Wang ZJ, Chu ZD, et al. A 12-week aerobic exercise program reduces hepatic fat accumulation and insulin resistance in obese, Hispanic adolescents. *Obesity.* 2010;18:384–90.

104. Sénéchal M, Rempel M, Duhamel TA, et al. Fitness is a determinant of the metabolic response to endurance training in adolescents at risk of type 2 diabetes mellitus. *Obesity.* 2015;23(4):823–32.

105. Bouchard C, An P, Rice T, et al. Familial aggregation of VO(2max) response to exercise training: results from the HERITAGE Family Study. *J Appl Physiol (1985).* 1999;87(3):1003–8.

106. García-Hermoso A, Cerrillo-Urbina AJ, Herrera-Valenzuela T, Cristi-Montero C, Saavedra JM, Martínez-Vizcaíno V. Is high-intensity interval training more effective on improving cardiometabolic risk and aerobic capacity than other forms of exercise in overweight and obese youth? A meta-analysis. *Obes Rev.* 2016;17(6):531–40.

107. Weston KL, Azevedo LB, Bock S, Weston M, George KP, Batterham AM. Effect of novel, school-based High-Intensity Interval Training (HIT) on cardiometabolic health in adolescents: project FFAB (Fun Fast Activity Blasts)—an exploratory controlled before-and-after trial. *PLoS One.* 2016;11(8):e0159116.

108. van der Heijden G-J, Toffolo G, Manesso E, Sauer PJJ, Sunehag AL. Aerobic exercise increases peripheral and hepatic insulin sensitivity in sedentary adolescents. *J Clin Endocrinol Metab.* 2009;94(11):4292–9.

109. Weaver CM, Gordon CM, Janz KF, et al. The National Osteoporosis Foundation's position statement on peak bone mass development and lifestyle factors: a systematic review and implementation recommendations. *Osteoporos Int.* 2016;27(4):1281–386.

110. Crabtree NJ, Arabi A, Bachrach LK, et al. Dual-energy x-ray absorptiometry interpretation and reporting in children and adolescents: the revised 2013 ISCD Pediatric Official Positions. *J Clin Densitom.* 2014;17(2):225–42.

111. Kim S, Valdez R. Metabolic risk factors in U.S. youth with low relative muscle mass. *Obes Res Clin Pract.* 2015;9(2):125–32.

112. Lamb MM, Ogden CL, Carroll MD, Lacher DA, Flegal KM. Association of body fat percentage with lipid concentrations in children and adolescents: United States, 1999–2004. *Am J Clin Nutr.* 2011;94(3):877–83.

113. Adegboye AR, Anderssen SA, Froberg K, et al. Recommended aerobic fitness level for metabolic health in children and adolescents: a study of diagnostic accuracy. *Br J Sports Med.* 2011;45(9):722–8.

114. Expert Panel on Integrated Guidelines for Cardiovascular Health and Risk Reduction in Children and Adolescents; National Heart, Lung, and Blood Institute. Expert panel on integrated guidelines for cardiovascular health and risk reduction in children and adolescents: summary report. *Pediatrics.* 2011;128(Suppl 5):S213–56.

115. Andersen K, Rasmussen F, Held C, Neovius M, Tynelius P, Sundström J. Exercise capacity and muscle strength and risk of vascular disease and arrhythmia in 1.1 million young Swedish men: cohort study. *BMJ.* 2015;351:h4543.

116. Juonala M, Viikari JSA, Ronnemaa T, Helenius H, Taittonen L, Raitakari OT. Elevated blood pressure in adolescent boys predicts endothelial dysfunction: the Cardiovascular Risk in Young Finns Study. *Hypertension.* 2006;48(3):424–30.

117. Juonala M, Viikari JS, Kahonen M, et al. Childhood levels of serum apolipoproteins B and A-I predict carotid intima-media thickness and brachial endothelial function in adulthood: the cardiovascular risk in Young Finns Study. *J Am Coll Cardiol.* 2008;52(4):293–9.

118. Davis PH, Dawson JD, Riley WA, Lauer RM. Carotid intimal-medial thickness is related to cardiovascular risk factors measured from childhood through middle age: the Muscatine Study. *Circulation.* 2001;104:2815–9.

119. Lauer RM, Lee J, Clarke WR. Predicting adult cholesterol levels from measurements in childhood and adolescence: the Muscatine Study. *Bull N Y Acad Med.* 1989;65(10):1127–42.

120. Frontini MG, Srinivasan SR, Xu J, Tang R, Bond MG, Berenson GS. Usefulness of childhood non-high density lipoprotein cholesterol levels versus other lipoprotein measures in predicting adult subclinical atherosclerosis: the Bogalusa Heart Study. *Pediatrics.* 2008;121:924–9.

121. Freedman DS, Patel DA, Srinivasan SR, et al. The contribution of childhood obesity to adult carotid intima-media thickness: the Bogalusa Heart Study. *Int J Obes (Lond).* 2008;32(5):749–56.

122. Freedman DS, Dietz WH, Tang R, et al. The relation of obesity throughout life to carotid intima-media thickness in adulthood: the Bogalusa Heart Study. *Int J Obes Relat Metab Disord.* 2004;28(1):159–66.

123. Lexell J, Downham DY. The occurrence of fibre-type grouping in healthy human muscle: a quantitative study of

cross-sections of whole vastus lateralis from men between 15 and 83 years. *Acta Neuropathol.* 1991;81(4):377–81.

124. Lexell J, Taylor CC, Sjostrom M. What is the cause of the ageing atrophy? Total number, size and proportion of different fiber types studied in whole vastus lateralis muscle from 15- to 83-year-old men. *J Neurol Sci.* 1988;84(2–3):275–94.

125. Lexell J, Downham D, Sjostrom M. Distribution of different fibre types in human skeletal muscles. Fibre type arrangement in m. vastus lateralis from three groups of healthy men between 15 and 83 years. *J Neurol Sci.* 1986;72(2–3):211–22.

126. Lindle RS, Metter EJ, Lynch NA, et al. Age and gender comparisons of muscle strength in 654 women and men aged 20–93 yr. *J Appl Physiol (1985).* 1997;83(5):1581–7.

127. Lynch NA, Metter EJ, Lindle RS, et al. Muscle quality. I. Age-associated differences between arm and leg muscle groups. *J Appl Physiol (1985).* 1999;86(1):188–94.

128. Folland JP, Williams AG. The adaptations to strength training: morphological and neurological contributions to increased strength. *Sports Med.* 2007;37(2):145–68.

129. Narici MV, Roi GS, Landoni L, Minetti AE, Cerretelli P. Changes in force, cross-sectional area and neural activation during strength training and detraining of the human quadriceps. *Eur J Appl Physiol Occup Physiol.* 1989;59(4):310–9.

130. Biolo G, Tipton KD, Klein S, Wolfe RR. An abundant supply of amino acids enhances the metabolic effect of exercise on muscle protein. *Am J Physiol.* 1997;273(1 Pt 1):E122–9.

131. Biolo G, Maggi SP, Williams BD, Tipton KD, Wolfe RR. Increased rates of muscle protein turnover and amino acid transport after resistance exercise in humans. *Am J Physiol.* 1995;268(3 Pt 1):E514–20.

132. Drummond MJ, Dreyer HC, Pennings B, et al. Skeletal muscle protein anabolic response to resistance exercise and essential amino acids is delayed with aging. *J Appl Physiol (1985).* 2008;104(5):1452–61.

133. Elliot TA, Cree MG, Sanford AP, Wolfe RR, Tipton KD. Milk ingestion stimulates net muscle protein synthesis following resistance exercise. *Med Sci Sports Exerc.* 2006;38(4):667–74.

134. Pennings B, Koopman R, Beelen M, Senden JM, Saris WH, van Loon LJ. Exercising before protein intake allows for greater use of dietary protein-derived amino acids for de novo muscle protein synthesis in both young and elderly men. *Am J Clin Nutr.* 2011;93(2):322–31.

135. Burd NA, Beals JW, Martinez IG, Salvador AF, Skinner SK. Food-first approach to enhance the regulation of post-exercise skeletal muscle protein synthesis and remodeling. *Sports Med.* 2019;49(Suppl 1):59–68.

136. Wirth J, Hillesheim E, Brennan L. The role of protein intake and its timing on body composition and muscle function in healthy adults: a systematic review and meta-analysis of randomized controlled trials. *J Nutr.* 2020;150(6):1443–60.

137. Snijders T, Trommelen J, Kouw IWK, Holwerda AM, Verdijk LB, van Loon LJC. The impact of pre-sleep protein ingestion on the skeletal muscle adaptive response to exercise in humans: an update. *Front Nutr.* 2019;6:17.

138. Morton RW, Murphy KT, McKellar SR, et al. A systematic review, meta-analysis and meta-regression of the effect of protein supplementation on resistance training-induced gains in muscle mass and strength in healthy adults. *Br J Sports Med.* 2018;52(6):376–84.

139. Hubal MJ, Gordish-Dressman H, Thompson PD, et al. Variability in muscle size and strength gain after unilateral resistance training. *Med Sci Sports Exerc.* 2005;37(6):964–72.

140. Pescatello LS, Devaney JM, Hubal MJ, Thompson PD, Hoffman EP. Highlights from the functional single nucleotide polymorphisms associated with human muscle size and strength or FAMuSS study. *Biomed Res Int.* 2013;2013:643575.

141. Kaminsky LA, Arena R, Myers J. Reference standards for cardiorespiratory fitness measured with cardiopulmonary exercise testing: data from the Fitness Registry and the Importance of Exercise National Database. *Mayo Clin Proc.* 2015;90(11):1515–23.

142. Kaminsky LA, Imboden MT, Arena R, Myers J. Reference standards for cardiorespiratory fitness measured with cardiopulmonary exercise testing using cycle ergometry: data from the Fitness Registry and the Importance of Exercise National Database (FRIEND) Registry. *Mayo Clin Proc.* 2017;92(2):228–33.

143. Trappe SW, Costill DL, Vukovich MD, Jones J, Melham T. Aging among elite distance runners: a 22-yr longitudinal study. *J Appl Physiol (1985).* 1996;80(1):285–90.

144. Billat V, Lepretre PM, Heugas AM, Laurence MH, Salim D, Koralsztein JP. Training and bioenergetic characteristics in elite male and female Kenyan runners. *Med Sci Sports Exerc.* 2003;35(2):297–304.

145. Jeukendrup AE, Craig NP, Hawley JA. The bioenergetics of world class cycling. *J Sci Med Sport.* 2000;3(4):414–33.

146. Tønnessen E, Sylta Ø, Haugen TA, Hem E, Svendsen IS, Seiler S. The road to gold: training and peaking characteristics in the year prior to a gold medal endurance performance. *PLoS One.* 2014;9(7):e101796.

147. Gormley SE, Swain DP, High R, et al. Effect of intensity of aerobic training on VO$_2$max. *Med Sci Sports Exerc.* 2008;40(7):1336–43.

148. Kim S, So WY, Kim J, Sung DJ. Relationship between bone-specific physical activity scores and measures for body composition and bone mineral density in healthy young college women. *PLoS One.* 2016;11(9):e0162127.

149. Callreus M, McGuigan F, Ringsberg K, Akesson K. Self-reported recreational exercise combining regularity and impact is necessary to maximize bone mineral density in young adult women: a population-based study of 1,061 women 25 years of age. *Osteoporos Int.* 2012;23(10):2517–26.

150. Mosti MP, Carlsen T, Aas E, Hoff J, Stunes AK, Syversen U. Maximal strength training improves bone mineral density and neuromuscular performance in young adult women. *J Strength Cond Res.* 2014;28(10):2935–45.

151. Zhao R, Zhao M, Zhang L. Efficiency of jumping exercise in improving bone mineral density among premenopausal women: a meta-analysis. *Sports Med.* 2014;44(10):1393–402.

152. Weaver CM, Teegarden D, Lyle RM, et al. Impact of exercise on bone health and contraindication of oral contraceptive use in young women. *Med Sci Sports Exerc.* 2001;33(6):873–80.

153. Jensen B, Moritoyo T, Kaufer-Horwitz M, et al. Ethnic differences in fat and muscle mass and their implication for interpretation of bioelectrical impedance vector analysis. *Appl Physiol Nutr Metab.* 2019;44(6):619–26.

154. Janssen I, Heymsfield SB, Wang ZM, Ross R. Skeletal muscle mass and distribution in 468 men and women aged 18–88 yr. *J Appl Physiol (1985).* 2000;89(1):81–8.

155. Melton LJ 3rd, Khosla S, Riggs BL. Epidemiology of sarcopenia. *Mayo Clin Proc.* 2000;75(Suppl):S10–2; discussion S12–3.

156. Melton LJ 3rd, Khosla S, Crowson CS, O'Connor MK, O'Fallon WM, Riggs BL. Epidemiology of sarcopenia. *J Am Geriatr Soc.* 2000;48(6):625–30.

157. Cherin P, Voronska E, Fraoucene N, de Jaeger C. Prevalence of sarcopenia among healthy ambulatory subjects: the sarcopenia begins from 45 years. *Aging Clin Exp Res.* 2014;26(2):137–46.

158. Larsson L. Morphological and functional characteristics of the ageing skeletal muscle in man. A cross-sectional study. *Acta Physiol Scand Suppl.* 1978;457:1–36.

159. Hakkinen K, Kraemer WJ, Newton RU, Alen M. Changes in electromyographic activity, muscle fibre and force production characteristics during heavy resistance/power strength training in middle-aged and older men and women. *Acta Physiol Scand.* 2001;171(1):51–62.

160. Fragala MS, Kenny AM, Kuchel GA. Muscle quality in aging: a multi-dimensional approach to muscle functioning with applications for treatment. *Sports Med.* 2015;45(5):641–58.

161. Ochala J, Frontera WR, Dorer DJ, Van Hoecke J, Krivickas LS. Single skeletal muscle fiber elastic and contractile characteristics in young and older men. *J Gerontol A Biol Sci Med Sci.* 2007;62(4):375–81.

162. Jozsi AC, Campbell WW, Joseph L, Davey SL, Evans WJ. Changes in power with resistance training in older and younger men and women. *J Gerontol A Biol Sci Med Sci.* 1999;54(11):M591–6.

163. Goodpaster BH, Kelley DE, Thaete FL, He J, Ross R. Skeletal muscle attenuation determined by computed tomography is associated with skeletal muscle lipid content. *J Appl Physiol (1985).* 2000;89(1):104–10.

164. Leskinen T, Sipila S, Kaprio J, Kainulainen H, Alen M, Kujala UM. Physically active vs. inactive lifestyle, muscle properties, and glucose homeostasis in middle-aged and older twins. *Age (Dordr).* 2013;35(5):1917–26.

165. Overend TJ, Cunningham DA, Paterson DH, Lefcoe MS. Thigh composition in young and elderly men determined by computed tomography. *Clin Physiol.* 1992;12(6):629–40.

166. Weigle DS, Sande KJ, Iverius PH, Monsen ER, Brunzell JD. Weight loss leads to a marked decrease in nonresting energy expenditure in ambulatory human subjects. *Metabolism.* 1988;37(10):930–6.

167. Gallagher D, Belmonte D, Deurenberg P, et al. Organ-tissue mass measurement allows modeling of REE and metabolically active tissue mass. *Am J Physiol.* 1998;275(2 Pt 1):E249–58.

168. Geisler C, Braun W, Pourhassan M, et al. Age-dependent changes in Resting Energy Expenditure (REE): insights from detailed body composition analysis in normal and overweight healthy caucasians. *Nutrients.* 2016;8(6):322.

169. Elia M, Ritz P, Stubbs RJ. Total energy expenditure in the elderly. *Eur J Clin Nutr.* 2000;54(Suppl 3):S92–103.

170. Alfonzo-Gonzalez G, Doucet E, Bouchard C, Tremblay A. Greater than predicted decrease in resting energy expenditure with age: cross-sectional and longitudinal evidence. *Eur J Clin Nutr.* 2006;60(1):18–24.

171. Borsheim E, Bahr R. Effect of exercise intensity, duration and mode on post-exercise oxygen consumption. *Sports Med.* 2003;33(14):1037–60.

172. Lytle JR, Kravits DM, Martin SE, Green JS, Crouse SF, Lambert BS. Predicting energy expenditure of an acute resistance exercise bout in men and women. *Med Sci Sports Exerc.* 2019;51(7):1532–7.

173. Williamson DL, Kirwan JP. A single bout of concentric resistance exercise increases basal metabolic rate 48 hours after exercise in healthy 59–77-year-old men. *J Gerontol A Biol Sci Med Sci.* 1997;52(6):M352–5.

174. Melby C, Scholl C, Edwards G, Bullough R. Effect of acute resistance exercise on postexercise energy expenditure and resting metabolic rate. *J Appl Physiol (1985).* 1993;75(4):1847–53.

175. Benton MJ, Swan PD. Effect of protein ingestion on energy expenditure and substrate utilization after exercise in middle-aged women. *Int J Sport Nutr Exerc Metab.* 2007;17(6):544–55.

176. Binzen CA, Swan PD, Manore MM. Postexercise oxygen consumption and substrate use after resistance exercise in women. *Med Sci Sports Exerc.* 2001;33(6):932–8.

177. Feldman HA, Longcope C, Derby CA, et al. Age trends in the level of serum testosterone and other hormones in middle-aged men: longitudinal results from the Massachusetts male aging study. *J Clin Endocrinol Metab.* 2002;87(2):589–98.

178. Fabbri E, An Y, Gonzalez-Freire M, et al. Bioavailable testosterone linearly declines over a wide age spectrum in men and women from the Baltimore Longitudinal Study of Aging. *J Gerontol A Biol Sci Med Sci.* 2016;71(9):1202–9.

179. Enea C, Boisseau N, Fargeas-Gluck MA, Diaz V, Dugue B. Circulating androgens in women: exercise-induced changes. *Sports Med.* 2011;41(1):1–15.

180. Couzinet B, Meduri G, Lecce MG, et al. The postmenopausal ovary is not a major androgen-producing gland. *J Clin Endocrinol Metab.* 2001;86(10):5060–6.

181. Vingren JL, Kraemer WJ, Ratamess NA, Anderson JM, Volek JS, Maresh CM. Testosterone physiology in resistance exercise and training: the up-stream regulatory elements. *Sports Med.* 2010;40(12):1037–53.

182. Balagopal P, Rooyackers OE, Adey DB, Ades PA, Nair KS. Effects of aging on in vivo synthesis of skeletal muscle myosin heavy-chain and sarcoplasmic protein in humans. *Am J Physiol.* 1997;273(4 Pt 1):E790–800.

183. Timmerman KL, Volpi E. Amino acid metabolism and regulatory effects in aging. *Curr Opin Clin Nutr Metab Care.* 2008;11(1):45–9.

184. Krentz AJ, Viljoen A, Sinclair A. Insulin resistance: a risk marker for disease and disability in the older person. *Diabet Med.* 2013;30(5):535–48.

185. Rutter MK, Sullivan LM, Fox CS, et al. Baseline levels, and changes over time in body mass index and fasting insulin, and their relationship to change in metabolic trait clustering. *Metab Syndr Relat Disord.* 2014;12(7):372–80.

186. Jensen GL. Inflammation: roles in aging and sarcopenia. *JPEN J Parenter Enteral Nutr.* 2008;32(6):656–9.

187. Haddad F, Zaldivar F, Cooper DM, Adams GR. IL-6-induced skeletal muscle atrophy. *J Appl Physiol (1985).* 2005;98(3):911–7.

188. Roubenoff R, Harris TB, Abad LW, Wilson PW, Dallal GE, Dinarello CA. Monocyte cytokine production in an elderly population: effect of age and inflammation. *J Gerontol A Biol Sci Med Sci.* 1998;53(1):M20–6.

189. Toth MJ, Matthews DE, Tracy RP, Previs MJ. Age-related differences in skeletal muscle protein synthesis: relation to

markers of immune activation. *Am J Physiol Endocrinol Metab.* 2005;288(5):E883–91.

190. Plomgaard P, Penkowa M, Pedersen BK. Fiber type specific expression of TNF-alpha, IL-6 and IL-18 in human skeletal muscles. *Exerc Immunol Rev.* 2005;11:53–63.

191. Wang Y, Pessin JE. Mechanisms for fiber-type specificity of skeletal muscle atrophy. *Curr Opin Clin Nutr Metab Care.* 2013;16(3):243–50.

192. Carlson SA, Fulton JE, Schoenborn CA, Loustalot F. Trend and prevalence estimates based on the 2008 Physical Activity Guidelines for Americans. *Am J Prev Med.* 2010;39(4):305–13.

193. Donges CE, Burd NA, Duffield R, et al. Concurrent resistance and aerobic exercise stimulates both myofibrillar and mitochondrial protein synthesis in sedentary middle-aged men. *J Appl Physiol (1985).* 2012;112(12):1992–2001.

194. Hakkinen K, Kallinen M, Izquierdo M, et al. Changes in agonist-antagonist EMG, muscle CSA, and force during strength training in middle-aged and older people. *J Appl Physiol (1985).* 1998;84(4):1341–9.

195. Benton MJ, Kasper MJ, Raab SA, Waggener GT, Swan PD. Short-term effects of resistance training frequency on body composition and strength in middle-aged women. *J Strength Cond Res.* 2011;25(11):3142–9.

196. Candow DG, Burke DG. Effect of short-term equal-volume resistance training with different workout frequency on muscle mass and strength in untrained men and women. *J Strength Cond Res.* 2007;21(1):204–7.

197. Doering TM, Jenkins DG, Reaburn PR, Borges NR, Hohmann E, Phillips SM. Lower integrated muscle protein synthesis in masters compared with younger athletes. *Med Sci Sports Exerc.* 2016;48(8):1613–8.

198. Izquierdo M, Hakkinen K, Ibanez J, Kraemer WJ, Gorostiaga EM. Effects of combined resistance and cardiovascular training on strength, power, muscle cross-sectional area, and endurance markers in middle-aged men. *Eur J Appl Physiol.* 2005;94(1–2):70–5.

199. Tzanis G, Philippou A, Karatzanos E, et al. Effects of high-intensity interval exercise training on skeletal myopathy of chronic heart failure. *J Card Fail.* 2017;23(1):36–46.

200. Blair SN, Kohl HW 3rd, Paffenbarger RS Jr, Clark DG, Cooper KH, Gibbons LW. Physical fitness and all-cause mortality. A prospective study of healthy men and women. *JAMA.* 1989;262(17):2395–401.

201. Barnett TA, Gauvin L, Craig CL, Katzmarzyk PT. Distinct trajectories of leisure time physical activity and predictors of trajectory class membership: a 22 year cohort study. *Int J Behav Nutr Phys Act.* 2008;5:57.

202. Fleg JL, Morrell CH, Bos AG, et al. Accelerated longitudinal decline of aerobic capacity in healthy older adults. *Circulation.* 2005;112(5):674–82.

203. Jackson AS, Sui X, Hebert JR, Church TS, Blair SN. Role of lifestyle and aging on the longitudinal change in cardiorespiratory fitness. *Arch Intern Med.* 2009;169(19):1781–7.

204. Wilson TM, Tanaka H. Meta-analysis of the age-associated decline in maximal aerobic capacity in men: relation to training status. *Am J Physiol Heart Circ Physiol.* 2000;278(3):H829–34.

205. Fitzgerald MD, Tanaka H, Tran ZV, Seals DR. Age-related declines in maximal aerobic capacity in regularly exercising vs. sedentary women: a meta-analysis. *J Appl Physiol (1985).* 1997;83(1):160–5.

206. Nes BM, Janszky I, Wisloff U, Stoylen A, Karlsen T. Age-predicted maximal heart rate in healthy subjects: the HUNT fitness study. *Scand J Med Sci Sports.* 2013;23(6):697–704.

207. Jackson AS, Beard EF, Wier LT, Ross RM, Stuteville JE, Blair SN. Changes in aerobic power of men, ages 25–70 yr. *Med Sci Sports Exerc.* 1995;27(1):113–20.

208. Ogawa T, Spina RJ, Martin WH 3rd, et al. Effects of aging, sex, and physical training on cardiovascular responses to exercise. *Circulation.* 1992;86(2):494–503.

209. Banks L, Sasson Z, Esfandiari S, Busato GM, Goodman JM. Cardiac function following prolonged exercise: influence of age. *J Appl Physiol (1985).* 2011;110(6):1541–8.

210. Hawkins SA, Marcell TJ, Victoria Jaque S, Wiswell RA. A longitudinal assessment of change in VO2max and maximal heart rate in master athletes. *Med Sci Sports Exerc.* 2001;33(10):1744–50.

211. Fleg JL, Lakatta EG. Role of muscle loss in the age-associated reduction in VO$_2$ max. *J Appl Physiol (1985).* 1988;65(3):1147–51.

212. Rosen MJ, Sorkin JD, Goldberg AP, Hagberg JM, Katzel LI. Predictors of age-associated decline in maximal aerobic capacity: a comparison of four statistical models. *J Appl Physiol (1985).* 1998;84(6):2163–70.

213. Porter C, Hurren NM, Cotter MV, et al. Mitochondrial respiratory capacity and coupling control decline with age in human skeletal muscle. *Am J Physiol Endocrinol Metab.* 2015;309(3):E224–32.

214. Short KR, Bigelow ML, Kahl J, et al. Decline in skeletal muscle mitochondrial function with aging in humans. *Proc Natl Acad Sci U S A.* 2005;102:5618–23.

215. Rooyackers OE, Adey DB, Ades PA, Nair KS. Effect of age on in vivo rates of mitochondrial protein synthesis in human skeletal muscle. *Proc Natl Acad Sci U S A.* 1996;93:15364–9.

216. Conley KE, Esselman PC, Jubrias SA, et al. Ageing, muscle properties and maximal O(2) uptake rate in humans. *J Physiol.* 2000;526(Pt 1):211–7.

217. Vigelso A, Prats C, Ploug T, Dela F, Helge JW. Higher muscle content of perilipin 5 and endothelial lipase protein in trained than untrained middle-aged men. *Physiol Res.* 2016;65(2):293–302.

218. Distefano G, Standley RA, Dube JJ, et al. Chronological age does not influence ex-vivo mitochondrial respiration and quality control in skeletal muscle. *J Gerontol A Biol Sci Med Sci.* 2017;72(4):535–42.

219. Carter HN, Chen CC, Hood DA. Mitochondria, muscle health, and exercise with advancing age. *Physiology (Bethesda).* 2015;30(3):208–23.

220. Bylund AC, Bjuro T, Cederblad G, et al. Physical training in man. Skeletal muscle metabolism in relation to muscle morphology and running ability. *Eur J Appl Physiol Occup Physiol.* 1977;36(3):151–69.

221. Catai AM, Chacon-Mikahil MP, Martinelli FS, et al. Effects of aerobic exercise training on heart rate variability during wakefulness and sleep and cardiorespiratory responses of young and middle-aged healthy men. *Braz J Med Biol Res.* 2002;35(6):741–52.

222. Valenzuela PL, Maffiuletti NA, Joyner MJ, Lucia A, Lepers R. Lifelong endurance exercise as a countermeasure against age-related V̇O$_2$ max decline: physiological overview and insights from masters athletes. *Sports Med.* 2020;50(4):703–16.

223. Heath GW, Hagberg JM, Ehsani AA, Holloszy JO. A physiological comparison of young and older endurance athletes. *J Appl Physiol Respir Environ Exerc Physiol.* 1981;51(3):634–40.

224. Pollock ML, Miller HS Jr, Wilmore J. Physiological characteristics of champion American track athletes 40 to 75 years of age. *J Gerontol.* 1974;29(6):645–9.

225. Grimby G, Saltin B. Physiological analysis of physically well-trained middle-aged and old athletes. *Acta Med Scand.* 1966;179(5):513–26.

226. Robinson S, Dill DB, Robinson RD, Tzankoff SP, Wagner JA. Physiological aging of champion runners. *J Appl Physiol.* 1976;41(1):46–51.

227. Dill DB, Robinson S, Ross JC. A longitudinal study of 16 champion runners. *J Sports Med Phys Fitness.* 1967;7(1):4–27.

228. Edholm P, Veen J, Kadi F, Nilsson A. Muscle mass and aerobic capacity in older women: impact of regular exercise at middle age. *Exp Gerontol.* 2021;147:111259.

229. Hautala AJ, Kiviniemi AM, Makikallio TH, et al. Individual differences in the responses to endurance and resistance training. *Eur J Appl Physiol.* 2006;96(5):535–42.

230. Sui X, Laditka JN, Church TS, et al. Prospective study of cardiorespiratory fitness and depressive symptoms in women and men. *J Psychiatr Res.* 2009;43(5):546–52.

231. Katzmarzyk PT, Craig CL, Gauvin L. Adiposity, physical fitness and incident diabetes: the physical activity longitudinal study. *Diabetologia.* 2007;50(3):538–44.

232. Szulc P, Seeman E. Thinking inside and outside the envelopes of bone: dedicated to PDD. *Osteoporos Int.* 2009;20(8):1281–8.

233. Trotter M, Hixon BB. Sequential changes in weight, density, and percentage ash weight of human skeletons from an early fetal period through old age. *Anat Rec.* 1974;179(1):1–18.

234. Riggs BL, Melton LJ III, Robb RA, et al. Population-based study of age and sex differences in bone volumetric density, size, geometry, and structure at different skeletal sites. *J Bone Miner Res.* 2004;19(12):1945–54.

235. Riggs BL, Melton LJ, Robb RA, et al. A population-based assessment of rates of bone loss at multiple skeletal sites: evidence for substantial trabecular bone loss in young adult women and men. *J Bone Miner Res.* 2008;23(2):205–14.

236. Garvey ME, Shi L, Gona PN, Troped PJ, Camhi SM. Age, sex, and race/ethnicity associations between fat mass and lean mass with bone mineral density: NHANES data. *Int J Environ Res Public Health.* 2021;18(23):16206.

237. Christiansen BA, Kopperdahl DL, Kiel DP, Keaveny TM, Bouxsein ML. Mechanical contributions of the cortical and trabecular compartments contribute to differences in age-related changes in vertebral body strength in men and women assessed by QCT-based finite element analysis. *J Bone Miner Res.* 2011;26(5):974–83.

238. Boskey AL, Coleman R. Aging and bone. *J Dent Res.* 2010;89(12):1333–48.

239. Wu F, Mason B, Horne A, et al. Fractures between the ages of 20 and 50 years increase women's risk of subsequent fractures. *Arch Intern Med.* 2002;162(1):33–6.

240. Kanis JA, Johnell O, Oden A, De Laet C, Jonsson B, Dawson A. Ten-year risk of osteoporotic fracture and the effect of risk factors on screening strategies. *Bone.* 2002;30(1):251–8.

241. Johnell O, Kanis JA, Oden A, et al. Predictive value of BMD for hip and other fractures. *J Bone Miner Res.* 2005;20(7):1185–94.

242. Ralston SH, Uitterlinden AG. Genetics of osteoporosis. *Endocr Rev.* 2010;31(5):629–62.

243. Khosla S. Pathogenesis of age-related bone loss in humans. *J Gerontol A Biol Sci Med Sci.* 2013;68(10):1226–35.

244. Greendale GA, Sowers M, Han W, et al. Bone mineral density loss in relation to the final menstrual period in a multiethnic cohort: results from the Study of Women's Health Across the Nation (SWAN). *J Bone Miner Res.* 2012;27(1):111–8.

245. Tang M, O'Connor LE, Campbell WW. Diet-induced weight loss: the effect of dietary protein on bone. *J Acad Nutr Diet.* 2014;114(1):72–85.

246. Sahni S, Broe KE, Tucker KL, et al. Association of total protein intake with bone mineral density and bone loss in men and women from the Framingham Offspring Study. *Public Health Nutr.* 2014;17(11):2570–6.

247. Mangano KM, Sahni S, Kiel DP, Tucker KL, Dufour AB, Hannan MT. Bone mineral density and protein-derived food clusters from the Framingham Offspring Study. *J Acad Nutr Diet.* 2015;115(10):1605–13.e1.

248. Darling AL, Manders RJF, Sahni S, et al. Dietary protein and bone health across the life-course: an updated systematic review and meta-analysis over 40 years. *Osteoporos Int.* 2019;30(4):741–61.

249. Vasquez E, Shaw BA, Gensburg L, Okorodudu D, Corsino L. Racial and ethnic differences in physical activity and bone density: National Health and Nutrition Examination Survey, 2007–2008. *Prev Chronic Dis.* 2013;10:E216.

250. Hardcastle SA, Gregson CL, Rittweger J, Crabtree N, Ward K, Tobias JH. Jump power and force have distinct associations with cortical bone parameters: findings from a population enriched by individuals with high bone mass. *J Clin Endocrinol Metab.* 2014;99(1):266–75.

251. Kopiczko A, Adamczyk JG, Gryko K, Popowczak M. Bone mineral density in elite masters athletes: the effect of body composition and long-term exercise. *Eur Rev Aging Phys Act.* 2021;18(1):7.

252. Shea KL, Barry DW, Sherk VD, Hansen KC, Wolfe P, Kohrt WM. Calcium supplementation and parathyroid hormone response to vigorous walking in postmenopausal women. *Med Sci Sports Exerc.* 2014;46(10):2007–13.

253. Mohr M, Helge EW, Petersen LF, et al. Effects of soccer vs swim training on bone formation in sedentary middle-aged women. *Eur J Appl Physiol.* 2015;115(12):2671–9.

254. Hinton PS, Nigh P, Thyfault J. Effectiveness of resistance training or jumping-exercise to increase bone mineral density in men with low bone mass: a 12-month randomized, clinical trial. *Bone.* 2015;79:203–12.

255. Souza D, Barbalho M, Ramirez-Campillo R, Martins W, Gentil P. High and low-load resistance training produce similar effects on bone mineral density of middle-aged and older people: a systematic review with meta-analysis of randomized clinical trials. *Exp Gerontol.* 2020;138:110973.

256. Nowak A, Straburzynska-Lupa A, Kusy K, et al. Bone mineral density and bone turnover in male masters athletes aged 40–64. *Aging Male.* 2010;13(2):133–41.

257. Gast U, Belavy DL, Armbrecht G, et al. Bone density and neuromuscular function in older competitive athletes depend on running distance. *Osteoporos Int.* 2013;24(7):2033–42.

258. Welch JM, Rosen CJ. Older women track and field athletes have enhanced calcaneal stiffness. *Osteoporos Int.* 2005;16(8):871–8.

259. Kemmler W, von Stengel S. Dose–response effect of exercise frequency on bone mineral density in post-menopausal, osteopenic women. *Scand J Med Sci Sports*. 2014;24(3):526–34.

260. Newman AB, Lee JS, Visser M, et al. Weight change and the conservation of lean mass in old age: the Health, Aging and Body Composition Study. *Am J Clin Nutr*. 2005;82(4):872–8; quiz 915–6.

261. Visser M, Pahor M, Tylavsky F, et al. One- and two-year change in body composition as measured by DXA in a population-based cohort of older men and women. *J Appl Physiol (1985)*. 2003;94(6):2368–74.

262. Rossi AP, Watson NL, Newman AB, et al. Effects of body composition and adipose tissue distribution on respiratory function in elderly men and women: the Health, Aging, and Body Composition Study. *J Gerontol A Biol Sci Med Sci*. 2011;66(7):801–8.

263. Batsis JA, Mackenzie TA, Lopez-Jimenez F, Bartels SJ. Sarcopenia, sarcopenic obesity, and functional impairments in older adults: National Health and Nutrition Examination Surveys 1999–2004. *Nutr Res*. 2015;35(12):1031–9.

264. da Silva AP, Matos A, Ribeiro R, et al. Sarcopenia and osteoporosis in Portuguese centenarians. *Eur J Clin Nutr*. 2017;71(1):56–63.

265. Murphy RA, Ip EH, Zhang Q, et al. Transition to sarcopenia and determinants of transitions in older adults: a population-based study. *J Gerontol A Biol Sci Med Sci*. 2014;69(6):751–8.

266. Shamliyan T, Talley KM, Ramakrishnan R, Kane RL. Association of frailty with survival: a systematic literature review. *Ageing Res Rev*. 2013;12(2):719–36.

267. Fried LP, Tangen CM, Walston J, et al. Frailty in older adults: evidence for a phenotype. *J Gerontol A Biol Sci Med Sci*. 2001;56(3):M146–56.

268. Marzetti E, Hwang AC, Tosato M, et al. Age-related changes of skeletal muscle mass and strength among Italian and Taiwanese older people: results from the Milan EXPO 2015 survey and the I-Lan Longitudinal Aging Study. *Exp Gerontol*. 2018;102:76–80.

269. Verdijk LB, Gleeson BG, Jonkers RA, et al. Skeletal muscle hypertrophy following resistance training is accompanied by a fiber type-specific increase in satellite cell content in elderly men. *J Gerontol A Biol Sci Med Sci*. 2009;64(3):332–9.

270. Clark BC, Manini TM. What is dynapenia? *Nutrition*. 2012;28(5):495–503.

271. Delmonico MJ, Harris TB, Visser M, et al. Longitudinal study of muscle strength, quality, and adipose tissue infiltration. *Am J Clin Nutr*. 2009;90(6):1579–85.

272. Visser M, Goodpaster BH, Kritchevsky SB, et al. Muscle mass, muscle strength, and muscle fat infiltration as predictors of incident mobility limitations in well-functioning older persons. *J Gerontol A Biol Sci Med Sci*. 2005;60(3):324–33.

273. Frisard MI, Broussard A, Davies SS, et al. Aging, resting metabolic rate, and oxidative damage: results from the Louisiana Healthy Aging Study. *J Gerontol A Biol Sci Med Sci*. 2007;62(7):752–9.

274. Geisler C, Braun W, Pourhassan M, et al. Gender-specific associations in age-related changes in Resting Energy Expenditure (REE) and MRI measured body composition in healthy Caucasians. *J Gerontol A Biol Sci Med Sci*. 2016;71(7):941–6.

275. Manini TM. Energy expenditure and aging. *Ageing Res Rev*. 2010;9(1):1–11.

276. Krems C, Luhrmann PM, Strassburg A, Hartmann B, Neuhauser-Berthold M. Lower resting metabolic rate in the elderly may not be entirely due to changes in body composition. *Eur J Clin Nutr*. 2005;59(2):255–62.

277. Melanson EL, Donahoo WT, Grunwald GK, Schwartz R. Changes in 24-h substrate oxidation in older and younger men in response to exercise. *J Appl Physiol (1985)*. 2007;103(5):1576–82.

278. Fatouros IG, Chatzinikolaou A, Tournis S, et al. Intensity of resistance exercise determines adipokine and resting energy expenditure responses in overweight elderly individuals. *Diabetes Care*. 2009;32(12):2161–7.

279. Hackney KJ, Engels HJ, Gretebeck RJ. Resting energy expenditure and delayed-onset muscle soreness after full-body resistance training with an eccentric concentration. *J Strength Cond Res*. 2008;22(5):1602–9.

280. Dolezal BA, Potteiger JA, Jacobsen DJ, Benedict SH. Muscle damage and resting metabolic rate after acute resistance exercise with an eccentric overload. *Med Sci Sports Exerc*. 2000;32(7):1202–7.

281. Carcaillon L, Blanco C, Alonso-Bouzon C, Alfaro-Acha A, Garcia-Garcia FJ, Rodriguez-Manas L. Sex differences in the association between serum levels of testosterone and frailty in an elderly population: the Toledo Study for Healthy Aging. *PLoS One*. 2012;7(3):e32401.

282. Hakkinen K, Pakarinen A, Kraemer WJ, Newton RU, Alen M. Basal concentrations and acute responses of serum hormones and strength development during heavy resistance training in middle-aged and elderly men and women. *J Gerontol A Biol Sci Med Sci*. 2000;55(2):B95–105.

283. Yuki A, Ando F, Otsuka R, Shimokata H. Low free testosterone is associated with loss of appendicular muscle mass in Japanese community-dwelling women. *Geriatr Gerontol Int*. 2015;15(3):326–33.

284. Welle S, Thornton C, Jozefowicz R, Statt M. Myofibrillar protein synthesis in young and old men. *Am J Physiol*. 1993;264(5 Pt 1):E693–8.

285. Yarasheski KE, Zachwieja JJ, Bier DM. Acute effects of resistance exercise on muscle protein synthesis rate in young and elderly men and women. *Am J Physiol*. 1993;265(2 Pt 1):E210–4.

286. Pitkanen HT, Oja SS, Kemppainen K, Seppa JM, Mero AA. Serum amino acid concentrations in aging men and women. *Amino Acids*. 2003;24(4):413–21.

287. Krok-Schoen JL, Archdeacon Price A, Luo M, Kelly OJ, Taylor CA. Low dietary protein intakes and associated dietary patterns and functional limitations in an aging population: a NHANES analysis. *J Nutr Health Aging*. 2019;23(4):338–47.

288. Wlazlo N, van Greevenbroek MM, Ferreira I, et al. Iron metabolism is prospectively associated with insulin resistance and glucose intolerance over a 7-year follow-up period: the CODAM study. *Acta Diabetol*. 2015;52(2):337–48.

289. Soriguer F, Colomo N, Valdes S, et al. Modifications of the homeostasis model assessment of insulin resistance index with age. *Acta Diabetol*. 2014;51(6):917–25.

290. Cesari M, Kritchevsky SB, Baumgartner RN, et al. Sarcopenia, obesity, and inflammation—results from the Trial of

Angiotensin Converting Enzyme Inhibition and Novel Cardiovascular Risk Factors study. *Am J Clin Nutr*. 2005;82(2):428–34.

291. Visser M, Pahor M, Taaffe DR, et al. Relationship of interleukin-6 and tumor necrosis factor-alpha with muscle mass and muscle strength in elderly men and women: the Health ABC Study. *J Gerontol A Biol Sci Med Sci*. 2002;57(5):M326–32.

292. Schaap LA, Pluijm SM, Deeg DJ, et al. Higher inflammatory marker levels in older persons: associations with 5-year change in muscle mass and muscle strength. *J Gerontol A Biol Sci Med Sci*. 2009;64(11):1183–9.

293. Garber CE, Blissmer B, Deschenes MR, et al. American College of Sports Medicine position stand. Quantity and quality of exercise for developing and maintaining cardiorespiratory, musculoskeletal, and neuromotor fitness in apparently healthy adults: guidance for prescribing exercise. *Med Sci Sports Exerc*. 2011;43(7):1334–59.

294. Nilwik R, Snijders T, Leenders M, et al. The decline in skeletal muscle mass with aging is mainly attributed to a reduction in type II muscle fiber size. *Exp Gerontol*. 2013;48(5):492–8.

295. Peterson MD, Rhea MR, Sen A, Gordon PM. Resistance exercise for muscular strength in older adults: a meta-analysis. *Ageing Res Rev*. 2010;9(3):226–37.

296. Peterson MD, Sen A, Gordon PM. Influence of resistance exercise on lean body mass in aging adults: a meta-analysis. *Med Sci Sports Exerc*. 2011;43(2):249–58.

297. Aagaard P, Magnusson PS, Larsson B, Kjaer M, Krustrup P. Mechanical muscle function, morphology, and fiber type in lifelong trained elderly. *Med Sci Sports Exerc*. 2007;39(11):1989–96.

298. Mikkelsen UR, Couppe C, Karlsen A, et al. Life-long endurance exercise in humans: circulating levels of inflammatory markers and leg muscle size. *Mech Ageing Dev*. 2013;134(11–12):531–40.

298a. Wroblewski AP, Amati F, Smiley MA, Goodpaster B, Wright V. Chronic exercise preserves lean muscle mass in masters athletes. *Phys Sportsmed*. 2011;39(3): 172-8. https://doi.org/10.3810/psm.2011.09.1933

299. Venturelli M, Schena F, Scarsini R, Muti E, Richardson RS. Limitations to exercise in female centenarians: evidence that muscular efficiency tempers the impact of failing lungs. *Age (Dordr)*. 2013;35(3):861–70.

300. Broskey NT, Greggio C, Boss A, et al. Skeletal muscle mitochondria in the elderly: effects of physical fitness and exercise training. *J Clin Endocrinol Metab*. 2014;99(5):1852–61.

301. Safdar A, Hamadeh MJ, Kaczor JJ, Raha S, Debeer J, Tarnopolsky MA. Aberrant mitochondrial homeostasis in the skeletal muscle of sedentary older adults. *PLoS One*. 2010;5(5):e10778.

302. Carrick-Ranson G, Hastings JL, Bhella PS, et al. The effect of lifelong exercise dose on cardiovascular function during exercise. *J Appl Physiol (1985)*. 2014;116(7):736–45.

303. Gram M, Vigelso A, Yokota T, et al. Two weeks of one-leg immobilization decreases skeletal muscle respiratory capacity equally in young and elderly men. *Exp Gerontol*. 2014;58:269–78.

304. Stratton JR, Levy WC, Cerqueira MD, Schwartz RS, Abrass IB. Cardiovascular responses to exercise. Effects of aging and exercise training in healthy men. *Circulation*. 1994;89(4):1648–55.

305. Vincent KR, Braith RW, Feldman RA, Kallas HE, Lowenthal DT. Improved cardiorespiratory endurance following 6 months of resistance exercise in elderly men and women. *Arch Intern Med*. 2002;162(6):673–8.

306. Tanaka H, Seals DR. Endurance exercise performance in Masters athletes: age-associated changes and underlying physiological mechanisms. *J Physiol*. 2008;586(1):55–63.

307. Coggan AR, Spina RJ, Rogers MA, et al. Histochemical and enzymatic characteristics of skeletal muscle in master athletes. *J Appl Physiol (1985)*. 1990;68(5):1896–901.

308. Katzel LI, Sorkin JD, Fleg JL. A comparison of longitudinal changes in aerobic fitness in older endurance athletes and sedentary men. *J Am Geriatr Soc*. 2001;49(12):1657–64.

309. Tanaka H, DeSouza CA, Jones PP, Stevenson ET, Davy KP, Seals DR. Greater rate of decline in maximal aerobic capacity with age in physically active vs. sedentary healthy women. *J Appl Physiol (1985)*. 1997;83(6):1947–53.

310. Connors MH, Sachdev PS, Kochan NA, Xu J, Draper B, Brodaty H. Cognition and mortality in older people: the Sydney Memory and Ageing Study. *Age Ageing*. 2015;44(6):1049–54.

311. Prince M, Bryce R, Albanese E, Wimo A, Ribeiro W, Ferri CP. The global prevalence of dementia: a systematic review and metaanalysis. *Alzheimers Dement*. 2013;9(1):63–75.e2.

312. Tarumi T, Zhang R. Cerebral hemodynamics of the aging brain: risk of Alzheimer disease and benefit of aerobic exercise. *Front Physiol*. 2014;5:6.

313. Tseng BY, Gundapuneedi T, Khan MA, et al. White matter integrity in physically fit older adults. *Neuroimage*. 2013;82:510–6.

314. Iso-Markku P, Waller K, Kujala UM, Kaprio J. Physical activity and dementia: long-term follow-up study of adult twins. *Ann Med*. 2015;47(2):81–7.

315. Larson EB, Wang L, Bowen JD, et al. Exercise is associated with reduced risk for incident dementia among persons 65 years of age and older. *Ann Intern Med*. 2006;144(2):73–81.

316. Young J, Angevaren M, Rusted J, Tabet N. Aerobic exercise to improve cognitive function in older people without known cognitive impairment. *Cochrane Database Syst Rev*. 2015;(4):CD005381.

317. Forbes D, Forbes SC, Blake CM, Thiessen EJ, Forbes S. Exercise programs for people with dementia. *Cochrane Database Syst Rev*. 2015;(4):CD006489.

318. Seeman E. Structural basis of growth-related gain and age-related loss of bone strength. *Rheumatology (Oxford)*. 2008;47(Suppl 4):iv2–8.

319. Szulc P, Maurice C, Marchand F, Delmas PD. Increased bone resorption is associated with higher mortality in community-dwelling men ≥50 years of age: the MINOS study. *J Bone Miner Res*. 2009;24(6):1116–24.

320. Szulc P, Samelson EJ, Kiel DP, Delmas PD. Increased bone resorption is associated with increased risk of cardiovascular events in men: the MINOS study. *J Bone Miner Res*. 2009;24(12):2023–31.

321. Durdin R, Parsons C, Dennison EM, et al. Inflammatory status, body coposition and ethnic differences in bone mineral density: the Southall and Brent Revisited Study. *Bone*. 2022;155:116286.

322. Nguyen TV, Center JR, Eisman JA. Osteoporosis in elderly men and women: effects of dietary calcium, physical activity, and body mass index. *J Bone Miner Res*. 2000;15(2):322–31.

323. Shams-White MM, Chung M, Du M, et al. Dietary protein and bone health: a systematic review and meta-analysis

from the National Osteoporosis Foundation. *Am J Clin Nutr*. 2017;105(6):1528–43.

324. Tarantino U, Piccirilli E, Fantini M, Baldi J, Gasbarra E, Bei R. Sarcopenia and fragility fractures: molecular and clinical evidence of the bone-muscle interaction. *J Bone Joint Surg Am*. 2015;97(5):429–37.

325. Pereira FB, Leite AF, de Paula AP. Relationship between pre-sarcopenia, sarcopenia and bone mineral density in elderly men. *Arch Endocrinol Metab*. 2015;59(1):59–65.

326. Go SW, Cha YH, Lee JA, Park HS. Association between sarcopenia, bone density, and health-related quality of life in Korean men. *Korean J Fam Med*. 2013;34(4):281–8.

327. Sjoblom S, Suuronen J, Rikkonen T, Honkanen R, Kroger H, Sirola J. Relationship between postmenopausal osteoporosis and the components of clinical sarcopenia. *Maturitas*. 2013;75(2):175–80.

328. Suominen H, Rahkila P. Bone mineral density of the calcaneus in 70- to 81-yr-old male athletes and a population sample. *Med Sci Sports Exerc*. 1991;23(11):1227–33.

329. Korhonen MT, Heinonen A, Siekkinen J, et al. Bone density, structure and strength, and their determinants in aging sprint athletes. *Med Sci Sports Exerc*. 2012;44(12):2340–9.

330. Marques EA, Mota J, Carvalho J. Exercise effects on bone mineral density in older adults: a meta-analysis of randomized controlled trials. *Age (Dordr)*. 2012;34(6):1493–515.

331. Kelley GA, Kelley KS, Kohrt WM. Exercise and bone mineral density in men: a meta-analysis of randomized controlled trials. *Bone*. 2013;53(1):103–11.

332. Shojaa M, von Stengel S, Kohl M, Schoene D, Kemmler W. Effects of dynamic resistance exercise on bone mineral density in postmenopausal women: a systematic review and meta-analysis with special emphasis on exercise parameters. *Osteoporos Int*. 2020;31(8):1427–44.

333. Kemmler W, Shojaa M, Kohl M, von Stengel S. Effects of different types of exercise on bone mineral density in postmenopausal women: a systematic review and meta-analysis. *Calcif Tissue Int*. 2020;107(5):409–39.

334. McDowell MA, Brody DJ, Hughes JP. Has age at menarche changed? Results from the National Health and Nutrition Examination Survey (NHANES) 1999–2004. *J Adolesc Health*. 2007;40(3):227–31.

335. Anderson SE, Must A. Interpreting the continued decline in the average age at menarche: results from two nationally representative surveys of U.S. girls studied 10 years apart. *J Pediatr*. 2005;147(6):753–60.

336. Freedman DS, Khan LK, Serdula MK, et al. The relation of menarcheal age to obesity in childhood and adulthood: the Bogalusa Heart Study. *BMC Pediatr*. 2003;3:3.

337. Solomon SJ, Kurzer MS, Calloway DH. Menstrual cycle and basal metabolic rate in women. *Am J Clin Nutr*. 1982; 36(4):611–6.

338. Melanson KJ, Saltzman E, Russell R, Roberts SB. Postabsorptive and postprandial energy expenditure and substrate oxidation do not change during the menstrual cycle in young women. *J Nutr*. 1996;126(10):2531–8.

339. Matsuo T, Saitoh S, Suzuki M. Effects of the menstrual cycle on excess postexercise oxygen consumption in healthy young women. *Metabolism*. 1999;48(3):275–7.

340. Henry CJ, Lightowler HJ, Marchini J. Intra-individual variation in resting metabolic rate during the menstrual cycle. *Br J Nutr*. 2003;89(6):811–7.

341. Benton MJ, Hutchins AM, Dawes JJ. Effect of menstrual cycle on resting metabolism: a systematic review and meta-analysis. *PLoS One*. 2020;15(7):e0236025.

342. Piers LS, Diggavi SN, Rijskamp J, van Raaij JM, Shetty PS, Hautvast JG. Resting metabolic rate and thermic effect of a meal in the follicular and luteal phases of the menstrual cycle in well-nourished Indian women. *Am J Clin Nutr*. 1995;61(2):296–302.

343. Zderic TW, Coggan AR, Ruby BC. Glucose kinetics and substrate oxidation during exercise in the follicular and luteal phases. *J Appl Physiol (1985)*. 2001;90(2):447–53.

344. Horton TJ, Miller EK, Glueck D, Tench K. No effect of menstrual cycle phase on glucose kinetics and fuel oxidation during moderate-intensity exercise. *Am J Physiol Endocrinol Metab*. 2002;282(4):E752–62.

345. Vaiksaar S, Jurimae J, Maestu J, et al. No effect of menstrual cycle phase on fuel oxidation during exercise in rowers. *Eur J Appl Physiol*. 2011;111(6):1027–34.

346. Suh SH, Casazza GA, Horning MA, Miller BF, Brooks GA. Luteal and follicular glucose fluxes during rest and exercise in 3-h postabsorptive women. *J Appl Physiol (1985)*. 2002;93(1):42–50.

347. Fukuba Y, Yano Y, Murakami H, Kan A, Miura A. The effect of dietary restriction and menstrual cycle on excess postexercise oxygen consumption (EPOC) in young women. *Clin Physiol*. 2000;20(2):165–9.

348. Giacomoni M, Bernard T, Gavarry O, Altare S, Falgairette G. Influence of the menstrual cycle phase and menstrual symptoms on maximal anaerobic performance. *Med Sci Sports Exerc*. 2000;32(2):486–92.

349. Burrows M, Bird SR. Velocity at $\dot{V}O_{2\,max}$ and peak treadmill velocity are not influenced within or across the phases of the menstrual cycle. *Eur J Appl Physiol*. 2005;93(5–6):575–80.

350. Vaiksaar S, Jurimae J, Maestu J, et al. No effect of menstrual cycle phase and oral contraceptive use on endurance performance in rowers. *J Strength Cond Res*. 2011;25(6):1571–8.

351. Sakamaki-Sunaga M, Min S, Kamemoto K, Okamoto T. Effects of menstrual phase-dependent resistance training frequency on muscular hypertrophy and strength. *J Strength Cond Res*. 2016;30(6):1727–34.

352. McNulty KL, Elliott-Sale KJ, Dolan E, et al. The effects of menstrual cycle phase on exercise performance in eumenorrheic women: a systematic review and meta-analysis. *Sports Med*. 2020;50(10):1813–27.

353. Chumlea WC, Schubert CM, Roche AF, et al. Age at menarche and racial comparisons in US girls. *Pediatrics*. 2003;111(1):110–3.

354. Marsh CA, Grimstad FW. Primary amenorrhea: diagnosis and management. *Obstet Gynecol Surv*. 2014;69(10):603–12.

355. Castelo-Branco C. Management of Turner syndrome in adult life and beyond. *Maturitas*. 2014;79(4):471–5.

356. Jones MR, Goodarzi MO. Genetic determinants of polycystic ovary syndrome: progress and future directions. *Fertil Steril*. 2016;106(1):25–32.

357. Fourman LT, Fazeli PK. Neuroendocrine causes of amenorrhea—an update. *J Clin Endocrinol Metab*. 2015;100(3):812–24.

358. Abou Sherif S, Newman R, Haboosh S, et al. Investigating the potential of clinical and biochemical markers to differentiate between functional hypothalamic amenorrhoea and polycystic ovarian syndrome: a retrospective observational study. *Clin Endocrinol (Oxf)*. 2021;95(4):618–27.

359. Barbarino A, De Marinis L, Tofani A, et al. Corticotropin-releasing hormone inhibition of gonadotropin release and the effect of opioid blockade. *J Clin Endocrinol Metab.* 1989;68(3):523–8.

360. Rabin DS, Johnson EO, Brandon DD, Liapi C, Chrousos GP. Glucocorticoids inhibit estradiol-mediated uterine growth: possible role of the uterine estradiol receptor. *Biol Reprod.* 1990;42(1):74–80.

361. Nattiv A, Loucks AB, Manore MM, et al. American College of Sports Medicine position stand. The female athlete triad. *Med Sci Sports Exerc.* 2007;39(10):1867–82.

362. De Souza MJ, Nattiv A, Joy E, et al. 2014 Female Athlete Triad coalition consensus statement on treatment and return to play of the Female Athlete Triad: 1st International Conference held in San Francisco, California, May 2012 and 2nd International Conference held in Indianapolis, Indiana, May 2013. *Br J Sports Med.* 2014;48(4):289.

363. Gibbs JC, Williams NI, De Souza MJ. Prevalence of individual and combined components of the female athlete triad. *Med Sci Sports Exerc.* 2013;45(5):985–96.

364. O'Donnell E, Goodman JM, Harvey PJ. Clinical review: cardiovascular consequences of ovarian disruption: a focus on functional hypothalamic amenorrhea in physically active women. *J Clin Endocrinol Metab.* 2011;96(12):3638–48.

365. Roupas ND, Georgopoulos NA. Menstrual function in sports. *Hormones (Athens).* 2011;10(2):104–16.

366. Lieberman EH, Gerhard MD, Uehata A, et al. Estrogen improves endothelium-dependent, flow-mediated vasodilation in post-menopausal women. *Ann Intern Med.* 1994;121(12):936–41.

367. Liu SL, Lebrun CM. Effect of oral contraceptives and hormone replacement therapy on bone mineral density in premenopausal and perimenopausal women: a systematic review. *Br J Sports Med.* 2006;40(1):11–24.

368. Frisch RE, McArthur JW. Menstrual cycles: fatness as a determinant of minimum weight for height necessary for their maintenance or onset. *Science.* 1974;185(4155):949–51.

369. Robinson L, Aldridge V, Clark EM, Misra M, Micali N. A systematic review and meta-analysis of the association between eating disorders and bone density. *Osteoporos Int.* 2016;27(6):1953–66.

370. Keen AD, Drinkwater BL. Irreversible bone loss in former amenorrheic athletes. *Osteoporos Int.* 1997;7(4):311–5.

371. Mountjoy M, Sundgot-Borgen JK, Burke LM, et al. IOC consensus statement on relative energy deficiency in sport (RED-S): 2018 update. *Br J Sports Med.* 2018;52(11):687–97.

372. Mountjoy M, Sundgot-Borgen J, Burke L, et al. The IOC consensus statement: beyond the Female Athlete Triad — Relative Energy Deficiency in Sport (RED-S). *Br J Sports Med.* 2014;48(7):491–7.

373. Elliott-Sale KJ, Tenforde AS, Parziale AL, Holtzman B, Ackerman KE. Endocrine effects of relative energy deficiency in sport. *Int J Sport Nutr Exerc Metab.* 2018;28(4):335–49.

374. Office on Women's Health. Stages of pregnancy. U.S. Department of Health & Human Services. 2019. Available from: https://www.womenshealth.gov/pregnancy/youre-pregnant-now-what/stages-pregnancy.

375. Simpson ER, MacDonald PC. Endocrine physiology of the placenta. *Annu Rev Physiol.* 1981;43:163–88.

376. Tan EK, Tan EL. Alterations in physiology and anatomy during pregnancy. *Best Pract Res Clin Obstet Gynaecol.* 2013;27(6):791–802.

377. Angueira AR, Ludvik AE, Reddy TE, Wicksteed B, Lowe WL Jr, Layden BT. New insights into gestational glucose metabolism: lessons learned from 21st century approaches. *Diabetes.* 2015;64(2):327–34.

378. Kiserud T, Piaggio G, Carroli G, et al. The World Health Organization fetal growth charts: a multinational longitudinal study of ultrasound biometric measurements and estimated fetal weight. *PLoS Med.* 2017;14(1):e1002220.

379. Lee SY, Chien DK, Huang CH, Shih SC, Lee WC, Chang WH. Dyspnea in pregnancy. *Taiwan J Obstet Gynecol.* 2017;56(4):432–6.

380. Torgersen KL, Curran CA. A systematic approach to the physiologic adaptations of pregnancy. *Crit Care Nurs Q.* 2006;29(1):2–19.

381. San-Frutos L, Engels V, Zapardiel I, et al. Hemodynamic changes during pregnancy and postpartum: a prospective study using thoracic electrical bioimpedance. *J Matern Fetal Neonatal Med.* 2011;24(11):1333–40.

382. Thabah M, Ravindran V. Musculoskeletal problems in pregnancy. *Rheumatol Int.* 2015;35(4):581–7.

383. Kovacs FM, Garcia E, Royuela A, Gonzalez L, Abraira V; Spanish Back Pain Research Network. Prevalence and factors associated with low back pain and pelvic girdle pain during pregnancy: a multicenter study conducted in the Spanish National Health Service. *Spine (Phila Pa 1976).* 2012;37(17):1516–33.

384. Wang SM, Dezinno P, Maranets I, Berman MR, Caldwell-Andrews AA, Kain ZN. Low back pain during pregnancy: prevalence, risk factors, and outcomes. *Obstet Gynecol.* 2004;104(1):65–70.

385. Ritchie JR. Orthopedic considerations during pregnancy. *Clin Obstet Gynecol.* 2003;46(2):456–66.

386. Ireland ML, Ott SM. The effects of pregnancy on the musculoskeletal system. *Clin Orthop Relat Res.* 2000;(372):169–79.

387. Kovacs CS. Calcium and bone metabolism during pregnancy and lactation. *J Mammary Gland Biol Neoplasia.* 2005;10(2):105–18.

388. Yamaga A, Taga M, Minaguchi H, Sato K. Changes in bone mass as determined by ultrasound and biochemical markers of bone turnover during pregnancy and puerperium: a longitudinal study. *J Clin Endocrinol Metab.* 1996;81(2):752–6.

389. Hreshchyshyn MM, Hopkins A, Zylstra S, Anbar M. Associations of parity, breast-feeding, and birth control pills with lumbar spine and femoral neck bone densities. *Am J Obstet Gynecol.* 1988;159(2):318–22.

390. Drinkwater BL, Chesnut CH 3rd. Bone density changes during pregnancy and lactation in active women: a longitudinal study. *Bone Miner.* 1991;14(2):153–60.

391. Black AJ, Topping J, Durham B, Farquharson RG, Fraser WD. A detailed assessment of alterations in bone turnover, calcium homeostasis, and bone density in normal pregnancy. *J Bone Miner Res.* 2000;15(3):557–63.

392. Butte NF, King JC. Energy requirements during pregnancy and lactation. *Public Health Nutr.* 2005;8(7A):1010–27.

393. Rasmussen KM, Catalano PM, Yaktine AL. New guidelines for weight gain during pregnancy: what obstetrician/gynecologists should know. *Curr Opin Obstet Gynecol.* 2009;21(6):521–6.

394. Martinez-Hortelano JA, Cavero-Redondo I, Alvarez-Bueno C, Garrido-Miguel M, Soriano-Cano A, Martinez-Vizcaino V. Monitoring gestational weight gain and prepregnancy BMI

using the 2009 IOM guidelines in the global population: a systematic review and meta-analysis. *BMC Pregnancy Childbirth.* 2020;20(1):649.

395. Pinheiro RL, Areia AL, Mota Pinto A, Donato H. Advanced maternal age: adverse outcomes of pregnancy, a meta-analysis. *Acta Med Port.* 2019;32(3):219–26.

396. Elchert J, Beaudrot M, DeFranco E. Gestational weight gain in adolescent compared with adult pregnancies: an age-specific body mass index approach. *J Pediatr.* 2015; 167(3):579–85.e1–2.

397. Kinnunen TI, Waage CW, Sommer C, Sletner L, Raitanen J, Jenum AK. Ethnic differences in gestational weight gain: a population-based cohort study in Norway. *Matern Child Health J.* 2016;20(7):1485–96.

398. Goldstein RF, Abell SK, Ranasinha S, et al. Gestational weight gain across continents and ethnicity: systematic review and meta-analysis of maternal and infant outcomes in more than one million women. *BMC Med.* 2018;16(1):153.

399. Cheikh Ismail L, Bishop DC, Pang R, et al. Gestational weight gain standards based on women enrolled in the Fetal Growth Longitudinal Study of the INTERGROWTH-21st Project: a prospective longitudinal cohort study. *BMJ.* 2016;352:i555.

400. Berggren EK, Groh-Wargo S, Presley L, Hauguel-de Mouzon S, Catalano PM. Maternal fat, but not lean, mass is increased among overweight/obese women with excess gestational weight gain. *Am J Obstet Gynecol.* 2016;214(6):745.e1–5.

401. Ruhstaller KE, Bastek JA, Thomas A, McElrath TF, Parry SI, Durnwald CP. The effect of early excessive weight gain on the development of hypertension in pregnancy. *Am J Perinatol.* 2016;33(12):1205–10.

402. Morisset AS, St-Yves A, Veillette J, Weisnagel SJ, Tchernof A, Robitaille J. Prevention of gestational diabetes mellitus: a review of studies on weight management. *Diabetes Metab Res Rev.* 2010;26(1):17–25.

403. Hedderson MM, Gunderson EP, Ferrara A. Gestational weight gain and risk of gestational diabetes mellitus. *Obstet Gynecol.* 2010;115(3):597–604.

404. Durst JK, Sutton AL, Cliver SP, Tita AT, Biggio JR. Impact of gestational weight gain on perinatal outcomes in obese women. *Am J Perinatol.* 2016;33(9):849–55.

405. Goldstein RF, Abell SK, Ranasinha S, et al. Association of gestational weight gain with maternal and infant outcomes: a systematic review and meta-analysis. *JAMA.* 2017;317(21):2207–25.

406. Godoy AC, Nascimento SL, Surita FG. A systematic review and meta-analysis of gestational weight gain recommendations and related outcomes in Brazil. *Clinics (Sao Paulo).* 2015;70(11):758–64.

407. Hung TH, Chen SF, Hsu JJ, Hsieh TT. Gestational weight gain and risks for adverse perinatal outcomes: a retrospective cohort study based on the 2009 Institute of Medicine guidelines. *Taiwan J Obstet Gynecol.* 2015;54(4):421–5.

408. Moehlecke M, Costenaro F, Reichelt AA, Oppermann ML, Leitao CB. Low gestational weight gain in obese women and pregnancy outcomes. *AJP Rep.* 2016;6(1):e77–82.

409. Elliott-Sale KJ, Barnett CT, Sale C. Exercise interventions for weight management during pregnancy and up to 1 year postpartum among normal weight, overweight and obese women: a systematic review and meta-analysis. *Br J Sports Med.* 2015;49(20):1336–42.

410. Muktabhant B, Lawrie TA, Lumbiganon P, Laopaiboon M. Diet or exercise, or both, for preventing excessive weight gain in pregnancy. *Cochrane Database Syst Rev.* 2015;(6): CD007145.

411. da Silva SG, Ricardo LI, Evenson KR, Hallal PC. Leisure-time physical activity in pregnancy and maternal-child health: a systematic review and meta-analysis of randomized controlled trials and cohort studies. *Sports Med.* 2017;47(2):295–317.

412. Poyatos-Leon R, Garcia-Hermoso A, Sanabria-Martinez G, Alvarez-Bueno C, Sanchez-Lopez M, Martinez-Vizcaino V. Effects of exercise during pregnancy on mode of delivery: a meta-analysis. *Acta Obstet Gynecol Scand.* 2015;94(10): 1039–47.

413. Di Mascio D, Magro-Malosso ER, Saccone G, Marhefka GD, Berghella V. Exercise during pregnancy in normal-weight women and risk of preterm birth: a systematic review and meta-analysis of randomized controlled trials. *Am J Obstet Gynecol.* 2016;215(5):561–71.

414. Sanabria-Martinez G, Garcia-Hermoso A, Poyatos-Leon R, Gonzalez-Garcia A, Sanchez-Lopez M, Martinez-Vizcaino V. Effects of exercise-based interventions on neonatal outcomes: a meta-analysis of randomized controlled trials. *Am J Health Promot.* 2016;30(4):214–23.

415. McDonald SM, May LE, Hinkle SN, Grantz KL, Zhang C. Maternal moderate-to-vigorous physical activity before and during pregnancy and maternal glucose tolerance: does timing matter? *Med Sci Sports Exerc.* 2021;53(12):2520–7.

416. Sundgot-Borgen J, Sundgot-Borgen C, Myklebust G, Solvberg N, Torstveit MK. Elite athletes get pregnant, have healthy babies and return to sport early postpartum. *BMJ Open Sport Exerc Med.* 2019;5(1):e000652.

417. Tenforde AS, Toth KE, Langen E, Fredericson M, Sainani KL. Running habits of competitive runners during pregnancy and breastfeeding. *Sports Health.* 2015;7(2):172–6.

418. Wowdzia JB, McHugh TL, Thornton J, Sivak A, Mottola MF, Davenport MH. Elite athletes and pregnancy outcomes: a systematic review and meta-analysis. *Med Sci Sports Exerc.* 2021;53(3):534–42.

419. Borodulin KM, Evenson KR, Wen F, Herring AH, Benson AM. Physical activity patterns during pregnancy. *Med Sci Sports Exerc.* 2008;40(11):1901–8.

420. Mottola MF, Campbell MK. Activity patterns during pregnancy. *Can J Appl Physiol.* 2003;28(4):642–53.

421. American College of Obstetricians and Gynecologists. Physical activity and exercise during pregnancy and the postpartum period: ACOG Committee Opinion, Number 804. *Obstet Gynecol.* 2020;135(4):e178–88.

422. Persinger R, Foster C, Gibson M, Fater DC, Porcari JP. Consistency of the talk test for exercise prescription. *Med Sci Sports Exerc.* 2004;36(9):1632–6.

423. U.S. Department of Health and Human Services. *Physical Activity Guidelines for Americans.* 2nd ed. Washington (DC): U.S. Department of Health and Human Services; 2018.

424. Coll CV, Domingues MR, Goncalves H, Bertoldi AD. Perceived barriers to leisure-time physical activity during pregnancy: a literature review of quantitative and qualitative evidence. *J Sci Med Sport.* 2017;20(1):17–25.

425. Bisson M, Marc I, Brassard P. Cerebral blood flow regulation, exercise and pregnancy: why should we care? *Clin Sci (Lond).* 2016;130(9):651–65.

426. Szymanski LM, Satin AJ. Strenuous exercise during pregnancy: is there a limit? *Am J Obstet Gynecol.* 2012;207(3):179.e1–6.

427. InterLACE Study Team. Variations in reproductive events across life: a pooled analysis of data from 505 147 women across 10 countries. *Hum Reprod.* 2019;34(5):881–93.

428. Velez MP, Alvarado BE, Rosendaal N, et al. Age at natural menopause and physical functioning in postmenopausal

women: the Canadian Longitudinal Study on Aging. *Menopause*. 2019;26(9):958–65.

429. Muka T, Oliver-Williams C, Kunutsor S, et al. Association of Age at onset of menopause and time since onset of menopause with cardiovascular outcomes, intermediate vascular traits, and all-cause mortality: a systematic review and meta-analysis. *JAMA Cardiol*. 2016;1(7):767–76.

430. Mondul AM, Rodriguez C, Jacobs EJ, Calle EE. Age at natural menopause and cause-specific mortality. *Am J Epidemiol*. 2005;162(11):1089–97.

431. Morris DH, Jones ME, Schoemaker MJ, Ashworth A, Swerdlow AJ. Familial concordance for age at natural menopause: results from the Breakthrough Generations Study. *Menopause*. 2011;18(9):956–61.

432. Murabito JM, Yang Q, Fox C, Wilson PW, Cupples LA. Heritability of age at natural menopause in the Framingham Heart Study. *J Clin Endocrinol Metab*. 2005;90(6):3427–30.

433. Morris DH, Jones ME, Schoemaker MJ, McFadden E, Ashworth A, Swerdlow AJ. Body mass index, exercise, and other lifestyle factors in relation to age at natural menopause: analyses from the breakthrough generations study. *Am J Epidemiol*. 2012;175(10):998–1005.

434. Dorjgochoo T, Kallianpur A, Gao YT, et al. Dietary and lifestyle predictors of age at natural menopause and reproductive span in the Shanghai Women's Health Study. *Menopause*. 2008;15(5):924–33.

435. Sun L, Tan L, Yang F, et al. Meta-analysis suggests that smoking is associated with an increased risk of early natural menopause. *Menopause*. 2012;19(2):126–32.

436. Eum KD, Weisskopf MG, Nie LH, Hu H, Korrick SA. Cumulative lead exposure and age at menopause in the Nurses' Health Study cohort. *Environ Health Perspect*. 2014;122(3):229–34.

437. Rothman MS, Carlson NE, Xu M, et al. Reexamination of testosterone, dihydrotestosterone, estradiol and estrone levels across the menstrual cycle and in postmenopausal women measured by liquid chromatography-tandem mass spectrometry. *Steroids*. 2011;76(1–2):177–82.

438. Shea KL, Gavin KM, Melanson EL, et al. Body composition and bone mineral density after ovarian hormone suppression with or without estradiol treatment. *Menopause*. 2015;22(10):1045–52.

439. Ley CJ, Lees B, Stevenson JC. Sex- and menopause-associated changes in body-fat distribution. *Am J Clin Nutr*. 1992;55(5):950–4.

440. Rosenfalck AM, Almdal T, Gotfredsen A, Hilsted J. Body composition in normal subjects: relation to lipid and glucose variables. *Int J Obes Relat Metab Disord*. 1996;20(11):1006–13.

441. Greendale GA, Han W, Finkelstein JS, et al. Changes in regional fat distribution and anthropometric measures across the menopause transition. *J Clin Endocrinol Metab*. 2021;106(9):2520–34.

442. Casey BA, Kohrt WM, Schwartz RS, Van Pelt RE. Subcutaneous adipose tissue insulin resistance is associated with visceral adiposity in postmenopausal women. *Obesity (Silver Spring)*. 2014;22(6):1458–63.

443. Peppa M, Koliaki C, Hadjidakis DI, et al. Regional fat distribution and cardiometabolic risk in healthy postmenopausal women. *Eur J Intern Med*. 2013;24(8):824–31.

444. Myint PK, Kwok CS, Luben RN, Wareham NJ, Khaw KT. Body fat percentage, body mass index and waist-to-hip ratio as predictors of mortality and cardiovascular disease. *Heart*. 2014;100(20):1613–9.

445. Cerhan JR, Moore SC, Jacobs EJ, et al. A pooled analysis of waist circumference and mortality in 650,000 adults. *Mayo Clin Proc*. 2014;89(3):335–45.

446. Douchi T, Yamamoto S, Yoshimitsu N, Andoh T, Matsuo T, Nagata Y. Relative contribution of aging and menopause to changes in lean and fat mass in segmental regions. *Maturitas*. 2002;42(4):301–6.

447. van Geel TA, Geusens PP, Winkens B, Sels JP, Dinant GJ. Measures of bioavailable serum testosterone and estradiol and their relationships with muscle mass, muscle strength and bone mineral density in postmenopausal women: a cross-sectional study. *Eur J Endocrinol*. 2009;160(4):681–7.

448. Brown M. Skeletal muscle and bone: effect of sex steroids and aging. *Adv Physiol Educ*. 2008;32(2):120–6.

449. Widrick JJ, Maddalozzo GF, Lewis D, et al. Morphological and functional characteristics of skeletal muscle fibers from hormone-replaced and nonreplaced postmenopausal women. *J Gerontol A Biol Sci Med Sci*. 2003;58(1):3–10.

450. Greising SM, Baltgalvis KA, Lowe DA, Warren GL. Hormone therapy and skeletal muscle strength: a meta-analysis. *J Gerontol A Biol Sci Med Sci*. 2009;64(10):1071–81.

451. Lowe DA, Baltgalvis KA, Greising SM. Mechanisms behind estrogen's beneficial effect on muscle strength in females. *Exerc Sport Sci Rev*. 2010;38(2):61–7.

452. Hodson L, Harnden K, Banerjee R, et al. Lower resting and total energy expenditure in postmenopausal compared with premenopausal women matched for abdominal obesity. *J Nutr Sci*. 2014;3:e3.

453. Chevalier S, Marliss EB, Morais JA, Lamarche M, Gougeon R. Whole-body protein anabolic response is resistant to the action of insulin in obese women. *Am J Clin Nutr*. 2005;82(2):355–65.

454. Chevalier S, Gougeon R, Choong N, Lamarche M, Morais JA. Influence of adiposity in the blunted whole-body protein anabolic response to insulin with aging. *J Gerontol A Biol Sci Med Sci*. 2006;61(2):156–64.

455. Finkelstein JS, Brockwell SE, Mehta V, et al. Bone mineral density changes during the menopause transition in a multiethnic cohort of women. *J Clin Endocrinol Metab*. 2008;93(3):861–8.

456. Svejme O, Ahlborg HG, Karlsson MK. Changes in forearm bone mass and bone size after menopause—a mean 24-year prospective study. *J Musculoskelet Neuronal Interact*. 2012;12(4):192–8.

457. Nguyen TV, Jones G, Sambrook PN, White CP, Kelly PJ, Eisman JA. Effects of estrogen exposure and reproductive factors on bone mineral density and osteoporotic fractures. *J Clin Endocrinol Metab*. 1995;80(9):2709–14.

458. Khosla S, Melton LJ 3rd, Riggs BL. The unitary model for estrogen deficiency and the pathogenesis of osteoporosis: is a revision needed? *J Bone Miner Res*. 2011;26(3):441–51.

459. Sowers MR, Zheng H, Greendale GA, et al. Changes in bone resorption across the menopause transition: effects of reproductive hormones, body size, and ethnicity. *J Clin Endocrinol Metab*. 2013;98(7):2854–63.

460. Lee SW, Jo HH, Kim MR, You YO, Kim JH. Association between obesity, metabolic risks and serum osteocalcin level in postmenopausal women. *Gynecol Endocrinol*. 2012;28(6):472–7.

461. Crandall CJ, Hovey KM, Andrews CA, et al. Bone mineral density as a predictor of subsequent wrist fractures: findings from the Women's Health Initiative Study. *J Clin Endocrinol Metab*. 2015;100(11):4315–24.

462. Sullivan SD, Lehman A, Thomas F, et al. Effects of self-reported age at nonsurgical menopause on time to first fracture and bone mineral density in the Women's Health Initiative Observational Study. *Menopause*. 2015;22(10):1035–44.

463. Ryan AS, Nicklas BJ, Berman DM. Hormone replacement therapy, insulin sensitivity, and abdominal obesity in postmenopausal women. *Diabetes Care.* 2002;25(1):127–33.

464. Marjoribanks J, Farquhar C, Roberts H, Lethaby A, Lee J. Long-term hormone therapy for perimenopausal and postmenopausal women. *Cochrane Database Syst Rev.* 2017;1: CD004143.

465. Sims ST, Larson JC, Lamonte MJ, et al. Physical activity and body mass: changes in younger versus older postmenopausal women. *Med Sci Sports Exerc.* 2012;44(1):89–97.

466. Straight CR, Ward-Ritacco CL, Evans EM. Association between accelerometer-measured physical activity and muscle capacity in middle-aged postmenopausal women. *Menopause.* 2015;22(11):1204–11.

467. Gao HL, Gao HX, Sun FM, Zhang L. Effects of walking on body composition in perimenopausal and postmenopausal women: a systematic review and meta-analysis. *Menopause.* 2016;23(8):928–34.

468. Green JS, Stanforth PR, Rankinen T, et al. The effects of exercise training on abdominal visceral fat, body composition, and indicators of the metabolic syndrome in postmenopausal women with and without estrogen replacement therapy: the HERITAGE family study. *Metabolism.* 2004;53(9):1192–6.

469. Zarins ZA, Johnson ML, Faghihnia N, et al. Training improves the response in glucose flux to exercise in postmenopausal women. *J Appl Physiol (1985).* 2009;107(1):90–7.

470. Santa-Clara H, Szymanski L, Ordille T, Fernhall B. Effects of exercise training on resting metabolic rate in postmenopausal African American and Caucasian women. *Metabolism.* 2006;55(10):1358–64.

471. Zarins ZA, Wallis GA, Faghihnia N, et al. Effects of endurance training on cardiorespiratory fitness and substrate partitioning in postmenopausal women. *Metabolism.* 2009;58(9):1338–46.

472. Taaffe DR, Sipila S, Cheng S, Puolakka J, Toivanen J, Suominen H. The effect of hormone replacement therapy and/or exercise on skeletal muscle attenuation in postmenopausal women: a yearlong intervention. *Clin Physiol Funct Imaging.* 2005;25(5):297–304.

473. Bea JW, Cussler EC, Going SB, Blew RM, Metcalfe LL, Lohman TG. Resistance training predicts 6-yr body composition change in postmenopausal women. *Med Sci Sports Exerc.* 2010;42(7):1286–95.

474. Nichols JF, Omizo DK, Peterson KK, Nelson KP. Efficacy of heavy-resistance training for active women over sixty: muscular strength, body composition, and program adherence. *J Am Geriatr Soc.* 1993;41(3):205–10.

475. Hakkinen K, Kraemer WJ, Pakarinen A, et al. Effects of heavy resistance/power training on maximal strength, muscle morphology, and hormonal response patterns in 60–75-year-old men and women. *Can J Appl Physiol.* 2002;27(3):213–31.

476. Thomas E, Gentile A, Lakicevic N, et al. The effect of resistance training programs on lean body mass in postmenopausal and elderly women: a meta-analysis of observational studies. *Aging Clin Exp Res.* 2021;33(11):2941–52.

477. van Gemert WA, Schuit AJ, van der Palen J, et al. Effect of weight loss, with or without exercise, on body composition and sex hormones in postmenopausal women: the SHAPE-2 trial. *Breast Cancer Res.* 2015;17:120.

478. van Gemert WA, Monninkhof EM, May AM, Peeters PH, Schuit AJ. Effect of exercise on insulin sensitivity in healthy postmenopausal women: the SHAPE study. *Cancer Epidemiol Biomarkers Prev.* 2015;24(1):81–7.

479. Martyn-StJames M, Carroll S. A meta-analysis of impact exercise on postmenopausal bone loss: the case for mixed loading exercise programmes. *Br J Sports Med.* 2009;43(12):898–908.

480. Kelley GA, Kelley KS, Kohrt WM. Effects of ground and joint reaction force exercise on lumbar spine and femoral neck bone mineral density in postmenopausal women: a meta-analysis of randomized controlled trials. *BMC Musculoskelet Disord.* 2012;13:177.

481. Kistler-Fischbacher M, Weeks BK, Beck BR. The effect of exercise intensity on bone in postmenopausal women (part 2): a meta-analysis. *Bone.* 2021;143:115697.

482. Ma D, Wu L, He Z. Effects of walking on the preservation of bone mineral density in perimenopausal and postmenopausal women: a systematic review and meta-analysis. *Menopause.* 2013;20(11):1216–26.

483. Baber RJ, Panay N, Fenton A; IMS Writing Group. 2016 IMS recommendations on women's midlife health and menopause hormone therapy. *Climacteric.* 2016;19(2):109–50.

484. Troiano RP, Berrigan D, Dodd KW, Masse LC, Tilert T, McDowell M. Physical activity in the United States measured by accelerometer. *Med Sci Sports Exerc.* 2008;40(1):181–8.

485. Dunniway DL, Camune B, Baldwin K, Crane JK. FRAX(R) counseling for bone health behavior change in women 50 years of age and older. *J Am Acad Nurse Pract.* 2012;24(6):382–9.

486. Cadmus-Bertram LA, Marcus BH, Patterson RE, Parker BA, Morey BL. Randomized trial of a fitbit-based physical activity intervention for women. *Am J Prev Med.* 2015;49(3):414–8.

487. Aparicio-Ting FE, Farris M, Courneya KS, Schiller A, Friedenreich CM. Predictors of physical activity at 12 month follow-up after a supervised exercise intervention in postmenopausal women. *Int J Behav Nutr Phys Act.* 2015;12:55.

488. Trappe S, Hayes E, Galpin A, et al. New records in aerobic power among octogenarian lifelong endurance athletes. *J Appl Physiol (1985).* 2013;114(1):3–10.

489. Burtscher M, Nachbauer W, Wilber R. The upper limit of aerobic power in humans. *Eur J Appl Physiol.* 2011;111(10):2625–8.

490. Ronnestad BR, Hansen J, Stenslokken L, Joyner MJ, Lundby C. Case Studies in Physiology: temporal changes in determinants of aerobic performance in individual going from alpine skier to world junior champion time trial cyclist. *J Appl Physiol (1985).* 2019;127(2):306–11.

491. Everman S, Farris JW, Bay RC, Daniels JT. Elite distance runners: a 45-year follow-up. *Med Sci Sports Exerc.* 2018;50(1):73–8.

492. Lepers R, Bontemps B, Louis J. Physiological profile of a 59-year-old male world record holder marathoner. *Med Sci Sports Exerc.* 2020;52(3):623–6.

493. Maud PJ, Pollock ML, Foster C, et al. Fifty years of training and competition in the marathon: Wally Hayward, age 70 — a physiological profile. *S Afr Med J.* 1981;59(5):153–7.

494. Karlsen T, Leinan IM, Baekkerud FH, et al. How to be 80 year old and have a $\dot{V}O_{2max}$ of a 35 year old. *Case Rep Med.* 2015;2015:909561.

495. Billat V, Dhonneur G, Mille-Hamard L, et al. Case Studies in Physiology: maximal oxygen consumption and performance in a centenarian cyclist. *J Appl Physiol (1985).* 2017;122(3):430–4.

496. Ingjer F. Maximal oxygen uptake as a predictor of performance ability in women and men elite cross-country skiers. *Scand J Med Sci Sports.* 1991;1(1):25–30.

497. Constantini N. Medical concerns of the dancer. In: *IMS World Congress of Sports Medicine.* Budapest, Hungary; 2011.

498. American College of Sports Medicine. *Guidelines for Exercise Testing and Prescription.* 10th ed. Philadelphia (PA): Wolters Kluwer; 2018.

Benefits and Risks Associated With Exercise and Physical Activity and Preexercise Evaluation

INTRODUCTION

This chapter reviews the benefits and risks of exercise and presents recommendations for preexercise health screening and evaluation. Several terms are used throughout, including physical activity, exercise, and physical fitness. Physical activity is defined as any bodily movement produced by the contraction of skeletal muscles that results in a substantial increase in caloric requirements over resting energy expenditure (1). Exercise is a type of physical activity consisting of planned, structured, and repetitive bodily movement done to improve and/or maintain one or more components of physical fitness (1). Physical fitness is a set of attributes or characteristics individuals have or achieve that relate to their ability to perform physical activity and activities of daily living (2). These attributes are commonly separated into health-related components (cardiorespiratory endurance, body composition, muscular strength, muscular endurance, flexibility) and skill-related components (agility, coordination, balance, power, reaction time, speed); however, these components of physical fitness may not be mutually exclusive as several skill-related components may contribute to health goals (2).

Participation in a program of regular physical activity and reducing sedentary time are recommended for nearly all adults, including those with chronic diseases and conditions (2–7). A physically active lifestyle can enhance physical fitness, positively effect physiological adaptations, and elicit many health benefits, including reducing chronic disease morbidity and delaying all-cause and disease-specific mortality (1, 2, 8). Reducing time spent in sedentary activities *in addition to* participating in exercise confers additional health benefits (6, 9–11).

Conversely, there are some associated risks of physical activity notwithstanding the considerable benefits (12). The most common risks of exercise are musculoskeletal injuries and untoward cardiovascular events (10, 13–16). These adverse consequences of exercise tend to be elevated in individuals who are insufficiently active, particularly when engaging in unaccustomed physical activities, and in individuals who engage in high-volume/high-intensity exercise routines (13, 17–19). Given that about three-fourths of the U.S. population and a substantial proportion of the global population fails to achieve recommended targets for physical activity (6, 20), improving physical activity in insufficiently active people can increase overall health, while at the same time reducing the acute risks of exercise (1, 6, 11, 21).

Evaluation of an individual's physical activity, fitness, health status, and risk factors prior to embarking on a new program of exercise, in addition to careful attention to elements of the exercise prescription, can reduce the risks of exercise (2, 16). This chapter reviews the benefits and risks of physical activity and then presents recommendations for preexercise evaluation with an eye to attenuate the inherent risks of exercise.

BENEFITS OF REGULAR PHYSICAL ACTIVITY AND EXERCISE

The health benefits of regular physical activity and exercise are substantial and irrefutable (1, 6). Increased levels of cardiorespiratory and muscular fitness, more healthful body composition, enhanced bone health, improved cognitive function, reduction of falls, and other health-related improvements result from regular physical activity and exercise (1, 2, 22). Regular exercise is a fundamental element of primordial, primary, and secondary disease prevention strategies and is recommended as a part of care by a number of respected health organizations including the

American Heart Association (AHA), the World Health Organization, the American Diabetes Association, and the American Cancer Society (3, 23–25). There is a dose-response relationship between physical activity and health benefits. Even small amounts of physical activity provide some benefits, whereas greater amounts of physical activity result in more substantial health benefits (1).

Regular physical activity and exercise reduce the risks of developing cardiometabolic diseases, such as coronary heart disease (CHD), Type 2 diabetes mellitus, obesity, some cancers, and their associated risk factors. Furthermore, physical activity is an important part of the management of cardiometabolic, musculoskeletal, and neuromuscular diseases; mental health disorders; and other diseases when they are present (23, 24, 26–34). Engaging in regular exercise and physical activity and having higher cardiorespiratory fitness (CRF) and muscular strength also confer a survival advantage; delay the onset of cardiovascular disease (CVD), diabetes, some cancers, and other diseases; and reduce the risks of some of the adverse sequelae of several diseases when present (10, 23, 35–41). A systematic review and meta-analyses by Nocon and colleagues (42) examining studies of physical activity reported reductions in all-cause mortality of 33% (95% confidence interval [CI]: 28%–37%) and 30% (95% CI 30%–40%) in CVD mortality. The benefits of a physically activity lifestyle extend to older adults as well. One systematic review of older adults found that all-cause mortality is reduced by 22% with regular moderate-to-vigorous physical activity, even if the recommended volumes of physical activity were not achieved (43).

The benefits of physical activity on all-cause mortality occur in a dose-response manner, as illustrated by one study that showed a 4% reduction in mortality occurring with every additional 15 minutes per day of moderate-to-vigorous physical activity, over the range of 15–100 minutes of exercise per day (44). When combined with other healthy lifestyle behaviors, a physically active lifestyle is estimated to confer an increased life expectancy of 7–8 years (13). Moreover, a meta-analysis of studies reporting instrument-measured physical activity by Ekelund et al. (45) showed that both exercise volume and intensity are associated with the risks of mortality. A nonlinear dose-response association with physical activity across all intensities has been demonstrated, with mortality risks lowered by 52%–73% when spanning the least active to the most active, respectively (45). In the same study, when looking at different intensities of physical activity (i.e., light, moderate, vigorous intensities), there was a reduced risk of mortality such that there was a dose-response

relationship; the risks of mortality decreased substantially with increasing volumes of physical activity within each of the three intensities (45).

The benefits of exercise extend to individuals with disease and may affect the trajectory of the disease. For example, a systematic review and meta-analysis by Morishita et al. (46) reported a 24% reduction in mortality in people with cancer and nearly 50% lower risk of cancer recurrence. A longitudinal study of people treated with kidney transplant showed that the most active individuals had a 24% lower risk of experiencing a cardiovascular event (e.g., myocardial infarction, stroke, coronary or lower extremity artery revascularization) adjusted for CVD and risk factors, and other health-related characteristics (37). Compared to the lowest tertile of physical activity, kidney transplant recipients in the highest tertile experienced a significantly lower risk of CVD events (hazard ratio 0.76; 95% CI 0.59–0.98), CVD mortality (hazard ratio 0.58; 95% CI 0.35–0.96), and all-cause mortality (hazard ratio 0.76; 95% CI 0.59–0.98) (37).

CRF and Mortality and Morbidity

CRF is a strong predictor of all-cause and disease-specific mortality and morbidity (13, 47–49). It is an equivalent or stronger predictor of the risk of CVD mortality and morbidity than are other traditional CVD risk factors such as smoking, dyslipidemia, hypertension, and diabetes, and this association is independent of physical activity (48–51).

Research supporting the association between CRF and all-cause mortality has produced a number of studies which show that individuals who have higher levels of CRF experience lower rates of all-cause mortality (51–53). For example, one study found that with every 1 metabolic equivalent (MET) increase in CRF there was a decrease in all-cause mortality of 16% in men and 17% in women (54).

Specifically, highly fit people have been shown to have a 50% decrease in 30-year risk of CVD mortality in comparison to low-fit people, irrespective of the presence of CVD risk factors (55). The benefits of higher CRF are not only limited to CVD mortality, as a study with 12,728 men who had a history of musculoskeletal conditions, such as arthritis, back pain, etc., found that those with higher CRF had lower all-cause (hazard ratio 0.50; 95% CI 0.23–1.10), CVD (hazard ratio 0.38; 95% CI 0.20–0.74), and cancer mortality (hazard ratio 0.40; 95% CI 0.20–0.80) (52). In a study with 120,705 patients who underwent exercise tests, individuals with higher CRF had lower all-cause mortality (hazard ratio 0.41; 95%

CI 0.39–0.42), with women having lower all-cause mortality compared with men, even though they had lower overall CRF levels than men (53). Additionally, when comparing participants across age- and sex-adjusted fitness groups (*i.e.*, low [<25th percentile], below average [25th–49th percentile], above average [50th–74th percentile], high [75th–97.6th percentile], and elite [≥97.7th percentile]), those with elite-level fitness had an 80% lower risk of mortality compared with individuals with low fitness (hazard ratio 0.20; 95% CI 0.16–0.24). Importantly, the risks decreased moving across low to high fitness categories, with no apparent upper limit of benefit, demonstrating that there are benefits across a range of fitness levels and moving from the lowest level of CRF can be beneficial to risk reduction (51).

Several studies have attempted to quantify if changes in CRF level can reduce one's risk for all-cause and disease-specific mortality (56). Studying 9,777 individuals who underwent CRF testing on multiple occasions, Blair et al. (56) reported that compared with participants who remained low fit, those who became more fit had a 44% reduction in age-adjusted all-cause mortality (relative risk [RR] 0.56; 95% CI 0.41–0.75) and a 52% lower age-adjusted CVD mortality (RR 0.48; 95% CI 0.31–0.74). These data translate into a 7.9% reduction in all-cause mortality with each 1-minute increase in fitness treadmill test duration over time. Imboden et al. (57) studied 833 men and women who underwent peak cardiopulmonary exercise tests on two occasions and found that with each 1 mL·kg^{-1}·min^{-1} improvement in CRF, there was an associated 11% reduction in all-cause mortality, a 15% reduction in CVD mortality, and a 16% reduction in cancer mortality.

In those who have known cardiovascular conditions, having low CRF levels increases risk for all-cause mortality in comparison to having a moderate or high fitness level (moderate fit: hazard ratio 0.54, 95% CI 0.42–0.69; high fit: hazard ratio 0.32, 95% CI 0.24–0.44) (58). But with improvement in CRF, as a result of attending a 12-week cardiac rehabilitation program, there was an associated reduction in all-cause mortality such that there was a 13 percentage point reduction with each MET increase in CRF, and the low fit at baseline realized a 30 percentage point reduction in mortality risk with improvement of CRF. By 1 year after program entry, for each MET increase in CRF, there was a 25 percentage point reduction in overall mortality (58).

Studies have shown that having a higher CRF reduces the risks of atrial fibrillation (59, 60), Type 2 diabetes mellitus (36, 61–63), and some cancers (52, 64–67).

Adding biological plausibility to these findings, a dose-response relationship exists between CRF and changes in disease-mediating biomarkers, such as adiposity, blood lipids, glucose and inflammatory markers, autonomic function, vascular and mitochondrial function, and many more alterations in the structure and function of multiple physiological systems occur (68–75).

HARMS OF SEDENTARY TIME

There is a growing concern with the effects of sedentary time on health-related outcomes. Sedentary behavior refers to any waking activity characterized by an energy expenditure 1.5 METs or less and a sitting or reclining posture, such as during television watching, electronic device use, driving, and reading (76). Insufficient physical activity encompasses two types of behaviors: (a) physical inactivity in which an individual does not do any walking, or moderate- to vigorous-intensity physical activity; and (b) physical activity that does not reach the levels required for health benefits (76). Insufficient physical activity, especially when combined with excessive sedentary time, is associated with higher risks of morbidity and mortality (77). The scientific literature suggests that sedentary behavior may be a risk factor *independent* of physical activity, although the evidence is not definitive because of conflicting results across different age groups and populations (78).

As a result of the growing interest in the effects of sedentary time, the 2018 U.S. Physical Activity Guidelines Advisory Committee examined the available studies in this area and rated the evidence as strong for the associations between high volumes of sitting time and the risk for all-cause and cardiovascular mortality, as well as CVD and Type 2 diabetes morbidity (1). They also reported strong evidence for a dose-response relationship between sedentary behavior and all-cause mortality, CVD mortality, and the incidence of CVD (1). Other studies have found significant associations between sedentary behavior and all-cause mortality, CVD, hypertension, obesity, Type 2 diabetes mellitus, metabolic syndrome, and increased waist circumference (9, 11, 50, 79).

Sedentary time can be difficult to measure via self-report, so more recent studies have focused on using instrumented measures of sedentary time to add to the understanding of the role of sedentary time in health. A study by Diaz et al. (80) showed that total sedentary time and prolonged uninterrupted bouts of sedentary behaviors were associated with elevated risks of all-cause mortality. A subsequent study reported that when sedentary time and prolonged sedentary time were replaced by light or moderate-to-vigorous physical activity, the risks of all-cause mortality were attenuated in the less active people, but not in those who were very active (~3.5 h per d of physical activity) (81). A harmonized meta-analysis of over 44,000 people who were followed for 4–14.5 years showed that mortality risks were augmented in individuals with greater time in sedentary behavior when accompanied by less moderate-to-vigorous physical activity compared to those with high physical activity and low sedentary time (79). However, for those who were in the highest tertile of moderate-to-vigorous physical activity (about 30–40 min per d), the mortality risks were similar across all tertiles of sedentary time, whereas the risks of death for the least active increased with increasing amounts sedentary time (lowest [hazard ratio 65%; 95% CI 1.25%–2.19%]; middle [hazard ratio 65%; 95% CI 1.24%–2.21%]; and highest [hazard ratio 263%; 95% CI 1.93%–3.57%]) (79). These findings are in contrast to the findings of studies using self-reported physical activity that have reported that, even in people who are regularly active, the risk of CVD can worsen with increasing durations of sedentary time, especially when periods of sedentary time are not broken up with short interludes of standing or light-intensity physical activity (6, 11). The linear associations between sedentary time and all-cause mortality appear to be mediated by CRF, although spending more than 10 hours per week in a car was associated with a 27% increase in mortality, even when controlling for CRF (82).

Intervention studies where sedentary time was broken up by physical activity have focused primarily on cardiometabolic biomarkers (77). A systematic review reported substantive evidence that breaking up sedentary time with physical activity has a positive impact on postprandial glucose, blood lipids, and other cardiometabolic biomarkers in people with Type 2 diabetes mellitus and those who were insufficiently active (83). Furthermore, these studies indicate that replacing sedentary time with light-intensity physical activity, and even standing, may be sufficient to engender these positive adaptations (83). A meta-analysis of the effects of protracted sitting time on cardiometabolic biomarkers found that uninterrupted sitting results in moderate elevations in postprandial glucose and insulin, but breaking up sedentary time results in decreases in postprandial glucose and delayed (~12–16 h later) decreases in plasma triglycerides (84). Moreover, the intensity of the physical activity during breaks in sitting did not alter the positive effects on these biomarkers.

Therefore, encouraging patients, especially those who are resistant to adopting a formal exercise program, to stand and move about regularly can confer some health benefits.

RISKS OF UNTOWARD CARDIOVASCULAR EVENTS DURING PHYSICAL ACTIVITY

Among the most serious complications associated with physical activity are acute myocardial infarction (AMI) and sudden cardiac death (SCD). Acutely, the risks of both AMI and SCD increase transiently during physical activity especially in sedentary individuals with diagnosed or occult CVD performing vigorous-intensity exercise (13). However, this risk is attenuated with higher levels of CRF and habitual participation in exercise (13, 85, 86). Even "weekend warriors" and those exercising less than 2 days per week realize risk reductions and benefits with exercise (13, 87).

Across several studies, the estimated elevated risks of SCD with vigorous exercise range from 6 to 17 times higher compared to time spent being sedentary (2, 13), whereas the likelihood of an AMI associated with vigorous exercise is estimated to increase by 2–10 times (13). However, although the RRs are higher during vigorous exertion, the absolute risks of these events are very low (88, 89).

There is a higher incidence of SCD and AMI with exertion in men compared with women, competitive versus recreational athletes, and in older (≥35 years) compared with younger (<35 years) people, and these risks may be affected by health status, personal characteristics, and the nature of the exercise (13). The risks of SCD and MI increase with age, although some studies report the highest number of exertion-related SCD in people ages 40–64 years (13, 90). The risks of SCD and AMI are disproportionally higher in inactive individuals who perform unaccustomed high-intensity exercise (13). For example, Mittleman et al. (44) found that the risk of AMI during or immediately following vigorous exercise was 50 times higher for habitually inactive people compared to those who regularly exercised for 1 hour for 5 or more days·per week.

Warning signs or symptoms may precede exercise-related cardiovascular events in some, but not all, individuals over the hours or even days and weeks before the acute cardiac event, as shown in Table 3.1 (13, 91). A sign is observable evidence of disease such as skin pallor

Table 3.1	Major Signs or Symptoms Suggestive of Cardiovascular Disease, Metabolic and Renal Disease[a]
Signs or Symptoms	**Clarification/Significance**
Pain; discomfort (or other anginal equivalent) in the chest, neck, jaw, arms, or other areas that may result from myocardial ischemia; or other recent-onset pain of unknown origin	One of the cardinal manifestations of cardiac disease; in particular, coronary artery disease
	Key features favoring an ischemic origin include the following: Character: constricting, squeezing, burning, "heaviness," or "heavy feeling"
	Location: substernal, across midthorax, anteriorly; in one or both arms, shoulders; in neck, cheeks, teeth; in forearms, fingers in interscapular region
	Provoking factors: exercise or exertion, excitement, other forms of stress, cold weather, occurrence after meals
	Key features against an ischemic origin include the following: character: dull ache; "knifelike," sharp, stabbing; "jabs" aggravated by respiration
	Location: in left submammary area; in left hemithorax
	Provoking factors: after completion of exercise, provoked by a specific body motion
Shortness of breath at rest or with mild exertion	Dyspnea (defined as an abnormally uncomfortable awareness of breathing) is one of the principal symptoms of cardiac and pulmonary disease. It commonly occurs during strenuous exertion in healthy, well-trained individuals and during moderate exertion in healthy, untrained individuals. However, it should be regarded as abnormal when it occurs at a level of exertion that is not expected to evoke this symptom in a given individual. Abnormal exertional dyspnea suggests the presence of cardiopulmonary disorders, in particular, left ventricular dysfunction or chronic obstructive pulmonary disease.
Dizziness or syncope	Syncope (defined as a loss of consciousness) is most commonly caused by a reduced perfusion of the brain. Dizziness and, in particular, syncope during exercise may result from cardiac disorders that prevent the normal rise (or an actual fall) in cardiac output. Such cardiac disorders are potentially life-threatening and include severe coronary artery disease, hypertrophic cardiomyopathy, aortic stenosis, and malignant ventricular dysrhythmias. Although dizziness or syncope shortly after cessation of exercise should not be ignored, these symptoms may occur even in healthy individuals as a result of a reduction in venous return to the heart.
Orthopnea or paroxysmal nocturnal dyspnea	Orthopnea refers to dyspnea occurring at rest in the recumbent position that is relieved promptly by sitting upright or standing. Paroxysmal nocturnal dyspnea refers to dyspnea, beginning usually 2–5 h after the onset of sleep, which may be relieved by sitting on the side of the bed or getting out of bed. Both are symptoms of left ventricular dysfunction. Although nocturnal dyspnea may occur in individuals with chronic obstructive pulmonary disease, it differs in that it is usually relieved following a bowel movement rather than specifically by sitting up.

(continued)

Table 3.1	Major Signs or Symptoms Suggestive of Cardiovascular Disease, Metabolic and Renal Disease[a] (*continued*)
Signs or Symptoms	**Clarification/Significance**
Ankle edema	Bilateral ankle edema that is most evident at night is a characteristic sign of heart failure or bilateral chronic venous insufficiency. Unilateral edema of a limb often results from venous thrombosis or lymphatic blockage in the limb. Generalized edema (known as anasarca) occurs in individuals with the nephrotic syndrome, severe heart failure, or hepatic cirrhosis.
Palpitations or tachycardia	Palpitations (defined as an unpleasant awareness of the forceful or rapid beating of the heart) may be induced by various disorders of cardiac rhythm. These include tachycardia, bradycardia of sudden onset, ectopic beats, compensatory pauses, and accentuated stroke volume resulting from valvular regurgitation. Palpitations also often result from anxiety states and high cardiac output (or hyperkinetic) states, such as anemia, fever, thyrotoxicosis, arteriovenous fistula, and the so-called idiopathic hyperkinetic heart syndrome.
Intermittent claudication	Intermittent claudication refers to the pain that occurs in the lower extremities with an inadequate blood supply (usually as a result of atherosclerosis) that is brought on by exercise. The pain does not occur with standing or sitting, is reproducible from day to day, is more severe when walking upstairs or up a hill, and is often described as a cramp, which disappears within 1–2 min after stopping exercise. Coronary artery disease is more prevalent in individuals with intermittent claudication. Patients with diabetes are at increased risk for this condition.
Known heart murmur	Although some may be innocent, heart murmurs may indicate valvular or other cardiovascular disease. From an exercise safety standpoint, it is especially important to exclude hypertrophic cardiomyopathy and aortic stenosis as underlying causes because these are among the more common causes of exertion-related sudden cardiac death.
Unusual fatigue or shortness of breath with usual activities	Although there may be benign origins for these symptoms, they also may signal the onset of or change in the status of cardiovascular disease or metabolic disease.

[a]These signs or symptoms must be interpreted within the clinical context in which they appear because they are not all specific for cardiovascular, metabolic, or renal diseases.

Reprinted from Liguori G, Feito Y, Fountaine C, Roy BA, editors. *ACSM's Guidelines for Exercise Testing and Prescription.* 11th ed. Baltimore (MD): Lippincott, Williams & Wilkins; 2022. 34 p.

(paleness), cyanosis (bluish color of the skin or mucous membranes), or a rash. A symptom is what the individual feels or perceives, such as chest discomfort or fatigue. One study reported that 36% of cases of SCD had typical CHD symptoms during the week preceding the event (91) and that 40% had prodromal symptoms before experiencing an AMI (86). This highlights the need for the clinical exercise physiologist (CEP) to educate their patients regarding the signs and symptoms associated with cardiac events (10).

The overall risks of SCD and MI associated with physical activity are low and the benefits of physical activity outweigh the risks in most people (1, 13). However, because of the gravity of the consequences, these risks merit close scrutiny in the processes of preexercise screening and risk assessment before prescribing exercise. These benefits and risks should play a role in decisions about the most appropriate setting and type of supervision indicated for each individual, so that safety of the participant is optimized.

Risks of SCD

Exercise-related SCD is defined as sudden death that occurs during or within 1 hour of cessation of exercise (12). The incidence of SCD associated with physical activity and exercise varies across age, sex, and other characteristics, and estimates of the incidence range from 3% to 26% of all SCD, with proportionally more exercise-related SCDs occurring in younger age groups (13). The risks of exertion-related SCD are 15–20 times lower in women compared with men (92–94). Most studies have examined the role of vigorous physical activity as a trigger for SCD; there is less known about the role of moderate-intensity exertion as a contributing factor (13).

SCD can occur from triggers other than exercise, but regardless of the trigger, studies of the incidence of SCD in the general population show that the risks of critical events are low. A study conducted in the Netherlands among SCD in people 10–90 years of age showed the incidence of SCD was 2.1 per 100,000 person-years, and in people 35 years of age or less it was 0.3 per 100,000 person-years (95). Additionally, Søholm et al. (96) found that the Charlson comorbidity index, an indicator of overall disease burden, was significantly lower in people with exercise-SCD (0; 95% CI 0–1) compared with SCD that was not associated with exercise (1; 95% CI 0–2), demonstrating a protective effect of physical activity and exercise.

When assessing risk for SCD during acute bouts of activity it has been shown that the absolute risk of SCD during a discrete exercise bout is quite low. Only 7% of people with SCD who were attended by the emergency medical system in Copenhagen over a 9-year period reported that the SCD was associated with exercise (96). In a meta-analysis, Dahabreh and Paulus (85) reported a nearly fivefold increased risk of incident SCD associated with physical activity (RR 4.98; 95% CI 1.47–16.91); however, the absolute risk of SCD was inversely associated with each additional hour of physical activity and projected to be 2–3 SCD per 10,000 person-years. Absolute risks were similarly low in retrospective data from 22,726,000 attendees of fitness programs, with 1 fatal cardiac event per 887,526 person-hours in fitness facilities and, in another study, absolute estimates of SCD were 1 per 2,897,057 person-hours of physical activity in YMCA facilities (89,97). Sports participation data, collected over 13 years, from the Oregon Sudden Unexpected Death Study of community, found that the incidence of SCD among people ages 35–65 years was 21.7 (95% CI 8.1–35.4) per 1 million per year (98). The estimates were somewhat higher in cardiac rehabilitation programs at 1 event per 58,000 patient hours, but still quite low (99), and as cardiac rehabilitation programs cater to a specific population, many of whom have experienced CVD and/or an adverse cardiac event, these data are not surprising. Table 3.2 provides a summary of contemporary exercise-based cardiac rehabilitation program complication rates.

Exercise-related SCD is more frequent in men compared with women (96, 100). For example, a retrospective analysis of individuals who presented with exercise-related

Table 3.2	Summary of Contemporary Exercise-Based Cardiac Rehabilitation Program Complication Rates					
Investigator	Year	Patient Exercise Hours	Cardiac Arrest	Myocardial Infarction	Fatal Events	Major Complications[a]
Van Camp and Peterson (203)	1980–1984	2,351,916	1/111,996[b]	1/293,990	1/783,972	1/81,101
Digenio et al. (204)	1982–1988	480,000	1/120,000[c]		1/160,000	1/120,000
Vongvanich et al. (205)	1986–1995	268,503	1/89,501[d]	1/268,503[d]	0/268,503	1/67,126
Franklin et al. (99)	1982–1998	292,254	1/146,127[d]	1/97,418[d]	0/292,254	1/58,451
Average			1/116,906	1/219,970	1/752,365	1/81,670

[a]Myocardial infarction and cardiac arrest.

[b]Fatal 14%.

[c]Fatal 75%.

[d]Fatal 0%.

Used with permission from Thompson PD, Franklin BA, Balady GJ, et al; American Heart Association, American College of Sports Medicine. Exercise and acute cardiovascular events placing the risks into perspective: a scientific statement from the American Heart Association Council on Nutrition, Physical Activity, and Metabolism and the Council on Clinical Cardiology. *Circulation.* 2007;115(17):2358–68.

SCD found that 82% were male (100). The incidence of SCD during marathon and half-marathon participation was more than five times higher in men (0.90 per 100,000; 95% CI 0.67–1.18) compared with women (0.16 per 100,000; 95% CI 0.07–0.31) (101). The Physician's Health study of 22,071 male physicians without CVD, followed for 12 years, reported an absolute risk of SCD of 1 SCD per 1.51 million episodes of vigorous physical activity (92). The absolute risk was lower in women in the Nurses' Health Study, where the absolute risk of sudden death with moderate-to-vigorous physical activity was 1 per 36.5 million hours of exertion (102).

The risk of exertion-related SCD is higher in individuals participating in strenuous sporting events. Although the risk of SCD is low in younger people (<35 years), the risks of SCD are more than fourfold higher in competitive athletes compared with recreational athletes (98). Data from France report an incidence rate of SCD in young athletes of 0.9 per 100,000 per year in young competitive athletes compared with 0.2 per 100,000 per year among young noncompetitive athletes; however, in absolute number, there are more SCDs in noncompetitive younger athletes (94). Data on marathon running and triathlon participation also show that the risks of SCD also are minimal (13). The incidence of SCD with marathon racers has been found to be 0.54 (95% CI 0.72–1.38) per 100,000 participants during full marathons and 0.27 (95% CI 0.17–0.43) per 100,000 participants during half marathons (101). Data collected from multiple sources including the U.S. National Registry of Sudden Death in Athletes were used to estimate the incidence of death and SCD in triathletes, and incident death or cardiac arrest was 1.74 per 100,000 participants (103). The incidence of SCD was elevated in men 60 or more years compared with younger men, and interestingly, the length of the triathlon did not affect the risks (103). The culmination of the data on SCD and exercise suggests that the benefits of being active far outweigh the risks of engaging in a regular exercise program.

Risks of AMI

AMI associated with exercise (*i.e.*, occurring during or within 1 h of exercise) is a relatively infrequent but potentially serious complication with exercise (13). A meta-analysis of studies using U.S. data showed a 3.45 (95% CI 2.33–5.13) increased risk of AMI with exertion (85). A case–crossover study of 530 survivors of AMI in Costa Rica reported a nearly fivefold risk of AMI associated with heavy exertion, with higher risks in people with low physical fitness or with high CVD risk profiles (104). Mittleman et al. (44) conducted interviews with 1,228 survivors of AMI within 4 days of their acute coronary event and asked about their physical activity the day before the onset of the AMI. Of these patients, 4.4% were engaging in heavy exercise 1 hour or less of the onset of the acute episode. The estimated RR of AMI with exertion was 5.9 (95% CI 4.6–7.7), although the risks were modulated when the participants exercised more days per week.

The Stockholm Heart Epidemiology Program interviewed 699 survivors of AMI in a case–referent study of vigorous exertion (*i.e.*, moving boulders, snow shoveling, running, etc.) and found that 5.7% of the AMI survivors experienced their event during or following exercise, and researchers estimated the rate of exercise-related AMI to be 1.5 per million person-hours and the RR of exertion-related AMI was 3.3 (95% CI 2.4–4.5) (86). Interestingly, 40% of the interviewees said that they had experienced symptoms before having the AMI, and 70% had at least one episode of chest pain (86). These data suggest that the risk of AMI is low for most people, but it is imperative that individuals who demonstrate any symptoms report these to a health care provider and get clearance prior to engaging in vigorous exercise.

Psychological factors may exacerbate one's risk for AMI if individuals are experiencing a level of high stress, including feeling angry or emotionally upset. Using the INTERHEART Study database comprised of 12,461 patients who experienced a first AMI, Smyth et al. (105) estimated the probability of exertion-related AMI and found the odds of having an AMI within 1 hour of exercise to be 2.31 (99% CI 1.96–2.72) compared with the same time frame the day prior to the AMI, and an attributable risk of 7.7% (99% CI 6.3–8.8). When exercise occurred along with anger or emotional upset, the RR of AMI increased to 3.05 (99% CI 2.29–4.07).

Intensity of activity may also play an important role in increasing the risk of AMI after exercise. Von Klot et al. (106), studying 1,301 cases of AMI that occurred within 2 hours of exertion, found a lower risk of AMI with moderate- (~5 METs) than higher-intensity (≥6 METs) exercise. The RR for higher-intensity and moderate-intensity exercise was 5.7 (95% CI 3.6–9.0) and 1.6 (95% CI 1.2–2.1), respectively, relative to very light or no exertion. When strenuous exertion occurred outside, the RR of AMI was four times higher than indoor exercise, which was not explained by temperature (106). Therefore, these data suggest it is vital that patients be educated on how to gauge the intensity of their exercise sessions.

Modification of Risks of SCD and AMI With Chronic Exercise

It is well known that the transient risk of exercise is considerably higher in inactive people compared with regularly active people who meet the recommended volumes of exercise. It has been reported that the risk of AMI during vigorous exercise was 50 times higher in people who were insufficiently active compared with exercisers who exercised on 5 or more days per week (44). Further, the researchers found that the RR of AMI with exertion decreased exponentially with each additional day of exercise in which the participants engaged per week (44). The RR of those exercising less than 1 day per week was 107 (95% CI 67–171), whereas moving to 1–2 days per week of exercise, the RR decreased to 19.4 (95% CI 9.9–38.1), further decreasing with 3–4 exercise days per week (RR 8.6; 95% CI 3.6–20.5) and was 2.4 (95% CI 1.5–3.7) when exercise was done on 5 or more days per week (44). Similarly, a meta-analysis demonstrated an inverse dose-response relationship between volumes of physical activity and SCD and AMI, such that a respective 30% decrease in risk of SCD (RR 0.70; 95% CI 0.50–0.99) and a 45% decrease in risk of AMI (RR 0.53; 95% CI 0.41–0.69) connected with exertion occurred with each additional episode of physical activity per week (85). The risk estimates for AMI ranged from 4.5 to 107 in the most inactive individuals compared to 0.86–3.3 in the most active individuals (85). Whang et al. (102), studying 69,693 participants without prior CVD followed up from 1986 to 2004, showed a transient increase in the risk of SCD during exercise (RR 2.38; 95% CI 1.23–4.60) compared with the risks during no exertion or less physical activity. With increasing amounts of moderate-to-vigorous physical activity, the risk of SCD decreased so that among those who exercised 2 or more hours per week, the risk was insignificant.

A systematic review by Aune et al. (107) examined the risk of SCD among 136,298 participants in eight prospective studies and found the risk of sudden death in the most active individuals was 52% (95% CI 45%–60%) lower than the least active. The analysis of a dose-response association in the same study found up to 20 MET-hours per week of physical activity, the risks of SCD decline by 32% (95% CI 14%–45%), and this risk plateaus around 20–25 MET-hours per week (107).

The limited data available also suggest an association between risk and physical fitness levels (86, 107). Aune et al. (107) found a 42% reduction in risk of SCD in the most fit compared with the lowest fit individuals, whereas Hallqvist et al. (86) showed a U-shaped association

between physical fitness and AMI so that risks of AMI increased at low and higher levels of estimated CRF.

Physical Activities Associated With Acute Coronary Events

A number of studies have described the types of activities and circumstances surrounding exercise-related SCD and AMI. However, there are no studies that have been conducted to identify physical activities that are "risky" in a methodical manner that include gathering information about the characteristics of the participants, participation rates, and the environmental and other circumstances surrounding the coronary event. However, it is often the case that the trigger for an acute MI or SCD is the individual engaging in unaccustomed vigorous or near maximal physical activity or activities that are performed under stressful environmental or psychological conditions (13). Studies of AMI and SCD have identified increased risks during running, racquet sports, sports with bouts of high-intensity exertion, marathons, triathlons, hiking, snow shoveling, downhill and cross-country skiing, and hunting (90, 103, 108–112). Frequently, individuals who experience an AMI or SCD have several CVD risks factors, known CVD, impaired cardiac function, and congenital heart diseases such as cardiomyopathies (13, 113). Environmental conditions such as altitude or cold conditions have been identified as contributory factors, as have exertion under stressful conditions and emotional upset or anger (105, 108, 114–116).

Not all SCDs are due to CHD. Finocchiaro et al. (117) examined a registry of SCD in the United Kingdom to determine the causes of SCD in athletes. Their findings showed that 42% of SCDs were due to sudden arrhythmic death syndrome; 40% had myocardial diseases including idiopathic left ventricular hypertrophy, myocardial fibrosis, arrhythmogenic right ventricular cardiomyopathy, and hypertrophic cardiomyopathy; 5% had anomalies of the coronary arteries. They found that older athletes (≥35 years old) commonly had myocardial diseases, whereas younger athletes more frequently had coronary artery anomalies (117). A meta-analysis of SCD in young athletes showed that 26.7% of SCDs occurred in youth with structurally normal hearts without identifiable cause and 10.3% SCDs were due to hypertrophic cardiomyopathy (118). Among marathoners experiencing SCD, the most common cause of death was known or suspected hypertrophic cardiomyopathy, and ischemic heart disease was frequently the cause among the survivors of SCD who were resuscitated (101). Nonacute coronary disease (60%)

and exercise-induced acute coronary syndrome (33%) are the most common causes of SCD, with coronary artery plaque rupture the second most common cause (98).

Potential Cardiovascular Harms of Exercise

Heart diseases such as CHD, cardiomyopathies, and channelopathies can increase the probability of sudden death and other adverse cardiovascular events, and in some diseases, exercise can worsen the disease (13, 119). Although the benefits of exercise are well understood in most cases of ischemic heart disease and heart failure, the recommendations are less clear in some other heart conditions (13, 113, 119–121).

Exercise can worsen certain types of CVD, such as congenital cardiomyopathies like arrhythmogenic right ventricular dysplasia (ARVD) and other inherited arrhythmogenic conditions with a higher risk of SCD (12, 122–124). Indeed, exercise increases the risks of ventricular tachycardia and fibrillation, heart failure, and ARVD in desmosomal mutation carriers (124). There is a lack of conclusive evidence that exercise causes harm in the presence of these cardiomyopathies; nevertheless, clinical guidelines recommend that exercise be avoided or greatly curtailed in these patients (125).

Some researchers have suggested that very large volumes of exercise, such as with long-distance endurance training performed consistently over a long period of time, may be associated with adverse cardiovascular events, including atrial and ventricular arrhythmias and an increased risk of CHD (13, 72, 126–128). Endurance training results in left and right ventricular remodeling and may result in elevations in creatine kinase-MB, troponins, β-type natriuretic peptides and other biomarkers, and cardiac dysfunction lasting for 1–2 days following competitive events (126, 127). Studies of endurance exercise in animals have reported evidence of ventricular fibrosis and inducible ventricular arrhythmias. Studies of human endurance athletes have found a higher prevalence of cardiac fatigue, right ventricular dysfunction, decreased ejection fraction, myocardial fibrosis, atherosclerosis, and atrial fibrillation (126, 127, 129).

Moderate volumes of exercise appear to be protective of the development of atrial fibrillation, whereas regular endurance training of greater volumes can increase the risks of developing atrial fibrillation by as much as fivefold, especially in men less than 60 years of age (129–132). On the other hand, having lower CRF is associated with a higher risk of atrial fibrillation, more commonly in people

with obesity (59, 60). The mechanisms for the increased incidence of atrial fibrillation in endurance athletes are not well known, but it is hypothesized that structural alterations and changes in autonomic tone and the presence of any arrhythmogenic atrial substrate may contribute to shortened refractory period, slower conduction, and heterogeneity of conduction (129). However, it should be emphasized that these results are neither well understood nor definitive, and significant evidence indicates that exercise modifies many CVD risk factors and even high-volume exercisers experience a very low rate of adverse CVD events, even in people with known heart disease (3, 13, 24, 126). Further, people with heart disease may be able to participate in competitive sports according to current recommendations for athletic participation for people with various types of cardiovascular abnormalities (133).

RISKS OF MUSCULOSKELETAL INJURY AND ACCIDENTS DURING PHYSICAL ACTIVITY

Risks of exercise include accidents and injuries, most commonly musculoskeletal injuries (14, 134–136). Data from the National Health Interview Survey (NHIS) reported that 7 million adults and children received medical attention because of a sports-related injury, with 25.9 injury episodes per 1,000 population (95% CI 24.4–27.4) (137). The majority (64%) of injuries occurred in people ages 5–24 years and there were twice as many injuries observed in females compared to males. The majority of injuries occurred in a sports facility (30.7%), followed by school (19.7) and in the home (16.5%) (137). Basketball, cycling, recreational sports, and exercising were noted as activities resulting in the greatest number of reported injuries (137). The cause of injury was direct contact by striking or collision (34%), falling (28%), and overexertion (13%), while the majority of injuries occurred in the upper (31.2%) and lower (38.9%) extremities, with strains and sprains accounting for 31% of the injuries. Head and neck injuries were involved in 1.1 million injury episodes.

In runners, the rate of injury is estimated to range from 37% to 50% (138), with the most prevalent running injuries being medial tibial stress syndrome (9.5%), Achilles tendinopathy (6.2%–9.5%), and plantar fasciitis (4.5%–10%) (139). Walking and moderate-intensity physical activities are associated with a very low risk of musculoskeletal complications when completed in a manner consistent with current recommendations (2, 6, 7). Walkers had about a 25% lower risk of musculoskeletal injury compared with runners in one study (134). Further, increasing the volume of walking did not result in greater incidence of injury in walkers, whereas larger volumes of running were associated with increased injuries. However, not all studies support the adverse effects of large volumes of running (140).

Often high-intensity interval training (HIIT) is perceived to have a high risk of injuries. In two small studies that reviewed the available literature, the incidence of reported injury ranged from 12% to 72%, with reported injury rates ranging from 0.27 to 3.3 per 1,000 training hours (141, 142). The most injured parts of the body were the shoulder, spine, and knee. The data are limited with varied methodology, which makes it difficult to make conclusions; however, the injury rates reported appear to be similar to a number of sports activities such as Olympic weightlifting, rugby, football, and similar sports (141, 142).

The more important factor in injury incidence may be the type and intensity of the activity, with the greatest rates of injury associated with higher-intensity effort and sports involving twisting, turning, or physical contact. Conditioning and appropriate training regimens are key to preventing injury (13, 14, 134, 143–146). Poor muscular strength and inadequate training regimens have also been implicated in greater rates of injury during sports and exercise (144, 146–148). Inordinate exercise demands, especially during the initial weeks of a physical conditioning regimen, often result in excessive muscle soreness, orthopedic injury, and attrition (10). For most adults, starting at a comfortable volume of light- to moderate-intensity exercise and progressing gradually is a prudent strategy. Once fitness is achieved, progression to more vigorous exercise and sports can occur as tolerated (10, 16, 149). Overuse and other musculoskeletal injuries can be avoided by engaging in a variety of exercises, sometimes termed cross-training, and warming up and cooling down before and after an exercise session.

PREEXERCISE EVALUATION

The preexercise evaluation consists of four steps that should be taken by the CEP before a new patient engages in physical activity. The preexercise evaluation consists of (a) informed consent, (b) exercise preparticipation health screening, (c) medical history, and (d) CVD risk factor analysis, which are described in detail.

The preexercise evaluation is designed to identify those individuals for whom it is safe to begin exercise without further medical evaluation. It will also help to identify individuals: (a) needing medical clearance prior to engaging in exercise (2, 16); (b) with clinically significant disease who may benefit from participating under the supervision of a CEP or in a medically supervised exercise program; or (c) with medical conditions that may require exclusion from an exercise program until those conditions are abated or better controlled (2). This information is also important in guiding the individualized decisions related to exercise testing and exercise prescription.

Informed Consent

The first step when working with a new patient is to obtain informed consent, a process designed to protect both the patient and CEP. Obtaining informed consent is both an ethical and legal obligation and should be completed before collection of any personal and confidential information, exercise testing, exercise prescription, and exercise participation. The content and extent of the informed consent process may vary. In general, informed consent is the process in which the CEP verbally explains the purpose(s) of screening and assessment, the nature of these procedures, and the risks and benefits associated with screening, assessment, expectations of the participant, and the exercise program. The consent form should also include a statement indicating that the patient has been given the opportunity to ask questions and that they are free to withdraw from participation at any time. Following the verbal explanation, the patient must provide written informed consent. Because this is a legal document, it may be wise for the CEP to consult with the legal office in writing an informed consent form to ensure all the necessary components are included. Maintaining confidentiality of medical and personal data is an ethical practice principle, guided by professional ethical codes of ethics, and laws such as the 1996 Health Insurance Portability and Accountability Act (HIPAA) and privacy laws, depending on the setting in which exercise services are provided.

EXERCISE PREPARTICIPATION HEALTH SCREENING

The overarching purpose of exercise preparticipation health screening is to identify individuals at risk for serious exercise-related cardiovascular events, including SCD and AMI. The risk of exercise-related SCD and AMI is highest among individuals who are physically inactive or those with known or occult coronary artery disease (CAD) who perform unaccustomed vigorous-intensity exercise (1, 2, 16, 44, 85, 89, 150). As discussed earlier in this chapter, the absolute risk of these events is very low, and exercise is safe for most people. Nonetheless, vigorous-intensity exercise is associated with an increased risk of acute adverse cardiovascular events, and reducing this risk in susceptible individuals is of paramount importance for the CEP (2, 16).

The exercise preparticipation health screening guidelines seek to balance the need for medical clearance with the safety of exercise for most people. As unnecessary referral to health care providers can be a barrier to adopting physical activity, may place a financial burden on the individual and the health care system, and can result in unnecessary diagnostic testing and follow-up (2, 16), the exercise preparticipation health screening guidelines attempt to identify those who would be at highest risk for exercise-associated adverse events.

American College of Sports Medicine (ACSM) exercise preparticipation health screening recommendations are not a replacement for sound clinical judgment, and all decisions about referral to a health care provider for medical clearance prior to initiating an exercise program should be made on an individual basis. ACSM exercise prescreening algorithm, described in Figure 3.1, is primarily used by exercise professionals working in a health fitness setting with a general, nonclinical population. In clinical settings, the CEP typically has access to a greater amount of participant information than is typically available in health fitness and other community-based settings. As discussed later in this chapter, CEPs can use this information to guide their decision-making with respect to necessary health risk appraisal, referrals to other health care providers, exercise testing, and the exercise prescription. However, ACSM preparticipation screening recommendations remain helpful in clinical settings because of their emphasis on current physical activity and signs and symptoms of disease that can indicate the need for further consultation with the referring physician or other health care providers (16).

How to Use ACSM Preparticipation Health Screening Algorithm

ACSM screening algorithm (Figure 3.1) begins by classifying individuals into six categories based on four risk modulators of adverse exercise-related cardiovascular events (2, 16):

- The individual's current level of physical activity
- Presence of signs or symptoms of cardiovascular, metabolic, or kidney disease
- Known cardiovascular, metabolic, or kidney disease
- The desired exercise intensity

Current Level of Physical Activity

The current level of participation in regular exercise or a structured physical activity program plays a key role in the exercise preparticipation screening process. Determining physical activity levels is essential because physically inactive individuals are at greater risk for adverse cardiovascular events compared to active individuals (1, 2, 13, 16, 44, 85, 150–152).

Current participation in regular exercise is defined as performing planned, structured physical activity for at least 30 minutes at moderate intensity on at least 3 days per week for at least the past 3 months. In most cases, exercise is self-reported, by either questionnaire or interview. People are not always proficient at estimating the amount of exercise that they perform and often inaccurately estimate physical activity levels (153). Therefore, the CEP is encouraged to discuss exercise habits with the participant to clarify current exercise levels. Once the level of exercise is determined, the participant should be placed in the appropriate branch of the algorithm.

Presence of Signs or Symptoms of Cardiovascular, Metabolic, or Kidney Disease

Adverse cardiovascular events often are preceded by warning signs or symptoms of cardiovascular, metabolic, or kidney disease (88, 91, 111). Thus, all participants should be screened for the presence or absence of signs and symptoms suggestive of these diseases (see Table 3.1). Careful screening for signs and symptoms is important because it is possible that a disease is present but has not been diagnosed. Nonspecific symptoms such as breathlessness, or dyspnea, can be challenging to interpret and may require the CEP to ask follow-up questions to help distinguish between an expected symptom, such as may occur with deconditioning, versus a pathological symptom, as may occur because of a pathological condition, for example, heart failure (2). When available, a recent medical history including test and laboratory results can be used to assist the CEP in interpreting signs and symptoms.

Participants may be unfamiliar with or ignore the signs and symptoms of cardiovascular, metabolic, and kidney disease; underestimate the importance of signs or symptoms; or mistakenly believe that symptoms they experience are due to some other cause (*i.e.*, "I am short of breath because I am out of shape.") (154). Educating exercise participants about the major signs and symptoms of cardiovascular, metabolic, and kidney disease is an important

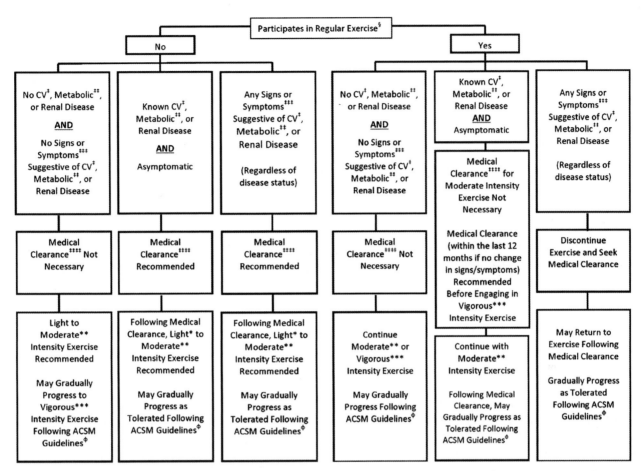

FIGURE 3.1 ACSM preparticipation screening algorithm. (Riebe D, Franklin BA, Thompson PD, et al. Updating ACSM's recommendations for exercise pre-participation health screening. *Med Sci Sports Exerc.* 2015;47(11):2473–9.) §Exercise participation performing planned, structured physical activity at least 30 min at moderate intensity on at least 3 days per week for at least the last 3 months. *Light-intensity exercise 30%–<40% HRR or $\dot{V}O_2R$, 2–<3 METs, RPE 9–11, an intensity that causes slight increases in HR and breathing. **Moderate-intensity exercise 40%–<60% HRR or $\dot{V}O_2R$, 3–<6 METS, RPE 12–13, an intensity that causes noticeable increases in HR and breathing. ***Vigorous-intensity exercise ≥60% HRR or $\dot{V}O_2R$, ≥6 METs, RPE ≥14, an intensity that causes substantial increases in HR and breathing. ‡Cardiovascular (CV) disease and cardiac, peripheral vascular, or cerebrovascular disease. ‡‡Metabolic disease Type 1 and 2 diabetes mellitus. ‡‡‡Signs and symptoms at rest or during activity. Includes pain, discomfort in the chest, neck, jaw, arms, or other areas that may result from ischemia; shortness of breath at rest or with mild exertion; dizziness or syncope; orthopnea or paroxysmal nocturnal dyspnea; ankle edema; palpitations or tachycardia; intermittent claudication; known heart murmur; unusual fatigue or shortness of breath with usual activities. ‡‡‡‡Medical clearance approval from a health care professional to engage in exercise. ΦACSM Guidelines: see Chapters 6, 7, 9, 10, and 11. ACSM, American College of Sports Medicine; HR, heart rate; HRR, heart rate reserve; MET, metabolic equivalent; RPE, rate of perceived exertion; $\dot{V}O_2R$, oxygen uptake reserve.

role of the CEP because it has the potential to decrease the incidence of acute cardiovascular events (10, 88).

Known Cardiovascular, Metabolic, or Kidney Disease

Next, individuals with known CVD (CHD, peripheral artery disease [PAD], cerebrovascular), metabolic (Type 1 and Type 2 diabetes mellitus), or kidney diseases should be identified. Participants should be asked if a physician or other qualified health care provider has ever diagnosed them with any of these conditions.

ACSM exercise preparticipation health screening recommendations do not require the CEP to automatically refer those with known pulmonary disease for medical clearance because pulmonary disease does not increase the risks of adverse cardiovascular events during or immediately following exercise (155). However, the CEP should pay careful attention to the signs and symptoms of CVD in patients with chronic obstructive pulmonary disease (COPD). Because they share the common risk factor of smoking, COPD and CVD are often comorbid conditions, and the presence of COPD in current or former smokers is an independent predictor of overall cardiovascular events (16, 156).

Desired Exercise Intensity

The desired exercise intensity for the initial exercise prescription is the final component in the preparticipation screening algorithm. Because vigorous-intensity exercise is more likely to trigger acute cardiovascular events (vs. light- to moderate-intensity exercise), it is important to identify the intensity at which a participant intends to exercise (44, 88).

Preparticipation Screening Algorithm Categories

Once information about the four risk modulators has been ascertained, participants are placed in one of six categories based on the exercise preparticipation screening algorithm. Table 3.3 provides a summary of the six categories, and Figure 3.2 provides a questionnaire that guides the CEP through the screening process (157).

ADDITIONAL CONSIDERATIONS FOR PREEXERCISE EVALUATION

As ACSM preexercise evaluation is more appropriate for health fitness settings, it is recommended that CEPs working with participants with known CVD or with CVD risk-equivalent diseases like diabetes mellitus or kidney disease (*i.e.*, kidney) use more in-depth risk stratification criteria from the American Association of Cardiovascular and Pulmonary Rehabilitation (AACVPR), the American College of Cardiology (ACC), the AHA, and the American College of Physicians (ACP) (158). The AACVPR criteria are identified in Box 3.1 (159).

MEDICAL HISTORY

Compared to preparticipation health screening, the medical history provides a more comprehensive overview of a participant's overall well-being. The information collected during the medical history can provide insight into goals, exercise history, and exercise preferences and can help to guide the CEP when designing an appropriately individualized exercise prescription.

Some health care providers provide CEPs with a comprehensive medical history when they refer participants to a facility, whereas others require that the CEP request this information. In some cases, the CEP will need to rely on the participant for this information. Communication

Table 3.3	The Six Categories for Use With the Preparticipation Screening Algorithm
Individuals Who Are Currently Inactive	**Individuals Who Are Currently Active**
Participants who are asymptomatic and without known CV, metabolic, or kidney disease can immediately, and without medical clearance, initiate an exercise program at light to moderate intensity and may progress gradually following ACSM guidelines.	Participants who are asymptomatic with no history of CV, metabolic, or kidney disease may continue with their current exercise program or progress as appropriate without medical clearance.
Participants who are asymptomatic but have a known history of CV, metabolic, or kidney disease should obtain medical clearance before initiating a structured exercise program of any intensity. Following medical clearance, the individual may embark on light- to moderate-intensity exercise and may gradually progress as tolerated following ACSM guidelines.	Participants who are asymptomatic but have a known history of CV, metabolic, or kidney disease (*i.e.*, are clinically "stable") may continue with moderate-intensity exercise without medical clearance. However, if these individuals desire to progress to vigorous-intensity aerobic exercise, medical clearance (within the last 12 mo) is recommended.
Symptomatic participants should seek medical clearance, regardless of disease status. If signs or symptoms are present with activities of daily living, medical clearance may be urgent. Following medical clearance, the individual may embark on light- to moderate-intensity exercise and may gradually progress as tolerated following ACSM guidelines.	Participants who experience signs or symptoms suggestive of CV, metabolic, or kidney disease (regardless of disease status) should discontinue exercise and obtain medical clearance before continuing exercise at any intensity.

ACSM, American College of Sports Medicine; CV, cardiovascular.

Data from Riebe D, Franklin BA, Thompson PD, et al. Updating ACSM's recommendations for exercise pre-participation health screening. *Med Sci Sports Exerc.* 2015;47(11):2473–9.

Exercise Preparticipation Health Screening Questionnaire for Exercise Professionals

Assess your client health needs by marking all true statements.

Step 1

SIGNS & SYMPTOMS
Does your client experience:
_____ chest discomfort with exertion
_____ unreasonable breathlessness
_____ dizziness, fainting, blackouts
_____ ankle swelling
_____ unpleasant awareness of a forceful, rapid, or irregular heart rate
_____ burning or cramping sensations in your lower legs when walking short distance
_____ known heart murmur

If you **did** mark any of the statements under the symptoms, **STOP**, your client should consult with a health care provider before engaging or resuming in exercise. Your client may need to use a facility with a **medically qualified staff.**

If you **did not** mark any symptoms, continue to Steps 2 and 3

Step 2

CURRENT ACTIVITY
Has your client performed planned, structured physical activity for at least 30 min at moderate intensity on at least 3 d per wk for at least the last 3 mo?

Yes ☐   No ☐

Continue to Step 3

Step 3

MEDICAL CONDITIONS
Has your client had or do they currently have:
_____ a heart attack
_____ heart surgery, cardiac catheterization, or coronary angioplasty
_____ pacemaker/implantable cardiac defibrillator/rhythm disturbance
_____ heart valve disease
_____ heart failure
_____ heart transplantation
_____ congenital heart disease
_____ diabetes
_____ renal disease

Evaluating Steps 2 and 3:
- If you **did not mark any of the statements in Step 3**, medical clearance is not necessary.
- If you marked Step 2 **"yes"** and **marked any of the statements in Step 3**, your client may continue to exercise at light to moderate intensity without medical clearance. Medical clearance recommended before engaging in vigorous exercise.
- If you marked Step 2 **"no"** and **marked any of the statements in Step 3,** medical clearance is recommended. Your client may need to use a facility with a **medically qualified staff.**

FIGURE 3.2 Exercise preparticipation health screening questionnaire for exercise professionals. (Used with permission from Magal M, Riebe D. New preparticipation health screening recommendations: what exercise professionals need to know. *ACSM's Health Fitness J.* 2016;20(3):22–7.)

| Box 3.1 | American Association of Cardiovascular and Pulmonary Rehabilitation (AACVPR) Risk Stratification Algorithm for Risk of Event |

Patient is at **HIGH RISK** if ANY ONE OR MORE of the following factors are present:
- Resting left ventricular ejection fraction <40%
- Survivor of cardiac arrest or sudden death
- Complex ventricular dysrhythmias (ventricular tachycardia, frequent [>6/min] multiform PVCs) at rest or with exercise
- MI or cardiac surgery complicated by cardiogenic shock, CHF, and/or signs/symptoms of postprocedure ischemia
- Abnormal hemodynamics with exercise, especially flat or decreasing systolic blood pressure or chronotropic incompetence with increasing workload
- Significant silent ischemia (ST depression 2 mm or greater without symptoms) with exercise or in recovery
- Signs/symptoms including angina pectoris, dizziness, light-headedness or dyspnea at low levels of exercise (<5.0 METs)[a] or in recovery
- Maximal functional capacity less than 5.0 METs[a]
- Clinically significant depression or depressive symptoms

Patient is at **LOW RISK** if ALL of the following factors are present:
- Resting left ventricular ejection fraction >50%
- No resting or exercise-induced complex dysrhythmias (ventricular tachycardia, frequent [>6/min] multiform PVCs)
- Uncomplicated MI, CABG, angioplasty, atherectomy, or stent
- Absence of CHF or signs/symptoms indicating postevent ischemia
- Normal hemodynamic and ECG responses with exercise and in recovery
- Asymptomatic with exercise or in recovery, including absence of angina
- Maximal functional capacity of at least 7.0 METs[a]
- Absence of clinical depression or depressive symptoms

Patient is at **INTERMEDIATE RISK** if they meet neither high-risk nor low-risk standards:
- Resting left ventricular ejection fraction = 40%–50%
- Signs/symptoms including angina at "moderate" levels of exercise (60%–75% of maximal functional capacity) or in recovery
- Mild-to-moderate silent ischemia (ST depression <2 mm) with exercise or in recovery

[a]If measured functional capacity is not available, this variable can be excluded from the risk stratification process.

CABG, coronary artery bypass grafting; CHF, congestive heart failure; ECG, electrocardiogram; MET, metabolic equivalent; MI, myocardial infarction; PVC, premature ventricular complex.

From American Association of Cardiovascular and Pulmonary Rehabilitation. Stratification algorithm for risk of event. Available from: https://registry.dev.aacvpr.org/Documents/AACVPR%20Risk%20Stratification%20Algorithm_June2012.pdf.

with the health care provider can also provide the CEP with the reason for referral to the program. Although some program participants have a clear understanding of why they are visiting the exercise facility, others need further encouragement and explanation for why engaging in an exercise program is the right next step for them. For example, an individual with Type 2 diabetes may have their blood glucose under control with the use of medication and may not understand that in addition to potentially helping them to reduce the amount of medication needed for blood glucose control, engaging in an exercise program is beneficial for their blood pressure (BP), cholesterol levels, weight control, and quality of life (27).

Common components included in a medical history are shown in Box 3.2. Figure 3.3 shows an example of a medical history questionnaire (160). There are additional online tools that the CEP may access including, but not limited to, the PARMed-X (http://eparmedx.com/) and Adult Pre-Exercise Screening System (APSS) tool from Exercise and Sports Science Australia (https://www.essa.org.au/Public/ABOUT_ESSA/Pre-Exercise_Screening_Systems.aspx).

Demographic Information

Demographic information includes variables such as age, sex, race, and ethnicity. Age is important to consider as the number of people diagnosed with chronic conditions increases with advancing age, and the prevalence of arthritis, CVD, chronic pulmonary disease, diabetes, and

---

Box 3.2   **Common Components of the Medical History**

The medical history may include the following:

- Demographic information:
  - Age
  - Sex
  - Race
  - Ethnicity
- Recent illness, hospitalizations, new medical diagnoses, or surgical procedures
- Medication use (including dietary/nutritional supplements) and drug allergies
- Previous medical diagnoses and history of medical procedures
  - Cardiovascular diseases, including:
    - hypertension
    - heart failure
    - valvular dysfunction (*e.g.*, aortic stenosis/mitral valve disease)
    - myocardial infarction and other acute coronary syndromes
    - percutaneous coronary interventions including angioplasty and coronary stent(s)
    - coronary artery bypass surgery
    - other cardiac surgeries such as valvular surgery
    - cardiac transplantation
    - pacemaker and/or implantable cardioverter defibrillator
    - ablation procedures for dysrhythmias
  - Obesity
  - Diabetes mellitus
  - Dyslipidemia
  - Peripheral vascular disease
  - Pulmonary diseases, including:
    - asthma
    - emphysema
    - bronchitis
  - Cerebrovascular diseases, including:
    - stroke
    - transient ischemic attacks
  - Blood disorders, including:
    - anemia
    - other blood dyscrasias (*e.g.*, lupus erythematosus)
  - Phlebitis
  - Deep vein thrombosis or emboli

- Cancer and course of treatment
- Pregnancy
- Mental health disorders, including:
  - anxiety
  - depression
  - eating disorders
- Musculoskeletal disorders and orthopedic conditions
  - Arthritis
  - Osteoporosis
  - Joint swelling
  - Any condition that would make ambulation or use of certain test modalities difficult
- Neuromuscular diseases
  - Parkinson disease
  - Multiple sclerosis
  - Huntington disease
- History of symptoms
  - Discomfort (*e.g.*, pressure, tingling sensation, pain, heaviness, burning, tightness, squeezing, numbness) in the chest, jaw, neck, back, or arms
  - Light-headedness, dizziness, or fainting
  - Temporary loss of visual acuity or speech
  - Transient unilateral numbness or weakness
  - Shortness of breath
  - Rapid heartbeat or palpitations, especially if associated with physical activity, eating a large meal, emotional upset, or exposure to cold (or any combination of these activities)
- Previous physical examination findings, including:
  - height
  - weight
  - blood pressure
  - murmurs, clicks, gallop rhythms, other abnormal heart sounds
  - other unusual cardiac and vascular findings
  - lung sounds
    - abnormal pulmonary findings (*e.g.*, wheezes, rales, crackles)
  - edema
- Laboratory findings, including:
  - plasma glucose
  - hemoglobin A1C
  - high-sensitivity C-reactive protein
  - serum lipids and lipoproteins

(continued)

Box 3.2	Common Components of the Medical History (*continued*)

- Family history of:
  - cardiac disease
  - pulmonary disease
  - metabolic disease
  - stroke
  - sudden death
  - cancer
  - other medical conditions
- Physical activity/exercise evaluation
  - Information on readiness for change and habitual level of activity

- Frequency, intensity, duration or time, and type (FITT) of exercise
- Work history with emphasis on current or expected physical demands, noting upper and lower extremity requirements
- Other lifestyle habits, including:
  - caffeine intake
  - alcohol use
  - tobacco use
  - recreational (illicit) drug use

HEALTH HISTORY QUESTIONNAIRE

NAME _____ AGE _____ DATE _____ DATE OF BIRTH _____

     First   M.I   Last   day/month/year   day/month/year

ADDRESS _____

           Street   City/State/Zip

TELEPHONE (home) _____ (business) _____ (oral) _____

OCCUPATION _____ PLACE OF EMPLOYMENT _____

MARITAL STATUS (select one)   SINGLE   MARRIED   DIVORCED   WIDOWED

SPOUSE: _____

EDUCATION   ELEMENTARY_____ HIGH SCHOOL _____COLLEGE _____

GRADUATE _____

ETHNICITY: _____ PERSONAL PHYSICIAN _____

LOCATION _____

Person for last doctor visit? _____ Date of last physician exam _____

Have you previously been tested for an exercise program?   YES ____   NO ____   YEAR(s) _____

LOCATION OF TEST _____

Person for contact in case of an emergency _____ Phone # _____

(relationship) _____

FIGURE 3.3 Sample medical history questionnaire (From American College of Sports Medicine. *ACSM's Resources for the Exercise Physiologist.* 3rd ed. Wolters Kluwer; 2021. p. 40–2.)

PLEASE CHECK YES OR NO

Past (Have you ever had?)		
	YES	NO
High blood pressure _____	☐	☐
Heart problems_____	☐	☐
Disease of arteries _____	☐	☐
Varicose veins_____	☐	☐
Lung disease_____	☐	☐
Asthma _____	☐	☐
Kidney disease _____	☐	☐
Hepatitis_____	☐	☐
Diabetes_____	☐	☐
Orthopedic problems_____	☐	☐
Arthritis_____	☐	☐

FAMILY (Has any immediate family member or grandparent had?)		
	YES	NO
Heart attacks _____	☐	☐
High blood pressure _____	☐	☐
High cholesterol_____	☐	☐
Stroke _____	☐	☐
Diabetes _____	☐	☐
Congenital heart default __	☐	☐
Heart operations_____	☐	☐
Early death _____	☐	☐
Other family illness_____		
_____		
_____		

PRESENT SYMPTOMS (Have you monthly had?)		
	YES	NO
Chest pain discomfort ___	☐	☐
Shortness of breath _____	☐	☐
Dizzy spells _____	☐	☐
Skipped heart beats_____	☐	☐
Trouble sleeping _____	☐	☐
Ankle swelling _____	☐	☐
Leg pain cramping _____	☐	☐
Frequent headaches ____	☐	☐
Frequent odds _____	☐	☐
Back pain _____	☐	☐
Orthopedic problems____	☐	☐

(FOR STAFF COMMENTS)

_____

_____

_____

HEALTH HISTORY QUESTIONNAIRE

Are you currently following a weight-reduction diet plan?   **Yes** _____   **No** _____   **Name:** _____

If so, how long have you been dieting? _____months   **Is the plan prescribed by your doctor? Yes** _____ **No** _____

Have you used weight-reduction diet in the past?   Yes _____   **No.** _____   **If yes, how often and which type(s)?**

_____

_____

Please indicate the reasons why you want to join the exercise program.

To lose weight _____ **Doctor's recommendation** _____ **For good health** _____ **Enjoyment** _____.

Release of tension _____ **Improve physical appearance** _____ **Other** _____

FOR STAFF USE

_____

_____

FIGURE 3.3 (*continued*)

HEALTH HISTORY QUESTIONNAIRE

HOSPITALIZATIONS: Please list recent hospitalizations (Woman: do not list normal pregnancies)

Year   Location   Person

_____

_____

_____

Any other medical problems or other concerns not already identified? Yes ___ No _____   (Please list below)

_____

_____

Have you ever had your cholesterol measured? Yes ___ No ____If yes, (value)_____(Date) _____

_____

Are you taking any prescription or nonprescription medications? Yes _____   No_____   (Include birth-control pills)

Medication   Reason for Taking   For How Long?

_____

_____

_____

Do you currently smoke?   Yes ___ No ___ If so, what? Cigarettes _____Cigars ____Pipe _____

How much per day: < 5 pack ____   0.5 to 1 pack _____ 1.5 to 2 packs _____ >2 packs _____

Have you ever quit smoking? Yes ___ No ___When? _____   How many years and how much did you smoke?

_____

Do you drink any alcoholic beverages? Yes _____   No _____   If Yes, how much in 1 week?

Beer_____ (cans)   Wine _____(glasses)   Hard liquor _____ (drinks)

Do you drink any caffeinated beverages?   Yes _____   No ____   If Yes, how much in 1 week?

Coffees _____(cups) Tea _____(glasses)   Soft drinks _____(cans)

_____

ACTIVITY LEVEL EVALUATION

What is your occupational activity level?   Secondary _____: light: _____ moderate ___: heavy _____

Do you currently engage in vigorous physical activity on a regular basis? Yes ____ No ____

If so, what type? _____ How many days per week? _____

How much time per day? (check one)   <15 min_____   15–30 min _____   30–45 min ____   >60 min _____

Do you ever have an uncomfortable shortness of breath during exercise? Yes ____ No ____

Do you ever have chest discomfort during exercise? Yes _____ No _____. If so, does it go away with rest? _____

Do you engage in any recreational or leisure-time physical activities on a regular basis? Yes _____ No _____

If so, what activities? _____

On average :   How often?_____times/week: For how long? _____time/session

FIGURE 3.3 (continued)

hypertension is highest among those 65 years and older (161). Moreover, aerobic fitness levels and muscular strength have been shown to decrease with age (2, 162, 163), especially among individuals with insufficient levels of physical activity. Personal factors such as age, sex, race, ethnicity, and other sociocultural variables may affect exercise preferences (164), and barriers to exercise participation can differ among age groups (164, 165), between males and females (164, 166, 167), and among racial/ethnic groups (168).

Recent Illness, Hospitalizations, New Medical Diagnoses, or Surgical Procedures

Information about recent illnesses, hospitalizations, new medical diagnoses, injuries, and/or recent surgical procedures often offers insight into the reason for participant referral to a program. For example, if a program participant has experienced a recent AMI and follow-up coronary artery bypass grafting (CABG), this information confirms the reason for referral, guides the health education and exercise program toward secondary prevention, and indicates the exercise prescription needs to avoid elements that interfere with healing.

Prescription and Over-the-Counter Medication Use

It is recommended that the CEP obtain a comprehensive list of prescription and over-the-counter medications (including recent changes in medications) and dietary supplements, as certain medications and supplements affect physiological responses to exercise (*e.g.*, β-blockers affect heart rate). To ensure accuracy, participants should bring to their first visit a list of their medications and supplements, including details regarding prescribed dose and frequency, as participants may not accurately recall this information. Alternatively, participants can bring their medications with them. Doing so allows the CEP to record medication information in full and get a sense of how well the participant adheres to the prescribed medication regimen. Drug and other allergies and intolerances should also be recorded.

Medical Diagnoses and History of Medical Procedures

Medical diagnoses and courses of treatment including, but not limited to, cardiovascular, cerebrovascular, metabolic, pulmonary, and neurologic diseases, musculoskeletal conditions, cancer, and/or any conditions that may be exercise limiting, should be recorded. Recently, the emergence of COVID-19 infections may be of interest to the CEP especially for those considered to have post-COVID-19 syndrome, who exhibit symptoms over months/years (169). As the symptoms of post-COVID-19 syndrome include myalgia, fatigue, dyspnea, brain fog/difficulty concentrating, and reduced physical function (169, 170), and also may involve abnormal sequelae affecting pulmonary (171), cardiovascular (172, 173), and other body systems (174), the CEP may need to address any concerns during the initial consult with the patient and proceed with the exercise prescription and education plan accordingly.

With all patients, it is especially important to discuss and identify all medical conditions that affect a participant's exercise preference and ability, as these will have a direct effect on the exercise prescription. For example, a history of cancer and related treatments may have a direct effect on the design of the exercise program, as adjuvant chemotherapy has been associated with loss of bone mineral density and subsequently increased risk for osteopenia and osteoporosis (175). In such a case, the CEP should be sure to include activities associated with increasing or maintaining bone density, while avoiding activities with increased risk of falls and subsequent fractures. Participants' cognitive abilities, hearing abilities, and visual acuity may also need assessment, specifically if any of these affects their ability to understand and follow directions. It may help to have several orientation sessions focused on familiarization with the facility's layout and equipment. For example, an individual with low vision may require extra time to explore each piece of equipment tactilely to ensure their comfort and safety when exercising.

History of Symptoms

History of current or past symptoms associated with documented medical conditions and their onset is important to record. Any reoccurrence of these symptoms should prompt the CEP to advise a participant to seek appropriate and timely medical attention. Symptoms associated with the onset of acute cardiac events (*e.g.*, if the client experienced a previous AMI, what, if any, signs and symptoms did they experience prior to the event) may be of special interest. Additionally, if a participant with Type 1 diabetes mellitus reports certain symptoms when hypoglycemic, having these noted in the participant's chart would allow facility staff to respond quickly to assist the participant in raising their blood glucose level if such symptoms should occur while the participant is exercising.

Physical Examination Findings and Laboratory Results

Body weight, height, resting BP, breath sounds, presence of abnormal heart sounds or unusual cardiac or vascular findings, evidence of edema, orthopnea, and the presence of neuropathies may be included in the medical history. Height and weight are used to calculate body mass index (BMI), which can be used as an indicator for increased risk of many chronic conditions, including CVD, and metabolic and joint diseases (2).

Documentation of baseline resting BP may provide the CEP with a way to track changes associated with program participation or changes in health status (Table 3.4) (176, 177). Additionally, if a participant has known neuropathies, programs can be designed to limit activities that may cause blistering or injury to areas with decreased sensation and to take precautions because of associated balance difficulties.

Baseline values of plasma glucose, hemoglobin A1C (HbA1C), serum lipids and lipoproteins, and high-sensitivity C-reactive protein (hs-CRP) allow for the identification of CVD risk factors and can help to document physiological improvements resulting from exercise participation (Tables 3.5 and 3.6) (206) and other interventions.

Family History

Heritable conditions in first-degree family members (parents, siblings, and children) are often recorded in the medical history. These medical conditions include, but are not limited to, CHD, diabetes, dyslipidemia, and cancer (2). When evaluating family history as a CVD risk factor, it is important to note that there is specific definition for this risk factor: myocardial infarction, coronary revascularization, or sudden death before 55 years in father or other male first-degree relatives or before 65 years in mother or other female first-degree relatives.

Physical Activity/Exercise Evaluation

A participant's medical history may contain information about exercise history, but the level of detail documented by health care providers may be limited. It is the responsibility of the CEP to augment the information provided in

Table 3.4	Classification and Management of Blood Pressure for Adults			
BP Classification	SBP (mm Hg)	DBP (mm Hg)	Lifestyle Modification	Treatment Recommendations
Normal	<120	And <80	Encourage	Promote optimal lifestyle habits; reassess yearly
Elevated	120–129	And <80	Yes	Nonpharmacological therapy; reassess in 3–6 mo.
Stage 1 hypertension	130–139	Or 80–89	Yes	Estimate 10-yr CVD risk. If <10% risk, start with healthy lifestyle recommendations; reassess in 3–6 mo. If ≥10% risk or ASCVD, DM, kidney disease, recommend lifestyle change and pharmacological treatment; reassess within 1 mo.
Stage 2 hypertension	≥140	Or ≥90	Yes	Nonpharmacological treatment and BP-lowering medication; follow-up monthly until BP is controlled.

Treatment determined by highest BP category.

ASCVD, atherosclerotic cardiovascular disease; BP, blood pressure; CVD, cardiovascular disease; DBP, diastolic blood pressure; DM, diabetes mellitus; SBP, systolic blood pressure.

From Whelton PK, Carey RM, Aronow WS, et al. 2017 ACC/AHA/AAPA/ABC/ACPM/AGS/APhA/ASH/ASPC/NMA/PCNA guideline for the prevention, detection, evaluation, and management of high blood pressure in adults: executive summary: a report of the American College of Cardiology/American Heart Association Task Force on Clinical Practice Guidelines. *Hypertension.* 2018;71(6):1269–324. doi:10.1161/HYP.0000000000000066.

Table 3.5	Classification of Cholesterol and Triglyceride Levels (mg·dL⁻¹)
Non-HDL-C	
<130	Desirable
130–159	Above desirable
160–189	Borderline high
190–219	High
≥220	Very high
LDL-C	
<100	Desirable
100–129	Above desirable
130–159	Borderline high
160–189	High
≥190	Very high
HDL-C	
<40 (men)	Low
<50 (women)	Low
Triglycerides	
<150	Normal
150–199	Borderline high
200–499	High
≥500	Very high[a]

To convert LDL, total cholesterol, and HDL from mg·dL⁻¹ to mmol·L⁻¹, multiply by 0.0259. To convert triglycerides from mg·dL⁻¹ to mmol·L⁻¹, multiply by 0.0113.

[a]Severe hypertriglyceridemia is another term used for very high triglycerides in pharmaceutical product labeling.

HDL-C, high-density lipoprotein cholesterol; LDL-C, low-density lipoprotein cholesterol; non-HDL-C, total cholesterol minus HDL-C.

Used with permission from Liguori G, Feito Y, Fountaine C, Roy BA, editors. *ACSM's Guidelines for Exercise Testing and Prescription.* 11th ed. Baltimore (MD): Lippincott, Williams & Wilkins; 2022. 51 p.

the medical history and obtain a comprehensive physical activity/exercise history, because the exercise history is an important component in developing the exercise prescription. The CEP should inquire about a participant's physical activity and exercise history, exercise preferences, barriers to exercise (*i.e.,* childcare, transportation, family responsibilities), and signs or symptoms that they currently or have previously experienced during exercise (*i.e.,*

chest discomfort, shortness of breath, knee pain, low back pain). The CEP should also record information related to the frequency, intensity, time, and types(s) of physical activity a participant has engaged in, both in the past and currently. Information on work history, with details of the physical demands of current or previous employment, may also be helpful when developing the exercise prescription. As some occupations are highly active and others highly sedentary, the participant's work history may affect components of the exercise prescription, including the mode and duration of activities that are appropriate or enjoyable.

Other Lifestyle Habits

Information pertaining to a participant's lifestyle habits, including diet and use of caffeine, alcohol, tobacco, or recreational drugs, is often included in the medical history (see Figure 3.3). Several lifestyle assessment tools are available, including the Fantastic Lifestyle Assessment (178) and the Healthy Lifestyle and Personal Control Questionnaire (179). Lifestyle assessments can be used as tools to assist with behavior modification and goal setting. Additionally, information to this end can indicate if specialized health education programs are recommended and/or if other members of the health care team, including dietitians, smoking cessation professionals, respiratory therapists, and specialized physicians, should be consulted. Adequate communication among members of the health care team regarding management of lifestyle factors contributes to a comprehensive approach to participant care.

CVD RISK FACTOR ASSESSMENT

As diseases of the heart remain the leading cause of death in the U.S., accounting for 23.1% of deaths in the U.S. in 2019 (180), identifying CVD risk factors is highly recommended, as it is central to developing an effective lifestyle modification plan for prevention and/or management of CVD and related conditions (181, 182). Additionally, the risk factor identification process can serve as a teaching tool, motivating the client to engage in lifestyle modification for the prevention and management of modifiable risk factors.

Positive CVD risk factors are associated with increased risk of development for CVD. These include age, family history, cigarette smoking, physical inactivity, BMI/waist circumference, BP, lipids, and blood glucose (2). In

Table 3.6	Typical Ranges of Normal Values for Selected Blood Variables in Adults			
Variable	Men	Neutral	Women	SI Conversion Factor
Hemoglobin (g·dL^{-1})	13.5–17.5		11.5–15.5	10 (g·L^{-1})
Hematocrit (%)	40–52		36–48	0.01 (proportion of 1)
Red cell count (×10^6·µL^{-1})	4.5–6.5 million		3.9–5.6 million	1 (×10^{12}·L^{-1})
Hemoglobin (whole blood)		30–35		10 (g·L^{-1})
Mass concentration (g·dL^{-1})				
White blood cell count (×10^3·µL^{-1})		4,000–11,000		1 (×10^9·L^{-1})
Platelet count (×10^3·µL^{-1})		150,000–450,000		1 (×10^9·L^{-1})
Fasting glucose[a] (mg·dL^{-1})		60–99		0.0555 (mmol·L^{-1})
Hemoglobin A1C		≤6%		N/A
Blood urea nitrogen (BUN; mg·dL^{-1})		4–24		0.357 (mmol·L^{-1})
Creatinine (mg·dL^{-1})		0.3–1.4		88.4 (µmol·L^{-1})
BUN/creatinine ratio		7–27		
Uric acid (mg·dL^{-1})		3.6–8.3		59.48 (µmol·L^{-1})
Sodium (mEq·dL^{-1})		135–150		1.0 (mmol·L^{-1})
Potassium (mEq·dL^{-1})		3.5–5.5		1.0 (mmol·L^{-1})
Chloride (mEq·dL^{-1})		98–110		1.0 (mmol·L^{-1})
Osmolality (mOsm·kg^{-1})		278–302		1.0 (mmol·kg^{-1})
Calcium (mg·dL^{-1})		8.5–10.5		0.25 (mmol·L^{-1})
Calcium, ion (mg·dL^{-1})		4.0–5.0		0.25 (mmol·L^{-1})
Phosphorus (mg·dL^{-1})		2.5–4.5		0.323 (mmol·L^{-1})
Protein, total (g·dL^{-1})		6.0–8.5		10 (g·L^{-1})
Albumin (g·dL^{-1})		3.0–5.5		10 (g·L^{-1})
Globulin (g·dL^{-1})		2.0–4.0		10 (g·L^{-1})
A/G ratio		1.0–2.2		10
Iron, total (µg·dL^{-1})		40–190	35–180	0.179 (µmol·L^{-1})

Table 3.6	Typical Ranges of Normal Values for Selected Blood Variables in Adults (*continued*)			
Variable	Men	Neutral	Women	SI Conversion Factor
Liver Function Tests				
Bilirubin (mg·dL^{-1})		<1.5		17.1 (μmol·L^{-1})
AST (U·L^{-1})	8–46		7–34	1 (U·L^{-1})
ALT (U·L^{-1})	7–46		4–35	1 (U·L^{-1})

For a complete list of Système International (SI) conversion factors, please see http://jama.ama-assn.org/content/vol295/issue1/images/data/103/DC6/JAMA_auinst_si.dtl.

Certain variables must be interpreted in relation to the normal range of the issuing laboratory.

[a]Fasting blood glucose 100–125 mg·dL^{-1} is considered impaired fasting glucose or prediabetes.

ALT, alanine transaminase (formerly SGPT); AST, aspartate transaminase (formerly SGOT); SGOT, serum glutamic-oxaloacetic transaminase; SGPT, serum glutamic-pyruvic transaminase.

Source: American College of Sports Medicine, Riebe D, Ehrman JK, Liguori G, Magal M. (2018). *ACSM's Guidelines for Exercise Testing And Prescription*. 10th ed. Philadelphia (PA): Wolters Kluwer.

addition to the positive risk factors, there is one negative risk factor: high high-density lipoprotein (HDL) cholesterol has been associated with some cardioprotective effects (2). Defining criteria for each of these risk factors are provided in Table 3.7 (2).

Modifiable risk factors are those that can be reduced through lifestyle changes and/or pharmacologic therapies. These include lipids, BP, blood glucose, BMI/waist circumference, physical inactivity, and cigarette smoking. Nonmodifiable risk factors for CVD include age, sex, and family history.

Prevalence of Cardiovascular Risk Factors

The prevalence of cardiovascular risk factors is of interest to the CEP because of the number of patients encountered with positive risk factors. Participating in screening for risk factors varies by age group in the U.S., with adults 65 years and over participating in screening more often, compared to younger individuals (183). Rates of screening for high blood cholesterol are increasing, and approximately 67% of men and 72% of women in the National Health and Nutrition Examination Survey (NHANES) study, aged 20 years and over, participated in cholesterol screening during 2011–2014 (184).

As noted earlier, Type 2 diabetes is a modifiable risk factor for CVD. The 2020 National Diabetes Statistics Report found that 13.0% of all U.S. adults (34.2 million people) had diabetes, with an estimated 26.8 million people diagnosed and 7.3 million people undiagnosed (185).

New diabetes diagnoses were higher among non-Hispanic blacks and people of Hispanic origin compared to non-Hispanic Asians and non-Hispanic whites, and it should be noted that of those newly diagnosed with diabetes, there were individuals who were also smokers (15%), were overweight (89%), and were physically inactive (38%) (185).

As obesity is a modifiable risk factor for both CVD and Type 2 diabetes, this outcome is regularly assessed among the U.S. population and recent data from the 2018 NHANES illustrate that the prevalence of both obesity and severe obesity among adults has increased from 1999 to 2018 (186). Data from 2017 to 2018 show that 42.4% are considered obese (BMI of ≥30 kg·m^{-2}), with a similar prevalence among men and women and by age group (186). Non-Hispanic black women have the highest prevalence of obesity (56.9%) compared to all other groups. Also of note, the prevalence of severe obesity in adults was 9.2% and was higher in women (11.5%) compared to men (6.9%).

Data from the NHANES (2017–2018) found the prevalence of hypertension was 45.4% among adults and was higher among men (51%) compared to women (39.7%) (187). Additionally, the prevalence of hypertension was higher among non-Hispanic black (57.1%) compared to non-Hispanic white (43.6%) or Hispanic (43.7%) adults. It is important to note that prevalence of hypertension increases with age: 22.4% among adults aged 18–39 years, 54.5% among those aged 40–50 years, and 74.5% among those aged 60 years and over (187). For example,

Table 3.7	Atherosclerotic CVD Risk Factors and Defining Criteria
Positive Risk Factors[a]	**Defining Criteria**
Age	Men $\geq$ 45 yr; women $\geq$ 55 yr
Family history	Myocardial infarction, coronary revascularization, or sudden death before 55 yr in father or other male first-degree relatives or before 65 yr in mother or other female first-degree relatives
Cigarette smoking	Current cigarette smoker or those who quit within the previous 6 mo or exposure to environmental tobacco smoke
Physical inactivity	Not meeting the minimum threshold of 500–1,000 MET-min of moderate-to-vigorous physical activity or 75–100 min·wk^{-1} of moderate- to vigorous-intensity physical activity
Body mass index/waist circumference	Body mass index $\geq$ 30 kg·m^{-2} or waist girth >102 cm (40 inches) for men and >88 cm (35 inches) for women
Blood pressure	Systolic blood pressure $\geq$130 mm Hg and/or diastolic blood pressure $\geq$80 mm Hg, based on an average of $\geq$2 readings obtained on $\geq$2 occasions, or on antihypertensive medication
Lipids	LDL cholesterol $\geq$130 mg·dL^{-1} (3.37 mmol·L^{-1}) or HDL[a] cholesterol <40 mg·dL^{-1} (1.04 mmol·L^{-1}) in men and <50 mg·dL^{-1} (1.30 mmol·L^{-1}) in men or non-HDL cholesterol <130 (3.37 mmol·L^{-1}) or on lipid-lowering medication. If total serum cholesterol is all that is available, use $\geq$200 mg·dL^{-1} (5.18 mmol·L^{-1}).
Blood glucose	Fasting plasma glucose $\geq$100 mg·dL^{-1} (555.5 mmol·L^{-1}) or 2-h plasma glucose values in OGTT $\geq$140 mg·dL^{-1} (7.77 mmol·L^{-1}) or HbA1C $\geq$ 5.7%
Negative risk factors	Defining criteria
HDL cholesterol[b]	$\geq$60 mg·dL^{-1} (1.55 mmol·L^{-1})

[a]If the presence or absence of a CVD risk factor is not disclosed or is not available, that CVD risk factor should be counted as a risk factor.

[b]High HDL cholesterol is considered a negative risk factor. For individuals having high HDL $\geq$60 mg·dL^{-1} (1.55 mmol·L^{-1}), one positive risk factor is subtracted from the sum of positive risk factors.

CVD, cardiovascular disease; HbA1C, hemoglobin A1C; HDL, high-density lipoprotein; LDL, low-density lipoprotein; MET, metabolic equivalent; OGTT, oral glucose tolerance test.

Used with permission from Liguori G, Feito Y, Fountaine C, Roy BA, editors. *ACSM's Guidelines for Exercise Testing and Prescription.* 11th ed. Baltimore (MD): Lippincott, Williams & Wilkins; 2022.

non-Hispanic black adults have higher rates of hypertension compared to non-Hispanic whites or Hispanics (187).

During 2015–2018, 11.4% of adults had high total cholesterol ($\geq$240 mg/dL), with similar prevalence by sex, race, and Hispanic origin (184). The overall prevalence of low HDL cholesterol (<40 mg/dL) was 17.2% but was significantly higher in men (26.6%) compared to women (8.5%), and was lowest in non-Hispanic black adults and higher in Hispanic adults (184).

Data summarizing the trends in major cardiovascular risk factors from 1999 to 2018 were recently published in the *Journal of the American Medical Association* by He et al. (188). Additionally, data from the NHIS reveal that 24.3% of adults meet the Physical Activity Guidelines for aerobic and muscle-strengthening activities, but these rates vary by geographic region (189). Men are more likely than women, and younger adults are more likely than older adults to meet the recommendations for aerobic activity, whereas non-Hispanic white adults are more likely than non-Hispanic black and Hispanic adults to meet the recommendations for both aerobic and muscle-strengthening activities (189). Physical inactivity is also higher among individuals with less education and those with a family income at or near the poverty level (189).

Researchers also estimate that 14.0% of U.S. adults currently smoke cigarettes. Smoking prevalence is higher among men, adults aged 25–44 years and 45–64 years, individuals with lower education levels, those who live below the poverty level, those without insurance or insured through Medicaid, those who live in the Midwest, individuals with a disability or limitation, and those who experience severe anxiety (190).

Evaluating CVD Risk

Practitioners commonly calculate the total number of risk factors to provide an overview of risk for CVD (see Table 3.7). It is standard practice that if the presence or absence of a CVD risk factor is not available or unknown, the CVD risk factor counts as a positive risk factor. For individuals having an HDL above 60 mg·dL^{-1} or more (1.55 mmol·L^{-1}), one positive risk factor is subtracted from the sum of positive risk factors.

The total number of risk factors is important when evaluating CVD risk because there is often a clustering of risk factors; moreover, the increase in the number of risk factors present is exponentially related to an increase in the estimated 10-year risk of CHD in both men and women (191). Global risk assessment tools can be helpful in identifying individuals who may warrant more careful observation for CVD signs and symptoms and may benefit from intensive risk factor reduction efforts (192). The ACC has a 10-year atherosclerotic CVD risk estimator assessment tool available for primary prevention. It is recommended that this risk estimator only be used in patients who do not currently have a diagnosis of atherosclerotic CVD: http://tools.acc.org/ascvd-risk-estimator/ (193, 194). Additionally, as seen in Table 3.8, there are several risk assessment tools that are readily available to the CEP and health care providers. The appropriate assessment tool may depend on the sex, race, and socioeconomic status of the patient; therefore, the CEP should take into consideration how these assessment tools were developed and the populations for whom they are most appropriate (194).

Evaluating CVD risk can also guide the CEP, and other members of the health care team, to implement the lifestyle changes that will serve the patient most effectively, including smoking cessation and dietary modification, in addition to implementing a program of regular physical activity and exercise (194). For some patients, pharmacotherapy may also be a prudent implementation, and discussion with their health care provider may be warranted.

Referring for Medical Clearance

In some cases, information gathered during the preexercise evaluation (*e.g.*, exercise preparticipation health screening, medical history) will result in the participant being referred for medical clearance. Medical clearance is defined as approval from a physician to engage in exercise. When medical clearance is warranted, such as in the case of individuals with CVD, pulmonary, metabolic, or kidney diseases, participants should be referred to their primary care physician. The breadth and depth of medical follow-up is left to the discretion and clinical judgment of the provider to whom the participant is referred.

Because there are no universally recommended medical screening recommendations, the type of procedures conducted during clearance may vary widely from provider to provider and may include verbal consultations, resting or stress electrocardiogram or echocardiogram, computed tomography for the assessment of coronary artery calcium, or even nuclear medicine imaging studies or angiography (2). CEPs may request written clearance along with special instructions or restrictions (*e.g.*, exercise intensity) for the participant in question. For the long-term health and safety of participants, continued communication between the CEP and the individual's health care providers is encouraged.

Ideal Cardiovascular Health

The AHA has identified health metrics to define and monitor "ideal cardiovascular health" (195), shifting attention toward the prevention of risk factors for CVD. This emphasis on prevention is important because, even when risk factors are well managed, CVD risk for these individuals remains elevated compared to those without risk factors (196). Ideal cardiovascular health exists in the presence of seven healthy behaviors and factors that include sufficient physical activity (meeting recommended targets for exercise), nonsmoking, healthy diet, BMI in normal range, normal BP, normal blood glucose, and normal blood lipoprotein levels (197). Ideal cardiovascular health is strongly associated with favorable CVD biomarkers and indicators of subclinical disease (195, 198), as well as a lower risk of long-term CVD mortality and non-CVD mortality (199). According to the AHA's 2018 heart disease and stroke statistics update, the prevalence of ideal status among U.S. adults was 77.1% for smoking, 60.3% for total cholesterol,

Table 3.8   Features of U.S.-Based Cardiovascular Risk Assessment Tools

Risk Assessment Tool	Variables Included	Outcomes Predicted	Derivation Sample	Features	Comments About Implementation
Pooled cohort equations http://tools.acc.org/ascvd-risk-estimator-plus/#!/calculate/estimate/	• Age • Sex • Race • Total cholesterol • HDL-C • SBP • Antihypertensive therapy • History of diabetes mellitus • Current smoking	Hard ASCVD (CHD death, nonfatal MI, fatal or nonfatal stroke)	Five community-based cohorts of white and black participants	Sex- and race-specific equations for four groups: white men, white women, black men, black women	• Available in apps/online and in some electronic health record platforms • Uncertain utility in other racial/ethnic groups • Data available for reclassification by CAC score
Framingham General CVD Risk Profile https://reference.medscape.com/calculator/framingham-cardiovascular-disease-risk	• Age • Sex • Total cholesterol • HDL-C • SBP • Antihypertensive therapy • History of diabetes mellitus • Current smoking	Total CVD (CHD death, MI, coronary insufficiency, angina, ischemic stroke, hemorrhagic stroke, transient ischemic attack, intermittent claudication, and heart failure)	Single community-based cohort of two generations	Sex-specific equations for whites	• Available online • Uncertain utility in other racial/ethnic groups • Uncertain calibration to hard ASCVD endpoint • Uncertain reclassification by CAC score
Reynolds Risk Score http://www.reynoldsriskscore.org/	• Age • Sex • Total cholesterol • HDL-C • SBP • Current smoking • hs-CRP level • Parental history of MI before age 60 yr	Expanded ASCVD (CHD death, nonfatal MI, fatal or nonfatal stroke, coronary revascularization)	Largely white health professionals enrolled in clinical trials	Sex-specific equations	• Available online • Uncertain utility in other racial/ethnic groups • Uncertain calibration to hard ASCVD endpoint • Uncertain reclassification by CAC score

ASCVD, atherosclerotic cardiovascular disease; CAC, coronary artery calcium; CHD, coronary heart disease; CVD, cardiovascular disease; HDL-C, high-density lipoprotein cholesterol; hs-CRP, high-sensitivity C-reactive protein; MI, myocardial infarction; SBP, systolic blood pressure.

Reprinted from Lloyd-Jones DM, Braun LT, Ndumele CE, et al. Use of risk assessment tools to guide decision-making in the primary prevention of atherosclerotic cardiovascular disease: a special report from the American Heart Association and American College of Cardiology. *J Am Coll Cardiol.* 2019;73(24):3153–67. doi:10.1016/j.jacc.2018.11.005. Erratum in: *J Am Coll Cardiol.* 2019 Jun 25;73(24):3234.

53.2% for fasting plasma glucose, 49.7% for physical activity, 45.4% for BP, 29.6% for BMI, and 1.1% for healthy diet (200). A large meta-analysis showed that 32.2% of the participants had an overall poor cardiovascular health status (*i.e.*, having 0–2 ideal metrics), whereas males have greater proportions of ideal total cholesterol and physical activity levels and females have higher estimates of ideal values for the other five metrics (201). Additionally, older adults displayed more than a doubled frequency of poor cardiovascular health compared to younger adults (201).

A strong linear dose-response relationship between ideal cardiovascular health metrics and both all-cause and CVD-related mortality was found in a recent meta-analysis (202). This study demonstrated that achieving only one additional ideal cardiovascular health metric significantly reduces mortality and for each additional ideal cardiovascular health metric an individual has, there was a 19% reduction in mortality from CVD and 11% decline in the risk of all-cause mortality (202).

As an essential member of the health care team, the CEP provides an exercise prescription that can help to prevent CVD risk factors and support the CVD prevention plan prescribed by the health care provider. The CEP may also inform health care providers when assessment suggests that risk factors may not be under good control, that there are problems with treatment adherence, or that adverse side effects are present.

Improving the Safety of Exercise for CVD Patients

A number of strategies can be used by the CEP to promote exercise safety and decrease the chance of an exercise-related adverse event. These include the following (16):

- Monitor participants for changes that may alter their preexercise evaluation and exercise recommendations. For example, a participant who initially declared no signs or symptoms of disease may develop them only after beginning an exercise program. In this case, the participant should discontinue exercise and see a health care provider for medical clearance.
- When prescribing exercise, incorporate a minimum of a 2- to 3-month transitional phase during which the duration and intensity of exercise are gradually increased as fitness improves.
- Incorporate proper warm-ups and cool-downs into exercise sessions.
- Educate participants about the warning signs and symptoms of cardiovascular, metabolic, and kidney diseases and the importance of reporting these immediately to their health care provider.
- Instruct physically inactive individuals to delay vigorous-intensity physical activities until they have gained sufficient physical fitness following the initial exercise training period.

SUMMARY

A substantial body of scientific evidence indicates that regular physical activity brings substantial health benefits to people of all ages. Although exercise is associated with an increased risk for cardiovascular complications, the benefits far outweigh the risk. Proper preparticipation health screening procedures help exercise professionals identify participants who may be at a higher risk for an exercise-related event so that they may be medically cleared prior to participation. Although ACSM preparticipation health screening procedures were designed primarily for nonclinical populations, they can also provide helpful guidance in the clinical setting, particularly when combined with the preparticipation exercise evaluation that consists of a comprehensive medical history and the identification of CVD risk factors. Exercise physiologists working with participants with known CVD can also employ more in-depth risk stratification procedures. Careful attention to these procedures helps to ensure that exercise training is initiated safely.

CHAPTER REVIEW QUESTIONS

1. Discuss the benefits and risks of engaging in a program of regular exercise and physical activity.
2. How does the design of ACSM exercise preparticipation health screening procedures promote increases in physical activity among those ready to participate?
3. Explain the differences between signs and symptoms of disease. Provide some examples of each.
4. Identify the signs and symptoms that should be screened for when conducting the exercise preparticipation screening process.

5. What is the risk of SCD or AMI during exercise in inactive people? How does this change with regular exercise training?
6. List the factors that modulate the risk of exercise-related cardiovascular events.
7. What are some strategies that can decrease the risk of CVD adverse events?

8. Identify the positive and negative risk factors associated with CVD and their defining criteria.
9. List the components of a comprehensive medical history.
10. List the factors associated with increased risk of injuries during exercise and how the exercise prescription might address these factors.

CASE STUDIES

Using the guide given later, determine the following for case studies one through three: (1) use ACSM preparticipation health screening algorithm to determine if medical clearance is needed; and (2) determine the CVD risk factors.

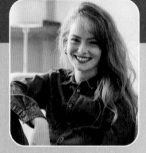

Case 3.1

A 24-year-old woman is joining a fitness center. Since graduating from college and becoming an architect 1 year ago, she no longer walks with her friends in the afternoon or plays intramural basketball. She reports no significant medical history and no symptoms of any diseases, even when running to catch the train. Her father was diagnosed with hypertension when he was 42 years and her 51-year-old mother has Type 2 diabetes. The client smokes socially on occasion (~5–10 cigarettes per week) and drinks alcohol one or two nights a week. She has the following: height: 165.1 cm (65 inches); weight: 74.8 kg (165 lb); BMI: 27.5 kg·m^{-2}; resting heart rate (RHR): 74 beats per minute (bpm); resting BP: 124/74 mm Hg; low-density lipoprotein cholesterol (LDL-C): 118 mg·dL^{-1}; HDL: 61 mg·dL^{-1}; fasting blood glucose (FBG): 106 mg·dL^{-1}. She wants to begin a walking program on a treadmill.

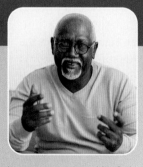

Case 3.2

A 65-year-old male nonsmoker recently decided to train for a 5-km fun run to raise money for muscular dystrophy. He hasn't exercised in years but used to participate in road races when he was younger. His father died of a heart attack at age 67 years and his mother died of breast cancer at age 89 years. Last year, he was diagnosed with Type 2 diabetes and currently takes metformin. He also reports taking a statin to lower his cholesterol. Height: 177.8 cm (70 inches); weight: 98.2 kg (216 lb); BMI: 31.0 kg·m^{-2}; RHR: 78 bpm; resting BP: 134/86 mm Hg; total serum cholesterol: 184 mg·dL^{-1}; HDL: 44 mg·dL^{-1}; FBG: 98 mg·dL^{-1}.

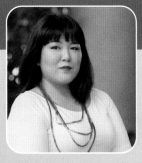

Case 3.3

A 45-year-old perimenopausal Asian American female elementary school teacher would like to start an exercise program as part of a weight management program. She takes a bus to work and walks about four blocks to and from the bus stop each day. She is married and has three children, ages 10, 7, and 5 years. She used to participate in Zumba and Yoga classes but quit after the birth of her second child because of lack of time. She reports no history of surgeries or chronic diseases, but admits to chronic fatigue and periods of depression. Her family history is significant with mother having breast cancer at age 48 years, and her father having long-term hypertension who developed chronic kidney disease and received a kidney transplant 1 year ago at age 65 years. Height: 157.5 cm (52 inches); weight: 70.8 kg (156 lb); BMI: 28.5 kg·m^{-2}; RHR: 82 bpm; resting BP: 130/80 mm Hg; total serum cholesterol: 210 mg·dL^{-1}; HDL: 40 mg·dL^{-1}; FBG: 88 mg·dL^{-1}.

CASE STUDY GUIDE

Preparticipation Health Screening

	Case 3.1	Case 3.2	Case 3.3
Currently participates in regular exercise?			
Known CV, metabolic, or kidney disease?			
Signs or symptoms suggestive of disease?			
Desired intensity?			
Medical clearance needed?			

CVD Risk Factors

Age?			
Family history?			
Cigarette smoking?			
Physical inactivity?			
BMI/waist circumference?			
Blood pressure?			
Lipids?			
Blood glucose?			
Negative risk factor — HDL ≥ 60 mg·dL^{-1}			
Number of CVD risk factors?			

REFERENCES

1. Physical Activity Guidelines Advisory Committee, *Physical Activity Guidelines Advisory Committee Scientific Report*. Washington (DC): U.S. Department of Health and Human Services; 2018.
2. American College of Sports Medicine. *ACSM's Guidelines for Exercise Testing and Prescription*. 11th ed. Philadelphia (PA): Wolters Kluwer; 2022.
3. Artinian NT, Fletcher GF, Mozaffarian D, et al; American Heart Association Prevention Committee of the Council on Cardiovascular Nursing. Interventions to promote physical activity and dietary lifestyle changes for cardiovascular risk factor reduction in adults: a scientific statement from the American Heart Association. *Circulation*. 2010;122(4):406–41.
4. Lane Cordova AD, Jerome GJ, Paluch AE, et al; Committee on Physical Activity of the American Heart Association Council on Lifestyle and Cardiometabolic Health. Supporting physical activity in patients and populations during life events and transitions: a scientific statement from the American Heart Association. *Circulation*. 2022;145(4):e117–28.

5. Patel AV, Friedenreich CM, Moore SC, et al. American College of Sports Medicine Roundtable Report on physical activity, sedentary behavior, and cancer prevention and control. *Med Sci Sports Exerc.* 2019;51(11):2391–402.

6. World Health Organization. WHO guidelines on physical activity and sedentary behavior. 2020. Available from: https://www.who.int/publications/i/item/9789240015128.

7. U.S. Department of Health and Human Services. *Physical Activity Guidelines for Americans.* 2nd ed. U.S. Department of Health and Human Services; 2018. Available from: https://health.gov/sites/default/files/2019-09/Physical_Activity_Guidelines_2nd_edition.pdf.

8. Hargreaves M. Exercise and health: historical perspectives and new insights. *J Appl Physiol (1985).* 2021;131(2):575–88.

9. Carter S, Hartman Y, Holder S, Thijssen DH, Hopkins ND. Sedentary behavior and cardiovascular disease risk: mediating mechanisms. *Exerc Sport Sci Rev.* 2017;45(2):80–6.

10. Garber CE, Blissmer B, Deschenes MR, et al. American College of Sports Medicine position stand. Quantity and quality of exercise for developing and maintaining cardiorespiratory, musculoskeletal, and neuromotor fitness in apparently healthy adults: guidance for prescribing exercise. *Med Sci Sports Exerc.* 2011;43(7):1334–59.

11. Young DR, Hivert MF, Alhassan S, et al; Physical Activity Committee of the Council on Lifestyle and Cardiometabolic Health; Council on Clinical Cardiology; Council on Epidemiology and Prevention; Council on Functional Genomics and Translational Biology; and Stroke Council. Sedentary behavior and cardiovascular morbidity and mortality: a science advisory from the American Heart Association. *Circulation.* 2016;134(13):e262–79.

12. Franklin BA. Cardiovascular events associated with exercise. The risk-protection paradox. *J Cardiopulm Rehabil.* 2005;25(4):189–95; quiz 196–7.

13. Franklin BA, Thompson PD, Al-Zaiti SS, et al; American Heart Association Physical Activity Committee of the Council on Lifestyle and Cardiometabolic Health; Council on Cardiovascular and Stroke Nursing; Council on Clinical Cardiology; and Stroke Council. Exercise-related acute cardiovascular events and potential deleterious adaptations following long-term exercise training: placing the risks into perspective-an update: a scientific statement from the American Heart Association. *Circulation.* 2020;141(13):e705–36.

14. Hootman JM, Macera CA, Ainsworth BE, Addy CL, Martin M, Blair SN. Epidemiology of musculoskeletal injuries among sedentary and physically active adults. *Med Sci Sports Exerc.* 2002;34(5):838–44.

15. Orsi C, Montomoli C, Otte D, Morandi A. Road accidents involving bicycles: configurations and injuries. *Int J Inj Contr Saf Promot.* 2017;24(4):534–43.

16. Riebe D, Franklin BA, Thompson PD, et al. Updating ACSM's recommendations for exercise preparticipation health screening. *Med Sci Sports Exerc.* 2015;47(11):2473–9.

17. Drew MK, Finch CF. The relationship between training load and injury, illness and soreness: a systematic and literature review. *Sports Med.* 2016;46(6):861–83.

18. Mittleman MA, Mostofsky E. Physical, psychological and chemical triggers of acute cardiovascular events: preventive strategies. *Circulation.* 2011;124(3):346–54.

19. Saint-Maurice PF, Troiano RP, Matthews CE, Kraus WE. Moderate-to-vigorous physical activity and all-cause mortality: do bouts matter? *J Am Heart Assoc.* 2018;7(6):e007678.

20. Whitfield GP, Hyde ET, Carlson SA. Participation in leisure-time aerobic physical activity among adults, National Health Interview Survey, 1998–2018. *J Phys Act Health.* 2021;18(S1):S25–36.

21. Guo L, Zhang S. Association between ideal cardiovascular health metrics and risk of cardiovascular events or mortality: a meta-analysis of prospective studies. *Clin Cardiol.* 2017;40(12):1339–46.

22. Bauman A, Merom D, Bull FC, Buchner DM, Fiatarone Singh MA. Updating the evidence for physical activity: summative reviews of the epidemiological evidence, prevalence, and interventions to promote "Active Aging". *Gerontologist.* 2016;56(Suppl 2):S268–80.

23. Campbell KL, Winters-Stone KM, Wiskemann J, et al. Exercise guidelines for cancer survivors: consensus statement from International Multidisciplinary Roundtable. *Med Sci Sports Exerc.* 2019;51(11):2375–90.

24. Claas SA, Arnett DK. The role of healthy lifestyle in the primordial prevention of cardiovascular disease. *Curr Cardiol Rep.* 2016;18(6):56.

25. Colberg SR, Sigal RJ, Yardley JE, et al. Physical activity/exercise and diabetes: a position statement of the American Diabetes Association. *Diabetes Care.* 2016;39(11):2065–79.

26. BaroneGibbs B, Hivert MF, Jerome GJ, et al; American Heart Association Council on Lifestyle and Cardiometabolic Health; Council on Cardiovascular and Stroke Nursing; and Council on Clinical Cardiology. Physical activity as a critical component of first-line treatment for elevated blood pressure or cholesterol: who, what, and how?: a scientific statement From the American Heart Association. *Hypertension.* 2021;78(2):e26–37.

27. Colberg SR, Albright AL, Blissmer BJ, et al; American College of Sports Medicine; American Diabetes Association. Exercise and type 2 diabetes: American College of Sports Medicine and the American Diabetes Association: joint position statement. Exercise and type 2 diabetes. *Med Sci Sports Exerc.* 2010;42(12):2282–303.

28. Marwick TH, Hordern MD, Miller T, et al; Council on Clinical Cardiology, American Heart Association Exercise, Cardiac Rehabilitation, and Prevention Committee; Council on Cardiovascular Disease in the Young; Council on Cardiovascular Nursing; Council on Nutrition, Physical Activity, and Metabolism; Interdisciplinary Council on Quality of Care and Outcomes Research. Exercise training for type 2 diabetes mellitus: impact on cardiovascular risk: a scientific statement from the American Heart Association. *Circulation.* 2009;119(25):3244–62.

29. Treat-Jacobson D, McDermott MM, Bronas UG, et al; American Heart Association Council on Peripheral Vascular Disease; Council on Quality of Care and Outcomes Research; and Council on Cardiovascular and Stroke Nursing. Optimal exercise programs for patients with peripheral artery disease: a scientific statement from the American Heart Association. *Circulation.* 2019;139(4):e10–33.

30. Deslandes A, Moraes H, Ferreira C, et al. Exercise and mental health: many reasons to move. *Neuropsychobiology.* 2009;59(4):191–8.

31. Bannuru RR, Osani MC, Vaysbrot EE, et al. OARSI guidelines for the non-surgical management of knee, hip, and polyarticular osteoarthritis. *Osteoarthritis Cartilage*. 2019;27 (11):1578–89.

32. Bonavita S. Exercise and Parkinson's disease. *Adv Exp Med Biol*. 2020;1228:289–301.

33. Kim Y, Lai B, Mehta T, et al. Exercise training guidelines for multiple sclerosis, stroke, and Parkinson disease: rapid review and synthesis. *Am J Phys Med Rehabil*. 2019;98(7):613–21.

34. Kolasinski SL, Neogi T, Hochberg MC, et al. 2019 American College of Rheumatology/Arthritis Foundation guideline for the management of osteoarthritis of the hand, hip, and knee. *Arthritis Care Res (Hoboken)*. 2020;72(2):149–62.

35. García-Hermoso A, Cavero-Redondo I, Ramírez-Vélez R, et al. Muscular strength as a predictor of all-cause mortality in an apparently healthy population: a systematic review and meta-analysis of data from approximately 2 million men and women. *Arch Phys Med Rehabil*. 2018;99(10):2100–13.e5.

36. Juraschek SP, Blaha MJ, Blumenthal RS, et al. Cardiorespiratory fitness and incident diabetes: the FIT (Henry Ford ExercIse Testing) project. *Diabetes Care*. 2015;38(6):1075–81.

37. Kang AW, Bostom AG, Kim H, et al. Physical activity and risk of cardiovascular events and all-cause mortality among kidney transplant recipients. *Nephrol Dial Transplant*. 2020;35(8):1436–43.

38. Laddu D, Parimi N, Cauley JA, et al. The association between trajectories of physical activity and all-cause and cause-specific mortality. *J Gerontol A Biol Sci Med Sci*. 2018;73(12):1708–13.

39. Li R, Xia J, Zhang XI, et al. Associations of muscle mass and strength with all-cause mortality among US older adults. *Med Sci Sports Exerc*. 2018;50(3):458–67.

40. Ozemek C, Laddu DR, Lavie CJ, et al. An update on the role of cardiorespiratory fitness, structured exercise and lifestyle physical activity in preventing cardiovascular disease and health risk. *Prog Cardiovasc Dis*. 2018;61(5–6):484–90.

41. Wahid A, Manek N, Nichols M, et al. Quantifying the association between physical activity and cardiovascular disease and diabetes: a systematic review and meta-analysis. *J Am Heart Assoc*. 2016;5(9):e002495.

42. Nocon M, Hiemann T, Müller-Riemenschneider F, Thalau F, Roll S, Willich SN. Association of physical activity with all-cause and cardiovascular mortality: a systematic review and meta-analysis. *Eur J Cardiovasc Prev Rehabil*. 2008;15(3):239–46.

43. Hupin D, Roche F, Gremeaux V, et al. Even a low-dose of moderate-to-vigorous physical activity reduces mortality by 22% in adults aged ≥60 years: a systematic review and meta-analysis. *Br J Sports Med*. 2015;49(19):1262–7.

44. Mittleman MA, Maclure M, Tofler GH, Sherwood JB, Goldberg RJ, Muller JE. Triggering of acute myocardial infarction by heavy physical exertion. Protection against triggering by regular exertion. Determinants of Myocardial Infarction Onset Study Investigators. *N Engl J Med*. 1993;329(23):1677–83.

45. Ekelund U, Tarp J, Steene-Johannessen J, et al. Dose-response associations between accelerometry measured physical activity and sedentary time and all cause mortality: systematic review and harmonised meta-analysis. *BMJ*. 2019;366:l4570.

46. Morishita S, Hamaue Y, Fukushima T, Tanaka T, Fu JB, Nakano J. Effect of exercise on mortality and recurrence in patients with cancer: a systematic review and meta-analysis. *Integr Cancer Ther*. 2020;19:1534735420917462.

47. Kaminsky LA, Arena R, Ellingsen Ø, et al. Cardiorespiratory fitness and cardiovascular disease — the past, present, and future. *Prog Cardiovasc Dis*. 2019;62(2):86–93.

48. Myers J, McAuley P, Lavie CJ, Despres JP, Arena R, Kokkinos P. Physical activity and cardiorespiratory fitness as major markers of cardiovascular risk: their independent and interwoven importance to health status. *Prog Cardiovasc Dis*. 2015;57(4):306–14.

49. Ross R, Blair SN, Arena R, et al; American Heart Association Physical Activity Committee of the Council on Lifestyle and Cardiometabolic Health; Council on Clinical Cardiology; Council on Epidemiology and Prevention; Council on Cardiovascular and Stroke Nursing; Council on Functional Genomics and Translational Biology; Stroke Council. Importance of assessing cardiorespiratory fitness in clinical practice: a case for fitness as a clinical vital sign: a scientific statement from the American Heart Association. *Circulation*. 2016;134(24):e653–99.

50. Despres JP. Physical activity, sedentary behaviours, and cardiovascular health: when will cardiorespiratory fitness become a vital sign? *Can J Cardiol*. 2016;32(4):505–13.

51. Mandsager K, Harb S, Cremer P, Phelan D, Nissen SE, Jaber W. Association of cardiorespiratory fitness with long-term mortality among adults undergoing exercise treadmill testing. *JAMA Netw Open*. 2018;1(6):e183605.

52. Lemes ÍR, Sui X, Fritz SL, et al. Cardiorespiratory fitness and risk of all-cause, cardiovascular disease, and cancer mortality in men with musculoskeletal conditions. *J Phys Act Health*. 2019;16(2):134–40.

53. Harb SC, Wang TKM, Cremer PC, et al. Associations between cardiorespiratory fitness, sex and long term mortality amongst adults undergoing exercise treadmill testing. *Int J Cardiol*. 2021;342:103–7.

54. Al-Mallah MH, Juraschek SP, Whelton S, et al. Sex differences in cardiorespiratory fitness and all-cause mortality: the henry ford exercise testing (FIT) project. *Mayo Clin Proc*. 2016;91(6):755–762.

55. Wickramasinghe CD, Ayers CR, Das S, de Lemos JA, Willis BL, Berry JD. Prediction of 30-year risk for cardiovascular mortality by fitness and risk factor levels: the Cooper Center Longitudinal Study. *Circ Cardiovasc Qual Outcomes*. 2014;7(4):597–602.

56. Blair SN, Kohl HW 3rd, Barlow CE, Paffenbarger RS Jr, Gibbons LW, Macera CA. Changes in physical fitness and all-cause mortality. A prospective study of healthy and unhealthy men. *JAMA*. 1995;273(14):1093–8.

57. Imboden MT, Harber MP, Whaley MH, et al. The association between the change in directly measured cardiorespiratory fitness across time and mortality risk. *Prog Cardiovasc Dis*. 2019;62(2):157–62.

58. Martin BJ, Arena R, Haykowsky M, et al; APPROACH Investigators. Cardiovascular fitness and mortality after contemporary cardiac rehabilitation. *Mayo Clin Proc*. 2013;88(5):455–63.

59. Qureshi WT, Alirhayim Z, Blaha MJ, et al. Cardiorespiratory fitness and risk of incident atrial fibrillation: results from the Henry Ford Exercise Testing (FIT) Project. *Circulation*. 2015;131(21):1827–34.

60. Xue Z, Zhou Y, Wu C, et al. Dose-response relationship of cardiorespiratory fitness with incident atrial fibrillation. *Heart Fail Rev.* 2020;25(3):419–25.

61. Holtermann A, Gyntelberg F, Bauman A, Jensen MT. Cardiorespiratory fitness, fatness and incident diabetes. *Diabetes Res Clin Pract.* 2017;134:113–20.

62. Kokkinos P, Faselis C, Narayan P, et al. Cardiorespiratory fitness and incidence of type 2 diabetes in United States veterans on statin therapy. *Am J Med.* 2017;130(10):1192–8.

63. Qiu S, Cai X, Yang B, et al. Association between cardiorespiratory fitness and risk of type 2 diabetes: a meta-analysis. *Obesity (Silver Spring).* 2019;27(2):315–24.

64. Ezzatvar Y, Ramírez-Vélez R, Sáez de Asteasu ML, et al. Cardiorespiratory fitness and all-cause mortality in adults diagnosed with cancer systematic review and meta-analysis. *Scand J Med Sci Sports.* 2021;31(9):1745–52.

65. Fardman A, Banschick GD, Rabia R, et al. Cardiorespiratory fitness and survival following cancer diagnosis. *Eur J Prev Cardiol.* 2021;28(11):1242–9.

66. Hillreiner A, Baumeister SE, Sedlmeier AM, Finger JD, Schlitt HJ, Leitzmann MF. Association between cardiorespiratory fitness and colorectal cancer in the UK Biobank. *Eur J Epidemiol.* 2020;35(10):961–73.

67. Vainshelboim B, Lima RM, Edvardsen E, Myers J. Cardiorespiratory fitness, incidence and mortality of lung cancer in men: a prospective cohort study. *J Sci Med Sport.* 2019;22(4):403–7.

68. Ashor AW, Lara J, Siervo M, et al. Exercise modalities and endothelial function: a systematic review and dose-response meta-analysis of randomized controlled trials. *Sports Med.* 2015;45(2):279–96.

69. Cartee GD, Hepple RT, Bamman MM, Zierath JR. Exercise promotes healthy aging of skeletal muscle. *Cell Metab.* 2016;23(6):1034–47.

70. da Silva VP, de Oliveira NA, Silveira H, Mello RG, Deslandes AC. Heart rate variability indexes as a marker of chronic adaptation in athletes: a systematic review. *Ann Noninvasive Electrocardiol.* 2015;20(2):108–18.

71. Fogelholm M. Physical activity, fitness and fatness: relations to mortality, morbidity and disease risk factors. A systematic review. *Obes Rev.* 2010;11(3):202–21.

72. Lavie CJ, O'Keefe JH, Sallis RE. Exercise and the heart — the harm of too little and too much. *Curr Sports Med Rep.* 2015;14(2):104–9.

73. Lin X, Zhang X, Guo J, et al. Effects of exercise training on cardiorespiratory fitness and biomarkers of cardiometabolic health: a systematic review and meta-analysis of randomized controlled trials. *J Am Heart Assoc.* 2015;4(7):e002014.

74. Phillips SA, Mahmoud AM, Brown MD, Haus JM. Exercise interventions and peripheral arterial function: implications for cardio-metabolic disease. *Prog Cardiovasc Dis.* 2015;57(5):521–34.

75. Wilson MG, Ellison GM, Cable NT. Basic science behind the cardiovascular benefits of exercise. *Heart.* 2015;101(10):758–65.

76. Tremblay MS, Aubert S, Barnes JD, et al. Sedentary Behavior Research Network (SBRN) — terminology consensus project process and outcome. *Int J Behav Nutr Phys Act.* 2017;14(1):75.

77. Owen N, Healy GN, Dempsey PC, et al. Sedentary behavior and public health: integrating the evidence and identifying potential solutions. *Annu Rev Public Health.* 2020;41:265–87.

78. de Rezende LF, Rodrigues Lopes M, Rey-López JP, Matsudo VK, Luiz Odo C. Sedentary behavior and health outcomes: an overview of systematic reviews. *PLoS One.* 2014;9(8):e105620.

79. Ekelund U, Tarp J, Fagerland MW, et al. Joint associations of accelerometer measured physical activity and sedentary time with all-cause mortality: a harmonised meta-analysis in more than 44 000 middle-aged and older individuals. *Br J Sports Med.* 2020;54(24):1499–506.

80. Diaz KM, Howard VJ, Hutto B, et al. Patterns of sedentary behavior in US middle-age and older adults: the regards study. *Med Sci Sports Exerc.* 2016;48(3):430–8.

81. Diaz KM, Duran AT, Colabianchi N, Judd SE, Howard VJ, Hooker SP. Potential effects on mortality of replacing sedentary time with short sedentary bouts or physical activity: a national cohort study. *Am J Epidemiol.* 2019;188(3):537–44.

82. Shuval K, Finley CE, Barlow CE, Nguyen BT, Njike VY, Pettee Gabriel K. Independent and joint effects of sedentary time and cardiorespiratory fitness on all-cause mortality: the Cooper Center Longitudinal Study. *BMJ Open.* 2015;5(10):e008956.

83. Benatti FB, Ried-Larsen M. The effects of breaking up prolonged sitting time: a review of experimental studies. *Med Sci Sports Exerc.* 2015;47(10):2053–61.

84. Saunders TJ, Atkinson HF, Burr J, MacEwen B, Skeaff CM, Peddie MC. The acute metabolic and vascular impact of interrupting prolonged sitting: a systematic review and meta-analysis. *Sports Med.* 2018;48(10):2347–66.

85. Dahabreh IJ, Paulus JK. Association of episodic physical and sexual activity with triggering of acute cardiac events: systematic review and meta-analysis. *JAMA.* 2011;305(12):1225–33.

86. Hallqvist J, Möller J, Ahlbom A, Diderichsen F, Reuterwall C, de Faire U. Does heavy physical exertion trigger myocardial infarction? A case-crossover analysis nested in a population-based case-referent study. *Am J Epidemiol.* 2000;151(5):459–67.

87. Lee IM, Sesso HD, Oguma Y, Paffenbarger RS Jr. The "weekend warrior" and risk of mortality. *Am J Epidemiol.* 2004;160(7):636–41.

88. Thompson PD, Franklin BA, Balady GJ, et al; American Heart Association Council on Nutrition, Physical Activity, and Metabolism; American Heart Association Council on Clinical Cardiology; American College of Sports Medicine. Exercise and acute cardiovascular events placing the risks into perspective: a scientific statement from the American Heart Association Council on nutrition, physical activity, and metabolism and the council on clinical cardiology. *Circulation.* 2007;115(17):2358–68.

89. Goodman JM, Burr JF, Banks L, Thomas SG. The acute risks of exercise in apparently healthy adults and relevance for prevention of cardiovascular events. *Can J Cardiol.* 2016;32(4):523–32.

90. Bohm P, Scharhag J, Meyer T. Data from a nationwide registry on sports-related sudden cardiac deaths in Germany. *Eur J Prev Cardiol.* 2016;23(6):649–56.

91. Franklin BA, Lavie CJ. Triggers of acute cardiovascular events and potential preventive strategies: prophylactic role of regular exercise. *Phys Sportsmed.* 2011;39(4):11–21.

92. Albert CM, Mittleman MA, Chae CU, Lee IM, Hennekens CH, Manson JE. Triggering of sudden death from cardiac causes by vigorous exertion. *N Engl J Med.* 2000;343(19):1355–61.

93. Kiyohara K, Sado J, Matsuyama T, et al. Out-of-hospital cardiac arrests during exercise among urban inhabitants in Japan: insights from a population-based registry of Osaka City. *Resuscitation.* 2017;117:14–7.

94. Marijon E, Tafflet M, Celermajer DS, et al. Sports-related sudden death in the general population. *Circulation.* 2011;124(6):672–81.

95. Berdowski J, de Beus MF, Blom M, et al. Exercise-related out-of-hospital cardiac arrest in the general population: incidence and prognosis. *Eur Heart J.* 2013;34(47):3616–23.

96. Søholm H, Kjaergaard J, Thomsen JH, et al. Myocardial infarction is a frequent cause of exercise-related resuscitated out-of-hospital cardiac arrest in a general non-athletic population. *Resuscitation.* 2014;85(11):1612–8.

97. Vander L, Franklin B, Rubenfire M. Cardiovascular complications of recreational physical activity. *Phys Sportsmed.* 1982;10(6):89–97.

98. Marijon E, Uy-Evanado A, Reinier K, et al. Sudden cardiac arrest during sports activity in middle age. *Circulation.* 2015;131(16):1384–91.

99. Franklin BA, Bonzheim K, Gordon S, Timmis GC. Safety of medically supervised outpatient cardiac rehabilitation exercise therapy: a 16-year follow-up. *Chest.* 1998;114(3):902–6.

100. Chappex N, Schlaepfer J, Fellmann F, Bhuiyan ZA, Wilhelm M, Michaud K. Sudden cardiac death among general population and sport related population in forensic experience. *J Forensic Leg Med.* 2015;35:62–8.

101. Kim JH, Malhotra R, Chiampas G, et al. Cardiac arrest during long-distance running races. *N Engl J Med.* 2012; 366(2):130–40.

102. Whang W, Manson JE, Hu FB, et al. Physical exertion, exercise, and sudden cardiac death in women. *JAMA.* 2006; 295(12):1399–403.

103. Harris KM, Creswell LL, Haas TS, et al. Death and cardiac arrest in U.S. triathlon participants, 1985 to 2016: a case series. *Ann Intern Med.* 2017;167(8):529–35.

104. Baylin A, Hernandez-Diaz S, Siles X, Kabagambe EK, Campos H. Triggers of nonfatal myocardial infarction in Costa Rica: heavy physical exertion, sexual activity, and infection. *Ann Epidemiol.* 2007;17(2):112–8.

105. Smyth A, O'Donnell M, Yusuf S; INTERHEART Investigators. Response by Smyth et al to Letters Regarding Article, "Physical activity and anger or emotional upset as triggers of acute myocardial infarction: the interheart study". *Circulation.* 2016;134(15):1059–67.

106. von Klot S, Mittleman MA, Dockery DW, et al. Intensity of physical exertion and triggering of myocardial infarction: a case-crossover study. *Eur Heart J.* 2008;29(15):1881–8.

107. Aune D, Schlesinger S, Hamer M, Norat T, Riboli E. Physical activity and the risk of sudden cardiac death: a systematic review and meta-analysis of prospective studies. *BMC Cardiovasc Disord.* 2020;20(1):318.

108. Burtscher M. Risk and protective factors for sudden cardiac death during leisure activities in the mountains: an update. *Heart Lung Circ.* 2017;26(8):757–62.

109. Burtscher M, Pachinger O, Mittleman MA, Ulmer H. Prior myocardial infarction is the major risk factor associated with sudden cardiac death during downhill skiing. *Int J Sports Med.* 2000;21(8):613–5.

110. Haapaniemi S, Franklin BA, Wegner JH, et al. Electrocardiographic responses to deer hunting activities in men with and without coronary artery disease. *Am J Cardiol.* 2007;100(2):175–9.

111. Northcote RJ, Ballantyne D. The influence of beta-adrenoceptor blockers with and without intrinsic sympathomimetic activity on heart rate, arrhythmias and ST-T segments, using ambulatory electrocardiography. *Br J Clin Pharmacol.* 1988;25(2):179–85.

112. Waite O, Smith A, Madge L, Spring H, Noret N. Sudden cardiac death in marathons: a systematic review. *Phys Sportsmed.* 2016;44(1):79–84.

113. Link MS, Estes NAM 3rd. Sudden cardiac death in the athlete: bridging the gaps between evidence, policy, and practice. *Circulation.* 2012;125(20):2511–6.

114. Burtscher M, Ponchia A. The risk of cardiovascular events during leisure time activities at altitude. *Prog Cardiovasc Dis.* 2010;52(6):507–11.

115. Cornwell WK 3rd, Baggish AL, Bhatta YKD, et al; American Heart Association Exercise, Cardiac Rehabilitation, and Secondary Prevention Committee of the Council on Clinical Cardiology; and Council on Arteriosclerosis, Thrombosis and Vascular Biology. Clinical implications for exercise at altitude among individuals with cardiovascular disease: a scientific statement from the American Heart Association. *J Am Heart Assoc.* 2021;10(19):e023225.

116. Franklin BA, George P, Henry R, Gordon S, Timmis GC, O'Neill WW. Acute myocardial infarction after manual or automated snow removal. *Am J Cardiol.* 2001;87(11):1282–3.

117. Finocchiaro G, Papadakis M, Robertus JL, et al. Etiology of sudden death in sports: insights from a United Kingdom regional registry. *J Am Coll Cardiol.* 2016;67(18):2108–15.

118. Ullal AJ, Abdelfattah RS, Ashley EA, Froelicher VF. Hypertrophic cardiomyopathy as a cause of sudden cardiac death in the young: a meta-analysis. *Am J Med.* 2016;129(5):486–96.e2.

119. El Masri I, Kayali SM, Blount C, Kirolos I, Khouzam JP, Kabra R. Is exercise helpful or harmful in dealing with specific arrhythmia. *Curr Probl Cardiol.* 2021;46(3):100740.

120. Balady GJ, Williams MA, Ades PA, et al; American Heart Association Exercise, Cardiac Rehabilitation, and Prevention Committee, the Council on Clinical Cardiology; American Heart Association Council on Cardiovascular Nursing; American Heart Association Council on Epidemiology and Prevention; American Heart Association Council on Nutrition, Physical Activity, and Metabolism; American Association of Cardiovascular and Pulmonary Rehabilitation. Core components of cardiac rehabilitation/secondary prevention programs: 2007 update: a scientific statement from the American Heart Association Exercise, Cardiac Rehabilitation, and Prevention Committee, the Council on Clinical Cardiology; the Councils on Cardiovascular Nursing, Epidemiology and Prevention, and Nutrition, Physical Activity, and Metabolism; and the American Association of Cardiovascular and Pulmonary Rehabilitation. *Circulation.* 2007;115(20):2675–82.

121. Taylor RS, Long L, Mordi IR, et al. Exercise-based rehabilitation for heart failure: Cochrane systematic review, meta-analysis, and trial sequential analysis. *JACC Heart Fail.* 2019;7(8):691–705.

122. Cerrone M. Exercise: a risky subject in arrhythmogenic cardiomyopathy. *J Am Heart Assoc.* 2018;7(12):e009611.

123. Goff ZD, Calkins H. Sudden death related cardiomyopathies — arrhythmogenic right ventricular cardiomyopathy, arrhythmogenic cardiomyopathy, and exercise-induced cardiomyopathy. *Prog Cardiovasc Dis.* 2019;62(3):217–26.

124. James CA, Bhonsale A, Tichnell C, et al. Exercise increases age-related penetrance and arrhythmic risk in arrhythmogenic right ventricular dysplasia/cardiomyopathy-associated desmosomal mutation carriers. *J Am Coll Cardiol.* 2013; 62(14):1290–7.

125. Al-Khatib SM, Stevenson WG, Ackerman MJ, et al. 2017 AHA/ACC/HRS guideline for management of patients with ventricular arrhythmias and the prevention of sudden cardiac death: a report of the American College of Cardiology/American Heart Association Task Force on Clinical Practice Guidelines and the Heart Rhythm Society. *J Am Coll Cardiol.* 2018;72(14):e91–220.

126. Eijsvogels TM, Fernandez AB, Thompson PD. Are there deleterious cardiac effects of acute and chronic endurance exercise? *Physiol Rev.* 2016;96(1):99–125.

127. Parry-Williams G, Sharma S. The effects of endurance exercise on the heart: panacea or poison? *Nat Rev Cardiol.* 2020;17(7):402–12.

128. Sharma S, Merghani A, Mont L. Exercise and the heart: the good, the bad, and the ugly. *Eur Heart J.* 2015;36(23): 1445–53.

129. Elliott AD, Linz D, Verdicchio CV, Sanders P. Exercise and atrial fibrillation: prevention or causation? *Heart Lung Circ.* 2018;27(9):1078–85.

130. Claessen G, Colyn E, La Gerche A, et al. Long-term endurance sport is a risk factor for development of lone atrial flutter. *Heart.* 2011;97(11):918–22.

131. Elosua R, Arquer A, Mont L, et al. Sport practice and the risk of lone atrial fibrillation: a case-control study. *Int J Cardiol.* 2006;108(3):332–7.

132. Molina L, Mont L, Marrugat J, et al. Long-term endurance sport practice increases the incidence of lone atrial fibrillation in men: a follow-up study. *Europace.* 2008;10(5): 618–23.

133. Maron BJ, Udelson JE, Bonow RO, et al; American Heart Association Electrocardiography and Arrhythmias Committee of Council on Clinical Cardiology, Council on Cardiovascular Disease in Young, Council on Cardiovascular and Stroke Nursing, Council on Functional Genomics and Translational Biology, and American College of Cardiology. Eligibility and disqualification recommendations for competitive athletes with cardiovascular abnormalities: task force 3: hypertrophic cardiomyopathy, arrhythmogenic right ventricular cardiomyopathy and other cardiomyopathies, and myocarditis: a scientific statement from the American Heart Association and American College of Cardiology. *Circulation.* 2015;132(22):e273–80.

134. Colbert LH, Hootman JM, Macera CA. Physical activity-related injuries in walkers and runners in the aerobics center longitudinal study. *Clin J Sport Med.* 2000;10(4): 259–63.

135. Gilchrist J, Jones BH, Sleet DA, Kimsey CD; CDC. Exercise-related injuries among women: strategies for prevention from civilian and military studies. *MMWR Recomm Rep.* 2000;49(RR-2):15–33.

136. Howard EN, DeFina LF, Leonard D, Custodio MA, Morrow JR Jr. Physical activity and musculoskeletal injuries in women: the women's injury study. *J Womens Health (Larchmt).* 2013;22(12):1038–42.

137. Conn JM, Annest JL, Gilchrist J. Sports and recreation related injury episodes in the US population, 1997–99. *Inj Prev.* 2003;9(2):117–23.

138. van Mechelen W. Running injuries. A review of the epidemiological literature. *Sports Med.* 1992;14(5):320–35.

139. Lopes AD, Hespanhol Júnior LC, Yeung SS, Costa LO. What are the main running-related musculoskeletal injuries? A systematic review. *Sports Med.* 2012;42(10):891–905.

140. Williams PT, Thompson PD. Dose-dependent effects of training and detraining on weight in 6406 runners during 7.4 years. *Obesity (Silver Spring).* 2006;14(11):1975–84.

141. Gardiner B, Devereux G, Beato M. Injury risk and injury incidence rates in crossfit. *J Sports Med Phys Fitness.* 2020;60(7):1005–13.

142. Klimek C, Ashbeck C, Brook AJ, Durall C. Are injuries more common with crossfit training than other forms of exercise? *J Sport Rehabil.* 2018;27(3):295–9.

143. Gabbett TJ, Kennelly S, Sheehan J, et al. If overuse injury is a 'training load erro', should undertraining be viewed the same way? *Br J Sports Med.* 2016;50(17):1017–8.

144. Gabbett TJ. The training-injury prevention paradox: should athletes be training smarter and harder? *Br J Sports Med.* 2016;50(5):273–80.

145. Hootman JM, Macera CA, Ainsworth BE, Martin M, Addy CL, Blair SN. Association among physical activity level, cardiorespiratory fitness, and risk of musculoskeletal injury. *Am J Epidemiol.* 2001;154(3):251–8.

146. Suchomel TJ, Nimphius S, Stone MH. The importance of muscular strength in athletic performance. *Sports Med.* 2016;46(10):1419–49.

147. Laursen JB, Andersen TE, Andersen LB. Strength training as superior, dose-dependent and safe prevention of acute and overuse sports injuries: a systematic review, qualitative analysis and meta-analysis. *Br J Sports Med.* 2018;52(24):1557–63.

148. Suchomel TJ, Nimphius S, Bellon CR, Stone MH. The importance of muscular strength: training considerations. *Sports Med.* 2018;48(4):765–85.

149. Knapik JJ. The importance of physical fitness for injury prevention: part 2. *J Spec Oper Med.* 2015;15(2):112–5.

150. Franklin BA, McCullough PA. Cardiorespiratory fitness: an independent and additive marker of risk stratification and health outcomes. *Mayo Clin Proc.* 2009;84(9):776–9.

151. Berlin JA, Colditz GA. A meta-analysis of physical activity in the prevention of coronary heart disease. *Am J Epidemiol.* 1990;132(4):612–28.

152. Powell KE, Thompson PD, Caspersen CJ, Kendrick JS. Physical activity and the incidence of coronary heart disease. *Annu Rev Public Health.* 1987;8:253–87.

153. Schuna JM Jr, Johnson WD, Tudor-Locke C. Adult self-reported and objectively monitored physical activity and sedentary behavior: NHANES 2005–2006. *Int J Behav Nutr Phys Act.* 2013;10:126.

154. Moser DK, Kimble LP, Alberts MJ, et al. Reducing delay in seeking treatment by patients with acute coronary syndrome

and stroke: a scientific statement from the American Heart Association Council on cardiovascular nursing and stroke council. *Circulation*. 2006;114(2):168–82.

155. Hill K, Gardiner PA, Cavalheri V, Jenkins SC, Healy GN. Physical activity and sedentary behaviour: applying lessons to chronic obstructive pulmonary disease. *Intern Med J*. 2015;45(5):474–82.

156. de Barros e Silva PG, Califf RM, Sun JL, et al. Chronic obstructive pulmonary disease and cardiovascular risk: insights from the NAVIGATOR trial. *Int J Cardiol*. 2014;176(3):1126–8.

157. Magal M, Riebe D. New preparticipation health screening recommendations: what exercise professionals need to know. *ACSM Health Fitness J*. 2016;20(3):22–7.

158. Williams SV, Fihn SD, Gibbons RJ. Guidelines for the management of patients with chronic stable angina: diagnosis and risk stratification. *Ann Intern Med*. 2001;135(7):530–47.

159. American Association of Cardiovascular and Pulmonary Rehabilitation. Stratification algorithm for risk of event. Available from: https://registry.dev.aacvpr.org/Documents/AACVPR%20Risk%20Stratification%20Algorithm_June2012.pdf.

160. American College of Sports Medicine. *ACSM's Resources for the Exercise Physiologist*. 3rd ed. Philadelphia (PA): Wolters Kluwer; 2021.

161. Bodenheimer T, Chen E, Bennett HD. Confronting the growing burden of chronic disease: can the U.S. health care workforce do the job? *Health Aff (Millwood)*. 2009;28(1):64–74.

162. Ades PA, Toth MJ. Accelerated decline of aerobic fitness with healthy aging. *Circulation*. 2005;112(5):624–6.

163. Walston JD. Sarcopenia in older adults. *Curr Opin Rheumatol*. 2012;24(6):623–7.

164. Booth ML, Bauman A, Owen N, Gore CJ. Physical activity preferences, preferred sources of assistance, and perceived barriers to increased activity among physically inactive Australians. *Prev Med*. 1997;26(1):131–7.

165. Schutzer KA, Graves BS. Barriers and motivations to exercise in older adults. *Prev Med*. 2004;39(5):1056–61.

166. Sequeira S, Cruz C, Pinto D, Santos L, Marques A. Prevalence of barriers for physical activity in adults according to gender and socioeconomic status. *Br J Sports Med*. 2011;45(15):A18–9.

167. Gallagher NA, Clarke PJ, Gretebeck KA. Gender differences in neighborhood walking in older adults. *J Aging Health*. 2014;26(8):1280–300.

168. August KJ, Sorkin DH. Racial/ethnic disparities in exercise and dietary behaviors of middle-aged and older adults. *J Gen Intern Med*. 2011;26(3):245–50.

169. Raveendran AV, Jayadevan R, Sashidharan S. Long COVID: an overview. *Diabetes Metab Syndr*. 2021;15(3):869–75.

170. Humphreys H, Kilby L, Kudiersky N, Copeland R. Long COVID and the role of physical activity: a qualitative study. *BMJ Open*. 2021;11(3):e047632.

171. Torres-Castro R, Vasconcello-Castillo L, Alsina-Restoy X, et al. Respiratory function in patients post-infection by COVID-19: a systematic review and meta-analysis. *Pulmonology*. 2021;27(4):328–37.

172. Mitrani RD, Dabas N, Goldberger JJ. COVID-19 cardiac injury: implications for long-term surveillance and outcomes in survivors. *Heart Rhythm*. 2020;17(11):1984–90.

173. Silva Andrade B, Siqueira S, de Assis Soares WR, et al. Long-COVID and Post-COVID health complications: an up-to-date review on clinical conditions and their possible molecular mechanisms. *Viruses*. 2021;13(4):700.

174. van Kessel SAM, Olde Hartman TC, Lucassen PLBJ, van Jaarsveld CHM. Post-acute and long-COVID-19 symptoms in patients with mild diseases: a systematic review. *Fam Pract*. 2022;39(1):159–67.

175. Shapiro CL, Manola J, Leboff M. Ovarian failure after adjuvant chemotherapy is associated with rapid bone loss in women with early-stage breast cancer. *J Clin Oncol*. 2001;19(14):3306–11.

176. Whelton PK, Carey RM, Aronow WS, et al. 2017 ACC/AHA/AAPA/ABC/ACPM/AGS/APhA/ASH/ASPC/NMA/PCNA guideline for the prevention, detection, evaluation, and management of high blood pressure in adults: a report of the American College of Cardiology/American Heart Association Task Force on Clinical Practice Guidelines. *Hypertension*. 2018;71(6):e13–5.

177. James PA, Oparil S, Carter BL, et al. 2014 Evidence-based guideline for the management of high blood pressure in adults: report from the panel members appointed to the Eighth Joint National Committee (JNC 8). *JAMA*. 2014;311(5):507–20.

178. Wilson DMC, Ciliska D. Lifestyle assessment. *Can Fam Physician*. 1984;30:1527–32.

179. Darviri C, Alexopoulos EC, Artemiadis AK, et al. The Healthy Lifestyle and Personal Control Questionnaire (HLPCQ): a novel tool for assessing self-empowerment through a constellation of daily activities. *BMC Public Health*. 2014;14:995.

180. Heron M. Deaths: leading causes for 2019. *Natl Vital Stat Rep*. 2021;70(9):1–114.

181. Eckel RH, Jakicic JM, Ard JD, et al. 2013 AHA/ACC guideline on lifestyle management to reduce cardiovascular risk: a report of the American College of Cardiology/American Heart Association Task Force on Practice Guidelines. *J Am Coll Cardiol*. 2014;63(25 Pt B):2960–84.

182. Goff DC Jr, Lloyd-Jones DM, Bennett G, et al. 2013 ACC/AHA guideline on the assessment of cardiovascular risk: a report of the American College of Cardiology/American Heart Association Task Force on Practice Guidelines. *J Am Coll Cardiol*. 2014;63(25 Pt B):2935–59.

183. Centers for Disease Control and Prevention. Trends in cholesterol screening and awareness of high blood cholesterol — United States, 1991–2003. *MMWR Morb Mortal Wkly Rep*. 2005;54(35):865–70.

184. Carroll M, Fryar C, Kit B. Total and high-density lipoprotein cholesterol in adults: United States, 2011–2014. In: *NCHS Data Brief*. Hyattsville (MD): National Center for Health Statistics; 2015.

185. Centers for Disease Control and Prevention. *National Diabetes Statistics Report, 2020*. Atlanta (GA): U.S. Department of Health and Human Services; 2020.

186. Hales CM, Carroll MD, Fryar CD, Ogden CL. Prevalence of obesity and severe obesity among adults: United States, 2017–2018. *NCHS Data Brief*. 2020;(360):1–8.

187. Ostchega Y, Fryar CD, Nwankwo T, Nguyen DT. Hypertension prevalence among adults aged 18 and over: United States, 2017–2018. *NCHS Data Brief*. 2020;(364):1–8.

188. He J, Zhu Z, Bundy JD, Dorans KS, Chen J, Hamm LL. Trends in cardiovascular risk factors in US adults by race and ethnicity and socioeconomic status, 1999–2018. *JAMA.* 2021;326(13):1286–98.

189. Whitfield GP, Carlson SA, Ussery EN, Fulton JE, Galuska DA, Petersen R. Trends in meeting physical activity guidelines among urban and rural dwelling adults — United States, 2008–2017. *MMWR Morb Mortal Wkly Rep.* 2019;68:513–8.

190. Cornelius ME, Wang TW, Jamal A, Loretan CG, Neff LJ. Tobacco product use among adults — United States, 2019. *MMWR Morb Mortal Wkly Rep.* 2020;69(46):1736–42.

191. Wong ND. Epidemiological studies of CHD and the evolution of preventive cardiology. *Nat Rev Cardiol.* 2014;11(5):276–89.

192. Arnett DK, Blumenthal RS, Albert MA, et al. 2019 ACC/AHA guideline on the primary prevention of cardiovascular disease: a report of the American College of Cardiology/American Heart Association Task Force on Clinical Practice Guidelines. *Circulation.* 2019;140(11):e596–646.

193. American College of Cardiology. ASCVD risk estimator plus. 2022. Available from: https://tools.acc.org/ASCVD-Risk-Estimator-Plus/#!/calculate/estimate.

194. Lloyd-Jones DM, Braun LT, Ndumele CE, et al. Use of risk assessment tools to guide decision-making in the primary prevention of atherosclerotic cardiovascular disease: a special report from the American Heart Association and American College of Cardiology. *J Am Coll Cardiol.* 2019;73(24):3153–67.

195. Maclagan LC, Tu JV. Using the concept of ideal cardiovascular health to measure population health: a review. *Curr Opin Cardiol.* 2015;30(5):518–24.

196. Daviglus ML, Lloyd-Jones DM, Pirzada A. Preventing cardiovascular disease in the 21st century: therapeutic and preventive implications of current evidence. *Am J Cardiovasc Drugs.* 2006;6(2):87–101.

197. Lloyd-Jones DM, Hong Y, Labarthe D, et al; American Heart Association Strategic Planning Task Force and Statistics Committee. Defining and setting national goals for cardiovascular health promotion and disease reduction: the American Heart Association's strategic impact goal through 2020 and beyond. *Circulation.* 2010;121(4):586–613.

198. Xanthakis V, Enserro DM, Murabito JM, et al. Ideal cardiovascular health: associations with biomarkers and subclinical disease and impact on incidence of cardiovascular disease in the Framingham Offspring Study. *Circulation.* 2014;130(19):1676–83.

199. Younus A, Aneni EC, Spatz ES, et al. A systematic review of the prevalence and outcomes of ideal cardiovascular health in US and Non-US populations. *Mayo Clin Proc.* 2016;91(5):649–70.

200. Benjamin EJ, Virani SS, Callaway CW, et al; American Heart Association Council on Epidemiology and Prevention Statistics Committee and Stroke Statistics Subcommittee. Heart disease and stroke statistics-2018 update: a report from the American Heart Association. *Circulation.* 2018;137(12):e67–492.

201. Peng Y, Cao S, Yao Z, Wang Z. Prevalence of the cardiovascular health status in adults: a systematic review and meta-analysis. *Nutr Metab Cardiovasc Dis.* 2018;28(12):1197–207.

202. Aneni EC, Crippa A, Osondu CU, et al. Estimates of mortality benefit from ideal cardiovascular health metrics: a dose response meta-analysis. *J Am Heart Assoc.* 2017;6(12):e006904.

203. Van Camp SP, Peterson RA. Cardiovascular complications of outpatient cardiac rehabilitation programs. *JAMA.* 1986;256(9):1160–3.

204. Digenio AG, Sim JG, Dowdeswell RJ, Morris R. Exercise-related cardiac arrest in cardiac rehabilitation. The Johannesburg experience. *S Afr Med J.* 1991;79(4):188–91.

205. Vongvanich P, Paul-Labrador MJ, Merz CN. Safety of medically supervised exercise in a cardiac rehabilitation center. *Am J Cardiol.* 1996;77(15):1383–5.

206. Riebe D, Ehrman JK, Liguori G, Magal M, editors. *ACSM's Guidelines for Exercise Testing and Prescription* 10th ed. Baltimore (MD): Lippincott, Williams & Wilkins; 2018.

Movement Prescription for Apparently Healthy Adults

INTRODUCTION

The benefits of regular physical activity, defined as meeting federal physical activity and public health guidelines for aerobic and muscle-strengthening activities, are well established for all ages and sectors of the global population. Unfortunately, in the U.S., only an estimated 20% of adults meet current physical activity guidelines (PAG) that include both aerobic and muscle-strengthening recommendations (1). Although not well documented, it is estimated that an even lower percentage of the adults would meet the comprehensive exercise guidelines provided by the American College of Sports Medicine (ACSM) (2) that include cardiorespiratory, muscular fitness, and flexibility recommendations. Additionally, most adults in the U.S. spend approximately 55% of most days in a seated position (1, 3), although this number will vary based on stage of life and occupation.

The overarching goal of this chapter is to provide a framework for exercise prescription for apparently healthy adults. This chapter reframes exercise prescription as a daily movement prescription that crosses the spectrums of (a) sedentary behaviors to moderate–vigorous physical activities as well as (b) physical activity behaviors and exercise behaviors, with the latter being more planned, structured, and intended to improve physical fitness. Additionally, the 24-hour movement paradigm is introduced as an evolving model that incorporates all movements along the continuum from sleep to sedentary behaviors to physical activity of various intensities. The contemporary perspective offered in this chapter can help individuals improve their personal behavior management toward the goal of enhancing longevity but, as importantly, preventing chronic disease and disability, thereby maximizing health span, functional fitness, and health-related quality of life. Moreover, this chapter summarizes the "best practice" advice of the evidence-based movement guidelines and identifies a variety of resources and tools that can

BOX 4.1 — Exercise Preparticipation Health Screening

As discussed in Chapter 3, adequate screening is imperative for moving safely, especially when working with clients who are beginning an exercise program, are increasing the intensity of their program, or have one or more chronic conditions.

assist the clinical exercise physiologist (CEP) who wishes to share this advice with clients (Box 4.1).

MOVEMENT PRESCRIPTION: A CONTEMPORARY PERSPECTIVE

The term *prescription* is often defined as a written order by a physician or clinician for the administration of medication or another intervention. More broadly, a prescription is simply a piece of advice. The term *exercise prescription* has been a staple of fitness and medical professional vocabularies for nearly 50 years, both within the literature and when consulting with clients and patients. It refers to a personalized plan of exercise or physical activity that considers the patient's current state of fitness and their therapeutic or performance goals. However, this traditional concept of exercise prescription for the apparently healthy adult has been updated. Currently, it would more accurately be referred to as a set of "movement guidelines" but also acknowledges the importance of sleep respecting the increased recognition of the 24-hour movement paradigm.

This shift toward "movement guidelines" and away from "exercise prescription" is supported by the social ecological model, which suggests that if we are going to incorporate consistent human movement into the behavioral patterns of all individuals in society, we will need to focus our attention and efforts on the behavioral choices of individuals within their environment. We need to acknowledge that humans belong to complicated social structures in an environment that has undergone rapid technological changes in the past 50 years that have effectively engineered the need for much, if any, human movement out of daily living. Ironically, at the same time technological advancements have removed our work energy expenditure opportunities through modern convenience, such as cars, elevators, washing machines, cooking appliances, and so forth, they have provided an array of gadgets to measure and track our activity patterns in real time, often termed wearable technologies (WTs). Technology has also given us numerous devices, often located in our pocket, to connect virtually to obtain information and ideas about exercise and physical activity and, likely more importantly, to receive coaching and social support to improve our adherence to our activity program. Increasing physical activity in all four of its domains (leisure time, household, occupational, and transportation) and reducing sedentary behavior must therefore become a focus of public health research and practice. In addition, intentional exercise (*e.g.*, resistance or functional training) is likely needed for most adults to preserve muscle mass, prevent joint and muscle pain (*e.g.*, low back pain), and maintain physical function, especially with advancing age.

Moreover, we need to refine our definition of fitness to reflect these dramatic societal and environmental changes. The current ACSM guidelines (2) provide the following definition for physical fitness: "although defined in several ways, physical fitness has generally been described as a set of attributes or characteristics individuals have or achieve that relate to their ability to perform physical activity or activities of daily living." Conventionally, the health-related components of fitness include cardiorespiratory fitness, body composition, muscular strength and endurance, and flexibility. The skill-related components include agility, coordination, balance, power, reaction time, and speed. Certainly, both the health- and skill-related components of physical fitness have direct application to athletic performance and certain occupational tasks (*e.g.*, firefighter, soldier, construction worker) as well as activities of daily living throughout the lifespan. Contemporary perspectives also recognize that these components may not be mutually exclusive for achieving health goals for many individuals (*e.g.*, balance activities are important for older adults).

However, what if most people do not need to perform daily physical activity to be productive and successful in life? Computers and devices, labor-saving machines for home and self-care, and automated transportation options all collectively remove the need to perform daily movement. Thus, applying the traditional definition and components of fitness to the daily lives of a typical human being in a technologically advanced, socially complex society may require a different conceptual frame. That is, our definition of fitness may need to include functional fitness, which emphasizes the physical, cognitive, and psychosocial challenges inherent in living a productive and meaningful life. An emphasis on functional fitness does not simultaneously de-emphasize the need for individuals to be physically active. Rather, it acknowledges that, in response to the evolution of our culture and environment, a conflict now exists between the level of physical activity needed for good health and what is required for daily living for most individuals.

Thus, this chapter focuses on the human movement paradigm, which encompasses all types of movement, including exercise, physical activity, and minimization of time spent in sedentary behaviors. The human movement paradigm provides a framework for movement prescription for apparently healthy adults, the prevention of chronic disease, and optimization of functional fitness. Figure 4.1 provides a conceptual model for the human movement paradigm. Figure 4.2 identifies terms related to this paradigm and functional fitness (as discussed later).

BENEFITS OF PHYSICAL ACTIVITY

ACSM guidelines (2) summarize the benefits of regular physical activity and/or exercise as follows:

- Improvement in cardiovascular and respiratory function
- Reduction in cardiovascular disease (CVD) risk factors
- Decreased morbidity and mortality most notably including lower incidence of:
  - CVD and coronary artery disease (CAD)
  - Type 2 diabetes mellitus (T2DM)
  - Cancer (breast, colon, bladder, endometrium, and lung)
  - Gallbladder disease
  - Osteoporotic fractures

Exercise
- Established Guidelines (ACSM)
- Cardiorespiratory, Resistance, and Flexibility Components
- Frequency, Intensity, Time, Type, Volume, Progression, Pattern
Human Movement Paradigm for Physical Movement Prescription
Physical Activity
- Established Guidelines (HHS-2018-PAG)
- Cardiorespiratory/ Aerobic and Resistance Components
Sedentary Behaviors
- No Comprehensive Detailed Guidelines
- Time spent in sedentary behavior should be limited

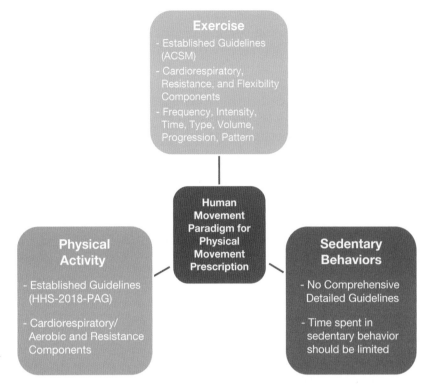

FIGURE 4.1 Human movement paradigm for physical movement prescription.

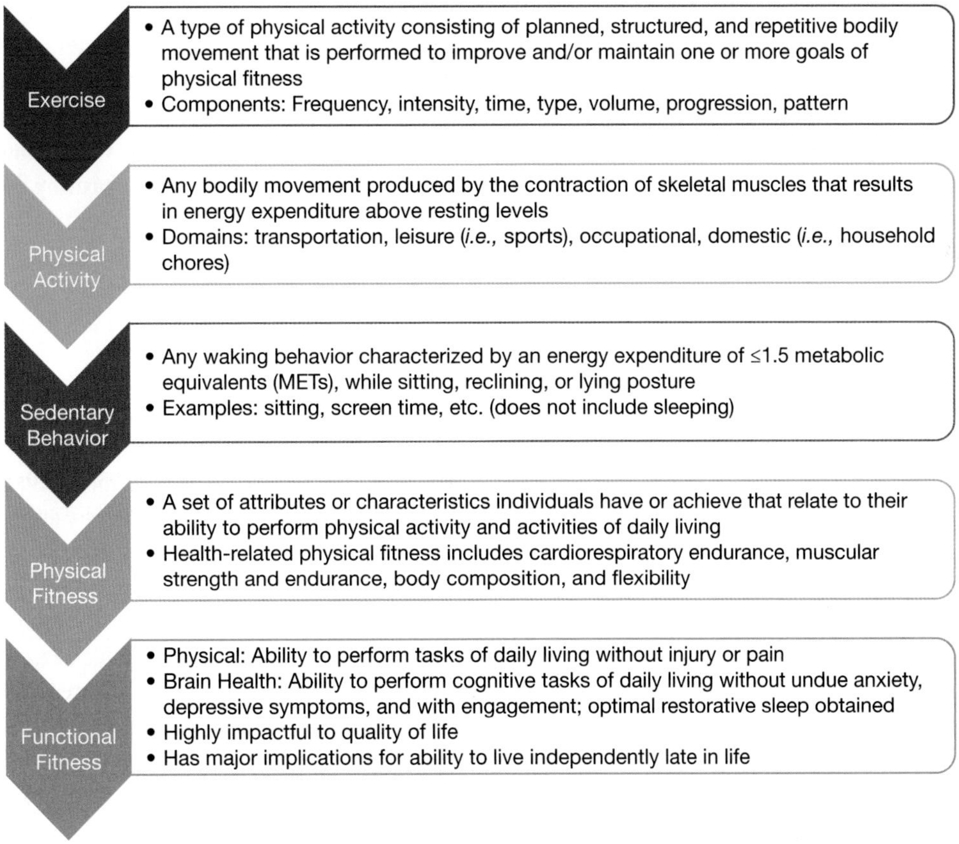

Exercise
• A type of physical activity consisting of planned, structured, and repetitive bodily movement that is performed to improve and/or maintain one or more goals of physical fitness
• Components: Frequency, intensity, time, type, volume, progression, pattern
Physical Activity
• Any bodily movement produced by the contraction of skeletal muscles that results in energy expenditure above resting levels
• Domains: transportation, leisure (i.e., sports), occupational, domestic (i.e., household chores)
Sedentary Behavior
• Any waking behavior characterized by an energy expenditure of ≤1.5 metabolic equivalents (METs), while sitting, reclining, or lying posture
• Examples: sitting, screen time, etc. (does not include sleeping)
Physical Fitness
• A set of attributes or characteristics individuals have or achieve that relate to their ability to perform physical activity and activities of daily living
• Health-related physical fitness includes cardiorespiratory endurance, muscular strength and endurance, body composition, and flexibility
Functional Fitness
• Physical: Ability to perform tasks of daily living without injury or pain
• Brain Health: Ability to perform cognitive tasks of daily living without undue anxiety, depressive symptoms, and with engagement; optimal restorative sleep obtained
• Highly impactful to quality of life
• Has major implications for ability to live independently late in life

FIGURE 4.2 Key terms of the human movement paradigm and conceptual links to functional fitness. (Based on information from US Department of Health and Human Services. Scientific report — 2018 physical activity guidelines — health.gov. February 2018 [cited 2019 Feb 12]. Available from: https://health.gov/paguidelines/second-edition/report/; American College of Sports Medicine. *ACSM's Guidelines for Exercise Testing and Prescription*. Eleventh, Spiral edition. Philadelphia (PA): Lippincott Williams & Wilkins; 2021; and Bull FC, Al-Ansari SS, Biddle S, et al. World Health Organization 2020 guidelines on physical activity and sedentary behaviour. *Br J Sports Med*. 2020;54(24):1451–62. doi:10.1136/bjsports-2020-102955.)

- Other benefits including the following:
  - Improved psychological constructs (anxiety, depression, well-being, quality of life)
  - Improved cognitive function
  - Improved sleep quality and efficiency
  - Enhanced physical functional performance (e.g., work, recreational, and sport activities)
  - For older adults specifically:
    - Reductions in functional limitations and enhanced physical function and independent living
    - Reduced risk of falls and fall-related injuries
    - Effective therapy for many chronic diseases

It is important to recognize that both primary modes of activity — cardiorespiratory/aerobic and muscular fitness/strengthening — contribute to many of the benefits listed earlier. In addition, for many of these diseases and health conditions, there is strong evidence of a dose–response relationship with physical activity and exercise. This implies that the benefits of exercise lie on a continuum, which means that even small amounts improve health with greater amounts of physical activity and exercise providing additional health benefits. These abundant benefits of physical activity/exercise might be distilled into the three primary categories of cardiorespiratory, metabolic, and functional fitness.

Improvements in Cardiorespiratory and Metabolic Fitness

Certainly, the strongest lines of evidence for the benefits of habitual physical activity and especially higher intensity aerobic exercise are the well-documented enhancements in cardiorespiratory function with a reduced physical stress for the same physical challenge (2). A reduction in primary and secondary risk factors for CVD in response to increased cardiorespiratory fitness is also well established (2). Physical activity, both cardiorespiratory and muscular fitness modes, also contributes to (a) metabolic fitness, improving the lipid profile, insulin action, and glucose tolerance, and (b) weight management and reduced abdominal and whole-body adiposity (2). Habitual physical activity also reduces chronic systemic inflammation (2), an important link to many chronic conditions prevalent in middle-aged and older adults (4). Moreover, the reduced risk of CVD, cancers, especially of the breast and colon, and other chronic conditions linked to physical activity is thought to be related to increased metabolic fitness.

Collectively, the positive effects of regular physical activity/exercise on the prevention of society's most prevalent chronic conditions — CVD, T2DM, cancer, and obesity — are well established (2). In sum, regular physical activity/exercise contributes to a reduced risk of morbidity and mortality, enhances quality of life, and increases both health span and lifespan. For additional information about the benefits of regular physical activity/exercise and the accompanying reduction in risk, please refer to Chapter 3.

Improvements in Functional Fitness

In addition, habitual movement can enhance functional fitness. Although ACSM (16) has conventionally defined functional fitness as "neuromotor fitness," which implies physical function (e.g., balance, agility, coordination), given the contemporary reframe of movement and fitness discussed earlier, a broader definition of function is encouraged. On a daily basis, functional fitness is of paramount importance to individuals, enabling them to perform physical, cognitive, and psychosocial tasks with greater productivity and well-being. Thus, this contemporary definition of functional fitness addresses our daily function "above the neck" along with physical function "below the neck." Indeed, improvements in response to human movement in brain health, as broadly defined and detailed later, are of increasing research interest and importance for optimal health and well-being. Notably, functional fitness is relevant to performing activities of daily living, work-related activity, recreational activities, and all levels of sports performance. It is also relevant to individuals throughout the lifespan, including children and adolescents, and young, middle-aged, and older adults.

Improvements in Physical Function

For many adults, physical fitness is needed for optimal physical functioning. For example, becoming physically fit helps correct posture mechanics, enabling an individual to endure long periods of sitting or standing without incurring musculoskeletal pain, especially low back, and hip pain. Physical fitness can also help prevent injury during semiregular leisure activity (e.g., weekend hiking) or when completing domestic chores and activities (e.g., lawn care or gardening, carrying groceries, or hobbies including home improvement activities; Figure 4.3). A large body of literature supports the critical role that physical activity and exercise, especially resistance training, play in maintaining functional capacity and independent living in older adults (5, 6). Notably, habitual physical activity offers protection against reduced physical function, which is linked to physical limitations and disability even in middle-aged adults (7).

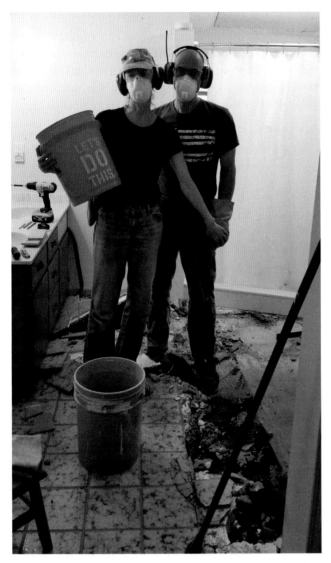

FIGURE 4.3 Physical fitness is needed to prevent injury when engaging in domestic chores and hobbies (photo provided by the authors).

negative ramifications as well, and these daily challenges to mental and cognitive capacities are among them. The recent 2018 *Physical Activity Guidelines for Americans* (2018-PAG) (1) clearly indicates the many benefits of physical activity to brain function in several distinct categories, including (a) cognition, (b) anxiety, mood, and depression, (c) sleep, and (d) quality of life. The benefits within the PAG (1) had a strong or moderate effect for the evidence grade.

Cognition

The literature regarding the beneficial effects of physical activity and exercise on cognitive ability is most conclusive in children and older adults. However, the importance of regular physical activity, including aerobic and resistance training, for cognitive function across the lifespan is of high public health importance and continues to be an active area of research. Regular physical activity reduces the risk of dementia including Alzheimer disease for adults, with adults older than 50 years also improving their cognition (executive function, attention, memory, crystallized intelligence, and processing speed). Notably, many of these improvements in cognition in response to aerobic exercise in older adults also demonstrated benefits in brain structure (8). A comprehensive review (9) reveals that, in addition to aerobic exercise, resistance training also improves brain and cognitive adaptations in older adults (Figure 4.4). These findings suggest that regular physical activity may help older adults remain productive, independent members of a knowledge- and information-based society for longer periods of life, successfully operating complex technologies like cell phones and computers.

Improvements in Brain Health

Our need to engage in challenging physical activity has been reduced in our daily lives as we physically move less to accomplish life tasks. However, the inverse has occurred for "cognitive fitness." Cognitive fitness is a state of optimized ability to reason, remember, learn, plan, and adapt. Many modern occupations involve knowledge or information work. Indeed, with social media and other Internet technologies continually increasing their processing speeds, individuals are frequently challenged to mentally process significant amounts of information. Although offering astonishing improvements to health care and other aspects of life, the modern technology-laden information age has

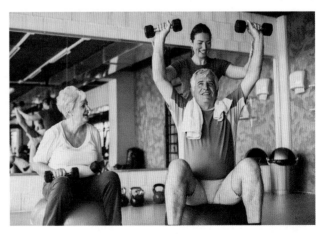

FIGURE 4.4 Older adults engaging in resistance training. (From wavebreakmedia/Shutterstock.)

Anxiety, Depression, Sleep, and Quality of Life

Like impairments in physical and cognitive functioning, impairments in psychosocial functioning such as anxiety or depression, or lacking vigor, vitality, or motivational energy also reduce an individual's functional fitness and quality of life. Unfortunately, contemporary society with all its modern advancements has also increased the prevalence of these challenges and afflictions, especially depression (10). For most individuals, remaining productive and emotionally balanced during an average day requires a great deal of stamina and the ability to manage a variety of stressors, including reduced sleep quantity and quality.

Fortunately, having a habitually physically active lifestyle, especially one including intentional exercise, can reduce the risk of mild anxiety, depressed mood, and depression. Acute physical activity also reduces short-term feelings of anxiety, termed *state anxiety* (1). Moreover, ample literature suggests that physical activity can improve mood, reduce fatigue, and enhance both physical and mental energy (11). Sleep quality and sleep outcomes are also positively influenced by physical activity and exercise habits (1). Indeed, poor sleep has been associated with decreased physical, cognitive, and psychosocial functioning, especially for middle-aged and older adults (12). Thus, having a higher level of physical activity, exercise, and physical fitness potentially enhances psychosocial fitness aspects of brain health, enhancing productivity and functioning in today's socially complex environment.

Summary of Benefits

The guidelines (1, 2) clearly summarize that habitual physical activity and exercise, perhaps accompanied by reductions in sedentary behavior, contribute to a reduced risk of morbidity and early mortality and enhance quality of life. Habitual movement can also enhance functional fitness, including physical, brain/cognitive, and psychosocial functioning, increasing the individual's daily capacity for productivity and well-being.

In summary, although increasing the likelihood of living a longer life free of chronic disease, regular physical activity will also help an individual feel and function better. As an example, targeted exercises can offset common occurrences of neuromuscular pain because of muscle imbalances caused by the sitting screen-based activities that make up a large portion of our daily lives. In this regard, corrective exercises can be considered an antidote to modern living. Essentially, by maintaining a lifestyle that consists of physical activity levels at or above federal

recommendations and limiting sedentary behaviors, individuals can greatly decrease their risk of morbidity and mortality (2). However, it also recognized that any physical activity, even if not meeting guidelines, is better than being sedentary.

MOVEMENT GUIDELINES FOR HEALTHY ADULTS

Given the myriad health benefits conferred by participation in regular physical activity and the detrimental effects of excessive sedentary behavior, ACSM, U.S. Department of Health and Human Services (HHS), and several nongovernmental public health organizations have issued movement guidelines for healthy adults. Here, we discuss the evolution and status of these guidelines.

ACSM Guidelines

Traditions often inform contemporary perspectives, and the history of exercise prescription in the U.S. is best provided by the updates of ACSM Position Stands (PSs; position stands are official statements from ACSM on topics related to sports medicine and exercise science) and *ACSM Guidelines for Exercise Testing and Prescription* (GETP), the latter currently in its 11th edition (2). Those in the field often refer to these documents as the best resources for exercise prescription information and standards.

ACSM PSs for Apparently Healthy Adults: 1978–2011

The various revisions of ACSM PSs provide a chronological record and contextualization for the evolution of exercise prescription. The first prominent ACSM PS, which was published in 1978, introduced the acronym FITT, which stands for Frequency (days per week), Intensity (% of heart rate reserve; repetitions and sets), Time (minutes per bout), and Type (mode) (13). This acronym proved useful in organizing the exercise prescription until it was expanded in the latest revisions of the PSs and guidelines, which are discussed later. The primary goal of the 1978 PS was to increase fitness in healthy adults with an exercise prescription most strongly concerned with cardiorespiratory fitness and the prevention of CVD. It advocated movements that involved large muscle groups and a continuous duration (15–60 min) undertaken with a moderate to high intensity, to be performed three to five times per week (13).

In 1990, a major revision occurred. The 1990 ACSM PS added resistance training (twice per week for all major muscle groups) to the initial cardiorespiratory training prescription (14). As exercise science continued to advance, the 1998 ACSM PS introduced more substantial changes (15). The prescription for cardiorespiratory exercise was given the time option of 20–60 continuous minutes or 10-minute bouts accumulating to 20–60 minutes. The resistance training prescription was altered to reflect different intensities for individuals younger or older than 50 years. Flexibility training was added as a new mode of exercise and was recommended on 2–3 days per week.

The most recent 2011 ACSM PS includes several updates based on expansions to the body of literature regarding exercise prescription for apparently healthy adults. First, neuromotor exercise training, involving motor skills, proprioceptive training, and multifaceted activities such as yoga, was added to the overall exercise prescription (16). These exercise recommendations encourage balance, agility, and coordination training on 2–3 days per week. Second, the recommendation for cardiorespiratory exercise training was updated to include moderate-intensity cardiorespiratory exercise training for ≥ 30 minutes per day on ≥ 5 days per week for a total of ≥ 150 minutes per week; or vigorous-intensity cardiorespiratory exercise training for ≥ 20 minutes per day on ≥ 3 days per week (≥ 75 min per wk); or a combination of moderate- and vigorous-intensity exercise to achieve a total energy expenditure of ≥ 500–$1,000$ metabolic equivalent (MET) minutes per week. (One MET = rate of energy expenditure while sitting at rest. For example, jogging is approximately 7 METs; jogging for 30 min per session three times per week = 630 MET min per wk.) Finally, the FITT acronym was expanded to include Volume and Progression (FITTVP). Volume is the product of exercise frequency, intensity, and time. Progression is adjusting exercise volume until a goal is reached. An additional P, which stands for Pattern, was also offered for the four modes of cardiorespiratory, resistance, flexibility, and neuromotor exercise training indicating how exercise could be spread out or accumulated in a session, day, or throughout the week.

ACSM PSs for Special Populations

Although the goal of this chapter is to examine exercise prescription for the apparently healthy adult, it should be appreciated that ACSM collaborates with numerous other agencies to promote guidelines for safe and effective exercise and physical activity for special populations. Over two decades ago, recommendations were provided for patients with CAD (17). Subsequent work focused on exercise and hypertension (18), bone health (19), and weight loss and weight regain prevention (20). In 2010, a joint PS with the American Diabetes Association on exercise and T2DM was published (21).

ACSM GETP: 1975–2021

With the growing interest in exercise training and prescription around the early 1970s, in 1972 ACSM formed a special subcommittee to develop GETP for both healthy and unhealthy adults. Published in 1975 (22), the work of this subcommittee culminated in the first edition of *ACSM's GETP* providing a concise summary of research-based recommendations for exercise testing and prescription, specifically for cardiac patients. The GETP is now one of the most used references for those in exercise and health-related fields.

For the nearly 50 years since its initial publication, each edition of the GETP has been developed by integrating guidelines and recommendations from ACSM PSs, scientific statements from other relevant organizations, as well as public health guidelines related to physical activity and health. Updated every 3–6 years, the GETP is now in its 11th edition (GETP-11) and covers exercise testing and prescription following the FITTVP principles for healthy populations as well as those with cardiovascular, pulmonary, metabolic, and other chronic diseases and brain-related disorders (2). It should be noted that intensity is often the most challenging of the FITTVP components to understand and implement. Table 4.1 identifies the recommended methods to prescribe cardiorespiratory or aerobic activity, with the heart rate reserve method being the most common for healthy adults.

Intensity for resistance training can also be relatively complicated to understand and prescribe. With this mode, intensity (*i.e.*, the load) refers to the weight lifted during a specific exercise. Intensity is often prescribed as a percentage of an individual's 1 repetition maximum (RM). However, to avoid risking injury during the 1 RM protocol, the amount of weight needed for overload is more often determined as the resistance/weight that causes safe failure (*i.e.*, inability to complete a repetition while simultaneously maintaining good form) and meets the goals of the program. Repetitions are highly dependent on the component of muscular fitness the individual desires to improve or maintain (*i.e.*, strength, endurance, power, or hypertrophy) and that will in turn influence the number of sets, weekly volume, etc. For general muscular fitness goals for most adults, a load aligning with 60–70% of the 1 RM, or a repetition range of 8–12, is effective (2). These intensity and repetition recommendations also align with the current PAG (1).

Table 4.1 Methods of Estimating Intensity of Cardiorespiratory Exercise

| Intensity | Relative Intensity | | | | Cardiorespiratory Endurance Exercise | | | | | | |
| | %HRR or %$\dot{V}O_2R$ | %HR_{max} | %$\dot{V}O_{2max}$ | Perceived exertion (rating on 6–20 RPE scale) | Intensity (%$\dot{V}O_{2max}$) Relative to Maximal Exercise Capacity in MET | | | Absolute Intensity | Absolute Intensity (MET) by Age | | |
					20 METs %O_{2max}	10 METs %O_{2max}	5 METs %O_{2max}	MET	Young (20–39 yr)	Middle age (40–64 yr)	Older (≥65 yr)
Very light	<30	<57	<37	Very light (RPE <9)	<34	<37	<44	<2.0	<2.4	<2.0	<1.6
Light	30–39	57–63	37–45	Very light to fairly light (RPE 9–11)	34–42	37–45	44–51	2.0–2.9	2.4–4.7	2.0–3.9	1.6–3.1
Moderate	40–59	64–76	46–63	Fairly light to somewhat hard (RPE 12–13)	43–61	46–63	52–67	3.0–5.9	4.8–7.1	4.0–5.9	3.2–4.7
Vigorous	60–89	77–95	64–90	Somewhat hard to very hard (RPE 14–17)	62–90	64–90	68–91	6.0–8.7	7.2–10.1	6.0–8.4	4.8–6.7
Near maximal to maximal	≥90	≥96	≥91	≥Very hard (RPE ≥ 18)	≥91	≥91	≥92	≥8.8	≥10.2	≥8.5	≥6.8

HR_{max}, maximal heart rate; HRR, heart rate reserve; MET, metabolic equivalent; RPE, rating of perceived exertion; $\dot{V}O_{2max}$, maximum oxygen consumption; $\dot{V}O_2R$, oxygen uptake reserve. (Based on information from American College of Sports Medicine. *ACSM's Guidelines for Exercise Testing and Prescription*. 11th, Spiral edition. Philadelphia (PA): Lippincott Williams & Wilkins; 2021.)

Although these are current guidelines, the prescribed exercise program should be modified according to an individual's habitual physical activity, physical functioning, health status, exercise responses, and stated goals. Finally, although the GETP-11 outlines optimal exercise training on a weekly basis for health benefits, some individuals may benefit from engaging in amounts of exercise less than recommended, either less days per week or perhaps only certain modes of exercise (*i.e.*, cardiorespiratory). Meeting some of the guidelines is better than none. The recommendations for the individualized exercise prescription for apparently healthy adults are summarized in Table 4.2.

Table 4.2	ACSM Recommendations for Individualized Exercise Prescription
Cardiorespiratory "aerobic" exercise	• **Frequency:** At least 3 d per wk; spreading sessions across 3–5 d per wk may be most conducive to reach recommended amounts of physical activity. • **Intensity:** Moderate and vigorous intensity is recommended for healthy adults, but light intensity can be beneficial for beginners. • **Time:** 30–60 min of moderate exercise or 20–60 min of vigorous, a combination of the two • **Type:** Aerobic exercise performed in a continuous or intermittent manner that involves major muscle groups • **Volume:** Accumulate 150 min per wk of moderate exercise, 75 min per wk of vigorous exercise, or an equivalent combination; aim to reach step count of >7,000 steps per d; expend ≥500–1,000 MET min per wk; some is better than none. • **Pattern:** No minimum bout duration • **Progression:** Gradual progression of FITT to avoid injury or cardiovascular event
Resistance exercise	• **Frequency:** Each major muscle group should be targeted at least 2 d per wk. • **Intensity:** Differs depending on exercise history and individual factors, especially muscular fitness component of interest (*e.g.*, strength, endurance, power, or hypertrophy); 60%–70% 1 repetition maximum (RM) is recommended for healthy adults. • **Time:** No amount of time specified • **Type:** Multijoint exercises targeting agonist and antagonist muscle groups; single-joint and core exercises can also be included. • **Volume (training sets per week):** 8–12 reps; range of repetition and set schemes are effective dependent on specific muscular fitness goals. • **Pattern:** Rest for 2–3 min between each set. • **Progression:** Gradually progress resistance, volume, or frequency.
Flexibility exercise	• **Frequency:** ≥2–3 d per wk; daily is most effective. • **Intensity:** Stretch to the point of tightness or slight discomfort. • **Time:** Holding a static stretch for 10–30 s is recommended; for proprioceptive neuromuscular facilitation stretching, 3–6 s light-to-moderate contraction followed by 10–30 s of assisted stretching is desired. • **Type:** Performing a series of flexibility exercises for each major muscle–tendon group is recommended. • **Volume:** 90 s of total stretching is recommended for each joint. • **Pattern:** Dynamic stretches are encouraged prior to exercise; static, ballistic, and/or proprioceptive neuromuscular facilitation stretching should not precede an exercise session. • **Progression:** Progress based on individual's level of discomfort and within their current range of motion

ACSM, American College of Sports Medicine; FITT, Frequency, Intensity, Time, and Type; MET, metabolic equivalent.

Source: Based on information from American College of Sports Medicine. *ACSM's Guidelines for Exercise Testing and Prescription.* 11th Spiral ed. Philadelphia (PA): Lippincott Williams & Wilkins; 2021.

Public Health Recommendations for Physical Activity

In addition to updating its own movement guidelines, ACSM has worked for decades in collaboration with public health agencies to develop recommendations for the general public.

Public Health Recommendations: 1995-2007

In 1995, Pate et al. (23) published a joint recommendation of the U.S. Centers for Disease Control and Prevention (CDC) and ACSM that every adult in the U.S. should accumulate 30 minutes or more of moderate-intensity physical activity on most, preferably all, days of the week. This joint CDC–ACSM statement was intended to increase public awareness of the importance of the health-related benefits of moderate-intensity physical activity.

The 1996 Surgeon General's Report on Physical Activity and Health (24) aligned with the CDC–ACSM statement, emphasizing that health benefits occur at a moderate level of physical activity (expending approximately 150 kcal per day). The Surgeon General's Report noted that, although physical activity need not be vigorous to provide health benefits, the amount of health benefit is related to the amount (volume) of physical activity (*i.e.*, the dose–response principle). Thus, lower-intensity activities needed to be performed for more time to obtain a similar health benefit. The Surgeon General's Report also emphasized adaptability and a lifestyle approach to enhance behavioral adherence, highlighting how leisure and recreational activity choices could be incorporated into a weekly plan.

In 2007, ACSM and the American Heart Association (AHA) issued updated recommendations for physical activity and health for adults 18–65 years old (25). These included the following:

- Moderate-intensity physical activity for 30 minutes on 5 days a week or vigorous-intensity aerobic activity for a minimum of 20 minutes, 3 days a week, was recommended.
- A combination of moderate- and vigorous-intensity activity was acceptable. Accumulated bouts of 10 minutes of moderate-intensity physical activity were also adequate.
- Activities that promote muscular strength and endurance on a minimum of 2 days a week were recommended.

Like the Surgeon General's Report, ACSM–AHA recommendations emphasized the dose–response relationship between physical activity and health, explaining that some individuals who desired greater fitness improvements, greater reductions in risk for chronic diseases or disabilities, or prevention of weight gain would need to exceed the minimum recommended amounts of physical activity. However, the variations in the different public health guidelines were confusing for many individuals. Even scholars called for better terminology to enhance research and public health efforts (26).

The PAG: 2008 and 2018

In 2008, HHS published the first edition of the *Physical Activity Guidelines for Americans* (2008-PAG) (27). Whereas ACSM exercise guidelines were written by scientists for fitness professionals, and are therefore comprehensive and detailed, the PAG sacrifice detail for enhanced readability. Indeed, a major goal of the 2008-PAG was to offer the general public a set of understandable recommendations for physical activity. The PAG documents are highly accessible, limit use of scientific terms, include ample resources for exercising safely and for specific exercises and activities, and offer behavioral management strategies. The PAG represent the recommended minimal amount of physical activity and not necessarily the ideal or optimal volume needed to realize benefits. Again, because there is a dose–response relationship between physical activity and health, greater amounts of physical activity will confer greater health benefits.

Notably, the content and structure of the PAG complement and align with the *Dietary Guidelines for Americans*, which is a joint effort of the HHS and the U.S. Department of Agriculture (USDA). The collective goal of the two documents is to provide guidance on the importance of being physically active and eating a healthy diet to promote good health and reduce the risk of chronic diseases. The *Dietary Guidelines for Americans* is updated every 5 years, whereas the PAG are updated every 10 years.

The 2008-PAG recommended the following:

- Adults should avoid inactivity and some activity is better than none.
- Adults should engage in 150 minutes of moderate-intensity aerobic activity per week, or 75 minutes of vigorous-intensity aerobic activity per week, or an equivalent combination of moderate and vigorous aerobic activity in bouts of 10 minutes or longer.
- For additional health benefits, adults should increase activity to 300 minutes per week of moderate-intensity

or 150 minutes per week of vigorous-intensity aerobic activity, or an equivalent combination.

■ Muscle-strengthening activities that are moderate or high intensity for all major muscle groups should be completed on 2 or more days per week.

Table 4.3 identifies a range of aerobic activities that vary in skill or physical fitness base. These activities along with physical work (*e.g.*, lawn or garden work) and other active leisure pursuits (*e.g.*, hiking) contribute to meeting the recommendations for aerobic activity.

Acknowledging the unique needs of various age groups, in addition to recommendations for the general adult population, the 2008-PAG included guidelines for children and adolescents as well as older adults.

The 2008-PAG recommended that children and adolescents engage in 60 minutes or more of physical activity daily and that most of that hour should be either moderate- or vigorous-intensity aerobic activity, including vigorous-intensity physical activity on at least 3 days a week. Muscle- and bone-strengthening physical activity on at least 3 days of the week was also recommended.

For older adults, the 2008-PAG reinforced the general guidelines for adults, but with the caveat that if health limitations prevent a person from accumulating 150 minutes of moderate-intensity aerobic activity a week, they should nevertheless strive to be as physically active as their abilities permit. Additionally, as the prevention of falling is of paramount importance among older adults, they were encouraged to engage in exercises that maintain or improve balance. These recommendations are well aligned with both ACSM PSs on Exercise and Physical Activity for Older Adults (5) and ACSM–AHA recommendations regarding Physical Activity and Public Health in Older Adults (28).

In 2018, HHS released the second edition of the PAG (2018-PAG) (1). New to the 2018-PAG are discussions of additional immediate and long-term health benefits of physical activity in the areas of brain health, cancer, fall-related injuries, sleep, physical functioning, and quality of life. Strategies to increase population levels of physical activity as well as a discussion of the health risks of sedentary behavior and its relationship to physical activity are also presented. The 2018-PAG are available at https:// health.gov/paguidelines/. Overall, the recommended amounts of physical activity for children and adolescents, adults, and older adults remain the same as those in the 2008-PAG. One major update is that the 2018-PAG state that physical activity in bouts of any length contribute to health benefits and therefore eliminates the previous requirement that aerobic physical activity of adults be accumulated in bouts of at least 10 minutes.

Additionally, the 2018-PAG expand upon the 2008-PAG to include specific physical activity recommendations for preschool-aged children (ages 3–5), women during pregnancy and the postpartum period, and

Table 4.3	Modes of Aerobic (Cardiorespiratory Endurance) Exercises to Improve Physical Fitness		
Exercise Group	**Exercise Description**	**Recommended for**	**Examples**
A	Endurance activities requiring minimal skill or physical fitness to perform	All adults	Walking, leisurely cycling, aqua-aerobics, slow dancing
B	Vigorous-intensity endurance activities requiring minimal skill	Adults (as per the preparticipation screening guidelines in Chapter 2) who are habitually physically active and/or at least average physical fitness	Jogging, running, rowing, aerobics, spinning, elliptical exercise, stepping exercise, fast dancing
C	Endurance activities requiring skill to perform	Adults with acquired skill and/ or at least average physical fitness levels	Swimming, cross-country skiing, skating
D	Recreational sports	Adults with a regular exercise program and at least average physical fitness	Racquet sports, basketball, soccer, downhill skiing, hiking

Source: Based on information from American College of Sports Medicine. *ACSM's Guidelines for Exercise Testing and Prescription.* 11th, Spiral ed. Philadelphia (PA): Lippincott Williams & Wilkins; 2021.

adults with chronic conditions or disabilities (1). For preschool-aged children, the 2018-PAG recommend engagement in physical activity throughout the day (1). Active play that includes a variety of different activities positively impacts growth and development at this age. The 2018-PAG recommend that women who are pregnant or in the postpartum period engage in at least 150 minutes of moderate-intensity aerobic activity per week (1). Further, women who regularly engaged in vigorous-intensity activity or were physically active prior to pregnancy can continue these activities. These women are encouraged to be under the care of a health care professional who can consult with them about how to adjust their physical activity during this time. Adults with chronic conditions or disabilities, who are able, should aim to meet the aerobic and muscle-strengthening guidelines for healthy adults as described in the 2008-PAG (1). When meeting these guidelines is not feasible, these individuals should engage in regular physical activity as their abilities allow and should avoid inactivity. These adults should also be under the care of a health care provider and can consult with their provider or a physical activity specialist to determine the appropriate types and amounts of activities for their abilities.

Sedentary Behavior

Our technologically advanced society has provided many highly beneficial tools and devices to save time and energy that have impacted our physical activity levels at work, at home, and in our social lives. However, reducing the time we spend in physical activity has created new health challenges and an urgent need to look at sedentary behavior as a major public health problem. Until recently, the term *sedentary behavior* — also called "sedentarism" or simply "sitting time" — has misleadingly been used as a synonym for not exercising. However, new research indicating that the harmful effects of prolonged sitting accrue even in those who exercise has led to new distinctions between the terms *physical inactivity* and *sedentary behavior* (29). The newly accepted definition of sedentary behavior is "any waking behavior characterized by an energy expenditure of ≤1.5 metabolic equivalents (METs), while in a sitting, reclining, or lying posture" (1, 29).

Health Effects of Sedentary Behavior

As previously mentioned, the general health risks of sedentary behavior are briefly discussed in the 2018-PAG (1). The guidelines state that more time spent in sedentary behavior increases an individual's risk for all-cause and

CVD mortality, CVD, T2DM, and cancers of the colon, endometrium, and lung (1). Although they are separate behaviors, the health risks associated with sedentary behavior are known to be dependent upon the level of moderate- to vigorous-intensity physical activity in which one engages. Those with high volumes of sedentary time can reduce their risk of all-cause mortality by engaging in high volumes of moderate- to vigorous-intensity activity. Additionally, low levels of sedentary behavior reduce, but do not eliminate the health risks associated with performing no moderate- to vigorous-intensity physical activity. Finally, replacing time spent in sedentary behavior with even light-intensity physical activity reduces the risk of all-cause mortality and the reduction is magnified if sedentary behavior is replaced with moderate- to vigorous-intensity physical activity (1). Because the majority of our population engages in high amounts of sedentary behavior and low levels of physical activity, most people will benefit from increasing their moderate- to vigorous-intensity activity in addition to reducing their sedentary behavior.

Public Health Recommendations for Sedentary Behavior

In 2020, the World Health Organization (WHO) released the *Guidelines on Physical Activity and Sedentary Behavior* (30). These guidelines recommend that persons of all ages and abilities limit the amount of time they spend in sedentary behavior. For children and adolescents, the guidelines specify limiting the amount of recreational screen time in which they engage. Adults, older adults, pregnant and postpartum women, as well as adults living with chronic disease and disability are encouraged to replace sedentary time with physical activity of any intensity, including light intensity. Beyond these general guidelines, the WHO indicates that currently there is insufficient evidence to specify recommendations for precise time limits or patterns of sedentary behavior in any age or population subgroup. For this same reason, neither ACSM nor HHS have endorsed any detailed recommendations for sedentary behavior.

The Future of Recommendations for Human Movement: 24-Hour Movement Guidelines

Developing research indicates that interactions among physical activity, sedentary behavior, and another important health behavior, sleep, are important for many aspects of health. Taken together, these behaviors comprise the 24-hour movement paradigm, which represents a new model for how we think about human movement (Figure 4.5). As such, some organizations have begun to incorporate physical activity, sedentary behavior, and sleep into comprehensive 24-hour movement guidelines. For example, the Canadian Society for Exercise Physiology has developed separate 24-hour movement guidelines for four population age groups (0–4 years, 5–17 years, 18–64 years, and 65+ years; https://csepguidelines.ca/) (31). Similarly, the Australian Council for Health, Physical Education, and Recreation released 24-Hour Movement Guidelines for Children and Young People in 2021 (32). As evidence supporting the interrelatedness of these behaviors and their impacts on health continues to accumulate, it is likely that we will see an increased adoption of 24-hour movement guidelines in the future.

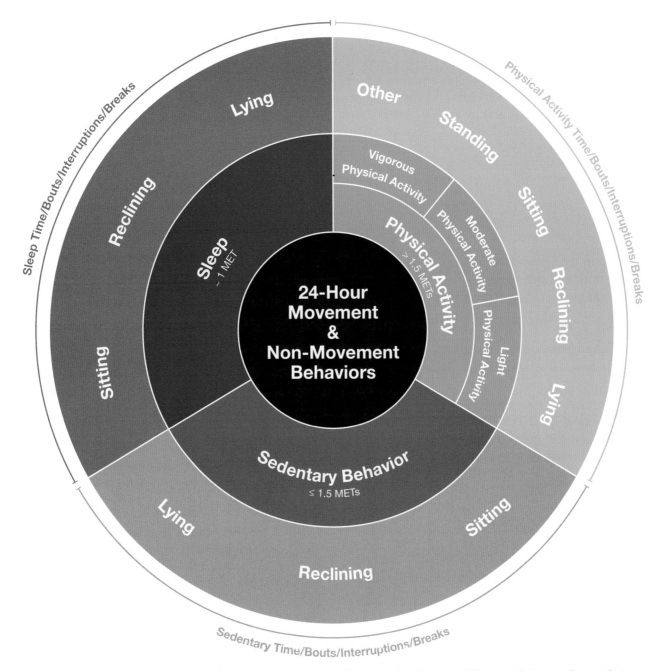

FIGURE 4.5 A conceptual model of the 24-hour movement paradigm. (Reprinted from Tremblay MS, Aubert S, Barnes JD, et al. Sedentary Behavior Research Network (SBRN)—Terminology Consensus Project process and outcome. *Int J Behav Nutr Phys Act.* 2017;14(1):75.)

Integration of the Recommendations: Key Messages

At first glance, the recommendations and guidelines provided by ACSM, HHS, and other public health agencies for physical activity and sedentary behavior might appear to be contradictory. However, upon closer examination, they converge to offer a set of key messages the CEP can use to frame a weekly movement prescription for the majority of apparently healthy adults.

The Benefits Are Well Established

A vast literature of scientific evidence supports the independent benefits of exercise training, physical activity, and reducing sedentary behavior on cardiorespiratory and metabolic health, neuromusculoskeletal health, brain and cognitive functioning, and psychological well-being including anxiety, depression, energy levels, and mood. Regular movement is a key to optimal functional fitness and a high health-related quality of life in contemporary society.

Risks Can Be Minimized With Appropriate Screening, Progression, and Modification

As described in Chapter 3, adequate screening is imperative for moving safely, especially when working with clients who are beginning an exercise program, are increasing the intensity of their program, or have one or more chronic conditions. As health benefits can be realized when progressing from a completely sedentary lifestyle to a minimally active lifestyle, it is appropriate to begin a program with lower intensity and progress slowly (2). Finally, the client's health status should always inform the modifications chosen to promote exercise safety. These modifications might include alterations in intensity for a cardiovascular condition, reducing impact to accommodate an orthopedic condition such as an arthritic knee or chronic low back pain, or choosing swimming or a stationary cycle as a mode for aerobic exercise to prevent falling because of balance challenges.

Cardiorespiratory and Resistance Training Are Both Important for Health

As noted earlier, the strongest evidence of the health benefits of habitual human movement is specific to cardiorespiratory (aerobic) and resistance (muscle-strengthening) training. Therefore, at a minimum, most adults should aim to meet the 2018-PAG recommendations for 150 minutes of moderate-intensity activity per week, or 75 minutes of vigorous-intensity aerobic activity per week, or an equivalent combination of moderate- and vigorous-intensity aerobic activity. The 2018-PAG guidelines of muscle-strengthening activities of moderate or greater intensity that involve all major muscles groups on 2 or more days a week should also be strongly encouraged for all adults, but especially middle-older individuals. The importance of resistance training and the resulting muscular fitness cannot be emphasized enough, especially in helping middle-older adults maintain their physical functional independence.

Moving More Promotes Greater Health Benefits

Meeting the minimum 2018-PAG guidelines is an important personal and population goal; however, increased movement — in terms of intensity or volume or perhaps mode (*e.g.*, adding flexibility training to an established aerobic training routine) — confers greater health benefits. Within the constraints presented by an individual's goals, health status, and willingness to allocate time and effort, more movement, within reason, is better.

Move Your Way

Although the human movement paradigm has framed the guidelines for moving for health, it is important to appreciate that there are many options to meet these guidelines. This is such an important message that the 2018-PAG is linked with the Move Your Way campaign (https://health.gov/our-work/nutrition-physical-activity/move-your-way-community-resources) to educate the public and offer suggestions as to how individuals can meet the guidelines in ways that work for their schedule, interests, and environment. As the guidelines and recommendations continue to reflect the growing body of scientific evidence, there will be more options than ever for a person to construct a weekly or perhaps daily movement plan, the latter being based on the 24-hour movement paradigm. This paradigm offers the opportunity for diversity within movement choices. For example, structured intentional exercise within a health club or fitness facility may be a primary choice for one individual. Another might primarily move outdoors, whether in physical labor or leisure activities such as hiking or walking a dog. Within a typical workday, parking further away from the building, taking stretching breaks, using the stairs instead of the elevator, or scheduling a walking meeting might be good options. Walking in the neighborhood with friends might also take the place of walking on the treadmill indoors, and simultaneously help maintain important social relationships. Gardening, carrying groceries, and housework are functional movement options that might take the place of resistance or flexibility training in a fitness facility. However, even given the endless options and opportunities to move, incorporating all portions of the human movement paradigm into daily living takes planning, effort, and a will to feel better by moving more and sitting less.

It's Never Too Late to Start

Although beyond the scope of this chapter, the scientific evidence clearly suggests that beginning habitual movement, especially aerobic exercise, early in life reduces the risk for numerous chronic conditions and helps maintain physical function in middle-older adulthood (8). However, individuals who become active later in life, even after a lifetime of physical inactivity and sedentary behavior, can still realize important health benefits. Moreover, chronic conditions are more prevalent in middle-older adulthood, and habitual exercise and physical activity play key roles in the management of most chronic conditions, including psychosocial challenges such as anxiety and depression, as discussed previously. Finally, habitual movement preserves an older adult's capacity for independent living and optimal social engagement.

Benefits Won't Accrue if Movement Is Not Habitual

Although the evidence is abundantly clear that movement is essential to health, the benefits cannot be realized if the behavior is not habitual. Both ACSM and HHS acknowledge that maintenance of movement behavior is challenging in most societies that have engineered most physical movement out of daily lives. Recall that only about 20% of adults in the U.S. adhere to the 2018-PAG (1). Alarmingly, in older adult cohorts, the prevalence of failing to meet the 2018-PAG is well over 90% (33). Thus, unlocking the behavioral keys to empower all individuals to be habitually active — for example, by impressing upon clients that physical activity does not have to take place in a fitness facility — is an important aspect of the CEP's treatment plan.

The Importance of Human Movement for Health Continues to Evolve

The literature regarding the importance of movement for health has evolved in a myriad of ways in the past 50+ years. Evidence of this evolution can be seen in the progression and expansion of ACSM GETP to include a variety of modes and supporting details for testing and prescription. This parallels the important changes in the past 10 years with the second edition of the PAG (2008–2018), especially regarding the new evidence of physical activity benefits for brain health, cancer, anxiety and depression, sleep, physical function, quality of life, and disease-specific mortality. Although research evidence and evidence-based applications and guidelines are important, they are of little value if they fail to increase habitual movement by members of society. Thus, a most salient area of interest for human movement and health is within the behavioral sciences; that is, we must find the keys (spanning from cell to society) to unlock the determinants of human movement behaviors. Only then will individuals be able to successfully navigate contemporary society as they are genetically programmed to be — engaged in daily moderate and intense physical movement and minimal sedentary behavior.

EMERGING TRENDS IN HUMAN MOVEMENT AND FITNESS

There is growing interest in health, wellness, physical activity, exercise, and fitness for the everyday consumer. Health, fitness, and exercise professionals have seen shifts in trends, notably many that were accelerated because of the COVID-19 global pandemic.

According to ACSM Fitness Trends for 2022 (34), the top fitness trends are (a) WT, (b) home exercise gyms, (c) outdoor activities, (d) strength training with free weights, (e) exercise for weight loss, (f) personal training, (g) high-intensity interval training, (h), body weight training, (i) online live and on-demand exercise classes, and (j) health and wellness coaching. A few important paradigm-shifting themes not to be missed are that (a) many individuals are choosing to complete their exercise and/or physical activity routines outside of conventional fitness facilities and centers (*e.g.*, at home, outside, online) and (b) individuals have an increased interest in strategies to enhance personal behavioral adherence (*e.g.*, WT, personal training, health and wellness coaching). These trends suggest a changing fitness paradigm that the CEP is encouraged to explore with their clients. More information can be found at https://www.acsm.org/education-resources/trending-topics-resources/acsm-fitness-trends. In this section, we will discuss two of these trends in relation to movement guidelines for the apparently healthy adult population. We will also discuss the Exercise is

Medicine (EIM) initiative, a long-standing initiative by ACSM to promote physical activity within the health care sector.

Wearable Technology

Paradoxically, the technological advances that engineered physical movement out of daily living can also assist the efforts of fitness professionals to improve the movement behaviors of their clients using personal WT. WT can be a device or application, typically wearable or portable, used to monitor activity metrics such as number of steps taken, distance walked/run, or kilocalories expended, or to remind the user to get up and move (Figure 4.6). Some apps include videos showing instructors demonstrating a particular exercise or leading an exercise class. Some WT is multidimensional, measuring other behaviors that affect a person's health and well-being beyond movement, such as sleep and stress. ACSM's annual fitness trends research study also named WT as the top trend for 2020 (35) and second top trend for 2021 (36). Market research indicates that the sales of WT has increased exponentially in recent years with sales of $35 billion in 2020, with expected sales to be nearly $115 billion by 2028 (37).

Emerging research demonstrates the impact WT has in promoting physical activity among an apparently healthy population, with Deloitte's 2021 Connectivity and Mobile Trends Survey reporting 39% of Americans own either a smartwatch or health and fitness tracker (38). Toth et al. (39) demonstrated that commercial trackers (*e.g.*, Garmin Vivofit 2, FitBit Charge) had minor step count errors (10%–15%) compared to research-grade trackers and are a suitable device to help

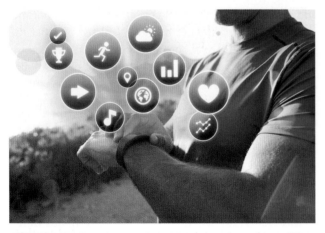

FIGURE 4.6 Wearable activity trackers are very popular. (From Shutterstock.)

individuals track physical activity. Wilson et al. (40) further demonstrated that WT coupled with an online weight loss program can predict improvements in weight loss, demonstrating the valuable role WT has in health promotion behaviors and outcomes.

Additionally, with the push to more online exercise classes and exercise-focused phone applications because of the COVID pandemic and shifting fitness trends, WT provides an innovative mechanism for the physical activity and exercise consumer to integrate technology into other aspects of physical activity promotion. For example, WT offers a personal yet objective accountability tool for physical activity, while facilitating social connection. Theoretically, personal WT promotes awareness, holds users accountable for movement goals, and records the movement in an easy and convenient manner. Also, when combined with social media and phone application interfaces, WT facilitates coaching and social support from trained fitness professionals or from family and friends. It is recognized that physical activity behaviors may change more successfully if theory-backed approaches are employed. The social cognitive theory posits that self-efficacy, self-monitoring, and social support are essential components for successful behavior change (41). These three factors can be targeted and manipulated using an innovative approach with WT. Finally, WT is a great strategy for integrating physical activity and movement throughout the day, which is critical to the 24-hour movement paradigm and reducing overall sedentary behavior while promoting activity.

Although the commercial landscape for WT is ever evolving, the CEP can employ some practical strategies to encourage clients to use WT effectively to reduce sedentary time and move more. Integrating the current recommended step counts for health, especially for sedentary individuals, is a start. Translation of step count data to daily movement suggests that 30 minutes per day of moderate to vigorous physical activity translates to approximately 7,900 steps per day for males and 8,300 steps per day for females, whereas 150 minutes per week of moderate to vigorous physical activity translates to approximately 7,000 steps per day or 49,000 steps per week (42). In order to encourage movement in clients with the lowest levels of physical activity while starting a program, teach them that inactive individuals are the population gaining the greatest initial improvement in health upon becoming habitually moderately active. A downside of WT, however, is that they may promote an "all or nothing" mindset so it is important to work with clients to ensure they understand all movement matters and contributes toward optimal health benefits (43). Finally, keep in mind that there are both benefits and challenges to all WT on the market. Researching and personally using emerging WT will help you foster an increase in the level of physical activity in your apparently healthy clients if they choose to use WT in their program.

Online Live and On-Demand Exercise Classes

In early 2020, the global COVID-19 pandemic upended society and affected all facets of life from travel to dining out to health care to the health fitness industry and beyond. An early target of the pandemic was the health fitness industry as health fitness clubs and facilities around the world were temporarily closed. As such, the health fitness industry was forced to pivot quickly and identify innovative strategies to deliver fitness classes and opportunities. One such strategy was providing exercise classes and instruction virtually. Online training uses "digital streaming technology to deliver group, individual, or instructional exercise programs online" (36). To add more flexibility and to encourage movement throughout the day, online training is available 24/7 and can be either live (synchronous) or prerecorded (asynchronous). Examples of online training platforms include Obe Fitness (www.obefitness.com), Openfit (www.openfit.com), and Class Pass (www.classpass.com). Online training platforms provide many of the benefits of an in-person class such as a certified, experienced trainer and social support along with different exercise options including yoga, Pilates, running, and walking to keep the consumer engaged. For individuals who are looking to become active in the convenience and privacy of their own home and are seeking more tailored programming, online training platforms can provide additional motivation to become active. Furthermore, online training platforms are changing the way consumers think about exercise and fitness. Online training platforms provide flexibility to consumers, allowing them to participate as their schedule allows, without having to leave work early to secure a spot in a high-demand fitness class. Subscriptions to these platforms are often comparable to the cost of a traditional fitness center membership.

Despite the push toward online training platforms, research examining the impact of online training on health outcomes is limited. Research conducted pre-COVID demonstrated that online group-based exercising was effective in motivating and enabling individuals who were less fit to train as much as fitter individuals and helped

older adults reduce feelings of loneliness (44). Postpandemic, one study (45) demonstrated that a virtual exercise program was safe for individuals with musculoskeletal conditions and improved their health outcomes while helping them feel more socially connected, which was especially critical during the time of COVID-19 mitigation measures. More research, however, should be conducted with a variety of populations, especially those prone to social isolation (*e.g.*, older adults), to examine both short-term and long-term impacts of online training platforms on physical activity levels along with health and well-being outcomes.

EIM Initiative

According to the 2018-PAG (1), there are nine sectors where physical activity should be promoted: (a) health care; (b) business and industry; (c) community recreation, fitness, and parks; (d) education; (e) faith-based settings; (f) mass media; (g) public health; (h) sports; and (i) transportation, land use, and community design. As such, the EIM initiative addresses the first sector of physical activity promotion and provides promising strategies to promote physical activity and reduce sedentary behavior within the population.

The health care system and health care providers can be important partners in educating and empowering patients to increase habitual movement in their daily lives, but effectiveness and access are limited in the current health care structure (46). The EIM initiative is a global initiative that is managed by ACSM and whose goal is to "make physical activity assessment and promotion a standard in clinical care, connecting health care with evidence-based physical activity resources for people everywhere and of all abilities." EIM is designed to improve patient health and well-being by encouraging health care providers to focus on physical activity as a vital sign, similar to heart rate and blood pressure (47).

Despite evidence that movement and physical activity may serve as a "miracle drug" (47) with a myriad of health benefits, it is typically not prescribed by health care providers compared to traditional pharmaceuticals. Health care providers, however, have the unique opportunity to facilitate behavior change by recommending this "miracle drug" through conversations with patients about personal movement behaviors. Notably, the majority of patients state their health care providers are primary sources of information for healthy behavior choices and they are more likely to adopt a behavior if it is recommended by their provider (48).

EIM is working to facilitate provider–patient conversations about physical activity and to provide written patient education materials that the client can take home. For example, an EIM physical activity prescription pad has been designed to enhance communication between providers and patients and to support patient motivation for behavior change. The EIM initiative also provides access to succinct patient educational materials for various common medical conditions — such as low back pain, T2DM, obesity, and anxiety/depression — that teach specific movements and exercise options helpful in managing these conditions. The reader is referred to the EIM Web site for a wealth of information (www.exerciseismedicine.org). Edbrooke et al. (49) provide guidance to health care providers on having these conversations with their patients. First, they recommend assessing the patient's current physical activity behaviors, including the number of days, minutes, and intensity. Next, health care providers should provide encouragement and tailoring of the patient's physical activity program as needed. Finally, health care providers should recommend patients to work with certified, physical activity professionals as needed for safety or health reasons.

Many health care providers report that a barrier to more effective health promotion is their discomfort in encouraging patients to engage in behaviors they themselves do not practice (50). However, this empathetic "me too" perspective can be used to enhance health behaviors; that is, a provider's own health behavior struggles, when shared with a patient during an impressionable time, can positively impact the patient's motivation (51). In addition, provider counseling is strongly related to their own health practices. Thus, increasing a health care provider's physical activity or other health behaviors may in turn increase their likelihood of engaging in health promotion counseling in their practice (52). Even active providers who prescribe physical activity to their patients, however, state they are unaware of what current guidelines to recommend (53). In short, when health care providers adopt healthier lifestyles, both they and their patients benefit. Adopting and reinforcing EIM practices result in health care providers also receiving more education and preparation in effective health promotion counseling. Therefore, utilizing the EIM tools is a logical place to start both personally and professionally for health care providers.

Research demonstrating the effectiveness of EIM to change patient movement behaviors is growing. One study, for example, followed a program called "Exercise as a Vital Sign" that had been implemented in four different medical centers. Data collected during outpatient visits indicated that participation in the program was associated with small but significant changes in exercise-related clinical processes and outcomes (54).

To become mainstream, EIM concepts will need to be integrated into provider training. Evidence in favor of establishing a required physical activity/exercise or kinesiology class into primary care medical education is growing in support, and medical schools are beginning to adopt the EIM content into their curricula. For example, EIM is being introduced into the curriculum for the University of South Carolina School of Medicine, Greenville, and a pilot study within the Greenville Health System evaluated the influence of the EIM program on patient care (55).

Assuming a health care provider models best practice for habitual physical movement and is skilled in assessing a patient's level of physical activity, the provider's next step is to educate and empower sedentary patients to become more physically active. Within the constraints of the health care system, patient contact time is limited, and referral is often the best course of action. Physical activity levels improve more when patients are referred to a qualified fitness professional specifically (56).

Although several models exist globally connecting physical activity prescription and referral within the health care system, one does not exist within the U.S. Whitsel et al. (57), however, propose an innovative model, the Physical Activity Care Continuum model, to be used within the U.S. The Physical Activity Care Continuum model connects patient screening, prescription, and referral within the clinical setting to community resources and a tailored physical activity plan (Figure 4.7). This model also incorporates a feedback loop to the health care provider about whether physical activity was initiated. The Physical Activity Care Continuum model proposes tailored physical activity counseling, data collection for evaluation, health care training, assessment measures, and an intentional equity focus. This model provides promise for more successful integration of physical activity prescription, referral, and follow-up within clinical settings for physical activity promotion and improvement in health outcomes.

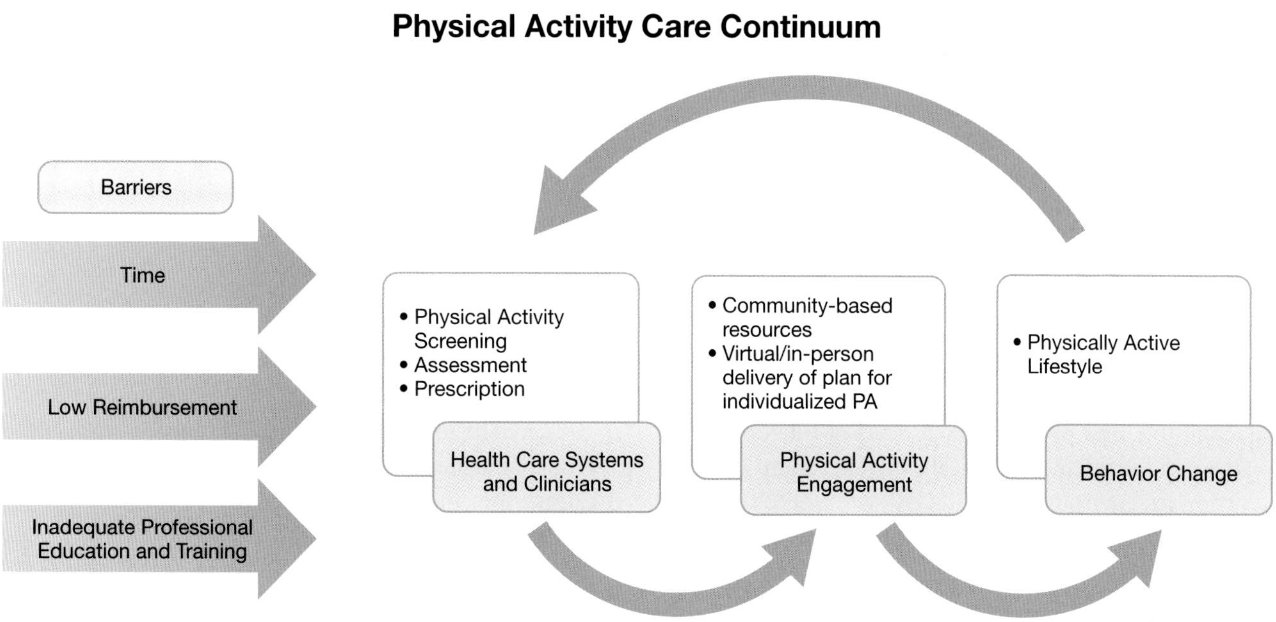

Physical Activity Care Continuum

FIGURE 4.7 The Physical Activity Care Continuum. (Reprinted from Whitsel LP, Bantham A, Jarrin R, Sanders L, Stoutenberg M. Physical activity assessment, prescription and referral in US healthcare: how do we make this a standard of clinical practice? *Prog Cardiovasc Dis.* 2021;64:84–95. doi:10.1016/j.pcad.2020.12.006.)

SUMMARY

The evidence base supporting the importance of habitual human movement for optimal health is extensive. Habitual human movement includes intentional exercise; physical activity in the broad domains of transportation, domestic chores, leisure, and occupation; and, in contrast, limiting time spent in sedentary behaviors. The human movement paradigm illustrates the important role of all three components for optimal human health. Indeed, the term *exercise prescription* is largely obsolete and should be replaced with the term *movement guidelines* to better capture contemporary perspectives. Looking into the future, an evolving literature base is focused on the 24-hour movement paradigm, inclusive of sleep, and health outcomes. The 24-hour movement paradigm will undoubtedly inform how we not only plan our weeks but also our days with respect to our patterns of movement and sedentary behaviors. Stay tuned for updated recommendations in the decades ahead. To reduce their chronic disease risk and enhance their daily functional fitness, individuals should meet the 2018-PAG; however, most individuals are challenged by both time and personal motivation, and only 20% of Americans currently do so. In this technologically advanced society, few occupations require significant physical activity; thus, habitual daily movement must be intentionally planned into the daily and weekly schedule. Paradoxically, technology can be used to foster human movement through increasingly popular personal WT, especially devices that link to social media and thereby may provide social support from friends and family. Finally, partnerships for personal health behavior management are essential for adherence. The EIM initiative is one such potential partnership where the focus is on physical activity as a vital sign from health care providers. However, an apparently healthy person does not need extensive medical clearance to be active. A simple prescreening is adequate to determine readiness to move. Individuals can utilize any of a variety of physical activity choices, locations, equipment, and resources to meet the recommendations without joining a fitness facility. Alternatively, they may seek the services of a qualified fitness professional to provide both guidance and motivation. Encourage all patients and clients to move most days if not every day and Move Your [Their] Way.

CHAPTER REVIEW QUESTIONS

1. How have ACSM PSs, which capture evidence-based guidelines for exercise, changed over the years since the inception of the 1978 version to the 2011 PSs?
2. What are the three main components of the human movement paradigm for optimal health, and how has this influenced the term *exercise prescription*?
3. Discuss the benefits of regular physical activity on cardiorespiratory, metabolic, and functional fitness. How does habitual movement enhance the physical, cognitive, and psychosocial aspects of functional fitness in today's technologically advanced and socially complex environment?
4. Compare and contrast the GETP-11 and the 2018-PAG.
5. Identify ACSM Fitness Trends for 2022 and the major paradigm-shifting themes that are found within these trends.
6. Identify some practical strategies for encouraging patients or clients to utilize a WT device with a social media interface to monitor their daily movement.
7. Describe the relationship between physical activity and sedentary behavior as they interact to influence health outcomes.
8. Identify the nine sectors where physical activity should be promoted according to the 2018-PAG.
9. What is ACSM EIM initiative, and how can its resources be located and utilized to encourage patients or clients to adopt a movement plan?
10. Describe the Physical Activity Care Continuum model and how it can play a role in promoting physical activity/movement in the health care sector.

CASE STUDIES

Case Study 4.1

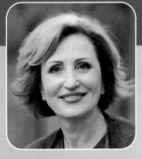

Angela is a middle-aged woman who presents at her yearly physical with a concern about mild intermittent low back pain. Also, although she is currently of normal weight, she is concerned about her increasing waistline. She is married to a man who also works full time, and they have two elementary school-aged children. She states she uses her treadmill almost daily for 30 minutes while she watches the morning news and drinks her coffee. Angela has never been involved in any strength training activities nor does she do any flexibility exercises. Her work requires long hours at a desk in front of a computer screen at a location where she parks close to the entrance, and she usually works through lunch so that she can leave early to meet her children from the bus after a lengthy commute. She cannot figure out why her waistline is expanding, as her eating patterns have not changed.

Angela is meeting the exercise guidelines for cardiorespiratory exercise, but she is not meeting them for muscular fitness and flexibility. Complimenting Angela on her cardiorespiratory activities would be important. Then, a short lesson on muscle balance and the importance of muscular fitness and resistance training should be provided. Muscle imbalances often present with chronic pain and, if left unchecked, lead to injury. They can be improved by incorporating appropriate muscular fitness and flexibility exercises. Thus, some potential items to discuss for Angela's lower back pain might be common muscle imbalances, their causes, and exercises to correct them.

Because most muscle imbalances arise from activities of daily living, keeping in mind what patients do when they are not exercising is important. Corrective exercises, typically a combination of muscular fitness exercises, especially of the core muscles group, and flexibility training can help participants improve overall functional fitness, especially to enhance performance of daily activities within their life.

The strategy for correcting muscle imbalances is to strengthen the weak muscles not used consistently in daily movements and to stretch the less flexible relatively strong muscles. For example, the rhomboid muscles get stretched all day from forward flexion of the spine sitting at desks. Strengthening the rhomboids by retracting the scapulae and sitting up tall while working at a desk might help Angela reduce the muscle imbalance caused by sitting at a desk with poor posture. Another example, likely pertinent to her low back pain, would be to encourage her to stretch her hip flexor muscle groups, which are in a chronically shortened position when sitting.

Other lifestyle modifications to help Angela would be to park her car further away from the door, have walking meetings, put her printer outside of her office, and get more movement in general in her day. To further encourage Angela to become more physically active, it will be important to remind her that she can meet the PAG and introduce some daily movement training in her workspace and her home and neighborhood, without needing to carve out time to go to a fitness facility. She can learn exercises to improve her muscular fitness and flexibility to improve her posture and functional fitness at home and potentially include her family. Likely as important, she will need to intentionally break up her sitting time.

Case Study 4.1 Questions

1. What are some additional ways that Angela can increase lifestyle physical activity throughout her days, specifically some ways that she can involve her family?
2. Because Angela is already in the habit of using the treadmill each morning, what are some ways you could progress her cardiorespiratory training overtime, while keeping her morning exercise sessions enjoyable?
3. Time is a commonly cited barrier to starting an exercise routine. When and how would you suggest that Angela fit her new strength and flexibility exercise sessions into her already busy routine?

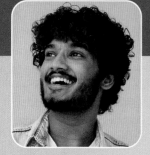

Case Study 4.2

Sam is a 27-year-old single man who has recently realized his pants are getting tighter in the waistband. Although his weight has not changed much since being a swimmer and diver throughout high school and college, he suspects his body composition has changed because of his expanding midsection. Sam works in the information technology industry for the local school system, so he spends much of his day sitting at a desk or attending meetings with the teachers. Outside of work, he helps his grandparents with farm chores, enjoys an occasional hike on the weekends with friends, walks his dog daily for approximately 15 minutes twice per day, is an avid sports watcher, and plays video games.

Sam is apparently healthy and has no definitive risk factors for cardiometabolic conditions, but at his yearly checkup for work, the physician asked Sam about his current exercise routine. After Sam responded with discontent about exercise, local gyms, and fitness fads, the physician recommended Sam consult with a fitness professional to create a plan for moving more and sitting less including:

■ Outdoor physical activity and exercise options,
■ Exercise options that do not require a facility or equipment, and
■ Ideas for changing his sitting time at work and during leisure pursuits.

Sam could also be advised to continue and perhaps increase the frequency, intensity, or duration of activities that he already enjoys, such as helping his grandparents on their farm, walking his dog regularly, and hiking on the weekends with friends. Hence his movement prescription could be related to his daily living setting. Because he accumulates enough moderate-intensity physical activity most weeks to meet the 2018-PAG through farming and hiking, strength training in nontraditional modes (*i.e.*, body weight exercises that require no special equipment, rock climbing, etc.) might be introduced. Sam should be encouraged to break up long bouts of sedentary behavior during the workday by walking upstairs to use the restroom, relying solely on the stairs rather than the elevator, or asking his supervisor for a standing desk. Workday breaks might also include stretching key muscle groups such as hip flexor and front shoulder muscle groups, which are often compromised by sitting and working at a computer. Finally, Sam should be encouraged to purchase a wearable device. Many current models synchronize wirelessly to a mobile device and provide up-to-the-minute feedback on movement. Additionally, many wearable devices have a setting to "alarm" the wearer when he/she has been sitting for over 1 hour. Because Sam likes technology, this may be a sensible way for him to self-monitor daily movement.

Case Study 4.2 Questions

1. If Sam expresses discontent about the cost of purchasing a wearable device, what are some other options you can suggest for using technology to track his ambulatory physical activity?

2. What are some physiological benefits of both regular exercise and reduced sitting time that you should explain to Sam when helping him move more and sit less?

3. Provide two examples of strength training exercises you may suggest to Sam that require no specialized equipment, so that he's able to incorporate them at home.

Case Study 4.3

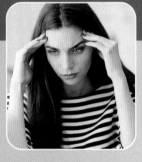

Monica is a 21-year-old cis-female who was attending an out-of-state school but transferred to be closer to home and is now enrolled in a local college pursuing a degree in accountancy. Monica's degree program utilizes a hybrid design where four out of her five classes are virtual. On some days, she spends almost the entire day in sitting positions, either attending classes or studying.

After feeling more tired and stressed than usual, she visits the Student Health Center to talk with her health care provider about the changes in her mood and how she suspects her schedule has impacted her quality of life. She has also noticed her grades are dropping and she isn't as engaged in many aspects of her life as she was before classes were in the virtual format.

Monica tells her health care provider that she played sports year-round in high school but is not active anymore because she works part-time to pay for school and could not afford the fees for intramural teams. Although she hasn't seen any noticeable changes in her weight, she reports feeling sluggish and burnt out. When asked about other factors in her life, Monica tells her health care provider that she is feeling overwhelmed because she is working part-time and has a full course load with many of those classes online, a modality that is not very comfortable or enjoyable. Because many of her classes are online and she is a transfer student, she has not met a lot of her classmates and feels isolated, which leads to increased feelings of anxiety and depression. She also describes that because of her busy schedule, she is only averaging about 4–5 hours of sleep per night. She

tries to catch up on sleep over the weekends, but still enters each week feeling exhausted. Despite her transition to virtual classes, she has managed to maintain a relatively stable diet and eating pattern with no large shifts in the number of meals or calories she consumes per day and no real differences in her dining-away-from-home habits.

According to the newly recognized 24-hour movement paradigm, Monica should be encouraged to (a) increase her level of physical activity, (b) reduce the amount of time she spends sitting, and (c) get adequate sleep on a regular basis. Regarding physical activity, Monica should be encouraged to use several strategies to help her meet PAG. For example, she could incorporate an activity tracker to monitor her physical activity each day and ensure she knows how much activity she is getting. She could also enroll in online fitness classes that she can work in during any spare time. Both strategies also provide the opportunity for interaction with others through online or social platforms, which may help Monica feel more connected to others and make it easier to maintain increased levels of physical activity. To reduce her sedentary behavior, Monica could create a standing desk where she can attend her online classes and do her schoolwork while standing instead of sitting all day. Additionally, Monica should be encouraged to take breaks in her class and study time to allow her to incorporate short bouts of physical activity. Finally, although not a focus of this chapter, Monica should aim to obtain an adequate amount of sleep on as many days of the week as possible. She should make sure that her sleep environment is conducive to restful sleep and should also maintain good sleep hygiene including a regular bedtime.

Case Study 4.3 Questions

1. What psychosocial benefits of movement should you explain to Monica to help her move more and sit less?
2. Discuss Monica's level of risk for health issues because of her sedentary behavior coupled with her inability to meet PAG. In the context of the 24-hour movement paradigm, what general recommendations would you offer

Monica related to her physical activity, sedentary behavior, and sleep?

3. Moving forward, as a CEP, how can you use the Physical Activity Care Continuum model to work more collaboratively with health care providers within the university health care system?

REFERENCES

1. US Department of Health and Human Services. Scientific report — 2018 physical activity guidelines — health.gov. February 2018 [cited 2019 Feb 12]. Available from: https://health.gov/paguidelines/second-edition/report/.
2. American College of Sports Medicine. *ACSM's Guidelines for Exercise Testing and Prescription*. Eleventh, Spiral edition. Philadelphia (PA): Lippincott Williams & Wilkins; 2021.
3. Ussery EN, Whitfield GP, Fulton JE, et al. Trends in self-reported sitting time by physical activity levels among US adults, NHANES 2007/2008–2017/2018. *J Phys Act Health*. 2021;18(SI):S74–S83. doi:10.1123/jpah.2021-0221.
4. Kasapis C, Thompson PD. The effects of physical activity on serum C-reactive protein and inflammatory markers: a systematic review. *J Am Coll Cardiol*. 2005;45(10):1563–9. doi:10.1016/j.jacc.2004.12.077.
5. American College of Sports Medicine; Chodzko-Zajko WJ, Proctor DN, Fiatarone Singh MA, et al. American College of Sports Medicine position stand. Exercise and physical activity for older adults. *Med Sci Sports Exerc*. 2009;41(7):1510–30. doi:10.1249/MSS.0b013e3181a0c95c.
6. Bauman A, Merom D, Bull FC, Buchner DM, Fiatarone Singh MA. Updating the evidence for physical activity: summative reviews of the epidemiological evidence, prevalence, and interventions to promote "active aging." *Gerontologist*. 2016;56(suppl 2):S268–80. doi:10.1093/geront/gnw031.
7. Hall KS, Cohen HJ, Pieper CF, et al. Physical performance across the adult life span: correlates with age and physical activity. *J Gerontol A Biol Sci Med Sci*. 2017;72(4):572–8. doi:10.1093/gerona/glw120.
8. Colcombe S, Kramer AF. Fitness effects on the cognitive function of older adults: a meta-analytic study. *Psychol Sci*. 2003;14(2):125–30. doi:10.1111/1467-9280.t01-1-01430.
9. Voss MW, Nagamatsu LS, Liu-Ambrose T, Kramer AF. Exercise, brain, and cognition across the life span. *J Appl Physiol (1985)*. 2011;111(5):1505–13. doi:10.1152/japplphysiol.00210.2011.
10. National Institute of Mental Health (NIMH). Major depression. Bethesda (MD): National Institute of Mental Health (NIMH); [cited 2022 Jan 6]. Available from: https://www.nimh.nih.gov/health/statistics/major-depression.
11. Puetz TW, O'Connor PJ, Dishman RK. Effects of chronic exercise on feelings of energy and fatigue: a quantitative

synthesis. *Psychol Bull*. 2006;132(6):866–76. doi:10.1037/0033-2909.132.6.866.
12. Kredlow MA, Capozzoli MC, Hearon BA, Calkins AW, Otto MW. The effects of physical activity on sleep: a meta-analytic review. *J Behav Med*. 2015;38(3):427–49. doi:10.1007/s10865-015-9617-6.
13. American College of Sports Medicine. American College of Sports Medicine Position statement on the recommended quantity and quality of exercise for developing and maintaining fitness in healthy adults. *Med Sci Sports*. 1978;10(3):vii–x.
14. American College of Sports Medicine. American College of Sports Medicine Position Stand: the recommended quantity and quality of exercise for developing and maintaining cardiorespiratory and muscular fitness in healthy adults. *Med Sci Sports Exerc*. 1990;22(2):265–74.
15. American College of Sports Medicine Position. American College of Sports Medicine Position Stand: the recommended quantity and quality of exercise for developing and maintaining cardiorespiratory and muscular fitness, and flexibility in healthy adults. *Med Sci Sports Exerc*. 1998;30(6):975–91. doi:10.1097/00005768-199806000-00032.
16. Garber CE, Blissmer B, Deschenes MR, et al. American College of Sports Medicine Position Stand: quantity and quality of exercise for developing and maintaining cardiorespiratory, musculoskeletal, and neuromotor fitness in apparently healthy adults: guidance for prescribing exercise. *Med Sci Sports Exerc*. 2011;43(7):1334–59. doi:10.1249/MSS.0b013e318213fefb.
17. American College of Sports Medicine. American College of Sports Medicine Position Stand: exercise for patients with coronary artery disease. *Med Sci Sports Exerc*. 1994;26(3):i–v.
18. Pescatello LS, Franklin BA, Fagard R, et al.; American College of Sports Medicine. American College of Sports Medicine Position Stand. Exercise and hypertension. *Med Sci Sports Exerc*. 2004;36(3):533–53. doi:10.1249/01.mss.0000115224.88514.3a.
19. Kohrt WM, Bloomfield SA, Little KD, Nelson ME, Yingling VR; American College of Sports Medicine. American College of Sports Medicine Position Stand: physical activity and bone health. *Med Sci Sports Exerc*. 2004;36(11):1985–96. doi:10.1249/01.mss.0000142662.21767.58.

20. Donnelly JE, Blair SN, Jakicic JM, Manore MM, Rankin JW, Smith BK; American College of Sports Medicine. American College of Sports Medicine Position Stand: appropriate physical activity intervention strategies for weight loss and prevention of weight regain for adults. *Med Sci Sports Exerc.* 2009;41(2):459–71. doi:10.1249/MSS.0b013e3181949333.

21. Colberg SR, Sigal RJ, Fernhall B, et al. Exercise and type 2 diabetes, The American College of Sports Medicine and the American Diabetes Association: joint position statement. *Diabetes Care.* 2010;33(12):e147–67. doi:10.2337/dc10-9990.

22. Stoedefalke K, Faulkner J. *Guidelines for Graded Exercise Testing and Exercise Prescription.* 1st ed. Philadelphia (PA): Wolters Kluwer; 1975.

23. Pate RR, Pratt M, Blair SN, et al. Physical activity and public health. A recommendation from the Centers for Disease Control and Prevention and the American College of Sports Medicine. *JAMA.* 1995;273(5):402–7. doi:10.1001/jama.273.5.402.

24. U.S. Department of Health and Human Services. Physical activity and health: a report of the Surgeon General. Atlanta (GA): Centers for Disease Control and Prevention; 1996. Available from: https://www.cdc.gov/nccdphp/sgr/pdf/sgrfull.pdf.

25. Haskell WL, Lee IM, Pate RR, et al. Physical activity and public health: updated recommendation for adults from the American College of Sports Medicine and the American Heart Association. *Med Sci Sports Exerc.* 2007;39(8):1423–34. doi:10.1249/mss.0b013e3180616b27.

26. Norton K, Norton L, Sadgrove D. Position statement on physical activity and exercise intensity terminology. *J Sci Med Sport.* 2010;13(5):496–502. doi:10.1016/j.jsams.2009.09.008.

27. U.S. Department of Health and Human Services. *2008 Physical Activity Guidelines for Americans.* Washington (DC): U.S. Department of Health and Human Services; 2008.

28. Nelson ME, Rejeski WJ, Blair SN, et al. Physical activity and public health in older adults: recommendation from the American College of Sports Medicine and the American Heart Association. *Med Sci Sports Exerc.* 2007;39(8):1435–45. doi:10.1249/mss.0b013e3180616aa2.

29. Tremblay MS, Aubert S, Barnes JD, et al.; SBRN Terminology Consensus Project participants. Sedentary Behavior Research Network (SBRN) — Terminology Consensus Project process and outcome. *Int J Behav Nutr Phys Act.* 2017;14(1):75. doi:10.1186/s12966-017-0525-8.

30. Bull FC, Al-Ansari SS, Biddle S, et al. World Health Organization 2020 guidelines on physical activity and sedentary behaviour. *Br J Sports Med.* 2020;54(24):1451–62. doi:10.1136/bjsports-2020-102955.

31. Ross R, Chaput JP, Giangregorio LM, et al. Canadian 24-hour movement guidelines for adults aged 18-64 years and adults aged 65 years or older: an integration of physical activity, sedentary behaviour, and sleep. *Appl Physiol Nutr Metab.* 2020;45(10 (Suppl. 2)):S57–S102. doi:10.1139/apnm-2020-0467.

32. Australian Government Department of Health and Aged Care. For infants, toddlers and preschoolers (birth to 5 years). Canberra, ACT (Australia): Australian Government Department of Health and Aged Care. January 14, 2021 [cited 2022 Jan 6]. Available from: https://www.health.gov.au/health-topics/physical-activity-and-exercise/physical-activity-and-exercise-guidelines-for-all-australians/for-infants-toddlers-and-preschoolers-birth-to-5-years.

33. Matthews CE, Chen KY, Freedson PS, et al. Amount of time spent in sedentary behaviors in the United States, 2003–2004. *Am J Epidemiol.* 2008;167(7):875–81. doi:10.1093/aje/kwm390.

34. Thompson WR. Worldwide survey of fitness trends for 2022. *ACSMs Health Fit J.* 2022;26(1):11–20. doi:10.1249/FIT.0000000000000732.

35. American College of Sports Medicine. Wearable tech named top fitness trend for 2020. ACSM_CMS. 2019 [cited 2022 Jan 6]. Available from: https://www.acsm.org/news-detail/2019/10/30/wearable-tech-named-top-fitness-trend-for-2020.

36. Thompson WR. Worldwide survey of fitness trends for 2021. *ACSMs Health Fit J.* 2021;25(1):10–9. doi:10.1249/FIT.0000000000000631.

37. Fortune Business Insights. Fitness tracker market size, share, growth & analysis. 2021 [cited 2022 Jan 6]. Available from: https://www.fortunebusinessinsights.com/fitness-tracker-market-103358.

38. Deloitte. Deloitte: how the pandemic stress-tested the increasingly crowded digital home. New York (NY): Deloitte United States. 2021 [cited 2022 Jan 6]. Available from: https://www2.deloitte.com/us/en/pages/about-deloitte/articles/press-releases/deloitte-pandemic-stress-tested-digital-home.html.

39. Toth LP, Park S, Pittman WL, et al. Validity of activity tracker step counts during walking, running, and activities of daily living. *Transl J Am Coll Sports Med.* 2018;3(7):52–9. doi:10.1249/TJX.0000000000000057.

40. Wilson KE, Harden SM, Kleppe L, McGuire T, Estabrooks PA. The impact of pairing a wearable movement tracker with an online community weight loss intervention. *Transl J Am Coll Sports Med.* 2020;5(4):29–38. doi:10.1249/TJX.0000000000000116.

41. Bandura A. *Social Foundations of Thought and Action: A Social Cognitive Theory.* 1st ed. Hoboken (NJ): Prentice Hall Inc; 1986.

42. Tudor-Locke C, Leonardi C, Johnson WD, Katzmarzyk PT, Church TS. Accelerometer steps/day translation of moderate-to-vigorous activity. *Prev Med.* 2011;53(1-2):31–3. doi:10.1016/j.ypmed.2011.01.014.

43. Achauer. Is it time to stop using your fitness tracker? *The Seattle Times.* December 21, 2021 [cited 2022 Jan 6]. Available from: https://www.seattletimes.com/life/is-it-time-to-stop-using-your-fitness-tracker/.

44. Baez M, Khaghani Far I, Ibarra F, Ferron M, Didino D, Casati F. Effects of online group exercises for older adults on physical, psychological and social wellbeing: a randomized pilot trial. *PeerJ.* 2017;5:e3150. doi:10.7717/peerj.3150.

45. American College of Rheumatology. Virtual exercise effective for people with arthritis and helps them stay socially connected too; [cited 2022 Jan 6]. Available from: https://www.newswise.com/articles/virtual-exercise-effective-for-people-with-arthritis-and-helps-them-stay-socially-connected-too.

46. Landro. The health-care industry is pushing patients to help themselves. *Wall Street Journal.* 2014 [cited 2022 Jan 6]. Available from: https://www.wsj.com/articles/the-

health-care-industry-is-pushing-patients-to-help-themselves-1402065145.

47. American College of Sports Medicine. *Exercise Is Medicine.* 2021 [cited 2022 Jan 6]. Available from: https://www.exerciseismedicine.org/home/.

48. Abramson S, Stein J, Schaufele M, Frates E, Rogan S. Personal exercise habits and counseling practices of primary care physicians: a national survey. *Clin J Sport Med.* 2000;10(1):40–8. doi:10.1097/00042752-200001000-00008.

49. Edbrooke L, Granger CL, Denehy L. Physical activity for people with lung cancer. *Aust J Gen Pract.* 2020;49(4):175–81. doi:10.31128/AJGP-09-19-5060.

50. Vickers KS, Kircher KJ, Smith MD, Petersen LR, Rasmussen NH. Health behavior counseling in primary care: provider-reported rate and confidence. *Fam Med.* 2007;39(10):730–35.

51. Frank E, Tong E, Lobelo F, Carrera J, Duperly J. Physical activity levels and counseling practices of U.S. medical students. *Med Sci Sports Exerc.* 2008;40(3):413–21. doi:10.1249/MSS.0b013e31815ff399.

52. Oberg E, Frank E. Physicians' health practices strongly influence patient health practices. *J R Coll Physicians Edinb.* 2009;39(4):290–1. doi:10.4997/JRCPE.2009.422.

53. Das BM, DuBose KD, Peyton A. Active health care providers' practices and views on counseling patients to be active. *Transl J Am Coll Sports Med.* 2018;3(24):190–5. doi:10.1249/TJX.0000000000000075.

54. Grant RW, Schmittdiel JA, Neugebauer RS, Uratsu CS, Sternfeld B. Exercise as a vital sign: a quasi-experimental analysis of a health system intervention to collect patient-reported exercise levels. *J Gen Intern Med.* 2014;29(2):341–8. doi:10.1007/s11606-013-2693-9.

55. Trilk JL, Phillips EM. Incorporating "Exercise is Medicine" into the University of South Carolina School of Medicine Greenville and Greenville Health System. *Br J Sports Med.* 2014;48(3):165–7. doi:10.1136/bjsports-2013-093157.

56. Heath GW, Kolade VO, Haynes JW. Exercise is Medicine™: a pilot study linking primary care with community physical activity support. *Prev Med Rep.* 2015;2:492–7. doi:10.1016/j.pmedr.2015.06.004.

57. Whitsel LP, Bantham A, Jarrin R, Sanders L, Stoutenberg M. Physical activity assessment, prescription and referral in US healthcare: how do we make this a standard of clinical practice? *Prog Cardiovasc Dis.* 2021;64:88–95. doi:10.1016/j.pcad.2020.12.006.

Cardiovascular Disease

INTRODUCTION

Cardiovascular disease (CVD) is the number one cause of death for men and women (~24% and 21%, respectively) in the U.S. Broadly defined as disorders affecting the heart or blood vessels, it includes acute coronary syndrome (ACS), heart failure (HF), peripheral artery disease (PAD), hypertension (HTN), stroke, and several other disorders. More than one in three American adults have at least one type of CVD and approximately 51% of these patients are 60 years of age or older (1). According to data from 2017 to 2018, the annual direct and indirect cost of CVD in the U.S. is an estimated $378.0 billion. This figure includes $226.2 billion in expenditures (direct costs, which include the cost of physicians and other professionals, hospital services, prescribed medications, and home health care but not the cost of nursing home care) and $151.8 billion in lost future productivity (indirect costs) attributed to premature CVD mortality in 2017–2018 (1) (Figure 5.1).

Given its prevalence and societal impact, it is not surprising that CVD is the most common disorder encountered by the clinical exercise physiologist (CEP). In the decades since CEPs began working in cardiac rehabilitation (CR) programs, the testing, exercise prescription, and programming for patients with CVD have evolved side by side with advancements in medical and surgical procedures and medications.

Although the evidence is overwhelming that a properly designed exercise regimen after diagnosis or intervention for CVD is beneficial, CEPs are at a crossroads.

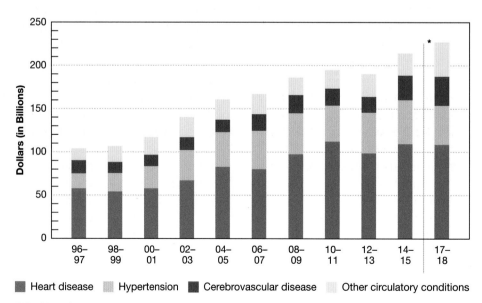

FIGURE 5.1 Estimated direct costs (in billions of dollars) of CVD, U.S., average annual (1996–1997 to 2017–2018). *International *Classification of Diseases, Ninth Revision* coding for 1996–2015; *International Classification of Diseases, 10th Revision* coding for 2016–2018. The 2016 data are omitted from this chart. (From Tsao CW, Aday AW, Almarzooq ZI, et al. Heart disease and stroke statistics-2022 update: a report from the American Heart Association. *Circulation.* 2022; 145(8):e153–639.)

The indications for referral to CR programs have expanded over recent years, and the number of people who can benefit from CEP services is not declining. At the same time, cardiac patients are more complex than ever. On average, they are getting older and coming to CR with more comorbidities and more medications than ever before; thus, the need to support their rehabilitation or CVD risk reduction is more imperative than ever (2, 3). Nevertheless, CR programs are struggling, and patients are spending less time overall in CR programs. Increased out-of-pocket costs to the patient, distance to travel to programs, the need to return to work sooner, and the availability of other potential sources for support with exercise may be factors. Moreover, perhaps because of our technologically advanced society, patients also seem to expect results more quickly, creating a culture of impatience that focuses on medications and procedures instead of changing behaviors to get at the root of the problem.

Success in CR is undoubtedly challenging. All CEPs can design an exercise regimen to increase the frequency, intensity, and time a patient exercises, but successfully helping patients adopt and maintain heart-healthy lifestyle choices including exercise and physical activity (PA) can be challenging. It takes attentive listening, appropriate evaluation, and a realistic prescription of exercise with just the right amount of support and follow-up. CEPs must bear in mind that their goals for patients may not be what the patients themselves are trying to achieve. Working toward a specific metabolic equivalent (MET) level may be a goal of the CEP, whereas the patient may simply want to "be more active" or "feel better" and "return to work."

Take for example a 62-year-old male security guard who had a myocardial infarction (MI) followed by a coronary stent procedure. He already walks about 8,000–10,000 steps a day while at work. What is the likelihood of convincing this patient to get an additional 150 minutes or more a week of moderately intense cardiovascular exercise? The CEP might be more successful in getting him to do 2 days a week of brisk cardiovascular exercise for 15–20 minutes and three to four strength exercises for 1–2 sets of 10–12 repetitions to complement his walking at work. CEPs need to understand the goals of their patients and be creative and flexible in their approach.

This chapter discusses the most common types of CVD that CEPs encounter. For each type of CVD listed, the pathophysiology, diagnosis, relation to exercise tolerance, treatment, and management, as well as the effects of exercise therapy, will be discussed.

First, an overview of cardiovascular anatomy and physiology is provided.

OVERVIEW OF CARDIOVASCULAR ANATOMY AND PHYSIOLOGY

In this section, a brief overview of the anatomy of the heart and circulatory system is provided. Specific anatomical features key to understanding cardiovascular physiology will be reviewed.

Heart

The heart is composed of a specialized type of muscle called the myocardium that is housed within a protective structure called the pericardium (Figure 5.2). The pericardial sac has two layers: The fibrous outer layer of the pericardium functions primarily to prevent overdistension of the myocardium. The thin inner layer of the pericardium, the epicardium, attaches to the myocardium, forming the outer wall of the heart. The space between these two pericardial layers contains a small amount of fluid, pericardial fluid, which allows the myocardium to move smoothly when contracting within the pericardium. The myocardium is the thick (middle) layer of the heart, which provides the contractile function. The inner wall of the heart, the endocardium, is composed of both a layer of endothelium and a layer of connective tissue.

The myocardium is organized into two sides, a right and a left, with both sides having two interior chambers, an upper atrium and a lower ventricle, which hold the blood that the heart circulates to the body (Figure 5.3). The atria and ventricles are connected by two valves, the tricuspid valve on the right side and the bicuspid (also known as mitral) valve on the left side, which allow blood to flow only in the direction from the atrium to the ventricle. Similarly, during ventricular relaxation, one-way valves prevent blood flow from the pulmonary artery (pulmonic valve) and aorta (aortic valve) to the right and left ventricles, respectively.

The myocardium has characteristics similar to those of skeletal muscle in that it contains actin and myosin myofilaments that attach via cross-bridges and function to create tension while shortening the myofibril. In comparison to skeletal muscle, though, the myocardium has a higher density of mitochondria (>33% of

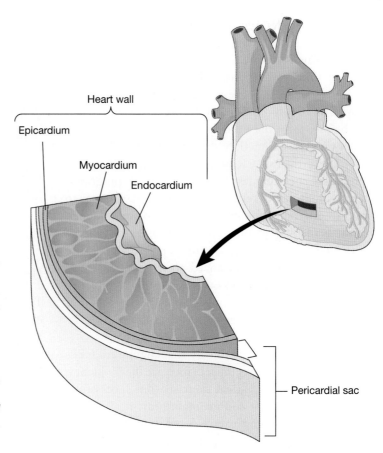

FIGURE 5.2 Layers of the heart and pericardium. The heart wall is composed of three layers: the epicardium (outer layer; epi- means "on top of"; cardi/o means "heart"), myocardium (heart muscle; my/o means "muscle"; cardi/o means "heart"), and endocardium (inner layer; endo- means "within"; cardi/o means "heart"). Notice the thickness of the myocardial or "muscle" layer. The pericardial sac is actually composed of two layers and has fluid in the space between the layers. This fluid helps to reduce friction when the heart beats. (Modified from Cohen BJ. *Memmler's the Human Body in Health and Disease.* 13th ed. Philadelphia (PA): Lippincott Williams & Wilkins; 2014.)

cell volume) and a higher myofibril-to-capillary ratio (1.0). The most distinct difference in the myocardium is the presence of intercalated discs, which are specialized portions of the cell membranes that connect individual cardiac muscle cells. The intercalated discs allow for specialized cellular communication as well as allowing the action potential to pass from one cell to the next adjoining cell, enabling the myocardium to contract as a functional unit, or actually two functional units—the atria and the ventricles.

The stimulus for myocardial contraction comes from a specialized structure called the sinoatrial (SA) node, commonly referred to as the pacemaker of the heart. From the SA node, the stimulatory impulse spreads through the heart via its electrical conduction system, which includes the atrioventricular (AV) node, the bundle of His, right and left bundle branches, and finally the diffuse terminal structures known as the Purkinje fibers (Figure 5.4). The primary feature of the heart's conduction system is its intrinsic ability to generate a stimulatory impulse. Although the impulse is usually generated from the SA node, which typically has a rate of discharge of approximately 75 times per minute, other myocardial tissues also have the capability of self-excitability. It

should be noted that there is a brief pause at the AV node (P-R interval on electrocardiogram [ECG]) to allow for ventricular filling.

Circulatory System

The heart functions as a pump to deliver oxygenated red blood cells to various organs and tissues in the body and then to return blood to the heart via a continuous network of blood vessels called the circulatory system. These blood vessels can be divided into three basic types: arteries, which carry blood to the tissues under high pressure; capillaries, which allow diffusion of gases and other substances through their thin walls; and veins, which return blood to the heart under low pressure. Both the arterial and venous parts of the circulation have smaller branches that deliver blood to (the arterioles) and collect blood from (the venules) the capillaries. The circulatory system functions primarily as a transportation network, carrying desired substances (*e.g.,* oxygen, glucose, hormones) to the tissues throughout the body and concurrently allowing tissues to dispose of unwanted substances (*e.g.,* carbon dioxide, lactic acid). The circulatory system actually consists of two separate

NORMAL HEART ANATOMY

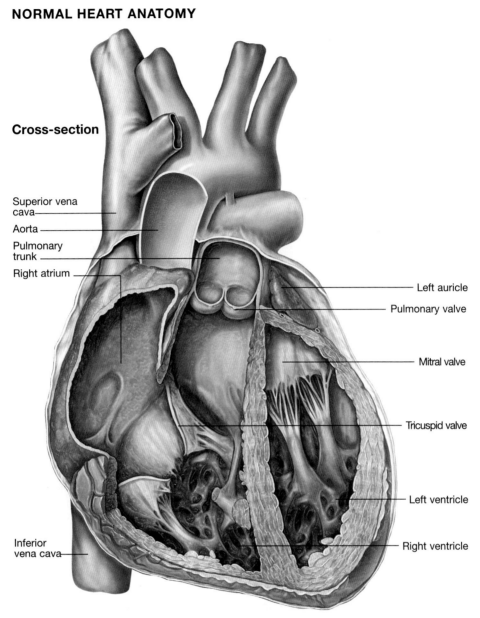

Cross-section

Superior vena cava

Aorta

Pulmonary trunk

Right atrium

Left auricle

Pulmonary valve

Mitral valve

Tricuspid valve

Left ventricle

Inferior vena cava

Right ventricle

FIGURE 5.3 Heart (cross-section). (Modified from Cohen BJ. *Memmler's the Human Body in Health and Disease.* 13th ed. Philadelphia (PA): Lippincott Williams & Wilkins; 2014.)

circulatory routes: the pulmonic circulation and the systemic circulation (Figure 5.5).

The pulmonic circulation carries blood from the right ventricle to the lungs via the pulmonary artery and then returns blood to the left atrium via the pulmonary vein. The pulmonic circulation serves the important functions of:

1. Removing carbon dioxide from the blood
2. Reoxygenating the blood via diffusion between the gases in the blood in the pulmonary capillaries and the gases in the alveoli

It is also important to recognize that in comparison to the systemic circulation, the pulmonic circulation requires less pressure to maintain blood flow because of the lower resistance in this branch of the circulation.

The systemic circulation carries blood from the left ventricle to the rest of the body via the aorta and then returns blood to the right atrium via the superior and inferior venae cavae. The aorta branches off numerous times to supply oxygenated blood and nutrients to the brain and to tissues throughout the body, and to collect carbon dioxide and other waste products from the same areas.

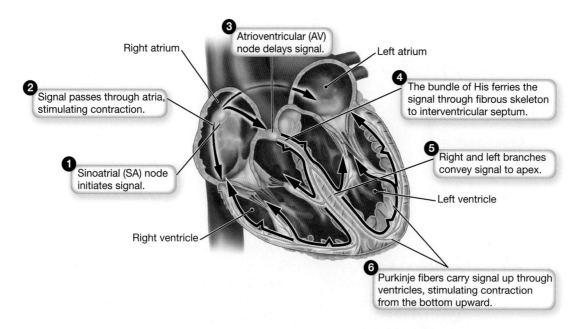

FIGURE 5.4 The cardiac conduction system (CCS). The anatomical components of the CCS and the steps involved in one heartbeat. The black arrows indicate the spread of electrical impulses through the conducting system. (Adapted with permission from McConnell TH, Hull KL. *Human Form Human Function: Essentials of Anatomy & Physiology*. Baltimore (MD): Wolters Kluwer Health; 2011.)

The heart has its blood supply delivered via the ascending aorta (Figure 5.6). The right coronary artery (RCA), which lies in the coronary sulcus, branches off to supply the right atrium and the right ventricle. Additionally, the RCA supplies blood to the anterior portion of the SA node (in 50%–60% of the population), the AV node (in 90% of the population), the ventricular septum, and the posterior wall of the left ventricle (in 70% of the population). The left coronary artery (LCA) immediately branches into two main divisions — the left circumflex coronary artery (LCx) and the left anterior descending (LAD) artery. The LCx, which lies in the anterior interventricular sulcus, provides the blood supply for the SA node (40%–50% of the population), the left atrium, and the lateral wall of the left ventricle; and it contributes to the supply of the posterior wall of the left ventricle. In approximately 10% of the population, the LCx is the dominant supplier of blood to the posterior wall of the left ventricle, and in approximately 20% of hearts, it shares equally in the supply of blood to this region. The LAD artery principally supplies blood to the wall of the left ventricle and the ventricular septum, with an additional role in providing some of the supply to the anterior wall of the right ventricle. After being distributed via an extensive capillary bed, blood drains from the thebesian veins (which then primarily empty into the right and left atria) and the anterior cardiac veins and coronary sinus (which both empty into the right atrium).

One other important anatomical feature of the circulatory system is the layer of endothelium that lines the blood vessels. It is important to note that the endothelium also lines the endocardium and the coronary blood vessels. Until recently, the function of the endothelium was not well understood. However, extensive research has revealed a number of important physiological roles of the endothelium (4). Some of these functions, which are related to coronary disease and exercise responses, are discussed in the following sections.

Cardiovascular Physiology

The heart will beat approximately three to four billion times during the average human's lifespan. With each beat of the heart, blood is ejected both to the lungs (pulmonic circulation) and to the rest of the body (systemic circulation), serving as the medium by which substances are transported throughout the body. It is essential that students interested in the primary and secondary prevention of CVD have a complete understanding of the physiological events that occur with each cycle of the heart. The first

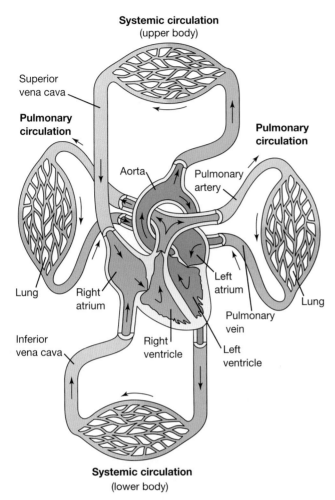

Systemic circulation
(upper body)

Superior
vena cava

**Pulmonary
circulation**

**Pulmonary
circulation**

Aorta

Pulmonary
artery

Lung

Right
atrium

Lung

Left
atrium

Pulmonary
vein

Inferior
vena cava

Right
ventricle

Left
ventricle

Systemic circulation
(lower body)

FIGURE 5.5 The pattern of circulation involves two circuits: the pulmonary circulation and the systemic circulation. In this diagram, red stands for oxygen-rich blood, and blue stands for oxygen-poor blood. Blood passes from the right ventricle into the pulmonary circulation. Once it is loaded up with oxygen, the blood returns to the left atrium, passes into the left ventricle, and is sent out to the rest of the body. This is the systemic circulation. (From Carter PJ, Goldschmidt WM. *Lippincott's Textbook for Long-Term Care Nursing Assistants*. Philadelphia (PA): Wolters Kluwer; 2009.)

comprehensive diagram of the events of the cardiac cycle was developed in 1915 and has been modified as shown in Figure 5.7. This figure describes the changes in pressure (aortic, ventricular, and atrial), left ventricular volume, and the ECG over the time period of one complete cardiac cycle. (The ECG is discussed in Chapter 6.) Notice that, although this figure illustrates events occurring in the left side of the heart, corresponding events are happening on the right side.

For the purpose of describing these events, the period toward the end of ventricular diastole is labeled phase 0. During this period, blood continues to flow into the left ventricle as noted by the increase in ventricular volume

as the mitral valve is open (atrial pressure > ventricular pressure) and the aortic valve is closed (aortic pressure > ventricular pressure). Before the myocardium can contract, it must be stimulated. The electrical activity of the heart is discussed in detail in the earlier ECG section.

Cardiac Output

Because the tissues depend on the heart to provide a continuous flow of fresh blood via the systemic circulation, it is important to understand the factors that allow this to happen and the ways these factors change in response to different demands of the tissues, such as those that occur during exercise. Cardiac output (CO or $\dot{Q}$) is defined as the total amount of blood that is ejected from the ventricle (usually measured from the left ventricle) into the circulation in 1 minute. Although this review concentrates on CO, it is important to remember that in order to maintain blood flow, an equal volume of blood must be returned (*i.e.*, the venous return) to the heart each minute.

The two primary determinants of CO are heart rate (HR) and stroke volume (SV). Thus, the heart can meet increased demands for blood flow from the tissues by increasing HR, SV, or both. At rest, CO averages about 4–5 L·min^{-1} for an adult. Two primary characteristics that affect CO are body size and age. Generally, CO is directly related to body size (*e.g.*, CO increases as body size increases), which accounts for most of the difference between the males and females. Also, after maturity, CO is inversely related to age (*e.g.*, as age increases, CO decreases). Thus, the expected CO for any given person should be adjusted based on that individual's characteristics.

Control of HR

As mentioned earlier, stimulation of the heart is intrinsically generated by the SA node. However, the rate of this stimulation can be affected by both neural and hormonal factors. The SA node is innervated by both the parasympathetic (cholinergic) and sympathetic (adrenergic) divisions of the autonomic nervous system. At rest, the HR is controlled by the relative dominance of the parasympathetic vagus nerve activity that decreases intrinsic firing rate of the SA node from 100 times per minute to 60–70 times per minute or even less (30–40 times/minute) is highly conditioned individuals. The vagus nerve releases acetylcholine, which binds to the muscarinic acetylcholine receptors (mAChRs) of the SA node membrane, which in turn causes the membrane to become hyperpolarized. In the membrane's hyperpolarized state, more

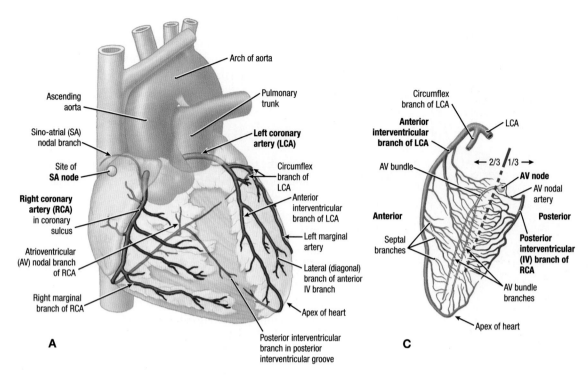

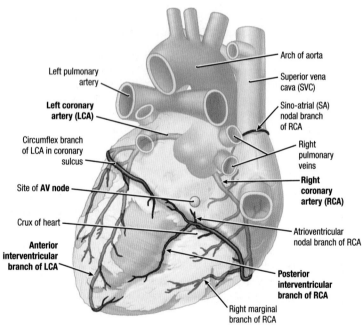

FIGURE 5.6 Coronary Arteries. **A.** Anterior view. **B.** Posteroinferior view. **C.** Arteries of isolated interventricular septum (from left side). In the most common pattern, the right coronary artery travels in the coronary sulcus to reach the posterior surface of the heart, where it anastomoses with the circumflex branch of the left coronary artery. Early in its course, it gives off the right atrial branch, which supplies the sinoatrial (SA) node via its sinoatrial nodal branch. Major branches are a marginal branch supplying much of the anterior wall of the right ventricle, an atrioventricular (AV) nodal branch given off near the posterior border of the interventricular septum, and a posterior interventricular branch in the interventricular groove that anastomoses with the anterior interventricular branch of the left coronary artery. The left coronary artery divides into a circumflex branch that passes posteriorly to anastomose with the right coronary artery on the posterior aspect of the heart and an anterior interventricular branch in the interventricular groove; the origin of the SA nodal branch is variable and may be a branch of the left coronary artery. The interventricular septum receives its blood supply from septal branches of the two interventricular (descending) branches: typically the anterior two-thirds from the left coronary and the posterior one-third from the right **(C)**. (From Agur AMR, Dalley AF. *Grant's Atlas of Anatomy*. 14th ed. Philadelphia (PA): Wolters Kluwer; 2016.)

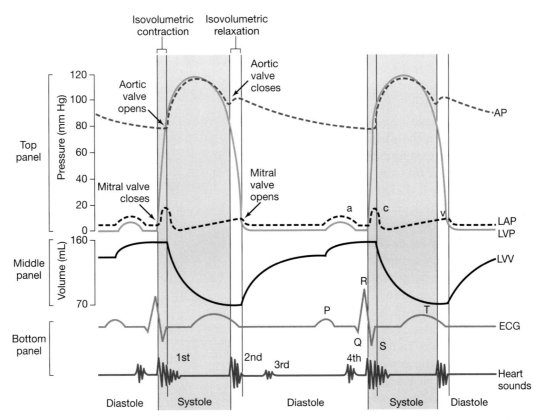

FIGURE 5.7 The Wiggers diagram: graphical representation of the cardiac cycle. This is a graphical representation of two cycles of diastole and systole (only left heart is shown). Top panel is left atrial pressure (LAP), left ventricular pressure (LVP), and aortic pressure (AP), and the panel includes the "a," "c," and "v" waves of the LAP tracing. Middle panel shows left ventricular volume (LVV). Also shown are the electrocardiogram (ECG) waves (P, QRS, and T—more on this in Chapter 6) as well as the heart sounds (first, second, third, and fourth heart sounds). (From Courneya CA, Parker MJ, Schwartzstein RM. *Cardiovascular Physiology*. Philadelphia (PA): Wolters Kluwer; 2010.)

time is needed for the membrane potential to reach the threshold required for an action potential; this results in a slowed rate of firing.

One of the primary mechanisms for increasing the HR is to reduce or remove the activity of the vagus nerve (*i.e.*, parasympathetic withdrawal). Without the influence of acetylcholine, the intrinsic rate of firing of the SA node can increase by up to 50%. Further increases in HR result from the adrenergic release of norepinephrine, which binds to the β1 receptors on the SA node and causes reduced membrane potential. This allows for an earlier depolarization of the SA node and a more rapid repolarization.

There can also be an indirect influence of adrenergic stimulation on HR. This response, which occurs during exercise, results from the release of the hormone epinephrine into the blood from the adrenal medulla, which is located on the kidney. The adrenal medulla is stimulated by the sympathetic nervous system as part of the body's reaction to stressful situations. The receptors on the SA

node can also bind with epinephrine from the circulation; this leads to further stimulation and a more rapid rate of firing. It should also be noted that many medications may influence HR.

Any factor that influences the HR may be referred to as a chronotropic factor. These factors are described as having a positive or a negative effect, depending on whether they increase or decrease HR, respectively.

Control of SV

As noted earlier, the second determinant of CO is SV. By increasing the volume of blood ejected with each contraction (*i.e.*, the SV), CO is increased. Similar to control of HR, changes in SV result both from intrinsic mechanisms and from neural and hormonal stimulation.

A review of terminology is in order. Preload is the load on the heart, measured as the pressure in the left ventricle immediately prior to ventricular contraction. The corresponding volume in the left ventricle at this time is the end-diastolic volume. Afterload is the force against which the left ventricle is working during contraction, measured as the pressure in the aorta at the end of diastole. In order for the aortic valve to open, pressure in the left ventricle must exceed that in the aorta. End-systolic volume represents the volume of blood remaining in the left ventricle immediately following ventricular contraction. SV represents the difference between end-diastolic volume and end-systolic volume. Finally, ejection fraction (EF) refers to the amount of blood ejected from the left ventricle as a percentage of the total volume in the left ventricle prior to contraction (*i.e.*, the end-diastolic volume).

The intrinsic mechanism for increasing SV is understood on the basis of observations made by two physiologists approximately one century ago and thus is named the Frank-Starling law. The underlying physiological mechanism that explains this response is the relationship between sarcomere length and cardiac muscle tension. As cardiac myocyte sarcomeres are lengthened (up to an optimal distance), more actin binding sites become available to the myosin cross-bridges to allow greater tension development. Thus, as ventricular volume is increased (principally via increased venous return, but also in response to atrial contraction), the wall of the ventricles becomes stretched, and this lengthens the sarcomeres (Figure 5.8). In the presence of dilated left ventricular chamber, the sarcomeres can be stretched too far and the ability of the myocytes to contract can be compromised, resulting in a reduced EF.

Essentially, the heart responds to an increase in ventricular volume by increasing its force of contraction, thereby generating a greater SV. Increasing the contractility of the ventricles via adrenergic stimulation further increases SV. This response, also known as a positive inotropic effect, results from a cascade of events in the myocardium that ultimately leads to an increase in its contractile force. Thus, at any given ventricular volume, increased contractility via adrenergic stimulation results in a decreased end-systolic volume. The same indirect effect of adrenergic stimulation (*i.e.*, release of epinephrine into the circulation by the adrenal medulla) mentioned earlier, in relation to control of HR, will also enhance contractility. In the entire heart, only the SA node has a density of adrenergic β1 receptors greater than that of the ventricles (5). Thus, adrenergic stimulation provides both positive chronotropic and inotropic effects.

Myocardial Oxygen Uptake

One of the most common measures in clinical exercise physiology is that of oxygen uptake ($\dot{V}O_2$), which is used to describe the energy expended by the body in meeting the

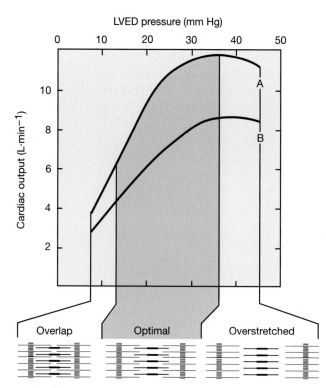

FIGURE 5.8 The Frank-Starling ventricular function curve in a normal heart. (Top) An increase in left ventricular end-diastolic (LVED) pressure produces an increase in cardiac output (curve B) by means of the Frank-Starling mechanism. The maximum force of contraction and increased stroke volume (SV) are achieved when diastolic filling causes the muscle fibers to be stretched about two- and one-half times their resting length. In curve A, an increase in cardiac contractility produces an increase in cardiac output without a change in LVED volume and pressure. (Bottom) Stretching of the actin and myosin filaments at the different LVED filling pressures. (From Hannon R. *Porth Pathophysiology*. 2nd ed. Philadelphia (PA): Wolters Kluwer; 2016.)

demands to perform work. Similarly, the demands placed on the heart to perform its work can be quantified by the measure of myocardial oxygen uptake ($m\dot{V}O_2$). Skeletal muscle can increase its uptake of oxygen both by increasing its extraction of oxygen from the blood and by obtaining a greater blood flow. The myocardium, on the other hand, extracts almost all of the oxygen from the blood when functioning at its basal level (*i.e.*, resting CO). Thus, when CO increases, and thus the work of the heart, all of the additional oxygen must come from increasing the rate of blood flow via the coronary arteries. Unlike the measurement of whole body, which can be obtained via the noninvasive method of open-circuit spirometry, determination of m would require invasive procedures to measure coronary blood flow and the difference between the amount of oxygen in the coronary arteries and the coronary veins (*i.e.*, the arteriovenous oxygen difference [a − vO₂ diff]). Because these invasive procedures are not practical, other indicators of myocardial work demands become important. Essentially, the two components of CO (HR and SV) determine m. Obviously, HR is easy to measure and quantify; however, SV — or more precisely the factors that determine SV — is more difficult to ascertain. Preload, afterload, and contractility all influence SV. A simple indicator of myocardial oxygen demand is the rate pressure product (also called the double product), which is derived from the product of HR and systolic blood pressure (BP). In patients with angina, in which myocardial demand exceeds myocardial blood supply, the rate pressure product is commonly used for clinical correlation.

CORONARY ARTERY DISEASE

Coronary artery disease (CAD) remains the No. 1 cause of death in the U.S. CAD accounted for approximately 13% of deaths in the U.S. in 2018, causing 365,744 deaths. Moreover, 26% of women will die within a year of an MI compared with 19% of men and by 5 years, 50% of women die, develop HF, or have a stroke compared with 36% of men (1). The good news is that from 2008 to 2018, the overall annual death rate attributable to CAD declined 27.9% and the actual number of deaths declined 9.8%. However, the societal burden and risk factors remain alarmingly high. The estimated direct and indirect cost of heart disease in 2016–2017 was $219.6 billion (1).

Pathophysiology

Given the high prevalence of CAD, an introduction to vascular pathophysiology is important for CEPs.

Atherosclerosis is the pathological process whereby lesions (or plaques) form within arteries, creating a narrowed lumen and thus impairing blood flow. Although the process also commonly takes place in the aorta, the cerebral arteries, the carotid arteries, and the femoral arteries, this review focuses on coronary artery atherosclerosis.

The most commonly accepted explanation for atherogenesis is the response-to-injury hypothesis. The atherogenic process begins when damage to the coronary artery endothelium occurs leading to inflammation within the artery. Many different factors have been associated with endothelial injury, including high BP, stress hormones, smoking, and high levels of circulating glucose and insulin. These major risk factors for CAD can directly promote endothelial damage. Once the damage has occurred, circulating platelets adhere to this portion

of the endothelium and are thereby stimulated to release a number of growth factors that trigger smooth muscle cell proliferation, monocyte binding, and low-density lipoprotein receptor activation. Monocytes are then able to infiltrate the damaged endothelium, where they become activated macrophages that accumulate cholesterol from low-density lipoproteins. As the macrophages accumulate cholesterol, they are transformed into foam cells that are capable of holding large amounts of lipids. The endothelial smooth muscle cells also are stimulated to release additional growth factors that lead to the development of fibrous connective tissue. The end result is the formation of a plaque or atheroma containing a variety of materials, characterized by an outer fibromuscular layer surrounding a cholesterol core. Initially, plaques can develop without affecting lumen size, but if the plaques continue to expand, they eventually result in narrowing of the coronary artery lumen (Figures 5.9 and 5.10).

Coronary artery plaque development can begin early in life, and atherosclerosis is generally thought to be a progressive disease. Lifestyle choices, especially smoking, level of PA, and dietary habits, play an important role in determining the progression of atherosclerosis. Plaques can remain stable for periods of time, grow slowly, or grow quite rapidly. Once formed, plaques are more susceptible to damage than other areas within the vessel.

Plaque rupturing causes most MIs. Rupture of the plaque is known to be precipitated by hemodynamic shear forces, as well as by vasoconstriction and possibly by some circulating substances. The size of the plaque

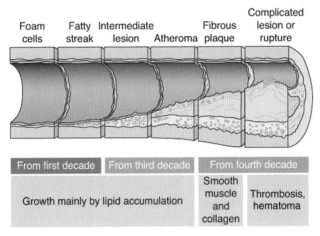

FIGURE 5.9 Progression of atheromatous plaque from initial lesion to complex and ruptured plaque. (Modified with permission from Grech ED. ABC of interventional cardiology: pathophysiology and investigation of coronary artery disease. *BMJ*. 2003;326(7397):1027–30, with permission from BMJ Publishing Group Ltd.)

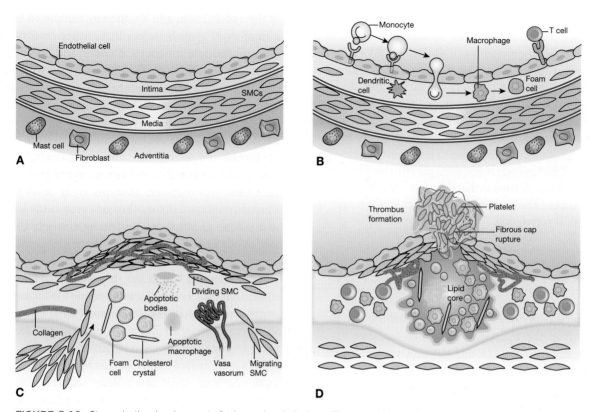

FIGURE 5.10. Stages in the development of atherosclerotic lesions. The normal muscular artery and the cell changes that occur during disease progression to thrombosis are shown. **A.** The normal artery contains three layers. The inner layer, the tunica intima, is lined by a monolayer of endothelial cells that is in contact with blood overlying a basement membrane. In contrast to many animal species used for atherosclerosis experiments, the human intima contains resident smooth muscle cells (SMCs). The middle layer, or tunica media, contains SMCs embedded in a complex extracellular matrix. Arteries affected by obstructive atherosclerosis generally have the structure of muscular arteries. The arteries often studied in experimental atherosclerosis are elastic arteries, which have clearly demarcated laminae in the tunica media, where layers of elastin lie between strata of SMCs. The adventitia, the outer layer of arteries, contains mast cells, nerve endings, and microvessels. **B.** The initial steps of atherosclerosis include adhesion of blood leukocytes to the activated endothelial monolayer, directed migration of the bound leukocytes into the intima, maturation of monocytes (the most numerous of the leukocytes recruited) into macrophages, and their uptake of lipid, yielding foam cells. **C.** Lesion progression involves the migration of SMCs from the media to the intima, the proliferation of resident intimal SMCs and media-derived SMCs, and the heightened synthesis of extracellular matrix macromolecules, such as collagen, elastin, and proteoglycans. Plaque macrophages and SMCs can die in advancing lesions, some by apoptosis. Extracellular lipid derived from dead and dying cells can accumulate in the central region of a plaque, often denoted the lipid or necrotic core. Advancing plaques also contain cholesterol crystals and microvessels. **D.** Thrombosis, the ultimate complication of atherosclerosis, often complicates a physical disruption of the atherosclerotic plaque. Shown is a fracture of the plaque's fibrous cap, which has enabled blood coagulation components to come into contact with tissue factors in the plaque's interior, triggering the thrombus that extends into the vessel lumen, where it can impede blood flow. (From Geschwind J, Dake M. *Abrams' Angiography.* 3rd ed. Philadelphia (PA): Wolters Kluwer; 2013.)

does not seem to be linearly related to the likelihood for rupture. Plaques that take up 40%–50% of the lumen are more likely to rupture than larger plaques (6). At the site of the rupture, a thrombus forms. The thrombus may then be incorporated into the plaque and/or may form a mural thrombus that partially protrudes into the lumen of the vessel. Mural thrombi may continue to increase in size and can rapidly progress to completely occlude the artery (Figure 5.11). When a coronary artery becomes occluded to the point at which oxygen supply cannot meet

oxygen demand (because of reduced blood flow), the region of the myocardium being supplied by this vessel is compromised. This condition is called myocardial ischemia. When it occurs, the myocardium must shift from its preferred aerobic energy production pathway (oxidation phosphorylation) to the anaerobic nonoxidative pathway (glycolytic), which releases by-products that cause cellular acidosis. The contractile ability of the myocardium becomes impaired, and systolic and diastolic functions deteriorate. This condition is recognizable both by signs

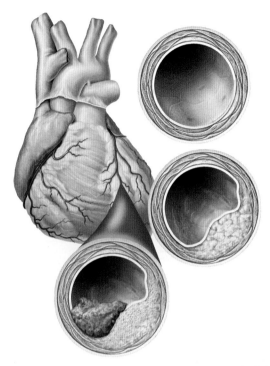

FIGURE 5.11 Atherosclerosis. In this example, a branch of the left coronary artery supplying the heart wall is shown in cross-section during three stages of atherosclerosis: no plaque present (top), well-formed plaque blocking 30% of the vessel lumen (middle), and formation of a thrombosis (lower). (Adapted with permission from Anatomical Chart Co. *Heart Disease Anatomical Chart*. 2nd ed. Philadelphia (PA): Wolters Kluwer; 2008.)

such as an abnormal ECG and by symptoms such as angina. Typically, ischemia does not occur until a coronary artery develops an obstruction of at least 50% of the luminal diameter, which is equivalent to a 75% reduction in cross-sectional area. If blood flow to the ischemic region is not restored within 30–60 minutes, necrosis of myocardial cells will begin and ultimately lead to an MI. Although the majority of cardiac myocyte death occurs during ischemia and the first few minutes of reperfusion, cell death does not stop there. In fact, necrosis and apoptosis, and potentially autophagy, can continue in the previously ischemic area for up to 3 days postreperfusion (7).

Although myocardial ischemia is commonly associated with atherosclerotic plaques that have significantly narrowed a coronary artery, it can also occur in vessels with little to no atherosclerosis. This happens when the smooth muscles surrounding a portion of a coronary artery are stimulated to contract intensely, resulting in vasospasm. Although the exact mechanisms that precipitate a coronary vasospasm for any given individual are not known, endothelial dysfunction and greater sensitivity to both neural and hormonal vasoconstrictive substances are believed to be factors.

Generally, ischemia is first recognized by the affected person during some stressful situation (*e.g.*, exercise, arousal, or anger). That is, at rest, the blood supply can meet the myocardial demands, but as the myocardial work increases to meet the demands of the stress, the reduced coronary artery lumen is unable to maintain sufficient blood supply. Unfortunately, some people do not develop angina during ischemia and thus lack a major warning signal that they have serious CAD. This condition, which can only be detected by an exercise test or other diagnostic procedure, is termed silent ischemia. If the ischemia occurs acutely during resting or occurs during activity and is not relieved with rest, it is possible that a thrombus has formed that has completely or almost completely occluded the coronary artery. Immediate emergency care is required in this situation to provide the patient with a percutaneous coronary intervention (PCI; angioplasty and stent) or a thrombolytic agent. The sooner this therapy begins, the more likely it is to eliminate or minimize the damage to the myocardium. However, it should be noted "reperfusion" of the myocytes may occur where the tissue damage caused when blood supply returns to tissue after a period of ischemia or lack of oxygen (anoxia or hypoxia). Investigations are underway to mitigate this type of cardiomyocyte injury and improve outcomes in patients with CAD.

Again, when ischemia goes untreated for more than 30–60 minutes, necrosis of myocardial cells (an MI) begins. The exact time frame for initiation of myocardial cell death depends on the severity of the ischemia (*i.e.*, whether it is precipitated by an incomplete or a complete occlusion of a coronary artery) and the extent of collateral coronary arteries supplying the affected area. Typically, the infarction starts in the endocardium, as coronary blood supply to this area is most remote. If the portion of the myocardium that is ischemic is large enough and is left untreated, the infarction can spread through the entire wall of the heart (*i.e.*, transmural: from endocardium to epicardium). Because of its characteristic ECG findings, this type of MI is called an ST-segment elevation myocardial infarction (STEMI). The irreversible nature of an MI is characterized by the rupture of the myocardial sarcolemma, which can be identified by levels of myocardial enzyme levels in the blood.

Diagnosis of CAD

When an individual presents with suspected myocardial ischemia, most commonly caused by CAD, there are a variety of diagnostic tests that can be utilized. Figure 5.12

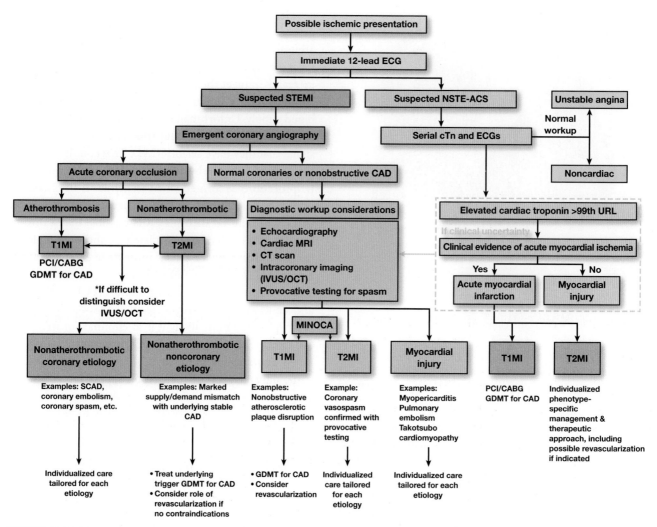

FIGURE 5.12 Diagnostic approach for patients with suspected acute myocardial ischemia. CABG, coronary artery bypass graft; CAD, coronary artery disease; CT, computed tomography; cTn, cardiac troponin; ECG, electrocardiogram; GDMT, guideline directed medical therapy; IVUS, intravascular ultrasound; MINOCA, myocardial infarction with non-obstructive coronary arteries; MRI, magnetic resonance imaging; NSTE-ACS, non ST-elevation acute coronary syndrome; OCT, optical coherence tomography; PCI, percutaneous coronary intervention; SCAD, spontaneous coronary artery dissection; STEMI, ST-segment elevation myocardial infarction; URL, upper range limit. (From Sandoval Y, Jaffe AS. Type 2 myocardial infarction: JACC review topic of the week. *J Am Coll Cardiol.* 2019;73(14):1846–60.)

describes the diagnostic approach that should be followed. Generally, the process of "ruling in or ruling out" an MI begins with obtaining a 12-lead ECG, as well as a detailed physical examination and history. When an ACS (acute MI) is suspected, cardiac enzymes including troponin C are obtained to determine if there is myocardial cell death (necrosis). Clinical evidence of myocardial ischemia (associated with imbalance of oxygen supply vs. demand) would then result in a diagnostic test and/or a revascularization intervention, either PCI or coronary artery bypass graft (CABG). As seen in Figure 5.13, there are several diagnostic tests that can be performed that can identify the pathophysiologic stages on the ischemic "cascade." The earliest stages of myocardial ischemia result in metabolic abnormalities of the cardiac myocytes. This requires the use of positron emission tomography (PET), which is not widely available and too expensive for clinical use. The next consequence of ischemia is the presence of myocardial perfusion abnormalities. This can be detected by perfusion scintigraphy (MPS), contrast echocardiography (MCE), or cardiac magnetic resonance imaging (CMR). All of these tests are widely available and routinely used for the detection of myocardial ischemia. Similarly, left ventricular systolic and/or diastolic abnormalities occur as the degree of ischemia progressed and can be detected with stress (induced pharmacologically or with exercise testing) echocardiography. Much further along the ischemia cascade would be the occurrence of ECG changes

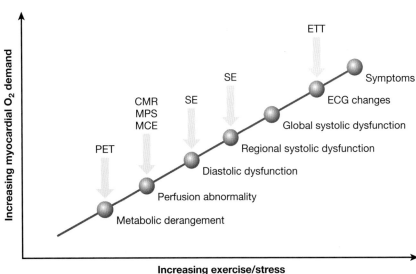

FIGURE 5.13 An illustration of the pathophysiological stages of the ischemic cascade along with the level of abnormality each functional imaging test is designed to detect. CMR, cardiac magnetic resonance; ECG, electrocardiogram; ETT, exercise treadmill test; MCE, myocardial contrast echocardiograph; MPS, myocardial perfusion scintigraphy; PET, positron emission tomography; SE, stress echocardiography. (From Shan BN, Senior R. Stress-induced myocardial ischaemia—perfusion contrast echocardiography to evaluate presence and severity of coronary artery disease. *Eur Cardiol.* 2011;7(3):172–6.)

(ST depression/elevation) that can be assessed during an exercise tolerance/stress test (ETT). Sensitivity or accuracy of the test in detecting myocardial ischemia is highest with PET (>90%) but decreases with MPS, CMR, and SE (~80%–90%) and further with ECG during ETT (~60%–70%). Although selecting a test with highest sensitivity is desirable, this must be balanced by the risk, complexity, and cost of these procedures.

Relation to Exercise Tolerance

Although many hospitals will get patients ambulating within a day or two after MI or surgery, exercise "stress" testing is often used to determine functional status, evaluate vocational readiness, and/or develop an individually based exercise prescription. For patients who have undergone successful and uncomplicated CABG, there appears to be little clinical benefit and unnecessary financial burden in routine exercise testing (8). If stress testing is performed in CABG patients, the most appropriate time is generally 3–4 weeks after surgery when most of the complications (sternal stability, incisional pain, rib soreness, hypovolemia, anemia, and muscle weakness) have resolved and the patient is able to give a near-maximal physiologic effort during the test.

Although some debate exists regarding the need and potential risks for exercise testing after PCI, many support the use of exercise testing 1–2 days postprocedure to evaluate the patient's functional status (9). More routinely, exercise testing is conducted 2–5 weeks and again at 6 weeks postprocedure. Testing at these intervals can help detect potential restenosis, assess functional capacity, provide advice concerning PA restrictions, and generate data for developing an exercise prescription (9).

Treatment and Management of CAD

CAD occurs through atherosclerotic and thrombotic processes, described in detail earlier in the chapter, and results in partial or complete occlusion of one or more coronary arteries. It can be prevented and generally well managed with the use of medications as well as lifestyle interventions (*i.e.*, diet, exercise, stress management, and tobacco cessation) that can reduce the presence/severity of CAD risk factors. Several studies have shown that CAD can be stabilized and even reversed with pharmacologic and/or aggressive lifestyle therapy (1, 10). Hambrecht et al. (11) demonstrated that CAD "regression" can occur in selected patients with CAD who accumulate more than 2,200 kcal per week in PA. However, in some patients, the coronary arteries become more severely and/or acutely obstructed, thus requiring an emergent revascularization procedure. The two procedures commonly used to "revascularize" a blocked coronary artery is to implant a stent in the area of the blockage or to entirely "bypass" the blocked segment of artery surgically. The trends in the use of these procedures are presented in Figure 5.14, and in 2014, an estimated 480,000 percutaneous transluminal coronary angioplasties (PCI), 371,000 inpatient coronary artery bypass (CABG) procedures, 1,016,000 inpatient diagnostic cardiac catheterizations, 86,000 carotid endarterectomies, and 351,000 pacemaker procedures were performed for inpatients in the U.S. According to the 2014 National Healthcare Cost and Utilization Project

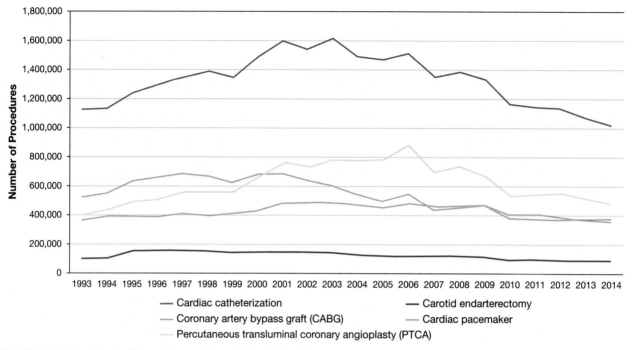

FIGURE 5.14 Trends in cardiovascular procedures, U.S., 1993–2014, inpatient procedures only. (From Tsao CW, Aday AW, Almarzooq ZI, et al. Heart disease and stroke statistics-2022 update: a report from the American Heart Association. *Circulation.* 2022;145(8):e153–639.)

statistics, the mean hospital charge for a cardiac revascularization surgery was $168,541, whereas for a PCI, it was $84,813.

ACUTE CORONARY SYNDROME

ACS is a group of characteristic signs and symptoms indicative of prolonged restricted coronary blood flow, which causes myocardial ischemia (Box 5.1). The characteristic symptoms include chest discomfort, angina (chest pain or pressure), arm pain, dyspnea, diaphoresis, jaw pain, nausea, and vomiting. Women with myocardial ischemia may present with completely atypical symptoms that are often overlooked or not associated with CVD. In a recent review, women were more likely than men to

Box 5.1	Symptoms of Angina and Other Forms of Concerning Heart Disease

Chest pain (pressure, tightness, heaviness), especially with exertion

Unusual shortness of breath

Seemingly sudden decreases in physical capacity to perform exercise

Palpitations, "skipped beats," fast or irregular heart rates

Syncope or near syncope

present atypical symptoms including neck, jaw, back pain, weakness, nausea, and fatigue, and less likely to survive a cardiovascular event (12). Clinical findings associated with ACS include unstable angina (UA), non-ST-segment elevation myocardial infarction (NSTEMI), and STEMI, all of which share common pathophysiological beginnings related to the progression of coronary plaque, instability, or rupture with or without luminal thrombosis and vasospasm (1).

CVD continues to be the leading cause of death for men and women in the U.S. Approximately more than 1 in 3 (~85.6 million) U.S. adults have at least one type of CVD with approximately 51% (~43.7 million) being 60 years of age or older (1). As of 2014, it is estimated that about 16.5 million Americans 20 years and older have been diagnosed with coronary heart disease (CHD) (13).

Every 40 seconds a U.S. adult will experience an acute coronary event (*e.g.*, UA, MI), with approximately 695,000 Americans experiencing a new acute coronary event and another 325,000 experiencing a repeat acute coronary event every year. Specifically, the annual estimate of those who experience an MI for the first time is 580,000 and 210,000 people with a recurrent MI (13).

The estimated prevalence for CHD between 2011 and 2014 in U.S. adult males 20 years and older identifies that Caucasians have a higher prevalence of ACS over Blacks, Hispanics, and Asians (7.7%, 7.1%, 5.9%, and 5.0%, respectively; 13). However, for U.S. females, the prevalence was highest among Hispanics compared to Blacks, Caucasians, and Asians (6.1%, 5.7%, 5.3%, and 2.6%, respectively; 13).

The cost to provide health care for people with ACS is on the rise. It is estimated that the cost of total heart disease in the U.S. between 2012 and 2013 was $199.6 billion, of which $11.5 billion was for treating patients with ACS (13). Medical costs to treat patients with CHD between 2013 and 2030 are projected to increase by roughly 100% (13).

Pathophysiology of ACS

ACS has been known to develop over a lifetime. Again, the events of atheroma growth leading to endothelial dysfunction are initiated by fatty deposits located in the innermost layer of the artery, known as the tunica intima, and have been shown to be present in infants and children (13a). Advancement of endothelial dysfunction is identified by the transition of an antiatherogenic to a proatherogenic atmosphere (14). The most common cause of ACS is the progressive $M\dot{V}O_2$ difference; that is, difference in myocardial oxygen demand versus supply. The outcome of myocardial oxygen demand being greater than supply is evident in ACS and can be explained by the detailed pathological process of atherosclerosis. In ACS, the occlusion of one or more coronary arteries is secondary to a cascade of events leading up to the blockage including breakdown of the endothelial lining (tunica intima), cell proliferation, disruption of atherosclerotic plaque, platelet aggregation, and subsequent thrombus formation leading to occlusion. The consequence of obstructed coronary blood flow can lead to a greater $M\dot{V}O_2$ difference progressing to myocardial ischemia, injury, and infarction.

The process of atherosclerosis begins with damage to the luminal endothelial lining of the tunica intima caused by controllable CVD risk factors including HTN, dyslipidemia, psychosocial stress, obesity, physical inactivity, and smoking. This endothelium becomes dysfunctional with a shift in the pattern of synthesis from the antiaggregant and vasodilatory nitric oxide and prostacyclin to the proaggregant and vasoconstrictor thromboxane (14). Over time, this damage causes white blood cells (leukocytes) to adhere to the luminal endothelial lining. The leukocytes eventually migrate through the intimal wall where accumulated lipoproteins are deposited. The leukocytes aggregate and transform into phagocytic macrophages that internalize the accumulated lipoproteins. This process initiates the development of foam cells that

eventually creates a fatty streak. As this process continues, the fatty streak can develop into dense fibrous plaque causing swelling and narrowing of the artery. As the process of swelling continues, a fibrous lesion (*i.e.*, thrombosis) develops and is provoked by a rupture of the fibrous cap. It is at this point that these particles in the blood adhere to the thrombus and a clot is formed. This clot can be large enough to partially or completely occlude the artery. Over time, the occluded artery with decreased oxygen-rich blood flow can initially develop into an ischemic response with identified hypokinesis, a response to injury with impaired function, and eventually an infarcted or akinetic result (Figure 5.10).

Diagnosis of ACS

Prolonged coronary occlusion, and eventual ventricular hypokinesis or akinesis, can result in physical symptoms collectively known as the patient's anginal equivalent. In the patient with ACS, when anginal symptoms are experienced with or without provocation (*i.e.*, while resting or during exertion), the patient may be diagnosed with UA. In contrast, anginal symptoms provoked only during exertion are diagnosed as stable angina. Some patients have silent ischemia; that is, they are asymptomatic and may not be aware that an ACS has occurred or is about to take place.

The density of the myocardium that is ischemic, injured, and/or infarcted is closely related to the percentage of lumen occlusion and the pressure differences across the artery stenosis. Diagnostic tests used to determine the extent of ischemia, injury, and/or infarction include the echocardiogram, ECG, cardiopulmonary stress tests, blood tests, and coronary artery catheterization. The kinetics of the left and right ventricular free walls can be observed and measured by echocardiogram. The ECG is useful in diagnosing ischemia (Figure 5.15) by observing transient horizontal or downsloping depression ($\geq$0.5 mm [$\geq$0.05 mV]) of the ST segment with anginal symptoms (15). ST-segment depression must be observed in two or more leads in the same anatomical position (*e.g.*, inferior leads II and III or II and aVF) to confirm ischemia. Myocardial ischemia can also be demonstrated with precordial T-wave inversion ($\geq$2 mm [$\geq$0.2 mV]), especially when critical stenosis is present in the left anterior descending coronary artery (LADCA; 15). However, as stated previously, ischemia is not always precipitated with angina (*e.g.*, silent ischemia) and angina does not always elicit ST-segment depression. In the setting of the NSTEMI, the ECG does not demonstrate changes in

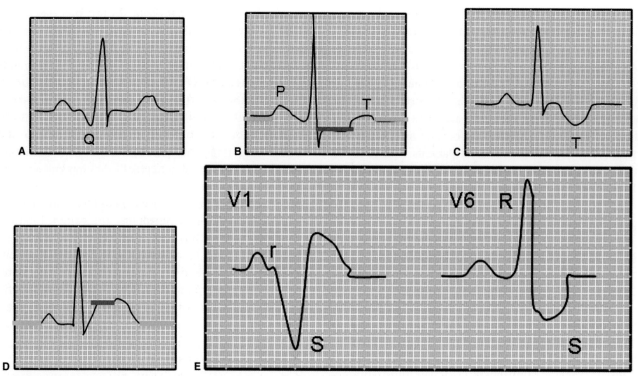

FIGURE 5.15 Electrocardiographic (ECG) features consistent with coronary artery disease. **A.** Q wave consistent with prior myocardial infarction. Significant Q waves are defined as any Q wave #30 ms in width or greater than 0.1 mV in depth or any QS complex. Q waves in two contiguous ECG leads are diagnostic for old infarction. Significant Q waves in leads V2 and V3 can be #20 ms wide. **B.** ST-segment depression consistent with subendocardial ischemia. Horizontal or downsloping ST depression #1 mm below baseline (the isoelectric T-P segment, green line) suggests ischemia. ST depression does not localize the ischemic territory well although the degree of ST depression correlates with the severity of occlusive coronary artery disease. **C.** T-wave inversion consistent with myocardial ischemia. Symmetric and deep T-wave insertion is suggestive of ischemia. Unlike ST depression, T-wave inversion can correlate with the diseased vessel. Deep, symmetric T-wave inversion across the precordial leads (termed Wellens pattern) is fairly specific for left anterior descending coronary ischemia. **D.** ST-segment elevation consistent with myocardial injury. Horizontal or upwardly concave ST elevation #1 mm above the baseline (the isoelectric T-P segment, green line) in the bipolar leads or #2 mm above the baseline in the precordial leads suggests injury or infarction. ST elevation in two contiguous ECG leads can localize the infarct-related artery and represents an indication for acute reperfusion therapy with either coronary intervention or fibrinolysis. **E.** Left bundle branch block (LBBB) pattern. Diagnostic features include QS or RS in lead V1, RS in lead V6, QRS duration >120 ms, and discordance between the direction of the QRS and T-wave vectors. The presence of LBBB indicates the presence of structural heart disease; when new and occurring in the context of chest pain, this finding is considered an ST elevation equivalent and represents an indication for acute reperfusion therapy with either coronary intervention or fibrinolysis. (From Stoller JK. *The Cleveland Clinic Foundation Intensive Review of Internal Medicine.* 6th ed. Philadelphia (PA): Wolters Kluwer; 2014.)

the ST segment and will appear normal. ST-segment depression, T-wave inversion, and intermittent ST-segment elevation may be demonstrated in, but are not required for, the diagnosis of NSTEMI (15). However, ST-segment depression of greater than or equal to 1 mm 2 ms past the J-point and/or T-wave inversion (≥1.0 mm) in two or more leads of the same anatomical direction (*i.e.*, leads II and III) are indicative of myocardial ischemia. During an STEMI or transmural MI, the ECG demonstrates greater than or equal to 1 mm elevation of the ST segment and anginal symptoms often occur prior to and during the event. Q waves are present following the evolving STEMI. When the clinician identifies prominent Q waves of at

least one-fourth to one-third the size of the following R waves, an STEMI has previously occurred, interpreted as an "old" MI. Suffice it to say, the CEP should always treat the patient first and then assess what is demonstrated on the ECG. Please refer to Chapter 6 for a discussion and clarification on ECG interpretation.

In an NSTEMI, the evolving MI cannot be identified on the ECG. Cardiac enzymes/biomarkers, such as troponin, creatine kinase-MB (CK-MB), and myoglobin, are measured to more specifically determine the presence and extent of injury or infarction. Troponin is the preferred biomarker of choice to determine myocardial injury/ infarction as it has a higher sensitivity and specificity for damage to myocardial cell. A positive troponin level is >0.04 ng·mL^{-1} and generally the higher amount of troponin released, the greater the damage to the myocardium. A primary limitation with biomarkers, including troponin, is that the biomarker may not always correlate with AMI.

Coronary catheterization is performed to determine the location of the occlusion (*i.e.*, angiography). It is also used to perform a procedure known as angioplasty to open and restore oxygen-rich blood flow, if necessary. Angioplasty involves inflating a balloon in the artery at the site of the occlusion to open the occlusion and allow blood to flow freely. A procedure known as coronary stenting involves the same process of inserting a balloon in the artery and inflating the balloon in the occlusion, but a stent around the outside of the balloon acts like a metal scaffolding to keep the lumen open. Restoration of blood from PCI is important but may also contribute to reperfusion injury.

Although diagnosis and treatment are performed by the primary care provider (PCP), it is imperative for the CEP to know and understand the procedures available to diagnose and treat ACS. In addition, the CEP must recognize when a patient complains of anginal symptoms and is in the throes of an evolving MI, whether it be an NSTEMI or STEMI.

Treatment and Management

The CEP may initially encounter patients with ACS in the inpatient setting. Prior to initiating contact, it is important for the CEP to review the patient's medical history. To do so, you will first need a referral from the patient's medical provider that documents the patient's underlying diagnosis.

Medical History Review

In the case of the patient diagnosed with ACS, your initial assessment should include a thorough review of the patient's medical record, including:

- History and physical
- Consultation
- Emergency department notes
- Physician progress notes
- Cardiac catheterization notes
- Blood tests/labs (*e.g.*, cardiac enzymes, lipid panel, glucose, and hemoglobin A1C)
- ECG results
- Echocardiography results
- Medication list

Essential information from the medical history includes the primary diagnosis, noncardiac comorbidities (*e.g.*, cancer, musculoskeletal and orthopedic injuries, neurological status) and risk factors (controllable and uncontrollable) for CVD, including smoking, HTN, dyslipidemia, diabetes, depression, psychosocial stress, obesity, physical inactivity, age, gender, and family history. It is also important to identify any other cardiovascular comorbidities (*e.g.*, peripheral vascular disease [PVD], HF, and cerebrovascular disease) in a patient diagnosed with ACS.

Once the underlying cardiac diagnosis has been determined and prior to scheduling the patient for their initial outpatient CR appointment, the CEP must review the patient's current insurance coverage status. The Centers for Medicare and Medicaid Services (CMS) states that in order for outpatient CR to be a covered benefit, the patient's discharge diagnosis must include at least one of the following diagnoses: current stable angina pectoris, acute MI (NSTEMI or STEMI) in the preceding 12 months, percutaneous transluminal coronary intervention (*e.g.*, angioplasty and/or stent procedure), CABG surgery, heart and/or lung transplant surgery, and/or stable, chronic HF, valve repair or replacement. Of note, UA is considered a contraindication for participation in outpatient CR. The CMS has defined stable, chronic HF as presenting with a left ventricular ejection fraction (LVEF) of 35% or less and New York Heart Association (NYHA) class II–IV symptoms despite being on optimal HF therapy for at least 6 weeks. Stable patients are defined as those who have not had recent (≤6 weeks) or planned (≤6 months) major cardiovascular hospitalizations or procedures. It is important to list the aforementioned diagnoses as the patient may have ACS secondary to UA, NSTEMI, or STEMI. The CEP must be aware of qualifying diagnoses for CR that are often concomitant with ACS.

Patient Interview

At the initial encounter with the patient, identify who you are and why you are meeting with them. In the hospital setting, initiate your conversation by addressing the patient by name and then providing them with your name, title/position, and department where you work. It is important to state that you are there by request of their physician(s). After initial rapport has been established with the patient, the CEP should identify the patient's own understanding of why they are in the hospital and what procedures were performed (*e.g.*, catheterization, cardiovascular surgery, and defibrillation). This initial meeting is useful to guide the CEP in introducing the changes the patient can make to prevent another cardiac event (*i.e.*, secondary prevention). The conversation may be very basic with certain patients or quite detailed with others. Depending on the patient's individual CVD risk factors, topics may include smoking cessation, stress management, improving nutrition by lowering sodium and saturated fat intake, and incorporating home exercise guidelines while adhering to temporary physical restrictions. Home exercise guidelines should include activities that the patient is physically capable of performing at their current state of health without causing symptoms associated with their anginal equivalent (*i.e.*, chest pain/pressure). Suggested activities include walking daily at a light to moderate intensity (rating of perceived exertion [RPE] 11–14 from a 6 to 20 Borg scale) over a progressively prolonged duration (*e.g.*, three 10-minute intervals or a total of 30 minutes daily). Detailed information/education regarding lifestyle modifications should be saved for when the CEP meets with the patient in the outpatient setting.

At the point of discharge from the inpatient admission, the patient will have a prescribed list of medications that include, but are not limited to, aspirin, an antiplatelet agent (*i.e.*, clopidogrel), a statin, a β-blocker, nitroglycerin, and an angiotensin-converting enzyme inhibitor (ACE-I). Depending on the patient and recommendations made by their provider, an angiotensin II receptor blocker (ARB) or a calcium channel blocker may be prescribed in lieu of or in addition to the above medications. This list of medications should be reviewed with the patient prior to discharge.

After establishing the initial contact and building rapport with the patient in the hospital setting, the CEP can discuss the details of and scheduling for an outpatient CR appointment. Outpatient facilities may refer to this appointment as the outpatient orientation, initial evaluation, or initial intake appointment. This appointment is designed to meet the patient in the outpatient setting to further evaluate their health status and begin a program of recovery known as phase II or outpatient CR. Prior to the CR orientation, the CEP will have taken the necessary time to review the patient's medical history, including comorbidities, in order to stratify risk of low, moderate, or high, according to the American College of Sports Medicine (ACSM) exercise preparticipation health screen recommendations (16). It is important to note that the patient's previous medical history may not provide enough information to design a safe and effective exercise prescription. A thorough initial interview by the CEP with the patient, and often the patient's family or friends, is the recommended approach prior to designing the exercise prescription and beginning CR in the outpatient setting.

During the interview, the CEP should incorporate active listening strategies to be more engaged in the conversation and allow the patient to be more open in discussing details of their health history. These strategies include demonstrating that you are primarily interested in what they have to say, demonstrating empathy, eliminating environmental noise, staying focused on the client, not interrupting, being attentive to body language, employing patience, acknowledging that you hear what is said, seeking clarification if necessary, and keeping your own emotions in check (17) incorporating these strategies allows the CEP to engage in deeper conversation and formulate a better understanding of the patient's needs and goals for recovery.

Active listening can also uncover the patient's state of readiness to make recommended changes in their lifestyle following their ACS event. It may be assumed that because their medication list was reviewed, home exercise guidelines were discussed, a smoking cessation handout was reviewed, nutritional advice was given, and ways to adhere to an exercise program were explained that the patient will incorporate these changes into their lifestyle. This is often a false assumption. It is recommended that the CEP review the stages of change in the transtheoretical model of behavior change to better understand the patient's stage of readiness to make changes to their health (see Chapter 15). These stages include precontemplation, contemplation, determination/preparation, action, maintenance, and relapse (18). The CEP may discover that the patient is not interested in making changes to improve their health or that they have already begun to make changes and just need some extra guidance and encouragement.

Effects of Exercise

Prior to initiating an exercise program, the CEP should consult with the patient's PCP or cardiologist to decide if exercise testing is necessary and safe. In some cases, as in orthopedic concerns or issues of frailty, the PCP may order a nonexercise or pharmacological stress test where the patient is injected with a radioisotope medication that mimics the effects of exercise on the heart and blood vessels. The ultimate approval for any test must come from the patient's PCP.

CR programs vary in deciding whether or not to obtain functional capacity data from graded exercise testing (GXT) prior to beginning an outpatient program. As there are various GXT protocols to assess cardiorespiratory fitness, the CEP must decide, together with the PCP/cardiologist, if the test is safe and appropriate for the patient. As a primary reference, the CEP should consider the absolute and relative contraindications for GXT as outlined by the *ACSM's Guidelines for Exercise Testing and Prescription* (16). Potential risk and safety concerns must always be paramount when considering assessment of cardiorespiratory function in the patient with ACS.

GXT may be cost prohibitive for some facilities and is not covered by all insurance plans. An alternative to GXT, and a standard practice by many cardiac rehabilitation programs, is to assess functional status with a 6-minute walk test (6MWT) or to orient the patient to the rehab exercise equipment during the initial CR appointment to establish their functional baseline. Even without availability of data from GXT, using Borg's RPE scale is the primary method for determining initial exercise intensities. Remember to always first consider what is best for the patient.

During the initial orientation, the CEP will need to identify exercise modalities that will be suitable for the patient. Factors to consider when deciding which modalities to incorporate in the exercise prescription include, but are not limited to:

- Underlying cardiovascular diagnosis
- Orthopedic limitations
- Metabolic disease history
- Fear from previous experiences
- Current emotional state and physical goals of the patient

As mentioned previously, patients with ACS tend to have multiple comorbidities and are not always physically capable of walking on the treadmill or riding a stationary bicycle.

The CEP must also take into consideration that the patient may not be able to attend the prescribed number of sessions each week. In fact, from large hospital systems to small rural programs, patient attendance and adherence is relatively poor. Common limiting factors include geographic distance to the facility, driving restrictions based on medical necessity, taking care of other family members, motivation/desire to participate, and financial limitations. Of these, the greatest factors that limit participation in an outpatient CR program are financial, and are typically due to lack of insurance coverage for CR, or a high deductible, high copayment, or insufficient coverage, and thus high out-of-pocket expenses. All patients have to meet certain specific qualifying diagnoses for insurance coverage. For patients diagnosed with ACS, most insurance carriers will cover participation in outpatient CR as long as the underlying diagnosis also meets CMS guidelines, as reviewed previously. However, CMS guidelines do not cover outpatient CR for patients with ACS diagnosed with UA alone. Generally, the patient with UA may have coronary catheterization with angioplasty and/or coronary stenting to correct the ischemic response. The patient with UA can be referred to a CR program as a covered benefit by their insurance if a coronary procedure (*i.e.,* angioplasty, coronary stenting, CABG surgery) is performed and/or if the patient has had an NSTEMI or STEMI. It is the responsibility of the CR program staff to know insurance coverage guidelines to attend CR. As most CR programs meet three times per week and copayments per individual session have skyrocketed, many patients find attending outpatient CR unaffordable. The CEP should be able to offer patients simple to somewhat complex home exercise recommendations, depending on the individual, if for any reason they state that they are unable to attend. Home-based CR is an alternative method for offering services that has become increasingly common. Home-based CR programs are managed by a third-party vendor with frequent contact by clinical program staff to prescribe exercise, monitor vital signs and progress, and provide progress reports to physicians.

CR Program, Follow-up, and Referrals

Some programs require the patient to first meet with their cardiology provider prior to beginning their outpatient CR sessions. This office visit is typically scheduled within 1–4 weeks after the patient has been discharged from their inpatient admission. The cardiologist's office will then contact CR program staff to request follow-up with the patient. The physician will sign an outpatient CR order form that allows the program staff to enroll the patient in CR. The patient is contacted by program staff and a CR orientation is scheduled.

After the initial orientation, the patient should be scheduled for their initial outpatient CR session. CR is considered an interdisciplinary field and most outpatient CR programs will be staffed with CEPs, registered nurse(s), a registered dietitian, and a licensed mental health professional. All patients are encouraged to take advantage of opportunities to meet with each member of the CR team to ask questions and become educated about their physical health, nutritional needs, and emotional well-being.

After the patient has begun attending CR sessions, they will have another appointment scheduled to meet with their cardiology provider as an outpatient. The CR program staff will prepare and send a progress report to the provider to update the patient's progress. Some programs will also forward progress reports to PCPs, cardiothoracic surgery, endocrinology, and pulmonology to name a few. This progress report should include all objective data collected including BPs, a confirmed list of medications the patient is taking, HRs and telemetry interpretations, and blood glucose readings, if necessary.

The progress report should also include subjective responses given by the patient as discussed with CR staff during their exercise and education sessions. CR staff should be attentive to any physical limitations the patient may demonstrate or have previously demonstrated as related to musculoskeletal, neurological, and orthopedic concerns from their current and/or previous health history.

The CEP must be aware of their scope of practice and know how and when to determine if the needs of their patient fall outside the discipline of clinical exercise physiology (*e.g.*, does the patient require physical therapy). This applies to all clinical staff on the CR team. The CEP should also know when to employ the services and expertise of their nursing staff. During the initial orientation, for example, the nurse may perform a physical assessment that may include examining the patient's catheterization or incision site for healing and signs of infection. It is vital that the CEP be intimately aware of their role and the roles of their clinical teammates in order to provide optimal patient care. This will also include knowing the number of CR sessions the patient's insurance will cover to optimally develop a tailored exercise prescription.

REVASCULARIZATION OF THE HEART

CAD occurs through the atherosclerotic process, described in detail earlier in the chapter, and results in partial or complete occlusion of one or more coronary arteries. It can be prevented and generally well managed with the use of medications as well as lifestyle interventions (*i.e.*, diet, exercise, stress management, and tobacco cessation) that can reduce the presence/severity of CAD risk factors. Several studies have shown that CAD can be stabilized and even reversed with pharmacologic and/or aggressive lifestyle therapy (1, 10).

Hambrecht et al. (11) demonstrated that CAD "regression" can occur in selected patients with CAD who accumulate more than 2,200 kcal per week in PA. However, in some patients, the coronary arteries become more severely and/or acutely obstructed, thus requiring an emergent revascularization procedure. The two procedures commonly used to revascularize a blocked coronary artery are to implant a stent in the area of the blockage or to entirely "bypass" the blocked segment of artery surgically. The trends in the use of these procedures are presented in Figure 5.14 and indicate that more than 900,000 revascularization procedures were performed on Americans in 2010 (1, 10).

The total number of inpatient cardiovascular operations and procedures increased by 28% between the years 2000 and 2010. Data on Medicare beneficiaries undergoing a coronary revascularization procedure between 2008 and 2012 indicate that the rapid growth in nonadmission PCI (from 60,405 to 106,495) has been more than offset by the decrease in PCI admissions (from 363,384 to 295,434). According to the 2012 National Healthcare Cost and Utilization Project statistics, the mean hospital charge for a cardiac revascularization surgery was $149,480, whereas for a PCI, it was $70,027 (1).

Revascularization Procedures

Two procedures are used to treat CAD.

Percutaneous Coronary Intervention

PCI is a minimally invasive procedure in which a catheter with an associated balloon is introduced via a peripheral artery (either the femoral artery in the groin or the radial artery at the wrist), thereby avoiding the need for surgery and general anesthesia. The balloon is inflated in the area of the blocked artery to dilate the lumen. In most patients, a coronary stent is then placed to prevent vascular recoil and restenosis (Figure 5.16).

Even with stent placement, approximately 15%–20% of patients will develop restenosis of the artery and require a repeat angioplasty procedure within 6–12 months. Newer drug eluting stents (DES) greatly reduce the risk of restenosis to less than 10% (19). In addition, to prevent clots from developing in the stent, patients are typically prescribed medications that inhibit blood platelets (usually aspirin plus an additional blood anticoagulant). These are needed for up to 1 year after the procedure.

Coronary Artery Bypass Graft

CABG surgery is a major surgical procedure requiring general anesthesia. In most patients, the procedure is performed after opening the chest through an incision through the sternum. Veins taken from the leg (saphenous

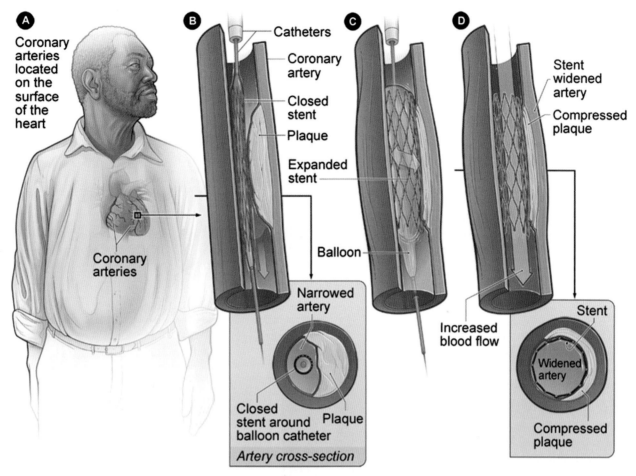

FIGURE 5.16 Stent placement. In **(A)**, the catheter is inserted across the lesion. In **(B)**, the balloon is inflated, expanding the stent and compressing the plaque. In **(C)**, the catheter and deflated balloon have been removed. In **(D)**, before-and-after cross-sections of the artery show the results of stent placement. (From National Heart, Lung, and Blood Institute. Stents. Available from: https://www.nhlbi.nih.gov/health-topics/stents.)

vein) and an artery taken from within the chest (internal thoracic or mammary artery) or the forearm (radial artery) are used to bypass the coronary artery blockages (Figure 5.17).

All bypass grafts are highly likely to remain patent (*i.e.*, open) for the first 5–8 years after the surgery. In fact, 95% of arterial bypass grafts are likely to remain open for 10+ years (19). However, within 10 years, about 50% of vein bypass grafts are significantly occluded. Although repeat CABG is possible, many patients with a blocked vein graft can be treated medically and/or with catheter-based interventions. Improving the coronary blood flow by either PCI or CABG may be needed emergently in patients with unrelenting myocardial ischemia or MI. Either procedure can be successful in eliminating angina, preventing myocardial injury, and improving the quality of life if performed rapidly. Patients who have had a recent MI have better survival if the blocked artery is opened early

after the event. In patients with damaged heart muscle and multiple blockages, CABG can prolong life even in the absence of symptoms (19).

Selection Criteria for PCI Versus CABG

As described earlier in this chapter, the heart has three major coronary arteries (and many smaller branches), each supplying a different area of the heart muscle. When a single artery is blocked, PCI is often preferred over surgery, as it is less invasive and allows faster recovery. When multiple arteries are blocked, a decision must be made between performing PCI to the multiple blockages or CABG. Sometimes arteries are blocked in such a way that only one revascularization choice is possible. For example, arteries that have been 100% occluded for years may not be amenable to PCI, and in this case, CABG may be the only option. In other cases, patients may be too frail to

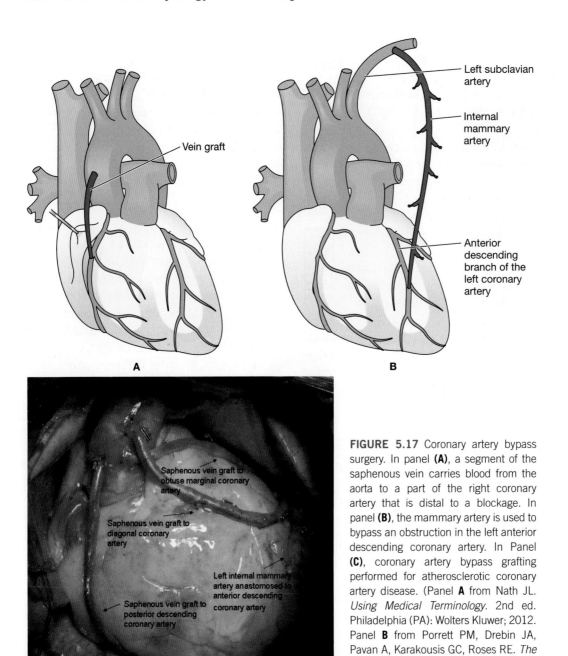

FIGURE 5.17 Coronary artery bypass surgery. In panel **(A)**, a segment of the saphenous vein carries blood from the aorta to a part of the right coronary artery that is distal to a blockage. In panel **(B)**, the mammary artery is used to bypass an obstruction in the left anterior descending coronary artery. In Panel **(C)**, coronary artery bypass grafting performed for atherosclerotic coronary artery disease. (Panel **A** from Nath JL. *Using Medical Terminology*. 2nd ed. Philadelphia (PA): Wolters Kluwer; 2012. Panel **B** from Porrett PM, Drebin JA, Pavan A, Karakousis GC, Roses RE. *The Surgical Review*. 4th ed. Philadelphia (PA): Wolters Kluwer; 2015.)

withstand CABG, but may be able to more safely undergo multivessel PCI. Until the last decade, vein grafts were the predominant conduit vessel of choice for CABG, but high graft failure has made arterial grafts more desirable (20).

In many patients with multivessel coronary disease, both PCI and CABG are technically feasible, but there continues to be a debate as to which procedure is best, especially for patients who also have diabetes mellitus (DM). Several studies have compared PCI and CABG in patients with multivessel CAD who were good candidates for either procedure. In one study involving patients without DM,

PCI and CABG provided similar control of chest pain and comparable survival over 5 years after the procedure (19). However, PCI-treated patients have a greater need for repeated procedures. An earlier study comparing PCI with CABG suggested that in patients with DM, CABG was associated with better long-term survival than PCI (21). This initial observation was confirmed in the largest ever study comparing PCI and CABG in patients with DM (22). This study showed that, compared with PCI, CABG improved survival in patients with DM by one-third over 5 years. The need for a repeat procedure was almost threefold greater in those who had PCI. The benefits of CABG came with the cost of an increased risk of stroke (5% vs. 2.5%) that usually occurred during or shortly after the surgery.

Neither CABG nor PCI completely eliminates the risk of MI in patients with stable CAD. However, CABG will often restore blood flow to a larger amount of heart muscle because not all coronary blockages are accessible by PCI. Recurrent narrowing of the artery is also more likely to occur after PCI. Bypass surgery is also thought to protect the heart and to prevent heart attack or sudden death even if a coronary artery suddenly occludes. For the patient with DM needing a revascularization procedure for multivessel coronary disease, CABG should usually be considered the procedure of choice. However, individualization of treatment needs to take into account the risk of CABG and patient preferences (Table 5.1).

After carefully weighing the evidence, PCI may be the choice for frail patients and those with a higher risk of stroke. Revascularization with either PCI or CABG does not change the atherosclerotic process, and lifestyle interventions are still essential for secondary prevention of CAD.

Medical Management Following PCI

Appropriate medical management of patients treated with PCI includes medications to prevent thrombosis during and after the procedure. Current recommendations from the American Heart Association (AHA)/American College of Cardiology (ACC) on secondary prevention of CAD suggest that after PCI with stent placement, aspirin should be prescribed for at least 6 months (10). In addition to aspirin, other anticoagulants are likely to be prescribed for PCI/stent patients.

Medical Management Following CABG

The management of CABG patients is dependent on the comorbid problems and the type of operative procedure performed. These operations are usually performed with extracorporeal circulation (bypass "pump" machine) as well as with a median sternotomy (separation of sternum). Anticoagulant therapy, including aspirin, is discontinued before CABG but is restarted and generally continued indefinitely postoperatively. The AHA/ACC guidelines on secondary prevention of CAD suggest that for CABG patients, aspirin "dosing regimens ranging from 100 to 325 mg per day appear to be efficacious" (10). The use of other more potent thrombolytic agents is dependent on the risk of thrombi and the presence of arrhythmias (*i.e.*, atrial fibrillation). Routine postoperative care, including early ambulation, usually results in discharge within 4–7 days postoperatively.

Table 5.1	Comparison of PCI and CABG in Patients With Diabetes Mellitus and Multivessel Coronary Artery Disease Who Are Candidates for Both Procedures	
Factor	PCI	CABG
Invasive	+	+++
Recovery time	+	+++
Procedural risk	+	++
Bleeding risk	++	+++
Ability to treat most blockages	+	+++
Need for repeat interventions	+++	+
Symptom control	+++	+++
Reduces risk of death	+	+++
Reduces risk of heart attack	+	++
Risk of stroke	+	++
Need for dual antiplatelet treatment	+++	+
Cost	++	+++
Need for long-term medications	+++	+++

CABG, coronary artery bypass graft; PCI, percutaneous coronary interventions.

In addition to antithrombotic therapy, β-blockers, ACE-Is, and/or ARBs are used depending on the degree of myocardial dysfunction (*i.e.*, reduced EF). HMG-CoA reductase inhibitors (statins) are widely used after revascularization due to their lipid-lowering and anti-inflammatory (also known as pleiotropic) effects as well as their ability to prevent and potentially reverse atherosclerotic lesions (23). The use of antiarrhythmic drugs, pacemakers, and implanted cardioverter defibrillator devices is considered individually in the revascularization patient depending on the type of arrhythmia and the degree of myocardial dysfunction.

The primary concerns for a patient who underwent a PCI are the potential recurrence of myocardial ischemia/angina and ensuring that the vascular incision site for catheter access has closed properly. Normally the catheter access site heals within 24–48 hours and the patient can resume normal activities soon thereafter. After PCI, there is a significant chance of restenosis of the treated vessel; therefore, the patient must be aware of the recurrence of symptoms and potential need for repeat PCI. For CABG patients, the focus will be on the healing of the sternum and the site where the blood vessel was removed for grafting.

In all patients with CAD who have undergone PCI or CABG, the control of risk factors is essential to prevent progressive atherosclerosis. Comprehensive rehabilitation programs that emphasize appropriate lifestyle modification and risk reduction have been shown to be highly beneficial (25).

Effects of Exercise Rehabilitation

Historically, CABG patients did not begin to exercise on their own or enter formal CR programs until 4–6 weeks after surgery, after approval by the surgeon (24). It has become more acceptable for uncomplicated CABG patients to begin CR as soon as possible after discharge (often within 1 week of surgery or less) as the benefits of light upper extremity range-of-motion (ROM) exercises and low-level ambulation have become more apparent (24).

Endurance Exercise Training

After appropriate screening for contraindications (16), endurance-type exercise training for the CABG patient can be guided initially by using resting HR + 30 beats per minute (bpm) or RPE 11–13 until more specific data from a symptom-limited exercise test are generated. When using any arbitrary approach to exercise prescription, however, the CEP must recognize that significant intersubject variability exists (24).

As the CABG patient progresses into and through outpatient CR, the CEP should develop a more traditional exercise prescription that specifies type, intensity, frequency, and duration tailored to the patient's needs (16). Some CABG patients may initially need lower intensity or other exercise modifications because of musculoskeletal discomfort (chest and back) or healing at the incision sites (sternum and legs).

For PCI patients, endurance-type exercise can begin almost immediately as long as the catheter access site, generally in the groin, has healed properly. The exercise prescription for PCI patients is generally similar to that for other cardiac patients; however, PCI patients may be able to progress more rapidly, particularly if there was no myocardial damage, and they are less likely to have had extended periods of physical inactivity pre- and postprocedure. As mentioned earlier, in the current era of stenting and aggressive pharmacotherapy, the risk for restenosis in PCI patients is reduced considerably. Nevertheless, the CEP should still observe the PCI patient closely throughout CR for potential recurrence of ischemic signs and symptoms indicative of restenosis (24).

Resistance and ROM Exercise Training

Even after just a few days of bed rest, a significant loss of lean body mass and cardiovascular function occurs. To counteract the deleterious effects of bed rest and other complications associated with CABG, ROM activities and resistance activities using very light (*i.e.*, 1–3 lb or 0.45–1.36 kg) hand weights are initiated while in the hospital or in the early outpatient setting. Stretching or flexibility activities can begin as early as 24 hours after CABG. Walking is a highly recommended and beneficial mode of exercise that can be initiated within a few days of the CABG or PCI procedure.

As indicated in Box 5.2, CABG patients should avoid traditional resistance training exercises (with moderate-to-heavy weights), until the sternum has healed sufficiently, which is generally by 3 months (16). It is also recommended that CABG patients should perform 3–4 weeks of aerobic exercise training before initiating traditional resistance exercise training (24). Surgery patients who experience sternal movement or wound complications should perform lower extremity exercises only. These lower body exercises may be initiated sooner than upper body exercises if the patient is progressing well. However, because significant soft tissue and bone damage of the chest wall can occur during surgery, upper body ROM exercise is essential. Otherwise, adhesions may develop and the musculature can become weaker

- Minimum of 5 wk after the date of MI or cardiac surgery, *including* 4 wk of consistent participation in a supervised CR endurance training program[a]
- Minimum of 3 wk following transcatheter procedure (PTCA, other), *including* 2 wk of consistent participation in a supervised CR endurance training program[a]
- No evidence of the following conditions:
  - Congestive heart failure
  - Uncontrolled dysrhythmias
  - Severe valvular disease
  - Uncontrolled hypertension. Patients with moderate hypertension (systolic BP > 160 mm Hg or diastolic BP > 100 mm Hg) should be referred for appropriate management, although these values are not absolute contraindications for participation in a resistance training program.
- Unstable symptoms

In this table, a resistance exercise program is defined as one in which patients lift weights 50% or greater of 1RM. The use of elastic bands, 1- to 3-lb hand weights, and light free weights may be initiated in a progressive fashion at phase II program entry, provided no other contraindications exist.

[a]Entry should be a staff decision with approval of the medical director and surgeon as appropriate.

AACVPR, American Association of Cardiovascular and Pulmonary Rehabilitation; BP, blood pressure; CR, cardiac rehabilitation; MI, myocardial infarction; PTCA, percutaneous transluminal coronary angioplasty.

From AACVPR Guidelines for Cardiac Rehabilitation and Secondary Prevention, 2013. *American Association of Cardiovascular and Pulmonary Rehabilitation. AACVPR Cardiac Rehabilitation Resource Manual.* Champaign (IL): Human Kinetics; 2013.

and shorter, accentuating postural problems and hindering strength gains. Because CABG patients typically have been sedentary during surgical convalescence, musculoskeletal soreness/fatigue is likely to be prominent in their recovery process.

For PCI patients, light resistance training with elastic bands and small hand weights can begin almost immediately for the upper body muscles and for the lower body if the catheter access site has healed properly (assuming the catheter access site was the leg). More aggressive resistance training for the PCI patient can be safely initiated 3 weeks (including 2 weeks of endurance activity) postintervention.

Addressing Behavioral Aspects

Because both CABG and PCI patients meet the CMS diagnostic criteria for CR participation and reimbursement, the primary objective of behavior change should initially focus on referral to these programs. In the CR program, a multidisciplinary team of health care providers will address various concerns related to the recovery/rehabilitation and secondary prevention efforts of the revascularized patient. Of course, obtaining an appropriate amount of PA is an essential part of this process.

At the initiation of a PA program, short- and long-term goals and priorities should be established with the patient, who must be an active participant in the process. The goals should be measurable and specific. The CEP can use the "SMART" acronym, which encompasses the key characteristics of an effective goal (see Chapter 15). Progress should be measured periodically, and the goals reassessed accordingly. This helps increase the patient's self-efficacy. The importance of planning and scheduling PA into the patient's daily routine needs to be emphasized. Finally, patient motivation is increased by committing to the goals verbally or in writing.

Follow-up and Referrals

Typically, CABG patients meet with their surgeon several times in the first 6 months postoperatively to ensure that appropriate sternal and wound healing has occurred. Thereafter, they typically resume seeing their PCP and/or cardiologist/internist on a regular basis (*i.e.*, every 6–12 months) unless problems arise. PCI patients will generally see their cardiologist within the first 3 months following the procedure and then regularly thereafter (3–6 months).

If the patient has participated in a CR program, there should be some type of follow-up (phone or in person) after one year of discharge from the program to assess long-term outcomes. Unfortunately, limited resources and lack of reimbursement often prevent this long-term follow-up from occurring. Unfortunately, among >300,000 Medicare fee-for-service beneficiaries eligible for CR in 2016, only 24.4% participated in the program and only 26.9% of these patients completed greater than or equal to

36 sessions. Participation decreased with increasing age and was lower in females, Hispanic people, Asian people, those eligible for dual Medicare/Medicaid coverage, and those with greater than or equal to 5 comorbidities.

HEART FAILURE

On the basis of data from the National Health and Nutrition Examination Survey (NHANES) from 2015 to 2018, approximately 6.0 million American adults had HF, which increased from approximately 5.7 million in 2009–2012 (25). The prevalence of HF is projected to continue to increase and affect more than 8 million people by 2030. Two main factors driving the increasing prevalence of HF are the aging population and increased presence of risk factors including diabetes and obesity. Trends show that the incidence of HF with preserved ejection fraction (HFpEF) is increasing and, in contrast, the incidence of HF with reduced ejection fraction (HFrEF) is decreasing, whereas both HF subtypes have similar all-cause mortality rates. Contemporary HFpEF with guideline-directed medical therapy is estimated to reduce the hazard of cardiovascular death or HF hospitalization by up to 62% compared with limited conventional therapy.

Many risk factors for HF and CAD are shared. These include advanced age, male sex, HTN, left ventricular hypertrophy, obesity, DM, smoking, dyslipidemia, poor diet, sedentary lifestyle, and psychological stress (26). Additionally, a previous MI, valvular heart disease, and alcohol abuse are considered risk factors for developing HF. In the U.S., it has been estimated that about 75% of the cases of HF in the adult population occurs in those with long-standing HTN (1). In fact, the lifetime risk for developing HF increases for those with higher BP or body mass index (BMI; highest for those with both HTN and obesity) regardless of age or race (27). From the Global Burden of Disease study, there were 17 primary causes of HF, but two-thirds of all cases could be attributed to four conditions: ischemic heart disease, chronic obstructive pulmonary disease (COPD), hypertensive heart disease, and rheumatic heart disease.

Pathophysiology of HF

HF is a complex and progressive clinical syndrome representing a common final stage of many different disorders of the heart with no absolute cure short of cardiac transplantation (26). The HF syndrome results from any structural or functional disorder that limits the ability of the left ventricle to relax and fill with blood (HFpEF) and/or contract and eject blood (HFrEF), which leads to neurohormonal and circulatory abnormalities that cause the characteristic signs and symptoms such as fluid retention, shortness of breath (SOB), and fatigue (28, 29). Physiological characteristics of HF include increased filling pressures and/or insufficient peripheral oxygen delivery (30). HF is associated with increased mortality, reduced quality of life, frequent hospitalizations, and complex medical management (30).

HF is a very heterogeneous disease and the pathophysiology is multifactorial. In the pathophysiology of HFrEF, there is an association between reduced myocyte function and alterations such as reduced Ca^{2+} sequestration by the sarcoplasmic reticulum (due to reduced function and expression of the sarcoplasmic reticulum Ca^{2+} ATPase) and upregulation of sarcolemmal Na^+/Ca^{2+} exchanger (both in function and in expression), a reduced affinity of troponin to Ca^{2+}, altered substrate metabolism, and impaired respiratory chain activity (31, 32). More recently, researchers have suggested that alterations in the degree of phosphorylation of cardiac myosin binding protein-C by protein kinase-A may contribute to the reduced myocyte function observed in HF. These collectively can lead to a decrease in the contractility of the heart and subsequently to reduced SV (reducing CO), reduced arterial pressure, and increased HR. Paradoxically, these alterations create changes in the force/frequency relationship that depress the Bowditch effect, such that contractile performance decreases with increasing HR (33). The decrease in mean arterial pressure (MAP) leads to decreased arterial baroreceptor activation, impairing the regulation of the HR by the vagus nerve, but the receptors maintain the ability to modulate sympathetic discharge (34). This control of the sympathetic discharge increases central (medullary cardiovascular centers) sympathetic outflow, causing a further downregulation of parasympathetic nervous system (32, 34).

The reduced MAP and increased sympathetic stimulation promote the release of renin from the kidneys, which converts angiotensinogen to angiotensin I (44; Figure 5.18). Angiotensin I is converted into the vasoconstrictor angiotensin II, which is enzymatically controlled by ACE. Angiotensin II also stimulates the release of aldosterone from the adrenal cortex. The decreased activation of the baroreceptors stimulates the release of vasopressin from the posterior pituitary, which (together with aldosterone) causes sodium retention and fluid absorption. Sympathetic stimulation of the adrenal medulla increases the release of epinephrine, which further contributes to vasoconstriction (32). The increased circulating epinephrine increases glycogenolysis by the liver, which increases

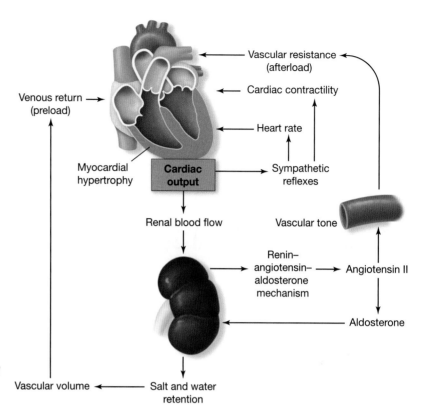

FIGURE 5.18 Compensatory mechanisms in heart failure. (From Braun C, Anderson C. *Applied Pathophysiology.* 3rd ed. Philadelphia (PA): Wolters Kluwer; 2016.)

blood glucose levels and raises extracellular osmolarity. This change in osmolarity and the reduced capillary hydrostatic pressure from the increased arterial constriction causes a shift of fluid from the interstitial and intracellular spaces into the intravascular space.

In response to the loss of CO from the reduced myocyte function, these changes are compensatory. They reflect a net balance between appropriate reflex responses to the reduced left ventricular function and the stimulus eliciting the adrenergic responses excessive to what is needed to achieve homeostasis (34). When a relatively normal SV and MAP can be maintained through increases in left ventricular diastolic volume, then the balance remains shifted toward appropriate compensatory reflexes, and plasma norepinephrine levels can be maintained (34). However, over time, the continued increased volume contributes to cardiac remodeling and further myocyte dysfunction. Furthermore, the chronic norepinephrine release causes a downregulation in cardiac β1 adrenergic receptors, altered β-receptor signal transduction, and a decrease in norepinephrine reuptake, tilting the balance toward the excessive adrenergic response (34). In other words, in the case of chronic HF, these changes can provide compensation early in the disease, but become pathologic, contributing to the progressive nature of HF (Figure 5.19).

Diagnosis of HF

An LVEF of less than 40% is most commonly associated with left ventricular chamber dilation (28–30). The reduced LVEF can be thought of as resulting from reduced squeezing of the heart muscle during systole. On the other hand, with HFpEF, the signs and symptoms of HF can exist in the presence of a normal LVEF (≥50%) and echocardiographic evidence of cardiac muscle dysfunction (28–30). This is most commonly associated with a nondilated left ventricle. Where HFrEF is associated with systolic dysfunction, HFpEF is associated with incomplete or abnormal relaxation during diastole, and in the past was referred to as diastolic HF (Figures 5.20 and 5.21).

Distinguishing between HFrEF and HFpEF is important in selecting appropriate treatment. The majority of patients enrolled in investigations of HF have been those with an HFrEF of less than 35%–40%, and treatments shown to be beneficial in HFrEF have not had the same efficacy in patients with HFpEF (28, 35).

Because HF evolves from another cardiovascular problem, it should never be a patient's only diagnosis, and the underlying cause should be sought (29). Frequently, HF is described as resulting from an ischemic etiology, which is damage to the myocardium related to an MI, and is

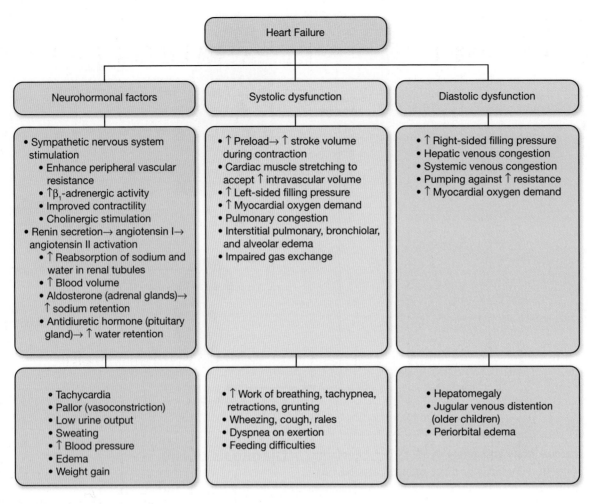

FIGURE 5.19 Pathophysiology of heart failure. (From Ricci S, Kyle T, Carman S. *Maternity and Pediatric Nursing.* 3rd ed. Philadelphia (PA): Wolters Kluwer; 2016.)

associated (most often) with the development of HFrEF. Nonischemic etiologies, which may lead to HFrEF or HFpEF, may be genetic (*i.e.*, neuromuscular disorders, familial, inborn errors of metabolism), lifestyle-related (*i.e.*, HTN, obesity, hygiene), or idiopathic (36, 37). From a clinical perspective, distinguishing the etiology of a patient's HF is helpful in determining the course of treatment and preventing further complications by the underlying disease.

Relation to Exercise Tolerance

Exercise capacity is dependent on both cardiac and peripheral mechanisms. It has been well established for some time that the relationship between peak oxygen consumption ($\dot{V}O_{2peak}$) and resting LVEF is poorly correlated in patients with HF (38). The measure of $\dot{V}O_{2peak}$ is dependent on HR, SV, and peripheral O_2 transfer as seen in the Fick equation: $= HR \times SV \times$ (arterial O_2 content $-$ venous O_2 content). In patients with HF, exercise capacity is

dependent on three factors: the cardiac reserve (amount of potential increase in HR and/or SV capable); O_2 transfer (peripheral vascular function); and O_2 utilization (mitochondrial number and function in skeletal muscle) (39). Other factors that influence exercise capacity include ergoreceptor activity and ventilatory efficiency.

Decreased CO (product of HR and SV) in patients with HF begins with a cascade of events by which the body attempts to maintain or improve CO. These events work to increase catecholamines, increase natriuretic peptide concentrations, and decrease nitric oxide bioavailability, all of which lead to increased vasoconstriction and decreased endothelial function and repair. When maintained chronically, the increased vasoconstriction and the decreased endothelial function increase ventricular afterload and reduce ventricular filling leading to reduced SV.

Additionally, consider the concept that MAP is the product of CO and total peripheral resistance (TPR); or MAP $=$ CO $\times$ TPR. This formula can be rewritten to

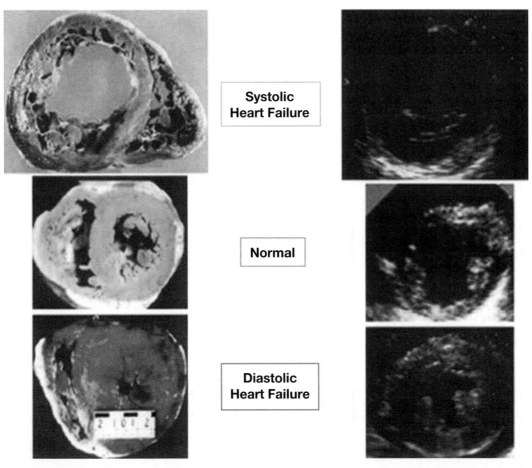

Systolic Heart Failure

Normal

Diastolic Heart Failure

FIGURE 5.20 Ventricular remodeling in systolic and diastolic heart failure. Left: Autopsy examples. Right: Cross-sectional two-dimensional echocardiographic views of systolic and diastolic heart failures compared with normal are illustrated. In systolic heart failure, the left ventricular cavity is markedly dilated and wall thickness is not increased. In diastolic heart failure, the cavity size is normal or decreased, and wall thickness is markedly increased. (Used with permission from Gabrielli A, Layon AJ, Yu M. *Civetta, Taylor and Kirby's Critical Care*. 4th ed. Philadelphia (PA): Wolters Kluwer; 2008. Top and bottom images in the left column are adapted with permission from Konstam MA. Systolic and diastolic dysfunction in heart failure? Time for a new paradigm. *J Card Fail*. 2003;9:1–3.)

demonstrate the relationship of CO to TPR, such that CO = MAP/TPR. So, maintaining MAP, an increase in TPR will result in a decrease in CO. Research indicates that 6 months of regular aerobic exercise training significantly reduces resting and exercise TPR in patients with HFrEF, with a significant inverse relationship between TPR and SV and improved agonist-mediated endothelium-dependent vasodilation in lower limb skeletal muscle vasculature (40). In the same study, there was evidence of reduced circulating epinephrine and norepinephrine at rest and during exercise in the exercise intervention group (40).

In 1996, Clark et al. (41) proposed the "muscle hypothesis," which suggested abnormalities in skeletal muscle as the cause for the symptoms (particularly dyspnea and fatigue) and reflex abnormalities experienced by patients with HF (42). In this review, Clark et al. provided evidence that demonstrated skeletal muscle in patients with HF is

histologically and functionally abnormal (41). Specifically, there is reduction in type I (fatigue-resistant) fibers with a shift toward type IIb fibers, which is accompanied by a reduction in the cross-sectional area of the muscle (atrophy) and the number of capillaries per fiber (41). There is also evidence that the number of mitochondria is reduced along with the surface area of the cristae within the available mitochondria (41), which limits the production of adenosine triphosphate (ATP) during aerobic exercise and contributes to the reduced exercise capacity.

In addition to these changes in the skeletal muscle structure and function, Clark et al. highlighted the role of ergoreceptors in the manifestation of exercise limitations (41). These receptors are responsible for the peripheral reflex that originates in skeletal muscle, and they are sensitive to the products of muscle work. Reduced skeletal muscle mass in the periphery is consistently associated

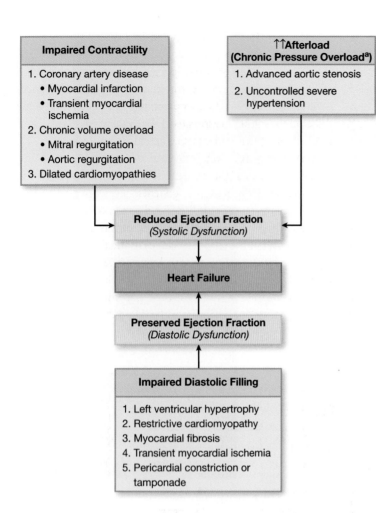

Impaired Contractility

1. Coronary artery disease
   • Myocardial infarction
   • Transient myocardial ischemia
2. Chronic volume overload
   • Mitral regurgitation
   • Aortic regurgitation
3. Dilated cardiomyopathies

↑↑Afterload (Chronic Pressure Overload[a])

1. Advanced aortic stenosis
2. Uncontrolled severe hypertension

Reduced Ejection Fraction *(Systolic Dysfunction)*

Heart Failure

Preserved Ejection Fraction *(Diastolic Dysfunction)*

Impaired Diastolic Filling

1. Left ventricular hypertrophy
2. Restrictive cardiomyopathy
3. Myocardial fibrosis
4. Transient myocardial ischemia
5. Pericardial constriction or tamponade

FIGURE 5.21 Conditions that cause left-sided heart failure through impairment of ventricular systolic or diastolic function. [a]In chronic stable stages, the conditions in this box (aortic stenosis, hypertension) may instead result in heart failure with preserved ejection fraction (EF) due to compensatory ventricular hypertrophy and increased diastolic stiffness (diastolic dysfunction). (From Lilly LS. *Pathophysiology of Heart Disease*. 6th ed. Philadelphia (PA): Wolters Kluwer; 2015.)

with overactivation of the ergoreflex response, exercise limitation, and progression of the HF syndrome (42, 43). The ergoreceptor reflex is an important contributor to the ventilatory response during exercise. Again, a common exercise testing finding in HF patients is an elevated ventilatory response to carbon dioxide ($\dot{V}E/\dot{V}CO_2$ slope), which is reflective of reduced ventilatory efficiency. Although pulmonary vascular resistance has been strongly correlated with slope (44), the degree of overactive ergoreceptor reflex has been linked to increased ventilation and reduced ventilatory efficiency (42, 43).

It seems then that these changes in skeletal muscle structure and function not only reflect the progression of the syndrome (a "vicious circle" that worsens symptoms) but also become their own "vicious circle" by causing discomfort with exercise (fatigue and dyspnea) that is interpreted as a warning or need to reduce exercise training and other incidental activities. This then causes an additional detraining effect that further reduces the patient's exercise tolerance. Endurance training, in contrast, has been shown to improve the surface density of the cristae of mitochondria in patients with HF, thereby improving the ability of mitochondria to produce ATP (45).

Exercise Testing

It is very helpful to base prescribed exercise training intensity ranges on the results of exercise testing. Ideally, the patient's exercise capacity would be assessed with cardiopulmonary exercise (CPX) testing. This testing is the gold standard for determining cardiorespiratory fitness, but other useful variables can be acquired from this test. These include prognostic indicators such as ventilatory efficiency and oscillatory breathing pattern, as well as documentation of symptoms, HR and BP responses, arrhythmia burden, and pacemaker response. If available, CPX testing should be done over other stress testing methods because of the wealth of information that can be obtained.

If CPX testing is unavailable, then standard GXT is acceptable, which can provide an estimate of exercise capacity and still account for symptoms, hemodynamic responses, and device response. A second alternative to assess functional capacity is the 6-minute walk test, which is moderately correlated with obtained from CPX testing and does provide prognostic information. However, the arrhythmia response evaluation and response of a pacemaker are more difficult to fully evaluate. When added to a battery of tests (*i.e.*, the Senior Fitness Test), the 6-minute walk test can be used to evaluate frailty and assessment of physical independence (46). Strength testing can be performed safely and reliably in patients with HF, including one repetition maximum or estimated one repetition maximum testing. Any of the mentioned testing should be done prior to starting CR and after completing CR, and all demonstrate changes reliably.

Treatment and Management of HF

Mortality declines have been attributed primarily to evidence-based approaches to treat HFrEF and the implementation of treatment with neurohormonal blockade, coronary revascularization, implantable cardioverter defibrillators, and cardiac resynchronization therapies. Initiation of contemporary guideline-directed medical therapy for HFrEF

(quadruple therapy with angiotensin receptor neprilysin inhibitors, β-blockers, mineralocorticoid receptor antagonists, and sodium–glucose cotransporter-2 inhibitors) is estimated to reduce the hazard of cardiovascular death or HF hospitalization by up to 62% compared with limited conventional therapy, resulting in estimated 1.4–6.3 additional years alive. A subset of HF patients can actually recover their native heart function following left ventricular assist device (LVAD) placement. In the future, exercise may play a crucial role in increasing recovery in these patients.

Because HF is a progressive disease, current practices are designed to reduce patient symptoms and to slow its progression. There are four stages in the development and progression in HF as seen in Figure 5.22. Treatments include medications (Figure 5.23), as well as cardiac rhythm management with an electronic pacemaker or implantable cardioverter defibrillator (ICD). Advanced therapies,

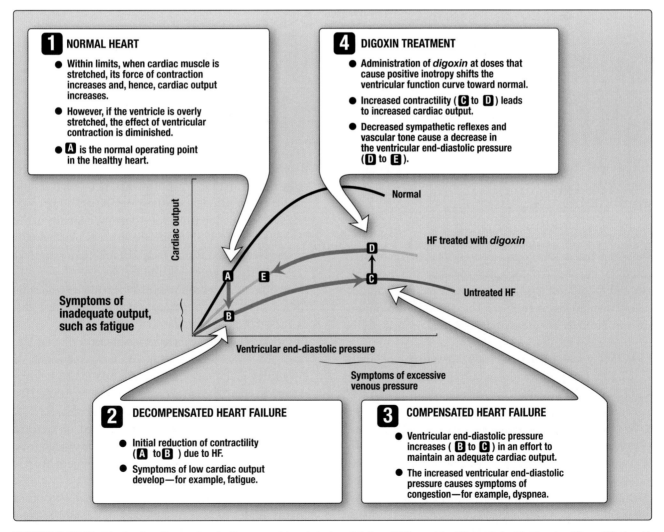

FIGURE 5.22 Ventricular function curves in the normal heart, in heart failure (HF), and in HF treated with digoxin. (From Whalen K. *Lippincott Illustrated Reviews: Pharmacology*. 6th ed. Philadelphia (PA): Wolters Kluwer; 2014.)

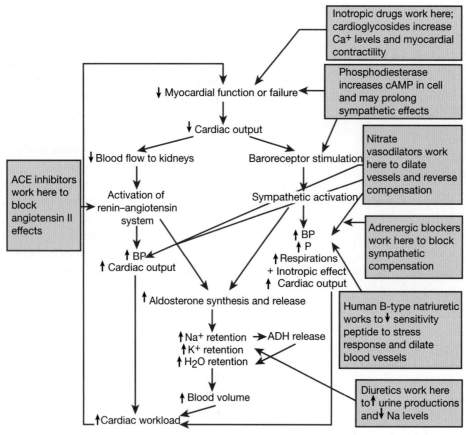

FIGURE 5.23 Sites of action of drugs used to treat heart failure (HF). (From Karch AM. *Focus on Nursing Pharmacology*. 7th ed. Philadelphia (PA): Wolters Kluwer; 2016.)

such as heart transplant or implantation of a ventricular assist device (VAD), are used in the treatment of end-stage HF (ESHF).

Pharmacological Management

The primary medical management of HF is targeted toward the control of the overactivated renin–angiotensin–aldosterone axis and the sympathetic adrenergic system along with resulting volume overload (29, 47). The following medications are considered part of the standard medical therapy for HF:

- ACE-Is — have been consistently shown to reduce hospitalizations, mortality, and slow the progression of HF (47).
- ARBs — recommended for patients who cannot tolerate ACE-I due to the side effects.
- Angiotensin receptor neprilysin inhibitor (ARNI) — approved in late 2015, a new drug combination of an ARB (valsartan) and a neprilysin inhibitor (sacubitril). ARNI has demonstrated a 20% improvement in the combined endpoint of cardiovascular mortality or HF-related hospitalization over enalapril (48). Evidence suggests this medication may replace ACE-I in the treatment of HF (49).

- β-Blocker therapy — improves 1-year mortality rates, reduces the number of hospitalizations, reduces the incidence of sudden cardiac death, and improves NYHA HF functional class and perceived quality of life (50, 51). In the U.S., there are three β-blockers approved by the Food and Drug Administration to treat HF: bisoprolol, carvedilol, and metoprolol.
- Loop diuretics — recommended for patients with continued signs and symptoms of volume overload and increased filling pressure.
- Isosorbide dinitrate/hydralazine combination — for African American patients with HF, the combination of long-acting oral nitrates and hydralazine should be considered standard therapy to reduce mortality, reduce HF-related hospitalizations, and improve quality of life (29, 52).
- Additional medications that can be used in the care and treatment of HF include aldosterone antagonists, digoxin, and a combination of oral nitrates and hydralazine (47).
- Further medical management should focus on other comorbidities such as dyslipidemia, DM, and/or concomitant pulmonary disease.

Nonpharmacological Management

Device therapy, such as implantation of an ICD with or without cardiac resynchronization therapy (CRT), is frequently used in the long-term management of HFrEF. Prophylactic use of ICDs for patients with LVEF ≤35% as protection against ventricular arrhythmic events was based primarily on the results of the Multicenter Automatic Defibrillator Implantation Trials (MADIT-I and MADIT-II; 48). Subanalysis of the results of MADIT-II indicated between 30% and 40% of patients with HFrEF (with an ischemic etiology) were found to have inducible ventricular tachycardia/fibrillation at baseline (53). During the course of the study, about 40% of these inducible patients received appropriate defibrillation treatment (53). Further analysis demonstrated that those with an LVEF <25%, widened QRS complex (>120 ms), or clinical HF received the most benefit (53).

About a third of patients with HFrEF have a left bundle branch block (LBBB) on their ECG, which is indicative of right and left ventricular dyssynchrony and is associated with worse clinical symptoms and left ventricular systolic function (54). This LBBB subpopulation is the target for CRT. These pacemaker devices are implanted with three lead wires, one of which is placed to stimulate the left ventricle to contract. These systems allow the device to time ventricular contraction after sensing atrial contraction, and to coordinate, or synchronize, the contraction of the left and right ventricles. Because ventricular arrhythmias occur in patients with HFrEF, cardiac resynchronization devices commonly have the ability to perform defibrillation. Several studies have consistently found reduced hospitalizations and survival benefit in those receiving CRT over those on optimal medical therapy alone or with ICD, but lower survival benefit from patients receiving CRT with defibrillation activated (55, 56).

Despite these advances in medical and device treatment for the management of HF, the best these treatments can do is to slow the progression of the disease. A large number of patients eventually require more advanced therapies, such as a heart transplant. The number of patients needing a heart transplant is much larger than the number of hearts available from donors. For example, in 2011, about 34% of U.S. patients on or added to the cardiac transplant waitlist received a transplanted heart and about 8% died while waiting (57). Optimizing the eligibility criteria, based on the severity of disease, the effect of comorbidities, the use of tobacco, alcohol, or illicit drugs, age, and psychosocial factors (58) and the introduction of new and improved antirejection therapies have improved posttransplant survival (59). For patients receiving heart transplant between 2002 and 2012, 1-year survival ranges between 84% and 85% (60). Heart transplant is discussed fully later in this chapter.

Traditionally, VADs have been used as a bridge-to-transplant (BTT) in certain patients waiting for a donor heart to become available. The VAD is a battery-powered mechanical pump that is used to transport blood from the left and/or right ventricle to the aorta or pulmonary artery, respectively. Advancements in VAD technology and durability and increased experience utilizing VAD systems are leading to wider use of these devices and beginning to improve 1-year survival to levels similar to that seen with heart transplant (61). Although heart transplantation (HT) still remains the best option for select patients with ESHF (57), the newest generation of VADs is beginning to be more widely used as destination therapy, providing an option for patients who do not qualify for transplant or who choose to defer it. However, the VAD must be implanted before irreversible end-stage organ disease has been reached (58). VADs can and have been "explanted" in patients who are determined to be "Responders" to the therapy. This has been shown to recover their heart function. A new category has been generated, which is called "Bridge to Recovery." VADs are discussed in more detail later in this chapter.

Medical History Review

Before beginning exercise training, HF patients should be stable and cleared to begin exercise by their PCP/cardiologist or the CR attending physician. The CMS advises that patients be on optimal, guideline-directed medical therapy for 6 weeks before beginning CR (62).

Once the patient is cleared to begin CR, the CEP reviews the medical history to determine what other comorbidities are present. Patients with HF are likely to have multiple comorbidities that may influence the exercise prescription or even the safety of exercising.

Common comorbidities among patients with HF include DM (40%–45% of patients), COPD (~33% of patients), anemia (15%–20% of patients), renal dysfunction (>50% of acute decompensated patients, no consistent data for patients with chronic HF), sleep-disordered breathing (>50% of patients), and atrial fibrillation (ranging from 10% to 50% depending on HF severity), along with other comorbidities like obesity and arthritis (63, 64). The patient's medical history is important in identifying potential limitations to exercise as well as the need to modify the exercise prescription.

Furthermore, the CEP should determine how many hospital admissions HF patients have had over the last

6–12 months and when their last HF-related admission occurred. This information can shed light on the patient's disease stability. Exploring with the patient any factors that might have led to the most recent HF-related hospitalization may provide insight into the patient's ability for self-care. Most HF-related hospitalizations can be attributed to poor self-care, including dietary indiscretion, medication nonadherence, or failure to realize or act upon signs and symptoms (65).

HF patients should be on guideline-directed medical therapy. Reviewing the patient's chart will help the CEP determine their medication regimen. If the patient is not on guideline-directed medical therapy, then determining the reason for this could provide important insight into the patient's disease severity and even, potentially, other lifestyle or comorbid factors.

The CEP should educate patients with HF on appropriate self-care measures. These include, for example, taking medications as prescribed, avoiding excessive fluid intake, limiting sodium intake, obtaining daily body weight, knowing when to contact a health care provider (*i.e.*, recognizing unexpected increases in weight, swelling, fatigue, and/or dyspnea as signs of worsening HF), and engaging in regular exercise (66).

Brief Physical Exam

In addition to reviewing the medical history, performing a brief physical exam can identify potential contraindications to exercise testing and training. The patient should undergo a brief physical exam prior to exercise testing. This should include the patient's weight, level of peripheral edema, and lung and heart sounds. A comparison of the data with previous assessments performed in the PCP's office will provide insight into the patient's stability since they were last seen. Moreover, the CEP should conduct a similar brief exam prior to the patient beginning exercise each day and compare the results to the baseline.

Body weight measurements vary with different scales and are unlikely to exactly match the reading on the patient's home scale; therefore, it's helpful for the CEP to ask the patient about any changes he or she may have noticed in body weight. A sudden increase in weight, for example, may indicate possible fluid retention and pending decompensation. The patient's PCP should be notified if the patient has gained 1.36 kg (3 lb) or more in the last 24 hours, 2.27 kg (5 lb) in the last week, or has been trending up for the last several days. Symptomatically, patients experiencing fluid retention will frequently express increased dyspnea. Furthermore, palpating peripheral edema in a patient is helpful for gauging weight gain as fluid retention. Listening to lung sounds can give insight into pulmonary congestion, which can occur in the absence of significant weight gain, but can increase the patient's dyspnea while exercising and may be an indicator that the patient is beginning to decompensate.

Any unusual findings should be reported to the attending physician and/or the physician who is managing the patient's HF. Any of these findings can indicate that exercise should be avoided unless a physician assesses and clears the patient to exercise (usually at decreased intensity or duration [or both] of exercise).

Personal Interview

When interviewing patients with HF prior to starting an exercise training program, several key elements need to be discussed. First and foremost, as with any patient beginning an exercise program, the CEP should determine the patient's stage of readiness to begin exercise, motivation, and goals. The CEP should point out any unrealistic goals and assist the patient in setting goals that are achievable. Although exercise training can improve many aspects of HF, it cannot cure HF, and this is an important point for patients to understand.

Another aspect of the interview should be to discuss the patient's resources. This includes social support, including family members or friends who can offer positive encouragement for the patient's exercise routine. It also includes the availability of physical resources that can help the patient exercise at or near their home. For example, does the patient have exercise equipment in the house? does the neighborhood have sidewalks and ample lighting? and are there any parks or walking paths nearby, and so on?

Motivational interviewing is an emerging trend in medicine, particularly with patients with chronic diseases needing lifestyle modification. This patient-centered interviewing style uses empathetic understanding to direct positive behavior change by helping patients explore and resolve barriers to change (67). Effective motivational interviewing includes an empathetic, reflective, and self-disclosing communication style in which the provider affirms the patient's efforts to change, and reframes patient statements in a way that acknowledges the patient's point of view on an issue, but allows the patient to reflect on their own perspective (67). Furthermore, the provider encourages positive self-talk, guiding the patient to identify personal strengths that will help them be successful at making a change, and uses humor to build rapport with the patient, allowing for more open discourse (67). Lastly, motivational interviewing actively involves patients in problem-solving in ways that make their personal goals truly attainable.

Research has demonstrated that motivational interviewing elicits goal setting, positive self-talk, and discussion of change (67). The CEP is encouraged to use motivational interviewing to guide goal setting in exercise training and progression toward those goals. In a recent study, a small group of minority adults with HF demonstrated greater improvements on exercise adherence and 6-minute walk testing when motivational interviewing was used (68).

Ideally, motivation interviewing will foster open dialogue and help establish a lasting relationship between the patient and CEP. It also should help the CEP to recognize areas of the patient's lifestyle modification that need to be referred to other health care experts. For example, it is very likely that the patient needs assistance with diet and nutrition and will benefit from referral to a registered dietitian nutritionist (RDN). Many patients will benefit from referral to clinical counseling services in order to address depression, anxiety, stress, or low self-esteem. Although patients commonly meet with a clinical counselor upon entering a CR program, they do not typically see a counselor regularly. Having a continuing, empathetic, open dialogue with the patient helps the CEP to recognize emotional or behavioral changes in the patient, who may require referral back to the clinical counselor.

Effects of Exercise

Prior to the 1980s, regular exercise was believed to be contraindicated in patients with HF, and patients were frequently prescribed bed rest. Evidence supporting ambulation in HF patients began to emerge in the late 1970s. However, up until the last decade or so, strenuous activity was still avoided because of patient reports of exercise intolerance. Currently, regular exercise (including cardiovascular and resistance training) is considered an important adjunctive treatment for patients with HF. Regular exercise has been shown to be safe and effective at reducing HF symptoms, reducing LV remodeling, improving depressive symptoms, improving quality of life, and increasing event-free survival (69–71). Currently, exercise training is supported and recommended in formal treatment guidelines, and the CMS covers CR to patients with HFrEF (28, 29, 62). Additionally, the majority of private insurance companies reimburse for CR, regardless of whether the patient has HFrEF or HFpEF (72).

Once the patient's medical and exercise history is understood, the patient's goals and understanding/expectations of exercise training are established, and exercise testing has been completed, the next step is to decide on the exercise prescription. The exercise prescription, including progression, should be approved by the attending physician. Likewise, if there is a need to change the exercise prescription (*e.g.*, patient progressing faster than expected or patient experiencing an HF decompensation), these changes should be approved by the attending physician.

The implementation and evaluation of the exercise prescription require the expertise of the CEP, who ensures that the prescription is written in a manner that progressively increases the components of the FITT principle (frequency, intensity, time [duration], and type [mode of exercise]). The volume of exercise (*i.e.*, frequency, intensity, and time) should progress to exercising most days of the week (4–6 days) with both supervised and independent exercise sessions. The exercise intensity should be mild, to begin with (55%–65% of the HR reserve or $\dot{V}O_2$ reserve) and progress to moderate intensity (70%–80% of HR reserve or $\dot{V}O_2$ reserve). The duration of exercise may include several short bouts of exercise (5–15 minutes) interspersed by short periods of rest. The duration can be increased progressively by increasing the length of the exercise bouts and shortening the rest periods. The duration of exercise should progress to a minimum of 30 minutes per day.

The patient's initial exercise capacity and level of frailty will dictate the initial exercise volume and rate of progression. For cardiorespiratory and vascular exercise training, the volume of exercise should be three to seven MET hours per week (73), and the combination of frequency, intensity, and duration should be used to progress and achieve this target. In many cases, patients may also need to "progress" to different modes of exercise. A patient may have a goal to walk around their block at home, but yet experience excessive dyspnea and leg fatigue with weight-bearing exercise. In this case, the patient could be started on a nonweight-bearing mode of exercise (*i.e.*, cycle ergometer or recumbent stepper) and progressed to increasingly longer bouts of treadmill exercise.

Resistance training should be incorporated into the exercise prescription for HF patients. Resistance training improves muscular strength and endurance and is an important adjunct to cardiovascular training to improve skeletal muscle function. Patients should only begin resistance training once they have demonstrated that they can tolerate the cardiovascular exercise. Most CRs programs will begin resistance training after the third to fourth week (9–12 sessions) of CR. However, beginning light resistance training earlier in stable patients who are too deconditioned to tolerate cardiovascular exercise may improve exercise tolerance. Like cardiovascular exercise, resistance training should begin at a lower intensity such as 40%–50% of the one repetition maximal (or estimated) or a resistance that the patient can perform 1–2 sets of 10–15 repetitions. Exercises should incorporate the major muscle groups of the upper and lower body and should be done at least 2 days per week. Progressing resistance training may take some time and should be based on the patient's accomplishments. A good guide for any particular exercise could be to increase resistance when the patient is able to achieve two sets of 15 repetitions.

Patients will achieve the most benefits of exercise training when they adhere to the exercise prescription and regularly attend CR sessions. The motivational interviewing discussed earlier is an ongoing process. Throughout CR, the CEP should identify and address the challenges to adherence for each patient and encourage the patient to be involved in problem-solving to address these challenges. This gives the patient ownership and an investment in implementing the solution, which may lead to greater adherence. Motivational interviewing also does not have to be a face-to-face exchange. Patients who stop coming to CR might be willing to have a conversation over the phone. Additionally, the CEP should regularly communicate with and follow up with other members of the interdisciplinary team. The electronic medical record and the increasing ability of health care organizations to view records between systems have made such communication easier. If the patient's health care provider sees notes of several missed CR sessions, this documentation may prompt a conversation about adherence at the patient's next office visit. There are many challenges to exercise adherence for those with and without chronic diseases. Although motivational interviewing techniques have proven efficacy, continued research addressing adherence is needed.

PERIPHERAL ARTERY DISEASE

PAD is caused by atherosclerotic lesions in the arteries of the lower extremities that restrict blood flow distally (74).

It is estimated that over 200 million people have PAD worldwide, and the prevalence is increasing (75). In the U.S. alone, more than 14.5% of individuals over age 70 years have developed PAD, making it the third leading cause of cardiovascular morbidity following heart attack and stroke (76). PAD is associated with an elevated risk of CAD, MI, and stroke, and can lead to amputation and even death (77).

Men and women are equally affected by PAD. In both groups, the prevalence of PAD tends to increase with age (78) as illustrated in Figure 5.24 (79). Blacks have a higher

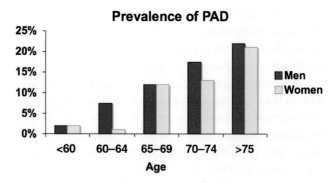

FIGURE 5.24 The prevalence of peripheral arterial disease. (Adapted from Criqui MH. The prevalence of peripheral arterial disease in a defined population. *Circulation.* 1985;71(3):510–5.)

risk of developing PAD than Caucasians, whereas Asians and Hispanics tend to have a lower risk (79).

Health care costs related to PAD are high. In 2001, a total of $4.37 billion was spent on PAD-related treatment among Medicare patients; 88% of the amount was for inpatient care (77). Moreover, the patients treated represented only 6.8% of the Medicare population. Considering that only about one-third of the population with PAD in the Hirsch et al. (77) study had detectable PAD, by symptom history and conventional testing, improved awareness and earlier detection strategies could potentially have a positive downstream impact on future health care costs, particularly in light of the favorable outcomes PAD patients have with exercise training.

Pathophysiology of PAD

The risk factors for PAD are similar to those for CAD and cerebrovascular disease, which share endothelial damage and atherosclerosis as underlying causes (80).

Cigarette smoking increases the risk of developing PAD by at least three times, and the number of pack years (the number of packs smoked per day multiplied by the number of years smoked) has a direct correlation with the severity of the disease (81). Although many other risk factors have been studied, cigarette smoking remains the most potent risk factor for developing PAD (79).

Severe or long-standing DM is strongly related to PAD. Moreover, some studies show that patients with diabetes with PAD are five times more likely to have an amputation than other patients with PAD (79). HTN is a risk factor for PAD; however, a consistently high systolic pressure is closely associated with PAD, but a high diastolic pressure is not (79). Studies have shown mixed results as to the significance of high cholesterol and triglycerides and the prevalence of PAD.

In PAD, endothelial damage and atherosclerosis result in stenosis or blockage of a peripheral artery. Ultimately, impaired blood flow can prompt symptoms that vary according to location, severity, and the number of blockages.

A typical symptom of PAD is claudication, which is pain in the legs—typically an ache or cramp—that occurs with exertion such as walking and is subsequently relieved by resting. Pain can also occur in the buttock, hip, thigh, or calf (82). Estimates suggest, however, that up to 40% of individuals with PAD have no leg pain.

Other signs of PAD that can be found in the lower extremities include muscle atrophy, hair loss, smooth shiny skin, skin that is cool to the touch, especially if accompanied by pain while walking, decreased or absent pulses in the feet, nonhealing ulcers or sores in the legs or feet, and cold or numb toes (82, 83).

PAD is associated with limited physical capacity and impaired functional status (84–86). The level of impairment can be similar to that of heart disease, but its nature is related to the symptoms of the conditions themselves (87). People with PAD are more limited by leg pains, discomfort,

and peripheral deconditioning, whereas patients with heart disease might be more limited by SOB, angina, and other cardiac-related symptoms. The type of leg symptoms can vary with PAD, and there is evidence that even those with presumed asymptomatic PAD can have significant impairments on objective measures of performance (85, 88). Along with significant impairments in functional capacity, patients with PAD have been found to have considerably lower health-related quality of life, similar to that found in populations with known heart disease (89).

Diagnosis of PAD

There are multiple tools to help confirm the diagnosis of symptomatic PAD. The easiest to use is the ankle/brachial systolic pressure index (ABI), a measure of the ratio between the systolic BP at the ankle and at the brachium (arm). It can be calculated by a trained CEP using a handheld Doppler device and BP equipment.

As seen in Figure 5.25, the measurement is taken with the patient in supine position. After the patient rests in

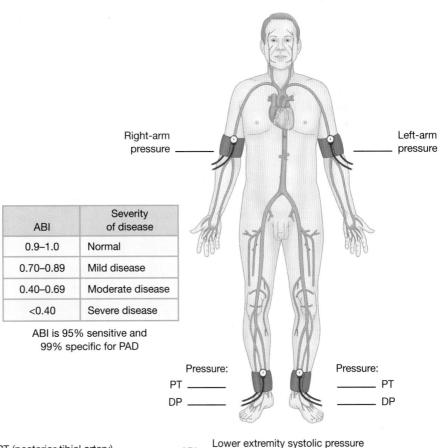

ABI	Severity of disease
0.9–1.0	Normal
0.70–0.89	Mild disease
0.40–0.69	Moderate disease
<0.40	Severe disease

ABI is 95% sensitive and 99% specific for PAD

FIGURE 5.25 Ankle/brachial systolic pressure index measurement to detect peripheral artery disease. (From Timby BK, Smith NE. *Introductory Medical-Surgical Nursing.* 12th ed. Philadelphia (PA): Wolters Kluwer; 2017.)

PT (posterior tibial artery)
DP (dorsalis pedis artery)
ABI (ankle/brachial systolic pressure index)

$$ABI = \frac{\text{Lower extremity systolic pressure}}{\text{Brachial artery pressure}}$$

supine position for about 5 minutes, the CEP measures the patient's BP. Using the Doppler device find the location of the blood flow, slowly inflate the cuff to about 20 points above which you no longer hear a pulse, then slowly deflate as you would for taking a regular BP. The corresponding number you read to the first sounds you hear should be recorded. This is repeated on both arms and both ankles. The highest number from each site on the foot is then divided by the highest number detected on the arms. Normal ranges are noted in Figure 5.25, but generally the ratio should be close to 1.0. Results less than 0.90 suggest some obstruction in blood flow to the lower extremities, whereas numbers above 1.3 suggest heavy, calcified, noncompressible arteries, which may also be a source of claudication symptoms.

A noninvasive vascular assessment (NIVA) may be ordered by a physician. This is typically done in a radiology or vascular surgeon's office. It combines an ABI with visual ultrasound to get a more accurate picture of where a lower extremity arterial occlusion may be located and what degree of severity may be present. In this case, pressure recordings will be done in multiple locations along the legs instead of just at the ankle.

If either the ABI or NIVA is positive, the next step is commonly a CT angiogram or even a lower extremity angiogram/catheterization to specifically delineate the anatomy and what options for revascularization are possible.

Treatment and Management of PAD

Medical History Review

PAD patients are often former or current smokers, over 50 years of age, and have multiple comorbidities that can affect their health and play a role in how the CEP designs the exercise prescription. One comorbidity of frequent concern is CAD. Many PAD patients already have CAD, but if it is not part of their medical history, because they have already developed plaque in their peripheral arteries, they are at considerably higher risk of developing it in their coronary arteries. Therefore, the CEP should carefully review any possible signs or symptoms of CAD during the initial interview and monitor PAD patients for CAD signs and symptoms as their exercise progresses.

Other key diseases/conditions to look for are any low back and lower extremity musculoskeletal or neuromuscular conditions, which may produce similar symptoms or exacerbate symptoms from PAD. Conditions such as arthritis and neuropathies from DM can also contribute to lower leg symptoms and need to be considered as a potential part of overall limitations.

Other conditions that can contribute to lower extremity pain and deconditioning should be noted. These can include, but are not limited to, arthritis and other musculoskeletal conditions, neuromuscular conditions, low back pain syndromes, and chronic pain syndromes such as fibromyalgia.

Careful review of medications is also important. Make sure you understand any potential effects on the exercise or exercise testing response that medications may have on your patient.

Patient Interview

The main symptoms to make sure you cover during your initial interview are those from PAD itself and those related to angina. This is important due to the significant risk of CAD in this patient population. How you phrase your questions can sometimes make the difference in picking up the right diagnosis or missing it completely. Make sure to avoid very general terms like "pain." This term can mean many different things to different people. Use more descriptive words such as pressure, tightness, and cramping to ensure you and your patient are communicating accurately. In reviewing for symptoms of claudication, make sure you cover the symptoms of the other possible comorbidities identified earlier (Figure 5.26).

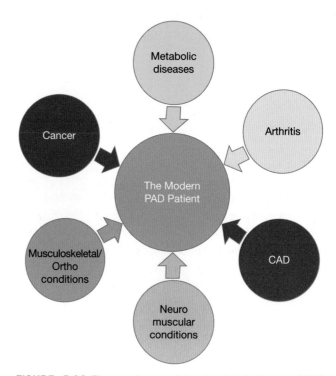

FIGURE 5.26 The modern peripheral arterial disease (PAD) patient. Notice the complex interactions with other comorbidities that must be considered when working with patients with PAD. CAD, coronary artery disease. (Original artwork by author: Mark A. Patterson, M.Ed., RCEP.)

The most typical symptoms of PAD include exertional cramping or tightness in the calf that might radiate up the leg with continued walking and resolves with rest. This pain is typically predictable and consistent with similar walking distances. Outside of the classroom and textbooks, the presentation of PAD symptoms can vary quite a bit. The pattern of how the symptoms occur is more important than how the symptoms are described. Look for lower extremity "discomforts" or weakness that comes in a predictable pattern. It could be as subtle as bilateral thigh fatigue, or as obvious as strong pain, or the patient may not be able to describe it clearly. Additional care should be taken with PAD patients, particularly when monitoring pain and to not exceed a tolerable pain threshold as this may become counterproductive.

Make sure to ask about any other activities or situations that might provoke the discomfort. If the patient develops the symptoms after sitting for long periods of time or after they have been standing and washing dishes at the sink, then the discomfort may be more musculoskeletal or neuromuscular in origin. Alternatively, the patient may have a musculoskeletal or neuromuscular condition and PAD at the same time.

In interviewing for any possible anginal symptoms, you must again watch out for falling into the trap of using just one approach. The words *chest pain* can mean different things to different people. By asking the patient, "Have you been experiencing chest discomfort, tightness, or pressure?" you may avoid missing something important.

Addressing Behavioral Aspects

Symptomatic PAD is a key barrier to starting and maintaining a consistent exercise regimen. The natural response to pain with walking is to avoid the pain, which in many cases means avoiding walking whenever possible. The pain can be excruciating and thus there is not much in the way of reward in their minds by pushing it and purposely causing the pain in order to get better. For this reason, behavioral barriers are probably the most important factor in designing an exercise regimen in this population.

Another significant barrier is time. Typically, the actual contact time the CEP has with a PAD patient is a single visit, with very few face-to-face contacts after that point. Even the most successful cardiac and pulmonary rehabilitation programs see a decline in patients' adherence to exercise after they run out of their allotted visits. If time has not been taken to work on behavior change, most likely the patient will return to their usual sedentary lifestyle, which brought them to your doorstep a few visits ago.

The first and most important step is to establish trust. Review as much of the patient's history as possible before they arrive. Greet them by looking in their eye and shaking their hand. Ask them how they are doing. Let them know that this session is about meeting their goals, not yours. Tell them: "I want to first understand the questions that you want answered today, any concerns you have, and what you want to get out of this visit." In the era of electronic medical records, it is also easy to try and interview a patient while typing on the computer. This is not the best way to perform active listening and communication skills. Make sure to turn and face them and give them verbal and physical cues that you are listening. This will typically allow the patient to open up and give you the truth about what is really going on and what their limitations are. They end up trusting that you are listening to them and really wanting to know what they need from this program. If you dive right in and just focus on their claudication symptoms and typical exercise regimens for PAD, you may miss out on some very important information and risk making the patient feel that they are being forced to do this.

At the end of the appointment, do not assume that the patient heard everything. Even if they were taking notes, they need to have the plan in writing from you. Give them diagrams of exercises when possible, and the follow-up plan in writing.

Remember that a person's emotions can contribute greatly to their pain. Regardless of whether it is due to physiology or psychology, it is their reality. You have to gain an understanding of all the possible factors that may be contributing to their pain even though you may not be able to address all of them with an exercise prescription. Lack of blood flow, arthritis, neuropathies, and personal and financial stressors may worsen the situation as much as any musculoskeletal or neuromuscular issue.

Follow-up and Referrals

The best way to follow up with this population will vary greatly depending on the resources and design of the precise program. CMS announced in 2017 that PAD is now an indication for attendance of a CR program. Although this is the case, an increasing issue is that many insurance companies may not cover typical cardiac and pulmonary rehabilitation services for PAD patients unless the patients also have a valid cardiac or pulmonary rehabilitation indication. Typically, this excludes these patients from programs unless there is a self-pay option that fits their budgets. Even if they are able to participate, the variance in the ability to get one-on-one counseling and help with exercise will have an impact on success rates weeks and months down the road. Generally, the longer you can work face-to-face with this population the better they will do. Some programs have a good case management component to them and allow for long-term follow-up. Even if follow-up is done with phone and e-mail communication, any continued contact is better than none.

Having a multifaceted, team approach is always better. Some programs have a team of allied health professionals on hand, whereas others refer out as necessary. Either way, it is important to have a network available to make sure the PAD patient gets the best outcomes possible. Having the ability to refer to a physical therapist (PT), RDN, behavior change specialist, and various physician specialists will go a long way to helping the patient succeed.

Effects of Exercise

The decision to perform exercise testing in this population is dependent on several factors. Most important are the available facilities, equipment, and personnel. Some facilities are set up to perform clinical exercise testing to screen for ischemic heart disease, whereas others may only be equipped to evaluate symptoms of claudication. Alternatively, the CEP may be part of a remote case management team and have to conduct some patient interactions via the phone or e-mail.

If you have the ability to perform ECG-monitored exercise testing, then you will need to make the decision if is truly necessary to do so or not. Keep in mind that performing exercise testing with an ECG has the potential for false-positive results and can create unnecessary downstream testing. If the patient has no documented history of CAD, but has considerable pretest likelihood of CAD or symptoms suggestive of CAD, you may want to proceed with ECG exercise testing. If the patient is asymptomatic for CAD, has low pretest likelihood of CAD, or has known CAD and has been followed closely by a cardiologist, then you might opt out of such testing.

The approach to the exercise prescription for this population must be carefully thought out. Considering only exercise(s) to reduce symptoms of claudication would be a mistake. As noted before, this population tends to have multiple comorbidities, which sometimes can actually be more limiting than the PAD, or can be a significant co-contributor to the patient's symptoms. Designing a program to address these comorbidities as well as the PAD is the best option. Always look at the entire picture with this population.

Keep in mind that many of these patients will have waited a great deal of time between their PCP's initial evaluation of their symptoms to their appointment with the CEP. The time required for testing/imaging, then typically a referral to vascular surgery to go over options, then a referral to a CEP can be weeks and even months. Significant deconditioning can take place during this time and can be more limiting than the PAD symptoms themselves (Figure 5.27).

Other considerations for the exercise prescription include the patient's past history of exercise, likelihood of sticking to any particular regimen moving forward, access to resources, and financial constraints. Outside of the actual physiology of their condition, one of the most important issues to address is the patient's need for counseling and behavior modification.

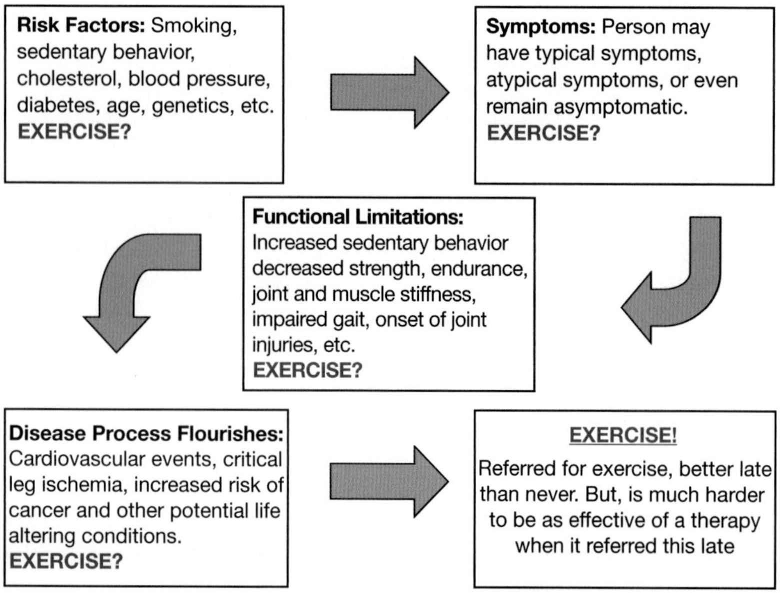

Risk Factors: Smoking, sedentary behavior, cholesterol, blood pressure, diabetes, age, genetics, etc. **EXERCISE?**

Symptoms: Person may have typical symptoms, atypical symptoms, or even remain asymptomatic. **EXERCISE?**

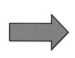

Functional Limitations: Increased sedentary behavior decreased strength, endurance, joint and muscle stiffness, impaired gait, onset of joint injuries, etc. **EXERCISE?**

Disease Process Flourishes: Cardiovascular events, critical leg ischemia, increased risk of cancer and other potential life altering conditions. **EXERCISE?**

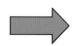

EXERCISE! Referred for exercise, better late than never. But, is much harder to be as effective of a therapy when it referred this late

FIGURE 5.27 The cascade of deconditioning and physiological consequences typical of patients with peripheral arterial disease (PAD) before they are normally sent for exercise training. (Original artwork by author: Mark A. Patterson, M.Ed., RCEP.)

HYPERTENSION

High blood pressure continues to be the leading cause of cardiovascular disease morbidity and mortality worldwide. Fortunately, HTN can be modified by lifestyle behaviors and pharmacological treatment that effectively reduce cardiovascular events and mortality.

Most hypertensives are initially asymptomatic, reducing the likelihood of early intervention. Left untreated, HTN causes significant remodeling in the cardiovascular and renal systems, perpetuating complications related to cardiovascular, cerebrovascular, and renal diseases. It is imperative to screen for and treat HTN as reductions in BP consistently attenuate or prevent the manifestation of these complications (16).

According to the Eighth Joint National Committee (JNC 8), HTN is the most common condition reported in medical care (90). Most recent data available from the NHANES 2015–2018) indicate that HTN affects approximately 121.5 million or more than 47% of Americans 20 years and over (91), with over $50 billion in estimated health care costs annually. HTN is more prevalent in adult males (51.7%) than females (42.8%), increases with age, and varies by ethnicity.

In the U.S., the prevalence of HTN is highest among non-Hispanic Black males (58.3%) and females (57.6%) compared to non-Hispanic Whites (51.0% males, 40.5% females), Hispanics (50.6% males, 40.8% females), and non-Hispanic Asians (51.0% males, 42.1% females) (91). Overall, awareness and treatment of HTN have increased over the past two decades, but only 21.6% of adults with HTN in the U.S. are controlled, which is decreased slightly from 2010. Among all adults with controlled HTN, non-Hispanic Whites reported the highest with 22.7%, followed by 19.7% non-Hispanic Blacks, 16.1% Hispanics, and 14.85% non-Hispanic Asians (91). The AHA projects the number of people with HTN to increase approximately 8% by the year 2030 (1), largely because of our aging population. These statistics alone strengthen the need for better understanding, identification, and treatment of HTN.

Pathophysiology of HTN

Approximately 90% of all hypertensive cases are classified as essential HTN (90). This definition implies that determinants of BP are highly variable; thus, no single cause can be deduced. The other 10% of hypertensive cases are classified as secondary HTN, which has a definitive cause such as renal failure, endocrine disorders, sleep apnea, neoplasms, and many more (92).

The etiology of HTN is multifactorial with the most frequently indicated causes of essential HTN including genetics, aging, psychosocial stress, obesity, DM, insulin resistance, alcohol abuse, sedentary lifestyle, high salt consumption, and low potassium consumption (93). These factors can work independently or synergistically to raise BP. Indeed, combinations of these factors are additive in nature, augmenting the vascular remodeling that eventually contributes to the development of CVD. Recent research has focused on vascular structural and functional disorders as they relate to this pathogenesis. Abnormalities such as oxidative stress, endothelial dysfunction, and arterial stiffness have gained traction as probable contributors to HTN.

Just like other bodily tissues, arterial blood vessels consist of living cells functioning collectively to serve the organism and adapt to stress. The "stress" from these risk factors comes in many forms but is mainly attributed to mechanical, inflammatory, dyslipidemic, and hyperglycemic stressors. These stressors instigate cellular and molecular processes that will strengthen the integrity of the vascular walls, affording the blood vessels enhanced physiological characteristics to withstand such pressures. However, the side effect of such adaptations is detrimental to the cardiovascular system, accelerating atherosclerosis and arteriosclerosis (thickening and stiffening of the arteries), ultimately attenuating vessel diameter and/or its ability to dilate.

The tunica media—the smooth muscle layer of arteries that ultimately controls vascular tone (Figure 5.28)— is regulated by several vasoactive agents including nitric oxide, angiotensin II, endothelin-1, aldosterone, proinflammatory cytokines, anti-inflammatory cytokines,

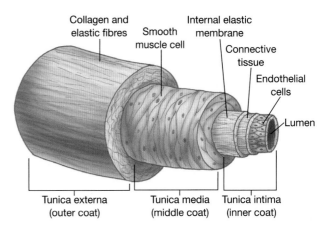

FIGURE 5.28 Diagram of a typical artery showing the tunica intima, tunica media, and tunica externa (tunica adventitia). (From Hannon R. *Porth Pathophysiology*. 2nd ed. Philadelphia (PA): Wolters Kluwer; 2016.)

and reactive oxygen species (ROS) (94). These agents are in constant flux as different environmental and behavioral situations influence their concentrations. Additionally, mechanical factors including shear stress (friction from blood flow) and increased pressure also modulate vascular tone. At any given moment, vasoconstrictive elements can outnumber vasodilatory elements, augmenting peripheral resistance. Thus, vascular tone is the total summation of all these factors that determine luminal diameter.

At its core, arterial BP is governed by the interactions between two variables: TPR and CO ($\dot{Q}$). TPR is heavily dependent on vascular tone or state of arterial dilation, whereas $\dot{Q}$ is determined by SV and HR. Because of physical properties that are beyond the scope of this review, pressure changes are most sensitive to diameter modulations; that is, reducing the lumen radius by a given percentage will increase BP. Thus, the following discussion of HTN risk factors will focus on their effect on vascular structural and functional changes.

Diagnosis of HTN

Given the widespread prevalence of HTN and well-established health ramifications, early detection is essential. HTN is currently defined as a systolic BP $\geq$ 130 mm Hg and/or diastolic BP $\geq$ 80 mm Hg while at rest in a seated position and confirmed by measurements taken on two separate days or by taking antihypertensive medication (95). Elevated BP is defined as a systolic BP 120–129 mm Hg

and diastolic BP $<$ 80 mm Hg within similar conditions (95). Individuals with elevated BP are at increased risk of developing HTN in the future. And normal BP is defined as a systolic and diastolic BP $<$120 and $<$80 mm Hg, respectively (95). The category of "prehypertension" is no longer classified or used in the current treatment algorithm. It is important to note there is no universal level of BP at which cardiovascular, cerebrovascular, and renal diseases begin to proliferate. However, in women, the risks of cardiovascular disease, MI, and HF are elevated at BP levels considered normal (96). Table 5.2 lists the classification and management of elevated BP and HTN.

The most recent recommendations from the U.S. Preventive Services Task Force support the use of office-based blood pressure in HTN screening despite major accuracy limitations (97). The accurate measure of BP is essential for HTN detection. Thus, it is important that standardized procedures are followed by training personnel, which are all-to-often not adhered to (98). Prior to measuring BP, it is important to allow the patient to rest in a seated position with feet flat on the floor for at least 5 minutes, but preferably 10 minutes, as catecholamine flux from moving, and the redistribution of blood flow during the act of sitting can modulate BP. All too often patients are rushed into the exam room, and their BP is measured before resting conditions have been reached. This can cause false-positive results and overtreatment. All patients are instructed to avoid caffeine, smoking, and exertional exercise within 30 minutes prior to BP measurements (95).

Table 5.2	Classification and Management of Elevated Blood Pressure and Hypertension				
				Initial Drug Therapy	
BP Classification	SBP (mm Hg)	DBP (mm Hg)	Lifestyle Modification	Without Compelling Indications	With Compelling Indications
Normal	<120	and <80	Encourage	No antihypertensive drug indicated	Drug(s) for compelling indications
Elevated	120–129	and <80	Yes		
Stage 1 hypertension	130–139	or 80–89	Yes	Thiazide-type diuretics for most; may consider other antihypertensive drugs or combination	Drug(s) for the compelling indications. *Other antihypertensive drugs as needed*
Stage 2 hypertension	≥140	or ≥90	Yes	Two-drug combination for most	

BP, blood pressure; DBP, diastolic blood pressure; SBP, systolic blood pressure.
From Writing Group, Whelton PK, Carey RM, et al. ACC/AHA/AAPA/ABC/ACPM/AGS/APhA/ASH/ASPC/NMA/PCNA guideline for the prevention, detection, evaluation, and management of high blood pressure in adults: a report of the American College of Cardiology/American Heart Association task force on clinical practice guidelines. *Hypertension.* 2017;71(6):e13–115. doi:10.1161/HYP.0000000000000065.

Additionally, BP varies from minute to minute and day to day because of its dependence on several acute and chronic intrinsic and extrinsic variables. Clinicians are advised to obtain several recordings during multiple sessions and calculate the mean in an effort to average the overall influence of these variables.

Risk Factors for HTN

Aging

Aging is the primary risk factor for HTN (Figure 5.29). The risk increases 10%–15% per decade of life beyond age 30 and over half of middle-aged adults and more than 75% of older adults having HTN (91). The high correlation between aging and HTN is likely due to chronic exposure to inflammation, stress, prehypertension, and renal disorders over time, which results in a greater chance of developing HTN.

Aging also results in characteristic anatomical and physiological changes in the vasculature. Arterial stiffness and endothelial dysfunction are thought to be significant manifestations in the aging and development of HTN (Figure 5.30).

The most pronounced age-related change is the stiffening of central elastic arteries such as the aorta, subclavians, and carotids. Stiffer arteries and damage to the vascular endothelial layer increase BP, increasing the risk for heart disease (Figure 5.31).

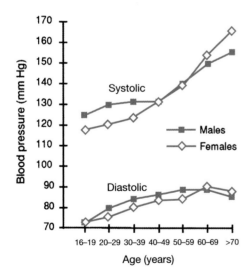

FIGURE 5.29 Relationship between blood pressure and age (*n* = 1,029) Systolic (upper curves) and diastolic (lower curves) values are shown. Notice that by age 60, the average systolic pressure of women exceeds that of men. (Modified from Kotchen JM, McKean HE, Kotchen TA. Blood pressure trends with aging. *Hypertension.* 1982;4(Suppl 3):111–29.)

As noted earlier, arterial stiffening is a compensatory mechanism as it strengthens arterial walls, affording arteries a better ability to withstand stressors like elevated BP and pro-inflammatory agents. However, stiffening also reduces the artery's natural ability to expand during systole and recoil during diastole. The loss of systolic expansion increases afterload and pushes stronger pulsatile flow deeper into the delicate capillaries. Left ventricular hypertrophy and tissue damage in end organs such as the kidney and brain are common clinical outcomes. Higher aortic pressures are physiologically more relevant to the pathogenesis of heart disease, kidney failure, and stroke (99, 100). Additionally, recoil of healthy elastic arteries generates enough kinetic energy to perfuse coronary circulation for the myocardium to receive 95% of its blood flow during diastole. The stiffening processes will attenuate arterial recoil and consequently create an ischemic environment within the myocardium (101).

Another clinically significant change with aging is morphological alteration within the endothelial layer of arterial blood vessels. This results in endothelial dysfunction. Under normal situations, the endothelial cells regulate vascular permeability, reduce platelet accumulation, and produce and react to vasoconstrictors and vasodilators that modulate the diameter of muscular arterioles in autocrine and paracrine fashion (102). With age, there is heightened exposure to oxidative compounds like ROS, a primary stimulant for endothelial dysfunction. Increased oxidative stress induces numerous pathological effects on the endothelium, but none more important than reducing its ability to synthesize nitric oxide, a very potent vasodilator (103). Additionally, the endothelium becomes more sensitive to vasoconstricting factors and less sensitive to vasodilatory factors, further perpetuating the problem (104). This process effectively induces TPR and increases systemic BP.

Obesity

Excessive adiposity, specifically visceral adiposity, is a major contributor to the development of HTN. There is a strong, linear relationship between BMI and BP (105). NHANES III reported that the risk for HTN was high for overweight individuals, but was significantly higher for individuals with obesity (106). Furthermore, epidemiological data show that an overweight phenotype predicts the future development of HTN. Approximately 70.4% of the American population is currently overweight or obese (107), with projections of alarming rates of severe obesity by 2030 (108). Taken together, clinically elevated body fat mass will continue to accelerate HTN risk until

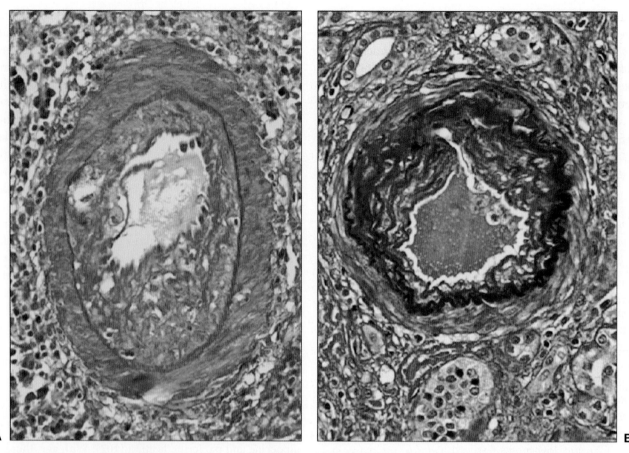

FIGURE 5.30 Comparison of chronic arterial sclerosis caused by aging/hypertension (arteriosclerosis) versus chronic rejection (transplant arteriopathy). **A.** Artery from a graft shows a neointima formation without increased elastic fibers and with a few scattered mononuclear cells. **B.** Artery from a native kidney shows neointima with marked duplication of the internal elastica (elastosis) and few or no inflammatory cells (Elastic tissue, ×400). (From Jennette JC, Olson JL, Schwartz MM, Silva FG. *Heptinstall's Pathology of the Kidney.* 7th ed. Philadelphia (PA): Wolters Kluwer; 2014.)

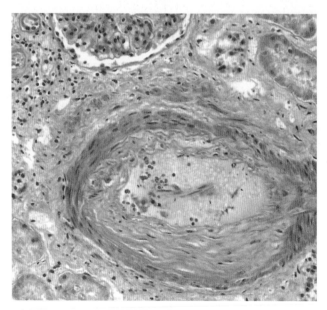

FIGURE 5.31 Hypertensive arteriosclerosis. The intimal thickness is greater than the medial thickness, indicative of severe hypertensive changes. (From Burke AP, Tavora F. *Practical Cardiovascular Pathology.* 6th ed. Philadelphia (PA): Wolters Kluwer; 2014.)

the commencement of significant lifestyle modifications and therapeutic interventions.

Obesity-related HTN is caused by several probable pathogenic mechanisms including increased sympathetic nervous system activity, overactive renin–angiotensin–aldosterone system (RAAS), and excessive production of pro-inflammatory cytokines acting on the endothelium. Working independently or in unison, these factors increase vascular tone and narrowing of the arterial lumen, thus contributing to the development of HTN and CVD.

High sympathetic nervous system activity has been demonstrated in individuals who are overweight and obese (109). Several studies have linked this increase to higher levels of circulating leptin (110, 111). Leptin stimulates the hypothalamic proopiomelanocortin (POMC) neurons causing activation of the melanocortin receptor 4 pathway, which has been shown to induce sympathetic activity (112). Elevated sympathetic activity increases vascular resistance via smooth muscle contraction, epinephrine release from the adrenals, and increase pressure natriuresis. There is also evidence of altered baroreflex sensitivity in obese hypertensives. In normotensive individuals, baroreflexors reset when exposed to higher BP and revert to normal settings when BP drops (113). However, higher sympathetic activity seems to inhibit resetting in individuals who are obese, causing greater CO and BP (114). Additionally, higher renal sympathetic activity induces sodium retention in the distal tubules (115). Elevated natriuretic processes function to increase water reabsorption with the renal tubular network causing elevated systemic blood volume, ultimately increasing BP.

Individuals who are obese can experience inappropriate activation of the RAAS, resulting in chronically elevated BP. Angiotensinogen, a hormone normally produced by hepatic cells in lean, healthy individuals, has also been found to be produced by adipocytes in individuals who are obese (112). Evaluated concentrations of angiotensinogen lead to increased production of the main effector, angiotensin II. Angiotensin II, by directly binding to its angiotensin II type 1 receptor, induces vasoconstriction in the peripheral arteries, vascular smooth muscle growth and proliferation, aldosterone release, natriuresis, and myocardial hypertrophy (94). Angiotensin II also stimulates ROS production in the vascular endothelium, further perpetuating endothelial dysfunction by reducing nitric oxide concentrations (116).

Chronic, low-grade inflammation, is another probable mechanism contributing to HTN in individuals who are obese. There is substantial evidence reporting a link between excessive visceral adiposity and increased vascular cytokine concentration, adaptive and innate immunity activity, and oxidative stress (117). Several current lines of research are continuing to discover and characterize inflammatory pathogenic mechanisms (118, 119). The main effects are summarized here.

Adipocytes produce many of the proteins involved in inflammation. Cytokines such as monocyte chemotactic protein-1 (MCP-1), tumor necrosis factor (TNF-α), and interleukins (IL-6, IL-8, and IL-10) are synthesized by adipose tissue. The systemic concentration of these cytokines varies according to fat mass: as visceral adiposity increases, a concurrent increase in pro-inflammatory cytokines also occurs. Additionally, many individuals who are obese also have elevated leptin concentrations. Higher leptin levels have been shown to increase inflammation by enhancing cytokine synthesis, macrophage activity, and oxidative stress (120). Pro-inflammatory cytokines and leptin have a significant role in promoting arterial stiffness, endothelial dysfunction, and atherosclerotic processes, thus accelerating the risk of HTN (121).

Another probable factor amplifying inflammation with obesity-related HTN is found in the gut. Consumption of high-calorie foods, one of several forces behind the obesity epidemic, can modulate intestinal concentration of the microflora. Firmicutes, the largest phylum, and Bacteroidetes are the two major types of gut bacterial microflora. When foods high in simple sugars and fatty acids are chronically consumed, the microflora concentrations shift to Bacteroidetes (122). Through mechanisms that are not entirely understood, as the Bacteroidetes increase in population, there is a concurrent weakening of the gap junctions between the intestinal cells. Inflammatory compounds produced by Bacteroidetes, such as lipopolysaccharide (LPS), are normally not absorbed by the body and pass into the stool. However, when the intestinal barrier is disrupted, inflammatory compounds can cross and circulate freely throughout the body (123). LPS stimulates cells, particularly adipocytes, to synthesize pro-inflammatory cytokines involved in vascular remodeling (124). Furthermore, LPS has been shown to change the phenotype of macrophages, an effect that augments the progression of atherosclerosis and increases BP (125).

Sedentary Lifestyle

Sedentary lifestyle is an independent risk factor for heart disease (16). There are, of course, many reasons for this, but its association with HTN is both clinically relevant and preventable. Several studies have shown physical inactivity to be associated with an increased incidence of HTN (126–129). Other studies have reported a decreased risk of HTN with active lifestyles (130, 131) and an inverse association between cardiorespiratory fitness and risk of HTN (132). Taken together, this evidence indicates a strong, inverse relationship between PA and the development of HTN.

Chronic sedentary lifestyles are associated with abdominal fat accumulation and development of chronic, low-grade inflammation (133, 134). Through the aforementioned mechanisms, excessive adiposity promotes a pro-inflammatory environment, which can initiate and support pathogenic pathways leading to arterial stiffness, endothelial dysfunction, and atherosclerosis. Together, these processes help shape systemic BP, eventually evolving into CVD.

Renal Failure

Renal failure can influence HTN through several different avenues and is a primary cause of HTN (Figure 5.32).

Increased resistance in afferent arterioles, reduced glomerular filtration, increased reabsorption of the tubular network, and nephron loss are pathological mechanisms involved in the development of HTN (92). These

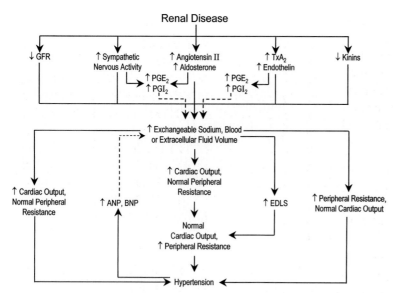

FIGURE 5.32 Pathophysiologic mechanisms responsible for the initiation of renal parenchymal hypertension and the hemodynamic patterns that sustain the elevated arterial pressure. Direct effect (↑); decreases or attenuates (↓). ANP, atrial natriuretic peptide; BNP, brain natriuretic peptide; EDLS, endogenous digitalis-like substance; GFR, glomerular filtration rate; PGE$_2$, prostaglandin E2; PGI$_2$, prostacyclin; TxA$_2$, thromboxane A2. (Modified from Smith MC, Dunn MJ. Hypertension in renal parenchymal disease. In: Laragh JH, Brenner BM, editors. *Hypertension: Pathophysiology, Diagnosis, and Management.* New York (NY): Raven Press; 1995. 2091 p.)

conditions may go undetected for many years, as the kidney has several compensatory mechanisms that can mask them. When abnormalities occur, other functional units increase working capacity to maintain normal glomerular filtration rate, creatinine clearance, and fluid balance. Like mechanical systems experiencing overload, these physiological systems eventually fail, leading to renal collapse and HTN.

Arterial stenosis and atherosclerosis are common causes of increased resistance in the afferent arterioles. Recall that the afferent arterioles deliver unfiltered blood to the glomerulus and are very sensitive to pressure changes. Blood flow to the glomerulus reduces as the arterial lumen narrows. Reduced blood flow through the preglomerular arteriole network stimulates renin release from the juxtaglomerular apparatus. As a result, the RAAS becomes activated and restores glomerular blood flow by increasing blood volume and afferent arteriole diameter. Therapies targeting preglomerular arteriole resistance have been found to reduce RAAS activity and lower BP (135). Reductions in glomerular filtration, likely the result of increased afferent arteriole resistance or glomerulonephritis, also cause renin release and vasodilation of the preglomerular arterioles by the macula densa cells. Together, these systems attempt to reestablish renal blood flow back to homeostatic levels while at the same time augmenting systemic BP.

Loss of functional nephrons is a clinical consequence of chronic HTN, uncontrolled DM, and glomerulonephritis (92). It is usually not the initial cause of HTN; however, it can contribute to and amplify the disease. When significant numbers of nephrons become infarcted, surviving nephrons must filter out larger amounts of water and solute to maintain blood volume. Additionally, increases

in the reabsorption of sodium by the tubular network of healthy nephrons can have severe consequences on BP. Elevated levels of angiotensin II and cortisol, known stimulants of sodium reabsorption, are commonly found in circulation of individuals with hypertension. As a direct result, these conditions eventually cause increased salt sensitivity and impaired natriuresis, which together act to elevate BP.

Insulin Resistance

Impaired glucose tolerance and insulin resistance are strongly correlated with arteriolopathy that develops into HTN. Indeed, individuals with Type 2 diabetes are at a significant risk of developing many of the pathologies associated with HTN (136, 137). Chronic hyperinsulinemia and hyperglycemia, both by-products of the diabetic phenotype, have been shown to induce the synthesis of advanced glycosylated end products (AGEs), stimulate generation of ROS within the vascular endothelium, and increase RAAS activity (138). The accumulation of circulating AGE impairs endothelial cell functionality, limiting their ability to regulate vascular diameter and permeability (103). Furthermore, AGE is a potent stimulator of the arterial stiffening process (139). AGE increases vascular smooth muscle cell (VSMC) growth factors, resulting in intimal–medial thickening, creating blood flow restrictions and higher pressures. AGE also stimulates the synthesis of matrix metalloproteinases (MMPs) by macrophages and neutrophils. Several MMPs that are largely involved in vascular remodeling have collagenolytic and elastinolytic properties and function to alter elastin-to-collagen ratios within the arterial wall culminating in reduced arterial extensibility (139–142). Increased collagen cross-linking and deposition at the expense of elastin fragmentation strengthens the arterial wall's ability to re-sist further damage; however, this phenotypic change can significantly augment vascular resistance and systemic BP as the artery loses the ability to buffer higher pressures. Taken together, insulin resistance leads to significant re-modeling within the vascular tunica, which in turn at-tenuates the arteries' ability to mediate vascular tone and pressure.

Stress

The physical manifestations of psychological stress are based on intrinsic and extrinsic events. Two systems involved in the stress response are the hypothalamic–pituitary–adrenocortical (HPA) axis and the sympatho-adrenomedullary (SAM) system. Together these systems orchestrate a variety of physiological responses, including increased cortisol production and sympathetic nervous system activation (105). Both of these systems regulate vascular tone and TPR, ultimately influencing systemic BP.

Stress can trigger the release of adrenocorticotropic hormone (ACTH) from the POMC neurons of the anterior pituitary gland. When released into systemic circulation, ACTH activates the production and release of cortisol, a mineralocorticoid, from the adrenal cortex. Chronically elevated levels of cortisol can have a wide range of effects on BP. Cortisol has been shown to inhibit nitric oxide synthesis, potentially contributing to endothelial dysfunction (143). It also inhibits the production of several other vasodilators such as histamine, prostaglandin, and bradykinin, creating an overall vasoconstriction effect (144). Higher levels of cortisol have also been found to increase sodium reabsorption by the kidneys and atrial natriuretic hormone concentration (145). Although this ultimately improves CO, BP is also significantly impacted.

Cortisol enhances the SAM system's influence on BP through different pathways. First, by increasing the enzymatic rate of phenylethanolamine-N-methyltransferase, a key enzyme involved in epinephrine synthesis, cortisol promotes sympathetic-derived vasoconstriction (146). Second, cortisol boosts the sensitivity of adrenergic receptors to neurotransmitters within the sympathetic nervous system, augmenting their influence on vascular tone (147). Increased sympathetic activity increases vasoconstriction of the renal capillaries, renin secretion, and sodium retention within the proximal and distal tubules. And finally, cortisol may increase HR and SV directly by stimulating the cardiovascular control centers in the medulla oblongata and hypothalamus (148). Taken together, there is substantial evidence linking exposure to chronic psychological stress and heightened hypertensive risk.

Genetics and Epigenetics

Despite an abundance of research into the genetic abnormalities associated with HTN in recent years, there has been limited success in identifying specific genes that significantly contribute to its development (92). Most genetic mutations involved in HTN are associated with renal salt handling within a nephron, impaired glucose tolerance, and genetic mutations like Liddle syndrome. However, most of the genetic influence on HTN occurs through the summation of multiple genetic variants that exert mild to moderate influences on systemic BP. New findings on epigenetic mechanisms linked to HTN have shown promise, though it may take years before its overall influence can be understood.

The initial evidence of a possible genetic link comes from twin studies showing that greater genetic relatedness between siblings is associated with greater BP similarities (149, 150). However, this relationship weakens after correcting for environmental influences. Thus, genetics alone cannot explain the development of HTN. It is a multifactorial disorder and dependent upon several behavioral and environmental factors operating independently and/or synergistically with genetics. Indeed, research into the environment's role in genetic expression has yielded evidence of viral/bacterial infections, smoking, activity level, and dietary history impacting genes at the transcriptional and translational level through DNA methylation, chromatin remodeling, and histone modification. Disturbances in the downstream patterns of protein synthesis can modulate cellular function and continue throughout the cell lineage. It is also important to note that epigenetic modifications can be inherited, which is a reason for inquiring about maternal and paternal lifestyle habits.

For example, studies using mouse models have found that consumption of a low-protein diet during pregnancy increases HTN risk in the offspring by elevating cortisol levels (151–153). Additionally, restricting protein intake during pregnancy reduces methylation of glucocorticoid receptor genes, resulting in the overexpression of cortisol receptors and increasing the sensitivity of organs to cortisol levels in the offspring (154). Prenatal stress levels can also influence HTN risk in the offspring (155). Although researchers have only begun to unravel a few potential epigenetic mechanisms related to HTN, this is another very important path to understanding the disease and developing effective therapeutic strategies.

High-Sodium Diet

Americans today consume eight times more sodium than in the past (156), with average daily sodium intake more than double the AHA recommended target of 1,500 mg/day (157). However, very little has changed in renal physiology since that time. This mismatch between the diet of our ancient ancestors and today has helped to create an HTN epidemic and health care crisis, especially within the African American community (158–160). Approximately 25% of the American population is "salt sensitive." These individuals experience hypertensive effects from acute and chronic sodium consumption (161). By definition, salt sensitivity is defined as a 10 mm Hg or greater increase in mean BP several hours after ingesting sodium (162). As a direct result, great efforts have been taken by ACSM and other organizations to educate the public about the hazards of excessive sodium consumption.

Two competing pathophysiologic mechanisms explain the strong correlation between sodium intake and BP: reduced renal clearance and endothelial dysfunction (163). According to the first mechanism, HTN is a consequence of impaired sodium excretion by damaged kidneys (92). Kidney injury can result from renal atherosclerosis or arteriosclerosis, genetic disorders, reduced RAAS responsiveness, uncontrolled DM, and HTN. These disorders can create ischemia within the renal system, eventually leading to tubulointerstitial disease and nephron infarction and shifting the balance to higher levels of sodium retention and blood volume (164).

A second mechanism has recently been proposed involving sodium's influence on vascular endothelial cells. High sodium concentrations in the blood cause greater sodium uptake by the endothelial cells (165). Excessive sodium retention by endothelial cells can disrupt cellular and enzymatic processes involved in nitric oxide production, resulting in elevated vascular tone and peripheral vascular resistance (166). As such, some have proposed excessive sodium consumption as a key contributor to endothelial dysfunction.

Effects of Exercise

HTN is a pervasive condition in adults, especially in those with other comorbidities. As a CEP, it is imperative to know the absolute and relative contraindications for exercise, the proper program design and progression model, the influence of antihypertensive drugs on exercise response, and other special considerations for this population. Individuals with diagnosed HTN but controlled resting BP do not require medical clearance before beginning light-to-moderate intensity exercise unless they have other comorbidities that warrant attention. Individuals with stage 2 HTN (systolic blood pressure [SBP] ≥ 140 mm Hg

or diastolic blood pressure [DBP] ≥ 90 mm Hg at rest) may require a medically supervised exercise test prior to beginning an exercise program, though most often CR is not reimbursable for HTN alone. If an exercise test is performed prior, it is recommended that medications be taken as normal and the CEP should be aware that any change in medication usage (type, dosage, etc.) may alter the hemodynamic response during exercise.

Resting systolic and diastolic BP must be below 200/110 mm Hg before the individual performs aerobic activity (16). If strength training, resting systolic and diastolic BP should be below 180/110 mm Hg (16). A lower threshold is indicated for strength training because the act of performing isometric and concentric contractions significantly increases systolic BP.

A normal hemodynamic response to exercise is a rise in systolic BP with no change or a slight reduction in diastolic BP. Systolic BP should increase linearly with workload at a rate of approximately 10 mm Hg per MET, although this may vary by age and sex (16). This is driven primarily by the sympathetic nervous system and is the product of an increase in CO and a decrease in TPR. However, individuals with hypertension are more likely to experience an exaggerated response to exercise resulting from any of several pathologies including endothelial dysfunction and neurovascular disorders. Exercise must be discontinued if the systolic and/or diastolic BP exceeds 250/115 mm Hg, as this pressure can injure the myocardium and arteries (16). Conversely, if during exercise the patient experiences a drop in systolic BP >10 mm Hg from baseline with increasing workload, exercise must be terminated immediately. Left ventricular failure is a primary cause of sudden decrease in systolic BP. In fact, a blunted hemodynamic response to exercise (defined as systolic BP < 140 mm Hg) is associated with an increased risk of all-cause mortality and future CVD (167, 168).

Upper- and lower body exercises can also produce altered hemodynamic responses depending on the workload and modality. Both submaximal and maximal arm exercises produce greater HR, SV, systolic BP, TPR, and sympathetic activity as compared to leg exercises when the power outputs are equal (169, 170). However, when the workloads are relative to maximal strength, the differences are negligible (171). The CEP should be cognizant of these differences when designing the exercise prescription.

The Valsalva maneuver, or the development of intraabdominal pressure to improve vertebral alignment, is a very popular technique used during resistance training. It also causes constriction of the abdominal aorta and inferior vena cava. Individuals with hypertension should avoid performing this maneuver during exercise, as it can cause dangerous spikes in BP. One study found that aortic pressure can reach 345/245 mm Hg during the upward phase of back squats (172). Although this is an extreme example, it indicates the importance of informing patients about the risks of holding their breath during resistance training. Instead, the focus should be on maintaining a continuous breathing pattern during exercise.

Lifestyle modification is a very potent therapy for hypertensive individuals. Chronically performed aerobic exercise can lead to more than 5 mm Hg reductions in resting systolic BP (173) whereas resistance exercise training may result in similar or even greater reductions in resting BP (174). ACSM recommends an exercise prescription and progression model very similar to that for a healthy adult (16). Individuals should perform aerobic training most days of the week along with 2–3 days of resistance training. Most individuals with hypertension should begin with moderate training intensity and should progress at a rate of 5%–10% each week until the maintenance phase is reached. Aerobic exercise should last 30–60 minutes. Resistance training should consist of at least one set of 8–12 repetitions with 8–10 major muscle groups. There are no restrictions on specific exercise modalities for individuals with hypertension.

A few special considerations unique to individuals with hypertension require the CEP's attention. Although these responses vary from person to person, it is important that CEPs are competent with their skills and have the ability to improvise should the need arise. With proper training techniques, appropriate patient education, and careful monitoring, the CEP can significantly improve patient safety and comfort while reaching outcome goals for each exercise session.

Postexercise hypotension response, or the reduction in BP below baseline levels, is a common physiological reaction to exercise and is viewed by many as a positive benefit of acute exercise. On average, systolic BP declines 5 mm Hg for 3–22 hours postexercise (173). There is little to no influence on diastolic BP. However, this reduction in systolic BP postexercise can be augmented in individuals with hypertension, especially those taking combination antihypertensive medications. A significant drop in BP can cause orthostasis and can increase the risk of falls and injury. Cooldown periods should therefore be extended for hypertensive individuals. Careful monitoring and rest is recommended for a period of time while the patient adjusts to this exercise response. A resting area and water should be provided until functional BP has been restored.

Education about the importance of a proper cooldown will improve adherence and safety.

Antihypertension medication is a very common therapy for people with HTN. The CEP will undoubtedly interact with patients taking single and combinatory medications that may modulate the exercise response. A few of the most commonly prescribed types of HTN medications are mentioned briefly here and are discussed in more detail in Chapter 7. With the exception of β-blockers, most common antihypertensive medications should not impact exercise tolerance. β-blockers reduce sympathetic influence on the heart, thus blunting HR and CO and causing BP to decrease. Individuals taking β-blockers will experience lower HR responses at submaximal and maximal intensities and thus should be accounted for in the exercise prescription. Additionally, vasodilatory agents such as ACE-Is and ARBs can produce an additive vasodilation effect when exercising in hot environments (*i.e.*, swimming in warm pools for arthritic relief, exercising during a high heat index) and produce a profound drop in BP. The CEP should advise patients to test and explore their exercise tolerance to these medications before exercising in hot environments. For more information on medications used in HTN, see Chapter 7.

Finally, the average BP reduction measured in individuals with hypertension following a period of chronic exercise training is approximately 5–8 mm Hg (95). Although this may not seem significant, it can have a substantial impact on risk reduction for CVD. In combination with other therapies such as weight loss, sodium and alcohol restriction, and smoking cessation, exercise can play a vital role in improving cardiovascular health while increasing lifespan in an unhealthy, sedentary population.

STROKE

A stroke (clinically known as a cerebrovascular accident or CVA) is the sudden death of brain cells following either ischemia or hemorrhage (Figure 5.33).

Stroke is a cause of death for about 150,000 Americans each year, accounting on average for about one out of every 20 deaths (91). Annually, nearly 800,000 people in the U.S. have a stroke, and 7.6 million Americans, or 2.7% of the adult population, have suffered a stroke (91). About 75% of those are first strokes and about 25% occur in people who have had a previous stroke (1). Stroke contributes to an estimated $52.8 billion (1, 91) in health care and productivity costs a year in the U.S. and is a leading cause of serious long-term disability (1).

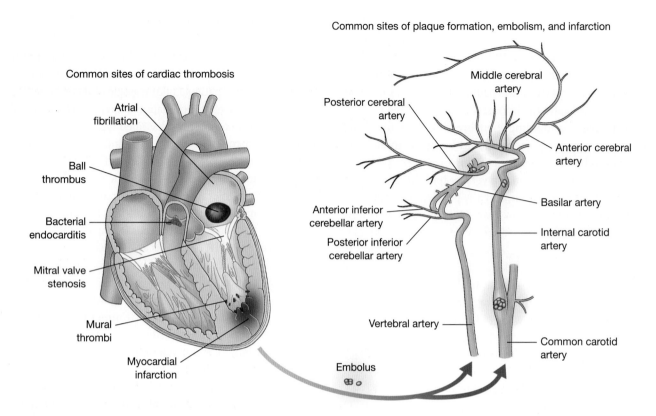

FIGURE 5.33 Illustrations of common areas of cardiac thrombosis, sites of plaque formation, embolism, and infarction. (From Honan L. *Focus on Adult Health.* 2nd ed. Philadelphia (PA): Wolters Kluwer; 2018.)

The risk of having a stroke is similar between males and females but varies by age and race and ethnicity. Generally, the risk of stroke increases with age (Figure 5.34). About two-thirds of people hospitalized for stroke are age 65 and above (175). Blacks and American Indians are more likely to suffer a stroke than are Hispanics and White Americans (176, 177). Blacks have also been found to be more likely to die following a stroke than White Americans (1). Over the past decade, crude stroke mortality rates have plateaued, regardless of age, as shown in Figure 5.35 (178).

Inactivity, smoking, and HTN are major risk factors for stroke. Nearly half of all Americans have at least one of these risk factors (176, 177). Other risk factors include

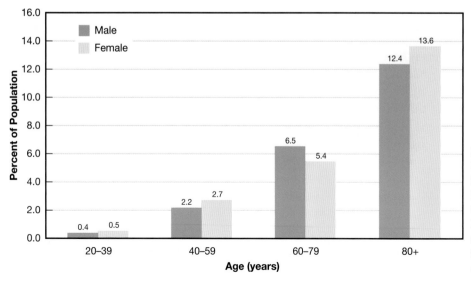

FIGURE 5.34 Prevalence of stroke, by age and sex, in the U.S. Data are from National Health and Nutrition Examination Survey, 2015–2018. (From Tsao CW, Aday AW, Almarzooq ZI, et al. Heart disease and stroke statistics-2022 update: a report from the American Heart Association. *Circulation.* 2022;145(8):e153–639.)

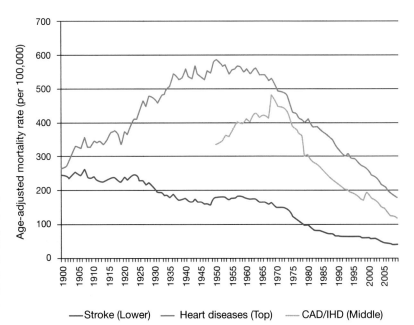

FIGURE 5.35 Stroke and heart disease mortality rates per 100,000 population for the U.S., 1900–2005, standardized to the USA2000 standard population. CAD, coronary artery disease; IHD, ischemic heart disease. (Reproduced from Lackland DT, Roccella EJ, Deutsch AF, et al. Factors influencing the decline in stroke mortality: a statement from the American Heart Association/American Stroke Association. *Stroke.* 2014;45(1):315–53.)

hyperlipidemia, DM, CAD or PAD, atrial fibrillation, metabolic syndrome, poor diet, alcohol abuse, and a history of prior transient ischemic attack (TIA), commonly referred to as a "mini-stroke."

Pathophysiology of Stroke

Strokes occur when blood flow to a part of the brain is obstructed, which can lead to loss of brain function and death. Strokes generally fall into two categories, ischemic or hemorrhagic. About 87% of strokes are ischemic, resulting from a thrombosis or embolism (Figure 5.36). About 10% are hemorrhagic, caused by a rupture of a vessel in the brain and leaking of blood into the brain tissue or cerebrospinal fluid (179).

As with the development of ischemia in CAD, an ischemic cascade occurs in an ischemic stroke (180). Although not every situation will adhere to this progression exactly, the cascade generally progresses as indicated in Box 5.3.

Approximately 25% of stroke victims die as a result of stroke, around 50% have moderate to severe residual health issues, whereas the remainder recover most or all of their prestroke health and function (179).

The faster the patients experiencing a stroke receive medical attention, the more likely they are to avoid irreversible damage.

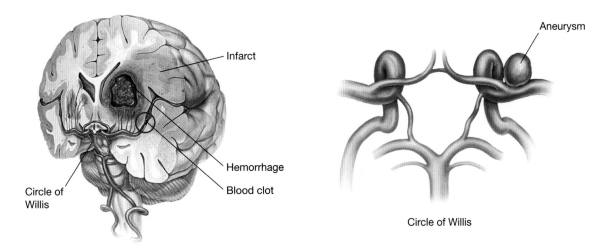

FIGURE 5.36 Mechanisms of stroke. Cross-section of brain showing hemorrhage, blood clot, and infarct. Shows circle of Willis with aneurysm. (From Anatomical Chart Company Staff. *Hypertension Anatomical Chart.* Philadelphia (PA): Wolters Kluwer; 2004.)

Box 5.3   Ischemic Cascade Characteristic of Ischemic Stroke

Lack of oxygen causes the neuron's normal process of making ATP for energy to fail.

The cell switches to anaerobic metabolism, producing lactic acid.

ATP-reliant ion transport pumps fail, causing the cell to become depolarized, allowing ions, including calcium (Ca^{++}), to flow into the cell and intracellular calcium levels to get too high.

Excess calcium entry overexcites cells and causes the generation of harmful chemicals in a process called excitotoxicity.

As the cell's membrane is broken down, more harmful chemicals flow into the cell.

Mitochondria break down, releasing toxins and apoptotic factors into the cell.

Cells start to die.

If the cell dies through necrosis, it releases glutamate and toxic chemicals into the environment around it. Toxins poison nearby neurons, and glutamate can overexcite them.

If and when the brain is reperfused, a number of factors lead to reperfusion injury.

An inflammatory response is mounted, and phagocytic cells engulf damaged but still viable tissue.

Harmful chemicals damage the blood–brain barrier.

Swelling of the brain occurs due to leakage of large molecules from blood vessels through the damaged blood–brain barrier. These large molecules pull water into the brain tissue after them by osmosis. This causes compression and damage to brain tissue.

ATP, adenosine triphosphate.

Neurological dysfunction after a stroke typically depends on the location and size of the lesion, as well as how quickly it might develop. It is possible to form collateral circulation if the blockage of blood flow forms slowly over time, which can lessen overall impairment. Typical poststroke impairments may include paralysis, motor control deficits, sensory disturbances (*i.e.*, pain, temperature, position/spatial awareness), speech and language deficits, memory loss, and emotional issues such as fear, anxiety, anger, and grief.

Treatment and Management

Medical History Review

The typical stroke patient is older, with more than one comorbidity and some coexisting impairment from the stroke, which are all factors that should be considered by the CEP. In the presence of an ischemic stroke, the risk of CAD must be assessed and taken into consideration if the decision is to perform any preexercise stress testing. Patients potentially may be on medications such as vasodilators, β-blockers, diuretics, and anticoagulants that need to be factored into clinical decision-making. The potential impact of other medications to manage symptoms such as seizures/spasticity, depression, or hypertonia may also need to be considered.

Patient Interview

Impairments following a stroke can vary greatly with regard to severity and therefore the CEP should avoid making assumptions regarding the patient's physical capacity before a proper assessment. With patients following a stroke, multiple factors might need to be addressed. It is important to be able to sit down and have enough time to speak with them, hear about their personal concerns, and be able to assess which concerns may be the most limiting and prioritize those that need to be addressed first. The CEP should also invite patients to share their personal goals and help them determine whether or not these goals seem achievable, given their condition. Take the time to get to know patients and their families, their work and home life, resources, and barriers. This will allow the CEP to understand how best to work with patients and, at the same time, gain their trust.

Considering the potential for neuromuscular issues that lead to inefficient movement, patients following a stroke may exhibit reduced exercise tolerance. Because these patients are at higher risk for CAD, the CEP should make sure to assess for signs and symptoms suggesting ACS or CAD. The CEP should make a determination if exercise testing is a reasonable next step after a comprehensive assessment.

Addressing Behavioral Aspects

The fact that the resultant condition of a person with stroke can range from complete recovery to biomechanical, speech, and emotional limitations, no standard exercise program can be applied in every situation. The CEP must individualize the program and must grasp all the factors that play a role in the patient's behavior change needs. Unlike many patients who have had an MI and stent, many patients with stroke have permanent physical disabilities or have a rehabilitation course that can take months or years.

Establishing trust with the patient is important regardless of the primary reason for seeing the CEP. Greet patients, look them in the eye when talking to them, and use active listening techniques. If the patient seems to veer off topic, the CEP might want to let the patient talk for a little while as it may reveal some other issues that could have an effect on how a program is developed. At times, the CEP needs to gently steer the patient back on track, always making sure they understand what is concerning the patient the most.

As with other cardiovascular disorders, make sure early in the process to assure the patient of your intention to focus on their needs and goals. For example, "I want to first understand the questions that you want answered today, any concerns you have, and what you want to get out of this visit." At the end of the appointment, even if the patient was taking notes, provide the exercise prescription in writing, with diagrams of exercises when possible, as well as the follow-up plan.

Follow-up and Referrals

Like patients with PAD, survivors of stroke may not have insurance coverage for prescribed exercise programs and may not be able to afford the CEP's services unless there is a self-pay option that fits their budgets. Even patients who are able to participate may not be able to afford multiple sessions. This is unfortunate because the longer the CEP can work with survivors of stroke, the better the outcome. Long-term follow-up, even if it is done through phone and/or e-mail, is helpful.

Depending on the level of physical impairment of the survivor of stroke, the CEP might want to consider involving physical therapy or occupational therapy to improve the efficiency of their movements and return them to normal ADLs. Patients may also need help from a speech language pathologist if they are having trouble recovering normal language skills. For patients who have residual impairments from the stroke, a relationship with a neurologist is typical, so the CEP will want to make contact with that health care provider. Having a multifaceted, team approach is always better when working with patients with stroke. Programs that do not have a team of allied health professionals available typically refer out as necessary. Either way, it is important to have a network available to help the patient with stroke achieve the best outcomes possible.

Effects of Exercise

PA and exercise are recommended for survivors of stroke and is a key component of poststroke care (181). However, the majority of survivors of stroke have impairments that impact functional capacity and lead to high rates of sedentary lifestyle. Lack of activity combined with the presence of other CVDs results in low cardiorespiratory fitness, which further compounds the ability to exercise. The primary objective of a poststroke exercise program should be a return to the activities of daily living (ADLs) followed by progression to improve functional capacity and fitness (16). As with all individuals, a comprehensive exercise prescription incorporating aerobic, muscle strengthening, and balance training is vital for individuals following a stroke.

Exercise testing maybe performed not only for developing an exercise prescription but also to screen for myocardial ischemia and CAD.

If a survivor of stroke does not have any poststroke impairments, then similar prescriptions can be followed as might be used for patients with CAD. If there are residual impairments from the stroke, then the exercise prescription becomes more complex. Working on all aspects of strength, endurance, and flexibility is important. Taking into consideration the patient's most limiting issues, the CEP may need to focus the approach on increasing endurance, efficiency of movement, strength, and balance to complete tasks at home and work. The CEP should be aware that not all impairments will be improved with exercise, and providing motivation to the patient in these situations will be paramount. The focus relies on the initial interview and understanding of perceived limitations as well as what was learned from any testing and evaluations performed. Of considerable importance with this population will be the setting and level of supervision needed. It is possible that a more traditional physical therapy or physical rehabilitation center setting is the best option.

HEART TRANSPLANTATION

HT is a surgical procedure performed to replace a poorly functioning heart with a healthy donor heart. Since the first allograft ("same species") orthotopic ("same position") HT was performed by Christiaan Barnard in 1967, HT has remained the gold standard treatment to improve survival and quality of life for patients with ESHF (Stage D). In 2020, 3,658 heart transplantations were performed in the U.S., the most per year to date (Figure 5.37). Of the recipients in 2020, 71.6% were male individuals, 59.4% were White people, 25.0% were Black people, 10.7% were Hispanic people, and 3.4% were Asian people. The largest proportion of these patients (41.8%) were between

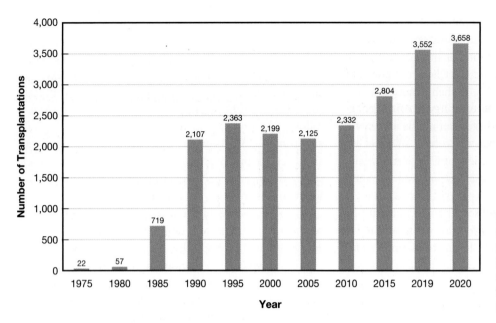

FIGURE 5.37 Trends in heart transplantations, U.S., 1975–2020. (From Tsao CW, Aday AW, Almarzooq ZI, et al. Heart disease and stroke statistics-2022 update: a report from the American Heart Association. *Circulation.* 2022;145(8):e153–639.)

50 and 64 years. For transplantations that occurred between 2008 and 2015, the 1-year survival rate was 90.5% for males and 91.1% for females; the 5-year survival rates based on 2008–2015 transplantations were 78.4% for males and 77.7% for females. Between 2011 and 2014, the median wait time for individuals in United Network for Organ Sharing heart status 1A was 87 days (95% CI, 80–94 days). As of February 21, 2021, 3,515 individuals were on the transplant waiting list for a heart transplant, and 49 people were on the list for a heart/lung transplant. The most common underlying diagnosis in adult patients undergoing HT was nonischemic cardiomyopathy. This was followed by ischemic cardiomyopathy, congenital heart disease, restrictive cardiomyopathy, hypertrophic cardiomyopathy, valvular heart disease, and "other" heart diseases. Patients in Stage D may also have a history of CAD or may have a diagnosed viral infection of the heart.

Pathophysiology of HT

Generally, patients with ESHF have a limited life expectancy and few options to improve longevity and quality of life. The patient's myocardium is weak and generally not responsive to medical therapies and lifestyle (*i.e.*, nutrition and PA) modifications designed to improve cardiac function. As the dysfunction of the myocardium progresses, the patient becomes more symptomatic and functional capacity progressively decreases, severely limiting the patient from participating in and performing ADLs. Most patients with left ventricular dysfunction (defined by an EF at or <20%) and impaired tissue oxygenation experience dyspnea, reduced functional capacity, and

increased generalized fatigue (182). If left untreated, the patient's physical and psychological status progressively worsens and the prognosis is poor.

Typically, the patient discusses available treatment options with the cardiologist. Current treatment options include medication, CABG, valve repair/replacement, ICD (Figure 5.38), CRT/biventricular pacing, mechanical circulatory support (MCS) via a VAD, and HT surgery.

The most common surgical method used in performing allograft orthotopic HT is the bicaval technique, in

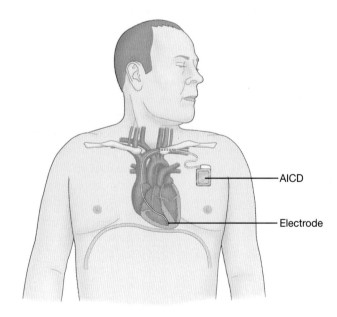

FIGURE 5.38 The automatic implanted cardioverter defibrillator (AICD). (From Timby BK, Smith NE. *Introductory Medical-Surgical Nursing.* 12th ed. Philadelphia (PA): Wolters Kluwer; 2017.)

which there is a greater emphasis on preserving the donor heart's right atrium (183). This technique reduces the onset of supraventricular arrhythmias by preventing late atrial dilation, the requirement of temporary pacing, and tricuspid regurgitation (183).

The CEP plays a key role in offering patients opportunities to improve their health and well-being following HT. Whereas exercise capacity and overall quality of life are reduced in ESHF, they are greatly improved with HT (Figure 5.39). It is imperative for the CEP to know and understand posttransplant physiology, pathophysiology, and treatment options available to the HT recipient in order to prescribe exercise and provide optimal patient care to improve functional capacity, quality of life, and survival.

Posttransplant Complications and Comorbidities

Although HT is a complicated and extremely involved surgery, the greatest risk for death does not primarily occur during surgery but as a result of complications following surgery. The primary causes of death following HT have consistently included the following:

- Acute rejection
- Graft failure
- Infection
- Cardiac allograft vasculopathy (CAV)
- Renal failure
- Malignancy (187)

Posttransplant Comorbidities

The most common comorbidities that occur following HT surgery include HTN, dyslipidemia, and DM. These comorbidities should be reviewed by the CEP and addressed to the patient as would be done with all patients for risk factor modification.

Prior to HT surgery, the patient with ESHF typically presents with more health concerns than just the physical effects of a low EF. The patient will undergo a pre-HT evaluation that includes obtaining measurements of functional capacity, hemodynamic data, NYHA classification, and exercise capacity as assessed by peak $\dot{V}O_2$ (184). Many patients diagnosed with ESHF have presented with underlying CAD, cardiomyopathy, and congenital heart disease (23). With underlying diagnoses come underlying comorbidities. Evaluation of comorbidities including age, obesity, diabetes, renal function, cerebral vascular disease, and PVD prior to and following HT is imperative to improve posttransplant outcomes (185).

With age, cardiac and vascular physiology change in ways that most commonly relate to progressively impaired function. For example, the elasticity of the vasculature decreases contributing to increased BP and poor perfusion. The aging process can also contribute to a loss in muscle mass, tone, and strength. Changes in energy metabolism also occur with age and commonly result in an accumulation of body fat. The body habitus of a potential recipient has been correlated with an increase in mortality following HT for patients with a BMI of >35 kg·m^{-2}, but not a convincing increase in mortality for patients with a BMI

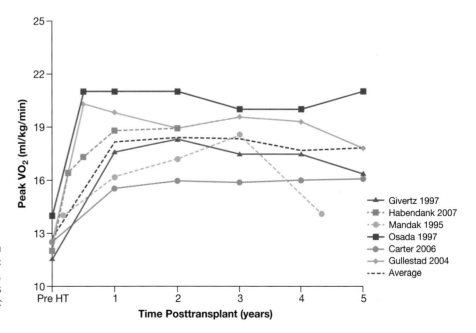

FIGURE 5.39 Time course of change in aerobic power (peak $\dot{V}O_2$) after cardiac transplant. (From Tucker W.I, Beaudry RI, Samuel TJ, et al. Performance limitations in heart transplant recipients. *Exerc Sport Sci Rev.* 2018;46(3):144–51.)

<35 kg·m^{-2} (185). Therefore, it is recommended for HT patients with a BMI >35 kg·m^{-2} to lose weight to achieve a BMI ≤ 35 kg·m^{-2} in order to decrease mortality following HT surgery.

Patients with diagnosed DM is a relative contraindication for HT, and the glycolated hemoglobin (HbA1C) must be assessed prior to surgery with a goal value of less than 7.5% or 58 mmol·mol^{-1} (185). Blood glucose control is imperative in maintaining vascular integrity. Poor glucose control and onset of disease under the age of 20 years are often associated with progressive target-organ dysfunction (i.e., renal failure) and coronary, cerebral, and PVD, with MI, stroke, PVD, and blindness in advanced cases (186). It is estimated that DM may be present in more than 40% of patients with HF, either as a primary cause of CAD and atherosclerosis or a common secondary comorbidity (1).

Kidney/renal dysfunction primarily affects BP control in the patient with ESHF and following HT as a result of impairment of the RAAS. When cardiac function becomes compromised, as in ESHF, there is a decrease in renal function and sympathetic stimulation that increases the secretion of renin. This release of renin triggers the conversion of angiotensinogen to angiotensin I and eventually angiotensin II. This cascade of events with increased release of renin leads to an increase in fluid volume and vasoconstriction. This increased fluid volume and vasoconstriction causes BP to rise and makes internal organs, including the heart, work harder. Adaptive mechanisms, as in compensated HF, may be helpful in the short term to improve cardiac function, but chronic stimulation of RAAS leads to adverse cardiovascular outcomes including ESHF (187).

As a consequence of other cardiovascular comorbidities, cerebrovascular diseases and/or PVDs are often experienced following HT and greatly affect the quality of life and survival (185). If the patient experienced a CVA following HT surgery, the CEP will need to discuss therapy options with the PT/occupational therapist (OT)/ speech language pathologist (SLP) in order to determine if the patient is appropriate to attend outpatient CR following discharge. PVD is often diagnosed concomitantly with CVD and is often part of the medical history of patients with ESHF. The patient with advanced PVD often experiences musculoskeletal pain in one or both gastrocnemius muscles, hips and thighs with ambulation, known as claudication. Symptomatic PVD, as experienced with claudication, is considered an independent risk factor for poor prognosis and a lower survival rate after HT (188).

Posttransplant Rejection

Following HT, the recipient's immune system does not recognize the transplanted heart as "self" and a deleterious process of rejection begins. From 2004 to 2010, with advances in immunosuppression, the incidence of all episodes of rejection as assessed from discharge to 1 year decreased from 32% to 25%, respectively (189). Rejection may not always be predicted and noticeable when the donor's heart is analyzed prior to HT.

There are four types of rejection:

- Hyperacute
- Acute cellular
- Acute vascular
- Cardiac allograft vasculopathy

Hyperacute rejection is a vigorous immune system response that takes place within minutes to hours and is a result of preformed donor-specific antibodies that, without retransplantation or total artificial heart support, is considered fatal (190). This type of rejection is relatively rare with today's advances in donor matching.

Acute cellular rejection is a T lymphocyte–mediated immune system response that promotes recipient tissue injury as a result of antibodies attacking the donor tissue. This response is commonly initiated months to years following heart transplant surgery. It occurs at least once in 50% of all HT and typically in the first 2–3 months (190).

In acute vascular rejection, the histological analysis of the donor's heart prior to HT may provide evidence of immunoglobulin and complement components in the microvasculature even in the absence of dysfunction (190). Damage to the vasculature can cause narrowing of the vasculature lumen and lead to impaired perfusion and decreased EF.

Prolonged vascular rejection causes the vascular lumen to narrow due to concentric endothelial cell proliferation secondary to prolonged tissue injury. This represents an accelerated form of CAD with prognosis for prolonged survival diminished. Coronary revascularization via percutaneous transluminal coronary intervention (coronary stent) and CABG is considered only palliative, with no long-term survival benefit (191).

It is important for the CEP and other clinical staff to monitor for signs of rejection, including SOB, fever, decreased urine output, retention of fluid, and weight gain. To monitor HT patients for signs of rejection, blood tests and biopsies of the heart are taken to inspect microscopically for damaged cells. Endomyocardial biopsy is the gold standard for diagnosing acute rejection following HT surgery. Typically, HT patients will be seen by the transplant cardiologist on a weekly basis for biopsy during the first 3–6 weeks following surgery, every 3 months for the first year, and then annually for the rest of their lives. This procedure involves a surgical cut in the neck, arm, or groin to allow access for a catheter to be inserted into an artery or vein and often takes about 30 minutes to complete.

Other Posttransplant Pathology

When the recipient's heart is surgically removed and the donor's heart is implanted, the nerves from the central nervous system that innervate the heart (cardiac plexus) from the recipient to the donor's heart are impaired electrically; sympathetic and parasympathetic activity is denervated. This causes chronotropic incompetence in which the patient experiences a higher resting HR and an impaired ability to lower HR after activity.

Following HT, the atrial remnant of the cardiac plexus from the recipient remains intact and the atria from the donor's heart generate the HR without receiving an impulse from the recipient's central nervous system (192). The electrophysiology from the recipient to the donor's heart may be impaired chronotropically, but inotropically remains physiologic. In the transplanted heart, the Frank-Starling mechanism remains intact due to an increase in SV (Figure 5.40), dependent on an increased left ventricular end-diastolic pressure and an increase in contractility secondary to an increased HR from circulating catecholamines (192, 193). A loss of vagus nerve

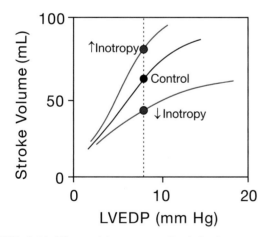

FIGURE 5.40 Effects of inotropy on Frank-Starling curves. An increase in inotropy shifts the Frank-Starling curve upward, whereas a decrease in inotropy shifts the Frank-Starling curve downward. Therefore, at a given preload (vertical dashed line), increased inotropy increases stroke volume, and decreased inotropy decreases stroke volume. LVEDP, left ventricular end diastolic pressure. (From Klabunde RE. *Cardiovascular Physiology Concepts.* 2nd ed. Philadelphia (PA): Wolters Kluwer; 2011.)

innervation (inhibited parasympathetic activity) impairs baroreceptor activity with an increase in catecholamine release causing an elevated resting HR. As a result of chronotropic incompetence, the resting HR of the HT recipient is typically above 100 bpm. As HR rises with exercise due to circulating catecholamines, the HR does not return to resting values as quickly as observed in the innervated heart. It may take minutes, not seconds, before return to resting values is observed.

Treatment and Management

Medications

The deleterious effects of HT rejection are numerous and can reduce the quality of life and survival. To help the patient physiologically tolerate the donor organ, immunosuppressants are prescribed. Immunosuppressive maintenance therapy for HT recipients is divided into three drug categories and administered as combination therapy. These categories include an antimetabolite (*e.g.*, azathioprine or sirolimus), antiproliferative (*e.g.*, cyclosporine or tacrolimus), and a steroid such as prednisone (194). Generally, patients remain on an antimetabolite and an antiproliferative for life, but take the steroid for approximately 1 year.

Some patients may need to take other medications following HT to treat common side effects of immunosuppressant therapy such as HTN, infection, dyslipidemia, impaired glucose tolerance, osteopenia/osteoporosis, nausea and vomiting, and depression. Medications prescribed to treat these common side effects include antihypertensives, antibiotics, statins, antidiabetics, bisphosphonates, proton pump inhibitors, and selective serotonin reuptake inhibitors (SSRIs), respectively. The CEP should be familiar with each of these drug classifications and review the patient's list of medications with the patient to ensure medication compliance and address any questions they have about their medications.

Mechanical Circulatory Support

Although approximately 6,000 HT surgeries are performed each year worldwide, there are more than 10 times more patients with ESHF awaiting surgery (195). Fortunately, advances in medical circulatory support technology have allowed patients with ESHF awaiting surgery as well as those who are not candidates for surgery to live longer. These therapies are thus used for BTT and as destination therapy (DT), respectively.

As noted earlier, the VAD is a battery-powered mechanical pump that is used to transport blood from the left and/or right ventricle to the aorta or pulmonary artery, respectively. The LVAD is inserted within the preperitoneal space of the abdomen with the inflow tract inserted in the apical region of the left ventricle (Figure 5.41). The pump component siphons blood from the left ventricle through a rotor, encased in housing, to a flexible tube extending to the aorta. The aortic valve constantly remains closed. The pump is powered by a battery pack located on the outside of the body. The battery pack is connected to a controller, which is connected to a driveline. The driveline is a cable that connects the controller to the LVAD.

In patients with an LVAD, BP cannot be assessed by standard methods with a stethoscope unless the pump is turned down/off. BP is therefore measured as MAP using a sphygmomanometer and locating nonpulsatile blood flow using a Doppler and conduction/ultrasound gel. A normal MAP range is 60–90 mm Hg.

A primary indication for MCS with LVAD implantation as a BTT is that the patient is listed for transplant. Criteria for transplant listing will be reviewed with the patient by their cardiologist, cardiothoracic surgeon, and MCS coordinators. Although quality of life and functional capacity can improve with MCS, the wait time from LVAD implant and recovery to HT surgery can take an emotional toll on the patient. Often, the MCS and HT teams will recommend that the BTT patient participate in outpatient CR to engage the patient physically and emotionally following MCS surgery. Participation can also prepare the patient physically and emotionally for HT surgery recovery.

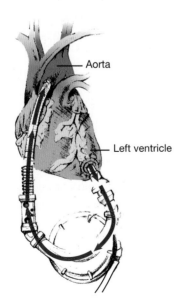

FIGURE 5.41 Left ventricular assist device. (Reprinted from Berg SM, Bittner EA, Zhao KH. *Anesthesia Review: Blasting the Boards.* Philadelphia (PA): Wolters Kluwer; 2016.)

LVAD may also be used as a bridge to recovery in some patients with HF. Patients with implanted LVAD may see improved cardiac function to the extent that the LVAD can be removed and transplantation avoided. Those patients with explanted LVAD have observed improved quality of life and exercise tolerance within the range of healthy adults (196). Thus, in some patients, combined with pharmacological therapy, LVAD may serve as a bridge to recovery, avoiding the need for HT.

The patient receiving MCS for DT does not meet the criteria for HT surgery and will be on MCS for life. The outpatient CR setting is just as important for these patients to engage them physically and emotionally.

In CR programs, the patient's heart rhythm is monitored with an ECG. This is an important feature for patients who receive an MCS device, who are prone to ventricular arrhythmias, and therefore have an ICD implanted prior to or during the MCS procedure. Recent guidelines suggest CR to be a class I recommendation following surgical placement of an MCS device (197). CR and exercise training in the patient with MCS are considered safe, but there are no specific guidelines to date for developing an exercise prescription in this population (198).

Medical History Review

Given the nature and severity of HT surgery, as well as the potential for infection and immediate signs of rejection, often the CEP will first encounter the allograft recipient in the inpatient setting. Prior to meeting the patient, the CEP will need to extensively review the patient's medical records and meet with their health care team (*i.e.*, nurse, PT, OT, physician) to determine if the patient's health status and acuity of illness is within the CEP's scope of practice.

Patient Interview

The CEP's initial patient contact is considered phase I CR or inpatient CR. Phase I CR will include reviewing sternal precautions, ROM activities for upper and lower extremities, bed mobility, transferring from sitting to standing, and ambulation. These activities are often performed with the PT and/or OT prior to or in combination treatment with the CEP. Prior to discharge from the hospital, the CEP will have had the opportunity to provide education regarding home exercise recommendations and details of phase II CR or outpatient CR. It is at this point the patient should be scheduled for their initial outpatient CR appointment.

During the initial interview, the CEP should begin by incorporating strategies that incorporate active listening to be more engaged in the conversation and allow the patient to be more open in discussing details of their health history. These strategies are similar to those listed in previous sections and include demonstrating interest in what patients have to say, demonstrating empathy, eliminating environmental noise, staying focused on the patient, not interrupting, being attentive to body language, employing patience, acknowledging that you hear what is communicated by the patient, seeking clarification when necessary, and keeping your own emotions in check (17). Incorporating these strategies allows the CEP to engage in deeper conversation and formulate a better understanding of the patient's needs prior to as well as during their recovery from surgery.

In the initial evaluation of the patient prior to HT surgery, the CEP and other health care providers may become aware of challenges the patient faces other than the expected physical consequences associated with ESHF. The psychological response can be complex at best for most patients during the period of time prior to anticipated cardiac surgery. The uncertainty in the waiting period prior to surgery can produce anxiety and impatience that is exhibited by uncharacteristic irritability, depression, and other mood changes. The CEP and other CR staff may be more aware of these changes in mood as there are more patients with ESHF being referred to the outpatient setting prior to the transplant. The CEP should take note of these changes and update the behavioral health specialist on staff or encourage the patient to talk with their PCP for referral to behavioral health counseling.

Following surgery, energy is compromised by decreased CO and physical inactivity, and patients typically need emotional support; thus, they are excellent candidates for comprehensive CR services (182). Early identification and treatment for depression in HT recipients are associated with outcomes similar to those for patients who are nondepressed (199). If a behavioral health specialist is not on staff and/or not accessible to the patient, the CEP and other clinical staff may incorporate the use of reliable and validated psychosocial screening tools for outpatient HT recipients such as the Patient Health Questionnaire 9-item scale (PHQ-9), Generalized Anxiety Disorder 7-item scale (GAD-7), and the Kessler Psychological Distress 10-item scale (K-10) (200). It would be advised to inform the patient's cardiologist and/or PCP if the results from these surveys indicate the need for behavioral health support.

Relation to Exercise Tolerance

The mechanisms underlying reduced exercise capacity after HT are multifactorial involving cardiac, vascular, and skeletal muscle limitations (Figure 5.42). Exercise training does effectively improve peak $\dot{V}O_2$ in HT patients, with the magnitude of increase being dependent on exercise intensity (201, 202). High-intensity interval training initiated shortly after HT (mean 11 weeks postsurgery) showed 25% improvements in peak $\dot{V}O_2$ after 9 months of training, which was greater than 15% improvements observed with moderate-intensity continuous training (203). Longer duration exercise training (>1 year) may result in HR and peak $\dot{V}O_2$ similar to or greater than age-predicted normative values (204–206). In fact, some HT recipients have gone on to complete marathons and Ironman triathlons, demonstrating the remarkable adaptability of the human body (200). More importantly, attending CR after HT is associated with improved clinical outcomes such as lower hospital readmission rates and longer survival (207).

The CEP may be involved in GXT prior to and/or following HT. Recent guidelines suggest GXT to guide transplant listing and recommend a maximal CPX test with a respiratory exchange ratio greater than 1.05, reaching an anaerobic threshold while the patient is on optimal medical therapy (185).

Following HT, GXT can be performed either with a treadmill or bicycle ergometer and should be performed at the implanting facility under observation by the patient's cardiologist. It may be recommended that the HT recipient participate in GXT after they have begun attending outpatient CR sessions to determine HR and BP response of maximal testing and post-HT outcomes. The CEP or other CR staff would make this recommendation to the patient's cardiologist. Keep in mind that the HT recipient may not even begin attending CR until 6–8 weeks post-HT surgery when the cardiologist deems it medically appropriate to begin. Although there are many benefits of GXT for the patient and clinical staff in assessing functional capacity, it may not always be necessary to put the patient through this type of functional testing.

Effects of Exercise

Data provided by GXT, including peak HR, BP response, and MET level, can be useful in designing the exercise prescription for starting or continuing a CR program. As discussed earlier, the HR response of the HT recipient differs from that of a normally innervated heart. The resting HR is usually between 90 and 110 bpm and will slowly rise with increased exercise intensity. In fact, the HR tends to be highest during the recovery phase following exercise. This is due primarily to the impaired sympathetic and parasympathetic responses of the denervated heart. The

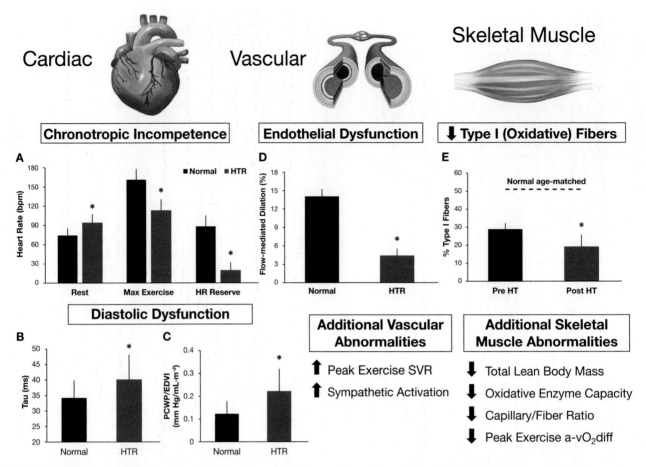

FIGURE 5.42 Central and peripheral mechanisms of exercise intolerance in heart transplant recipients (HTR). **A.** Chronotropic incompetence characterized by elevated resting heart rate (HR), reduced peak HR, and severely reduced HR research compared with normal age-matched controls. **B.** Delayed time constant of left ventricular pressure decay (tau). **C.** Reduced left ventricular (LV) compliance (increased LV stiffness). **D.** Impaired endothelial function measured by brachial artery flow-mediated dilation. E. Reduced percentage of type I (oxidative) fibers in vastus lateralis muscle pre-HT with further decline post HT. *Indicates significant ($P < 0.05$) between HTR and normal individuals (except (**E**), which indicates difference pre and post-HT). (From Tucker WJ, Beaudry RI, Samuel TJ, et al. Performance limitations in heart transplant recipients. *Exerc Sport Sci Rev.* 2018;46(3):144–51.)

HT recipient's ECG will demonstrate what looks like a bundle branch block (BBB) with normal PR intervals, often with two P waves, and widened QRS intervals. Please refer to Chapter 6 of this book for a description of ECG interpretation. The CEP and other CR staff should therefore allow the patient a longer warm-up period to progressively reach a steady state and a prolonged cooldown period to allow for HR to return to at or near their initial resting HR. Obtaining data from GXT will provide indications of HR response with increased intensities. However, as there are no specific target heart rate (THR) guidelines with exercise for this patient population, the CEP should use the original Borg RPE scale (6–20) to prescribe exercise workloads. The patient's RPE should stay between fairly light (11 of 20) and somewhat hard (14 of 20). The CEP and other CR staff need to use their best clinical judgment regarding HR response when prescribing an exercise routine.

Resistance training can be incorporated into the exercise prescription as skeletal muscle atrophy and bone loss can be consequences of glucocorticosteroid use in immunosuppressive therapy. Activities to engage slow and fast twitch muscle fibers should be focused on major muscle groups using both static and dynamic exercises. Static activities should be prescribed at a low to moderate intensity and be limited in time to less than 10 seconds to avoid increasing thoracic pressure and thus afterload and systemic pressure. Dynamic activities should also be performed at a low to moderate intensity. The CEP should advise the patient to avoid holding their breath (*i.e.*, the Valsalva maneuver) with all activities. Rubber tubing is a practical and effective tool as it comes in various resistance levels, can be used for upper and lower extremity activities, and is portable. CR staff should be in direct communication with the patient's primary cardiologist and review exercise prescriptions with their medical director prior to initiating an exercise program.

Post-HT Follow-up and Referrals

Following HT, as deconditioning is secondary to physical inactivity and a compromised CO, HT recipients should be offered the opportunity to address their physical and psychological needs. Comprehensive CR programs include exercise, education, and nutritional and psychosocial counseling. CR also provides HT recipients the opportunity to interact with other HT recipients who have had similar experiences and can provide a sense of familiarity when very little following HT seems familiar. Thus, CR programs offer HT recipients the opportunity to improve physically and emotionally in company with other cardiac patients and trained professionals who act as the eyes and ears of their medical team. That is, CR staff provide not only exercise testing and prescription but also detailed progress reports to the patient's medical team.

Most private insurance companies follow CMS guidelines for CR coverage allowing HT recipients' participation in up to 36 sessions within 36 weeks. All clinical CR staff should be certified in basic life support (BLS) and advanced cardiac life support (ACLS) as well as receive ECG interpretation training prior to working with all patients in CR, including HT recipients.

Throughout CR, HT recipients are encouraged to follow up with their PCP and primary cardiologist for regular follow-up appointments. Together with CR staff, the cardiologist and PCP can address underlying health concerns that may prevent the HT recipient from progressing physically and emotionally. Management of preexisting cardiovascular risk factors such as HTN, dyslipidemia, and DM is imperative for successful outcomes following HT surgery including quality of life and survival. Some patients may benefit from services beyond the scope of practice of the CEP and other CR staff. CR staff may need to refer the HT recipient to PT/OT services to address physical and occupational limitations preventing the patient from participating in outpatient CR, exercising at home, and ADLs. HT recipients also benefit from meeting with an RDN because they typically have specific nutritional needs including increasing protein intake to aid in improving muscular strength in response to steroid-induced skeletal muscle atrophy and fatigue.

Although HT improves the patient's CO and perfusion, the recipient is challenged by compromised immune function, functional intolerance, chronotropic incompetence, and other limitations on long-term survival after the surgery. Considering the various medications prescribed to improve immune function and prevent infection, the associated comorbidities often experienced as a consequence of these prescribed medications, and the physical and emotional toll of HT surgery, the HT recipient needs skilled and empathetic support. The CEP is uniquely positioned to offer this support throughout the course of the patient's recovery. Optimal care following HT surgery can only come from an interdisciplinary effort made by all members of the HT team including the patient, medical providers, and all members of the comprehensive CR team.

SPONTANEOUS CORONARY ARTERY DISSECTION

Spontaneous coronary artery dissection (SCAD) is defined as a sudden separation between the layers of a coronary artery wall that creates an intimal tear (or "flap") or an intramural hematoma (IMH) that obstructs blood flow (Figure 5.43). Although CAD can serve as a potential origin for dissection (208), SCAD can occur in the absence of CAD.

The first reported case study from 1931 described coronary dissection and rupture on the autopsy of a young woman with sudden death following repetitive retching and vomiting (209). In the 1980s, advances in coronary artery angiography allowed SCAD to be diagnosed without

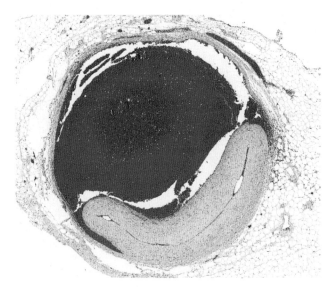

FIGURE 5.43 Spontaneous coronary artery dissection. A histologic cross-section showing the eccentric hematoma between the media and the adventitia. (From Burke AP, Aubry MC, Maleszewski J, Alexiev B, Tavora F. *Practical Thoracic Pathology.* 1st ed. Philadelphia (PA): Wolters Kluwer; 2016.)

autopsy (210), and recent innovations in high-resolution intracoronary imaging (especially optical coherence tomography [OCT]) have improved the ability to recognize and treat SCAD (211, 212).

The prevalence of SCAD in the general population appears to be around 4% of those presenting with ACS (212). SCAD is a significant cause of MI in young (25- to 55-year-old), apparently healthy individuals. The typical age range is 42–52 years, with patients as young as 14 years to well over 60 years. Previously, SCAD was thought to be rare, but diagnosis is increasing, possibly because of heightened awareness and improved diagnostic techniques.

Patients with SCAD are typically young women (an estimated 80%–90% of all SCAD patients) without traditional risk factors for atherosclerosis. In women under 50 years, SCAD has been reported to cause 22%–43% of cases of MI (212). Approximately 18%–25% of cases occur when the patient is in the postpartum period (211, 212). All races can be affected, but reports from the U.S. and Canada demonstrate 81%–83% are Caucasians (213).

A retrospective single-center report (214) identified 87 patients with angiographically confirmed SCAD. Incidence, clinical characteristics, treatment modalities, in-hospital outcomes, and long-term risk of SCAD recurrence or major adverse cardiac events were evaluated. The mean age of the subjects was 43 years, and 82% were female. Extreme exertion at SCAD onset was more frequent in men (7 of 16 vs. 2 of 71; $P < 0.001$), and postpartum status was observed in 13 of 71 women (18%). Presentation was STEMI in 49% of the patients. Multivessel SCAD was noted in 23% (214). Although long-term survival after SCAD is better than in patients with atherosclerotic ACS, 10-year recurrence rates are as high as 29% (211, 214).

Pathophysiology of SCAD

The specific etiology of SCAD remains unknown and is considered multifactorial. Several potential contributing factors to SCAD include fibromuscular dysplasia, pregnancy-related SCAD, recurrent pregnancies, connective tissue disorders, systemic inflammatory disease, hormonal therapy, coronary spasm, and recreational drug use (212, 215, 216) (Figure 5.44). Potential triggers or precipitating stressors might include intense exercise, intense emotional stress, labor and delivery, intense Valsalva-type activities, recreational drugs, intense hormonal therapy, and a rare case of the PCI procedure itself (212).

Arterial dissection with SCAD can occur within or between any of the three layers (intima, media, or adventitia) of the coronary artery wall (Figure 5.45). Two potential

Potential Predisposing and Precipitating Factors for SCAD	
Predisposing Factors	**Precipitating Factors**
Fibromuscular Dysplasia	Intense Exercises: Isometric or Aerobic
Pregnancy Related: antepartum, early post-partum, late post-partum, very late post-partum	Intense Emotional Stress
Recurrent Pregnancies: multiparity or multigravida	Labor and Delivery
Connective Tissue Disorder: Marfan Syndrome, Loeys-Dietz Syndrome, Ehler-Danlos syndrome type 4, cystic medial necrosis, alpha-1 antitrypsin deficiency, polycystic kidney disease	Intense Valsalva-Type Activities: *e.g.,* retching, vomiting, bowel movement, coughing
Systemic Inflammatory Disease: systemic lupus erythematosus, Chron Disease, ulcerative colitis, polyarteritis nodosa, sarcoidosis, Churg-Strauss Syndrome, Wegener granulomatosis, rheumatoid arthritis, Kawasaki, Giant Cell arteritis, celiac disease	Recreational Drugs: *e.g.,* cocaine, amphetamines, methemphetamines
Hormonal Therapy: oral contraceptive, estrogen, progesterone, beta-HCG, testosterone, corticosteroids	Intense Hormonal Therapy: *e.g.,* beta-HCG injections, corticosteroid injections
Coronary Artery Spasm	
Idiopathic	

FIGURE 5.44 Predisposing and precipitating etiologies of spontaneous coronary artery dissection. HCG, human chorionic gonadotropin. (Reprinted from Saw J, Mancini JGB, Humphries KH. Contemporary review on spontaneous coronary artery dissection. *J Am Coll Cardiol.* 2016;68(3):297–312 with permission from Elsevier.)

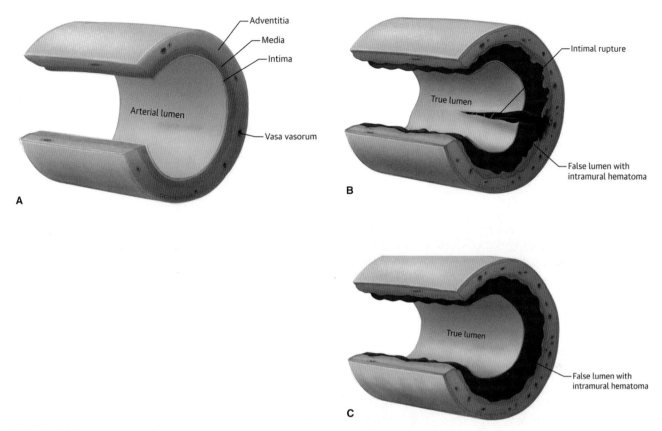

FIGURE 5.45 Mechanisms of spontaneous coronary artery dissection. **A.** Normal coronary artery. **B.** Intimal rupture initiating tear, with intramural hematoma formation. **C.** Spontaneous bleeding into the arterial wall, creating a false lumen filled with intramural hematoma. (Reprinted from Saw J, Mancini JGB, Humphries KH. Contemporary review on spontaneous coronary artery dissection. *J Am Coll Cardiol.* 2016;68(3):297–312 with permission from Elsevier.)

mechanisms for the separation of the arterial wall have been proposed (217). The first of these mechanisms is the intimal tear hypothesis, in which a primary disruption in the intimal/luminal interface creates an entry point for IMH accumulation inside of a false lumen, leading to separation of the arterial wall. The second mechanism is the medial hemorrhage hypothesis, in which a hemorrhage into the arterial wall is the primary mechanism (212).

Regardless of the mechanism, SCAD then causes accumulation of blood within the false lumen, which can compress the true lumen and lead to significant myocardial ischemia or even MI. Studies have demonstrated the presence of thrombi in either the true or false lumen, but were thought to be not significant and secondary to the dissection itself (212, 218). Once the ischemic episode due to SCAD is repaired, the resultant reperfusion may cause injury. Another concern with SCAD is the potential for significant propagation of the dissection proximally and distally from the initial tear. This may be the result of a weakening of the arterial wall (213). Coronary angiography typically reveals dissections that can vary from multiple long ones to a single short one. A discrete flap or false lumen within the coronary artery is not always apparent, and therefore the

diagnosis may be missed. Saw et al. (219) proposed an angiographic classification of SCAD describing three possible presentations (Figure 5.46): type 1 with arterial wall strain; type 2 with diffuse stenosis of varying severity; and type 3, which mimics atherosclerosis. Invasive coronary artery imaging, such as OCT or intravascular ultrasound, can be used to diagnose SCAD when it is not apparent on angiography. This can prove valuable in determining the magnitude and type of dissection (220).

The LADCA represents the most frequent site of SCAD (220). Eleid et al. (221) posited that features of coronary tortuosity are more frequent among SCAD patients compared with matched controls, and the presence of severe tortuosity is associated with recurrent SCAD (see Figure 5.47).

Diagnosis of SCAD

Accurate diagnosis of ACS due to SCAD is crucial because the recommended approaches to management can be different. Patients with nonatherosclerotic SCAD usually present with signs and symptoms characteristic of an acute MI. Chest pain, shoulder pain, syncope, dyspnea, diaphoresis, and nausea are common presenting symptoms (214, 222).

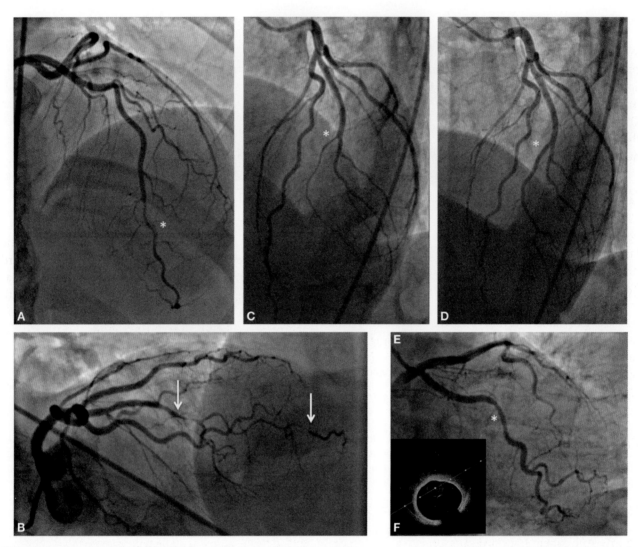

FIGURE 5.46 Angiographic classifications of SCAD. **A.** Type 1 spontaneous coronary artery dissection (SCAD) of distal left anterior descending (LAD) artery with staining of artery wall (*). **B.** Type 2A SCAD of mid-distal LAD (between arrows). **C.** Type 2B SCAD of diagonal branch (*), which healed 1 year later (* in **D**). **E.** Type 3 SCAD of mid-circumflex artery (*), with corresponding optical coherence tomography showing intramural hematoma in (**F**). (Reprinted from Saw J, Mancini JGB, Humphries KH. Contemporary review on spontaneous coronary artery dissection. *J Am Coll Cardiol.* 2016;68(3):297–312 with permission from Elsevier.)

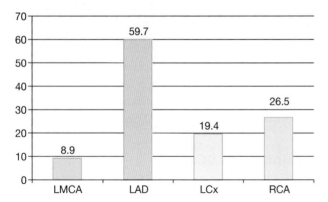

FIGURE 5.47 Spontaneous coronary artery dissection distribution in the coronary tree. LAD, left anterior descending; LCx, left circumflex artery; LMCA, left main coronary artery; RCA, right coronary artery. (Reprinted from Giacoppo D, Capodanno D, Dangas G, et al. Spontaneous coronary artery dissection. *Int J Cardiol.* 2014;175(1):8–20 with permission from Elsevier.)

Treatment of SCAD varies according to underlying pathology. PCI may be indicated; however, success rates of PCI are markedly reduced compared with success rates for ACS (62% vs. 92%). In a group of young women with SCAD during pregnancy or the postpartum period and treated with PCI, dissection propagation requiring additional stenting occurred in up to 50% of patients (223). In contrast, the relatively rapid rate of spontaneous vascular healing of SCAD (212, 224), to be as brief as 26 days (225), suggests a role for conservative management in stable patients with SCAD who have preserved coronary artery flow (226). Therefore, recommendations are to revascularize acute SCAD if the patient has hemodynamic instability or poor coronary artery blood flow and to medically treat acute SCAD if the patient is stable and has normal, or near-normal, coronary artery blood flow (227).

Treatment and Management of SCAD

Whereas most CR programs and traditional exercise prescription methods for a patient with recent MI may be appropriate for those with SCAD, a younger and more physically active population can present a challenge for CEPs. Challenging patients within this group include those with a recent history of vigorous PA or those who have occupations that require high levels of PA.

Medical History Review

The SCAD patient is typically an apparently healthy young person, without significant heart disease risk, and busy with family and career. As indicated in Figure 5.44, multiple emerging risk factors can help explain what has happened, but there are times when essentially very little is presented in a patient's medical history review. Regardless, the CEP should review with the patient the traditional heart disease risk factors and the risks for SCAD or recurrent SCAD and make sure patients have discussed these with their PCP and/or cardiologist. The CEP should also ensure that the patient understands their medications or other aspects of their plan of care. Because exercise is more widely becoming accepted as a vital sign, this too should be reviewed in detail.

Patient Interview

Initial interviews with SCAD patients have the potential to be very emotional. The CEP should strongly consider allowing the patient to bring a support person with them to the initial appointment. The more people in their support group that clearly understand how to help them along with exercise and PA recommendations, the better.

As with any patient with CVD, the CEP will want to discuss if the patient had been having any cardiac symptoms well prior to or after the acute event or any other cardiac symptoms of concern. Patients with CVD tend to be hypersensitive to just about any discomforts and sensations around the chest, even if clearly not related to the heart. SCAD patients will be no different, if not more sensitive. The CEP may be able to help them distinguish the type of symptoms that are of concern.

Outside of discussing any possible cardiac symptoms, CEPs need to discuss prior exercise history, current level of PA since leaving the hospital, any other physically limiting matters, financial resources, and social support, as has been stressed in prior sections of this chapter. The CEP should strongly encourage the SCAD patient to get in touch with community support groups and the multiple support groups now available online, and participate in SCAD registry such as the one conducted by the Mayo Clinic (228).

Exercise Testing

The CEP should strongly consider the use of some type of exercise stress testing as part of the evaluation of the SCAD patient for the development of the exercise prescription. Although this is not logistically easy for some programs, it has the potential to help build confidence and self-esteem in these patients. Currently, there are no specific guidelines for post-SCAD exercise testing, but a reasonable approach would be to use those established for patients following MI in the *Guidelines for Exercise Testing and Prescription* (16) published by ACSM.

The choice of submaximal, symptom-limited, or perhaps simply a practice exercise session depends on the specific needs of the patient to move forward toward rehabilitation. Considering the differing rates of spontaneous healing when medical management is used with this population, the CEP may still uncover an ischemic and/or anginal threshold during testing, which can be valuable in setting exercise intensities, but also for education of the SCAD patient in how they should proceed with PA outside of any monitored setting. Keep in mind that performing exercise testing with an ECG has the potential for false-positive results and can trigger unnecessary downstream testing.

Exercise Prescription

Similar to exercise testing, there are no established guidelines for the development of exercise prescription specific to the SCAD population. Again, a reasonable approach would be to use guidelines that have been established for the post-MI patient as developed by ACSM (16).

This population can present as two extremes — those who are afraid to exercise or return to exercise and those who want to jump right back into their prior exercise and PA regimen. Patients whose trigger for the SCAD event was a bout of exercise typically will be a bit more hesitant to return, but all patients are individuals and will respond to their SCAD event differently.

Multiple sources have suggested that entrance into CR programs post-SCAD is safe and beneficial (229–231). Krittanawong et al. (230) suggested that the biggest barrier to participation was lack of referrals to a program. Of those who did participate, 82% perceived physical health benefits and 75% reported positive emotional health benefits. However, given that intense exercise can be a trigger for a SCAD event, what is the best approach for patients wanting to return to higher intensity exercise?

Research evidence supports a traditional approach to CR similar to that used with patients who have suffered an MI from CAD. The Vancouver General Hospital dedicated

SCAD CR program (229), for example, used such an approach. All participants had initial exercise testing. Based on those results, the exercise intensity was set at 50%–70% of HR reserve for cardiovascular exercise, and the systolic BP during exercise was limited to less than 130 mm Hg. As exercise progressed during this 6-month program, HR was adjusted to subjective measures of "moderate to somewhat difficult." Resistance training was initiated with 0.91 kg (2 lb) to 5.44 kg (12 lb) free weights, and patients were to avoid lifting more than 9.1 kg (20 lb). The thresholds of exercise intensity were designed to limit possible excessive shear stress on artery walls. Although exercise prescriptions were fairly conservative, results were still very favorable from this approach. Those who participated in the program had an overall major adverse cardiovascular event (MACE) rate of 4.3%, whereas those who did not participate had a MACE rate of about 26.2%. The authors admitted that the rather conservative thresholds used for exercise intensity were not based on any literature that suggests exercising above this intensity would in any way bring harm to the patients.

As noted in the Krittanawong study in 2016, some patients cease participating in CR because they do not perceive any benefit (230). This perception was reflected by comments in their survey such as I found it too slow for me and left the program; my own workout routine was more than the rehab program; and I tried going and did not think it was worthwhile. Given this, a program with a more aggressive approach, such as the program used at the Mayo Clinic (231), may allow the CEP to work safely with patients who want to return to higher intensity exercise. Silber et al. (231) studied nine patients with SCAD who started CR at an average of 12 days after discharge. A typical exercise prescription for patients with MI was used, which also incorporated high-intensity interval training with perceived exertions of 15–17 on a 20-point perceived exertion scale. Results demonstrated safety and effectiveness, with improvements of 18% for peak and 22% in 6-minute walk distance. An older but relevant study (232) demonstrated the relationship of the relative risk of MI associated with vigorous exertion ($\geq$6 METs) according to the habitual frequency of vigorous exertion. The results demonstrated those without a history of prior vigorous exertion were at significantly more risk of MI during harder (higher intensity) efforts. The CEP could apply this logic when deciding how quickly to return any one particular SCAD patient to more intense activities.

For strength training specifically, there are no specific weight limit restrictions post-SCAD except for those the first few days post angiogram to let the puncture site from the angiogram heal. Weight limitations are at best arbitrary and should be developed relative to the individual's prior ability. A reasonable precaution would be to warn against any significant Valsalva maneuver when lifting weights and avoiding significant strain associated with efforts where only four to six repetitions can be complete. Isometric exercise modalities such as yoga, in which proper breathing techniques are used, should not pose a significant risk to the post-SCAD patient and the potential benefit outweighs any possible risk. Despite the limited data on the effects of PA on SCAD, general PA guidelines have been proposed (233). The recommendations include physical activities of moderate intensity for 30–40 minutes in duration, 5–7 days per week. Lower resistance and higher repetition strength training is also encouraged provided proper breathing and lifting techniques are followed. Appropriate warm-up is recommended as is avoidance of abrupt, prolonged and/or exhaustive high-intensity exercise, and environmental conditions considered extreme. Further, a scientific statement on SCAD from the AHA supports moderate-intensity exercise that starts low and gradually increases as demonstrated in the Vancouver General Hospital SCAD CR program (234). Much remains to be understood with exercise and SCAD, so sound clinical judgment and reasonable precautions are advised.

Addressing Behavioral Aspects

Working with SCAD patients can be both rewarding and frustrating. Patients who are ready to get back to being physically active progressing them at a reasonable rate is a critical challenge for the CEP. On the other hand, SCAD patients can be timid to exercise again and require multiple sessions to understand the benefits of exercise for their condition. Fortunately, for the SCAD patient who participates in a more traditional, monitored CR program, there will not only be an introductory session, but at least a few monitored sessions with rehabilitation personnel available to help meet the patient's physical and emotional needs. The most contemporary CR programs should be able to work well with this population.

Another barrier to engaging in CR is that many SCAD patients do not feel comfortable in the CR setting (235). They may feel awkward in a facility where they may be the youngest (by over a decade or more), or the experience could contribute to depression. Outside of this fact, there are other typical barriers to participation in a monitored CR program such as location of facilities, costs of visits, and need to return to work (235).

Again, the CEP should be mindful of the more athletic patients in the rehabilitation setting and individualize the patient's program relative to their abilities. If the CEP simply follows the usual post-MI guidelines, these patients may not see the value of continuing with sessions as progress will likely be too slow. If patients are more sedentary or deconditioned, then the usual post-MI progression may work very well for them.

If patients are unable to attend multiple sessions, the CEP will want to make sure to gain their trust quickly so they will feel more comfortable allowing the CEP to guide their progress. As has been advised in previous sections of this chapter, use active listening skills at the first meeting, and try to let the patient lead the conversation. Get to know what is most important for them at this point. Determine their resources and support so that you can provide the most appropriate advice in progressing with their exercise independently. Set reasonable goals and firm follow-up guidelines, stressing how the program will be of help to them over the coming weeks or months. As always, give them the plan in writing, and ask if they need any clarification. Never assume they heard everything. Make sure they know how best to communicate with you and encourage them to contact you. Many people assume that the CEP would be bothered to hear from them. Instead, let them know that frequent communication is a positive thing and increases your ability to help them progress to their goals.

Follow-up and Referrals

As with all patients with CVD, the closer the follow-up, the better. The type of program will of course dictate some of the communication. Having a multifaceted, team approach with PTs, RDNs, behavior change specialists, and physician specialists improves success. It is important to have a network available to make sure the SCAD patient achieves the best outcomes possible.

SUMMARY

The burden of CVD is growing. Whether the disease is experienced firsthand, through a family member, and/or through a friend or neighbor, it reaches us all. The greatest medicine we have today is not in seeking a cure for CVD but in prevention. The CEP is strategically positioned to promote and provide primary and secondary CVD prevention education. This approach should focus on addressing controllable CVD risk factors including HTN, dyslipidemia, psychosocial stress, obesity, smoking, and physical inactivity. It is well accepted that PA helps to reduce the signs and symptoms of CVD associated with these controllable risk factors.

To reach this goal, we need to remove the barriers that keep so many patients from accessing effective CVD prevention and treatment, including financial, geographical, and behavioral hurdles. In America today, more citizens have accepted the opportunity and responsibility of being medically insured. However, even insured patients often find the cost to participate in CVD prevention education and CR prohibitive. Furthermore, most CEPs are employed in health care facilities located in large cities and are less likely to reach people in rural regions far from a hospital. The expanding field of home-based CR offers CVD prevention education and support by incorporating telephone and Internet-based connections. The most successful outcomes incorporate behavioral interventions that address ambivalence and intrinsic motivation. The CEP plays a pivotal role in overcoming these hurdles by providing comprehensive CVD prevention education and targeted exercise prescription and support and is thus a vital member of the health care team.

CHAPTER REVIEW QUESTIONS

1. What is the most common cause of ACS?
2. Taking into consideration that PAD tends to be underdiagnosed in the general population, what approaches can be taken to better diagnose people at an earlier stage in the disease process where lifestyle modifications may be more effective in a shorter period of time?
3. If your patient is not eligible or is not able to participate in a regular CR visit schedule, what might be some reasonable ways to help ensure they can progress more independently?
4. What should be the main focus of early rehabilitation with survivors of stroke?
5. What are the common diagnoses requiring HT?
6. What is the role of the VAD in patients with ESHF?
7. Describe the interdisciplinary medical team approach, including the CEP, in providing care for the HT recipient after surgery.
8. Prior to measuring BP, why is it important to allow the patient to rest for at least 5 minutes, but preferably 10 minutes?
9. Compare/contrast the physiological differences between systolic and diastolic HF.
10. What are the general guidelines for generating an exercise prescription for a SCAD patient?

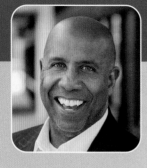

Case Study 5.1

John, a 45-year-old man who works full-time, has a history of Type 2 DM (noninsulin dependent), frequent heartburn/acid reflux, current tobacco use, increased emotional stress, and a strong family history of CAD. He presented to the emergency department with acute onset of substernal chest pain radiating to his left arm and lasting 1 hour in duration. He rated the pain a 10/10 (on a 10-point pain scale), described it as achy and sharp in character, and stated that it occurred while watching television. He reported having had similar chest pain the previous week while mowing the lawn, but it resolved on its own. His current medications include aspirin, Glucophage, and omeprazole. He has no known medication allergies.

An initial ECG demonstrated sinus rhythm with T-wave inversion in leads II, III, and aVF (see Chapter 6). Initial troponin was elevated at 1.55 ng·mL^{-1}. BP was 150/90 mm Hg. John was admitted for suspicion of acute NSTEMI. He was then transported to the catheterization lab for coronary angiography. The catheterization report indicated an 85% occlusion in his RCA. Dr. Murphy, the interventional cardiologist, decided John needed a coronary stent placed in the distal region of his RCA. Nonobstructive disease was found in his left circumflex (LCx) and LADCA. After his catheterization, he was transported to the cardiovascular care unit (CVCU), where he was cared for and monitored by nursing staff.

Dr. Murphy ordered CR. Thus, while in the CVCU, John was visited by a CR staff member, who provided CVD risk factor education and discussed components of outpatient CR. John expressed the concern that it would be difficult for him to attend CR as he would have to return to work as soon as possible. He admitted that he has not been in the habit of checking his blood sugar on a routine basis. He also stated he previously only had to take three medications and wanted to know why he had to take so many now. Acknowledging that his cardiologist recommended that he participate in CR after he goes home, he agreed to go ahead and schedule an initial CR orientation. John was discharged to home the following day.

Diagnosis:

NSTEMI, elevated troponin I level of 1.55 ng·mL^{-1}, hypertension

Current tobacco use

Stress

DM Type 2, noninsulin dependent

Assessment:

Single-vessel obstructive CAD with 85% stenosis of the distal RCA

Stenting of the proximal RCA with a DES

Nonobstructive disease of the LCx and LADCA.

Plan:

Medications: Aspirin 81 mg once daily, clopidogrel 75 mg once daily, metoprolol 25 mg twice daily, Glucophage 500 mg twice daily, Lisinopril 20 mg once daily, atorvastatin 10 mg once daily, omeprazole 60 mg one tab before every meal, and sublingual nitroglycerin 0.4 mg as needed for anginal symptoms.

Aggressive risk factor modification and secondary prevention through participation in outpatient CR program.

Case Study 5.1 Questions

1. How should the CEP and other CR staff approach providing information and support to John for secondary prevention following his ACS diagnosis?

2. What would the CEP need to be aware of regarding John's diagnosis and previous medical history when he participates in outpatient CR?

Case Study 5.2

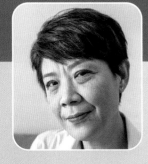

Claire, a 67-year-old woman with a history of hypertension and osteoporosis, presented to the Cardiovascular Institute for a routine nuclear pharmacological ("nonexercise") stress test prior to planned right total hip arthroplasty. Approximately 3 minutes after the radioactive tracer was injected, she experienced severe mid-scapular back pain radiating to her neck and right jaw rated at a 9/10 (nine on a 10-point scale). Current medications include aspirin, Lisinopril, Glucophage, and atorvastatin. She has medication allergy to angiotensin-converting enzyme inhibitors. Her ECG demonstrated a sinus rhythm with ST-segment elevation in frontal plane leads I and aVL as well as precordial leads V_{1-3} (see Chapter 6). Blood test demonstrated an elevated troponin at 25.6 ng·mL^{-1}. BP was 174/84 mm Hg. The interventional cardiologist was contacted, and the patient was emergently transported to the catheterization laboratory with diagnosed STEMI. Claire was given sublingual nitroglycerin and morphine and placed on supplemental oxygen.

The catheterization report documented a complete (100%) occlusion in her LADCA. No other obstruction was found. The interventional cardiologist, Dr. Smith, placed a DES in the proximal LADCA. Following her catheterization, she was transported to the CVCU for care and observation. That afternoon, Dr. Smith visited Claire on his rounds. He told her that although she originally presented for preoperative evaluation for surgery to replace her right hip, she would not be able to have this surgery for a while as she was now on aspirin and clopidogrel. He encouraged her to follow up with the outpatient CR team to assist in improving her cardiovascular health prior to being evaluated again for hip surgery.

Although disappointed, she reluctantly agreed to do whatever Dr. Smith asked her to do. Dr. Smith placed an order for inpatient CR, and a member of the CR staff visited Claire. The CR staff member began by introducing himself and asked her what her understanding was about what had happened during her stress test. She stated that she was confused and couldn't believe she had had a major heart attack. The CR staff member explained why Dr. Smith recommended that she follow up with CR upon discharge and also discussed Claire's entire health history including that she needed her right hip replaced. Because she lived independently and would like to feel better, Claire agreed to be scheduled for an outpatient CR orientation. She remained asymptomatic and was discharged to home the next morning.

Diagnosis:
  STEMI
  Elevated troponin I level at 25.6 ng·mL^{-1}
  Hypertension
  Osteoporosis
Assessment:
  Single-vessel obstructive CAD with 100% stenosis of the proximal LADCA
  Stenting of the proximal LADCA with a DES
  No other coronary disease
Plan:
  Medications: Aspirin 81 mg once daily, clopidogrel 75 mg once daily, metoprolol 25 mg twice daily, atorvastatin 80 mg once daily, and sublingual nitroglycerin 0.4 mg as needed for anginal symptoms.
  Participate in outpatient CR for CVD risk factor modification and secondary prevention with a physician-approved exercise prescription considering right hip discomfort and limited ROM.

Case Study 5.2 Questions

1. Explain the significance of the different troponin levels of John and Claire as associated with their diagnoses.
2. Briefly describe the difference in symptoms experienced by John versus Claire.
3. Briefly list the cascade of events in atherosclerosis that lead to occlusion and subsequent diagnosis of ACS.

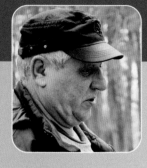

Case Study 5.3

Randy is a 62-year-old (BMI 36 kg·m^{-2}) man who was obese with a history of elevated cholesterol, hypertension, and obstructive sleep apnea (non-compliant with continuous positive airway pressure [CPAP] use). Prior to his MI, he was not prescribed any medications, consumed two to three cans of beer a day, and smoked 0.5 packs of cigarettes a day (ongoing for the last 40 years). He reports no illicit drug use, does no formal exercise, and has not seen a physician in the last 5 years. He is a semiretired tenured college professor in mechanical engineering.

In June, Randy suffered an STEMI. The patient was driving to the beach for a family summer vacation when he noticed some left shoulder and upper left chest pain. The patient arrived at his hotel at 6:00 AM and took three antacids and 800 mg of ibuprofen before lying down. The patient woke about 3 hours later feeling some nausea, SOB, and continued left chest pain. After some encouragement from his family, the patient went to the nearest emergency room (~10 hours from the time his symptoms started). He was diagnosed with an STEMI and was given tissue plasminogen activator, stabilized, and life-flighted to another hospital for cardiac catheterization. He was found to have severe obstruction in three vessels (proximal LAD artery, obtuse marginal and distal right coronary arteries) and subsequently underwent triple bypass surgery the next day. LVEF by ventriculography during his catheterizations was measured at 15%. On the day of discharge, a two-dimensional transthoracic echocardiogram was performed, which demonstrated a mildly dilated left ventricle with apical akinesis and an LVEF of 25%. The patient's length of stay was 5 days. He was discharged breathing comfortably, afebrile, no erythema or drainage from incision, and ambulating independently. The patient was also fitted for a wearable defibrillator prior to being discharged home and cleared to begin phase II CR.

One week after discharge, the patient was seen by a cardiologist in his hometown. During this visit, his chest wall was noted as healing well. The patient reported that he tried to slowly walk outside (back and forth several times on his flat driveway) for a couple of days, but had to stop frequently for dyspnea and leg fatigue (denies chest pain). He is fearful of exercising because of this and has not done much walking since. The patient hates wearing the wearable defibrillator and wants to know when he can stop wearing it. He admits that he is fearful of what it will feel like if he is shocked. The patient's cardiologist ordered a cardiopulmonary exercise test (results in box below) to be performed prior to starting CR and a repeat transthoracic ECG to be done in 3 months.

During intake into CR, the patient admitted that he has been unable to quit smoking, but has decreased his alcohol consumption to one can of beer a day. He remains noncompliant with his CPAP, stating that the mask makes him look silly and is a little uncomfortable. He has been compliant with his medications, which include Lisinopril 20 mg once daily, carvedilol 6.25 mg twice daily, furosemide 20 mg once daily, potassium chloride 20 mEq once daily, and simvastatin 20 mg once daily. His wife has been very helpful in getting his medication routine organized.

Exercise Test Results:

Variable	Predicted Value	Measured Value
Age (years)		62
Sex		Male
Height (cm)		171
Weight (kg)		105
Peak oxygen consumption (mL·kg^{-1}·min^{-1})	22.2	15.5
Maximum heart rate	158	112
Resting blood pressure (mm Hg)		110/70
Peak blood pressure (mm Hg)		150/68
Oxygen-pulse (mL per beat)	14.8	14.5
Peak ventilation (L·min^{-1})		78
Pulse oximetry (%)		95% rest, 96% exercise

Case Study 5.3 Questions

1. What are the benefits of having the patient perform a cardiopulmonary exercise test prior to starting CR?
2. Given the patient's medical and personal history, what other comorbidities might Randy be at risk for that might be contributing to his dyspnea and fatigue with exercise?
3. Considering the concepts of motivational interviewing, what aspects of the patient's lifestyle and self-care should the CEP affirm? What strategies can the CEP use to help the patient in areas where he has not been able to make changes?
4. Based on the exercise test results, what should be the patient's initial intensity for cardiorespiratory exercise?

Toward what level of intensity should the CEP progress his cardiorespiratory exercise?
5. Should this patient participate in resistance training? If not, why not? If so, then when should resistance training begin?
6. If the patient arrives at the CR unit on Wednesday with a 4-lb weight gain since he was last in CR on Monday, should the attending physician of CR be notified? Should the patient exercise?
7. Prior to the 3-month follow-up ECG, the patient experiences ventricular fibrillation and subsequent shock from his wearable defibrillator. The patient then has an ICD implanted. Once cleared to resume CR, would the patient's exercise plan be changed? If so how?

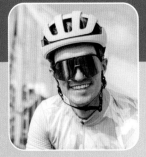

Case Study 5.4

Bill is a 26-year-old professional cyclist. He has no prior clinical history of any significant disease or conditions, does not have any concerning risk factors for any specific clinical disease or conditions, and is not on any medications. Four months ago, he started to notice left leg pain starting in the thigh while cycling. This would take 10–15 minutes to set in and if he continued to cycle or if he would increase his intensity or go up hills the pain would intensify and radiate down his leg and eventually his foot would go numb and he would be forced to stop cycling. The pain would resolve in a few minutes and he could resume cycling, but if he would go a similar distance and intensity, it would return consistently and predictably. Interestingly enough, when walking or running, the symptoms could not be reproduced. He initially went to see his primary care physician (PCP). Multiple tests were ordered including x-ray and MRI of the affected leg, which were both within normal limits. After further conversations with Bill, the physician decided to try simple bedside ABI. Results were 1.05 on the right and 1.09 on the left, both within normal limits. Because the PCP knew that simple bedside ABIs can be misleading, she ordered a NIVA. ABIs during that test were again normal at 1.04 on the right and 1.07 on the left, and ultrasound did not reveal any hemodynamically significant findings. Because the pattern of the symptoms seemed fairly typical and the location of the symptoms started up higher, the physician suspected PAD, but because the NIVA is limited in evaluating inflow disease, she consulted with a vascular surgeon. It

was decided to move forward and perform a lower extremity arteriogram while in supine position. This did not show any significant obstruction that could be causing his symptoms. Again, because the symptoms still seemed to make sense for a reduction of blood flow to the lower extremities, the vascular surgeon ordered an exercise ABI test to assess the possibility of a mechanical obstruction of flow during exercise. The CEP called Bill and went over testing options. Typically, a treadmill or stationary exercise bike would be used, but because symptoms seemed very positional specific, he was asked if he had an indoor trainer for his bike and to bring it in for testing. Bill also had a watts meter so he could better quantify power output in relation to his symptoms. The CEP assessed initial resting ABIs at 1.04 (125/120) on the right and 1.08 (127/118) on the left. Bill then got on his bike and indoor trainer and started to ride at a comfortable cadence. Initial power output was to be 30 W and to increase 30 W every 2 min. Bill noted onset of symptoms at 270 W and was able to continue until about 360 W before he needed to stop due to claudication symptoms. He was quickly placed in a supine position again, and ABIs were again determined. His right ABI postexercise was noted to be 0.97 (145/150) and considered normal, but his left ABI was 0.51 (78/152). An absolute drop of 20 mm Hg or more pre- to postexercise is considered abnormal. Bill's drop of 49 points was considered significantly abnormal. In this particular case, because so many of the previously conducted tests were normal, Bill asked to repeat the test to see if it produced similar results. Again, resting ABI on the left leg preexercise was 1.05, and postexercise was 0.49 with a similar 48-point drop.

(continued)

Case Study 5.4 (*continued*)

Bill was referred back to the vascular surgeon, who decided to repeat the lower extremity angiogram. This time, the test started in a supine position, then the vascular surgeon had Bill turn to his side and flex his leg to a similar position that would occur while biking. It was noted that, in this position, his left iliac artery would occlude. Different interventions were discussed including surgical options, but ultimately Bill decided to retire from professional cycling and pursue other career options.

Generally, the tried and true method of walking till the pain stops you, rest till gone, repeat over and over for 50 minutes is no longer the only approach, nor is it necessarily the best approach for all PAD patients suffering from lifestyle-limiting claudication. The application of exercise should encompass not only a focus on claudication symptoms but any functional limitations and health risk reduction. Thoroughly review the medical history, listen attentively to the patient's main concerns, and address not only their PAD symptoms but other potentially equally limiting factors. This patient-centered approach will help you gain trust from the patients you see and increase the likelihood that they will take your advice and give it a fair chance to work.

Case Study 5.4 Questions

1. What was the key finding in Bill's symptom history that led to continued testing and evaluation despite all initial testing for PAD being normal?

2. Is a postexercise drop in ABI to 0.49 considered moderate or severe?

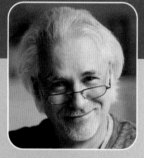

Case Study 5.5

Brendan is a 62-year-old man. He is 175.3 cm (69 inches) tall and weighs 90.7 kg (200 lb) with a BMI of 29.5. He has PAD, diagnosed by computed tomography angiography with serial left common femoral stenosis of 70%–75%, total occlusion of the left proximal popliteal artery with established collateral flow, and reconstitution to distal left lower leg. He also has Type 2 diabetes and hypertension and is a former smoker who quit last year with a 25 pack-year history. Of note is the fact that he also has degenerative disc disease of his lumbar spine, which can contribute to some sciatica pain in his left lower extremity.

His medications include an ACE-I for his hypertension, an oral antidiabetic for his diabetes, and a daily 81-mg aspirin. His recent labs revealed cholesterol of 208 mg·dL^{-1} (high-density lipoprotein of 38 mg·dL^{-1}, low-density lipoprotein [LDL] of 175 mg·dL^{-1}), BP of 134/84 mm Hg at rest, blood glucose of 134 mm Hg, and glycolated hemoglobin of 7.2.

He recently retired from his job in local utilities as a lineman, which he performed for 30 years.

When Brendan was interviewed about his symptoms, he stated that for the past 3–4 months he had noticed a fairly typical cramping and tightness in his left calf with walking. Specifically, he could walk about one to one and a half blocks before onset of the pain, then had to stop at about two blocks. Over the past 2–3 weeks, however, this worsened to the point at which he experienced onset of pain within half block and stopped at one block of walking. Walking uphill or when carrying heavy objects worsened the pain. The tightness/cramping resolved with 2–3 minutes of rest, but then he experienced an aching pain that encompassed his entire left leg and lasted for 30–45 minutes, sometimes longer. Brendan stated that the same pain would occur if he sat too long or if he stood and performed any tasks for too long. He denied chest pain.

When asked if he had been experiencing any chest pains, Brendan said he had not. He continued to talk about his various leg symptoms and how much they limited his quality of life.

The CEP decided to pursue a monitored exercise stress test using 12-lead ECG monitoring and typical constant speed PAD protocol with 3-minute stages (2.0 mph per 0% grade, increase grade by 3.5% every 3 minutes).

Resting measures revealed HR of 72 bpm, resting BP of 148/90 mm Hg, ECG sinus with regular rate and rhythm, and no concerning baseline changes.

Testing was started, and Brendan appeared initially comfortable with speed and movement on treadmill. By 30 seconds of testing, there was start of some ST-segment elevation in V1, V2, and V3 leads. A few seconds later, Brendan started to move his hands to his chest and was in obvious discomfort. Testing was stopped by 38 seconds, and Brendan was moved back to the exam room table. The supervising physician was called into the room, oxygen at 2 L·min^{-1} was started, and the nurse on call brought in the department urgent care kit that included appropriate medications and IV start kit. A single dose of sublingual nitroglycerin was administered, an IV was started, and ECG and chest discomforts resolved in about 3 minutes. Brendan remained stable from that point.

An ambulance was called to the clinic for transport to the local hospital for further evaluation. In the interim, the physical and CEP talked further with Brendan. Brendan still denied having any chest pains prior to testing today, but then elaborated and said he had been having symptoms of chest pressure and dyspnea with walking over the past week. In fact, he reported stopping three times today walking in from the parking lot to the clinic to catch up on his breath.

Brendan had a cardiac catheterization performed on the same day. It revealed distal left main stenosis of about 80%, mild to moderate mid-left circumflex disease, proximal 85% stenosis of his LADCA, and mid to distal right CAD of about 70%. Brendan had urgent CABG surgery the next day.

Case Study 5.5 Questions

1. What critical feature of the symptom assessment prior to the exercise test was missed in this case?

2. What do you feel was this patient's pretest likelihood of having significant CAD?

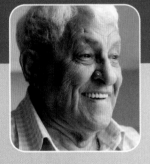

Case Study 5.6

Eddie is 67 years old and recently retired from his position as town sheriff. His former job kept him active most days of the week, but he now has a sedentary lifestyle. He currently weighs 102 kg (244 lb), has 28.6% body fat, and a BMI of 35 kg·m^{-2}. His last blood glucose recording on the glucometer read 220 mg·dL^{-1}. His fasting blood lipid profile is as follows: high-density lipoprotein was 55 mg·dL^{-1}, low-density lipoprotein was 188 mg·dL^{-1}, and total cholesterol was 283 mg·dL^{-1}. Eddie has been treating his hypertension with a daily regimen of bystolic (20 mg) and sodium restriction for the past 20 (or more) years. His average resting BP is 132/85 mm Hg and has a resting HR of 84 bpm. He denies any alcohol consumption or tobacco use. He has a family history of heart disease: his mother died from an MI at the age of 53 years. Finally, Eddie has an old knee injury that is aggravated by weight-bearing exercise.

Eddie has been referred to the CEP by his PCP. His PCP has cleared him for exercise. Eddie's case of hypertension is truly a pathology caused by multiple factors working independently and synergistically to bring about one of the most common symptoms of CVD. Treatment for hypertension involves aggressive lifestyle modifications and several pharmaceutical options. Chronic aerobic exercise is a potent therapeutic option as it has been shown to reduce both systolic and diastolic resting BP by approximately 5–10 mm Hg. Hypertensive individuals generally experience similar responses and adaptations to exercise training as compared to healthy counterparts; however, special considerations must be monitored when working with this population.

Case Study 5.6 Questions

1. According to current research, how much percent body weight does Eddie need to lose for clinically significant changes to occur to his resting BP? Using the ideal body weight equation and assuming all weight loss was due to reductions in adiposity, how many pounds (or kilograms) will Eddie need to lose to reach the desired percent body fat?

2. Identify at least three mechanisms by which chronic aerobic exercise training reduces BP in hypertensive individuals independent of weight loss.

3. Identify at least five special considerations for individuals with hypertension that the CEP must address before designing and implementing the exercise prescription plan for Eddie.

Case Study 5.7

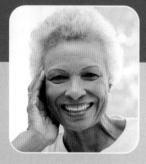

Nicole is a 72-year-old woman with a history of hypertension and a 30 pack-year history of smoking. She quit 10 years ago. She had a stroke about 2 months ago that left her with right-sided hemiplegia, mild speech impairment, and some emotional struggles as of late. She was evaluated by physical therapy while in the hospital and was referred to a skilled nursing facility for about a month, during which time she had daily physical therapy and progressed to the point at which she could again perform her normal daily activities and walk a couple of blocks in the neighborhood independently. She lives alone but has a daughter in the area. She was referred to an outpatient rehab facility to continue to work on strength and conditioning.

During her interview with the CEP, she mentioned that she has a regular card game each week with some friends and a happy hour on Fridays as well, but has been reluctant to attend these social activities lately. She denied being depressed, but the CEP noticed during the interview that she was struggling a bit about losing her independence and having others see her as weak. Different options for therapy

were discussed, and Nicole was scheduled to come in on Tuesdays and Thursdays when class sizes were smaller and she could get more one-on-one attention.

There were no concerning cardiac symptoms and, considering that testing her prior to starting an exercise regimen might make her feel even weaker, the CEP decided to evaluate Nicole's "endurance" while she was walking on the track and using a treadmill. More emphasis was placed on strength training in her case because of her repeated reports of feeling concerned about being weak.

Nicole was started on treadmill for 10 minutes, then continued through a general strengthening circuit for upper and lower body for one set of 12 repetitions to address her muscular fatigue. This was followed by another 10 minutes on the treadmill. Each week, 2 minutes were added to treadmill time. Weight was adjusted as she got stronger to maintain the 12 repetitions to fatigue. After 6 weeks, Nicole progressed to 20 minutes on the treadmill before and after her strengthening exercises and increased to two sets of 12 repetitions on her strengthening exercises. After 12 weeks, she mentioned that she had returned to all her usual social activities and was planning on a guided walking trip along the Appalachian Trail.

Case Study 5.7 Questions

1. What ultimately was the best mode of exercise to focus on for this individual and why?

2. Do you agree or disagree with the choice to not perform exercise testing prior to prescribing exercise and why?

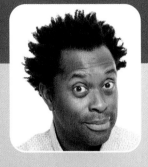

Case Study 5.8

Andy is a 40-year-old man with a history of hypertension, sedentary lifestyle, obesity, and "social" smoking. Last year, he suffered a hemorrhagic stroke. He had a complicated hospitalization and initial rehabilitation course of care. He struggled for 3–4 months with adjusting BP medications to get more optimal control and did not start any physical therapy until 6 months poststroke.

After his stroke, he quit smoking and has been adhering to his medication regimen as prescribed. He has a residual right foot drop with walking that may be a lifelong issue. When he tries to walk long distances, his abnormal gait causes premature fatigue and he sometimes feels as if he will lose his balance and fall, although he does not report any specific issues with falling at this point.

He tries to get in a walk about 2–3 days a week. He walks about 1 mile total but has to stop three to four times to let his right leg rest. He states that he has been consistent with his prescribed physical therapy exercises, feels pretty strong overall, but is concerned that he cannot get in adequate cardiovascular exercise to help with secondary prevention measures.

The CEP meets with Andy to perform preparticipation exercise testing. Although he is rather young and has a lower risk for CAD at this point, he does have multiple risk factors and had a stroke, so it seems reasonable to perform exercise testing to get an idea of his HR and BP response to exercise and of course to screen for any possible premature CAD. The CEP has Andy perform his stress test using a bike ergometer using a 20-W ramped protocol to volitional fatigue. He was on his usual medication regimen, which included metoprolol tartrate 50 mg bid. He was able to complete 8 minutes (160 W). There were no concerning changes on the ECG and no concerning symptoms. Andy stopped due to SOB and leg fatigue. His HR increased from 76 bpm at rest to 141 bpm at peak effort (78% of predicted maximal effort). His BP increased from 124/68 to 202/76 mm Hg at peak effort. Recovery period was unremarkable, and HR and BP recovery was normal.

His exercise prescription was to include continuing with daily physical therapy exercises 2 days a week of large muscle group strength training (two sets of 12 repetitions avoiding a Valsalva maneuver), exercise bike 3 days a week for 20 minutes at an HR zone of 115–125 bpm (65%–70% of predicted maximum) and close monitoring of exercise BP.

Case Study 5.8 Questions

1. Why did the CEP choose an exercise bike for exercise testing?

2. What are the main concerns regarding BP with exercise for this individual?

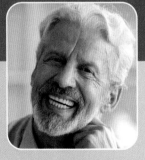

Case Study 5.9

Jim, a 52-year-old man, presented to the emergency department complaining of increased SOB and worsening fatigue. He reported that his feet have been swollen and his breathing has been labored for the past 2 weeks. The attending emergency physician noticed his previous medical history included an STEMI with a resulting EF of 20% occurring approximately 1 year ago. His medications included aspirin 81 mg daily, atorvastatin 40 mg daily, carvedilol 3.25 mg twice daily, clopidogrel 75 mg daily, furosemide 40 mg daily, and Lisinopril 40 mg daily. The physician put in an order

for an echocardiograph and performed a physical exam. He noted severe bilateral ankle edema and diminished lung sounds. The echocardiogram demonstrated an EF of 18%. Because of his previous cardiac history and his current health status, Jim was referred to the heart failure clinic and given a diagnosis of severe ischemic cardiomyopathy. He was discharged to home on optimal medical therapy and agreed to attend regular follow-up appointments in the heart failure clinic for the next 6 weeks. After 6 weeks of optimal medical therapy, Jim was referred to the outpatient CR program and participated for approximately 5 weeks before experiencing another bout of progressively increasing SOB, fatigue, and bilateral lower extremity edema.

(continued)

Case Study 5.9 (*continued*)

Jim had a follow-up appointment with his cardiologist who talked with him about his symptoms and ultimately referred him for HT. Shortly after this appointment, he participated in a pretransplant evaluation that revealed no specific contraindication for HT. Jim was listed for HT and experienced successful orthotopic HT the following year. Within days following his HT, his physicians placed an order for CR staff to meet with Jim as an inpatient. They had him begin to learn how to transfer from lying in bed to sitting at the edge of his bed to standing all while observing precautions to protect his chest incision. Jim began to walk during his second day following surgery, demonstrating good physical tolerance to this activity with a resting HR of 102 bpm and a BP of 124/66 mm Hg. His HR was elevated during his

walk; it would remain elevated for approximately 6 minutes following when resting in his chair. The CEP educated Jim on his new HR response and on pacing himself using the rating of perceived exertion scale with all activity. The CEP also reviewed components of home exercise following his discharge and encouraged him to be up and on his feet walking for a total of 30 minutes daily at a moderate intensity as tolerated. Jim progressed well through recovery and eventually was able to walk around the CVCU four times daily with improved tolerance. Prior to discharge, the CEP scheduled Jim for his initial outpatient CR orientation. He was discharged to home approximately 1 month after his HT surgery. His medications at discharge included azathioprine, cyclosporine, prednisone (immunosuppression), and atorvastatin.

Case Study 5.9 Questions

1. When Jim begins CR, what should the CEP and all CR staff be aware of regarding potential complications following his HT surgery?

2. As if you were addressing Jim, explain how and why his HR remains elevated following exercise and what he should include with every session of physical activity.

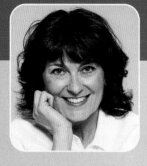

Case Study 5.10

Glenda, a 45-year-old woman, presented to the emergency department last night complaining of increased SOB and fatigue. HR was 112 bpm and BP was 176/92 mm Hg. Previous medical history includes tobacco use (one pack of cigarettes per day), hypertension, and an MI with a resulting EF of 45% about 10 years ago. Current medications include furosemide 80 mg daily, Lisinopril 20 mg daily, and aspirin 81 mg daily. Given her previous medical history and current symptoms, an echocardiogram was ordered by the attending physician with results of an EF of 15%. Blood test demonstrated a blood urea nitrogen (BUN) and creatinine of 23 and 1.2 mg·dL^{-1}, respectively. Glenda was referred to the heart failure team for evaluation.

She was told that her heart was very weak and that she needed to be listed for heart transplant. She was told she would have to quit smoking and make lifestyle changes to improve her BP. Glenda agreed.

She underwent HT surgery approximately 6 months after being placed on the heart transplant list. Immediately following surgery, her BUN and creatinine were 28 and 1.0 mg·dL^{-1}, respectively. She was started on cyclosporine 4.2 mg·kg^{-1} per day, azathioprine 1 mg·kg^{-1} per day, and prednisone 1 mg·kg^{-1} per day. She was also started on antibiotics including erythromycin. While in the intensive care unit, her systolic BPs ranged from 85 to 95 mm Hg and gradually increased to 110–120 mm Hg after about the fourteenth day following her HT. At this point in her recovery, blood tests for BUN and creatinine revealed continued elevation in both values despite optimal BPs. Concomitantly, her urine output dropped significantly in a 24-hour period. Her BUN and creatinine rose to 110 and 4.6 mg·dL^{-1}, respectively. Given her history and the rapid decline in the health of her kidneys, hemodialysis was ordered by her physician. Glenda reported nausea, decreased appetite, and muscle cramping. Due to this onset of renal failure, her cyclosporine was discontinued for 3 days. Her urine output began to improve after the third day of being off cyclosporine, and this medication was reinstituted. Her nausea decreased and her appetite improved.

Prior to discharge, her physician recommended she stay on dialysis given her previous medical history. Her physician also placed an order for her to follow up with outpatient CR upon discharge. Her dialysis appointments were on Tuesdays, Thursdays, and Saturdays, and her CR appointments were on Mondays, Wednesdays, and Fridays. CR sessions lasted 75 minutes including 15 minutes for warm-up, 45 minutes for aerobic exercises,

and 15 minutes for cooldown. The CEP designed an exercise prescription for her taking into account her previous medical history including HT surgery and dialysis therapy. Resistance exercises were incorporated at approximately 10 weeks following her HT surgery and were incorporated into her warm-up targeting her upper and lower body. Her aerobic exercise routine included 15 minutes on the treadmill, 15 minutes on the recumbent stepper, and 15 minutes on the recumbent elliptical. The cooldown portion included standing and sitting stretching with a different group education topic discussed daily. She met with the program's registered dietitian nutritionist to discuss nutrition needs, considering her renal and cardiovascular function. She was also able to meet with the program behavioral health specialist to discuss anxiety and depression following HT. She never returned to smoking, her BPs remained within normal limits, and her body weight remained stable.

Case Study 5.10 Questions

1. Briefly describe the denervated heart as a result of HT surgery.
2. Including Glenda's medical history, list the primary causes of death following HT surgery.
3. List common side effects associated with immunosuppressive therapy that should be noted by the CEP prior to Glenda beginning CR sessions.

REFERENCES

1. Mozaffarian D, Benjamin EJ, Go AS, et al; American Heart Association Statistics Committee; Stroke Statistics Subcommittee. Heart disease and stroke statistics—2016 update: a report from the American Heart Association. *Circulation.* 2016;133(4):e38–360.
2. Ozemek C, Babu AS, Arena R, Bond S; HL-PIVOT Network. Strategies to achieving the national 70% cardiac rehabilitation enrollment rate. *J Cardiopulm Rehabil Prev.* 2021;41(5):E14-5.
3. Grace SL, Kotseva K, Whooley MA. Cardiac rehabilitation: under-utilized globally. *Curr Cardiol Rep.* 2021;23(9):118.
4. Hill JM, Zalos G, Halcox JP, et al. Circulating endothelial progenitor cells, vascular function, and cardiovascular risk [Reprint in *Can J Cardiol.* 2004;20(Suppl B):44B–48B]. *N Engl J Med.* 2003;348(7):593–600.
5. Rodefeld MD, Beau SL, Schuessler RB, Boineau JP, Saffitz JE. Beta-adrenergic and muscarinic cholinergic receptor densities in the human sinoatrial node: identification of a high beta 2-adrenergic receptor density. *J Cardiovasc Electrophysiol.* 1996;7(11):1039–49.
6. Finn AV, Nakano M, Narula J, Kolodgie FD, Virmani R. Concept of vulnerable/unstable plaque. *Arterioscler Thromb Vasc Biol.* 2010;30:1282–92.
7. Baines CP. How and when do myocytes die during ischemia and reperfusion: the late phase. *J Cardiovasc Pharmacol Ther.* 2011;16(3–4):239–43.
8. Fletcher GF, Ades PA, Kligfield P, et al; American Heart Association Exercise, Cardiac Rehabilitation, and Prevention Committee of the Council on Clinical Cardiology, Council on Nutrition, Physical Activity and Metabolism, Council on

Cardiovascular and Stroke Nursing, and Council on Epidemiology and Prevention. Exercise standards for testing and training: a scientific statement from the American Heart Association. *Circulation.* 2013;128(8):873–934.

9. Riebe D, Ehrman JK, Liguori G, Magal M. *ACSM's Guidelines for Exercise Testing and Prescription.* 10th ed. Philadelphia (PA): Wolters Kluwer; 2018.

10. Smith SC, Benjamin EJ, Bonow RO, et al; World Heart Federation and the Preventive Cardiovascular Nurses Association. AHA/ACCF secondary prevention and risk reduction therapy for patients with coronary and other atherosclerotic vascular disease: 2011 update: a guideline from the American Heart Association and American College of Cardiology Foundation [Erratum appears in *Circulation.* 2015;131(15):e408].*Circulation.* 2011;124(22):2458–73.

11. Hambrecht R, Niebauer J, Marburger C, et al. Various intensities of leisure time physical activity in patients with coronary artery disease: effects on cardiorespiratory fitness and progression of coronary atherosclerotic lesions. *J Am Coll Cardiol.* 1993;22(2):468–77.

12. Garcia M, Mulvagh SL, Merz CN, Buring JE, Manson JE. Cardiovascular disease in women: clinical perspectives. *Circ Res.* 2016;118(8):1273–93.

13. Benjamin EJ, Blaha MJ, Chiuve SE, et al; American Heart Association Statistics Committee; Stroke Statistics Subcommittee. Heart disease and stroke statistics—2017 update: a report from the American Heart Association. *Circulation.* 2017;135(10):e146–603.

13a. Napoli C, D'Armiento FP, Mancini FP, et al. Fatty streak formation occurs in human fetal aortas and is greatly enhanced by maternal hypercholesterolemia: intimal accumulation of low density lipoprotein and its oxidation precede monocyte recruitment into early atherosclerotic lesions. *J Clin Invest.* 1997;100:2680–90.

14. Santos-Gallego CG, Picatoste B, Badimon JJ. Pathophysiology of acute coronary syndrome. *Curr Atheroscler Rep.* 2014;16(4):401.

15. Amsterdam EA, Wenger NK, Brindis RG, et al. 2014 AHA/ACC guideline for the management of patients with non-ST-elevation acute coronary syndromes: a report of the American College of Cardiology/American Heart Association Task Force on Practice Guidelines [Erratum appears in *J Am Coll Cardiol.* 2014;64(24):2713–4. Dosage error in article text]. *J Am Coll Cardiol.* 2014;64(24):e139–228.

16. Liguori G, Feito Y, Fountaine C, Roy BA. *ACSM's Guidelines for Exercise Testing and Prescription.* 11th ed. Philadelphia (PA): Wolters Kluwer/Lippincott Williams & Wilkins; 2022.

17. Huffman M, Miller C. *Evidence-Based Health Coaching for Healthcare Providers.* 3rd ed. Winchester (TN): Miller & Huffman Outcome Architects, LLC; 2013. p. 40–1.

18. Prochaska JO, Johnson S, Lee P. The transtheoretical model of behavior change. In: Shumaker SA, Ockene JK, Riekert KA, editors. *The Handbook of Health Behavior Change.* New York (NY): Springer Publishing Co; 2009. p. 59–84.

19. Fitchett DH, Gupta M, Farkouh ME, Verma S. Cardiology patient page: coronary artery revascularization in patients with diabetes mellitus. *Circulation.* 2014;130(12):e104–6.

20. Shavadia J, Norris CM, Graham MM, Verma S, Ali I, Bainey KR. Symptomatic graft failure and impact on clinical outcome after coronary artery bypass grafting surgery: results from the Alberta Provincial Project for Outcome Assessment in Coronary Heart Disease Registry. *Am Heart J.* 2015;169(6):833–40.

21. Farkouh ME, Domanski M, Sleeper LA, et al; FREEDOM Trial Investigators. Strategies for multivessel revascularization in patients with diabetes. *N Engl J Med.* 2012;367(25):2375–84.

22. Verma S, Farkouh ME, Yanagawa B, et al. Comparison of coronary artery bypass surgery and percutaneous coronary intervention in patients with diabetes: a meta-analysis of randomised controlled trials. *Lancet Diabetes Endocrinol.* 2013;1(4):317–28.

23. Anderson L, Nguyen TT, Dall CH, Burgess L, Bridges C, Taylor RS. Exercise-based cardiac rehabilitation in heart transplant recipients. *Cochrane Database Syst Rev.* 2017;(4):CD012264.

24. American Association of Cardiovascular & Pulmonary Rehabilitation. *AACVPR Cardiac Rehabilitation Resource Manual: Promoting Health and Preventing Disease.* Chicago (IL): Human Kinetics; 2006.

25. Dunlay SM, Roger VL. Understanding the epidemic of heart failure: past, present, and future. *Curr Heart Fail Rep.* 2014;11(4):404–15.

26. Bui AL, Horwich TB, Fonarow GC. Epidemiology and risk profile of heart failure. *Nat Rev Cardiol.* 2011;8(1):30–41.

27. Huffman MD, Berry JD, Ning H, et al. Lifetime risk for heart failure among white and black Americans: cardiovascular lifetime risk pooling project. *J Am Coll Cardiol.* 2013;61(14):1510–7.

28. McMurray JJ, Adamopoulos S, Anker SD, et al; ESC Committee for Practice Guidelines. ESC guidelines for the diagnosis and treatment of acute and chronic heart failure 2012: the task force for the diagnosis and treatment of acute and chronic heart failure 2012 of the European Society of Cardiology. Developed in collaboration with the Heart Failure Association (HFA) of the ESC [Erratum appears in *Eur Heart J.* 2013;34(2):158]. *Eur Heart J.* 2012;33(14):1787–847.

29. Yancy CW, Jessup M, Bozkurt B, et al. 2013 ACCF/AHA guideline for the management of heart failure: a report of the American College of Cardiology Foundation/American Heart Association Task Force on Practice Guidelines. *J Am Coll Cardiol.* 2013;62(16):e147–239.

30. Lindenfeld J, Albert NM, Boehmer JP, et al; Heart Failure Society of America. HFSA 2010 comprehensive heart failure practice guideline. *J Card Fail.* 2010;16(6):e1–194.

31. Just H. Pathophysiological targets for beta-blocker therapy in congestive heart failure. *Eur Heart J.* 1996;17(Suppl B):2–7.

32. Mohrman DE, Heller LJ. *Cardiovascular Physiology.* 7th ed. New York (NY): McGraw-Hill Medical; 2010.

33. Tong CW, Wu X, Liu Y, et al. Phosphoregulation of cardiac inotropy via myosin binding protein-C during increased pacing frequency or β1-adrenergic stimulation. *Circ Heart Fail.* 2015;8(3):595–604.

34. Floras JS. Sympathetic nervous system activation in human heart failure: clinical implications of an updated model. *J Am Coll Cardiol.* 2009;54(5):375–85.

35. Borlaug BA, Redfield MM. Diastolic and systolic heart failure are distinct phenotypes within the heart failure spectrum. *Circulation.* 2011;123(18):2006–13; discussion 2014.

36. Pettersen MD. Cardiomyopathies encountered commonly in the teenage years and their presentation. *Pediatr Clin North Am.* 2014;61(1):173–86.

37. Towbin JA, Lowe AM, Colan SD, et al. Incidence, causes, and outcomes of dilated cardiomyopathy in children. *JAMA.* 2006;296(15):1867–76.

38. Franciosa JA, Park M, Levine TB. Lack of correlation between exercise capacity and indexes of resting left ventricular performance in heart failure. *Am J Cardiol.* 1981;47(1):33–9.

39. Malhotra R, Bakken K, D'Elia E, Lewis GD. Cardiopulmonary exercise testing in heart failure. *JACC Heart Fail.* 2016;4(8):607–16.

40. Hambrecht R, Gielen S, Linke A, et al. Effects of exercise training on left ventricular function and peripheral resistance in patients with chronic heart failure: a randomized trial. *JAMA.* 2000;283(23):3095–101.

41. Clark AL, Poole-Wilson PA, Coats AJ. Exercise limitation in chronic heart failure: central role of the periphery. *J Am Coll Cardiol.* 1996;28(5):1092–102.

42. Piepoli MF, Kaczmarek A, Francis DP, et al. Reduced peripheral skeletal muscle mass and abnormal reflex physiology in chronic heart failure. *Circulation.* 2006;114(2):126–34.

43. Kaczmarek A, Jankowska EA, Witkowski T, et al. Chronic heart failure. The relationship between increased activity of skeletal muscle ergoreceptors and reduced exercise tolerance. *Kardiol Pol.* 2004;60(4):322–32; discussion 333–4.

44. Guazzi M, Myers J, Peberdy MA, Bensimhon D, Chase P, Arena R. Maximal dyspnea on exertion during cardiopulmonary exercise testing is related to poor prognosis and echocardiography with tissue Doppler imaging in heart failure. *Congest Heart Fail.* 2009;15(6):277–83.

45. Hambrecht R, Fiehn E, Yu J, et al. Effects of endurance training on mitochondrial ultrastructure and fiber type distribution in skeletal muscle of patients with stable chronic heart failure. *J Am Coll Cardiol.* 1997;29(5):1067–73.

46. Rikli RE, Jones CJ. Development and validation of criterion-referenced clinically relevant fitness standards for maintaining physical independence in later years. *Gerontologist.* 2013;53(2):255–67.

47. Yancy CW, Jessup M, Bozkurt B, et al. 2016 ACC/AHA/HFSA focused update on new pharmacological therapy for heart failure: an update of the 2013 ACCF/AHA guideline for the management of heart failure: a report of the American College of Cardiology/American Heart Association Task Force on Clinical Practice Guidelines and the Heart Failure Society of America. *J Am Coll Cardiol.* 2016;68(13):1476–88.

48. McMurray JJ, Packer M, Desai AS, et al; PARADIGM-HF Investigators and Committees. Angiotensin-neprilysin inhibition versus enalapril in heart failure. *N Engl J Med.* 2014;371(11):993–1004.

49. Macdonald PS. Combined angiotensin receptor/neprilysin inhibitors: a review of the new paradigm in the management of chronic heart failure. *Clin Ther.* 2015;37(10):2199–205.

50. Fiuzat M, Wojdyla D, Pina I, Adams K, Whellan D, O'Connor CM. Heart rate or beta-blocker dose? Association with outcomes in ambulatory heart failure patients with systolic dysfunction: results from the HF-ACTION trial. *JACC Heart Fail.* 2016;4(2):109–15.

51. Edelmann F, Musial-Bright L, Gelbrich G, et al; CIBIS-ELD Investigators and Project Multicenter Trials in the Competence Network Heart Failure. Tolerability and feasibility of beta-blocker titration in HFpEF versus HFrEF: insights from the CIBIS-ELD trial. *JACC Heart Fail.* 2016;4(2):140–9.

52. Taylor AL, Ziesche S, Yancy C, et al; African-American Heart Failure Trial Investigators. Combination of isosorbide dinitrate and hydralazine in blacks with heart failure [Erratum appears in *N Engl J Med.* 2005;352(12):1276]. *N Engl J Med.* 2004;351(20):2049–57.

53. Moss AJ. MADIT-I and MADIT-II. *J Cardiovasc Electrophysiol.* 2003;14(9 Suppl):S96–8.

54. Shenkman HJ, Pampati V, Khandelwal AK, et al. Congestive heart failure and QRS duration: establishing prognosis study. *Chest.* 2002;122(2):528–34.

55. Abraham WT, Young JB, Leon AR, et al; Multicenter InSync ICD II Study Group. Effects of cardiac resynchronization on disease progression in patients with left ventricular systolic dysfunction, an indication for an implantable cardioverter-defibrillator, and mildly symptomatic chronic heart failure. *Circulation.* 2004;110(18):2864–8.

56. Moss AJ, Hall WJ, Cannom DS, et al; MADIT-CRT Trial Investigators. Cardiac-resynchronization therapy for the prevention of heart-failure events. *N Engl J Med.* 2009;361(14):1329–38.

57. Colvin-Adams M, Smithy JM, Heubner BM, et al. OPTN/SRTR 2012 annual data report: heart. *Am J Transplant.* 2014;14(suppl 1):113–38.

58. Slaughter MS, Pagani FD, Rogers JG, et al; HeartMate II Clinical Investigators. Clinical management of continuous-flow left ventricular assist devices in advanced heart failure. *J Heart Lung Transplant.* 2010;29(4 Suppl):S1–39.

59. Wilhelm MJ. Long-term outcome following heart transplantation: current perspective. *J Thorac Dis.* 2015;7(3):549–51.

60. Lund LH, Edwards LB, Dipchand AI, et al; International Society for Heart and Lung Transplantation. The Registry of the International Society for Heart and Lung Transplantation: thirty-third adult heart transplantation report—2016; focus theme: primary diagnostic indications for transplant. *J Heart Lung Transplant.* 2016;35(10):1158–69.

61. Colvin M, Smith JM, Skeans MA, et al. Heart. *Am J Transplant.* 2016;16(Suppl 2):115–40.

62. Jacques L, Jensen TS, Schafer J, McClain S, Chin J. Decision memo for intensive behavioral therapy for obesity (CAG-00423N). 2014. Available from: https://www.cms.gov/medicarecoverage-database/view/ncacaldecisionmemo.aspx?proposed=Y&NCAId=253

63. Mentz RJ, Kelly JP, von Lueder TG, et al. Noncardiac comorbidities in heart failure with reduced versus preserved ejection fraction. *J Am Coll Cardiol.* 2014;64(21):2281–93.

64. Maisel WH, Stevenson LW. Atrial fibrillation in heart failure: epidemiology, pathophysiology, and rationale for therapy. *Am J Cardiol.* 2003;91(6A):2D–8D.

65. Ades PA, Keteyian SJ, Balady GJ, et al. Cardiac rehabilitation exercise and self-care for chronic heart failure. *JACC Heart Fail.* 2013;1(6):540–7.

66. Riegel B, Moser DK, Powell M, Rector TS, Havranek EP. Nonpharmacologic care by heart failure experts. *J Card Fail.* 2006;12(2):149–53.

67. Riegel B, Dickson VV, Garcia LE, Masterson Creber R, Streur M. Mechanisms of change in self-care in adults with heart failure receiving a tailored, motivational interviewing intervention. *Patient Educ Couns.* 2017;100(2):283–8.

68. McCarthy MM, Dickson VV, Katz SD, Chyun DA. An exercise counseling intervention in minority adults with heart failure. *Rehabil Nurs.* 2017;42(3):146–6.

69. Blumenthal JA, Babyak MA, O'Connor C, et al. Effects of exercise training on depressive symptoms in patients with chronic heart failure: the HF-ACTION randomized trial [Erratum appears in *JAMA.* 2012;308(17):1742]. *JAMA.* 2012;308(5):465–74.

70. Hollriegel R, Winzer EB, Linke A, et al. Long-term exercise training in patients with advanced chronic heart failure:

sustained benefits on left ventricular performance and exercise capacity. *J Cardiopulm Rehabil Prev.* 2016;36(2):117–24.

71. Laoutaris ID, Adamopoulos S, Manginas A, et al. Benefits of combined aerobic/resistance/inspiratory training in patients with chronic heart failure. A complete exercise model? A prospective randomised study. *Int J Cardiol.* 2013;167(5):1967–72.

72. Thirapatarapong W, Thomas RJ, Pack Q, Sharma S, Squires RW. Commercial insurance coverage for outpatient cardiac rehabilitation in patients with heart failure in the United States. *J Cardiopulm Rehabil Prev.* 2014;34(6):386–9.

73. Keteyian SJ, Pina IL, Hibner BA, Fleg JL. Clinical role of exercise training in the management of patients with chronic heart failure. *J Cardiopulm Rehabil Prev.* 2010;30(2):67–76.

74. Womack CJ, Gardner AW, Nael R. Peripheral artery disease. In: Durstine JL, editor. *ACSM's Exercise Management for Persons with Chronic Diseases and Disabilities.* 3rd ed. Champaign (IL): Human Kinetics; 2009. p. 114–9.

75. Criqui MH, Aboyans V. Epidemiology of peripheral artery disease. *Circ Res.* 2015;116(9):1509–26.

76. Panaich SS, Arora S, Patel N, et al. Comparison of inhospital outcomes and hospitalization costs of peripheral angioplasty and endovascular stenting. *Am J Cardiol.* 2015;116(4):634–41.

77. Hirsch AT, Hartman L, Town RJ, Virnig BA. National health care costs of peripheral arterial disease in the Medicare population. *Vasc Med.* 2008;13(3):209–15.

78. Allison MA, Ho E, Denenberg JO, et al. Ethnic-specific prevalence of peripheral arterial disease in the United States [Erratum appears in *Am J Prev Med.* 2014;47(1):103]. *Am J Prev Med.* 2007;32(4):328–33.

79. Criqui MH, Fronek A, Barrett-Connor E, Klauber MR, Gabriel S, Goodman D. The prevalence of peripheral arterial disease in a defined population. *Circulation.* 1985;71(3):510–5.

80. Bonow RO, Mann DL, Zipes DP, Libby P. *Braunwald's Heart Disease: A Textbook of Cardiovascular Medicine.* 9th ed. Philadelphia (PA): Elsevier Health Sciences; 2011.

81. Tadej M. A service pathway for patients at risk of peripheral arterial disease. *Br J Community Nurs.* 2013;18(4):168–72.

82. Creager MA, Loscalzo J. Vascular diseases of the extremities. In: Fauci AS, Braunwald E, Kasper DL, editors. *Harrison's Principles of Internal Medicine.* New York (NY): McGraw Hill; 2008. p. 1568–75.

83. Rooke TW, Wennberg PW. Diagnosis and management of diseases of the peripheral arteries and veins. In: Fuster V, O'Rourke RA, Walsh RA, Poole-Wilson P, editors. *Hurst's The Heart.* 12th ed. New York (NY): McGraw Hill; 2008. p. 2361–79.

84. Guyatt GH, Feeny DH, Patrick DL. Measuring health-related quality of life. *Ann Intern Med.* 1993;118(8):622–9.

85. McDermott MM, Greenland P, Liu K, et al. Leg symptoms in peripheral arterial disease: associated clinical characteristics and functional impairment. *JAMA.* 2001;286(13):1599–606.

86. Revicki DA. Health-related quality of life in the evaluation of medical therapy for chronic illness. *J Fam Pract.* 1989;29(4):377–80.

87. Regensteiner JG, Hiatt WR, Coll JR, et al. The impact of peripheral arterial disease on health-related quality of life in the peripheral arterial disease awareness, risk, and treatment: new resources for survival (PARTNERS) program. *Vasc Med.* 2008;13(1):15–24.

88. McDermott MM, Liu K, Greenland P, et al. Functional decline in peripheral arterial disease: associations with the ankle brachial index and leg symptoms. *JAMA.* 2004;292(4):453–61.

89. Marrett E, DiBonaventura M, Zhang Q. Burden of peripheral arterial disease in Europe and the United States: a patient survey. *Health Qual Life Outcomes.* 2013;11:175.

90. James PA, Oparil S, Carter BL, et al. 2014 evidence-based guideline for the management of high blood pressure in adults: report from the panel members appointed to the Eighth Joint National Committee (JNC 8) [Erratum appears in *JAMA.* 2014;311(17):1809]. *JAMA.* 2014;311(5):507–20.

91. Tsao CW, Aday AW, Almarzooq ZI, et al. Heart disease and stroke statistics-2022 update: a report from the American Heart Association. *Circulation.* 2022;145(8):e153–639.

92. Hall JE, Granger JP, do Carmo JM, et al. Hypertension: physiology and pathophysiology. *Compr Physiol.* 2012;2(4):2393–442.

93. Rao MS. Pathogenesis and consequences of essential hypertension. *J Indian Med Assoc.* 2003;101(4):251–3.

94. Oparil S, Zaman MA, Calhoun DA. Pathogenesis of hypertension. *Ann Intern Med.* 2003;139(9):761–76.

95. Whelton PK, Carey RM, Aronow WS, et al. 2017 ACC/AHA/AAPA/ABC/ACPM/AGS/APhA/ASH/ASPC/NMA/PCNA guideline for the prevention, detection, evaluation, and management of high blood pressure in adults: a report of the American College of Cardiology/American Heart Association Task Force on Clinical Practice Guidelines. *Hypertension.* 2018;71(6):e13–115.

96. Hongwei JI, Niiranen TJ, Fader F, et al. Sex differences in blood pressure associations with cardiovascular outcomes. *Circulation.* 2021;143(7): 761–3.

97. Guirguis-Blake JM, Evans CV, Webber EM, Coppola EL, Perdue LA, Weyrich MS. Screening for hypertension in adults: updated evidence report and systematic review for the US Preventive Services Task Force. *JAMA.* 2021;325(16):1657–69.

98. Muntner P, Shimbo D, Carey RM, et al. Measurement of blood pressure in humans: a scientific statement from the American Heart Association. *Hypertension.* 2019;73(5):e35–66.

99. Roman MJ, Devereux RB, Kizer JR, et al. Central pressure more strongly relates to vascular disease and outcome than does brachial pressure: the strong heart study. *Hypertension.* 2007;50(1):197–203.

100. Safar M, O'Rourke MF. *Arterial Stiffness in Hypertension.* New York (NY): Elsevier; 2006.

101. Laurent S, Cockcroft J, Van Bortel L, et al; European Network for Non-invasive Investigation of Large Arteries. Expert consensus document on arterial stiffness: methodological issues and clinical applications. *Eur Heart J.* 2006;27(21):2588–605.

102. Veerasamy M, Bagnall A, Neely D, Allen J, Sinclair H, Kunadian V. Endothelial dysfunction and coronary artery disease: a state of the art review. *Cardiol Rev.* 2015;23(3):119–29.

103. Marti CN, Gheorghiade M, Kalogeropoulos AP, Georgiopoulou VV, Quyyumi AA, Butler J. Endothelial dysfunction, arterial stiffness, and heart failure. *J Am Coll Cardiol.* 2012;60(16):1455–69.

104. Csiszar A, Ungvari Z, Edwards JG, et al. Aging-induced phenotypic changes and oxidative stress impair coronary arteriolar function. *Circ Res.* 2002;90(11):1159–66.

105. Hall JE. *Guyton and Hall Textbook of Medical Physiology.* 13th ed. Philadelphia (PA): Elsevier; 2016.

106. Must A, Spadano J, Coakley EH, Field AE, Colditz G, Dietz WH. The disease burden associated with overweight and obesity. *JAMA.* 1999;282(16):1523–9.

107. Centers for Disease Control and Prevention. *Obesity and Overweight.* Hyattsville (MD): National Center for Health Statistics; 2016. Available from: https://www.cdc.gov/nchs/fastats/obesity-overweight.htm.

108. Ward ZJ, Bleich SN, Cradock AL, et al. Projected US state-level prevalence of adult obesity and severe obesity. *N Engl J Med.* 2019;381(25):2440–50.

109. Davy KP, Orr JS. Sympathetic nervous system behavior in human obesity. *Neurosci Biobehav Rev.* 2009;33(2):116–24.

110. Carlyle M, Jones OB, Kuo JJ, Hall JE. Chronic cardiovascular and renal actions of leptin: role of adrenergic activity. *Hypertension.* 2002;39(2 Pt 2):496–501.

111. do Carmo JM, da Silva AA, Sessums PO, et al. Role of Shp2 in forebrain neurons in regulating metabolic and cardiovascular functions and responses to leptin. *Int J Obes.* 2014;38(6):775–83.

112. Hilzendeger AM, Morgan DA, Brooks L, et al. A brain leptin-renin angiotensin system interaction in the regulation of sympathetic nerve activity. *Am J Physiol Heart Circ Physiol.* 2012;303(2):H197–206.

113. Chapleau MW, Hajduczok G, Abboud FM. Mechanisms of resetting of arterial baroreceptors: an overview. *Am J Med Sci.* 1988;295(4):327–34.

114. Grassi G, Dell'Oro R, Facchini A, Quarti Trevano F, Bolla GB, Mancia G. Effect of central and peripheral body fat distribution on sympathetic and baroreflex function in obese normotensives. *J Hypertens.* 2004;22(12):2363–9.

115. Wofford MR, Hall JE. Pathophysiology and treatment of obesity hypertension. *Curr Pharm Des.* 2004;10(29):3621–37.

116. Szasz T, Bomfim GF, Webb RC. The influence of perivascular adipose tissue on vascular homeostasis. *Vasc Health Risk Manag.* 2013;9:105–16.

117. DeMarco VG, Aroor AR, Sowers JR. The pathophysiology of hypertension in patients with obesity. *Nat Rev Endocrinol.* 2014;10(6):364–76.

118. Mathieu P, Poirier P, Pibarot P, Lemieux I, Despres JP. Visceral obesity: the link among inflammation, hypertension, and cardiovascular disease. *Hypertension.* 2009;53(4):577–84.

119. Pietri P, Vlachopoulos C, Tousoulis D. Inflammation and arterial hypertension: from pathophysiological links to risk prediction. *Curr Med Chem.* 2015;22(23):2754–61.

120. Lago R, Gomez R, Lago F, Gomez-Reino J, Gualillo O. Leptin beyond body weight regulation: current concepts concerning its role in immune function and inflammation. *Cell Immunol.* 2008;252(1–2):139–45.

121. Dixit VD. Adipose-immune interactions during obesity and caloric restriction: reciprocal mechanisms regulating immunity and health span. *J Leukoc Biol.* 2008;84(4):882–92.

122. Cani PD, Delzenne NM, Amar J, Burcelin R. Role of gut microflora in the development of obesity and insulin resistance following high-fat diet feeding. *Pathol Biol.* 2008;56(5):305–9.

123. Geurts L, Lazarevic V, Derrien M, et al. Altered gut microbiota and endocannabinoid system tone in obese and diabetic leptin-resistant mice: impact on apelin regulation in adipose tissue. *Front Microbiol.* 2011;2:149.

124. Hersoug LG, Moller P, Loft S. Gut microbiota-derived lipopolysaccharide uptake and trafficking to adipose tissue: implications for inflammation and obesity. *Obes Rev.* 2016;17(4):297–312.

125. Creely SJ, McTernan PG, Kusminski CM, et al. Lipopolysaccharide activates an innate immune system response in human adipose tissue in obesity and type 2 diabetes. *Am J Physiol Endocrinol Metab.* 2007;292(3):E740–7.

126. Barengo NC, Hu G, Kastarinen M, et al. Low physical activity as a predictor for antihypertensive drug treatment in 25–64-year-old populations in eastern and south-western Finland. *J Hypertens.* 2005;23(2):293–9.

127. Haapanen N, Miilunpalo S, Vuori I, Oja P, Pasanen M. Association of leisure time physical activity with the risk of coronary heart disease, hypertension and diabetes in middle-aged men and women. *Int J Epidemiol.* 1997;26(4):739–47.

128. Montoye HJ, Metzner HL, Keller JB, Johnson BC, Epstein FH. Habitual physical activity and blood pressure. *Med Sci Sports.* 1972;4(4):175–81.

129. Pereira MA, Folsom AR, McGovern PG, et al. Physical activity and incident hypertension in black and white adults: the Atherosclerosis Risk in Communities Study. *Prev Med.* 1999;28(3):304–12.

130. Blair SN, Goodyear NN, Gibbons LW, Cooper KH. Physical fitness and incidence of hypertension in healthy normotensive men and women. *JAMA.* 1984;252(4):487–90.

131. Paffenbarger RS Jr, Wing AL, Hyde RT, Jung DL. Physical activity and incidence of hypertension in college alumni. *Am J Epidemiol.* 1983;117(3):245–57.

132. Kokkinos P. Cardiorespiratory fitness, exercise, blood pressure. *Hypertension.* 2014;64(6):1160–4.

133. Lee S, Kuk JL, Katzmarzyk PT, Blair SN, Church TS, Ross R. Cardiorespiratory fitness attenuates metabolic risk independent of abdominal subcutaneous and visceral fat in men. *Diabetes Care.* 2005;28(4):895–901.

134. Wong SL, Katzmarzyk P, Nichaman MZ, Church TS, Blair SN, Ross R. Cardiorespiratory fitness is associated with lower abdominal fat independent of body mass index. *Med Sci Sports Exerc.* 2004;36(2):286–91.

135. Laragh JH, Brenner BM. *Hypertension: Pathophysiology, Diagnosis, and Management.* 2nd ed. New York (NY): Raven Press; 1995.

136. Grinnan D, Farr G, Fox A, Sweeney L. The role of hyperglycemia and insulin resistance in the development and progression of pulmonary arterial hypertension. *J Diabetes Res.* 2016;2016:2481659.

137. Rao A, Pandya V, Whaley-Connell A. Obesity and insulin resistance in resistant hypertension: implications for the kidney. *Adv Chronic Kidney Dis.* 2015;22(3):211–7.

138. Shirwany NA, Zou MH. Arterial stiffness: a brief review. *Acta Pharmacol Sin.* 2010;31(10):1267–76.

139. Sell DR, Monnier VM. Molecular basis of arterial stiffening: role of glycation: a mini-review. *Gerontology.* 2012;58(3):227–37.

140. Cattell MA, Anderson JC, Hasleton PS. Age-related changes in amounts and concentrations of collagen and elastin in normotensive human thoracic aorta. *Clin Chim Acta.* 1996;245(1):73–84.

141. Reiser K, McCormick RJ, Rucker RB. Enzymatic and nonenzymatic cross-linking of collagen and elastin. *FASEB J.* 1992;6(7):2439–49.

142. Watanabe M, Sawai T, Nagura H, Suyama K. Age-related alteration of cross-linking amino acids of elastin in human aorta. *Tohoku J Exp Med.* 1996;180(2):115–30.

143. Kelly JJ, Mangos G, Williamson PM, Whitworth JA. Cortisol and hypertension. *Clin Exp Pharmacol Physiol Suppl.* 1998;25:S51–6.

144. Lip GYH, Hall JE. *Comprehensive Hypertension*. Philadelphia (PA): Mosby Elsevier; 2007.

145. Williamson PM, Kelly JJ, Whitworth JA. Dose-response relationships and mineralocorticoid activity in cortisol-induced hypertension in humans. *J Hypertens Suppl*. 1996;14(5):S37–41.

146. Yamori Y, Matsumoto M, Yamabe H, Okamoto K. Augmentation of spontaneous hypertension by chronic stress in rats. *Jpn Circ J*. 1969;33(4):399–409.

147. Davies AO, Lefkowitz RJ. Regulation of beta-adrenergic receptors by steroid hormones. *Annu Rev Physiol*. 1984;46:119–30.

148. al'Absi M, Arnett DK. Adrenocortical responses to psychological stress and risk for hypertension. *Biomed Pharmacother*. 2000;54(5):234–44.

149. Cui J, Hopper JL, Harrap SB. Genes and family environment explain correlations between blood pressure and body mass index. *Hypertension*. 2002;40(1):7–12.

150. Longini IM Jr, Higgins MW, Hinton PC, Moll PP, Keller JB. Environmental and genetic sources of familial aggregation of blood pressure in Tecumseh, Michigan. *Am J Epidemiol*. 1984;120(1):131–44.

151. Bogdarina I, Welham S, King PJ, Burns SP, Clark AJ. Epigenetic modification of the renin-angiotensin system in the fetal programming of hypertension. *Circ Res*. 2007;100(4):520–6.

152. Lillycrop KA, Phillips ES, Jackson AA, Hanson MA, Burdge GC. Dietary protein restriction of pregnant rats induces and folic acid supplementation prevents epigenetic modification of hepatic gene expression in the offspring. *J Nutr*. 2005;135(6):1382–6.

153. Lillycrop KA, Phillips ES, Torrens C, Hanson MA, Jackson AA, Burdge GC. Feeding pregnant rats a protein-restricted diet persistently alters the methylation of specific cytosines in the hepatic PPAR alpha promoter of the offspring. *Br J Nutr*. 2008;100(2):278–82.

154. Erhuma A, McMullen S, Langley-Evans SC, Bennett AJ. Feeding pregnant rats a low-protein diet alters the hepatic expression of SREBP-1c in their offspring via a glucocorticoid-related mechanism. *Endocrine*. 2009;36(2):333–8.

155. Darnaudery M, Maccari S. Epigenetic programming of the stress response in male and female rats by prenatal restraint stress. *Brain Res Rev*. 2008;57(2):571–85.

156. Eaton SB, Eaton SB 3rd, Konner MJ, Shostak M. An evolutionary perspective enhances understanding of human nutritional requirements. *J Nutr*. 1996;126(6):1732–40.

157. Harnack LJ, Cogswell ME, Shikany JM, et al. Sources of sodium in US adults from 3 geographic regions. *Circulation*. 2017;135(19):1775–83.

158. Falkner B, Kushner H. Effect of chronic sodium loading on cardiovascular response in young blacks and whites. *Hypertension*. 1990;15(1):36–43.

159. Luft FC, Miller JZ, Grim CE, et al. Salt sensitivity and resistance of blood pressure. Age and race as factors in physiological responses. *Hypertension*. 1991;17(1 Suppl):I102–8.

160. Weinberger MH, Miller JZ, Luft FC, Grim CE, Fineberg NS. Definitions and characteristics of sodium sensitivity and blood pressure resistance. *Hypertension*. 1986;8(6 Pt 2):II127–34.

161. Carey RM, Schoeffel CD, Gildea JJ, et al. Salt sensitivity of blood pressure is associated with polymorphisms in the sodium-bicarbonate cotransporter. *Hypertension*. 2012;60(5):1359–66.

162. Weinberger MH. Salt sensitivity of blood pressure in humans. *Hypertension*. 1996;27(3 Pt 2):481–90.

163. Choi HY, Park HC, Ha SK. Salt sensitivity and hypertension: a paradigm shift from kidney malfunction to vascular endothelial dysfunction. *Electrolyte Blood Press*. 2015;13(1):7–16.

164. Cowley AW Jr. Long-term control of arterial blood pressure. *Physiol Rev*. 1992;72(1):231–300.

165. Oberleithner H, Riethmuller C, Schillers H, MacGregor GA, de Wardener HE, Hausberg M. Plasma sodium stiffens vascular endothelium and reduces nitric oxide release. *Proc Natl Acad Sci U S A*. 2007;104(41):16281–6.

166. Olde Engberink RH, Rorije NM, Homan van der Heide JJ, van den Born BJ, Vogt L. Role of the vascular wall in sodium homeostasis and salt sensitivity. *J Am Soc Nephrol*. 2015;26(4):777–83.

167. Hedman K, Lindow T, Cauwenberghs N, et al. Peak exercise SBP and future risk of cardiovascular disease and mortality. *J Hypertension*. 2022;40(2):3000–309.

168. Hedman K, Kaminsky LA, Sabbahi A, et al. Low but not high exercise systolic blood pressure is associated with long-term all-cause mortality. *BMJ Open Sport Exerc Med*. 2021;7(2):e001106.

169. Toner MM, Sawka MN, Levine L, Pandolf KB. Cardiorespiratory responses to exercise distributed between the upper and lower body. *J Appl Physiol Respir Environ Exerc Physiol*. 1983;54(5):1403–7.

170. Vokac Z, Bell H, Bautz-Holter E, Rodahl K. Oxygen uptake/heart rate relationship in leg and arm exercise, sitting and standing. *J Appl Physiol*. 1975;39(1):54–9.

171. Faria EW, Faria IE. Cardiorespiratory responses to exercises of equal relative intensity distributed between the upper and lower body. *J Sports Sci*. 1998;16(4):309–15.

172. Palatini P, Mos L, Munari L, et al. Blood pressure changes during heavy-resistance exercise. *J Hypertens Suppl*. 1989;7(6):S72–3.

173. Pescatello LS, Franklin BA, Fagard R, et al. American College of Sports Medicine position stand. Exercise and hypertension. *Med Sci Sports Exerc*. 2004;36(3):533–53.

174. Pescatello LS, Buchner DM, Jakicic JM, et al.; 2018 Physical Activity Guidelines Advisory Committee. Physical activity to prevent and treat hypertension: a systematic review. *Med Sci Sports Exerc*. 2019;51(6):1314–23.

175. Hall MJ, Levant S, DeFrances CJ. Hospitalization for stroke in U.S. hospitals, 1989–2009. *NCHS Data Brief*. 2012;(95):1–8.

176. Centers for Disease Control and Prevention. Prevalence of stroke—United States, 2006–2010. *MMWR Morb Mortal Wkly Rep*. 2012;61(20):379–82.

177. Centers for Disease Control and Prevention. Vital signs: awareness and treatment of uncontrolled hypertension among adults—United States, 2003–2010. *MMWR Morb Mortal Wkly Rep*. 2012;61:703–9.

178. Lackland DT, Roccella EJ, Deutsch AF, et al; American Heart Association Stroke Council; Council on Cardiovascular and Stroke Nursing; Council on Quality of Care and Outcomes Research; Council on Functional Genomics and Translational Biology. Factors influencing the decline in stroke mortality: a statement from the American Heart Association/American Stroke Association. *Stroke*. 2014;45(1):315–53.

179. Palmer-McLean K, Harbst K. Stroke and brain injury. In: Durstine JL, editor. *ACSM's Exercise Management for Persons*

with Chronic Diseases and Disabilities. 3rd ed. Champaign (IL): Human Kinetics; 2009. p. 287–8.

180. Hinkle JL, Bowman L. Neuroprotection for ischemic stroke. *J Neurosci Nurs*. 2003;35(2):114–8.

181. Billinger SA, Arena R, Bernhardt, et al; American Heart Association Stroke Council; Council on Cardiovascular and Stroke Nursing; Council on Lifestyle and Cardiometabolic Health; Council on Epidemiology and Prevention; Council on Clinical Cardiology. Physical activity and exercise recommendations for stroke survivors: a statement for healthcare professionals from the American Heart Association/American Stroke Association. *Stroke*. 2014;45(8):2532–53.

182. Squires RW. Cardiac rehabilitation issues for heart transplantation patients. *J Cardiopulm Rehabil Prev*. 1990;10(5):159–68.

183. Toscano G, Bottio T, Gambino A, et al. Orthotopic heart transplantation: the bicaval technique. *Multimed Man Cardiothorac Surg*. 2015;2015:mmv035.

184. Alraies MC, Eckman P. Adult heart transplant: indications and outcomes. *J Thorac Dis*. 2014;6(8):1120–8.

185. Mehra MR, Canter CE, Hannan MM, et al; International Society for Heart Lung Transplantation (ISHLT) Infectious Diseases, Pediatric and Heart Failure and Transplantation Councils. The 2016 International Society for Heart Lung Transplantation listing criteria for heart transplantation: a 10-year update. *J Heart Lung Transplant*. 2016;35(1):1–23.

186. Miller L. Heart transplantation in patients with diabetes. *Circulation*. 2006;114(21):2206–7.

187. Unger T, Li J. The role of the renin-angiotensin-aldosterone system in heart failure. *J Renin Angiotensin Aldosterone Syst*. 2004;5(Suppl 1):S7–10.

188. Silva Enciso J, Kato TS, Jin Z, et al. Effect of peripheral vascular disease on mortality in cardiac transplant recipients (from the United Network of Organ Sharing Database). *Am J Cardiol*. 2014;114(7):1111–5.

189. Lund LH, Edwards LB, Kucheryavaya AY, et al; International Society for Heart and Lung Transplantation. The Registry of the International Society for Heart and Lung Transplantation: thirtieth official adult heart transplant report—2013; focus theme: age. *J Heart Lung Transplant*. 2013;32(10):951–64.

190. Yamani MH, Taylor DO. *Heart Transplantation*. Cleveland (OH): Cleveland Clinic Center for Continuing Education; 2010.

191. Schmauss D, Weis M. Cardiac allograft vasculopathy: recent developments. *Circulation*. 2008;117(16):2131–41.

192. Ramakrishna H, Jaroszewski DE, Arabia FA. Adult cardiac transplantation: a review of perioperative management part-I. *Ann Card Anaesth*. 2009;12(1):71–8.

193. DiNardo JA. *Anesthesia for Cardiac Surgery*. 2nd ed. Stamford (CT): Appleton & Lange; 1998. p. 213–14, 219–20.

194. Lindenfeld J, Miller GG, Shakar SF, et al. Drug therapy in the heart transplant recipient: part I: cardiac rejection and immunosuppressive drugs. *Circulation*. 2004;110(24):3734–40.

195. Khush KK, Hsich E, Potena L, et al; International Society for Heart and Lung Transplantation. The International Thoracic Organ Transplant Registry of the International Society for Heart and Lung Transplantation: Thirty-eighth adult heart transplantation report-2021; focus on recipient characteristics. *J Heart Lung Transplant*. 2021;40(10):1035–49.

196. Jakovljevic DG, Yacoub MH, Schueler S, et al. Left ventricular assist device as a bridge to recovery for patients with advanced heart failure. *J Am Coll Cardiol*. 2017;69(15):1924–33.

197. Feldman D, Pamboukian SV, Teuteberg JJ, et al; International Society for Heart and Lung Transplantation. The 2013 International Society for Heart and Lung Transplantation Guidelines for mechanical circulatory support: executive summary. *J Heart Lung Transplant*. 2013;32(2):157–87.

198. Loyaga-Rendon RY, Plaisance EP, Arena R, Shah K. Exercise physiology, testing, and training in patients supported by a left ventricular assist device. *J Heart Lung Transplant*. 2015; 34(8):1005–16.

199. Okwuosa I, Pumphrey D, Puthumana J, Brown R, Cotts W. Impact of identification and treatment of depression in heart transplant patients. *Cardiovasc Psychiatry Neurol*. 2014; 2014:747293.

200. Conway A, Sheridan J, Maddicks-Law J, et al. Accuracy of anxiety and depression screening tools in heart transplant recipients. *Appl Nurs Res*. 2016;32:177–81.

201. Tucker WJ, Beaudry RI, Samuel J, et al. Performance limitations in heart transplant recipients. *Exerc Sport Sci Rev*. 2018;46(3):144–51.

202. Dall CH, Snoer M, Christensen S, et al. Effect of high-intensity training versus moderate training on peak oxygen uptake and chronotropic response in heart transplant recipients: a randomized crossover trial. *Am J Transplant*. 2014;14(10):2391–9.

203. Nytrøen K, Rolid K, Andreassen AK, et al. Effect of high-intensity interval training in de novo heart transplant recipients in Scandinavia. *Circulation*. 2019; 139:2198–211.

204. Richard R, Verdier JC, Duvallet A, et al. Chronotropic competence in endurance training heart transplant recipients: heart rate is not a limiting factor for exercise capacity. *J Am Coll Cardiol*. 1999;33(1):192–7.

205. Pokan R, Von Duvillard SP, Ludwig J, et al. Effect of high-volume and -intensity endurance training in heart transplant recipients. *Med Sci Sports Exerc*. 2004;36(12):2011–6.

206. Haykowsky MJ, Halle M, Baggish A. Upper limits of aerobic power and performance in heart transplant recipients: legacy effect of prior endurance training. *Circulation*. 2018;137(7):650–2.

207. Bachmann JM, Shah AS, Duncan MS, et al. Cardiac rehabilitation and readmissions after heart transplantation. *J Heart Lung Transplant*. 2018;37(4):467–76.

208. Alfonso F, Bastante T, Rivero F, et al. Spontaneous coronary artery dissection. *Circ J*. 2014;78(9):2099–110.

209. Pretty HC. Dissecting aneurysm of coronary artery in a woman aged 42: rupture. *Br Med J*. 1931;1(3667):667.

210. Lodha A, Mirsakov N, Malik B, Shani J. Spontaneous coronary artery dissection: case report and review of literature. *South Med J*. 2009;102(3):315–7.

211. Hayes SN. Spontaneous coronary artery dissection (SCAD): new insights into this not-so-rare condition. *Tex Heart Inst J*. 2014;41(3):295–8.

212. Saw J, Mancini GBJ, Humphries KH. Contemporary review on spontaneous coronary artery dissection. *J Am Coll Cardiol*. 2016;68(3):297–312.

213. Saw J, Mancini GB, Humphries K, et al. Angiographic appearance of spontaneous coronary artery dissection with intramural hematoma proven on intracoronary imaging. *Catheter Cardiovasc Interv*. 2016;87(2):E54–61.

214. Tweet MS, Hayes SN, Pitta SR, et al. Clinical features, management, and prognosis of spontaneous coronary artery dissection. *Circulation*. 2012;126(5):579–88.

215. Koul AK, Hollander G, Moskovits N, Frankel R, Herrera L, Shani J. Coronary artery dissection during pregnancy and the postpartum period: two case reports and review of literature. *Catheter Cardiovasc Interv.* 2001;52(1):88–94.

216. Steinhauer JR, Caulfield JB. Spontaneous coronary artery dissection associated with cocaine use: a case report and brief review. *Cardiovasc Pathol.* 2001;10(3):141–5.

217. Maehara A, Mintz GS, Castagna MT, et al. Intravascular ultrasound assessment of spontaneous coronary artery dissection. *Am J Cardiol.* 2002;89(4):466–8.

218. Alfonso F, Paulo M, Gonzalo N, et al. Diagnosis of spontaneous coronary artery dissection by optical coherence tomography. *J Am Coll Cardiol.* 2012;59(12):1073–9.

219. Saw J, Ricci D, Starovoytov A, Fox R, Buller CE. Spontaneous coronary artery dissection: prevalence of predisposing conditions including fibromuscular dysplasia in a tertiary center cohort. *JACC Cardiovasc Interv.* 2013;6(1):44–52.

220. Giacoppo D, Capodanno D, Dangas G, Tamburino C. Spontaneous coronary artery dissection. *Int J Cardiol.* 2014;175(1):8–20.

221. Eleid MF, Guddeti RR, Tweet MS, et al. Coronary artery tortuosity in spontaneous coronary artery dissection: angiographic characteristics and clinical implications. *Circ Cardiovasc Interv.* 2014;7(5):656–62.

222. Mortensen KH, Thuesen L, Kristensen IB, Christiansen EH. Spontaneous coronary artery dissection: a Western Denmark Heart Registry study. *Catheter Cardiovasc Interv.* 2009;74(5):710–7.

223. Ito H, Taylor L, Bowman M, Fry ET, Hermiller JB, Van Tassel JW. Presentation and therapy of spontaneous coronary artery dissection and comparisons of postpartum versus nonpostpartum cases. *Am J Cardiol.* 2011;107(11):1590–6.

224. Alfonso F, Paulo M, Lennie V, et al. Spontaneous coronary artery dissection: long-term follow-up of a large series of patients prospectively managed with a "conservative" therapeutic strategy. *JACC Cardiovasc Interv.* 2012;5(10):1062–70.

225. Al-Hussaini A, Adlam D. Spontaneous coronary artery dissection. *Heart.* 2017;103(13):1043–51.

226. Tweet M, Hayes S, Lerman A, et al. Percutaneous coronary intervention for acute spontaneous coronary artery dissection is associated with reduced rates of technical success: abstract 17969. *Circulation.* 2012;126(Suppl 21):A17969.

227. Tweet MS, Eleid MF, Best PJ, et al. Spontaneous coronary artery dissection: revascularization versus conservative therapy. *Circ Cardiovasc Interv.* 2014;7(6):777–86.

228. Mayo Foundation for Medical Education and Research. Spontaneous coronary artery dissection (SCAD): overview. Rochester (MN): Mayo Foundation for Medical Education and Research; 2017. Available from: https://www.mayoclinic.org/diseasesconditions/spontaneous-coronaryartery-dissection/symptoms-causes/syc-20353711.

229. Chou AY, Prakash R, Rajala J, et al. The first dedicated cardiac rehabilitation program for patients with spontaneous coronary artery dissection: description and initial results. *Can J Cardiol.* 2016;32(4):554–60.

230. Krittanawong C, Tweet MS, Hayes SE, et al. Usefulness of cardiac rehabilitation after spontaneous coronary artery dissection. *Am J Cardiol.* 2016;117(10):1604–9.

231. Silber TC, Tweet MS, Bowman MJ, Hayes SN, Squires RW. Cardiac rehabilitation after spontaneous coronary artery dissection. *J Cardiopulm Rehabil Prev.* 2015;35(5):328–33.

232. Mittleman MA, Maclure M, Tofler GH, Sherwood JB, Goldberg RJ, Muller JE. Triggering of acute myocardial infarction by heavy physical exertion. Protection against triggering by regular exertion. Determinants of Myocardial Infarction Onset Study Investigators. *N Engl J Med.* 1993;329(23):1677–83.

233. Tweet MS, Olin JW, Bonikowske AR, Adlam D, Hayes SN. Physical activity and exercise in patients with spontaneous coronary artery dissection and fibromuscular dysplasia. *Eur Heart J.* 2021;42:3825–8.

234. Hayes SN, Kim ESH, Saw J, et al. Spontaneous coronary artery dissection: current state of the science. A scientific statement from the American Heart Association. *Circulation.* 2018;137:e523–57.

235. Patterson MA, Hayes SN, Squires RW, Tweet MS. Home-based cardiac rehabilitation in a young athletic woman following spontaneous coronary artery dissection. *J Clin Exerc Physiol.* 2016;5(1):6–11.

CHAPTER

6

Electrocardiography

INTRODUCTION

An electrocardiogram (abbreviated ECG or EKG from the German "kardio") is a recording of the electrical activity of the heart. For decades, the ECG has been an important tool in the clinical laboratory for the diagnosis of heart disease. For the clinical exercise physiologist (CEP) working in stress testing, cardiac rehabilitation, or related fields, the ability to accurately interpret an ECG is one of the most important skills to master. This chapter covers all the major areas of ECG interpretation. After describing mechanisms within the normal ECG, it introduces pacemakers and selected pathologies the CEP is likely to encounter. The chapter concludes with a discussion of the exercise stress test and exercise ECGs.

MEASUREMENT OF BASIC EVENTS OF THE NORMAL CARDIAC CYCLE

The purpose of this chapter is practical, to teach skills of ECG analysis. Electrophysiological concepts are discussed when they facilitate ECG interpretation; however, it is more productive to think in terms of the basic underlying electrical events than to simply memorize criteria for the various abnormalities.

ECG Paper and Calibration

As shown in Figure 6.1, the paper that is normally used to record ECGs has a grid pattern consisting of thin lines every millimeter in both the horizontal and vertical planes, with thicker lines every 5 mm. On the horizontal or *x* axis, each of these 1-mm boxes represents 40 ms (0.04 s) of elapsed time. Thus, five of these "small" (1 mm) boxes, or one "big" (5 mm) box is equivalent to 200 ms (0.20 s). On the vertical, or *y* axis, each 1-mm box represents 0.1 mV of

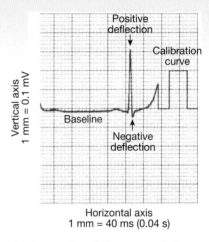

FIGURE 6.1 ECG paper. Each "thin" line equals 1 mm. Each "thick" line equals 5 mm. The calibration box is 10-mm tall (1.0 mV).

voltage, resulting in 10 mm of upward deflection (10 "little" or 2 "big" boxes) being equivalent to 1 mV (10 × 0.1 mV). By convention, upward deflections are referred to as positive and those moving downward are called negative.

All ECG machines provide some indication of calibration. The standard calibration mark is a 10-mm (1-mV) box (see Figures 6.1 and 6.2) or the printing of a phrase such as "1 cm = 1 mV" on the paper. Very large complexes may run off the paper and require the calibration to be changed to half (1 mV = 5 mm); conversely, very small ECG complexes can be enlarged for closer inspection by setting the calibration to 2× (1 mV = 20 mm). The effect of varying calibration is shown in Figure 6.2. To avoid misinterpretation of the magnitude of positive or negative deflections (*e.g.*, ST-segment elevation or depression), any deviation from the standard calibration voltage must be indicated on the ECG.

Paper speed can also be varied. Standard paper speed is 25 mm·s⁻¹, resulting in each 1-mm box representing 40 ms (0.04 s) of elapsed time on the *x* axis. Most machines also can be set to run at half (12.5 mm·s⁻¹) speed or double (50 mm·s⁻¹) speed. Under these conditions, 1 mm will

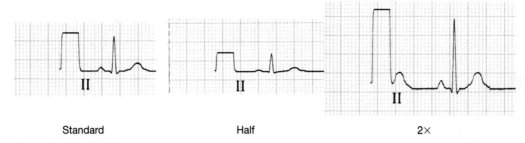

Standard   Half   2×

FIGURE 6.2 Calibration.

represent 80 ms (0.08 s) and 20 ms (0.02 s), respectively, instead of the usual 40 ms. Paper speed is often written on the top or bottom of the ECG paper. Any alteration in paper speed from normal (25 mm·s⁻¹) must be reported on the ECG.

P Wave and PR Segment

Normally, the first electrical event of a cardiac cycle is the depolarization of the atria. It begins in the sinoatrial (SA) node and spreads through the atria from cell to cell. Because the atria are relatively small, thin-walled chambers, the ECG will typically show a rather small waveform, termed the *P wave* (Figure 6.3). The normal P wave should be less than 120 ms (3 mm or 3 small squares) in duration and less than 0.25 mV (2.5 mm or 2.5 small squares) in amplitude. The normal ranges for a variety of ECG parameters are listed in Box 6.1.

A brief pause in the electrical impulse called the PR segment occurs after the P wave. The PR segment represents the electrically quiet period between atrial and ventricular depolarization. Intervals include both waves and segments; thus, the PR interval is the duration from the beginning of the P wave to the beginning of the QRS

complex and includes both the P wave and the PR segment (Figure 6.4). The PR interval is discussed in more detail shortly.

QRS Complex

Normally, the QRS complex follows the PR segment. The normal QRS complex should be less than 100 ms (2.5 mm or 2.5 small squares) in duration.

Figure 6.5 shows variations of QRS complexes. Often, the QRS complex consists of three distinct deflections. If the QRS complex begins with a downward (negative) deflection, it is called a Q wave. An upward (positive) deflection in the QRS complex is called an R wave. A deflection coming back toward baseline from below baseline is called an S wave.

If the QRS complex consists of only a positive deflection that then returns to baseline (without ever being below baseline), then the QRS complex consists solely of an R wave. If the first deflection is negative and is followed by a positive deflection, then the QRS complex consists of Q and R waves. Sometimes, the QRS complex has a second R wave after the S wave; this is called an R′ (pronounced "R prime").

A small wave is indicated with a lowercase letter. Thus, a QRS complex consisting of a small Q wave followed by a large R wave and a small S wave might be written as qRs.

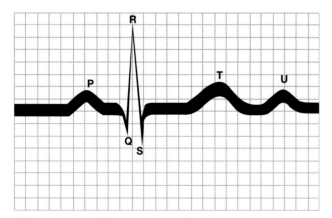

FIGURE 6.3 ECG waves.

Box 6.1	Normal Ranges for Selected ECG Parameters	
P-wave duration	≤120 ms (0.12 s) (3 mm)
P-wave amplitude	≤0.25 mV (2.5 mm)
PR interval	120–200 ms (0.12–0.20 s) (3–5 mm)
QRS duration	<100 ms (0.10 s) (2.5 mm)
QTc	<480 ms (0.440 s) (11 mm)
Heart rate	60–100 beats per minute

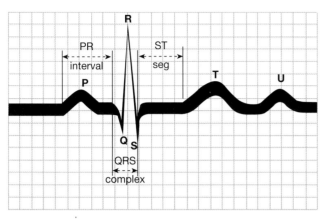

FIGURE 6.4 Waves, intervals, and segments.

T Wave, U Wave, and ST Segment

The last major electrical event of the normal cardiac cycle is ventricular repolarization, which appears on the ECG as the T wave (see Figure 6.3).

Sometimes a small complex known as the U wave follows the T wave (see Figure 6.3). The U wave is believed to represent the terminal stages of ventricular repolarization, possibly the repolarization of the Purkinje network.

The segment between the end of the QRS complex and the beginning of the T wave is called the ST segment (Figure 6.4). The term *ST segment* is used even in cases where the QRS complex lacks an S wave.

Under most normal circumstances, the ST segment is isoelectric, meaning that it should be on the baseline. Notice in Figure 6.4 that the line between the end of the P wave and the beginning of the QRS complex (the PR segment) is at roughly the same height as the line after the T wave (called the TP segment, as another P wave appears to be starting with the next cardiac cycle). Either the PR segment or the TP segment can be used as the isoelectric baseline. In Figure 6.4, the choice would not matter much as they are both at about the same level. Sometimes, however, the PR and TP segments are not at the same level. This situation can cause some difficulty in determining the magnitude of parameters such as ST-segment

depression and elevation. Strategies to overcome this are discussed later in the chapter.

MEASUREMENT OF INTERVALS AND DURATIONS

Recall that the grid of 1- and 5-mm boxes on the ECG paper can be used to quantify various ECG events. The measurements described subsequently assume normal calibration (1 mV = 10 mm, paper speed = 25 mm·s^{-1}).

Before proceeding to the next few sections, the student may find it helpful to have a cursory understanding of lead systems. Simply put, a lead is an electrical view of the heart. The standard ECG consists of 12 of these views (leads), each measuring the same electrical events of myocardial depolarization and repolarization from different points of reference. The electrical events are the same but viewed from different angles, they result in differing appearance of the P waves, QRS complexes, T waves, and other events. Leads are discussed in detail later in this chapter.

PR Interval

Figure 6.6 shows show measurement of a PR interval, which, as noted earlier, begins at the beginning of the P wave and ends at the beginning of the QRS complex. The measurement starts where the P wave leaves the baseline, whether the initial deflection of the P wave is positive or negative (usually, as in this case, it is positive). Measurement of the PR interval ends where the QRS complex begins, regardless of whether the QRS begins with a positive (R) or a negative (Q) wave.

The vertical lines under the "P" and "R" in Figure 6.6 show where to begin and end the measurement. A normal PR interval is between 120 and 200 ms (0.12–0.20 s). This is equivalent to three to five of the small (40 ms) boxes. Typically, the PR interval is measured in Lead II but can be seen in every one of the 12 ECG leads.

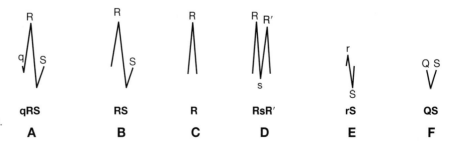

FIGURE 6.5 QRS complex morphologies.
A. qRS. **B.** RS. **C.** R. **D.** RsR. **E.** rS. **F.** QS.

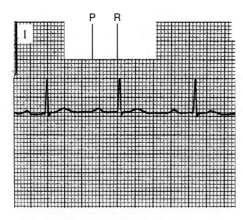

FIGURE 6.6 PR interval. The PR interval shown here is 280 ms (0.28 s).

QRS Duration

Measurement of the QRS duration (Figure 6.7) starts wherever the initial deflection of the QRS begins, whether it is positive (R wave) or negative (Q wave). The endpoint for the QRS is the end of the S wave if an S wave is present or the end of the R wave if an S wave is not present. Normally the QRS duration should be less than 100 ms (2.5 small boxes) in all ECG leads.

QT Interval

The QT interval (Figure 6.8) is measured from the beginning of the QRS complex to the end of the T wave. The length of the QT interval will normally vary with heart rate (HR), so one normal value cannot be described. Standard tables for rate-specific values can be consulted or the QT interval can be "corrected" for HR. A rate-corrected QT interval is abbreviated QT_c. The Bazett formula, shown here, is often used to calculate a QT_c. Although this formula is commonly applied to both sexes, some authorities recommend slightly different QT adjustments for males and females. The QT interval should be measured in whichever lead it is longest.

It is often difficult to accurately measure the QT interval, as determination of the precise ending of the T wave is

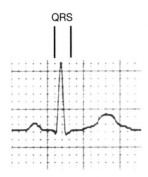

FIGURE 6.7 QRS duration. The QRS duration shown here is 80 ms (two small boxes).

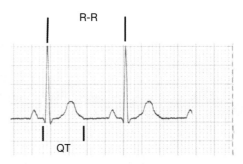

FIGURE 6.8 QT and R–R intervals. The figure shows a QT interval of 440 ms (0.44 s) and an R–R interval of 880 ms (0.88 s).

often difficult. This is particularly true if a U wave merges with the T wave. In such cases, an accurate QT interval cannot be determined.

Given here is the Bazett formula (in which QT is the QT interval in seconds and R–R is the time from one R wave to the next R wave in seconds):

$$QT_C = \frac{QT}{\sqrt{R-R}}$$

Note: With this formula, the values must be entered in seconds, not milliseconds.

The QT_c should be less than 440 ms (0.44 s).

MEASUREMENT OF HR

One of the most basic (yet critical) measurements made on virtually all ECGs is the assessment of HR. The normal range of resting HR is between 60 and 100 beats per minute (bpm). Most ECG machines will measure the average HR and usually print it on the ECG, so it might seem superfluous to measure rates by other methods. It is necessary, however, for two reasons. First, the rate measured by the ECG machine can be inaccurate. Second, when HR is varying, it is often necessary to know the rate at different time points on a single ECG, yet ECG machines only provide the average rate. To cover the full range of possibilities, the CEP should know several ways to measure HR. The method used to measure HR depends on whether the rhythm is regular or irregular. A regular rhythm is one in which the interval between R waves (R–R interval) is consistent. An irregular rhythm is one in which the R–R interval varies from beat to beat. Although some variance in the R–R interval is normal, a variation of greater than 0.08 seconds (two small squares) between beats can be used to define an irregular rhythm.

In cases when the rate is irregular, it is sometimes useful to describe the lowest and highest rates as well as the average. For example, the CEP might report that HR varied between 60 and 80 bpm, with an average rate of 70 bpm.

1500 Method

The 1500 method of determining HR is often used when very accurate determinations are needed. A 6- or 10-second strip can be run and the rate for each R–R interval determined, and then averaged. At normal calibration (paper speed of 25 mm·s^{-1}), there are 1500 mm or small squares in 1 minute. Thus, 1500 divided by the R–R interval in mm yields the HR. For example, if the R–R interval is 22 mm, the HR is approximately 68 bpm (1,500/22 = 68.18).

If the R–R intervals are fairly consistent, one measurement can yield a good estimation of the average rate. If the R–R intervals vary, several R–R intervals can be measured and the average rate determined. For greatest accuracy, every R–R interval on the ECG strip is measured and the average rate determined. This is typically not done as that degree of precision is beyond what is required for most clinical situations. This method is illustrated in Figure 6.9.

Triplets

Triplets is a handy method as it is very quick and easy to perform, and — if the rhythm is regular — provides an estimation of HR accurate enough for most clinical purposes. First, establish that the QRS complexes are coming along at regular intervals (*i.e.*, the R–R interval is consistent). This is important because, in the presence of varying R–R intervals, the estimation of rate by the triplet method will vary depending on which R–R was chosen for measurement. The triplets can still be used in this situation but, for accurate rate estimation, several representative R–R intervals would have to be measured and averaged.

The easiest way to use the triplets method is to find an R wave (or S wave) that falls on a thick (200 ms) line. The distance in big (200 ms) boxes to the next R wave (or S if an S wave was used initially) is then counted off using the following "triplets":

300-150-100   75-60-50

As shown in Figure 6.10A, if the next R wave fell on the first thick line from the reference R wave, then HR would be 300 bpm. If it fell on the second thick line, HR would be 150 bpm; on the third thick line 100 bpm; and so on. Figure 6.10B shows an example in which the next

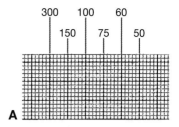

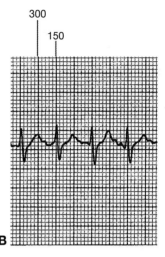

FIGURE 6.10 Heart rate triplets method. **A.** The triplets. **B.** Begin counting at the next thick line and continue until the next QRS complex.

R wave falls on the second thick line, making the HR approximately 150 bpm.

In the example shown in Figure 6.11, the reference R wave falls on a thick line and the next R wave falls on the first thin line following the fourth thick line. If the second R wave had fallen exactly on the fourth thick line, the HR would have been 75 bpm, and if it had fallen on the fifth thick line, the HR would have been 60 bpm. Therefore, we know that the rate is between 75 and 60 bpm. For some situations, it is accurate enough to say that the rate is "between 60 and 75." If more precision is desired, interpolation is simple. Because 75 − 60 = 15, and there are five small boxes between these thick lines, estimate that each small (1 mm) box represents about 3 bpm (15/5 = 3). Because the R wave in question is one small box short of the thick line representing 75 bpm and each box in this case is equivalent to 3 bpm, estimate that the HR is 72 bpm (75 − 3 = 72). The value assigned to each small (40 ms) box will vary. For example, if we have

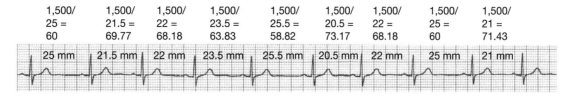

| 1,500/ 25 = 60 | 1,500/ 21.5 = 69.77 | 1,500/ 22 = 68.18 | 1,500/ 23.5 = 63.83 | 1,500/ 25.5 = 58.82 | 1,500/ 20.5 = 73.17 | 1,500/ 22 = 68.18 | 1,500/ 25 = 60 | 1,500/ 21 = 71.43 |

FIGURE 6.9 Heart rate 1,500 method. The average heart rate here is about 66 beats per minute.

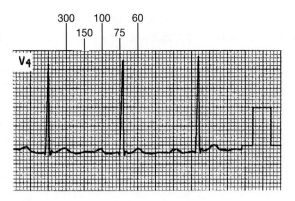

FIGURE 6.11 Heart rate triplets method. The approximate heart rate here is 72 beats per minute.

rates between 60 and 50, each small box represents 2 bpm (60 − 50 = 10, 10 ÷ 5 = 2), whereas if HR is between 150 and 100, each small box represents 10 bpm (150 − 100 = 50, 50 ÷ 5 = 10). The triplets are fairly accurate, particularly at rates less than 150 bpm but some accuracy is sacrificed for the sake of expedience at faster HRs.

6-Second Method

The 6-second method is a preferred method if the rhythm is irregular or, in other words, the R–R interval varies from beat to beat. This method will yield an average HR. Most ECG papers have marker lines on the bottom of the paper every 3 seconds (or sometimes every second), making it quite easy to measure a 6-second time interval. To estimate HR, count the number of full cardiac cycles (R–R intervals) in 6 seconds, then multiply

by 10. For example, in Figure 6.12, 6.5 R–R intervals are present in 6 seconds (note the vertical 3-second markers on the bottom of the strip); therefore, the HR is approximately 65 bpm. Note that it is R–R intervals that are counted, not R waves.

Different Atrial and Ventricular Rates

Normally, a QRS complex follows each P wave; thus, the atrial and ventricular rates normally are identical. Sometimes, as shown in Figure 6.13, atrial and ventricular rates are not the same. In this example, more than one P wave appears for each QRS complex. In such cases, it may be appropriate to measure and record both the atrial HR and the ventricular HR. The atrial rate (using P waves) can be measured using the same techniques described earlier for measurement of ventricular rates (using R waves). A definitive point needs to be chosen on the P wave as a reference point. The beginning of the P wave (where it leaves the baseline) or the peak of the P wave usually makes a good reference point.

SUPRAVENTRICULAR RHYTHMS

Rhythm is the pattern of the complexes, waves, and intervals; the regularity, or irregularity, of their occurrence; and the relationships among these constituents. Disturbances or irregularities of rhythm are usually called arrhythmias. A perhaps more accurate but less common term for the same phenomenon is dysrhythmia. A supraventricular rhythm is any rhythm originating above the ventricles of the heart.

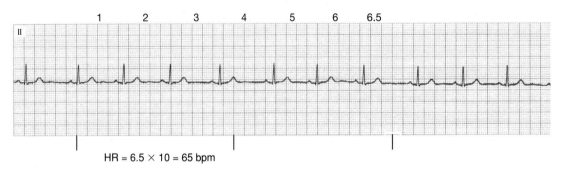

HR = 6.5 × 10 = 65 bpm

FIGURE 6.12 Heart rate 6-second method.

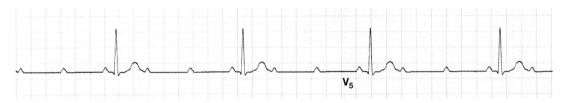

FIGURE 6.13 Differing atrial and ventricular rates. The atrial rate here is 107 beats per minute and the ventricular rate is 35 beats per minute.

Inspection of more than one ECG lead is necessary for many diagnoses (and can sometimes be of great help in determining the rhythm) but often only one lead is needed to determine the rhythm. In the interest of simplicity and clarity, assume that the ECGs used in this section are recorded using Lead II. Lead II is one of several bipolar leads, so named because these leads possess positive and negative sensing electrodes. For this discussion, the important point is that electrical current heading toward the positive pole of a lead will result in positive (rising above the baseline) deflections on the ECG and electrical events heading away from the positive pole (and therefore toward the negative pole) will result in negative (below baseline) deflections. A current traveling perpendicular to the axis of a lead will result in a waveform with roughly equal positive and negative components. Depending on various factors, either the positive or the negative component may come first, or the current may manifest as a flat line. Figure 6.14 illustrates these concepts in relation to P waves. The same concepts apply to other ECG waves as well.

As the positive pole of Lead II is placed on the left leg, and the negative pole is located on the right arm, Lead II is in line with the normal plane of key electrical events because depolarization normally tends to propagate through the heart from upper right to lower left and therefore toward the positive pole of Lead II.

Sinus Rhythms

As shown in Figure 6.15, the SA node is normally the first area of the heart to depolarize. This and similar figures throughout the book are not anatomically correct representations of the heart but rather diagrammatic illustrations of the conduction system. From the SA node, current spreads in many directions (as illustrated by the black arrows in Figure 6.15). The standard ECG measures the average (net) vector of all of the currents. As the SA node is located in the right upper portion of the right atrium (RA), the net current, or vector of atrial depolarization, spreads from the SA node toward the AV node. Depolarization normally begins spontaneously in the SA node (Figure 6.15). The normal spread of depolarization in the heart is shown in Figure 6.16. The intracellular fluid of the atrial cells is in contact with that of neighboring cells via gap junctions, allowing the depolarization to spread from cell to cell from the SA node (A) throughout the atria (B). This results in the P wave of the ECG. The atrioventricular (AV) node is surrounded by atrial tissue; therefore, the wave of depolarization spreading throughout the atria reaches the AV node. Normally, the tissue separating the atria from the ventricles does not conduct current; therefore, the only normal pathway for the depolarizing current to reach the ventricles is through the AV node and the next portion of the conduction system, which is known as the bundle of His (pronounced "hiss"). The tissue of the AV node conducts current at a much slower rate than other portions of the conduction system (because of tissue density), resulting in what appears to be a slight "delay" before the current reaches the ventricles (C). Physiologically, this delay permits time for the atria to contract and further fill the ventricles with blood before ventricular depolarization (and subsequent contraction). The area where the AV node and the bundle of His meet is called the AV junction.

Normal Impulse Origin and Pattern of Conduction

The normal pacemaker of the heart is the SA node. In this context, the term *pacemaker* refers to intrinsic areas of the heart that have the property of automaticity — that is, a regular pattern of depolarization in the absence of

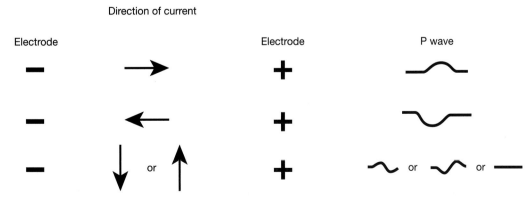

FIGURE 6.14 P waves resulting from current flow with differing orientation to electrodes.

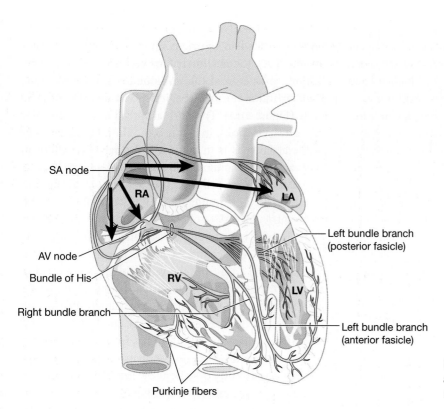

SA node —

RA

LA

AV node —

Bundle of His —

Right bundle branch —

Purkinje fibers

Left bundle branch (posterior fasicle)

RV

LV

Left bundle branch (anterior fasicle)

FIGURE 6.15 Atrial depolarization. LA, left atrium; LV, left ventricle; RA, right atrium; RV, right ventricle; SA, sinoatrial.

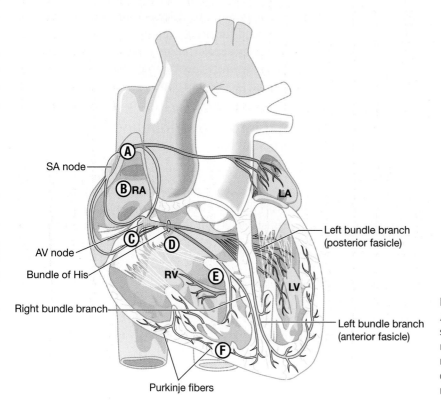

SA node —

(A)

(B) RA

LA

AV node —

(C)

(D)

Bundle of His —

Right bundle branch —

RV

(E)

LV

(F)

Purkinje fibers

Left bundle branch (posterior fasicle)

Left bundle branch (anterior fasicle)

FIGURE 6.16 Steps of the conduction system. *A,* SA node depolarizes. *B,* depolarization spreads throughout the atria. *C,* delay at the AV node. *D,* bundle of His depolarizes. *E,* left and right branches depolarize. *F,* Purkinje fibers depolarize. LA, left atrium; LV, left ventricle; RA, right atrium; RV, right ventricle; SA, sinoatrial.

external influence (although various factors including the autonomic nervous system can alter the rate of these depolarizations). Battery-operated electronic pacemakers, which are often used to pace the heart of patients with very slow rates and other conditions, are a separate issue and are discussed later in this chapter. In this context, the term *pacemaker* refers to the naturally occurring pacemakers.

As is the case with several areas of the heart, the SA node depolarizes regularly in the absence of external stimuli. Normally, the SA node depolarizes at a faster rate than the subsidiary pacemakers located in the AV node and the ventricles. Thus, the subsidiary pacemakers remain quiescent; that is, they are "reset" by the depolarizing current that arises from the SA node before they get a chance to fire. In the absence of depolarizations arising from the SA node, the subsidiary pacemakers can take control of pacing the heart. Usually, the lower pacemakers (*i.e.*, those located in the ventricles) have slower inherent rates; therefore, the higher pacemakers (*e.g.*, AV node) will typically take over pacing if the SA node fails to depolarize or does so at too slow a rate. Even if the SA node is firing at a normal rate, numerous factors can excite subsidiary pacemakers, resulting in beats that do not arise from the SA node.

Following the "delay" at the AV node, electrical current spreads down the bundle of His (D), and then down the left and right bundle branches (E). The bundle of His and the bundle branches are areas of tissue specialized for the conduction of current (*i.e.*, they function as "wires" rapidly bringing the current down into the ventricles). The left bundle branch bifurcates (splits) into two branches known as the anterior and posterior fascicles, but for the present, it is sufficient to simply think of the right bundle branch bringing the current down through the interventricular septum into the right ventricle and the left bundle branch bringing the current down through the interventricular septum into the left ventricle. It is important to note that branches from the left bundle branch depolarize the interventricular septum — thus, the septum depolarizes left to right. This is the second vector of depolarization.

The bundle branches travel down the interventricular septum toward the apex of the heart and then up the walls of the left and right ventricles. This causes the ventricles to depolarize from the bottom up and from the inside out. Because the left ventricle has a thicker ventricular wall, the third vector representing ventricular depolarization is from the interventricular septum toward the apex of the left ventricle.

Sprouting off the bundle branches are the smallest "wires" of the conduction system, the Purkinje fibers (F). Purkinje fibers are well dispersed throughout the ventricular myocardium, but do not reach every cell. Cells that are not directly in contact with Purkinje fibers are depolarized by neighboring cells because, as in the atria, the intracellular fluid of ventricular cells is in contact with that of adjoining cells via cellular connections known as gap junctions.

Because ventricular cells are linked together electrically by gap junctions, depolarizing electrical currents reaching the ventricles (or arising from the ventricles) can spread without using the conduction system but would spread more slowly and in a less organized manner. The purpose of the conduction system is to cause a more rapid and organized ventricular depolarization. Depolarizing current that spreads via the normal conduction system usually results in a "narrow" QRS complex (*i.e.*, <100 ms) because it travels quickly. Depolarizations that do not go through the conduction system normally, but instead spread by the slower cell-to-cell pathways, result in a "wide" (*i.e.*, ≥100 ms) QRS complex.

Normal Sinus Rhythm

Several requirements must be met for the designation of normal sinus rhythm (NSR). A "normal" HR has been somewhat arbitrarily designated as between 60 and 100 bpm. As the "sinus" part of the name indicates, in an NSR it is assumed that the SA node is pacing the heart. The net electrical current (vector) representing atrial depolarization from the SA node toward the AV node is pointing toward the positive pole of Lead II on the left leg. Therefore, a positive P wave (representing atrial depolarization) should be present in Lead II. In addition to these requirements, the rhythm must be regular, and one P wave must precede each QRS complex, and a QRS complex must follow each P wave. Figure 6.17 shows examples in which all these conditions are met. The two short strips in Figure 6.17A show simultaneous recordings of Lead II and a lead called aVR. Notice that the P waves are positive in Lead II and negative in Lead aVR. The positive pole of Lead aVR is located on the right arm; therefore, net electrical current (vector) representing atrial depolarization is traveling away from the positive pole of aVR, so there will be a negative P wave in aVR. If NSR is present, the P waves should be positive in Lead II and negative in Lead aVR. The longer Lead II strip in Figure 6.17B illustrates the regularity of the rhythm and the consistent presence of one P wave for each QRS complex. Longer ECGs such as this one are commonly referred to as rhythm strips.

Sinus Arrhythmia

If the other conditions for NSR are present (HR between 60 and 100 bpm, positive P waves in Lead II and one P wave for each QRS complex) but the rhythm is irregular (*i.e.*, the R–R interval is varying), then sinus arrhythmia is present. Compare Figures 6.17 and 6.18. Notice that with NSR (Figure 6.17) the R–R interval shows little variation. In other words, the rhythm is regular. Contrast this with Figure 6.18, in which the R–R interval varies significantly. One commonly used definition of significant variation is a difference of at least 80 ms (two small boxes) between the shortest and longest R–R intervals (see section on Measurement of HR).

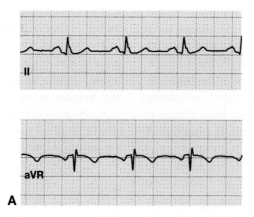

FIGURE 6.17 Normal sinus rhythm. **A.** P waves are positive in Lead II and negative in Lead aVR. **B.** Rhythm is regular with a heart rate (HR) between 60 and 100 beats per minute. PR intervals are consistent, with one P wave for each QRS.

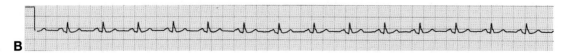

FIGURE 6.18 Sinus arrhythmia. The R–R interval varies significantly (one commonly used definition of significant variation is a difference of at least 80 ms or two small boxes between the shortest and longest R–R intervals).

Sinus Tachycardia and SA Nodal Reentrant Tachycardia

If all the conditions for NSR are present, with the exception that the HR is greater than 100 bpm, then sinus tachycardia is present (Figure 6.19). This term simply indicates that HR is faster than the criteria (60–100 bpm) for a normal sinus rate. As the HR increases, it may become more difficult to identify P waves. In Figure 6.19A, P waves are clearly visible. In Figure 6.19B, the rate is faster, the P waves have begun to merge with the T waves of the preceding beats, and thus are more difficult to distinguish.

If Figure 6.19B were recorded during exercise, it would be reasonable to assume that it represented sinus tachycardia. However, if this tracing were obtained under resting conditions, it likely would represent another sinus rhythm, SA nodal reentrant tachycardia, an abnormal depolarizing current that spins rapidly around in the area of the SA node, resulting in a fast HR. A current that circles around, repeatedly reentering the SA node, is called a reentrant current or circuit current. Because the initial depolarizations come from the SA node, the P waves appear normal. The rate is typically greater than 100 bpm and the rhythm is regular.

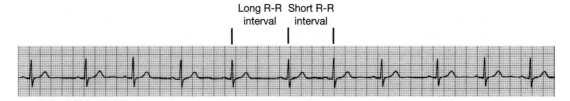

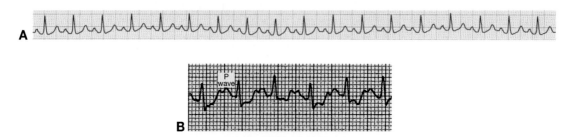

FIGURE 6.19 Sinus tachycardia. **A.** The heart rate is approximately 123 beats per minute. **B.** The heart rate is approximately 150 beats per minute.

Sinus tachycardia usually comes on gradually; for example, the rate may increase from 70 to 80 to 90, and so on, until it exceeds 100 bpm. It also shows a gradual decline in rate when returning to NSR. In contrast, SA nodal reentrant tachycardia has a sudden onset and a sudden cessation. For example, the rate may jump in one beat from 70 to 150 bpm. The termination is equally abrupt. Thus, when the onset or termination of the tachycardia is witnessed, the diagnosis is simplified.

If the onset is not witnessed, the rate and regularity offer important clues. Higher rates and constant R–R intervals are more typical of SA nodal reentrant tachycardia, whereas lower rates and R–R variability favor a diagnosis of sinus tachycardia. When the rhythm cannot be discerned with certainty, the word *versus* is often inserted between the possibilities, so Figure 6.19B might be described as "Sinus tachycardia versus SA nodal reentrant tachycardia."

The term *supraventricular tachycardia (SVT)* is sometimes used to describe narrow QRS complex tachycardia. An SVT with a sudden onset and termination may be referred to as paroxysmal atrial tachycardia (PAT) or paroxysmal supraventricular tachycardia (PSVT). These terms are rather vague, as the appearance of and mechanisms causing the various SVTs differ. It is preferable to differentiate between the various types of SVT.

Sinus Bradycardia

Sinus bradycardia (Figure 6.20) is simply a slow HR, usually defined as less than 60 bpm. The term *marked sinus bradycardia* is sometimes used when the rate is very low, as shown in Figure 6.20B. Sinus bradycardia can be a physiological adaption to regular exercise (as stroke volume increases, HR decreases to maintain the same cardiac output) or due to certain medications such as β-blockers. The CEP should carefully use the medical history and medication review to determine the cause of sinus bradycardia.

Sinus Pause

A delay occurring before the appearance of a P wave (Figure 6.21) may be caused by several mechanisms.

These include failure of the SA node to depolarize and an SA "block" that does not permit the depolarization to escape from the SA node. Notice in Figure 6.21A, that after the pause, the rhythm resumes with a P wave that looks normal. In Figure 6.21B the rhythm resumes with a normal-appearing QRS that is not preceded by a P wave. As discussed in the following sections, this implies that the beat does not originate in the SA node.

Pauses can be quantified. For example, Figure 6.21A could be described as "Sinus rhythm with a sinus pause of 1.16 s." The length of the pause is measured from the beginning of the P wave of the beat preceding the pause, to the beginning of the P wave of the beat following the pause (in this case, 29 little boxes, which is equivalent to 1,160 ms or 1.16 s).

Premature Atrial Complex

A premature atrial complex (PAC) is an early (premature) beat arising from somewhere above the ventricles other than the SA node (*i.e.*, in the atria or the AV junction). In general, depolarizations arising in areas of the heart other than the normal pacemaker (SA node) are referred to as ectopic. The site of origin of these ectopic depolarizations is termed an *ectopic focus*.

A PAC is sometimes referred to as a premature atrial contraction (although contraction is a mechanical term and not an electrical term). Other terms used to describe these beats include *atrial premature contraction (APC)*, *atrial premature depolarization (APD)*, and *atrial premature beat (APB)*. The term *junctional premature complex (JPC)* is also sometimes used to describe certain supraventricular beats.

Typical Conduction of the PAC

A PAC starts in an ectopic focus somewhere in the atria or the AV junction. Because the P wave represents atrial depolarization, it follows that depolarizations arising in areas of the atria other than the SA node will typically have P waves that differ in appearance from the sinus P waves. They will usually also take a different amount of time to travel through the atria and down into the ventricles; thus,

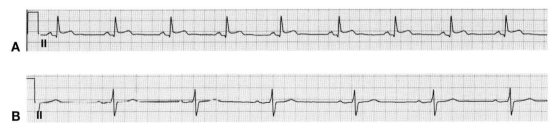

FIGURE 6.20 Sinus bradycardia. **A.** The heart rate is approximately 55 beats per minute. **B.** The heart rate is approximately 42 beats per minute.

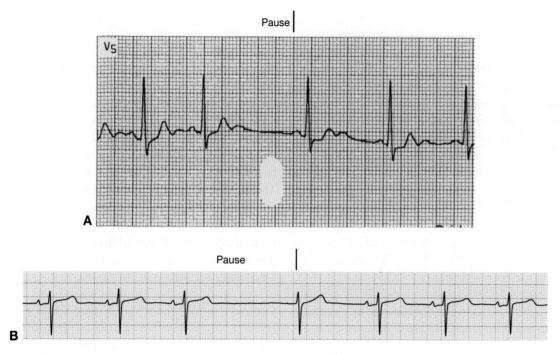

FIGURE 6.21 Sinus pause. **A.** The rhythm resumes with the sinus P wave. **B.** The rhythm resumes with the ectopic beat.

the PR interval of PACs will usually differ from that of sinus beats. A PAC originating in the upper or middle parts of the atria may still result in an upright P wave in Lead II. This is because the mean electrical vector of atrial depolarization is generally heading toward the positive pole of Lead II (Figure 6.22). The defining characteristic of a PAC is a premature beat: Notice that the P–P interval of the PAC shown in Figure 6.23 is shorter than the other P–P intervals. This is just a way of indicating that this P wave came early.

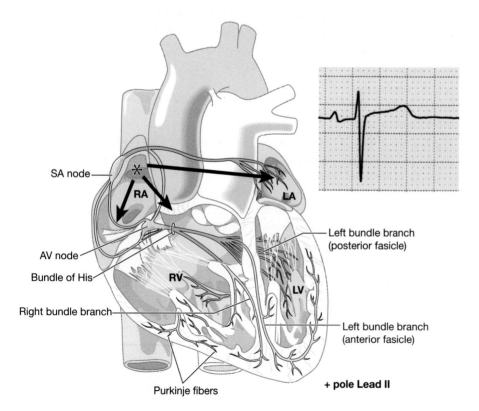

FIGURE 6.22 Atrial ectopic focus. The corresponding ECG is shown at the top right of this figure (asterisk indicates the ectopic focus). LA, left atrium; LV, left ventricle; RA, right atrium; RV, right ventricle; SA, sinoatrial.

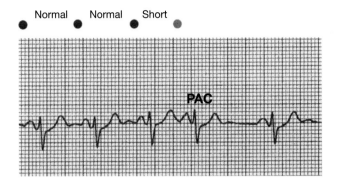

Normal   Normal   Short

PAC

FIGURE 6.23 Premature atrial complex (PAC). P–P intervals are shown at the top left of the strip.

Typically, a PAC is conducted normally through the AV node and ventricles, resulting in a QRS complex that appears normal. This is because conduction throughout the ventricles follows the normal path (AV node, bundle of His, bundle branches, and Purkinje fibers). The only abnormality is in atrial conduction. Cases where PACs lead to abnormal (aberrant) ventricular conduction are discussed later in this chapter. Sometimes a PAC is not conducted through the ventricles at all, usually because the AV node is still in a refractory period; this is called a blocked or nonconducted PAC (Figure 6.24). Notice how the P wave of the nonconducted PAC in Figure 6.24 merges with the T wave of the preceding beat. This P wave came so early that it failed to conduct down into the ventricles, probably because the rest of the conduction system was still in a refractory period. The P waves in this example are biphasic as this strip was recorded using Lead V$_1$, a lead that normally has biphasic P waves.

Atypical Conduction of the PAC

When an early beat arises lower in the atria or at the AV junction, the resulting wave of depolarization typically spreads through the atria in the opposite direction of beats originating in the SA node (Figure 6.25). In other words, these PACs may spread through the atria from bottom to top. In this case, atrial depolarization is spreading away from the positive pole of Lead II, resulting in a negative P wave in that lead. The depolarization also typically spreads down into the ventricles; however, here the impulse is usually conducted normally, resulting in a QRS complex that appears normal. Depending on exactly where the PAC arises and the prevailing conditions in the atria, junction, and ventricles, the atria may depolarize ahead of the ventricles (but backward, also called retrograde, in that the impulse spreads from bottom to top), at roughly the same time as the ventricles, or after the ventricles have finished depolarizing.

If the depolarization spreads through the atria first, then a negative P wave will be seen before the QRS complex (Figure 6.26A). If the depolarization spreads through the ventricles first, and then through the atria, a negative P wave will be seen after the QRS complex (Figure 6.26B). If the depolarization of atria and ventricles occurs at roughly the same time, no P wave may be visible (Figure 6.26C), as the much larger electrical events of ventricular depolarization (QRS complex) obscure the relatively small events of atrial depolarization (P wave). Beats originating low in the atria or at the AV junction may have negative P waves before or after the QRS complex or no P wave at all.

Junctional Premature Complexes

Figure 6.27 shows a PAC with a negative P wave before the QRS complex. Premature beats with negative or missing P waves are sometimes referred to as JPCs, as many of them arise at or near the AV junction.

Atrial Bigeminy, Trigeminy, and Quadrigeminy

Atrial bigeminy (Figure 6.28A) refers to a situation wherein every second beat is a PAC. Atrial trigeminy

P   P   P (nonconducted PAC)

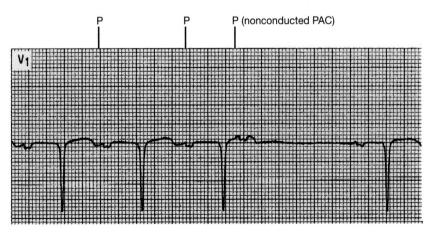

V$_1$

FIGURE 6.24 Nonconducted (blocked) premature atrial complex.

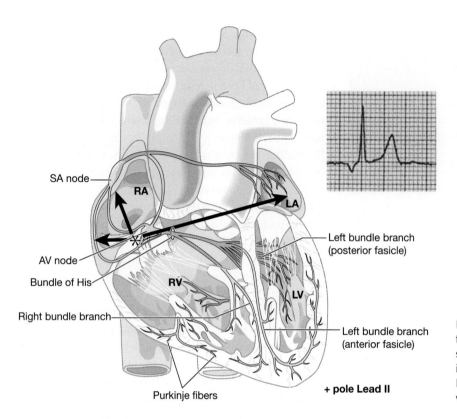

FIGURE 6.25 Atrial ectopic focus near the AV node. The corresponding ECG is shown at the top right of this figure (asterisk indicates the ectopic focus). LA, left atrium; LV, left ventricle; RA, right atrium; RV, right ventricle; SA, sinoatrial.

(Figure 6.28B) and atrial quadrigeminy (Figure 6.28C) are used to describe conditions wherein every third or fourth beat, respectively, is a PAC.

Ectopic Atrial Tachycardia

Three or more PACs occurring consecutively is defined as atrial tachycardia. Recall that an ectopic depolarization originates in an area other than the SA node; thus, ectopic atrial tachycardia describes a tachycardia that originates from the atria, but not from the sinus node. Two examples are shown in Figure 6.29. It is sometimes difficult to distinguish sinus tachycardia from ectopic atrial tachycardia. As previously discussed, ectopic beats usually have P waves and/or PR intervals that differ from what is considered normal. Even if the normal PR interval and P wave morphology are known, sinus tachycardia may affect the shape of the P waves and the time needed for AV conduction.

If the initiation or termination of the tachycardia is witnessed, diagnosis is much easier because ectopic atrial tachycardias typically have a sudden onset and

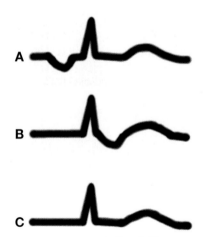

FIGURE 6.26 P waves with retrograde conduction. **A.** Negative P wave before QRS. **B.** Negative P wave after QRS. **C.** No visible P wave.

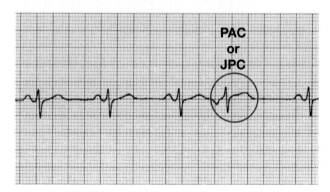

FIGURE 6.27 Ectopic beat arising at or near the atrioventricular junction. JPC, junctional premature complex; PAC, premature atrial complex.

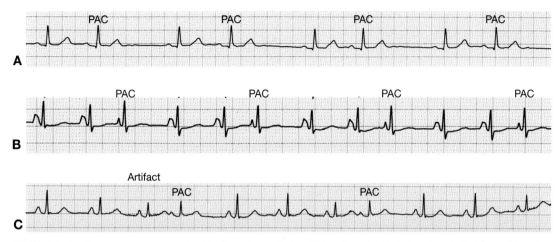

FIGURE 6.28 Premature atrial complex (PAC) patterns. **A.** Atrial bigeminy. **B.** Atrial trigeminy. **C.** Atrial quadrigeminy.

termination. Notice in Figure 6.29B how the rate abruptly changes. The initial rhythm is sinus tachycardia. A PAC then initiates a short run of ectopic atrial tachycardia. Notice how the P wave of the first ectopic beat merges with the T wave of the preceding beat. The P waves are then not readily apparent (but are present on top of the T waves) until the sinus P waves reemerge toward the end of the strip. Sinus tachycardia typically has a more gradual onset and termination. An exception to this is the previously described SA nodal reentrant tachycardia, which has a sudden onset. The P waves of an SA nodal reentrant tachycardia usually resemble sinus P waves (as they originate in the SA node), whereas the P waves of an ectopic atrial tachycardia typically differ in appearance from sinus P waves. Electrical alternans, a phenomenon in which the height (amplitude) of the R waves regularly alternates, commonly occurs with ectopic atrial tachycardia but is not typical in SA nodal reentrant tachycardia. Figure 6.29A shows this phenomenon.

Inspection of R–R variability (the variation between R–R intervals) can also be helpful. In ectopic atrial tachycardia and SA nodal reentrant tachycardia, the R–R interval is often very constant, whereas in sinus tachycardia, variation is typically seen. Normal ventilation can alter HR (*i.e.,*

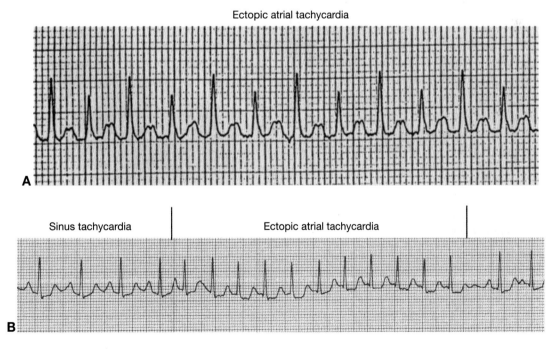

FIGURE 6.29 Ectopic atrial tachycardia. **A.** Note the alteration in the height of the R waves (electrical alternans). **B.** The sudden change in rate at the onset and termination helps distinguish this ectopic atrial tachycardia from sinus tachycardia.

the R–R interval changes coincidentally with inhalation and exhalation). If ventilation causes changes in the R–R interval, the diagnosis is more likely to be a sinus tachycardia as ectopic atrial tachycardia and SA nodal reentrant tachycardia are usually not significantly affected by ventilation.

HR can also provide ECG clues. Ectopic atrial tachycardia and SA nodal reentrant tachycardia are often exhibited as rates greater than 160 bpm. The higher the rate, the less likely that it is sinus tachycardia. The setting is also relevant. The previous discussion assumes that the patient is at rest. During strenuous exercise, sinus rates as high as 180–200 bpm are commonly observed in younger people but it is unusual (although possible) for sinus tachycardia to have a rate of greater than 140–160 bpm at rest.

Atrioventricular Nodal Reentrant Tachycardia

Current can rapidly circulate around the AV node, similar to what happens near the SA node in SA nodal reentrant tachycardia. If the reentry is occurring around the AV node, the resulting tachycardia is called AV nodal reentrant tachycardia (AVNRT). In AVNRT, the P waves are usually not seen or are negative and follow the QRS complex.

Figure 6.30 shows an ectopic atrial tachycardia (A) and two variations of AVNRT (B and C). Notice that the ectopic atrial tachycardia has negative P waves visible before the QRS complexes (recall that ectopic atrial tachycardia can have positive or negative P waves). Contrast this with the two AVNRTs, in which the P waves either are not visible (Figure 6.30C) or are negative and follow the QRS complexes (B). It is common practice to refer to any of these three rhythms as junctional tachycardia.

However, as the mechanisms underlying the rhythms are different, it is preferable to distinguish between ectopic atrial tachycardia and AVNRTs.

Junctional Escape

Areas near the AV junction possess the ability to spontaneously depolarize. If left alone, the AV junction will rhythmically depolarize at a rate of around 40–60 times per minute. Usually, the SA node depolarizes at a faster rate. Because each sinus depolarization resets the other pacemakers of the heart, secondary pacemakers such as the AV junction will not typically become apparent unless the SA node fails to depolarize or does so at an abnormally slow rate.

The morphology of junctional escape beats is identical to that described earlier for premature beats arising from or near the AV junction. The difference is that these depolarizations are not early; in fact, they could be thought of as late, as they usually only occur if the SA node fails to depolarize. This is a protective mechanism; in the event that the SA node fails to depolarize the heart in a timely manner, these and other subsidiary pacemakers can take over.

Depolarizations arising at or near the AV junction typically have a normal QRS complex and (a) no apparent P wave, (b) a negative P wave before the QRS complex, or (c) a negative P wave after the QRS complex. The QRS complexes are typically normal, as ventricular depolarization occurs through the normal ventricular conduction system. These are sometimes referred to as junctional escape beats.

Figure 6.31A shows a single junctional escape beat (the underlying rhythm is sinus bradycardia). In this case, an isolated delay in sinus depolarization has occurred. The delay is long enough to allow the AV junctional pacemaker to fire.

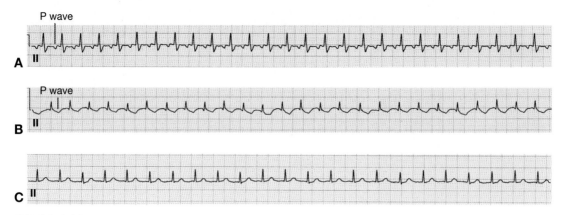

FIGURE 6.30 Junctional tachycardia. **A.** Ectopic atrial tachycardia shows negative P waves before QRS. **B.** Atrioventricular nodal reentrant tachycardia shows negative P waves after QRS. **C.** The atrioventricular nodal reentrant tachycardia here shows no visible P waves.

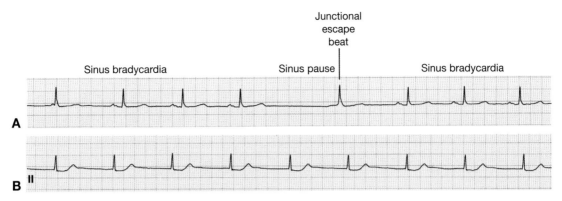

FIGURE 6.31 A. Junctional escape beat. **B.** Junctional escape rhythm.

In Figure 6.31B, the sinus pacemaker has either failed or slowed sufficiently that a junctional pacemaker has assumed control of the rhythm. This is usually referred to as a junctional escape rhythm. The HR in a junctional escape rhythm is generally less than 60 bpm.

Accelerated Junctional Rhythm

Rhythms that appear to be originating at or near the AV junction (narrow QRS complexes and negative or absent P waves) and have rates between 60 and 100–120 bpm are typically called accelerated junctional rhythms. The term simply indicates that the rate is faster than the junctional escape rate, yet slower than a junctional (ectopic atrial) tachycardia. Two examples are shown in Figure 6.32. As with other junctional rhythms, P waves may be absent or negative.

Atrial Fibrillation

In atrial fibrillation (A-Fib), electrical activity is so chaotic that no organized contractile activity is occurring in the atria.

Hundreds of areas of the atria are depolarizing independently and in various directions, so the ECG shows no signs of regularly occurring, organized atrial electrical activity. The atria are quivering rather than contracting and the normal contribution of atrial contraction to ventricular filling is lost. A normal P wave comes from the organized spread of electrical activity throughout the atria; thus, the P wave is also lost. Instead of P waves, fibrillatory (or "f" waves), may be seen. These f waves (Figure 6.33) may vary from very fine undulations (A), where the baseline appears almost flat, to coarse waves that may occasionally look almost like P waves (B).

A major determinant of clinical status in the patient with A-Fib is the ventricular rate, which is determined by how many of the hundreds of atrial impulses are able to depolarize the AV node. Because the impulses are coming at the AV node from a variety of directions, and at random times, conduction down into the ventricles is quite haphazard. However, when the AV node is depolarized, conduction from that point will usually occur through the normal mechanisms (AV node, bundle of His, etc.); therefore, the QRS complexes will generally be normal in appearance in A-Fib.

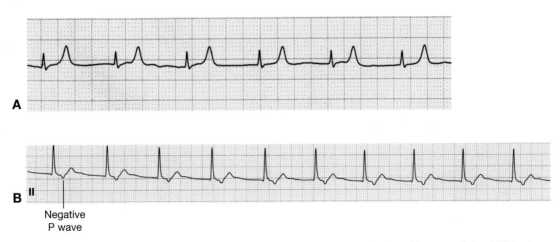

FIGURE 6.32 Accelerated junctional rhythms. **A.** An accelerated junctional rhythm with a rate of about 70 beats per minute and no apparent P waves. **B.** An accelerated junctional rhythm with a rate of about 64 beats per minute and negative P waves after QRS.

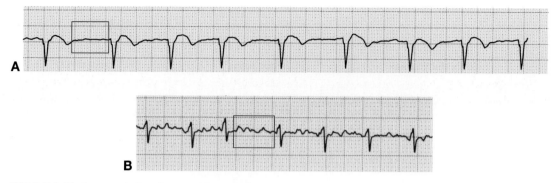

FIGURE 6.33 F waves. **A.** Fine F waves. **B.** Coarse F waves.

Regardless of the average rate of AV nodal (and, therefore, ventricular) depolarization, the rhythm will be irregular. An unusual term, *irregularly irregular*, is often used to describe the pattern of ventricular depolarizations that occur with A-Fib. Examine Figure 6.34. Notice that the ventricular rate (response) can vary from slow (Figure 6.34A), to moderate (B), to rapid (C). However, in each of these cases, the ventricular rhythm is very irregular. In contrast, in many dysrhythmias, the rhythm is not regular but is irregular in a predictable manner. For example, in atrial trigeminy, every third beat is early. Thus, the pattern in atrial trigeminy could be called regularly irregular, in that the irregularity is occurring in a pattern. Contrast this with the examples in Figure 6.34, where no predictable pattern of ventricular activity is present.

Sometimes this irregularity is not initially obvious at faster rates. On first glance, the pattern of QRS complexes in Figure 6.34C may appear fairly regular. Careful measurement of the R–R intervals will reveal that this is not the case; the pattern is, in fact, quite irregular. The faster rate simply makes it somewhat more difficult to immediately discern this. Checking the regularity of the R–R intervals is critical in distinguishing A-Fib from other rhythms.

Atrial Flutter

During atrial flutter, the atria are depolarized in an organized cyclical manner and at a very high rate, resulting in a distinctive "saw-tooth" pattern. The "F" waves of the atrial flutter are shown in Figure 6.35. A-Fib has fibrillatory waves, abbreviated with a lowercase "f," whereas an uppercase "F" is used to abbreviate the saw-tooth flutter waves of atrial flutter.

During atrial flutter, the atrial rate is often close to 300 bpm. The ventricular rate may vary. In some cases, a consistent fraction of the F waves conduct down into the ventricles; Figure 6.35A, B, and C shows consistent patterns of every fourth (4:1) or second (2:1) atrial impulse being conducted. Sometimes the AV conduction varies, as is seen in Figure 6.35D and E.

Atrial and ventricular rates can be described separately. For example, in Figure 6.35C, the atrial rate is about 300 bpm and the ventricular rate is about 75 bpm. Measuring the atrial and ventricular rates is a good way to double-check the ratio of atrial to AV conduction. In this example, the presence of 4:1 conduction is confirmed, as the atrial rate (300 bpm) is four times the ventricular rate (75 bpm). Simple inspection might lead to mistaking this strip for 3:1 flutter, as the fourth F wave is merging with the QRS complex and could be missed.

Although the 12 leads of the standard ECG have not been discussed in detail yet, it should be noted that the classic pattern of atrial flutter shows F waves in Leads II, III, and aVF (known collectively as the "inferior" leads as they electrically view the bottom of the heart).

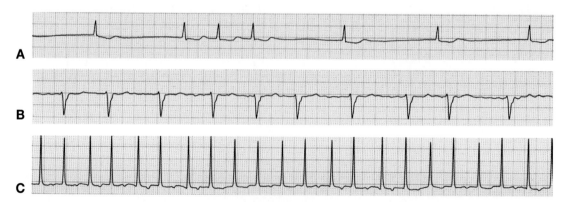

FIGURE 6.34 Atrial fibrillation. **A.** Slow ventricular response. **B.** Moderate ventricular response. **C.** Rapid ventricular response.

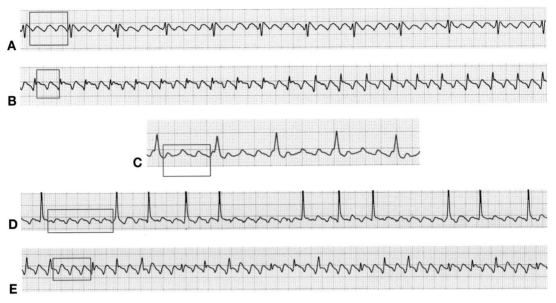

FIGURE 6.35 Atrial flutter. The boxes in **(A)** through **(E)** show the F waves. **A** and **C.** 4:1 atrioventricular conduction. **B.** 2:1 atrioventricular conduction. **D** and **E.** Variable atrioventricular conduction.

Figure 6.36 shows two 12-lead examples of atrial flutter. Note that F waves are present in Leads II, III, and aVF but may not be readily apparent in all leads.

Wandering Atrial Pacemaker and Multifocal Atrial Tachycardia

Although they differ in rate, wandering atrial pacemaker and multifocal atrial tachycardia have a similar ECG pattern. In both cases, several areas of the atria serve as pacemakers (thus, the pacemaker is "wandering" or "multifocal"). As would be expected in this situation, the P waves differ in appearance; in fact, a commonly accepted criterion for these rhythms is the presence of three or more different P-wave morphologies. Some of the different P-wave shapes are circled in Figure 6.37. The PR intervals may also vary for the same reasons described previously for PACs. These rhythms could be thought of as special cases of "frequent PACs."

Owing to the multiple foci, the rhythm tends to be irregular, perhaps even irregularly irregular. In contrast to A-Fib, P waves are consistently seen in these rhythms.

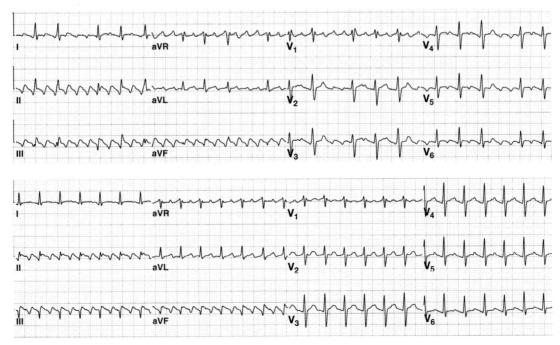

FIGURE 6.36 Atrial flutter. Two examples of a 12-lead ECG are shown here. Note the F waves in Leads II, III, and aVF.

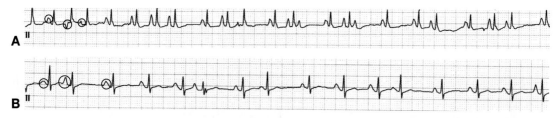

FIGURE 6.37 **A.** Multifocal atrial tachycardia. **B.** Wandering atrial pacemaker. Circles indicate different P-wave morphologies.

In keeping with general terminology, a rate greater than 100 bpm is usually considered a tachycardia. Thus, Figure 6.37A would be called multifocal atrial tachycardia, whereas (B) would be considered a wandering atrial pacemaker (as the rate is <100 bpm).

VENTRICULAR RHYTHMS

Recall that in previous sections in which various atrial arrhythmias were discussed, the QRS complex often had a normal (narrow) appearance because the depolarizations would reach the ventricular myocardium via the normal conduction system (AV node, bundle of His, bundle branches, and Purkinje fibers). For example, even during A-Fib, wherein the atrial myocardium is electrically unstable and functionally useless, the depolarizations that did reach the ventricles were assumed to result in normal QRS complexes.

Now imagine a situation in which a depolarization originates from an ectopic focus in the ventricles. As the ventricular myocardial cells are electrically connected via gap junctions, this depolarization spreads throughout the ventricles; however, because these currents are not spreading through the normal conduction pathways, they spread more slowly and in a less organized manner. A QRS complex resulting from currents that spread via these mechanisms has an appearance that is often described as "wide and bizarre"; wide (usually defined as >100 ms) because the spread of current is slower than normal and bizarre (as compared to the normal QRS morphology) because the electrical activity is not spreading via the normal routes (Figure 6.38).

Premature Ventricular Complexes

Examine the QRS complexes in Figure 6.39A. The QRS in the box is wider and different in appearance from the others. Several different terms, including *premature ventricular*

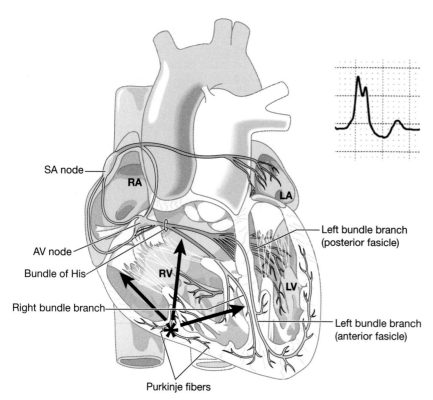

FIGURE 6.38 Ventricular ectopic focus. Asterisk indicates the ectopic focus. The corresponding ECG is shown at the top right of the figure. AV, atrioventricular; LA, left atrium; LV, left ventricle; RA, right atrium; RV, right ventricle; SA, sinoatrial.

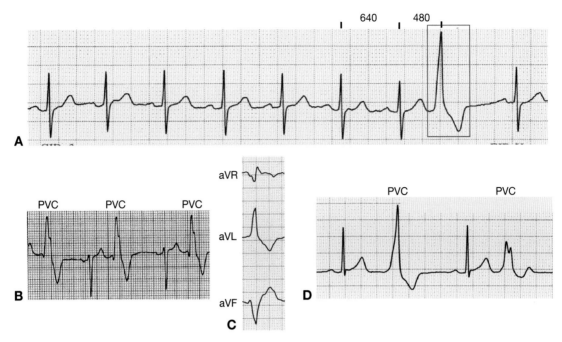

FIGURE 6.39 Premature ventricular complexes (PVCs). **A.** R–R intervals (ms). **B.** Uniform PVCs. **C.** Same PVC in three different leads. **D.** Multiform PVCs.

complex (PVC), ventricular premature depolarization (VPD), and *ventricular extrasystoles (VESs),* are used interchangeably to describe these types of events. PVC, the most common term, is apt because these beats are early (premature) and appear to arise in the ventricles (ventricular complexes).

By definition, PVCs must occur earlier than the next expected cardiac cycle. Notice in Figure 6.39A that the normal R–R interval is about 640 ms. The PVC (enclosed in the box) is early; the R–R interval from the previous normal beat to the PVC is only 480 ms. Notice also that the PVC is wide (QRS duration >100 ms) and has a different morphology (form or shape) than the other QRS complexes. It is also common with PVCs for the QRS complexes and the T waves to be oriented in opposite directions. In this example, the QRS complex is positive, whereas the T wave is negative.

Uniform and Multiform PVCs

Uniform PVCs look alike. Three PVCs of similar appearance (uniform) are shown in Figure 6.39B. Figure 6.39D shows two PVCs with different appearances in the same lead; these are called multiform PVCs. Panel C shows one PVC as seen in three different ECG leads. Notice that a given PVC will look different when viewed in different ECG leads, whereas multiform PVCs look different from each other in the *same* ECG lead.

Uniform PVCs look the same because they arise from the same ectopic focus; therefore, they are sometimes called unifocal PVCs. Multiform PVCs may arise from different areas of the ventricle, so they are sometimes

called multifocal. This may not be an appropriate term because it has been found that PVCs that differ in appearance (in the same lead) may actually arise from the same ectopic focus. Thus, the term *multiform* is preferred, as it does not imply multiple ectopic foci.

Compensatory Pauses and Interpolated PVCs

Compare the PVCs in Figure 6.40. In Figure 6.40A, the PVC is followed by a pause, and then the next P–QRS–T comes when it would have normally occurred had the PVC not intervened. This is an example of a PVC with a compensatory pause. The pause after the PVC results in the next R wave coming on time — in other words, two normal R–R intervals after the last normal R wave. Now examine the PVC in Figure 6.40B. In this case, the PVC falls right in the middle of a normal R–R interval and has no effect on the regularity of the other beats (no compensatory pause). This is called an interpolated PVC. Some interpolated PVCs do subtly alter the rhythm but the change is much less pronounced than a compensatory pause.

Ventricular Bigeminy, Trigeminy, and Quadrigeminy

Patterns of PVCs can be described using terminology similar to that used for PACs (Figure 6.41). Ventricular bigeminy (Figure 6.41A) is said to exist when every second beat is a PVC. Ventricular trigeminy (Figure 6.41B) occurs when every third beat is a PVC. In ventricular quadrigeminy (Figure 6.41C), every fourth beat is a PVC.

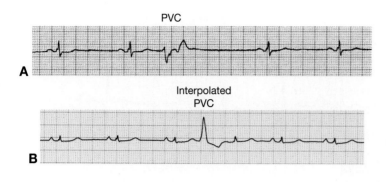

FIGURE 6.40 Ventricular ectopy. **A.** A compensatory pause after the premature ventricular complex (PVC). **B.** An interpolated PVC.

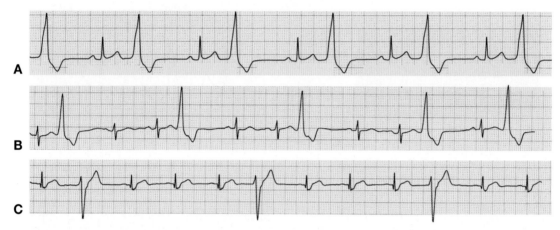

FIGURE 6.41 Ventricular ectopy. **A.** Ventricular bigeminy. **B.** Ventricular trigeminy. **C.** Ventricular quadrigeminy.

Ventricular Couplet and Tachycardia

The occurrence of two consecutive PVCs is called a ventricular couplet. By definition, a string of three or more consecutive PVCs is ventricular tachycardia (V-Tach). Examples of a couplet, and some "short runs" of V-Tach, are shown in Figure 6.42. Runs of V-Tach lasting less than 30 seconds are usually described as short, nonsustained, or self-terminating, whereas V-Tach lasting more than 30 seconds is described as sustained V-Tach.

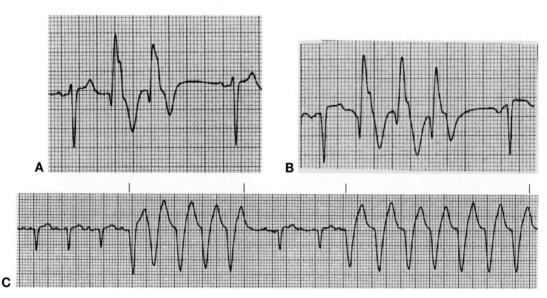

FIGURE 6.42 Ventricular ectopy. **A.** Ventricular couplet. **B.** Ventricular triplet (short run of ventricular tachycardia). **C.** Two runs of ventricular tachycardia.

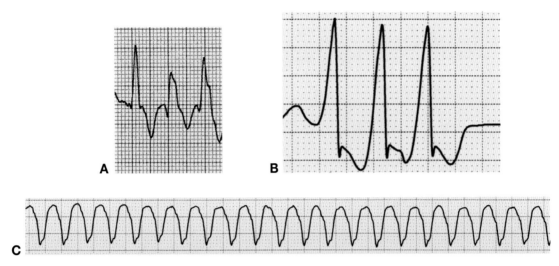

FIGURE 6.43 Ventricular tachycardia. **A.** Nonsustained polymorphic ventricular tachycardia (triplet). **B.** Nonsustained monomorphic ventricular tachycardia (triplet). **C.** Sustained monomorphic ventricular tachycardia.

V-Tach can be further described in terms of the morphology of the QRS complexes. For example, the pattern in Figure 6.43B and C could be described as monomorphic V-Tach because a relatively consistent pattern of QRS complexes is seen. Contrast this with the short run of polymorphic V-Tach shown in Figure 6.43A and the example in Figure 6.44; in these cases, the PVCs do not all appear the same.

Torsade de Pointes

An important subclass of polymorphic V-Tach is torsade de pointes ("twisting of points"), in which the polarity of the QRS complexes repetitively shifts. Notice in Figure 6.44 that the "point" of the QRS complexes alternately points downward and upward. Recognition of torsade de pointes as a specific subtype of V-Tach is important, as the cause (*e.g.*, electrolyte abnormalities and certain medication effects) may be reversible.

R-on-T PVCs

When a PVC falls on the T wave of the preceding beat, it is much more likely to lead to a serious arrhythmia such as ventricular fibrillation (V-Fib) or V-Tach. This is not to say that these so-called R-on-T PVCs always lead to dangerous arrhythmias; most often they do not. However, there is a much greater statistical likelihood of an R-on-T PVC initiating a serious arrhythmia as compared to other PVCs. Figure 6.45A shows an R-on-T PVC that did not initiate any further arrhythmias and Figure 6.45B shows one that did.

Accelerated Idioventricular Rhythm

Again, a tachycardia is usually considered to be an HR exceeding 100 bpm. Notice that the rhythms in Figure 6.46 show several examples of what appear to be three or more consecutive PVCs. Recall that three or more PVCs in a row is, by definition, V-Tach. Notice, however, in Figure 6.46B that the rate during the run of the apparent "PVCs" is clearly less than 100 bpm. Careful measurement of the runs of wide and bizarre beats in Figure 6.46A also reveals that the rate is slightly less than 100 bpm. Therefore, it is not strictly correct to refer to these events as tachycardia.

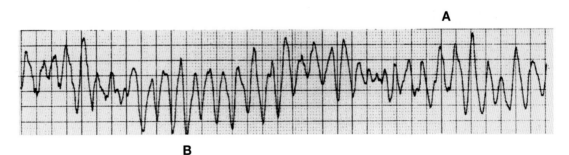

FIGURE 6.44 Torsade de pointes. A, Points up; B, points down.

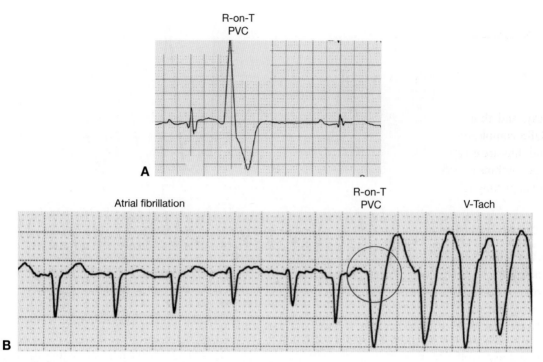

FIGURE 6.45 R-on-T premature ventricular complex (PVC). V-Tach, ventricular tachycardia. **A.** R-on-T PVC that does not cause further ectopy. **B.** R-on-T PVC (circled) initiating V-Tach.

Instead, these ventricular rhythms with normal rates are known as accelerated idioventricular rhythm (AIVR or slow V-Tach). Because, except for the rate, the appearance is just like V-Tach, the term *slow V-Tach* is also sometimes used.

(Idio)Ventricular Escape Rhythm

A ventricular escape rhythm (also known as an idioventricular escape rhythm) is usually seen in situations when higher pacemakers (SA node, AV node, etc.) have failed

to depolarize the ventricles. Thus, these rhythms can be protective; without them, the heart would cease to beat.

The appearance of the QRS complex is the same as that of a PVC (as these beats also arise in the ventricles); however, they are not PVCs. Escape beats and rhythms are not early (premature); they appear only when the normal pacemakers of the heart have failed. The QRS complexes of PVCs and of ventricular escape beats appear wide and bizarre for the same reason: they are not conducted through the ventricles via the normal conduction system. However, the wide and bizarre QRS complexes in Figure 6.39

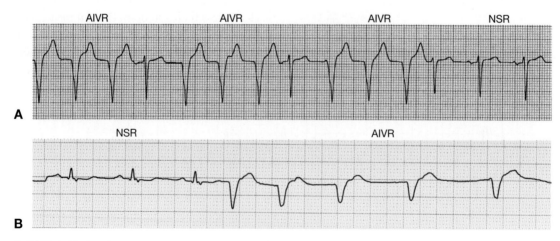

FIGURE 6.46 Accelerated idioventricular rhythm (AIVR). **(A)** and **(B)** are two examples of AIVR. NSR, normal sinus rhythm.

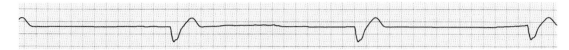

FIGURE 6.47 Idioventricular escape rhythm.

come early, and thus are PVCs, whereas the wide and bizarre QRS complexes in Figure 6.47 come after a long pause, and thus are escape beats. The HR during ventricular escape rhythms is usually quite slow and often inadequate for supporting reasonable perfusion of vital organs.

Ventricular Fibrillation

In V-Fib, the ventricles become electrically incoherent and numerous areas of the ventricular myocardium rapidly depolarize in a disorganized manner. The heart ceases to function as a pump and cardiac output drops to immeasurable levels. Examples of V-Fib are shown in Figure 6.48A. The upper strip shows larger undulations, sometimes called "coarse" V-Fib. The lower strip of Figure 6.48A has smaller

undulations, sometimes referred to as "fine" V-Fib. In both cases, the electrical activity is of low amplitude and appears chaotic, almost like artifact. In any type of V-Fib, the patient is pulseless and unresponsive, with essentially no cardiac output. If the ECG shows a pattern that appears to be V-Fib but the patient is alert and oriented or has a pulse and measurable blood pressure, then the rhythm cannot be V-Fib and what is seen on the monitor must be artifact. It is always important to observe the patient as well as the ECG.

Asystole

Asystole, shown at the end of the lower panels of Figures 6.48 and 6.49, is the lack of a rhythm; that is, the apparent absence of any electrical activity of the heart. In this situation,

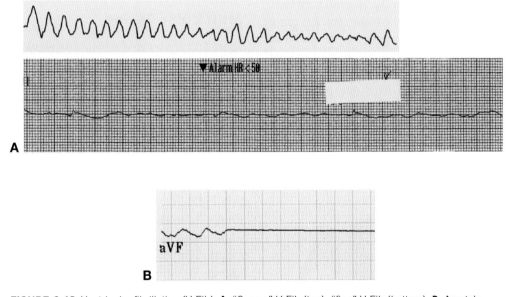

FIGURE 6.48 Ventricular fibrillation (V-Fib). **A.** "Coarse" V-Fib (top); "fine" V-Fib (bottom). **B.** Asystole.

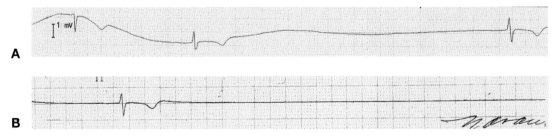

FIGURE 6.49 **A.** Agonal rhythm. **B.** Asystole.

all myocardial pacemakers have failed and the heart is not depolarizing. The appearance, therefore, is of a "flat line," as if the patient were not connected to the ECG machine at all. Patients in asystole will have no cardiac output and therefore will be pulseless and unresponsive.

ELECTRONIC PACEMAKERS

When a patient's intrinsic pacemakers (*e.g.*, SA node) fail to properly pace the heart, an electronic pacemaker is often implanted. The usual procedure involves subcutaneous placement of a small box containing a battery and a microchip that controls the device (Figure 6.50). From this box, wires lead to one or more chambers of the heart.

Fixed-Rate Versus Modern Pacemakers

Early transvenous electronic pacemakers were simple devices that continuously paced at a set rate. The first units used a pacing electrode, which was attached by wire to the controlling box and implanted on the epicardial surface. Over time, the endocardium of the right ventricle came to be the preferred pacing site, largely for practical reasons; for example, pacing electrodes in the left ventricle frequently caused blood clots to form.

Impulses generated in these fixed-rate pacemakers traveled down the wire and depolarized the area of the

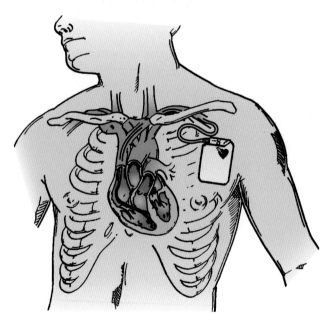

FIGURE 6.50 Electronic pacemaker.

ventricle near the electrode. This depolarization then spread throughout the ventricles using the electrical connections between the cells (gap junctions). As the depolarization did not spread via the normal conduction pathways, the ensuing QRS complexes were wide and bizarre. The HR was constant (*e.g.*, 72 bpm) and the pacemaker functioned monotonously with no regard for the intrinsic electrical activity of the heart.

Virtually all modern pacemakers are more sophisticated than the original fixed-rate pacemakers described earlier. For example, newer pacemakers sense the electrical activity of the heart and take over pacing only when the inherent rate is too low. The term *demand* pacemaker is often used to describe them, as they function only when needed (*i.e.*, when a "demand" is present). Many of the newer pacemakers are also capable of increasing HR in response to increased physical activity, which is sensed by various means such as accelerometers. Some pacemakers have the ability to automatically defibrillate if necessary, and/or to "overdrive" pace the heart in order to break certain arrhythmias.

Ventricular Pacing

Figure 6.51 shows an electronic pacemaker that is pacing the heart by depolarizing the ventricles. The dot in the right ventricle represents the pacemaker electrode. This electrode senses the electrical activity of the heart and remains quiescent unless the inherent HR drops below a threshold rate programmed into the pacemaker.

In the upper ECG strip of Figure 6.51, the first four beats are paced beats, depolarizations initiated by the pacemaker electrode. Each of these four wide and bizarre QRS complexes is preceded by a pacemaker spike (labeled "s"). The HR for these paced beats (which can be measured using the normal techniques for rate) is 60 bpm. The fifth QRS complex, and those following it in Figure 6.51, is not preceded by a pacemaker spike and has a normal (narrow) morphology. This is because the inherent rate has exceeded the pacemaker threshold settings (~60 bpm in this case); the pacemaker's sensor is sensing this and the pacemaker's pacing electrode is not depolarizing. For these beats, the heart is depolarized by the normal inherent mechanisms. The pacemaker only actively paces when the heart's native rate becomes too low.

The ECG in the lower panel of Figure 6.51 is from a different patient. The first five beats are paced (note the pacemaker spikes followed by wide and bizarre QRS complexes). The last four are not paced — they are normal

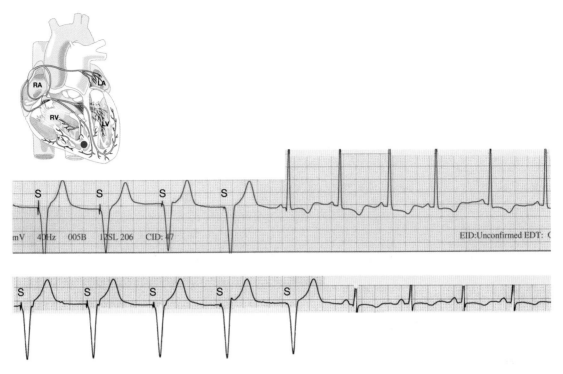

FIGURE 6.51 Ventricular pacing. LA, left atrium; LV, left ventricle; RA, right atrium; RV, right ventricle; S, spike.

QRS complexes preceded by P waves. Again, the pacemaker is only pacing the heart when the inherent rate drops below the rate programmed into the pacemaker (again about 60 bpm).

Atrial and Dual-Chamber Pacing

In the upper panel of Figure 6.52, a pacemaker spike ("S") precedes the P wave, not the QRS complex. This is an example of atrial pacing. In this case, a sensing and pacing electrode (represented by the dot) is located in the atrium. It senses electrical activity in the atria and fires if the atrial rate drops below the threshold, setting off the pacemaker. In this example, all the beats are paced.

Pacemaker spikes followed by a P wave are pacing the atria, whereas spikes followed by a QRS complex are pacing the ventricles. Notice that the QRS complexes in the upper panel of Figure 6.52 are normal in appearance (narrow). This normal appearance reflects the fact that, although the pacemaker depolarizes the atria, the current then spreads down into the ventricles using the normal conduction system (AV node, bundle of His, bundle branches, and Purkinje fibers). Figure 6.52B shows a pacemaker with pacing and sensing electrodes in both the atrium and the ventricle. An atrial pacemaker spike ("A") precedes the P waves and a ventricular pacemaker

spike ("V") precedes wide and bizarre QRS complexes. This type of pacemaker senses the inherent atrial rate, pacing the atria when needed, and also senses the ventricular rate, pacing the ventricles when needed. In this strip, all the beats show both atrial and ventricular pacing.

Letter codes are used to describe the various types of pacemakers. Up to five letters are used in the code, with the last two letters for more advanced functions such as rate-adaptive pacing. The basic functions are explained by the first three letters shown in Box 6.2.

Pacemaker Malfunctions

A variety of factors, including low batteries, displaced wires, fractured wires, and fibrous tissue growth near the area of insertion, can cause pacemakers to malfunction. Two of the major types of malfunction, failure to sense and failure to pace, are described here.

Failure to Sense

Several of the pacemaker spikes in panel A of Figure 6.53 are inappropriate for a "demand" pacemaker. The second, third, fourth, and fifth spikes come immediately after a native QRS complex. The depolarization of the heart by a

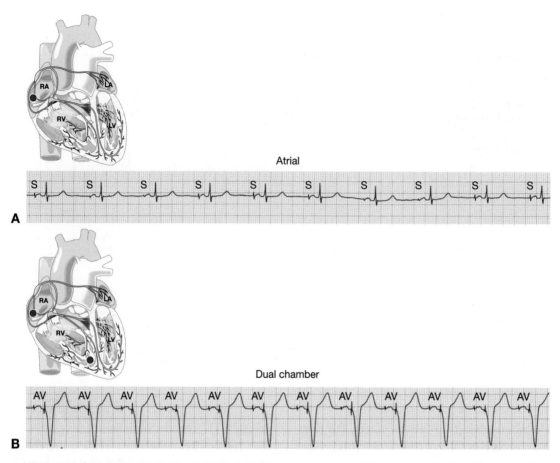

FIGURE 6.52 Electronic pacemakers. **A.** Atrial. **B.** Dual chamber. A, atrial pacemaker spike; LA, left atrium; LV, left ventricle; RA, right atrium; RV, right ventricle; S, spike; V, ventricular pacemaker spike.

native mechanism (likely the SA node, as these QRS complexes are preceded by a small P wave) should have been sensed and the pacemaker should not have fired. The pacemaker is failing at times to sense the inherent activity of the heart. Some of the native QRS complexes in this

ECG are not followed by pacing spikes; this indicates that the pacemaker is sensing some of the native beats.

Failure to Pace

Panels B and C of Figure 6.53 show examples of pacemaker spikes that are not followed by QRS complexes. The pacemaker has fired appropriately but failed to depolarize the heart.

In panel B, some of the pacemaker spikes are followed by QRS complexes and some are not; the failure to pace is intermittent. In panel C (from a different patient), the pacemaker is firing regularly but no QRS complexes follow. The electronic pacemaker is totally failing in its efforts to pace the heart. Neither is any inherent activity present; this patient is in asystole.

ATRIOVENTRICULAR BLOCK

An AV block is an interruption in, or complete obstruction of, impulse conduction from the atria to the ventricles. First-, second-, and third-degree AV blocks represent the varying degrees of obstruction.

Box 6.2	Pacemaker Codes

Letters

- Chamber paced (A = atrium, V = ventricle, D = dual)
- Chamber sensed (A = atrium, V = ventricle, D = dual, O = none)
- Response (I = inhibited, T = triggered, D = dual, O = none)

Examples

VVI = ventricular pacing, ventricular sensing, inhibited by inherent activity

DDD = dual pacing, dual sensing, dual responses

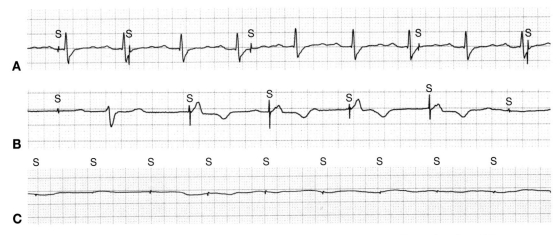

FIGURE 6.53 Electronic pacemaker failures. **A.** Failure to sense. **B.** Failure to pace (intermittent). **C.** Failure to pace.

First-Degree AV Block

Despite its name, first-degree AV "block" is simply a delay in the conduction of depolarization from the atria to the ventricles. In all other forms of AV block, at least some of the atrial depolarizations are truly blocked in that they fail to reach the ventricles. With first-degree AV block, PR intervals are consistently long (≥200 ms) but all the atrial depolarizations do reach the ventricles. If the PR interval is exactly 200 ms, the term *borderline* first-degree AV block is sometimes used.

Figure 6.54 shows some examples of first-degree AV block. Notice that every P wave is followed by a QRS complex and the PR intervals are consistent. The only abnormality is that the PR intervals are abnormally long (≥200 ms). In Figure 6.54B, the P waves are climbing onto the T waves of the previous beat.

Second-Degree AV Block

In second-degree AV block, some P waves are followed by a QRS complex but some are not. Two major types exist: Mobitz type I (also known as Wenckebach) and Mobitz type II.

Second-Degree AV Block Mobitz Type I (Wenckebach)

This phenomenon consists of a progressive lengthening of the PR interval, culminating in a P wave that does not conduct down into the ventricles and therefore is not followed by a QRS complex. The missing (often referred to as "dropped") QRS causes a break in the rhythm that leads to a characteristic appearance of groups of P–QRS–Ts with spaces in between. This is sometimes referred to as a "group beating" pattern.

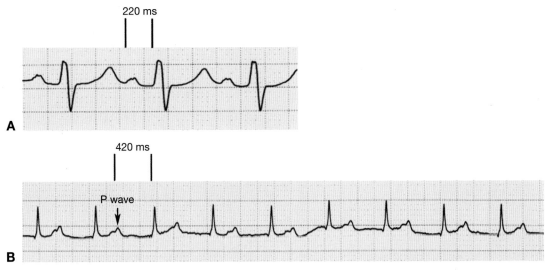

FIGURE 6.54 First-degree atrioventricular block. In **(A)** and **(B)**, PR intervals are between the vertical lines.

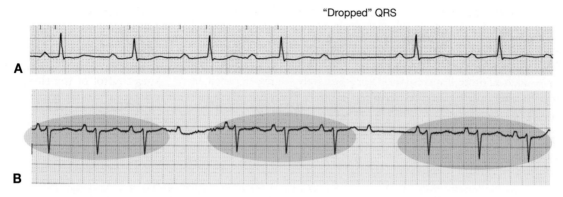

FIGURE 6.55 A. Second-degree atrioventricular block. **B.** Groups of QRS complexes (shaded).

Notice in Figure 6.55A how the PR interval becomes longer with each succeeding cycle until a P wave is not followed by a QRS complex. After the space caused by the missing QRS, the pattern begins again. In Figure 6.55B, the "groups" are shaded. Groups of QRS complexes may appear with other arrhythmias; therefore, to identify second-degree AV block Mobitz type I, the CEP must observe progressively lengthening PR intervals leading to a P wave that is not followed by a QRS complex. Nevertheless, the appearance of grouped beating should greatly raise the index of suspicion for second-degree AV block Mobitz type I.

The Mobitz type 1 pattern may be persistent or may occur intermittently. The ratio of P waves to QRS complexes may vary or remain constant. In Figure 6.55B, a consistent pattern of four P waves for every three QRS complexes is seen. This can be referred to as a 4:3 pattern. In many cases, a variation in the pattern occurs (e.g., sometimes 3:2, sometimes 4:3).

Second-Degree AV Block Mobitz Type II

This type of AV block results in multiple P waves per QRS complex. It may occur occasionally or be persistent

for long periods of time. Figure 6.56A shows a consistent pattern of three P waves per QRS complex, which might therefore be described as "second-degree AV block Mobitz type II with 3:1 conduction." In contrast, the pattern in the middle of the strip shown in Figure 6.56B could be described as having 2:1 conduction (and also is occurring only intermittently). Conduction patterns may vary — for example, between 3:1 and 4:1. Notice in these examples that, for the P waves that do conduct through to the ventricles, the resulting PR intervals are consistent.

2:1 AV Block

A pattern of two P waves per QRS complex could represent a Mobitz type I (Wenckebach) pattern, wherein the first P wave is the one associated with the "dropped" QRS complex. In such cases, the typical grouped beating pattern of Wenckebach does not occur. A pattern of two P waves per QRS complex could also be a Mobitz type II with 2:1 conduction.

Because it is often difficult to tell which pattern is present, some clinicians refer to a pattern of two P waves

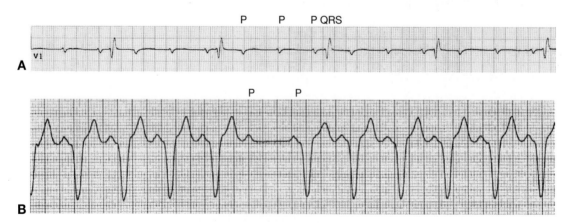

FIGURE 6.56 Second-degree atrioventricular block Mobitz type II. **A.** Second-degree atrioventricular block Mobitz type II 3:1. **B.** Intermittent second-degree atrioventricular block 2:1.

per QRS complex as a second-degree AV block without specifying whether it is a Mobitz I or a Mobitz II. If the rhythm is observed for some time, it may be possible to discern that it is in fact a Mobitz I, as a different pattern of periodicity — such as three P waves (with a progressively lengthening PR interval) to two QRS complexes (3:2) — may intermittently emerge.

Third-Degree AV Block (Complete Heart Block)

Third-degree AV block represents a complete electrical dissociation between the atria and the ventricles and therefore is also called complete heart block. Although it can be transient, the condition is often permanent and usually requires the implantation of an electronic pacemaker.

Because the atria and the ventricles are not communicating electrically, the resulting ECG appears as if an atrial ECG had been superimposed over a ventricular ECG. The atria might be in any atrial rhythm from NSR (Figure 6.57D) to A-Fib (Figure 6.57C). Irrespective of the atrial rhythm, it is independent from that of the ventricles. Although the atria are depolarizing (and may even be in NSR), as these depolarizations are not reaching the ventricles, some subsidiary pacemaker must take over for the ventricles, just as if the atria were not depolarizing at all. Usually, a junctional escape or idioventricular rhythm is pacing the ventricles. In the former case, the QRS complexes will typically be narrow, whereas in the

latter, the rate will tend to be very slow and the QRS complexes wide. These concepts are consistent with the escape rhythms. In previous discussions of escape rhythms, the higher pacemakers (*e.g.*, SA node) had failed, leading to lower pacemakers taking control of the rhythm. In the case of complete (third-degree) heart block, again, the higher pacemakers may be operating but the depolarizations are not reaching the ventricles.

As the atrial and ventricular rhythms are independent in this type of heart block, they must each be described in order to define the overall rhythm. For example, Figure 6.57B might be described as "sinus arrhythmia with third-degree AV block and a junctional escape rhythm." In this example, the P waves are coming along at a normal rate and have a normal morphology but significant variation is occurring in the P–P interval; thus, the atrial rhythm appears to be sinus arrhythmia. The QRS complexes are narrow and the ventricular rate is regular and slightly less than 50 bpm, consistent with a junctional escape rhythm. Figure 6.57B also illustrates the fact that P waves are often obscured in complete heart block. Notice that the second P wave is "missing" and likely buried in the T wave; the third is merging with a QRS complex; and the sixth and ninth P waves fall in with the ST segments.

In common with complete heart block, both types of second-degree AV block also have more P waves than QRS complexes. However, in second-degree AV block, a relationship exists between the atrial and ventricular rhythms. In Mobitz I, the pattern of progressively

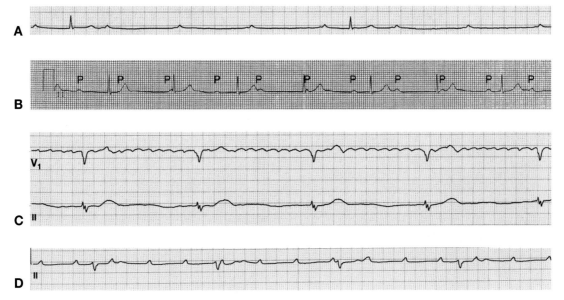

FIGURE 6.57 Third-degree (complete) atrioventricular block. **A.** Sinus bradycardia with complete heart block and a slow junctional escape rhythm. **B.** Sinus arrhythmia with complete heart block and a junctional escape rhythm. **C.** Atrial fibrillation with complete heart block and an idioventricular escape rhythm. **D.** Normal sinus rhythm with complete heart block and an idioventricular escape rhythm.

increasing PR intervals followed by a "dropped" QRS can be found, whereas in Mobitz II, the PR intervals of the beats that do conduct are consistent and, even if the conduction is varying (*e.g.*, between 2:1 and 3:1), a relationship between atrial and ventricular activity is present. In complete heart block, although patterns may occasionally appear to resemble something else (*e.g.*, progressive lengthening of the PR interval), careful inspection will reveal no consistent relationship between the atrial and ventricular rhythms. A long rhythm strip may be helpful in cases where the rhythm is not readily apparent.

Finally, in true third-degree AV block, the atrial rate must be faster than the ventricular rate. If the atria and ventricles are functioning independently, but the ventricular rate is faster than the atrial rate, the rhythm is called AV dissociation.

AV Dissociation

The terminology concerning third-degree AV block (a serious and often permanent condition) and AV dissociation (a transient and usually innocuous condition) can be confusing. During both conditions, the atria and the ventricles are dissociated — they are functionally electrically independently. Therefore, the term *AV dissociation* often comes up during discussions of third-degree AV block. Unfortunately, the term is also used to refer to a distinct situation in which the ECG is similar in all respects to third-degree AV block with the exception that the ventricular rate is faster (often very slightly so) than the atrial rate. This condition may occur in apparently healthy people during sleep. This typically benign type of AV dissociation often occurs when the supraventricular (usually sinus) rate has slowed and a lower pacemaker (junctional or idioventricular) begins to pace the ventricles. When the atrial rate increases, the ventricles are "captured" and

AV dissociation is no longer present; thus, this condition is typically transient.

Notice at the beginning of the ECG shown in Figure 6.58A that the atrial rate is slightly slower than the ventricular rate and the atrial and ventricular rhythms are distinct (dissociated). Some of the P waves (*e.g.*, the fifth) merge partially with the QRS complexes and therefore are partially obscured. Other P waves (*e.g.*, the seventh) are not visible because atrial and ventricular depolarizations are occurring concurrently and the QRS is therefore obliterating the P wave. At the end of the ECG, the atria appear to have "captured" the ventricles. The ventricular rate has slowed, facilitating the return to sinus rhythm.

Figure 6.58B shows another example of AV dissociation. Again, several of the P waves merge with QRS complexes. In this example, the ventricular rate is somewhat irregular and a PVC falls in the middle of the ECG.

ECG LEADS

The standard ECG has 12 different leads formed by the placement of 10 electrodes. Each of the 12 leads represents a different electrical view of the heart. Additional leads (*e.g.*, right sided) are sometimes used but most CEPs use the standard leads. The 12 standard ECG leads are identified in Box 6.3.

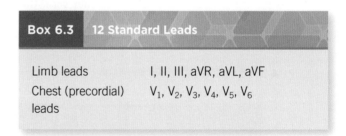

Box 6.3	12 Standard Leads
Limb leads	I, II, III, aVR, aVL, aVF
Chest (precordial) leads	V_1, V_2, V_3, V_4, V_5, V_6

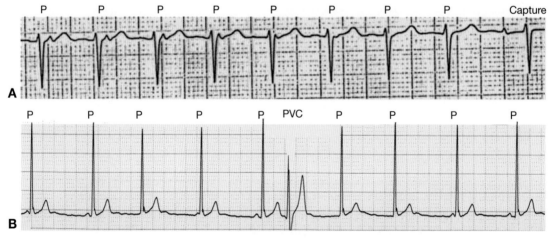

FIGURE 6.58 Atrioventricular (AV) dissociation. **A** and **B.** Two examples of AV dissociation.

Limb Leads

Leads I, II, and III are among the easiest to understand. They have two poles, designated positive and negative. The basic concepts of bipolar leads were introduced earlier in this chapter.

Figure 6.59 shows where the positive and negative poles of these leads are located. For example, the left arm electrode functions as the positive pole of Lead I and the right arm electrode as the negative pole. Notice that for Lead III the left arm electrode functions as the negative pole and the left leg electrode is the positive pole. A given electrode can be made to function as either pole (positive or negative) depending on which lead is being recorded. This also illustrates that electrodes are not leads. Electrodes are the conductive patches attached to the patient. The ECG machine uses the currents detected by these electrodes to obtain the various ECG leads.

Figure 6.59 also shows a triangle formed by Leads I, II, and III. Known as the Einthoven triangle, for the physiologist and Nobel laureate Willem Einthoven, who invented the modern ECG machine, this triangle diagrams the relationships between these leads. The three short ECG strips in Figure 6.59 show ECGs recorded simultaneously in these leads. Notice that the same electrical events appear quite different when viewed in the different leads (this is why different leads are used; they provide additional information).

Given the orientation of Leads I, II, and III, the voltage in Lead II at a given point in time should equal the sum of that obtained in Leads I and III. This relationship is sometimes expressed as I + III = II. This has some practical utility, as it is one way to verify whether the limb lead wires were placed in the correct positions. For instance, if the P waves in Lead II are negative, this may represent an ectopic rhythm or it may simply indicate misplacement of the wires. If the patient is present, the CEP should check that the wires are correctly attached to the electrodes, as it is a common mistake to reverse the right- and left-side wires (*e.g.*, RA and LA). If the patient is not present, one method of verifying proper limb lead wire placement is to ascertain whether I + III = II (this method catches some types of error, but not all). This is done quite simply; deflections above the baseline are given positive values, whereas deflections below the baseline are assigned negative values. For instance, a 2-mm deflection below the baseline would be counted as a −2 mm (or −0.2 mV), whereas a 2-mm upward deflection would be counted as +2 mm (or +0.2 mV). At a given time point, the sum of I + III should equal II. If not, it is likely that the wires were misplaced. In different leads, the peak of the R wave or other events may not occur at exactly the same time, so it is important to measure at the same time in the different leads. If the peaks of the R waves are not simultaneous, a ruler placed vertically so that it crosses Leads I, II, and III at a given time point can assist in measurement. Figure 6.60 shows an example where I + III does equal II, thus providing evidence that

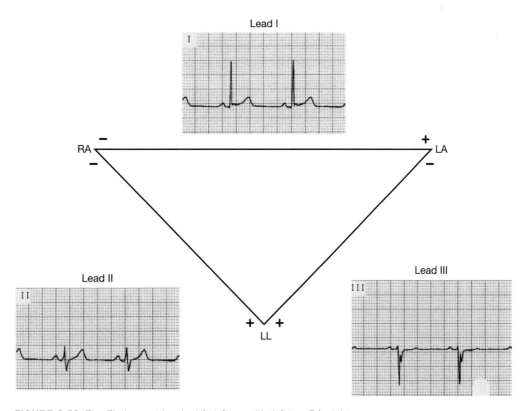

FIGURE 6.59 The Einthoven triangle. LA, left arm; LL, left leg; RA, right arm.

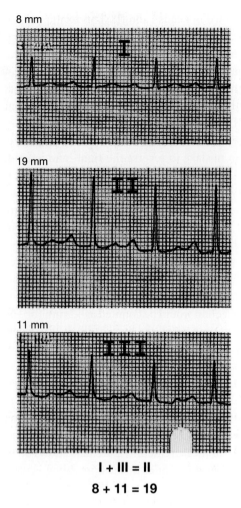

$$I + III = II$$
$$8 + 11 = 19$$

FIGURE 6.60 I + III = II.

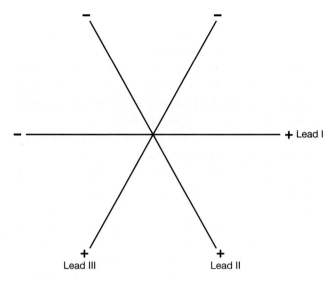

FIGURE 6.62 Triaxial diagram.

the wires were properly placed. One can also confirm the correct lead wire placement if the wave forms are pointed in the right direction for each lead. For example, as you will read later, the wave forms in Lead II should all be positive and the wave forms in aVR should all be negative.

It is helpful for many purposes to think of the leads of the Einthoven triangle as meeting at a central point.

In Figures 6.61 and 6.62, Leads I, II, and III are shown pushed inward, resulting in what is sometimes called a triaxial diagram. The utility of this will become apparent later. For now it is important to begin thinking of these leads as shown in Figure 6.62.

Although a great deal of information can be obtained from the original three leads (I, II, and III), it became clear over time that additional electrical views (*i.e.*, leads) would be helpful. The next three leads invented were aVR, aVL, and aVF. The "a" indicates that the voltage recorded by these leads is augmented and the last two letters indicate where the positive pole is: VR for vector right arm, VL for vector left arm, and VF for vector foot (actually between the two feet).

Neither the augmented limb leads nor the chest leads are simple bipolar leads. For example, leads aVR, aVL, and aVF have their voltage increased to increase clarity and neither these leads nor the chest leads have a single electrode functioning as a negative pole. Because of this,

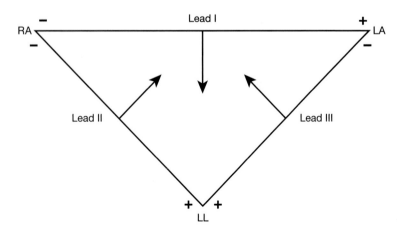

FIGURE 6.61 Collapsing the triangle. LA, left arm; LL, left leg; RA, right arm.

they are sometimes referred to as unipolar leads. A technical discussion of the nature of these leads is beyond the scope of this chapter. Fortunately, detailed knowledge of the technical aspects of these issues is not needed to successfully interpret ECGs; moreover, for conceptual purposes, it is quite useful (although technically incorrect) to think of all 12 leads as simple bipolar leads.

Figure 6.63 shows all six limb leads arranged to meet at a central point in what is often called a hexaxial diagram. The name of the lead (*e.g.*, I) is placed at the positive pole and the negative pole of each lead is labeled with a minus sign. The six limb leads are all obtained using only four electrodes (right arm, left arm, right leg, and left leg). The right leg electrode functions only as the electrical ground, so actually only three of these four electrodes come directly into play in obtaining the six leads. Inputs from the limb electrodes are manipulated by the ECG machine to construct the three augmented leads. All the limb leads are recorded in the frontal plane.

Chest Leads

The chest or "V" leads (V_1–V_6) are different from the limb leads in at least two respects. The chest leads record electrical activity from the perspective of the transverse (horizontal) plane and each lead has a distinct electrode that functions as the positive pole of that lead. Although no distinct electrode functions as the negative pole of these leads, it is useful to imagine a negative pole in the middle of the thorax. Figure 6.64 shows the chest lead electrode placement from an anterior view (V_6 cannot be seen in Figure 6.64).

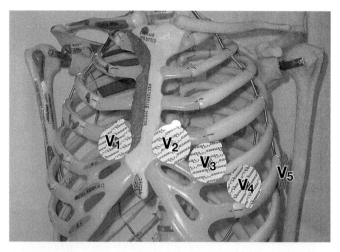

FIGURE 6.64 Anterior view of chest leads.

The V lead furthest to the right, V_1, is located just to the right of the sternum in the fourth intercostal space (space between the fourth and fifth ribs). Although the most rightward, obviously this lead is close to the centerline of the chest (midsagittal line). The standard ECG is mainly focused on the left ventricle, so relative to the left side of the heart this lead is "rightward." The V leads then proceed to the left. The lead furthest to the left, V_6, is in line with the middle of the axilla on the left side. For a general orientation, it is useful to conceive of V_1 and V_2 as close to the interventricular septum, V_3 and V_4 as "anterior" in relation to the left ventricle, and V_5 and V_6 as "lateral" in relation to the left ventricle. The specific placement of all the electrodes for a 12-lead ECG is identified in Box 6.4.

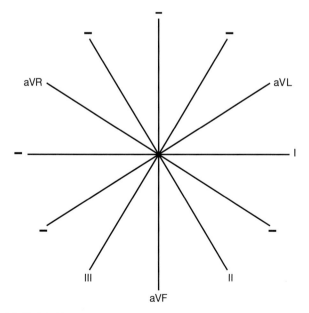

FIGURE 6.63 Hexaxial diagram.

Box 6.4	Electrodes
RA	Right arm
LA	Left arm
RL	Right leg
LL	Left leg
V_1	Fourth intercostal space just right of the sternum
V_2	Fourth intercostal space just left of the sternum
V_3	Midway between V_2 and V_4
V_4	Fifth interspace left midclavicular line
V_5	Left anterior axillary line on the same level as V_4
V_6	Left midaxillary line on the same level as V_4 and V_5

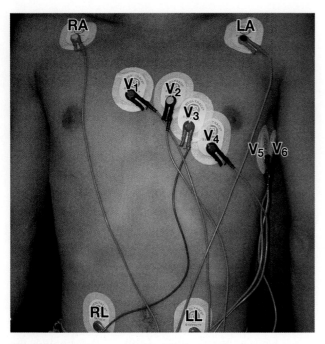

FIGURE 6.65 Mason–Likar (modified) electrode placement.

Modifications of Electrode Placement

The placement described is for resting supine ECGs. Unless otherwise indicated, resting ECGs are assumed to be recorded in the supine position with the electrodes in the standard placement. If the ECG is taken under other conditions (*e.g.*, standing), it should be labeled as such.

Some situations dictate different electrode placement. For example, when the ECG is recorded during an exercise stress test, the limb leads must be moved as they present a tripping hazard, and the tracing would be unreadable due to artifact. In such cases, the chest electrodes are placed in the normal positions but the limb electrodes are moved on to the torso in the Mason–Likar placement

shown in Figure 6.65 and described in Box 6.5. If a nonstandard placement such as the Mason–Likar is used, it should be noted on the ECG. Thus, an ECG recorded with the modified placement and patient standing might be marked, "Standing Mason–Likar."

Often, moving the limb electrodes to the modified placement has little effect on the ECG. However, as illustrated in Figure 6.66, significant ECG changes may occur. It may therefore be best to record an ECG with standard electrode placement and the patient supine to use for comparison if nonstandard postures and electrode placements will subsequently be done. A comparison of these ECGs can assist in determining whether changes on the ECG reflect important physiological phenomena or are simply artifacts from nonstandard conditions.

Localization of Leads

Certain leads typically offer better "views" of certain areas of the heart (Figures 6.67 and 6.68, and Box 6.6). As the positive poles of Leads II, III, and aVF all point downward (straight down in the case of aVF, and obliquely downward in the cases of II and III), these leads together are known as the inferior leads. Leads I and aVL are oriented (left) laterally, so they are included with V_5 and V_6 (V_6 cannot be seen in Figure 6.67) as lateral leads. Leads V_1 and V_2 are close to the interventricular septum and V_4 and V_5 are near the anterior surface of the left ventricle. Lead aVR has a unique perspective and therefore does not belong to a "group" as the other leads do.

Leads that view the same area of the heart are "contiguous leads." For example, Leads II, III, and aVF are contiguous inferior leads. This is important because ECG abnormalities such as ST-segment elevation and depression associated with ischemia/infarct in an area of the heart will appear in multiple contiguous leads.

Box 6.5	Mason–Likar Lead Placement (Also Known as the Modified or Exercise Lead Placement)
LA	Left subclavicular fossa
RA	Right subclavicular fossa
RL[a]	Right anterior abdominal wall at the point where an imaginary line coming laterally from the umbilicus would intersect with an imaginary line coming inferiorly from the middle of the right clavicle
LL[a]	Left anterior abdominal wall at the point where an imaginary line coming laterally from the umbilicus would intersect with an imaginary line coming inferiorly from the middle of the left clavicle

[a]Other placements have been described for RL and LL. We describe one that is acceptable and easy to objectively determine.

LA, left arm; LL, left leg; RA, right arm; RL, right leg.

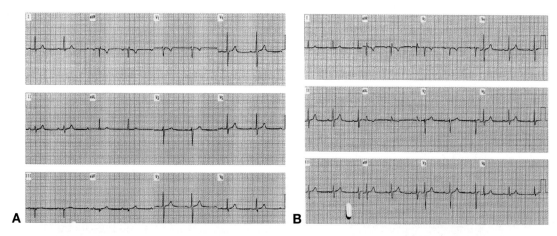

FIGURE 6.66 ECG changes from modified lead placement. **A.** Standard. **B.** Mason–Likar.

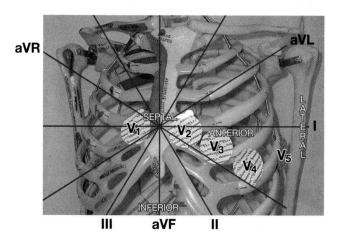

FIGURE 6.67 Leads.

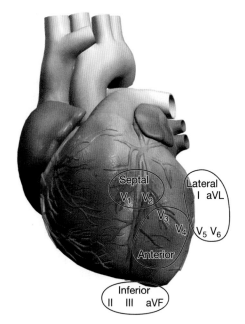

FIGURE 6.68 Approximate areas of the heart associated with different leads.

Box 6.6   Localization of Leads

Area	Leads
Inferior	II, III, aVF
Lateral	I, aVL, V_5, V_6
Septal	V_1, V_2
Anterior[a]	V_3, V_4

[a]Some classifications consider V_1, V_2, V_3, and V_4 to be the "anterior" leads. Leads depicting the same area of the heart are "contiguous leads."

Normal Patterns of the 12 Leads

The patterns that appear in the various leads will vary depending on numerous factors such as the mean electrical axis of the heart, so it is difficult to fully describe what is normal in each of the leads. Some general principles can, however, be described.

As previously discussed, if NSR is present, the P waves should be upright (positive) in Lead II and negative in Lead aVR. In fact, if NSR is present, the P waves should be upright in Leads I, II, V_5, and V_6. If the P waves are not positive in all these leads, the term *unusual P-wave axis* is sometimes used. This implies that the rhythm is not sinus in origin and likely is an ectopic atrial rhythm.

Some general concepts concerning the morphology of the QRS complexes in the chest leads are very useful in interpreting ECGs. Normally, the first portion of the ventricles to depolarize is the interventricular septum, which in most people is activated first by a portion of the left bundle branch. Normally, the septum depolarizes from left to right — in other words, toward the positive poles of V_1 and V_2 (this is at least partially due to the anterior

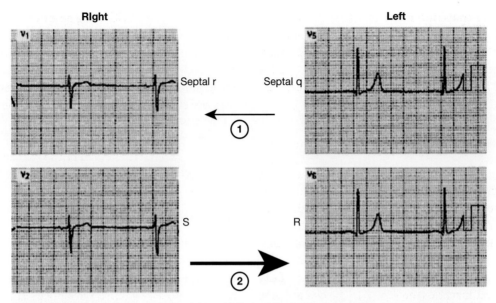

FIGURE 6.69 Normal patterns in the right and left chest leads. The interventricular septum depolarizes first (1), followed by depolarization of the rest of the ventricles (2). Arrows indicate the relative size and direction of the net current.

vector of depolarization) and away from the positive poles of V_5 and V_6. Therefore, a small r wave of short duration is seen in the right chest leads (V_1 and V_2) and a very small q wave of short duration in the left chest leads (V_5 and V_6). Because this is caused by septal activation, the small r in the right chest leads is often referred to as a septal r wave and the small q in the left chest leads as a septal q wave. Following septal activation, the bulk of the right and left ventricles depolarize more or less simultaneously. Because the left ventricle has so much more mass than the right, the mean vector of current is flowing toward the left chest leads and away from the right chest leads. This results in large R waves in V_5 and V_6 and large S waves in V_1 and V_2. Figure 6.69 illustrates these concepts.

The same electrical event of ventricular depolarization results in different recordings in the various leads because of their position and orientation. Leads V_3 and V_4 are in the middle between the right and left chest leads; therefore, the QRS seen in these leads normally has a morphology somewhere in between the rS of V_1 and the qR of V_6. The increase in R-wave amplitude from V_1 across to the left chest leads is called R-wave progression. The size of the R waves in the middle chest leads (V_4 and V_5) is typically intermediate, whereas both lateral chest leads (V_5 and V_6) should normally show relatively large R waves (although it is common for V_5 to have a larger R than V_6).

As the pattern shifts from an rS in the right chest leads to a qR in the left chest leads, somewhere, typically in V_3 and V_4, the height of the R wave becomes greater than the depth of the S wave. The point (lead) where the R wave becomes as large as or larger than the S wave is called the transition zone (Figure 6.70). Early transition occurs when the R wave is as large as or larger than the S wave in V_1 or V_2. A transition that does not occur until V_5 or V_6 is called late transition. Ectopic beats are not included in these determinations, so in the late transition example of Figure 6.70, the second QRS complex with the large R wave in Lead V_3 would not be counted because it is a PVC.

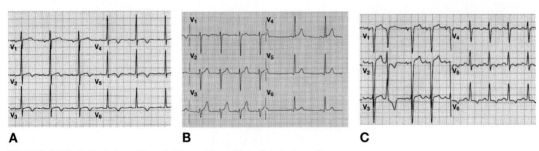

A **B** **C**

FIGURE 6.70 A. Early transition. **B.** Normal transition. **C.** Late transition.

Abnormalities of transition may indicate various conditions, to be discussed later in this chapter. Sometimes the height of the r waves does not increase significantly moving across from the right to the left chest leads. This is abnormal and is referred to as poor R-wave progression.

AXIS

Axis is a term used to describe the net direction (or net vector) that the current of ventricular depolarization is traveling in the frontal plane. It can be normal or deviated to the left or right. Axis deviations may indicate significant clinical conditions such as myocardial infarction, congenital heart defects, or pulmonary disease, and thus are important to understand. Many contemporary ECG machines will estimate axis; however, CEPs need to know how to make the necessary observations and calculations and not rely on any machine.

Depolarization of the ventricles is a complex event, occurring in three dimensions with current traveling in numerous directions simultaneously. The net direction of this current (in the frontal plane) can be determined from a standard 12-lead ECG using an extension of some basic principles described previously. Recall that current moving toward the positive pole of a lead will result in a positive deflection, current moving away from the positive pole (toward the negative pole) of a lead is recorded as a negative deflection, and current moving perpendicular to the orientation of a lead causes a deflection with a net voltage of zero (either a flat line or a complex with equal positive and negative components). These principles can be used to determine the net vector of electrical currents recorded on an ECG.

Normal Axis

For many purposes, the CEP needs to determine only whether the axis is normal, deviated to the left or right, or extremely deviated (to the right). A normal axis can usually be determined very readily by simple inspection of Leads I and aVF. If the overall QRS complexes in these leads are positive, then the axis is normal. The QRS complexes of Leads I and aVF in Figure 6.71 are very positive, consisting mainly of relatively large R waves. This implies that the net vector of ventricular depolarization is traveling toward the positive poles of these leads. The axis need

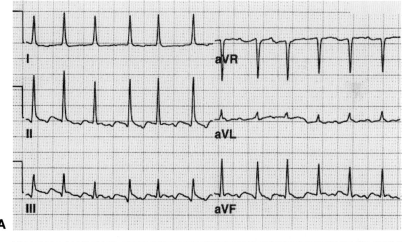

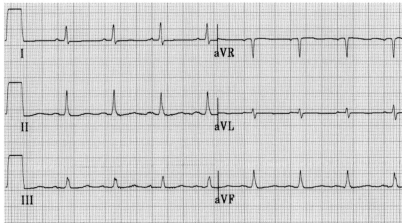

FIGURE 6.71 Normal axes. **(A)** and **(B)** are just two examples with a normal axis.

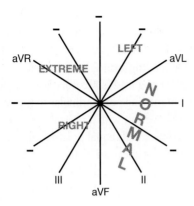

FIGURE 6.72 Axis quadrants.

not be heading directly at the positive pole and, obviously, could not simultaneously be heading directly at the positive poles of both leads, but rather is oriented more toward their positive poles than away from them. If this is the case for Leads I and aVF, the net vector (axis) of the electrical current falls within the normal axis range.

Depolarization of the heart normally proceeds down and to the left. This is the basis for the normal axis quadrant (Figure 6.72). With many ECGs, this simple, cursory inspection of Leads I and aVF to establish that the QRS complexes are more positive than negative is usually all that is needed to establish that the axis is normal.

Axis Quadrant

More precise descriptions of the axis are sometimes needed. As indicated in Box 6.7, the first step is establishing in which "quadrant" the axis is directed. A simple way to determine this is illustrated in Figure 6.73. This technique uses the arms in a kind of semaphore flag signaling system. Because the positive pole of Lead I is on the left arm, the left arm is extended out to the left if the QRS in Lead I is generally positive. Conversely, if the overall

---

Box 6.7   Determining Axis

- Determine quadrant by inspecting Leads I and aVF.
- Find the limb lead with the most isoelectric QRS complex.
- The axis is perpendicular to the lead with the isoelectric QRS complex and falls in the quadrant previously determined.

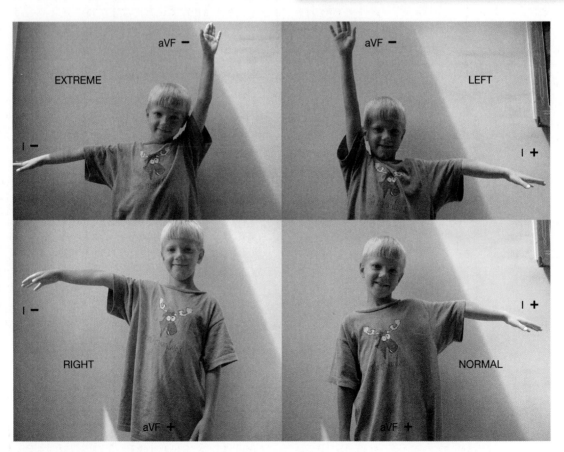

FIGURE 6.73 Method for determining axis quadrant.

QRS complex in Lead I is generally negative, extend the right arm out to the right (away from the positive pole). On the basis of the hexaxial diagram, the positive pole of aVF can be imagined as between the two feet. Therefore, if the QRS is generally positive in Lead aVF, extend an arm straight down; if the QRS in aVF is negative, extend the arm up. In between the arms is the quadrant wherein the axis lies. For example, if the QRS is generally negative in Lead I and positive in Lead aVF, the axis lies in the right quadrant. If the QRS is negative in both I and aVF, the axis lies in the extreme quadrant. Using this method, one can quickly determine the quadrant. As previously noted, this is often all that is of interest to the CEP. An axis in the right quadrant is said to exhibit right axis deviation (RAD), one in the left quadrant left axis deviation (LAD), one in the extreme quadrant an extreme axis deviation (or extreme RAD), and an axis in the normal quadrant is said to have a normal axis.

Figure 6.74 is the hexaxial diagram previously described. The name of each lead is placed by the positive pole of the lead. An additional feature is that the circle described by this diagram has been subdivided into four parts: normal, left (axis deviation), right (axis deviation), and extreme (axis deviation). Notice that the four axis quadrants are not equal; the normal quadrant is expanded. Many apparently normal individuals have an axis that falls in the left quadrant slightly above the positive pole of Lead I, so it is common to expand the normal axis zone as shown. This complicates matters slightly as it is possible for an axis in the left quadrant to be considered normal. Some authorities use zones of equal size to avoid this problem. In such a system, the normal quadrant is not expanded and any axis in the left quadrant would be considered LAD. The expanded normal quadrant (+90 to −30 degrees) is used for the purposes described for CEPs.

Quantitative Description of Axis (Degrees)

The axis can also be described numerically using a system shown in Figure 6.74. The axis circle is divided into 360 degrees. By convention, there are +180 degrees and −180 degrees, with the positive pole of Lead I designated as 0 degrees. If the net current of ventricular depolarization in a particular patient travels directly toward the positive pole of Lead II (+60), this should result in the QRS complex in Lead II largely consisting of a positive deflection (*i.e.*, R wave). The orientation of Lead aVL is perpendicular to Lead II; therefore, the QRS complex in Lead aVL should be largely isoelectric.

The axis can be determined by building upon these principles. The first step is to establish the quadrant. (Notice that the chest leads are not used, as these leads are not aligned in the frontal plane.) The QRS complexes in Leads I and aVF of Figure 6.75 are more positive than negative; therefore, the axis must fall in the normal quadrant. Next, determine which of the limb leads shows an isoelectric QRS complex (one that has equal positive and negative components). In Figure 6.75, the positive R wave of aVL is almost identical in height to the depth of the negative S wave; thus, the net QRS is essentially isoelectric. Applying these findings, if Lead aVL is isoelectric, then the axis should be perpendicular to it. The axis is in the normal quadrant, so it must be +60 degrees.

The QRS complex in Figure 6.76 in Lead I is largely positive, whereas that in Lead aVF is mostly negative. Therefore, the axis must fall in the left quadrant. None of the limb leads is truly isoelectric (positive and negative components of the QRS complex canceling out to zero). This is often the case and necessitates selection of the lead that is closest to isoelectric. Although the positive and negative components of the QRS complex in Lead aVR are not identical, the QRS in this lead is closer to isoelectric than the QRS in the other limb leads. This means that the axis is close to, but not exactly perpendicular to, this lead (either −60 degrees or +120 degrees). Because the axis is in the left quadrant, the axis must be closest to −60 degrees. As the QRS complex in Lead aVR is not exactly isoelectric, the axis is not exactly perpendicular to this lead; however, the exact axis should be within 15 degrees of the axis obtained using this method. This approximation is useful for most clinical purposes. The axis in Figure 6.76 can be described qualitatively as LAD and quantitatively as −60 degrees.

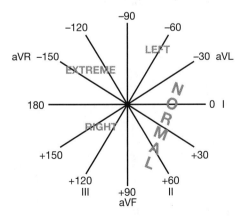

FIGURE 6.74 Axis degrees. Normal (−30 to +90 degrees), right axis deviation (+90 to 180 degrees), extreme right axis deviation (180 to −90 degrees), and left axis deviation (−30 to −90 degrees).

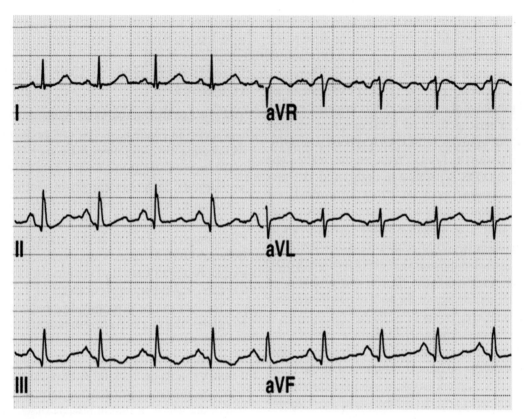

FIGURE 6.75 Normal axis (+60 degrees).

If the expanded normal quadrant is used, it is possible for the axis to be in the left quadrant, yet still be considered normal. In Figure 6.77, the QRS complex is mostly positive in Lead I and negative in Lead aVF; therefore, the axis is in the left quadrant. Of the limb leads, Lead II is the closest to isoelectric. If the axis is in the left quadrant and roughly perpendicular to Lead II, it must be close to −30 degrees. This axis is quantitatively described as

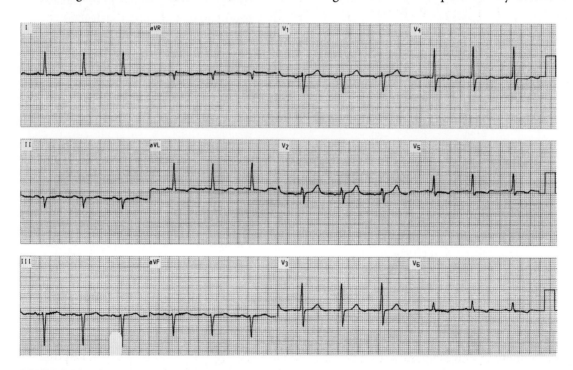

FIGURE 6.76 Left axis deviation (−60 degrees).

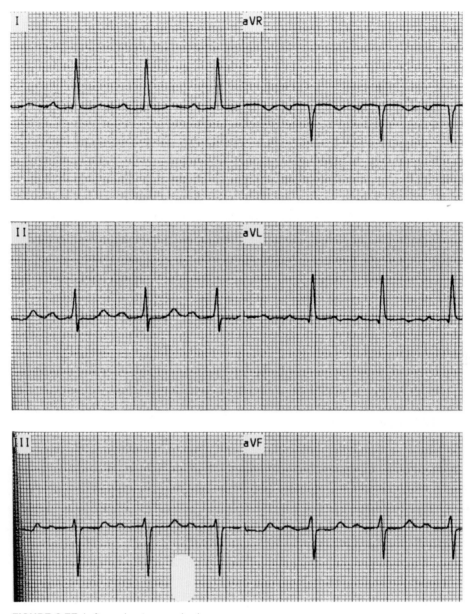

FIGURE 6.77 Left quadrant, normal axis.

−30 degrees. If the QRS complex in Lead II were perfectly isoelectric, the axis would be exactly −30 degrees and therefore normal; however, because Lead II is not exactly isoelectric, the axis is close to, but not exactly, −30 degrees. If the axis were slightly more negative than −30 degrees, then it would be considered LAD, whereas if it were slightly more positive than −30 degrees, it would be a normal axis. A little reasoning can resolve this dilemma. If the QRS complex in Lead II is more positive than negative, which it is in this case, then the axis must be pointing a little more toward the positive pole of Lead II (+60 degrees) and therefore falls into the normal quadrant. If

the QRS complex in Lead II were more negative than positive, then the axis would be directed a little more toward the negative pole of Lead II (−120 degrees) and therefore LAD would be present.

In Figure 6.78, the axis is roughly perpendicular to Lead aVF (aVF has the most isoelectric QRS complex). Because aVF is used with Lead I in determining the quadrant, this might seem to be a problem. In reality, the axis in this case is quite easy to estimate as it must be roughly perpendicular to Lead aVF and oriented toward Lead I (as the QRS in Lead I is clearly more positive than negative), and therefore must be approximately 0 degrees. Because

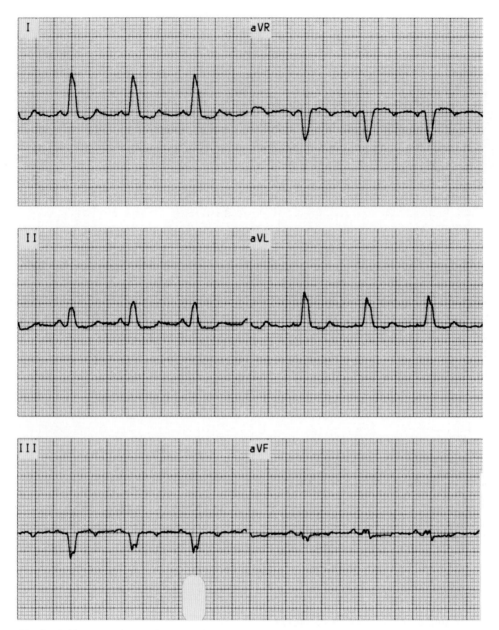

FIGURE 6.78 Horizontal axis (0 degrees).

0 degree falls within the normal quadrant, the axis is normal. Similarly, if Lead I had the most isoelectric QRS complex, then the axis would be roughly perpendicular to Lead I. In such cases, if the QRS complex in Lead aVF were positive, the axis would be +90 degrees, and if the QRS complex in aVF were negative, the axis would be −90 degrees.

Figure 6.79 is an ECG from a patient in A-Fib. The net QRS complexes in Lead I are negative and those in aVF are positive; thus, the axis lies in the RAD quadrant. Clearly, Lead aVR is the most isoelectric as it has essentially no QRS complexes (because the axis lies directly perpendicular to the orientation to this lead). As it has

been established that the axis is in the right quadrant, numerically the axis must be +120 degrees.

Indeterminate Axis

In the case illustrated in Figure 6.80, notice that most of the limb leads exhibit isoelectric QRS complexes. This is because the mean electrical axis of this patient's heart is not in the frontal plane; in fact, the axis is perpendicular to the frontal plane. Normal methods cannot be used in such cases and the axis is usually simply described as indeterminate.

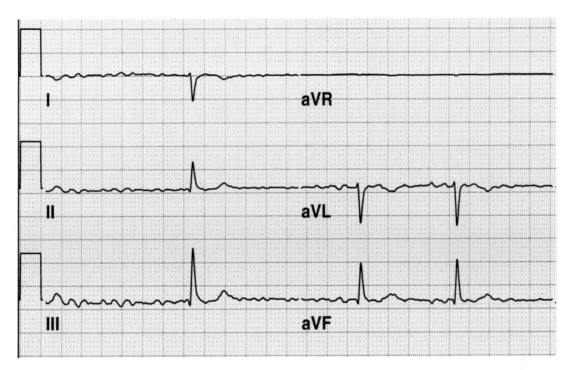

FIGURE 6.79 Right axis deviation (+120 degrees).

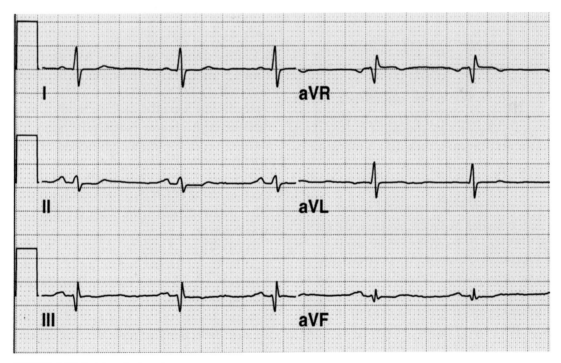

FIGURE 6.80 Indeterminate axis.

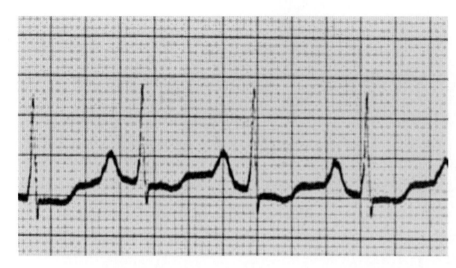

FIGURE 6.81 Right atrial abnormality (enlargement).

ECG FINDINGS IN CARDIAC PATHOLOGIES

This section discusses the ECG patterns found with the most common cardiac pathologies, including myocardial hypertrophy, conduction defects, and ischemia and infarct, as well as pericarditis, electrolyte imbalances, and other conditions.

Myocardial Hypertrophy

The patterns seen in myocardial hypertrophy may be summarized as follows: hypertrophy of the atria leads to larger P waves, whereas hypertrophy of the ventricles leads to larger QRS complexes. Of course, a few specifics must be learned but the basic premise is that simple.

Right Atrial Abnormality

As the SA node is located in the RA, normally the RA begins to depolarize slightly before the left atrium (LA). An enlarged RA takes longer to depolarize and therefore a significant portion of the electrical activity of an enlarged RA occurs as the LA is depolarizing. These electrical signals (right and left atrial) add together resulting in an abnormally tall and often pointy ("peaked") P wave (Figure 6.81) typically found in Lead II. A P wave greater than or equal to 0.25 mV (2.5 mm) is considered abnormally tall. Because the LA depolarizes normally and the lengthened depolarization of the RA occurs more or less concurrently, the overall time of atrial depolarization is not changed.

Sometimes the ECG shows normal P waves when the RA is, in fact, enlarged; moreover, sometimes the P waves are abnormally tall when the atria are of normal size. Therefore, the term *right atrial abnormality* (RAA) is preferable to the term *right atrial enlargement* (RAE), as the former indicates an ECG finding but does not assert that particular morphological changes have occurred. Because RAA is often seen with pulmonary disease, this pattern of tall P waves is commonly referred to as P pulmonale.

Left Atrial Abnormality

When the RA is of normal size, but the LA is enlarged, a wide P wave, often with a notch in the middle, may be seen typically in Lead II. The first part of this wide P wave represents the normal electrical activity of the normal RA (because the RA begins to depolarize before the LA). The enlarged LA then takes longer to depolarize; therefore, the latter part of the P wave lengthens, resulting in the abnormally long ($\geq$120 ms) P wave in Lead II (Figure 6.82). A common cause of left atrial abnormality (LAA) is mitral valve disease; therefore, the pattern is commonly referred to as P mitrale.

Lead V_1 must also be inspected. Normally, the P wave in V_1 is biphasic, consisting of an initial positive deflection representing the depolarization of the RA (the vector of which is largely oriented anteriorly and therefore toward the positive pole of V_1) followed by a negative deflection that represents the depolarization of the LA (which is oriented posteriorly and therefore away from the positive pole of V_1). As would be expected, the negative portion of the P wave in V_1 may be altered if the LA is enlarged. "A box wide and a box deep" is a common way to refer to the LAA pattern in Lead V_1; that is, the negative part of the P wave in V_1 must be at least 40 ms (one small box) in width and 0.1 mV (one small box) in depth (Figure 6.82C).

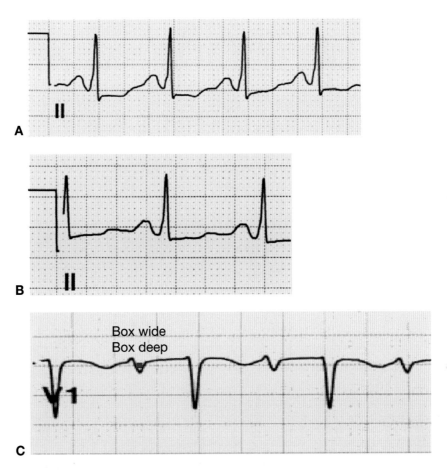

FIGURE 6.82 Left atrial abnormality (enlargement). **A** and **B.** Wide P waves in Lead II. **C.** Wide and deep terminal negative component of P wave in Lead V_1.

The appearance of either pattern — a wide P wave in Lead II or a "box wide and a box deep" pattern for the negative part of the P wave in V_1 — is sufficient to diagnose LAA. The term *left atrial enlargement (LAE)* is also used for this condition but, again, it is not preferable as this implies a morphological finding that may not be present.

Right Ventricular Hypertrophy

Of the chest leads, V_1 is the most rightward and therefore closest to the right ventricle. As such, an increase in the size of the right ventricle often leads to an abnormally large R wave in this lead. This change may be easy to miss, as the resulting R wave may not actually appear very large. This is because the usual pattern in V_1 is a very small r wave followed by a large S wave. The usual criterion for a "large" R wave in V_1 is that the R wave be the same height or greater than the depth of the S wave. In Figure 6.83, the r wave is not very large in V_1. However, it is the same size or greater than the s wave and so is abnormally large.

Similar to the situation with the atria, the ECG patterns described earlier may be seen when actual enlargement of the ventricle has not occurred; therefore, a phrasing such as "probable right ventricular hypertrophy (RVH)" is preferable to stating definitely that RVH has occurred based solely on ECG findings. Other findings suggestive of RVH include a persistent s wave in V_6, an axis shifted to the right, or the presence of RAA (factors leading to an enlarged right ventricle also commonly affect the RA). The changes associated with RVH are often subtle and good numerical criteria are not available.

Left Ventricular Hypertrophy

Normally the right chest leads (V_1 and V_2) show a small r wave from septal depolarization followed by a large S wave associated with the simultaneous depolarization of the left and right ventricles, whereas the left chest leads (V_5 and V_6) show septal depolarization as a small q wave followed by a large R wave associated with depolarization

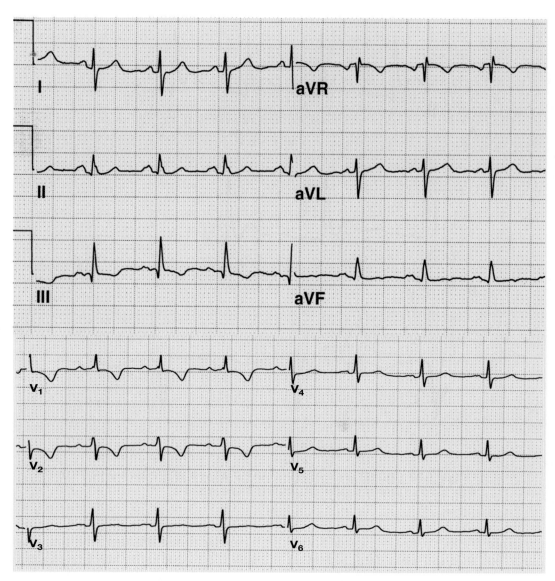

FIGURE 6.83 Right ventricular hypertrophy.

of the ventricles. These patterns occur because the left ventricle has so much more mass than the right ventricle and therefore is electrically predominant, resulting in the net vector of depolarization of the ventricles being directed toward the positive poles of V_5 and V_6 and away from the positive poles of V_1 and V_2. When the left ventricle is enlarged, this pattern is exaggerated: the R waves in Leads V_5 and V_6 and the S waves in Leads V_1 and V_2 become even larger.

One commonly accepted criterion for left ventricular hypertrophy (LVH) is to add the height of the tallest R wave in V_5 or V_6 to the depth of the deepest S wave in V_1. If the result is greater than 3.5 mV (35 mm), then "voltage for LVH" is said to be present (Figures 6.84 and 6.85). Usually, this criterion is only used for patients 35 years and older. For patients younger than 35 years, a total of 50 or 55 mm is often substituted for 35 mm. Another common formula for LVH voltage is the R in Lead I + the S in Lead III > 25 mm.

LVH is not always pathological. The ECG shown in Figure 6.84 is from a former Olympic rower. In this case, the left ventricle likely hypertrophied as a normal response to a long history of intense exercise and chronic volume overload and not chronic pressure overload seen in patients with pulmonary disease. Box 6.8 compares the ECG findings in the different types of hypertrophy.

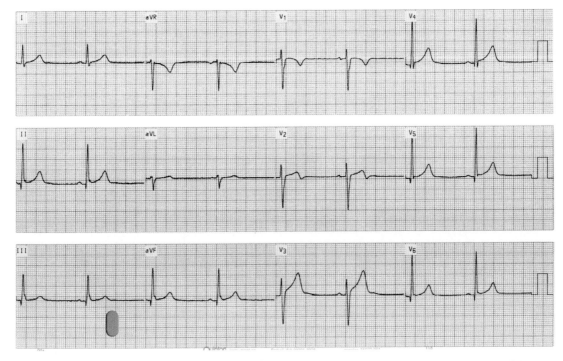

FIGURE 6.84 Voltage for a left ventricular hypertrophy.

Repolarization Abnormalities ("Strain Pattern")

Enlargement of the left ventricle commonly results in abnormal repolarization, causing a characteristic pattern of T-wave inversion and ST-segment depression seen in the leads with tall R waves (visible in V_5–V_6 in Figure 6.85). These ST-T-wave abnormalities are often referred to as a strain pattern, although the term *repolarization abnormality* is preferable. If repolarization abnormalities are present, it is much more likely that LVH is actually present. Other findings that support the presence of LVH include LAA and widening of the QRS complex.

Repolarization abnormalities have important implications for exercise testing. As discussed later in this

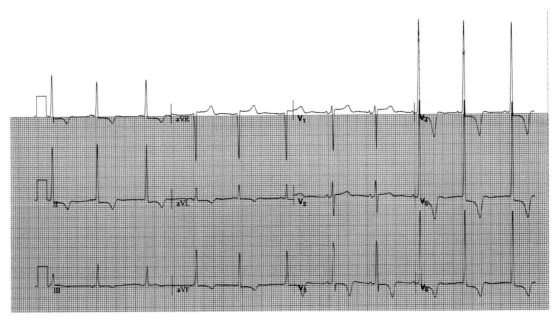

FIGURE 6.85 Voltage for a left ventricular hypertrophy with "strain."

Box 6.8	ECG Findings in Hypertrophy
RAA	P wave in Lead II taller than/equal to 2.5 mm
LAA	P wave in Lead II (usually notched) wider than/equal to 120 ms
	and/or
	Negative part of P wave in Lead V_1 1 mm wide and 1 mm deep
RVH	R in $V_1 \geq$ S in V_1
LVH[a]	R wave in Lead V_5 or V_6 + S wave in $V_1 \geq 35$ mm
	and/or
	R wave in Lead AVL $\geq$ 12 mm
	and/or
	R wave in Lead I + S wave in Lead III > 25 mm

[a]Many different criteria for LVH have been described; we list three common ones. It should be recognized that other criteria may be used. LAA, left atrial abnormality; LVH, left ventricular hypertrophy; RAA, right atrial abnormality; RVH, right ventricular hypertrophy.

chapter, ST-segment depression and T-wave inversion are indicative of ischemia. Their presence on the resting ECG renders an ordinary (ECG only) stress test inaccurate ("nondiagnostic") for myocardial ischemia. In such cases, it may be preferable to perform a test using imaging, such as a nuclear stress test or stress echocardiography.

As the positive pole of Lead aVL is leftward, increases in the size of the left ventricle may also result in large R waves in this lead, with "large" often defined as greater than or equal to 1.2 mV (12 mm). Figures 6.86 and 6.87 show examples of these tall R waves in Lead aVL. The ECG in Figure 6.87 also shows repolarization abnormalities in Lead aVL.

Multichamber Hypertrophy

Multiple chambers of the heart may be enlarged simultaneously. In this case, the ECG may show patterns characteristic of more than one type of hypertrophy. For example, in Figure 6.88A, the P waves are both wide and tall. Thus, the criteria for both RAA and LAA are present. This pattern is often called biatrial abnormality. Figure 6.88B shows wide and tall P waves in Lead II and the terminal negative component of the P wave in V_1 is a box wide and a box deep. The height of the R waves in V_5 or V_6 added to the depth of the S waves in V_1 is greater than 35 mm. Therefore, this ECG exhibits biatrial abnormality and voltage for LVH.

As previously mentioned, findings on the ECG do not always correlate precisely with the physical size of the heart's chambers. For example, the patient whose ECG is shown in Figure 6.89 had significant hypertrophy of the left ventricle as determined by transesophageal echocardiography but the ECG does not meet any of the criteria for LVH. This is why descriptions limited to the ECG findings, such as "voltage for LVH," are preferred.

Conduction Defects

A simple way to conceptualize problems with the conduction system (Figure 6.90) is to imagine the right and left bundle branches as wires. Because the cells of the ventricular myocardium are linked together electrically by gap junctions, if one of these wires were to be cut, the spread of current through the ventricles would still occur; however, it would take longer and would be less organized. Keeping in mind that the function of the ventricular conduction system is to facilitate a rapid and organized depolarization, it should be logical that defects in the system will result in a slower and less organized electrical activation of the ventricles. The slower activation will typically appear on the ECG as a wider QRS complex in many

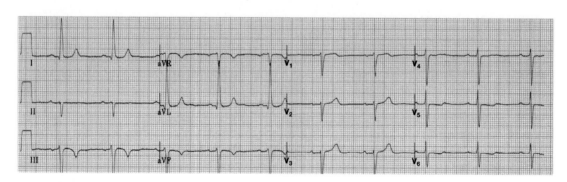

FIGURE 6.86 Voltage for left ventricular hypertrophy in Lead aVL.

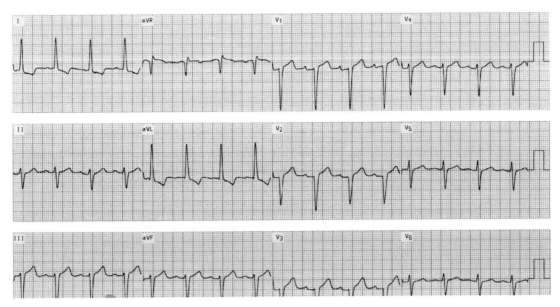

FIGURE 6.87 Voltage for a left ventricular hypertrophy in Lead aVL with "strain."

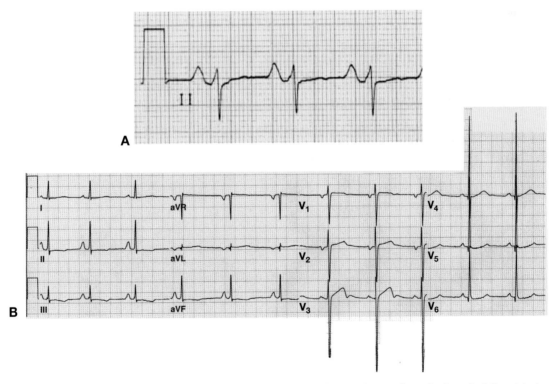

FIGURE 6.88 Multichamber hypertrophy. **A.** Biatrial abnormality. **B.** Biatrial abnormality and voltage for left ventricular hypertrophy.

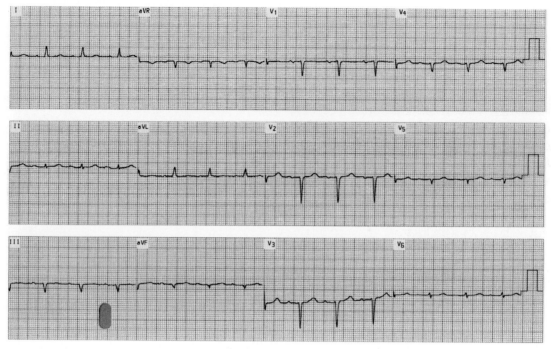

FIGURE 6.89 Hypertrophy present without ECG evidence.

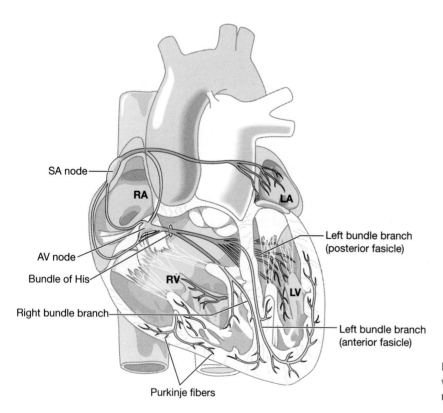

SA node

RA

LA

AV node

Bundle of His

Right bundle branch

RV

LV

Left bundle branch
(posterior fasicle)

Left bundle branch
(anterior fasicle)

Purkinje fibers

FIGURE 6.90 Conduction system. AV, atrio-ventricular; LA, left atrium; LV, left ventricle; RA, right atrium; RV, right ventricle; SA, sinoatrial.

leads, whereas the abnormal patterns of current flow will be apparent by an altered QRS morphology. Using some basic principles, the resultant changes in the QRS are quite understandable.

Right Bundle Branch Block

Imagine that the left bundle branch is functioning normally but the right bundle branch has somehow been cut. In actuality, part of the system may be ischemic or have suffered degenerative changes; however, thinking of it simply as a cut wire is helpful in understanding the resultant ECG patterns. The initial event of ventricular activation is depolarization of the interventricular septum. Typically, the septum is activated by fibers that originate from the left bundle branch. This being the case, septal activation is usually not affected by a right bundle branch block (RBBB). Septal depolarization occurs from left to right and therefore results in a small r wave in leads V_1 and V_2 and a small q wave in leads V_5 and V_6.

Following septal depolarization, normally the left and right ventricles would depolarize simultaneously. As noted earlier, the left ventricle is electrically dominant, resulting in the net vector of current heading toward the left, seen on the ECG as a large R wave in V_5 and V_6 and a large S wave in V_1 and V_2. In RBBB, conduction occurs normally in the left ventricle but is delayed in the right ventricle (as the right bundle branch is not functional). That is, as both ventricles are depolarizing, the net current is directed toward the left as usual, resulting in an S wave in V_1 and V_2 and an R wave in V_5 and V_6. The left ventricle finishes depolarization in a normal time frame but the right ventricle continues to depolarize. The vector of this late current is toward the right and anteriorly, and therefore results in an R' wave in V_1 and V_2 and an s wave in V_5 and V_6 (in the absence of RBBB, the left chest leads usually do not have s waves). Putting this series of events together, the classic RBBB pattern consists of wide QRS complexes with an rSR' in leads V_1 and V_2 and a qRs pattern in leads V_5 and V_6 with a longer than normal S wave (Figure 6.91A).

For various reasons, this classic pattern is not always observed. In Figure 6.91, the notched r of panel B (the latter part of the r wave is not an r' as the downward deflection never goes below the baseline) and the wide r of panel C are typical of other patterns sometimes seen with RBBB. Note that in all cases, the QRS is wide (>120 ms in duration) and the R waves are larger than would normally be seen in the right chest leads.

Left Bundle Branch Block

Imagine that the right bundle branch is functioning normally but the left bundle branch has somehow been cut.

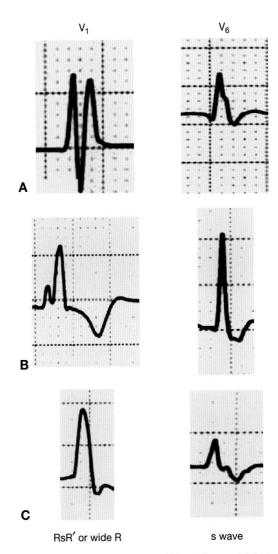

FIGURE 6.91 **A**, **B**, and **C** represent different forms of right bundle branch block patterns.

The right ventricle should depolarize quickly and normally but the left ventricle will be activated by the slower cell-to-cell pathways. Also, septal activation will usually be affected, as the septum is typically depolarized by fibers that originate from the left bundle branch. Therefore, the normal initial (septal) r waves in V_1 and V_2 will be lost, as will the normal initial (septal) q waves of V_5 and V_6. Instead of the septum activating first, the initial event will be depolarization of the right and left ventricles, with the net vector of this current directed toward the more massive left ventricle. Because of the direction of current flow, this will be seen on the ECG as an R wave in Leads V_5 and V_6 and a Q wave in Leads V_1 and V_2. The right ventricle will finish depolarizing in a normal amount of time but the completion of the left ventricular depolarization will take longer than usual, causing a continued (wide) R wave in the left chest leads. The resultant pattern

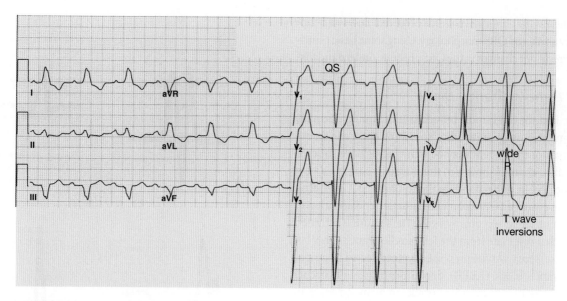

FIGURE 6.92 Left bundle branch block.

of a left bundle branch block (LBBB) is typically a wide (>120 ms in duration) and sometimes notched R wave in Leads V_5 and V_6 and a wide QS pattern in Leads V_1 and V_2 (Figure 6.92). Leads I and aVL also typically show wide R waves as these leads are also leftward.

Complete and Incomplete Bundle Branch Blocks

In both RBBB and LBBB, ventricular depolarization takes longer than normal because part of the conduction system is disabled. This prolongs the QRS complexes in certain leads. A normal QRS duration is less than 100 ms (2.5 small boxes). During a bundle branch block, a QRS duration greater than or equal to 100 but less than 120 ms is often called an incomplete bundle branch block (or intraventricular conduction delay). In contrast, a QRS duration greater than or equal to 120 ms is a complete bundle branch block. For example, a QS in V_1 and a wide R in V_6 (LBBB pattern) accompanied by a QRS duration slightly greater than 100 ms might be referred to as an incomplete LBBB.

The QRS duration usually is not prolonged in all leads. Some authorities suggest using the QRS duration in V_1 for RBBB and in V_6 for LBBB but as bundle branch blocks were first described before the chest leads came into use (only the limb leads existed at the time), others use the widest QRS of the limb leads as the benchmark.

Secondary ST-T Changes From Bundle Branch Blocks

The abnormal depolarization patterns of RBBB and LBBB result in abnormal repolarization, which is manifested in ST-segment and T-wave abnormalities. With LBBB, the ST segments in the left chest leads are typically depressed and the T waves inverted, whereas the ST segments in the right chest leads are typically elevated. With RBBB, ST-segment depressions and T-wave inversions are seen in the right chest leads, whereas the left chest leads are typically unaffected (other than the presence of the s waves previously described). These changes are shown in Figure 6.93 and are referred to as secondary ST-T changes because they are secondary to the abnormal depolarization occurring because of the bundle branch block. In later sections of

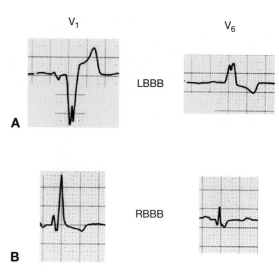

FIGURE 6.93 Secondary ST-T changes. With left bundle branch block (LBBB) **(A)**, there is ST elevation in V_1 and ST depression/T-wave inversion in V_6. With right bundle branch block (RBBB) **(B)**, we see ST depression/T-wave inversion in V_1.

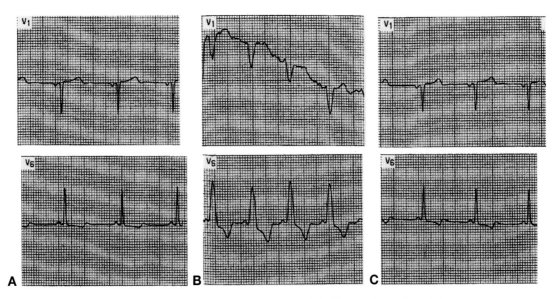

FIGURE 6.94 Rate-related left bundle branch block: **(A)** at rest, **(B)** with exercise, and **(C)** during recovery.

this chapter, primary ST-T changes (*e.g.*, from myocardial infarction) are described.

Exercise-Induced (Rate-Related) Bundle Branch Blocks

Figure 6.94 shows ECGs (Leads V_1 and V_5) from the same patient under three conditions: rest, exercise, and after recovery from exercise. The QRS complex in Lead V_6 is not wide at rest or during recovery but shows an LBBB pattern during the stress of exercise. In some patients, because of degenerative changes, ischemia, or other factors, the conduction system functions normally (or fairly normally) during low stress conditions but temporary bundle branch blocks occur when the HR increases. If this occurs during exercise, the phenomenon is sometimes called an exercise-induced bundle branch block. Because these transient blocks coincide with increases in HR and may occur at rest if the HR is high enough, they may also be called rate-related bundle branch blocks. The V_1 exercise strip in Figure 6.94 also shows a type of artifact known

as wandering baseline, which can be caused by patient movement.

Intraventricular Conduction Defect

Sometimes a conduction problem exists but the ECG pattern suggests neither RBBB nor LBBB. In such cases, the term *intraventricular conduction defect (IVCD)* may be used. In Figure 6.95, for example, the QRS duration is abnormally long (*i.e.*, ≥100 ms) but neither the RBBB nor the LBBB pattern is present. IVCD recognizes a conduction defect that fits neither the RBBB nor the LBBB pattern. The term *intraventricular conduction delay* is also used.

Fascicular (Hemi) Blocks

Although the left bundle branch is often spoken of as if it were one "wire," the human conduction system is better conceptualized as trifascicular, consisting of one right bundle branch and a left bundle branch with two major fascicles. Figure 6.90 shows the anterior and posterior

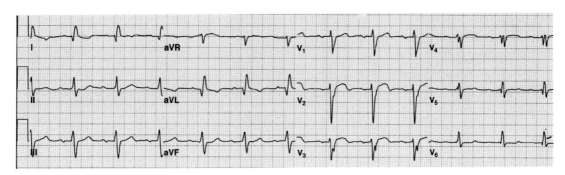

FIGURE 6.95 Intraventricular conduction defect (delay).

fascicles of the left bundle branch. The anterior and posterior designations are used in this book but these fascicles are sometimes referred to as superior (for anterior) and inferior (for posterior).

Occasionally, one of these fascicles functions normally while the other does not. Failure of one of the fascicles is called a fascicular block or hemiblock. Oddly, failure of one fascicle only mildly prolongs the QRS duration; a more significant effect is a shift of the axis.

In the case of a left anterior fascicular block, the axis shifts to the left and becomes −45 degrees or more negative. Thus, an axis of −45 degrees or more negative (*e.g.*, −60 degrees) is considered presumptive evidence of left anterior fascicular block. An easy way to recognize this is if the S wave in Lead aVF is deeper than the R wave in Lead I is tall. Notice that in Figure 6.96 the S wave in Lead aVF is about 7 mm deep, whereas the R wave in Lead I is only about 5 mm tall. This is simply a quick method of recognition; the usual methods of axis determination will also reveal whether the axis meets the criteria for this type of conduction defect. Abnormal septal activation must be ruled out to properly diagnose left anterior fascicular block. Therefore, small q waves of brief duration in two of the three Leads I, aVL, and V_6 (evidence of normal septal activation) as well as an axis of −45 degrees or more negative must be present. The criteria for a left anterior

fascicular block should not be applied in the presence of an inferior wall myocardial infarction, as these infarcts shift the QRS axis.

In the case of a left posterior fascicular block, which is less common, the axis is shifted well to the right and will be greater than 120 degrees (Figure 6.97). Many factors can shift the axis to the right, so an axis greater than 120 is only assumed to represent left posterior fascicular block when other causes (*e.g.*, pulmonary disease) are ruled out. The finding may therefore be described as a *possible* left posterior fascicular block.

Bifascicular Blocks

The trifascicular conduction system (right bundle branch and anterior and posterior fascicles of the left bundle branch) can suffer failure of two of the three constituent pieces. (If all three parts fail, then complete heart block is present.) If the two fascicles of the left bundle branch fail, then LBBB is present. If the right bundle branch and one of the fascicles of the left bundle branch fail, then a bifascicular block is present. Figure 6.98 shows the two possible combinations of bifascicular block. In both cases, the RBBB pattern is seen. In Figure 6.98A, the axis meets criteria for a left posterior fascicular block, whereas in Figure 6.98B, the axis is representative of left anterior fascicular block.

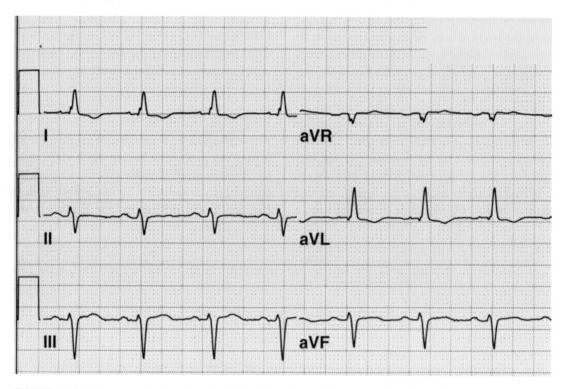

FIGURE 6.96 Left anterior fascicular hemiblock. Note that the axis is more negative than −45 degrees, and there is a Q wave in aVL.

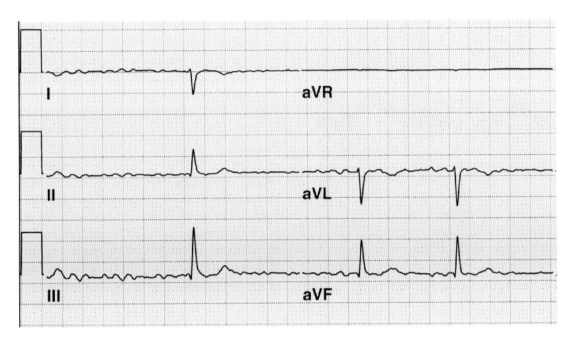

FIGURE 6.97 Left posterior fascicular hemiblock. The rhythm here is atrial fibrillation. The axis is greater than 120 and other causes have been ruled out.

Ischemia and Infarcts

Myocardial ischemia, a lack of oxygen to the myocardium, is typically due to an inadequate supply of blood, which in turn is due to the blockage of a coronary artery. If prolonged,

ischemia leads to increasing damage to and eventual death of myocardial tissue. This condition is clinically known as a myocardial infarction or, in layman's terms, a heart attack.

Myocardial ischemia and infarction cause distinctive changes in the ECG, with many of these changes affecting

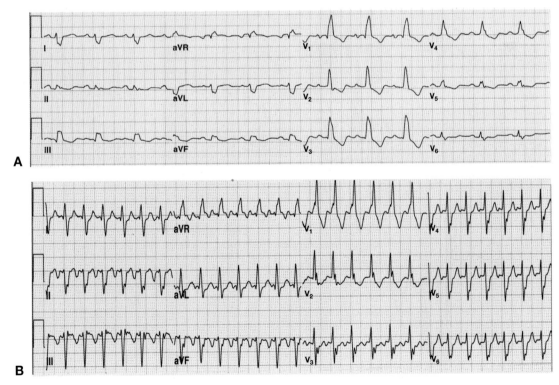

FIGURE 6.98 Bifascicular blocks. **A.** Right bundle branch block and left posterior fascicular block. **B.** Right bundle branch block and left anterior fascicular block.

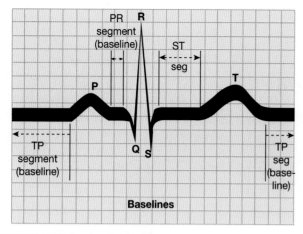

FIGURE 6.99 Isoelectric points.

the ST segment and/or the T wave. Recall that the ST segment begins at the end of the QRS complex and ends at the beginning of the T wave and should be isoelectric (*i.e.*, on the baseline), as shown in Figure 6.99. Significant displacement, whether elevation or depression, of the ST segment is often defined as greater than or equal to 1 mm (0.1 mV) of displacement from the baseline, with the P-R or T-P segment serving as the baseline.

In the past, elevation of the ST segment was thought to be indicative of ischemia of the whole thickness of a segment of myocardium from subendocardium to subepicardium (transmural ischemia). This was referred to as a transmural

infarct. In contrast, depression of the ST segment was thought to result from ischemia of roughly the inner half of a segment of myocardium (the subendocardium) and was called a subendocardial infarct. More recently, it was appreciated that the situation regarding ischemia and resultant ECG changes does not always coincide with these transmural and subendocardial designations. Considering this, current terminology recognizes ST-segment elevation myocardial infarction (STEMI) and non–ST-segment elevation myocardial infarction (NSTEMI), avoiding any assumptions about which layers of the myocardium are involved. It is currently thought that complete occlusion of a coronary artery results in ST-segment elevation, whereas partial occlusion results in ST-segment depression and/or T-wave inversion. Some typical patterns of ST-segment elevation and depression are shown in Figure 6.100.

ST-Segment Elevation Myocardial Infarction

If no intervention such as thrombolytic therapy or percutaneous coronary intervention is performed in a timely manner, STEMI infarcts typically progress through a three-phase series of ECG changes designated acute, evolving, and old. Three examples of the three phases are shown in Figure 6.101.

The acute phase is characterized by significant ST-segment elevations sometimes accompanied by the onset

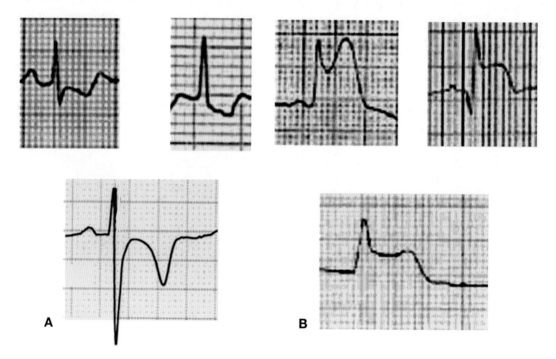

FIGURE 6.100 ST changes with ischemia. **A.** Partial occlusion showing ST depression and T-wave inversion. **B.** Complete occlusion showing ST elevation.

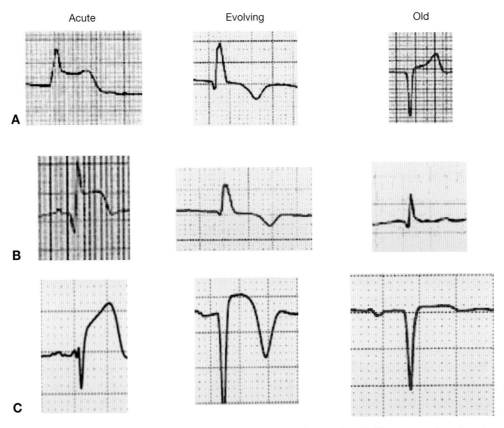

FIGURE 6.101 ST-segment elevation myocardial infarction phases. **A** to **C.** Three examples of acute, evolving, and old phases of a STEMI.

of new Q waves. However, the first ECG change of this type of infarct is often very tall, peaked T waves that are sometimes referred to as hyperacute T waves (Leads V_1–V_3 in Figure 6.102). These are brief and often gone by the time an ECG is performed, so ST-segment elevations are usually the first pattern encountered clinically during a STEMI. The ST elevations may last for several hours or more.

The ST-segment elevations are typically followed by an evolving pattern characterized chiefly by a return of the ST segments toward baseline (although still possibly elevated) and the inversion of T waves. New Q waves may also appear during this phase if they had not appeared in the acute phase. The evolving phase lasts for hours to days or longer.

The evolving phase is often followed by a so-called old pattern that primarily consists of Q waves. During the old phase, the ST segments and T waves may have normalized and the only evidence of the infarct remaining may be Q waves.

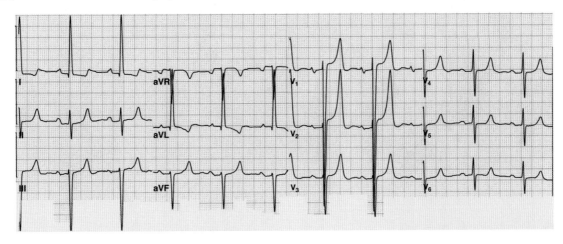

FIGURE 6.102 Hyperacute T waves.

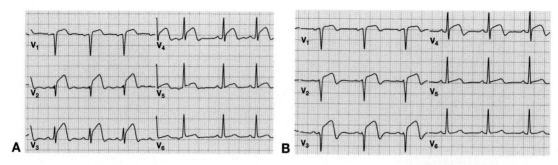

FIGURE 6.103 Serial ECGs of an ST-segment elevation myocardial infarction patient upon presentation **(A)** and a day later **(B)**.

Figure 6.103 shows ECGs taken on the same patient during the acute and evolving phases of a STEMI. Notice that the first ECG shows significant ST-segment elevations in the chest leads. By the next day, these ST elevations were returning toward the baseline (although still significantly elevated in many leads), whereas T-wave inversions have begun to appear in some of these leads (V_2–V_4).

Figure 6.104 shows two ECGs from a patient who did not come to the hospital until his infarct had already progressed to the evolving phase. Because he attributed his substernal sensation of pressure to "indigestion," this patient waited several hours until seeking medical attention. Presumably an ECG taken earlier would have revealed large ST-segment elevations in many of the chest leads. This can be inferred by the patterns of modest ST elevations combined with T-wave inversions in V_1–V_5 (which should come after the acute phase of very significant ST

elevation). Four days later, some residual ST elevations remain but the main abnormality is the presence of significant Q waves. In this case, the T waves are no longer inverted.

Significance of Q Waves

The appearance of significant Q waves following an infarct suggests that a significant amount of myocardium has died. Because this dead area (necrosis) is no longer electrically active, the ECG appears to have almost an electrical "hole"; that is, the Q waves represent electrical current in other areas of the heart, which has now become apparent because of a lack of activity in the damaged area. For example, new Q waves in the inferior leads (II, III, and aVF) can be seen following an inferior wall STEMI. These Q waves represent depolarization of other areas of myocardium unbalanced by activity of the inferior wall.

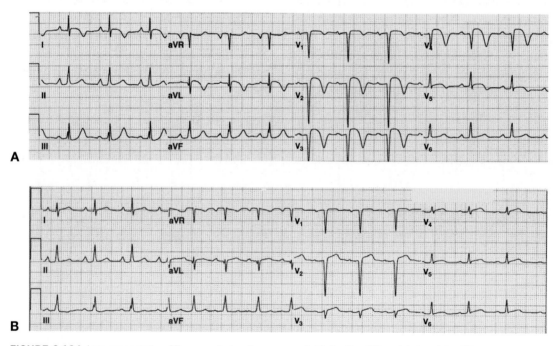

FIGURE 6.104 Late presentation ST-segment elevation myocardial infarction **(A)** and 4 days later **(B)**.

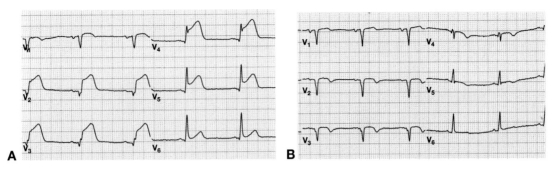

FIGURE 6.105 Acute and old stages of ST-segment elevation myocardial infarction upon presentation **(A)** and 3 months later **(B)**.

This electrical activity seems to be moving away from the inferior wall, resulting in negative deflections (Q waves). In order to be considered significant, Q waves should be at least 40 ms (0.04 s) in duration. An infarction that has resulted in the appearance of significant Q waves is often referred to as a Q-wave infarction.

Figure 6.105 shows ECGs from the same patient taken roughly 3 months apart. The first ECG was taken during the acute phase of a STEMI. Notice the significant ST elevations in most of the chest leads. Four months later, V_5 and V_6 reveal little evidence of the event (although the R-wave amplitude is decreased and some nonspecific ST-T-wave changes are present), whereas V_1–V_4 show the telltale Q waves indicating an old STEMI.

Indeterminate Age Infarct

Commonly, an ECG will show a pattern that is a combination of the evolving and old STEMI patterns. Modest but significant ST-segment elevations may persist for months or even years following an infarct. A pattern of residual ST elevation accompanied by Q waves is often referred to as an indeterminate age infarct, as it is a hybrid of the

evolving and old patterns and therefore the approximate age of the infarct cannot be determined. Figure 6.106 (Leads V_1–V_3) shows an infarct of indeterminate age.

Non–ST-Segment Elevation Infarction

The ECG changes during an NSTEMI do not follow a three-phase course as seen with a STEMI. During an acute NSTEMI, the ST segments are significantly depressed (≥ 1 mm) and/or the T waves are inverted. Figure 6.107 shows ECG changes consistent with a lateral wall NSTEMI (Leads V_4–V_6).

After the acute phase, no definitive ECG evidence may remain, although it is common for the height of R waves in affected areas to decrease and for varying degrees of T-wave inversion and/or ST-segment depression to remain. Necrotic tissue can lead to Q waves with a STEMI, whereas the loss of viable myocardium during an NSTEMI can lead to decreases in R-wave amplitude. The term *poor r-wave progression* is used to describe failure of the r waves to significantly increase in amplitude across the chest leads. This finding can be due to an infarct or other causes.

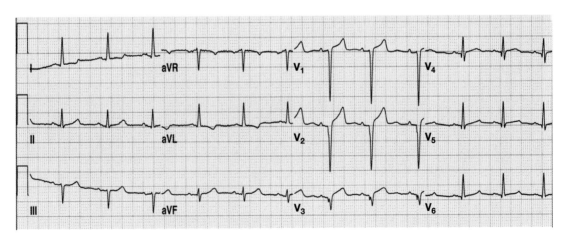

FIGURE 6.106 Indeterminate age infarct.

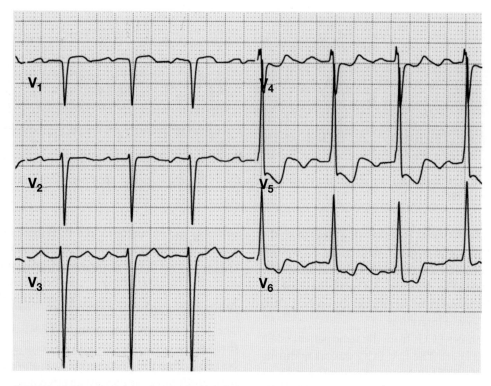

FIGURE 6.107 Non–ST-segment elevation myocardial infarction.

Comparison with previous ECGs may be useful to ascertain whether such findings are new and thus presumably due to an NSTEMI or were preexisting. Figure 6.108 shows two ECGs from the same patient. The ECG in Figure 6.108A was taken during an NSTEMI that occurred 5 years previously. Although the ECG shown in Figure 6.108B was suspicious for acute ischemia/infarction (possible NSTEMI), the availability of the previous

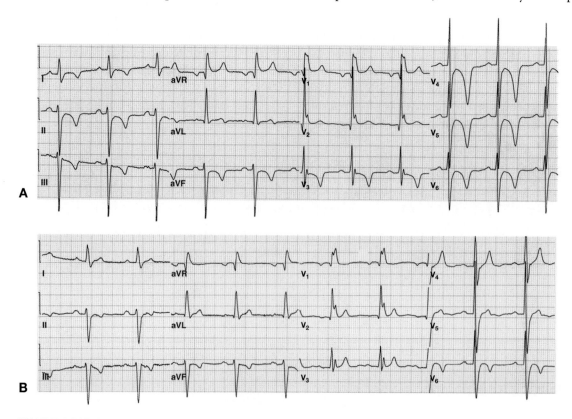

FIGURE 6.108 A. A patient with non–ST-segment elevation myocardial infarction. **B.** The same patient 5 years later.

ECG (Figure 6.108A) assisted clinicians in determining that the ST-T changes seen in Figure 6.108B were likely preexisting and not due to an acute ischemic event.

If no previous ECGs are available, and sometimes even if they are, it may be difficult or impossible to diagnose an NSTEMI from the ECG after it has resolved. This is in contrast to STEMI postinfarct Q waves that can persist for years and sometimes for life, allowing diagnosis of a previous STEMI long after the event.

Localization of Infarcts

The different leads are positioned to electrically "view" different areas of the heart. A given myocardial infarction typically affects only one or two areas of the heart; therefore, ECG changes associated with an infarct are often confined to a few leads. ECG changes associated with ischemia/infarct appear in multiple contiguous leads (see Box 6.6) For example, a lateral wall STEMI results in ST-segment elevations in Leads V_5 and V_6 and/or I and aVL, whereas an inferior wall NSTEMI causes ST depression and/or T-wave inversions in Leads II, III, and aVF.

Combinations of areas can also be described. For example, significant ST-segment elevations in V_1, V_2, V_3, and V_4 would be indicative of an anteroseptal STEMI (anterior and septal walls). Another patient with ST-segment depressions and T-wave inversions in II, III, aVF, V_5, and V_6 could be said to be suffering an inferolateral NSTEMI (inferior and lateral walls).

"Reciprocal" Changes/Remote Ischemia

Sometimes during a STEMI (which, by definition, is associated with ST-segment elevations), ST-segment depressions are seen in a different area of the heart. Figure 6.109 A reveals an inferior wall STEMI (with right ventricular involvement as shown in Figure 6.109B) with typical ST elevations in the inferior leads. Notice that the ST segments are depressed in Leads I and aVL of the same ECG. It had been believed that such ST depressions seen in an area distant from the ST elevations were simply a sort of mirror image of the STEMI. In other words, the same area of ischemia/infarct (inferior wall in this example) would appear as ST elevations in leads covering the affected area and ST depressions in leads focused on the "opposite" side of the heart (the lateral wall in this case). This concept has generally been discredited and it is now believed that ST depressions occurring during a STEMI represent ischemia in another area of the heart. In this model, the ST elevations seen in Leads II, III, and aVF of Figure 6.109 are indicative of an inferior wall STEMI and the ST depressions in Leads I and aVL represent ischemia of the lateral wall (sometimes referred to as remote ischemia as it is distant from the site of the infarct). The theory is that changes in myocardial function and, therefore, myocardial perfusion due to an infarct in one area of the heart can cause another area of the heart to become ischemic.

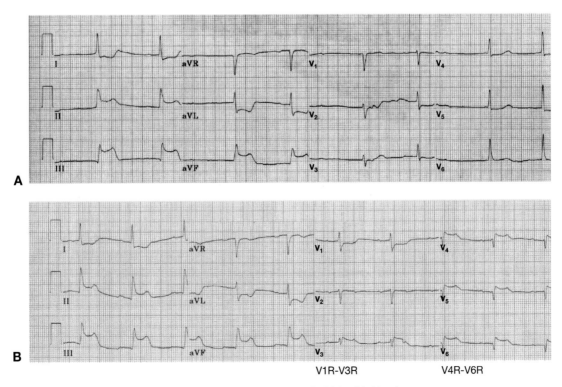

FIGURE 6.109 Right-sided leads. **A.** Standard lead placement. **B.** Right-sided leads.

Right Ventricular Infarctions

Although the septal leads (V_1 and V_2) are often referred to as "right" chest leads, this is in relation to the left ventricle. A standard 12-lead ECG has very limited coverage of the right ventricle. If a right ventricular infarction is suspected, additional leads can be placed on the right side of the chest. Figure 6.109 shows a standard 12-lead ECG (A) and an ECG with the chest leads shifted to the right (B). For a right-sided ECG, the normal V_2 becomes Lead V_{1R}, the normal V_1 becomes V_{2R} and the electrodes for V_{3R}–V_{6R} are placed in the normal anatomical locations, but on the right rather than the left side of the chest. The ECG should then be labeled in some way to make it clear that this placement has been used. This can be done by labeling each lead (V_{1R}, etc.) or by simply indicating "right-sided leads."

Notice that an acute inferior wall STEMI is evident in both ECGs but the ST changes of the concurrent right ventricular infarction are seen only in Figure 6.109B (ST elevations in V_{3R}–V_{6R}). With the usual anatomical distributions of the coronary arteries, right ventricular infarctions often accompany inferior wall infarctions.

Posterior Wall Infarctions

Although no leads of the standard 12-lead ECG are positioned on the posterior thorax, posterior wall infarctions (for historical reasons sometimes referred to as *true* posterior wall infarctions) can be detected by inspection of Leads V_1 and V_2. These leads are positioned roughly over the interventricular septum. As such, they are on the opposite side of the heart from the posterior wall. Because of this, posterior wall infarctions are seen as a mirror image in V_1 and V_2. Figure 6.110 shows two different examples (A and B) of posterior wall infarcts as seen in a septal lead. The left-hand images show the ECG as it appears in the septal lead, whereas the images on the right are mirror images. Notice that the mirror images show Q waves and ST-segment elevations consistent with a STEMI. Perform any one of the following to appreciate these changes on the original ECG:

- View Leads V_1 and V_2 in a mirror (with the mirror at a 90-degree angle to the paper).
- Flip the ECG over, hold it up to a light, and read it through the paper.
- Imagine the tracing as it would appear upside down (R waves imagined as Q waves, and ST depressions pictured as ST elevations).

If relatively large R waves appear in V_1 and/or V_2, one of these techniques should be used to search for a posterior wall infarct. As the normal pattern in these leads is a small r and a large S wave, an R wave that is about the same size as the s wave or larger is considered relatively large. Therefore, an r wave of only a few millimeters (Figure 6.110B) could be considered "large" in the septal leads. Box 6.9 is helpful for reviewing the heart area and leads associated with that area.

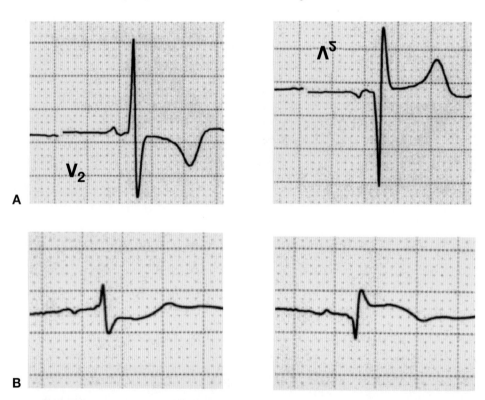

FIGURE 6.110 Posterior wall infarct. This figure shows the septal lead appearance (left) and the mirror image (right). **(A)** and **(B)** are two examples.

Box 6.9	Heart Area and Leads Associated With That Area

Area	Leads
Inferior	II, III, aVF
Lateral	I, aVL, V_5, V_6
Septal	V_1, V_2
Anterior	V_3, V_4
Posterior	V_1, V_2 (mirror image)

Infarctions and Bundle Branch Blocks

Recall that LBBBs usually result in T-wave inversions and ST-segment depressions in the left chest leads and Q waves and ST elevations in the right chest leads, whereas RBBBs cause ST depressions and T-wave inversions in the right chest leads. Such changes are secondary to the abnormal depolarization and repolarization patterns associated with bundle branch blocks. These secondary changes sometimes present a challenge when attempting to diagnose infarction.

In the presence of RBBB, myocardial ischemia/infarction generally still results in the usual ECG changes in leads other than V_1 and V_2, and Q waves in V_1 and V_2 retain their diagnostic significance. For example,

Figure 6.111A shows the typical rSR′ with secondary T-wave inversions seen in the septal leads (V_1 and V_2) with RBBB. Figure 6.111B shows the inferior leads (II, III, and aVF) from the same ECG. The QS patterns shown are indicative of an old STEMI (a Q-wave infarct), even in the presence of an RBBB. Other infarct patterns such as ST depression or elevation in leads other than V_1 or V_2 would also retain their usual diagnostic significance in the presence of RBBB.

When an infarct involves the septum (the area associated with V_1 and V_2), the situation is slightly more involved. Figure 6.112 shows ECGs from two different patients with RBBB and infarcts that involved the septum. In Figure 6.112B, the ST-segment elevations of the STEMI are more apparent, particularly in Lead V_2. In Figure 6.112A (from a different patient), the ST elevations are more subtle but still apparent. In both cases, the T waves are upright, not inverted. This might appear to be normal but, in fact, is due to the infarct. Keeping in mind that T waves in the septal leads should be inverted in the presence of an RBBB (secondary ST-T changes), the upright T waves seen here are abnormal and represent primary ST-T changes from the septal infarct. Essentially, upright T waves in these leads in the presence of a bundle branch block are in many ways equivalent to T-wave inversions in the absence of a bundle branch block.

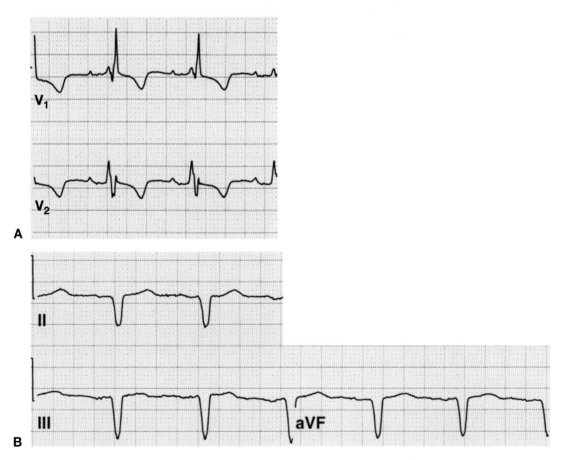

FIGURE 6.111 Old inferior wall infarction with right bundle branch block. **A.** Septal leads. **B.** Inferior leads.

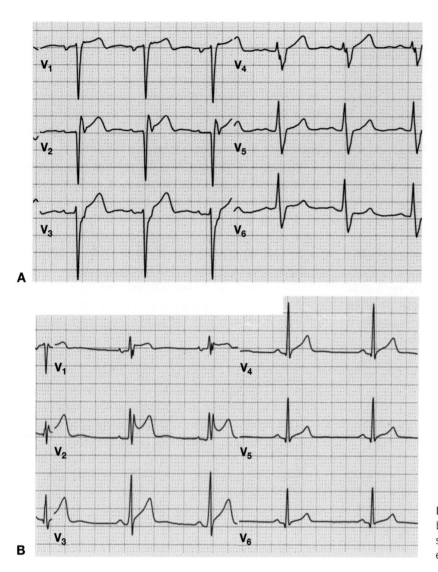

FIGURE 6.112 Septal infarct with right bundle branch block. **A.** Note subtle ST elevations in septal leads. **B.** More pronounced septal ST elevations.

LBBB also complicates diagnosis of an infarct. A new or presumably new LBBB in and of itself greatly raises the index of suspicion for an infarct. This is because infarctions often damage the conduction system and lead to LBBB. With a pre-existing LBBB, secondary ST-T changes should be present; thus, as with RBBB, the primary ST-T changes lead to upright or nearly upright T waves. In Figure 6.113, the T waves in the lateral leads are not inverted, although they should be from the LBBB. This is because a lateral wall infarct is also occurring. The infarct causes them to invert and become upright. The changes are present in both panels, although they are more subtle in Figure 6.113A. The Q waves and ST-segment elevations in the right chest leads with LBBB are another complicating factor. These changes make it difficult or impossible to diagnose a septal infarct in the presence of LBBB.

ST-T-Wave Changes Not Due to Ischemia/Infarct

There are several ST-T wave changes that are not due to ischemia or infarction. For example, the ST-T-wave changes secondary to bundle branch blocks have been described previously. Hypertrophy patterns are also associated with ST-T-wave changes. For example, the tall R waves seen in the lateral precordial leads and/or Leads I and aVL with LVH may be accompanied by ST-segment depression and T-wave inversion in a so-called strain pattern. It can be extremely challenging or impossible to accurately diagnose ischemic changes in leads showing a "strain" pattern, as the ST depressions and T-wave inversions may be secondary to the hypertrophy or may be due to ischemia (primary changes). In leads not exhibiting the tall R waves associated with hypertrophy, ST-segment depressions and T-wave inversions retain their usual diagnostic significance as in ischemia and/or NSTEMI. In leads that previously showed a "strain" pattern, the return to an upright configuration (pseudonormalization) for previously inverted T waves is suggestive of ischemia. This is analogous to the reversion to an upright pattern for T waves previously inverted in conjunction with bundle branch blocks. ST-segment elevations retain their usual diagnostic significance in the presence of hypertrophy patterns.

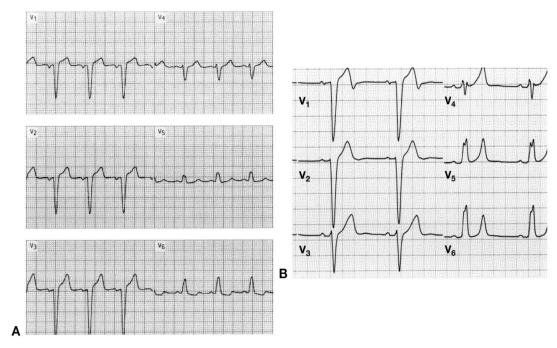

FIGURE 6.113 Left bundle branch block primary ST-T changes. **A.** Modest upright T waves in left chest leads. **B.** More robust positive T waves in V₅ and V₆.

Miscellaneous Effects and Conditions

Artifact

Patient movement, failure to properly prepare the skin, and use of ECG electrodes that have been stored improperly or are past the expiration date are some common causes of ECG artifact. Modern ECG machines typically offer various mechanisms to reduce artifact but it can still render a tracing difficult or impossible to interpret properly.

Artifact is particularly common when a patient is exercising. During exercise ECGs, the lead wires are a common source of artifact. Securing a belt or tight mesh shirt around or over the patient can keep lead wires from moving around.

The various ECG leads often are not uniformly distorted by artifact. Figure 6.114A shows an erratic baseline caused by improper storage of an electrode that dried its conductive gel. The electrode in question was placed in the left leg position and therefore caused artifact in Leads II and III. Other leads (not shown) were unaffected. Recalling which electrodes are active for the various leads can be useful. In this example, rather than re-prepping and

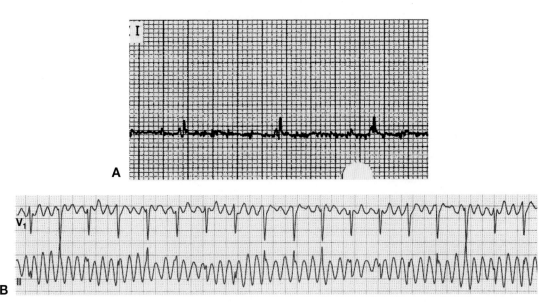

FIGURE 6.114 A. Artifact from dry electrode. **B.** Artifact simulating ventricular tachycardia in Lead II.

replacing all the electrodes, the CEP solved the problem by simply replacing the left leg electrode. In addition, a proper skin preparation can reduce the amount of artifact.

Figure 6.114B shows a patient's ECG viewed simultaneously in Leads V_1 and II. Notice that in Lead II the rhythm appears to be V-Tach. This strip is from an obese patient who was ambulating. The electrodes were all on the torso in the modified (Mason–Likar) placement and the artifact was from subcutaneous fat moving as the patient walked. A comparison of the two leads reveals that most of what appear to be wide QRS complexes in Lead II are not QRS complexes at all. Inspection of multiple leads can often help in determining the actual rhythm.

Digitalis Effect

Excessive digitalis (digitalis toxicity) can cause a variety of arrhythmias and types of heart block but even normal therapeutic doses commonly result in a characteristic and often shallow "U-shaped" depression of the ST segment (Figure 6.115). This is known as digitalis effect. The presence of digitalis effect does not imply an overdose of the medication but rather a common finding in patients taking this medication. Digitalis effect complicates ECG interpretation because ST-segment depressions due to digitalis can be difficult or impossible to distinguish from ST changes due to ischemia.

Pericarditis

Pericarditis (inflammation of the pericardium) results in ST-segment elevations that may initially appear similar to those of STEMI. However, the ST elevations of pericarditis differ in several ways from those of an acute infarct.

Given the fact that the pericardium surrounds the heart, pericarditis typically results in ST elevations in all leads except aVR. In contrast, it is rare for an infarct to cause ST elevations in leads associated with more than one or two regions. Also, as noted earlier, the ST-segment elevations associated with STEMI change rapidly ("evolve"), with Q waves commonly developing over time. The ST elevations from pericarditis are more persistent and the evolution is much slower. It involves changes in T-wave morphology; however, the T waves are not tall and peaked as they are with STEMI. Further, there is no development of Q waves. The PR segments in many leads are depressed below baseline; this does not occur during STEMI. Also, recall that, during a STEMI, it is common to see ST-segment depression in some leads because of remote ischemia. With pericarditis, all leads except for aVR typically show ST elevations.

Figure 6.116 is from a patient with pericarditis. Notice that the ST segments are elevated significantly in almost all leads (exceptions are III and aVR) and the PR segments in several leads are mildly depressed (using the TP segment as baseline). These ST changes persisted for several days and did not go through the evolutionary changes typical of STEMI.

Early Repolarization

Elevation of ST segments does not always indicate infarction or pericarditis. Many apparently healthy individuals

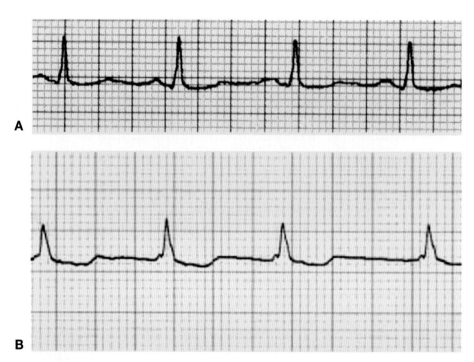

FIGURE 6.115 Digitalis effect. **(A)** and **(B)** are two examples of the digitalis effect.

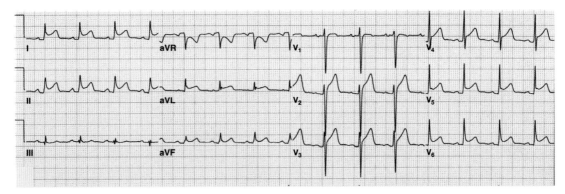

FIGURE 6.116 Pericarditis.

show significant (>1 mm) ST elevations that appear to be a normal variant and are thought to be due to unusually fast repolarization of the ventricles. A characteristic feature of early repolarization is a brief upward deflection in one or more leads at the J point (where the QRS complex ends and the ST segment begins). Although subtle, this upward deflection can be seen clearly at the beginning of the ST segment in Lead V_3 in the area circled in Figure 6.117 and is also visible in the inferior leads and V_5 and V_6. These changes are not typically seen globally as in pericarditis, although they often occur in multiple leads. The ST elevations of early repolarization do not change over time as those of STEMI do.

A somewhat simplistic but useful observation is that ST-segment elevations associated with occlusion of coronary arteries tend to have a somewhat convex appearance said to resemble a frown. In contrast, the normal variant types tend to be slightly concave and are likened to a smile (Figure 6.118).

Low Voltage

In some instances, the electrical activity of the heart is less than normal. Low voltage many be seen, for example, in patients with hypothyroidism or in those who have had a large infarct that results in the death of numerous myocardial cells.

In other cases, the heart's electrical activity is within normal limits but the current recorded by the surface electrodes used in a standard ECG is below normal as a result of resistance to current flow. This resistance can be

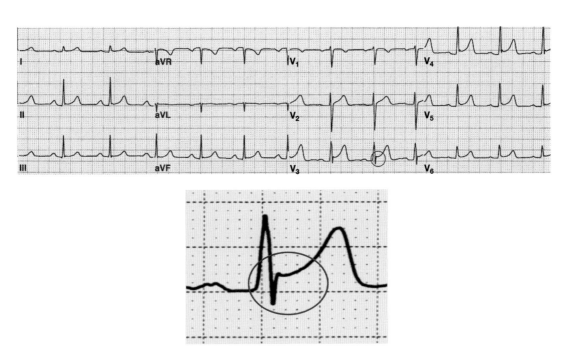

FIGURE 6.117 Early repolarization. Note the small "notch" at the J point (circled).

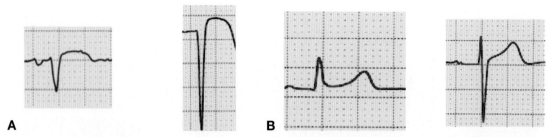

FIGURE 6.118 Ischemic and benign ST elevation. **A.** Ischemic (convex). Looks like a "frown." **B.** Normal variant (concave). Looks like a "smile."

due to a large amount of subcutaneous fat or to increased intrathoracic air volume (*e.g.,* as seen with emphysema).

Various definitions of low voltage are in clinical use. One criterion is a total QRS voltage of less than or equal to 5 mm (0.5 mV) in each of the limb leads. In Figure 6.119, no QRS has a total voltage (including positive and negative deflections) of 5 mm (0.5 mV) or greater in any of the limb leads (I, II, III, aVR, aVL, aVF). Another criterion is that no chest lead has a total voltage (R and S together) of greater than 15 mm (1.5 mV). Both criteria should be met (total QRS voltage of less than or equal to 5 mm in each limb lead and ≤15 mm in each chest lead).

Because these ECG findings may be due to diverse causes, a specific diagnosis cannot be made depending on the ECG alone and such tracings may simply be described as low voltage QRS complex.

Hypocalcemia and Hypercalcemia

Both high and low plasma calcium levels are associated with specific ECG findings. Hypercalcemia decreases the QT interval and hypocalcemia prolongs it (Figure 6.120). It is difficult to provide universally applicable numerical cutoffs for what constitutes a short QT interval; however, when the ST segment is essentially not present (the beginning of the T wave comes right after the QRS complex), it

is reasonable to assume that the QT is short and that hypercalcemia is a likely cause. Prolongation of the QT interval is determined by the usual methods; however, hypocalcemia is only one possible cause of a prolonged QT interval.

Hyperkalemia

Hyperkalemia (elevated plasma potassium) causes a variety of changes on the ECG depending on how high the elevation is. The initial and, arguably, the most important finding is the appearance of tall, peaked T waves (Figure 6.121). As serum potassium levels continue to rise, the T waves remain tall and peaked and an unusual rhythm develops. This appears to be an idioventricular rhythm but is a sinoventricular rhythm, which is unique to hyperkalemia (Figure 6.121). Patients at this or later stages of hyperkalemia would be too sick to appear in an exercise stress testing laboratory or cardiac rehabilitation facility.

Nonspecific ST-T Abnormalities

Specific T-wave patterns are associated with unique abnormalities. For instance, deep asymmetrical T-wave inversions occurring in conjunction with tall R waves suggestive of ventricular hypertrophy represent the repolarization abnormality pattern (strain pattern). Many

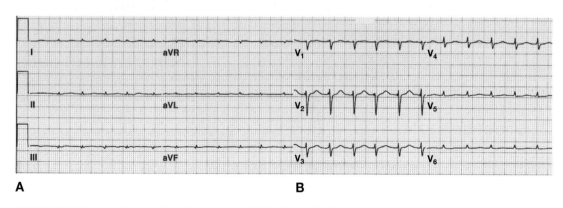

FIGURE 6.119 Low voltage. **A.** Limb leads with no QRS >5 mm. **B.** Chest leads with no QRS >15 mm.

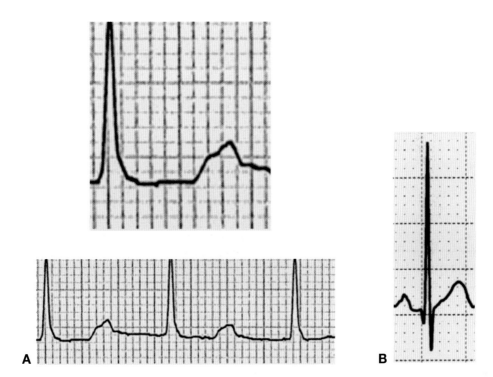

FIGURE 6.120 A. Hypocalcemia (long QT). **B.** Hypercalcemia (short QT).

patients will exhibit subtle T-wave and/or ST-segment changes that deviate from normal but are not robust enough to be diagnostic of any particular condition. For example, the ST segment may be slightly elevated or depressed but not enough to reach specific diagnostic criteria (typically 1 mm). Similarly, T waves may be abnormal in that they are positive but very small, or very subtly inverted. They may even be nonexistent. None of these situations meets any specific diagnostic criteria, yet each is a deviation from what is considered normal. Collectively, such findings are referred to as nonspecific ST-T abnormalities (or nonspecific ST-T changes).

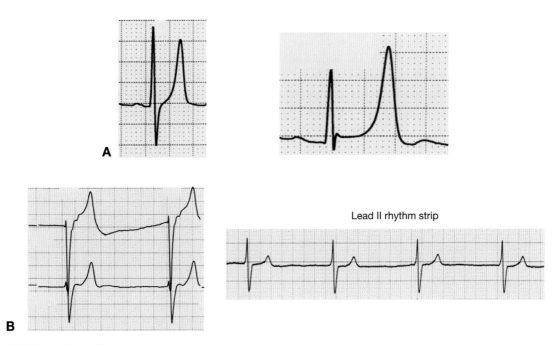

Lead II rhythm strip

FIGURE 6.121 A. Early hyperkalemia. **B.** Progressing hyperkalemia.

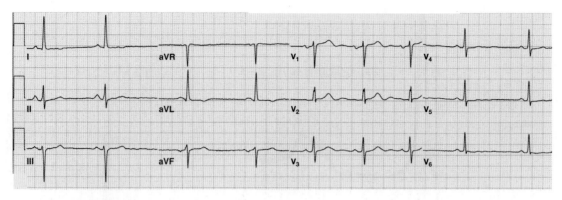

FIGURE 6.122 Nonspecific ST-T-wave abnormalities.

In Figure 6.122, the T waves are very small (II, III, aVF) or virtually nonexistent (V_4–V_6) in certain leads and some ST segments are mildly elevated (V_1 and V_2) or mildly depressed (V_4 and V_5). Any of these would qualify as nonspecific abnormalities.

Preexcitation Syndromes

Preexcitation is characterized by an abnormally short delay between the beginning of atrial depolarization and the beginning of ventricular depolarization. In some types of preexcitation, such as Lown–Ganong–Levine (L-G-L) syndrome, the only ECG finding is a PR interval less than 120 ms (0.12 s). It is not possible to tell from a standard 12-lead ECG whether a short PR interval is the result of L-G-L or is simply a normal variant, so when interpreting such an ECG, it may be appropriate to simply indicate that the PR interval is short.

A common preexcitation syndrome is Wolff–Parkinson–White (WPW). In addition to the normal AV node/bundle of His electrical pathway connecting the atria and ventricles, patients with WPW have an extra AV "wire" — an accessory pathway. This pathway may be active

regularly, in which case ECG evidence will be visible, or it may be a "concealed" pathway that is not active at all times. When the pathway is concealed, the ECG may appear normal.

When active, the accessory pathway of WPW allows depolarizations to travel from atria to ventricles via two paths — the normal AV node/bundle of His pathway and an accessory pathway known as the bundle of Kent. The accessory pathway does not have the "delay" inherent in the AV node, so depolarizations travel rapidly from atria to ventricles. Although the accessory pathway is allowing a more rapid AV conduction, the normal depolarizations are also proceeding. These rapid and normal (and slightly slower) depolarizations join together at the beginning of ventricular depolarization. This physiology explains the three features (triad) of WPW (Figure 6.123). First, early repolarization of the ventricles via an accessory pathway results in a short PR interval. Second, merging of the early and normal depolarizing currents widens the beginning of the QRS complex. Third, this widening is distinctive, with the base of the QRS said to resemble the Greek letter Delta (a Delta wave). Figure 6.124 shows two 12-lead ECGs from patients with WPW. The triad of a short PR

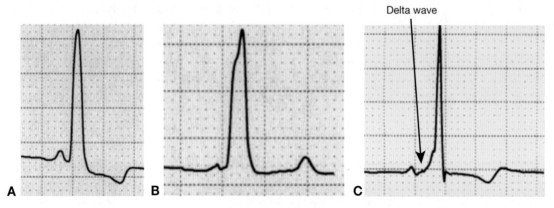

FIGURE 6.123 Wolff–Parkinson–White triad. **A.** Short PR interval. **B.** Wide QRS complex. **C.** Delta wave.

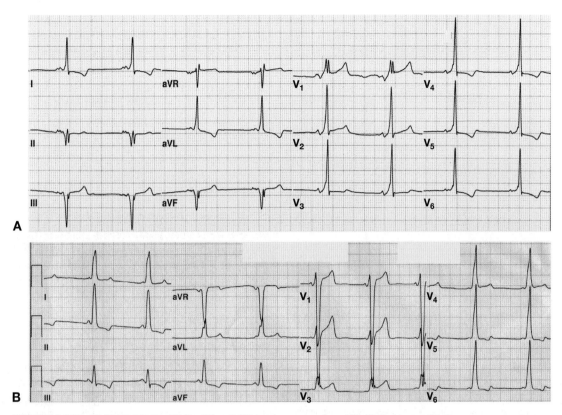

FIGURE 6.124 Wolff–Parkinson–White. **(A)** and **(B)** are two examples of Wolff–Parkinson–White.

interval, wide QRS complex, and a Delta wave can be located in each cardiogram; however, these changes will not be found in all leads.

These accessory pathways are of more than academic concern as they can serve as a conduit for reentry tachycardia. Figure 6.125 shows two ECGs from the same patient. In Figure 6.125A, the classic triad of WPW can be seen. Figure 6.125B shows a reentrant tachycardia facilitated by the accessory pathway.

Situs Inversus

Occasionally an ECG similar to that shown in Figure 6.126 is encountered. The P waves are negative in Lead II and positive in aVR, the axis is extremely deviated (in fact, the opposite from the norm), and the r waves are tiny in the leftward leads (I, aVL, V_5, V_6). In many respects, this ECG exhibits findings opposite from what would normally be expected. Thus, it would be appropriate to check that the lead wires are attached to the proper electrodes or established by other means (voltage in I + III = II, etc.) and that these findings are not due to technical error.

In Figure 6.126, the cause of this "backward" ECG is not technical error but a congenital condition known as situs inversus, which is characterized by a reversal of the

position and orientation of the viscera known. Because the heart and other major organs are reversed relative to normal — as in a mirror image, the electrical activity of the heart is largely opposite. Reversing the placement of the arm and leg leads (RA placed on LA, etc.) and placing the chest leads on the right side of the chest (as described previously for right-sided infarcts) will allow appropriate recording of an ECG for these patients.

Pediatric ECGs

This chapter has been concerned with the interpretation of adult ECGs. The normal and abnormal ECG patterns of pediatric patients differ in important ways from that of adults. Even a brief inspection of the normal pediatric (neonatal) ECG shown in Figure 6.127 should illustrate this concept. Note, for example, the fast rate, the relatively tall R waves in the rightward chest leads, and the narrowness (i.e., short duration) of the QRS complexes.

Pulmonary Pattern

Acute overload of the right side of the heart can result in a distinctive ECG pattern variously referred to as a pulmonary pattern, cor pulmonale, or right heart strain

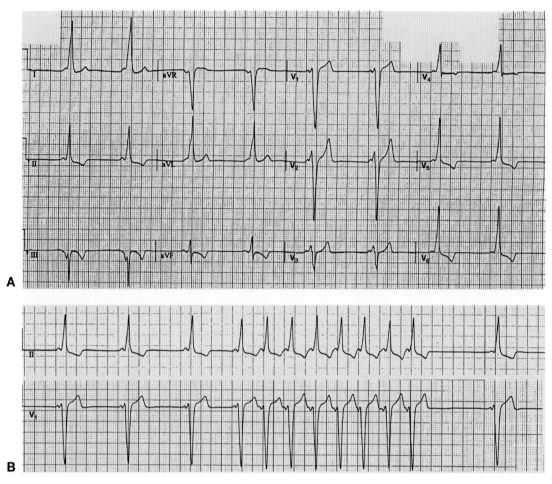

FIGURE 6.125 A. Sinus rhythm. **B.** Supraventricular tachycardia associated with Wolff–Parkinson–White.

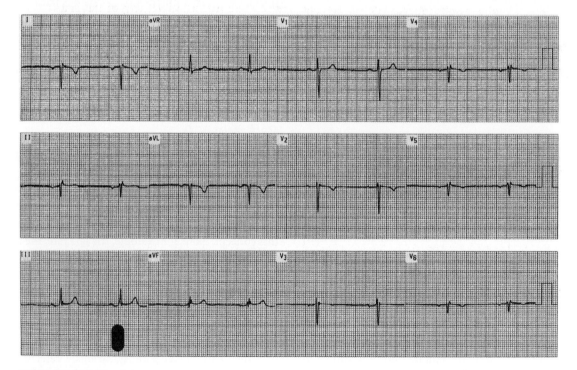

FIGURE 6.126 Situs inversus.

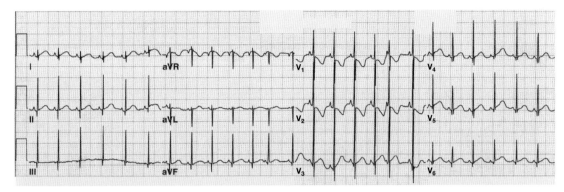

FIGURE 6.127 Pediatric ECG.

(Figure 6.128). The hallmarks of the pattern are an S wave in Lead I and Q waves and T-wave inversions (usually shallow) in Lead III. This combination is commonly referred to in shorthand as "S1-Q3-T3." Various lung disorders, including pulmonary embolism, can cause an S1-Q3-T3.

Prinzmetal Angina

Complete occlusion of a coronary artery is associated with ST-segment elevation. During a STEMI, arterial occlusions are typically caused by a thrombus. ST elevations will persist and eventually undergo the evolutionary pattern unless ischemia is relieved by interventions such as thrombolytic therapy or angioplasty. In contrast, a condition variously known as Prinzmetal angina, vasospastic angina, or variant angina results in transient ST-segment elevations caused by contraction of the smooth muscle surrounding a coronary artery typically not occurring with exertion but when the patient is at rest. The ST elevations typically only last for a few minutes (Figure 6.129), as blood flow is restored when the smooth muscle relaxes.

Pulseless Electrical Activity

In some conditions (*e.g.*, cardiac tamponade), the electrical activity of the heart may be normal (or fairly normal) even though mechanical functioning is severely impaired. Usually, the ECG recording of electrical activity is closely coupled with contractile activity; however, the two are not synonymous. If what should be a perfusing rhythm is seen on the ECG, but the patient has no pulse or measurable blood pressure, pulseless electrical activity (PEA) is present. As such, PEA cannot be identified solely by ECG findings but requires correlation with clinical observations.

The term *electromechanical dissociation (EMD)* was formerly used to describe this situation. Although the newer term PEA is now preferred, both terms are instructive as the electrical activity of the heart is dissociated from the mechanical and, because of the low or nonexistent cardiac output, no pulse is present. The ECG may show virtually any rhythm including NSR, but without intervention, the lack of meaningful cardiac output will quickly lead to severe clinical deterioration and death.

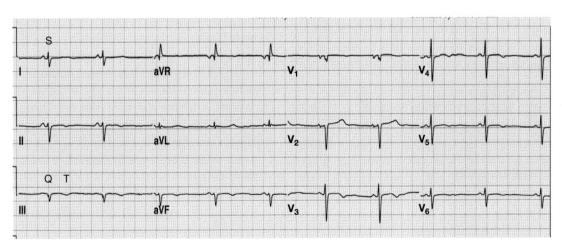

FIGURE 6.128 S1-Q3-T3 (pulmonary pattern).

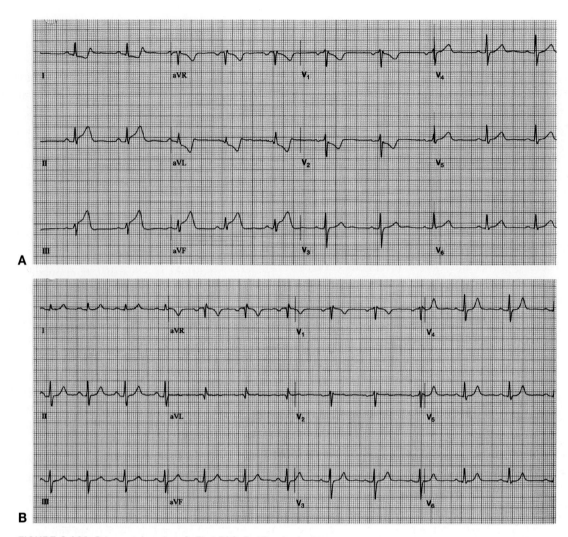

FIGURE 6.129 Prinzmetal angina. **A.** First ECG. **B.** After 4 minutes.

PRESTRESS TEST ECGS

As noted earlier, unless otherwise indicated, an ECG is assumed to have been recorded with the patient supine and at rest with the electrodes in the normal positions. Before an exercise test, it is best to run properly labeled resting 12-lead ECGs under the three conditions described in the following.

■ Supine (with standard electrode positioning). As it is taken under standard conditions, this resting ECG can be fairly compared with previous and future resting ECGs. For pharmacological stress tests (*e.g.*, dipyridamole), this is the only resting ECG needed, as the patient will remain in the supine, resting position throughout the test.

■ Supine Mason–Likar. For exercise tests, the limb electrodes must be moved onto the torso. In some patients, the Mason–Likar electrode placement causes changes on the ECG. Comparison of this ECG with the standard supine ECG will establish which, if any, changes are caused by electrode positioning. In many patients, no changes will occur.

■ Standing Mason–Likar. In some patients, standing causes ECG changes. Comparison of this ECG with the supine Mason–Likar will test for such changes. In many patients, however, the ECG will not change with the standing position. In either case, the standing Mason–Likar is an appropriate baseline ECG to perform before treadmill exercise, to enable the CEP to evaluate ST-segment changes for ischemia. For cycle ergometer exercise, a resting ECG performed with the patient seated on the ergometer may be substituted for a standing ECG.

A variety of technical problems can occur during the prestress test ECG. If artifact is present at rest, it almost certainly will worsen with exercise. Many modern ECG machines have a built-in system for testing whether the "prep" was properly done. This may be of help but tracings should also be inspected manually for technical adequacy. If needed, re-prepping or other measures to correct technical problems should be done before exercise. Once the technical problems are resolved, the resting ECGs should be redone.

Negative P waves in Lead II, positive waves in aVR, an abnormal R and S wave progression in the chest leads, or other unusual findings such as severe axis deviation should prompt the CEP to check wire placement, as it is common to misplace wires (*e.g.*, the LA wire placed on the RA electrode). It is also common for resting tracings to have artifact from patient movement, coughing, and so on. If this occurs, the source of the artifact should be identified and corrected and a "clean" tracing obtained before proceeding.

EXERCISE ECGS

The exercise ECG is one of the more powerful ways to diagnose cardiovascular disease and at the same time determine the patient's exercise tolerance. Simultaneously, the physician and the CEP can work together to determine the presence or absence of disease and to develop an exercise prescription based on the results of the exercise test. This section discusses how to record and monitor the exercise ECG.

ECG Recording and Monitoring

When an ECG is recorded during exercise, the type, intensity, and time of exercise should be recorded. Most modern systems will automatically label ECGs but in some cases it must be done manually. For example, "Treadmill 1.7 minutes per hour per 10% grade 2:00 minutes" or "Cycle ergometer 50 W stage time 2:00 minutes, total exercise time 4:00" make it clear what the conditions were when the ECG was recorded. For pharmacological tests, ECGs should be labeled with the protocol time and dosage and type of medication. For example, "Dobutamine, 6:00 minutes, 20 $\mu g \cdot kg^{-1} \cdot min^{-1}$." ECGs recorded during the postexercise period should also be labeled with specific information. For example, "2:00 Recovery" is a common

way to indicate that the recording was made 2 minutes into the postexercise (or other stress) period.

Although minimized by good skin preparation, even under the best of circumstances, some motion artifact will often be present on the ECG during an exercise stress test. It is important that at least one lead give a clean enough tracing to monitor the rhythm. Typically, three leads are monitored continuously with 12-lead ECGs run at predetermined intervals and additional rhythm ECGs printed when needed. Commonly, Leads II, V_1, and V_5 are monitored continuously, as this allows views of the inferior, septal, and lateral walls. In addition, Lead II is in line with the usual P-wave axis and can therefore be used for rhythm monitoring and V_1 and V_5 are well positioned to demonstrate rate-related bundle branch blocks. Monitoring these three leads increases the likelihood that the CEP will observe any important changes that may arise. Other leads also may be used; for example, if it appears that the ST segments are becoming depressed in V_5, it may be useful to monitor, at least temporarily, other lateral leads.

The ECG machine will usually be programmed to print 12-lead ECGs every minute (or minimally every stage) and at peak exercise during stress, as well as every 2–3 minutes during recovery. If ectopic beats or other events of interest occur, additional ECGs (often 3-lead rhythm strips) should be run as needed. The 12-lead ECG run at peak exercise often shows a great deal of motion artifact, so it may be useful to run an additional 12-lead or a long 3-lead rhythm strip shortly after peak exercise. As the patient enters the recovery period, motion artifact usually is reduced but any ischemic changes should still be present.

ST-Segment Changes

The interpretation of ST-segment changes is of great interest during exercise stress testing. An artery significantly narrowed by coronary artery disease (CAD) is often still capable of supplying enough blood and therefore oxygen to meet the metabolic demands of the heart at rest and so the resting ECG in such patients may be normal. Adding stress through exercise or other mechanisms increases the metabolic demands on the heart. A narrowed coronary artery may be unable to supply sufficient blood in this setting, rendering the subendocardium ischemic with resultant ST-segment depressions on the ECG.

To quantify ST-segment changes, a baseline must be established. The PR or TP segments can be used as baselines for ST-segment measurements. During exercise stress testing, it is recommended that the PR segment be used. The typical ECG finding indicating myocardial ischemia during stress is significant depression of the ST segment. The most common definition of "significant" depression is an ST segment that is 0.1 mV (1 mm) or more below the baseline. Depressions of less than 0.1 mV (1 mm) may be noted but are not usually considered indications of a "positive" (indicating the presence of disease) test result. Because the patient is moving during an exercise stress test, motion artifact often complicates interpretation. For example, sporadic artifact ST depressions often appear. Because of this, it is common to require three or more consecutive complexes showing ST depression before accepting it as a true finding.

ST-segment depressions occur in three patterns (Figure 6.130). An ST segment that is depressed but flat is called horizontal depression (Figure 6.130A). Depression that becomes greater over the course of the ST segment is called downsloping (Figure 6.130B). Depression that lessens over the course of the ST segment is called upsloping (Figure 6.130C). With horizontal depression, it does not matter where the depth of the depression is measured as it will yield the same result, but with upsloping or downsloping, the magnitude of the ST depression will vary depending on the measurement point. One commonly used measurement point is 80 ms (0.08 s; 2 mm or 2 small squares) after the J point (where the QRS complex ends and the ST segment begins). Other measurement points have been used, so it is good policy to state not only the magnitude of the depression but

also where the ST measurement was made. For example, one might describe a particular ST segment as having "0.2 mV of downsloping ST depression 80 ms post J point." It is common to use mm instead of mV, sec instead of ms and "post QRS complex" instead of "post J point," so the same findings could be described as "2 mm of downsloping ST-segment depression 0.08 s post QRS complex."

Using the terminology just described, the ST changes shown in Figure 6.130 could be reported as follows:

1. "0.1 mV (or 1 mm) of horizontal ST-segment depression" With horizontal depression, it is not critical to state where it was measured as the value is the same at all points of the ST segment.
2. "0.15 mV (or 1.5 mm) of downsloping ST-segment depression 80 ms post J point" The amount of depression varies depending on where it is measured. At a point 80 ms (two small boxes) past the end of the QRS complex, the ST segment is about 1.5 mm below the PR-segment baseline.
3. "Upsloping, but isoelectric 80 ms post J point" Initially the ST segment is depressed, but with upsloping, the depression lessens over time. In this instance, the ST segment has essentially returned to the baseline by 80 ms post QRS complex. ST segments on the baseline are often referred to as isoelectric.

Figure 6.131 shows resting and stress ECGs from a treadmill exercise test. At rest, the ST segments in all leads were isoelectric. During exercise, ST depression occurred in multiple leads. A complete description of the results of this test should include a description of the magnitude of the changes, which leads they

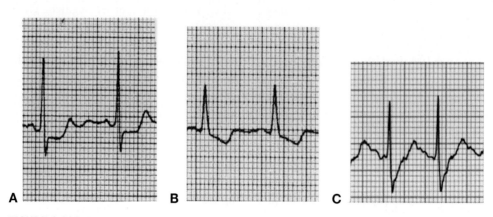

FIGURE 6.130 Patterns of ST-segment depression: horizontal **(A)**, downsloping **(B)**, and upsloping **(C)**.

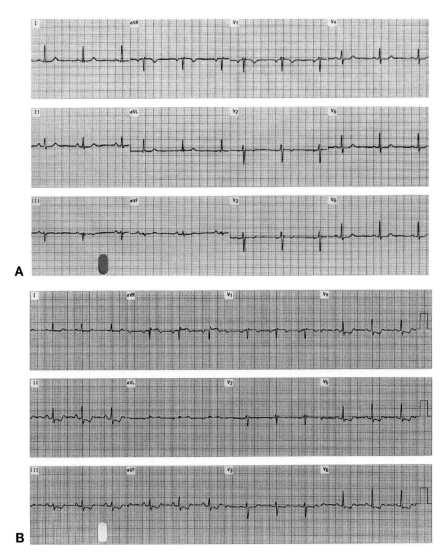

FIGURE 6.131 ST depression during exercise stress. **A.** At rest. **B.** During stress.

occurred in, and what exercise intensity elicited the changes. Often ST depression occurs during exercise. During this test, the patient exercised to an estimated intensity of 6.2 METs (metabolic equivalent of tasks) but the ST segments did not become depressed until the recovery (postexercise) period. Thus, these ECG changes could be described as "0.1 mV of downsloping ST-segment depression in the inferior leads and V_4–V_6 during recovery from 6.2 METs."

If changes occur during exercise, it is best to describe when they initially became significant and any worsening. For example, changes that were significant in V_5 and V_6 at 5 METs but worsened as the test progressed might be described as "0.1 mV of horizontal ST-segment depression in the lateral precordial leads at 5 METs progressing to 1.5 mV of horizontal depression

at 7 METs." It is also important to indicate how long it took for depressed ST segments to return to baseline (*e.g.*, "ST segments returned to baseline 5 minutes into recovery").

ST Depressions Occurring Only in the Inferior Leads

To be considered indicative of a "positive" test, ST-segment changes must occur in two or more contiguous leads (see Box 6.6). In this setting, *contiguous* means leads grouped together and associated with a certain area of the heart. For example, V_5, V_6, I, and aVL are contiguous, as they are all associated with the lateral wall. Leads II, III, and aVF are contiguous and associated with the inferior wall.

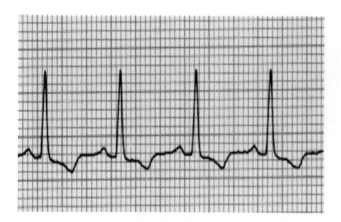

FIGURE 6.132 Stress T-wave inversion.

T-Wave Inversions

Stress-induced T-wave inversions (Figure 6.132), whether occurring in isolation or accompanied by ST-segment depressions, may also be evidence of ischemia. If T-wave inversions are not associated with ST-segment depressions, they are not usually considered strong enough evidence to consider a test positive but they should be noted. As these changes are sometimes caused by hyperventilation, some authorities recommend that, after the T waves return to baseline in the recovery period, the patient be asked to hyperventilate for a few minutes to see whether the

T-wave inversions recur. It they do, presumably ischemia is not the cause. Hyperventilation should be performed with the patient seated as a precaution in case dizziness occurs.

Arrhythmias

The type and relative frequency of arrhythmias should be described. For example, a phrase such as "frequent PVCs including multiform couplets" could be used to describe Figure 6.133. The ECG shown in Figure 6.134 is from a test that was stopped because of the onset of V-Tach. The report of this test might include a phrase such as, "The test was terminated due to monomorphic ventricular tachycardia."

ST-Segment Elevations

Although rare, elevation of the ST segment (presumably due to transmural ischemia) is sometimes seen during stress and is an indication to stop the test. Notice the ST-segment elevations in Figure 6.135. This ECG was recorded in a patient for whom coronary angiography later revealed 99% occlusion of a major coronary artery. In addition to severe occlusions of a major coronary artery, ST elevations can be caused by vasospasm.

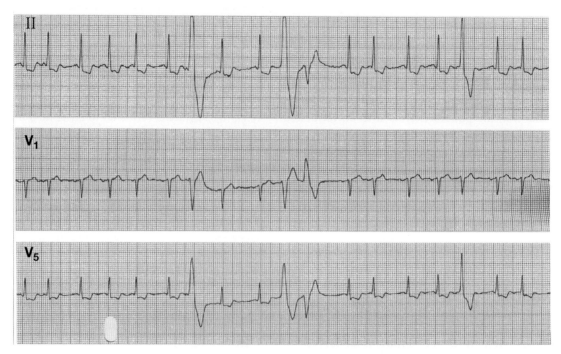

FIGURE 6.133 Arrhythmias during stress.

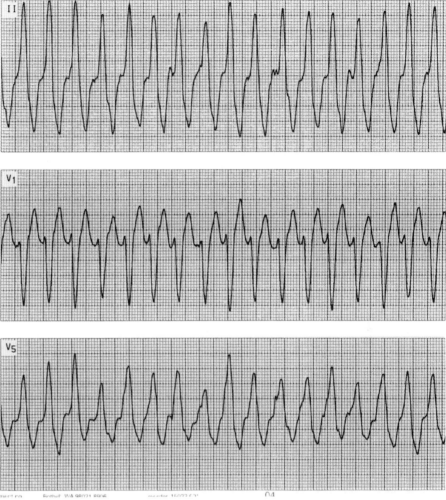

FIGURE 6.134 Ventricular tachycardia during stress.

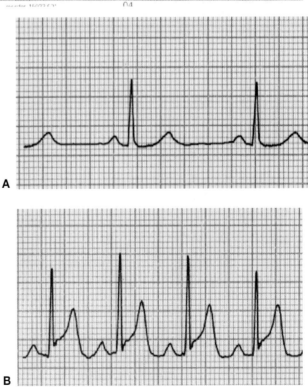

FIGURE 6.135 Stress ST elevation. **A.** At rest. **B.** During exercise.

SUMMARY

The ECG has been the most utilized tool in the clinical laboratory for the diagnosis of heart disease for many decades. Depending on the precise data needed, the physician and CEP may accompany or replace the ECG with other diagnostic techniques; however, the ECG alone is often an appropriate choice. For example, some patients with a new onset of chest pain may be better off with a stress ECG rather than with a more expensive invasive test. Or, if the new symptom has been accompanied by other signs, such as hypertension, again the stress ECG may be selected. Regardless of its use, the CEP will find that an ability to read and interpret ECGs is an essential skill to master.

CHAPTER REVIEW QUESTIONS

1. Which part of the ECG is most important when looking for myocardial ischemia, injury, or acute infarction?

2. In a right ventricular bundle branch block or left ventricular bundle branch block, which part of the ECG is affected?

3. By definition, ventricular tachycardia is diagnosed when how many premature ventricular contractions occur in succession?

4. When a patient is subjected to chronic pulmonary hypertension, what kinds of ECG changes would be expected?

5. Digitalis, a drug typically used to increase myocardial contractility in patients who have been diagnosed with congestive heart failure, creates what kinds of changes on the resting ECG?

6. What part of the ECG is typically affected when a patient experiences a complete occlusion of the proximal portion of the left anterior descending coronary artery?

7. A sudden onset of an accelerated rhythm originating in the atria can cause shortness of breath and some patients may lose consciousness. What is this rhythm called?

8. Toward the completion of a graded exercise test, it is not abnormal for the HR to exceed 180 bpm. At this kind of rate, the T-P interval becomes so short that the T-wave and P-wave appear to merge. The ECG then takes on the appearance of an SVT. How do you know the difference between a normal rhythm and an SVT during a graded exercise test at an HR over 180 bpm?

9. Virtually all ECG machines provide a standard for calibration. What is the standard for both voltage and time?

10. Premature ventricular contractions occur frequently and most are benign. However, when a PVC occurs every other myocardial contraction, what is it called?

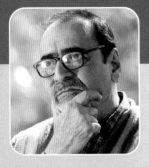

Case Study 6.1

Wendell is a 64-year-old teacher who had experienced some chest pain in the past couple of weeks. It seems to get worse after physical exertion. The last time he had this kind of pain was when the elevator was not working in his classroom building and he had to climb two sets of stairs to get to the third floor. Because of what seemed to be exertional chest pain, he was given a graded exercise test. At 3.30 minutes of the treadmill test, the following ECG was taken.

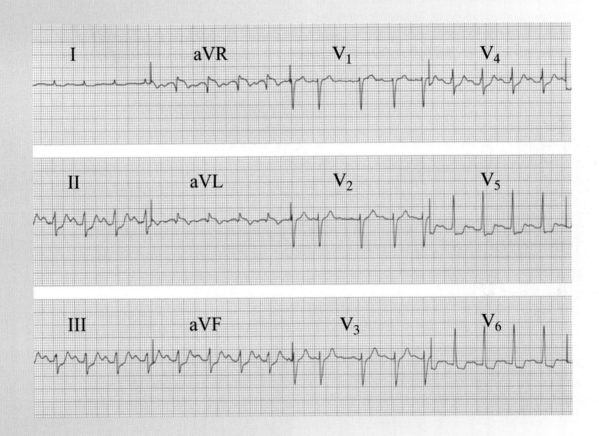

Case Study 6.1 Questions

1. Is the ECG normal or abnormal?

2. If abnormal, what is the abnormality?

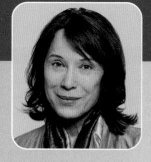

Case Study 6.2

Maria is a 55-year-old attorney who has been in that stressful occupation for 30 years. She was diagnosed 18 years ago with hypertension and was told to lose weight and get some exercise, all of which she ignored. She stopped taking the medication prescribed by her doctor because it made her nauseous and at times sleepy. She could not afford either of those conditions because of her occupation. She needed to always remain sharp. As a result of a new management in her law firm, all attorneys were required to have a routine physical examination including an ECG regardless of the absence of any symptoms. Given here is Maria's ECG. Her blood pressure at the time was 186/110 mm Hg.

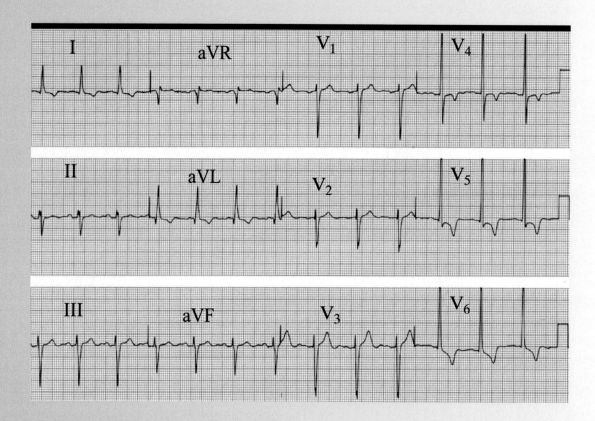

Case Study 6.2 Questions

1. Is the ECG normal or abnormal?

2. If abnormal, what is the abnormality?

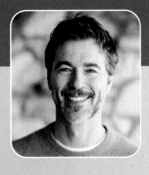

Case Study 6.3

Nico is a 37-year-old construction worker who experienced severe crushing chest pain while working on a roof. After sitting down for a while, the pain was not relieved by rest. His coworkers managed to get him off the roof and when the pain did not subside, a coworker drove him to the local hospital. While in the emergency department and learning that his father had died of an acute myocardial infarction at the age of 40 years, an ECG was taken.

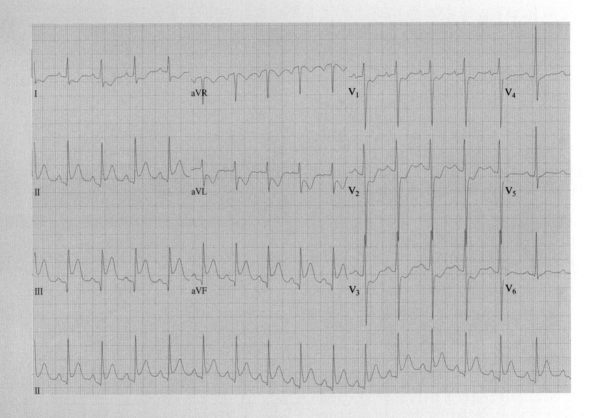

Case Study 6.3 Questions

1. Is the ECG normal or abnormal?

2. If abnormal, what is the abnormality?

CHAPTER

7

Pharmacology

INTRODUCTION

Pharmacology is the study of the effects of prescribed (or illegal) drugs on living organisms and physiological systems. There are two divisions of the study of pharmacology — pharmacodynamics and pharmacokinetics. Pharmacodynamics is the study of a drug's molecular, biochemical, and physiological effects or actions. Pharmacokinetics is the study of what the body does to a drug or how a drug moves through the body. Four main processes are included: absorption, distribution, metabolism, and excretion. Additionally, pharmacokinetics depends on an individual's age, sex, illnesses, and so on, and on the drug's chemical characteristics. This chapter is restricted to describing the pharmacodynamics of all drugs discussed. Research into the effects of exercise and a specific drug's pharmacokinetics is limited, and little is currently known (1). Clinical exercise physiologists (CEPs) play an important role in patient care. With proper knowledge and resources, CEPs can assist patients with medication compliance, review instructions related to their medication regimen, and explain the purpose of each medication relative to the management of their chronic health conditions. CEPs also need to be aware of potential medication side effects as they care for the patient in their setting. It is very helpful for patients to bring their current medications or a list with them to initial testing or rehabilitation program appointments. CEPs can review the medications with the patient and their caregiver(s), if they have one (Figure 7.1). Electronic medical records (EMRs) have allowed patients to carry their medication list with them (*i.e.*, Epic MyChart app on their smartphone), and CEPs can usually access medication lists electronically. Those patients seeking care between multiple providers are best served by bringing current medication lists because not all EMRs "talk to each other." For instance, if a patient goes outside their typical health provider network for care, the new network may not use the same EMR; the

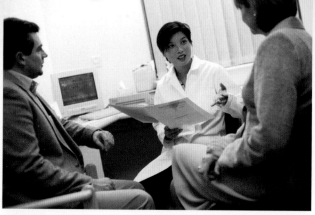

FIGURE 7.1 CEP reviewing medications with patient and caregiver. CEP, clinical exercise physiologist. (From Mohr WK. *Psychiatric-Mental Health Nursing*. 8th ed. Philadelphia (PA): Wolters Kluwer; 2012.)

chance medication lists and provider notes are available on the new provider's EMR is decreased.

Some medications discussed in this chapter may not be currently available or approved in the U.S.; however, in other countries, some medications may be available and/or could have different commercial names. The generic names are the same. Medications, either available or not, are included because they may still be seen on medical records, and practitioners should be familiar with what they are and how they function. New medications are put on the market each year, and some generic medications are newly produced once a trade name comes off patent. CEPs are challenged to keep up with changing knowledge of common medications and to learn new medications; new findings and medications are regularly published. It is important for CEPs to continue professional development activities including clinical patient care and medications.

It is also imperative CEPs are aware of potential drug–drug interactions, which can increase or decrease the effectiveness of the interacting medications and cause drug toxicity if drug absorption, clearance, or half-life is affected. Even though the rate of drug–drug interactions is thought to be less than 5%, each interaction could result in hospitalization and more expense to the patient, hospital, and insurer (if insured). CEPs can work with clients and their providers to discuss potential changes in therapy because of drug–drug interactions.

Physicians use standard abbreviations for prescribing medication dosages. These include qd (daily), bid (twice daily), tid (three times daily), qid (four times daily), and qw (once a week). These abbreviations are used in this chapter as well.

Organization of medications can be helpful with medication compliance. There are many versions of "pill boxes" in the market. Figure 7.2 shows a few ways to organize medications. CEPs can assist with this when a need is identified.

This chapter covers medications from five clinical areas (*e.g.*, cardiovascular, pulmonary, metabolic, orthopedic, and neuromuscular) in which CEPs commonly practice; however, the chapter does not discuss all medications in those clinical areas. Each medication class will cover medication names (both brand name and generic),

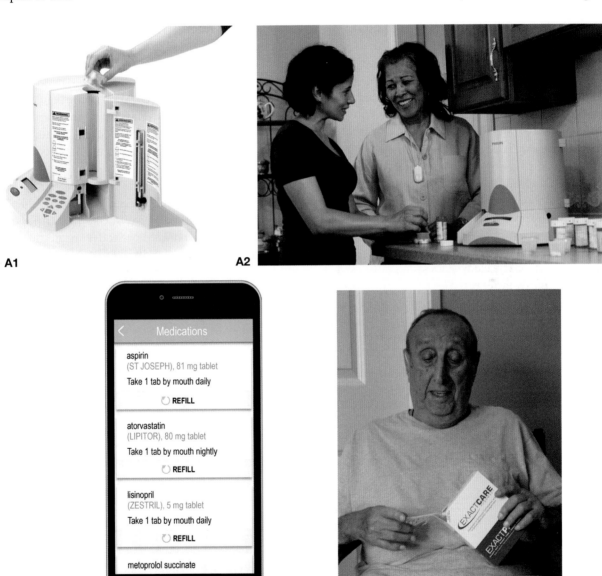

FIGURE 7.2 Examples of devices and systems designed to improve medication adherence and independence. **A1.** An automatic pill dispenser with a tamper-proof locking system and an audible alarm, with 28 compartments that can be programmed for taking medications up to four times a day. **A2.** Healthcare provider showing patient how to use automatic pill dispenser. **B1.** Medication list through smartphone app or healthcare provider online medical record. **B2.** Individualized dosing system for prescription and nonprescription medications, for use in homes and institutions, with each tear-apart compartment printed with patient name, date and time of administration, medication name and dose, and pill description. (Courtesy of and modified from Eblis/Shutterstock; Phovoir/Shutterstock; ExactCare Pharmacy. Available from: ExactCarepharmacy.com.)

therapeutic uses, mechanism of actions, side effects, drug interactions, and the effect of the medication class on heart rate (HR), blood pressure (BP), electrocardiogram (ECG), and exercise tolerance. All medication classes covered in the *American College of Sports Medicine (ACSM) Guidelines for Exercise Testing and Prescription* (2, 3) are not included in this chapter.

CARDIOVASCULAR DRUGS

Management of cardiovascular disease (CVD) and its risk factors includes multiple components: control of BP, support of cardiac function, antithrombotic therapy as needed, lipid control, diabetes mellitus (DM) management as needed, and exercise, reduced sodium intake, and smoking cessation if appropriate. This section discusses all classes of cardiovascular medications covered in ACSM guidelines book (2, 3). It is not inclusive of all medications in these classes, but does include some older, many common, and some newer ones. Medications that affect BP are presented first, followed by those that support cardiac function and help decrease angina and other symptoms. Antilipemic agents and blood modifiers (*e.g.*, anticoagulants and antiplatelets) are the last two medication types covered in this section.

Medications That Affect BP

Many cardiovascular medications help control BP. This reduces the cardiovascular event risk of cerebrovascular accident (CVA) and acute myocardial infarction (AMI), both fatal and nonfatal.

β-Blockers

β-Blockers are receptor antagonists that block receptor sites for epinephrine and norepinephrine (adrenergic β receptors) in the sympathetic nervous system. Typically used as second-line BP medications in primary prevention of hypertension (HTN), β-blockers (β-adrenergic blocking agents) are primary medications for HTN treatment. They are also used for angina pectoris, heart failure (HF) because of systolic dysfunction — part of goal-directed medical therapy (GDMT), and irregular heart rhythms including supraventricular tachycardia and atrial fibrillation. In addition, β-blockers are sometimes prescribed to treat migraine headaches, anxiety, and essential tremors.

β-Blockers are split into two categories, cardioselective and noncardioselective, as can be seen in Table 7.1. Those that are cardioselective affect the cardiovascular system, whereas noncardioselective medications can affect multiple systems of the body.

Table 7.1	β-Blockers First Through Third Generations		
Drug (Generic) Name	Brand (Trade) Name	Cardioselective	Noncardioselective
Acebutolol hydrochloride[a]	Sectral	Second	
Atenolol	Tenormin	Second	
Betaxolol hydrochloride	Kerlone	Second	
Bisoprolol fumarate	Zebeta	Second	
Esmolol hydrochloride	Brevibloc	Second	
Metoprolol succinate	Toprol XL	Second	
Metoprolol tartrate	Lopressor, Lopressor SR	Second	
Nebivolol	Bystolic	Third, also nitrate oxide–mediated vasodilation	
Carvedilol[b]	Coreg, Coreg CR		Third, also nitrate oxide–mediated vasodilation
Labetalol[b]	Trandate, Normodyne		Third, also nitrate oxide–mediated vasodilation
Nadolol	Corgard		First

Table 7.1	β-Blockers First Through Third Generations (*continued*)		
Drug (Generic) Name	Brand (Trade) Name	Cardioselective	Noncardioselective
Penbutolol	Levatol		First
Pindolol[a]	Visken		First
Propranolol	Inderal, Inderal LA, Betachron, InnoPran		First
Sotalol	Betapace, Sorine		First
Timolol	Blocadren, Timolide		First

[a]β-Blockers with intrinsic sympathomimetic activity.

[b]Combined αβ-blocker.

Therapeutic Use

β-Blockers are used to decrease HR, BP, and the heart's contractility. These effects result in a decreased myocardial oxygen demand and ischemia. Recent data show O_2 pulse — a surrogate of stroke volume — doesn't decrease during exercise; perceived exertion and dyspnea are also decreased during peak exercise as compared to non-beta blockade (4). They are expected to be used indefinitely, unless contraindicated once started in patients who have had an MI, acute coronary syndrome (ACS), or left ventricular dysfunction with or without HF symptoms (5).

β-Blockers are known to increase survival rate and reduce angina attacks. They are used as secondary prevention in patients following an MI and in patients with ACS to reduce cardiac workload. β-Blockers are also used to control HR in patients with atrial fibrillation and mitral stenosis and many other cardiac conditions (6). Patients with a reduced left ventricular ejection fraction (LVEF) should be placed on β-blockers — part of GDMT (7). β-Blockers are started at low doses and titrated up until the patient cannot tolerate an increase in further dosage. When the β-blocker dose is too high, symptoms can include hypotension, excessive bradycardia, fatigue, and heart block may occur.

Mechanism of Action

β-Blockers block the neurotransmitters epinephrine and norepinephrine from binding to β receptors (β_1 and/or β_2) in cells. Epinephrine and norepinephrine are responsible for increasing the HR and myocardial contractility and cause similar effects in other organs. With these receptors blocked, the effects of epinephrine and norepinephrine are not realized.

β-Blockers have three different generations (see Table 7.1) and differing mechanisms of action. First-generation β-blockers are noncardioselective (*e.g.*, propranolol, sotalol). They block both the β_1 (cardiac) and β_2 (noncardiac) receptors, causing a reduced cardiac output as well as reduced renal output and reduced function in the gastrointestinal (GI) tract, liver, lungs, skeletal muscle, vascular smooth muscle, and other areas. Second-generation β-blockers (*e.g.*, atenolol, metoprolol) are cardioselective and only block the β_1 receptors, reducing cardiac output. Third-generation β-blockers (*e.g.*, nebivolol) are either cardioselective or noncardioselective and also have other effects (*e.g.*, nitrate-mediated vasodilation (8)).

Side Effects

There are common side effects of β-blockers; however, many people experience only mild side effects or none at all. The most common include fatigue, cold hands or feet, diarrhea, and weight gain. Few people realize shortness of breath, depression, or trouble sleeping because of β-blockers. Asthmatics are not usually prescribed first-generation β-blockers because they can trigger potentially severe asthma attacks. Moreover, noncardioselective β-blockers have side effects on patients with bronchospastic obstructive pulmonary disease. β-Blockers may also mask signs of hypoglycemia, so regular blood glucose monitoring is vitally important. β-Blockers can also detrimentally decrease HR in those with sinus bradycardia or reduce the conduction of electrical signals through the atrioventricular (AV) node.

Related Drug Interactions

β-Blockers, like all medications, can interact with other medications. Cardioselective β-blockers used in conjunction with verapamil can have additive effects that potentially decrease HR and BP to unsafe levels. β-Blockers taken with clonidine can see increases in BP. Noncardioselective β-blockers used along with β-agonists (*e.g.*, albuterol, levalbuterol, salmeterol) could cause bronchospasm. The interaction between β-blockers and barbiturates reduces blood plasma levels of β-blockers and thereby their effectiveness.

Effects on HR, BP, ECG, and Exercise

Because β-blockers reduce cardiac output, both HR and BP (systolic and diastolic) will be reduced at rest and with exercise. One would also expect a blunted HR and BP response with increases in workloads. There should be no changes to the heart rhythm with β-blockers, which actually confer a reduction in sudden cardiac death. Long-term use of β-blockers has been shown to reduce cardiac volume (9), so hypertrophic ECG changes should not be seen with serial ECGs. It is especially important to look at the ECG of a patient with atrial fibrillation, as β-blockers can help control the rate and rhythm. Patients should be able to exercise without limitations unless they realize symptoms. Electrocardiography is discussed in detail in Chapter 6.

Angiotensin-Converting Enzyme Inhibitors

The renin–angiotensin–aldosterone system (RAAS) is the primary target for renal protection and has been so for many years (10). Angiotensin-converting enzyme inhibitors (ACE-I), the first class of medications to target the RAAS, help decrease the progression of renal failure because of HTN. They are also used to treat HTN and HF because of systolic dysfunction, diabetes nephropathy, or cerebrovascular disease. ACE-I, β-blockers, and diuretics are commonly used in combination to treat HF — part of GDMT (7). As seen in Table 7.2, ACE-I are often used alone or can be combined with hydrochlorothiazide (HCTZ) or calcium channel blockers (CCBs) to reduce BP.

Therapeutic Use

ACE-I are indicated for treating HTN and systolic HF along with chronic renal failure, DM, and peripheral artery disease (11). Patients with MI are prescribed ACE-I and should be instructed to take them indefinitely as long as they are tolerated. ACE-I have been shown to decrease mortality after heart attacks and decrease cardiac remodeling from high BP. Patients with HF receive ACE-I to decrease the onset of HF symptoms. Captopril has been found to decrease the progression of kidney problems in patients with insulin-dependent diabetes mellitus (IDDM) or HTN.

In addition to being primary medications for the abovementioned CVDs, ACE-I are used to treat chronic kidney disease (CKD). CKD treatment targets the renin–angiotensin system, and ACE-I are one mainstay of the regimen. They have been shown to decrease glomerular

Table 7.2	Angiotensin-Converting Enzyme Inhibitors		
Drug (Generic) Name	Brand (Trade) Name	Combination ACE-I + HCTZ	ACE-I + CCB
Benazepril	Lotensin	Lotensin HCT	Lotrel (+amlodipine)
Captopril	Capoten	Capozide	
Enalapril	Vasotec	Vaseretic	Lexxel (+felodipine)
Fosinopril	Monopril	Monopril HCT	
Lisinopril	Zestril, Prinivil	Prinzide, Zestoretic	
Moexipril	Univasc	Uniretic	
Perindopril	Aceon		Prestalia (+amlodipine)
Quinapril	Accupril	Accuretic	
Ramipril	Altace		
Trandolapril	Mavik		Tarka (+verapamil)

ACE-I, angiotensin-converting enzyme inhibitors; CCB, calcium channel blocker; HCTZ, hydrochlorothiazide, a thiazide diuretic.

Source: From American College of Sports Medicine. *ACSM's Guidelines for Exercise Testing and Prescription.* 10th ed. Baltimore (MD): Lippincott Williams & Wilkins; 2017.

HTN and protein excretion in the urine independently of their cardiovascular effects (10).

Mechanism of Action

The RAAS plays a significant role in HTN, MI, HF, renal failure, and diabetes nephropathy. Smooth muscle surrounds the endothelial lining of blood vessels. When vascular smooth muscle contracts, BP increases. Contraction occurs when angiotensin II is formed.

The RAAS begins with the release of the enzyme renin by the kidneys. Renin converts angiotensinogen, a blood protein secreted by the liver, to angiotensin I. Angiotensin I is then converted to angiotensin II with the assistance of angiotensin-converting enzyme. In response to angiotensin II, the blood vessel walls decrease in diameter, and BP therefore increases.

ACE-I act to decrease the conversion of angiotensin I to angiotensin II. Inhibiting the RAAS allows the blood vessels to dilate or remain the same diameter; thus, a lower BP is typically realized. This in turn allows the heart to pump against a lower pressure. Long-term benefits can be realized as well because, without ACE-I treatment, cardiac remodeling typically progresses, leading to cardiac and vascular hypertrophy, as well as collagen development by cardiac fibroblasts (12).

ACE-I combined with HCTZ (see Table 7.2) work to reduce BP by decreasing the conversion of angiotensin I to angiotensin II and to reduce blood volume, thereby helping to treat HF. HCTZ will be further discussed later in this chapter. ACE-I combined with CCBs (see Table 7.2) help decrease BP and to block calcium channels that vasoconstrict vascular smooth muscle. CCBs will be discussed in detail later in this chapter.

Side Effects

Even though ACE-I are usually tolerated well, there are side effects. The most common include abnormal taste (like a metallic or salty taste), cough, dizziness, drowsiness, headache, rash, weakness, and increased sun sensitivity. Other side effects are hyperkalemia (elevated blood potassium levels), low BP, chest pain, increased uric acid levels, and increased blood urea nitrogen (BUN) and creatinine levels (a sign of decreased kidney function). Some people complain of a dry cough when taking ACE-I. Switching to another ACE-I typically does not alleviate the cough. It usually takes about 1 month for the cough to go away after ceasing to take the ACE-I (13). ACE-I are contraindicated for patients who have angioedema, are pregnant, have hyperkalemia, or have bilateral renal artery stenosis. Patients with angioedema can have worsening swelling of tissues with ACE-I. Pregnant women are not prescribed ACE-I because the drugs can cause birth defects. Patients with hyperkalemia can see exacerbated decreases in liver function if put on ACE-I. Patients with bilateral renal artery stenosis can experience worsening kidney function as seen with increased BUN and creatinine levels.

Related Drug Interactions

Concomitant use of ACE-I and thiazide or loop diuretics can lead to hypotension in those with depleted sodium or blood volume levels. Likewise, it is imperative to monitor blood potassium levels in those using potassium supplements, salt substitutes containing potassium, and other drugs that can increase potassium levels (14). ACE-I can exacerbate acute renal failure in those who are taking nonsteroidal anti-inflammatory drugs (NSAIDs). These medications include aspirin (acetylsalicylic acid [ASA]), ibuprofen, indomethacin, and naproxen. The BP-lowering effects of ACE-I can also be decreased with NSAIDs (14). Lithium blood concentrations may be increased with ACE-I usage. Eskalith and Lithobid are two drugs that contain lithium. Side effects from lithium toxicity include confusion, poor memory, or lack of awareness, fainting, fast or slow HR, frequent urination, increased thirst, irregular pulse, stiffness of the arms or legs, excessive shortness of breath with exertion, unusual fatigue, and weight gain (14).

Effects on HR, BP, ECG, and Exercise

ACE-I help decrease BP but have no direct effect on HR. They have been shown to increase oxygen extraction (15), which may lead to an increase in exercise capacity in those without HF. Exercise capacity has been shown to be increased with ACE-I use (16) in patients with HF. ACE-I have no known direct effect on the ECG. As long as patients are not symptomatic from hypotension, ACE-I may allow patients to exercise with a lower BP for a longer period of time.

Angiotensin II Receptor Blockers

Angiotensin II receptor blockers (ARBs) are similar to ACE-I and used instead of ACE-I in patients who do not tolerate ACE-I well. They are indicated in patients with HTN, diabetic nephropathy, and HF. ARBs are associated with a reduced occurrence of side effects, mostly the dry cough associated with ACE-I (17). They are formulated alone, in combination with CCBs, in combination with diuretics (HCTZ or chlorthalidone), or in combination with both CCBs and diuretics (see Table 7.3).

Table 7.3	Angiotensin II Receptor Blockers			
Drug (Generic) Name	Brand (Trade) Name	Combination ARB + Diuretic (HCTZ[a] or Chlorthalidone[b])	Combination ARB + HCTZ + CCB[c]	Combination ARB + CCB[d]
Azilsartan	Edarbi	Edarbyclor[b]		
Candesartan	Atacand	Atacand HCT[a]		
Eprosartan	Teveten	Teveten HCT[a]		
Irbesartan	Avapro	Avalide[a]		
Losartan	Cozaar	Hyzaar[a]		
Olmesartan	Benicar	Benicar HCT[a]	Tribenzor	Azor
Telmisartan	Micardis	Micardis HCT[a]		Twynsta
Valsartan	Diovan	Diovan HCT[a]	Exforge HCT	Exforge

[a]ARB + HCTZ for use in HTN and HF.

[b]ARB + Chlorthalidone for use in HTN.

[c]ARB + HCTZ + CCB for use in HTN.

[d]ARB + CCB for use in HTN.

ARB, angiotensin II receptor blocker; CCB, calcium channel blocker; HCTZ, hydrochlorothiazide, a thiazide diuretic.

Source: From American College of Sports Medicine. *ACSM's Guidelines for Exercise Testing and Prescription.* 10th ed. Baltimore (MD): Lippincott Williams & Wilkins; 2017.

Therapeutic Use

Studies comparing ARBs and ACE-I showed no difference in cardiovascular mortality or outcomes between them (17). ARBs, like ACE-I, are used to treat HTN with systolic HF (in those patients who do not tolerate ACE-I well), proteinuric chronic renal failure, or DM. ARBs are not indicated for use in patients following an MI with an ejection fraction (EF) 40% or greater, or for peripheral artery disease treatment, much like ACE-I. ARBs combined with CCBs (see Table 7.3) block the angiotensin II type I receptor and the calcium channels that help vasoconstrict blood vessels. Those formulated in combination with diuretics (HCTZ or chlorthalidone; Table 7.3) work to reduce vasoconstriction and blood volume. The diuretic works along with the ARB to decrease blood volume in two places — vascular smooth muscle with the ARB and kidneys with the diuretic. Those combined with CCBs and diuretics (see Table 7.3) work through the three pathways described above.

Mechanism of Action

ARBs are similar to ACE-I because they act on the vascular smooth muscle; however, they have slightly different pathways. Instead of blocking the conversion of angiotensin I to angiotensin II, ARBs work by blocking the angiotensin II type I receptor in cardiac, renal, and vascular smooth muscle cells (9). Activation of these receptors is responsible for causing vasoconstriction and fluid retention. Blocking them in turn blocks the chemical reaction that takes place to cause constriction of the blood vessel (12). ARBs are helpful in patients following an MI with an EF below 40% because they reduce BP and also help to reduce blood volume, an important therapeutic goal with HF.

Side Effects

ARBs are contraindicated in the same groups as ACE-I and have the same side effects.

Related Drug Interactions

ARBs and ACE-I should not be taken together, because this combination increases the risk of hypotension, hyperkalemia, and renal impairment.

Effects on HR, BP, ECG, and Exercise

ARBs have the same effect on HR, BP, and ECG and the same benefits/hindrance to exercise as ACE-I.

Angiotensin Receptor-Neprilysin Inhibitors

The first-in-class medication Entresto combines the ARB valsartan and the neprilysin inhibitor sacubitril to treat patients with reduced ejection fraction heart failure (HFrEF) (Table 7.4). Its primary action is to help patients avoid hospitalizations and potentially help them to live longer.

Therapeutic Use

Entresto contains two active ingredients that work in different ways. As discussed above, valsartan, is used to treat HF by reducing vascular constriction, whereas sacubitril relaxes blood vessels and decreases sodium and fluids in the body (18).

Mechanism of Action

Neprilysin (https://www.rxlist.com/neprilysin/definition.htm) inhibitors are a class of drugs used to treat HTN (https://www.rxlist.com/high_blood_pressure_hypertension_medications/drug-class.htm) and congestive heart failure (CHF) (https://www.rxlist.com/heart_failure/definition.htm) peptides, thereby, promoting the removal of sodium from the blood. Without natriuretic peptides, sodium levels would increase promoting HTN (19).

Neprilysin also plays a role in the degradation of vasoactive peptides such as bradykinin. Bradykinin is a vasodilator that allows vasodilation facilitating the free flow of blood in the vessels. In the absence of bradykinin, the blood vessels may not relax and may cause an increase in BP. Neprilysin inhibitor increases the availability of bradykinin to achieve vasodilation and natriuresis (excretion of sodium), thus, helping to lower BP (19).

Side Effects

Common side effects include dizziness, light-headedness, or cough. Serious side effects may include hyperkalemia, hypotension, and renal failure. Angiotensin receptor-neprilysin inhibitors (ANRIs) are also contraindicated in patients with DM and those with end-stage renal disease (ESRD). Pregnant women should not use an ARNI (18).

Related Drug Interactions

Entresto should not be taken within 36 hours before or after taking any other ACE-I. An individual with DM or ESRD should not use Entresto together with any medication that contains aliskiren such as Tekturna or Tekamlo (18).

Effects on HR, BP, ECG, and Exercise

Entresto improved BP, exercise tolerance, LVEF, peak $\dot{V}O_2$, and ventilatory efficiency. Further studies are necessary to better clarify the underlying mechanisms of this functional improvement (20).

Direct Renin Inhibitors

The only direct renin inhibitor (DRI) on the market is aliskiren (brand name: Tekturna). It is also formulated in combination with HCTZ to treat HTN (Table 7.5).

Therapeutic Use

Aliskiren, or Tekturna, is used to treat HTN and may have beneficial effects on renal disease because of HTN (10). Tekturna is combined with HCTZ to further decrease BP through the addition of a diuretic. The combination is also shown to decrease the progression of renal failure (10).

Table 7.4	Angiotensin Receptor-Neprilysin Inhibitors
Drug (Generic) Name	Brand (Trade) Name
Valsartan + sacubitril	Entresto

Table 7.5	Direct Renin Inhibitor	
Drug (Generic) Name	Brand (Trade) Name	Combination DRI + HCTZ[a]
Aliskiren	Tekturna	Tekturna HCT

[a]DRI + HCTZ for use in HTN.

DRI, direct renin inhibitor; HCTZ, hydrochlorothiazide, a thiazide diuretic.

Source: From American College of Sports Medicine. *ACSM's Guidelines for Exercise Testing and Prescription.* 10th ed. Baltimore (MD): Lippincott Williams & Wilkins; 2017.

Mechanism of Action

As their name implies, DRIs inhibit the RAAS at the start of the process; that is, they act to inhibit the release of renin, the enzyme responsible for the conversion of angiotensinogen to angiotensin I by the kidneys.

Side Effects

Common side effects include those seen with ACE-I and ARBs as well as dizziness, headache, nausea, and a stuffy nose. DRIs are contraindicated in the same populations for whom ACE-I are contraindicated. They are also contraindicated in patients with DM and those with stage 3 ESRD or worse (18). Pregnant women should not use a DRI.

Related Drug Interactions

Aliskiren should not be used in combination with ACE-I or ARBs, as doing so could worsen hyperkalemia (21).

Effects on HR, BP, ECG, and Exercise

DRIs have the same effect on HR, BP, and ECG and the same benefits/hindrance to exercise as ACE-I.

Calcium Channel Blockers

CCBs are medications that block the entry of calcium into cardiac myocytes and vascular smooth muscle cells. They help decrease the myocardial and peripheral oxygen demand. CCBs affect preload and afterload, and some also influence cardiac rhythm through their effect on the sinoatrial (SA) and AV nodes. CCBs are classified into two groups: dihydropyridines and nondihydropyridines.

Therapeutic Use

Dihydropyridines are used to treat patients with isolated systolic HTN (Table 7.6). They are also used to treat angina pectoris because of a mismatch between myocardial oxygen demand and supply, Prinzmetal angina because of coronary spasms, and ischemic heart disease. Nondihydropyridines are indicated for HTN, as well as for angina, paroxysmal supraventricular tachycardia, and other arrhythmias (Table 7.7).

Mechanism of Action

Muscle contraction is triggered by the entry of calcium (Ca^{2+}) into a cell through a calcium channel. CCBs preferentially bind to the Ca^{2+} channels and slow entry of Ca^{2+} into the cardiac and vascular smooth muscle cells. Blocking this entry can relax both cardiac and vascular smooth muscle, thereby reducing BP, symptoms of ischemic heart disease, and cardiac arrhythmias.

Calcium channels are divided into subtypes (L, N, and T), and dihydropyridines and nondihydropyridines link to different calcium channel receptor sites. The L-type channel, for example, is specific and sensitive to dihydropyridine CCBs (12). In this way, the dihydropyridines

Table 7.6	Dihydropyridines — Calcium Channel Blockers
Drug (Generic) Name	**Brand (Trade) Name**
Amlodipine	Norvasc
Clevidipine (intravenous formulation only)	Cleviprex
Felodipine	Plendil
Isradipine	DynaCirc, DynaCirc CR
Nicardipine	Cardene, Cardene SR
Nifedipine long-acting[a] and short-acting[b]	Adalat CC,[a] Afeditab CR,[a] Nifediac CC, Procardia,[b] Procardia XL[a]
Nimodipine	Nymalize, Nimotop
Nisoldipine	Sular

[a]Long-acting nifedipine.

[b]Short-acting nifedipine.

Source: Modified from: American College of Sports Medicine. *ACSM's Guidelines for Exercise Testing and Prescription.* 10th ed. Baltimore (MD): Lippincott Williams & Wilkins; 2017.

Table 7.7	Nondihydropyridines — Calcium Channel Blockers
Drug (Generic) Name	Brand (Trade) Name
Diltiazem	Cardizem
Diltiazem, extended-release	Cardizem CD or LA, Cartia XT, Dilacor XR, Dilt CD or XR, Diltia XT, Diltzac, Taztia XT, Tiadylt ER, Tiazac
Verapamil	Calan, Verelan, Covera HS, Isoptin
Verapamil, controlled- and extended-release	Calan SR, Covera HS, Isoptin SR, Verelan, Verelan PM
Verapamil + trandolapril	Tarka

Source: Modified from: American College of Sports Medicine. *ACSM's Guidelines for Exercise Testing and Prescription*. 10th ed. Baltimore (MD): Lippincott Williams & Wilkins; 2017.

and nondihydropyridines act somewhat differently; however, both types have the same general effect of reducing preload and afterload along with symptoms of ischemic heart disease and cardiac arrhythmias. Reducing afterload allows the myocardium to generate less force and contributes to a lower systolic BP. Arterial tone and vascular resistance are reduced in the vascular system, whereas atrial and ventricular contraction are reduced in cardiac myocytes. CCBs are also known to reduce excitability and increase the membrane potential necessary to invoke electrical stimulation and subsequent contraction (22).

Side Effects

Common side effects of CCBs include constipation, dizziness, excessive bradycardia, fatigue, flushed feeling, headache, hypotension, nausea, palpitation, and peripheral edema (23). Some side effects are more common with specific CCBs (*e.g.*, dizziness, edema, flushing, headache, and palpitation are more common with nifedipine). Diltiazem, nifedipine, and verapamil can exacerbate HF, because they reduce the heart's contractility, and they are not commonly prescribed when patients have HF and HTN (24).

Related Drug Interactions

Certain drug interactions involving CCBs can have harmful effects. Verapamil and diltiazem are known to slow the excretion of and increase the concentration of carbamazepine, simvastatin, atorvastatin, and lovastatin in the blood (25). Several CCBs (*e.g.*, diltiazem and felodipine) have been shown to increase the blood concentration of cyclosporine in those taking cyclosporine. Digoxin levels can increase in those taking verapamil and nifedipine. These

effects can result in drug toxicity. Verapamil has been shown to increase pancreatic β cell secretion of insulin in patients with DM, thus helping to control blood glucose (26). In contrast, CCBs affect patients without DM by decreasing insulin secretion and can have deleterious effects if not controlled.

Dihydropyridines, except amlodipine, have been shown to negatively interact with grapefruit or grapefruit juice. Consumption of grapefruit or grapefruit juice while taking dihydropyridines (within 1 h of consumption) typically increases the plasma concentration of the medications. There is a wide difference among dihydropyridines, but the increased concentration can cause drug toxicity (27).

Effects on HR, BP, ECG, and Exercise

All CCBs decrease BP, whereas CCBs have varied effects on HR, ECG, and exercise tolerance. Nondihydropyridines have little direct effect on exercise tolerance (27, 28). Some CCBs are antiarrhythmic agents and help to control the heart's rhythm — and indirectly control the HR (see section on Antiarrhythmic Agents, for more information).

Diuretics

Diuretics are drugs that increase the body's excretion of fluids. They are used to decrease HF symptoms, modify disease progression, and prolong survival. The combination of ACE-I, β-blockers, and diuretics is currently considered the best practice for HF treatment (7); this regimen has been shown to improve survival in patients with HF (9). Many different types of diuretics exist, and their mechanisms of action will be discussed separately below (see Table 7.8, for the diuretic types and names).

Table 7.8	Diuretics		
Drug (Generic) Name	Brand Name		
Thiazides			
Bendroflumethiazide	(+Nadolol) Corzide		
Chlorothiazide	Diuril		
Hydrochlorothiazide (HCTZ)	Hydrodiuril, Microzide, Oretic		
Hydroflumethiazide	Saluron		
Methyclothiazide	Enduron		
Polythiazide	Renese		
Trichlormethiazide	Naqua		
Thiazide-Like			
Chlorthalidone	Hygroton, Thalitone, (+Atenolol) Tenoretic		
Indapamide	Lozol		
Metolazone	Mykrox, Zaroxolyn		
Quinethazone	Hydromox		
Loop Diuretics			
Bumetanide (taken once daily by mouth or continuously by intravenous)	Bumex		
Ethacrynic acid (taken bid by mouth or continuously by intravenous)	Edecrin		
Furosemide (taken bid by mouth or continuously by intravenous)	Lasix		
Torsemide (taken by mouth only)	Demadex		
Potassium-Sparing Diuretics			**Combined With HCTZ**
Amiloride	Midamor		Moduretic, Hydro-ride
Triamterene	Dyrenium		Dyazide, Maxzide
Mineralocorticoid (Aldosterone) Receptor Blockers			**Combined With HCTZ**
Eplerenone	Inspra		
Spironolactone	Aldactone		Aldactazide
Canrenone	Not available in the U.S.		
Potassium canrenoate	Not available in the U.S.		

Source: Modified from American College of Sports Medicine. *ACSM's Guidelines for Exercise Testing and Prescription*. 10th ed. Baltimore (MD): Lippincott Williams & Wilkins; 2017.

Therapeutic Use

Diuretics are indicated for patients with edema, HTN, HF, and certain kidney disorders. Thiazides are usually the first-line diuretic unless another diuretic agent is indicated, or drug resistance occurs (29, 30). They are used either alone or in combination with other medications (ACE-I, ARB, or CCB) to treat mild or moderate HTN and have a beneficial effect on morbidity and mortality (cardiovascular and cerebrovascular systems (31)). Diuretics decrease preload and extracellular volume to reduce symptoms of HF and treat HTN. They increase the urine flow rate and the natriuretic rate (rate of NaCl excretion). Sodium restriction is also important in those sensitive to sodium. However, if preload is decreased too quickly, cardiac output could be decreased and create side effects. Volume overload from increased Na^+ results in pulmonary edema, whereas volume depletion from insufficient Na^+ can result in cardiovascular failure. Patients with HF are best kept in a euvolemic status to reduce side effects and symptoms (12).

Mechanism of Action

Thiazides and thiazide-like diuretics increase salt excretion through inhibition of the Na^+–Cl^- transport at the distal convoluted tubule. This results in an increased urinary excretion of NaCl. They also increase K^+ and uric acid excretion, but at a lower rate than loop diuretics (12). Thiazides also are sometimes used to treat osteoporosis because they decrease Ca^{2+} excretion.

Loop diuretics inhibit the Na^+–K^+–$2Cl^-$ ion transport protein in the thick ascending limb of the loop of Henle, increasing Na^+ and fluid delivery to the distal fluid segment. K^+ secretion is also improved, especially when combined with mineralocorticoid (aldosterone) receptor blockers. Bumetanide and furosemide, as compared to torsemide, have short half-lives and are typically prescribed bid (12). Torsemide is taken once daily.

Potassium-sparing diuretics decrease excretion of K^+ from the body while decreasing extracellular body fluids and blood volume through increases in NaCl excretion. Amiloride or triamterene taken along with spironolactone are commonly referred to as "potassium-sparing diuretics" (12). They work at the late distal tubule and collecting duct levels of the kidney, where K^+ is maintained in the bloodstream, instead of being excreted in the urine.

Mineralocorticoid receptor blockers (aldosterone antagonists) inhibit salt and water retention and decrease K^+ and H^+ excretion. They act in the late distal tubule and collecting duct decreasing the aldosterone binding to the mineralocorticoid receptor. This increases diuresis (12).

Side Effects

Typical side effects seen with diuretic use are increased urination, dizziness, headaches, light-headedness, nausea, and vomiting. Some people report tinnitus, vertigo, and hearing disturbances. The side effects typically worsen with an increased dosage or frequency. Dehydration and electrolyte depletion are seen with excessive dosages. Potassium replacement aids (e.g., KDur) are commonly prescribed to decrease the risk of electrolyte depletion, including hypokalemia, and cardiac arrhythmias associated with electrolyte

imbalances (e.g., frequent premature ventricular contractions and nonsustained ventricular tachycardia).

Loop diuretic overdosage could lead to hyponatremia along with depletion of extracellular fluids. Signs of this include hypotension, decreased glomerular filtration rate (GFR), thromboembolisms, hepatic encephalopathy (in patients with liver disease), and circulatory collapse (12). Some patients taking loop diuretics experience hyperuricemia (leading to gout), hyperglycemia (potentially leading to DM), or increased low-density lipoprotein cholesterol (LDL-C) and triglyceride (TRIG) levels along with reduced high-density lipoprotein cholesterol (HDL-C) levels. Ethacrynic acid (Edecrin) is only recommended for those with sulfonamide allergies or who cannot tolerate other loop diuretics.

Thiazide and thiazide-like diuretics lead to erectile dysfunction more commonly than other diuretics and many other HTN medications. The side effects of potassium-sparing diuretics, thiazide, and thiazide-like diuretics are similar to those of loop diuretics. Thiazide and thiazide-like diuretics can also increase glucose intolerance and thereby uncover DM in patients who didn't know they had it. Those with cirrhosis are also at risk of developing metabolic acidosis while taking mineralocorticoid receptor blockers (12).

Related Drug Interactions

Loop diuretics when taken with a variety of other medications can have side interactions. Specifically, loop diuretics are known to increase anticoagulant activity, increase arrhythmias from digitalis, increase lithium blood levels, increase propranolol blood levels, increase blood glucose with sulfonylureas, increase risk of ototoxicity with cisplatin, decrease diuretic response with probenecid, promote excessive diuresis with thiazide diuretics, and increase electrolyte imbalance and nephrotoxicity with amphotericin B (12).

Patients taking quinidine along with thiazide diuretics need to be monitored for hypokalemia because the QT interval on the ECG can become prolonged and cause torsades de pointes (see Chapter 6). Hyperkalemia is the most serious side effect of potassium-sparing diuretics. Patients with renal failure, taking ACE-I, or taking potassium supplements should not take potassium-sparing diuretics (11). In contrast, both thiazide and loop diuretics can cause life-threatening hypokalemia.

Effects on HR, BP, ECG, and Exercise

Diuretics do not affect HR or ECG; however, they decrease BP. Spironolactone has been shown to increase exercise tolerance in patients with HF with preserved EF (HFpEF (32)).

Vasodilating Agents and Other Medications That Support Cardiac Function

The medications discussed here support cardiac function, including contractility and electrophysiology/rhythm maintenance, and help decrease angina and other symptoms. Many of these medications have vasodilatory properties.

Nitrates and Nitrites

Nitrates, including nitroglycerin (NTG), and nitrites are organic nitric oxide compounds that have been used in the treatment of CVD for over a century. They are used for angina (both stable and unstable), MI or history of MI, HF and other low cardiac output syndromes, and HTN. Nitrates and nitrites dilate blood vessels, allowing blood to flow through them with less resistance.

Therapeutic Use

Nitrates and nitrites are used to increase the lumen size of blood vessels and treat the symptoms of angina pectoris (Table 7.9). The resistance of blood flow is directly related to the lumen size, which is inversely proportional to the fourth power of the lumen's radius. Myocardial ischemia causes angina pectoris and is because of a mismatch of oxygen availability and demand. When the lumen size is decreased because of atherosclerosis or other disease, or when the oxygen demand is greater than availability, angina can occur. This can occur at rest or with exertion. Patients having angina attacks because of coronary spasms are excellent candidates for nitrate/nitrite use. The medications dilate the affected areas and epicardial coronary arteries.

Mechanism of Action

In the cardiovascular system, nitrates and nitrites lead to smooth muscle relaxation through the release of nitric oxide (NO). NO increases the levels of cyclic guanylyl monophosphate (GMP), which dephosphorylates the myosin light chain and reduces the cellular Ca^{2+} concentration, leading to the relaxation of smooth muscle cells surrounding blood vessels. Vasodilation of blood vessels increases the lumen's radius, thus decreasing the resistance and increasing the blood supply to the tissues. Nitrates and nitrites decrease venous return, preload, and afterload. Systemic pressure decreases along with pulmonary vascular resistance. These effects can correct the oxygen demand imbalance.

Table 7.9	Nitrates and Nitrites	
Drug (Generic) Name	**Brand Name**	**Short- or Long-acting**
Amyl nitrite (inhaled)	Amyl Nitrite	Long
Isosorbide mononitrate	Monoket	Long
Isosorbide dinitrate	Dilatrate SR, Isordil	Long
Isosorbide dinitrate + hydralazine HCl	BiDil	Long
Nitric oxide (inhaled)	INOmax	Short
Nitroglycerin, capsules ER	Nitro-Time, Nitroglycerin Slocaps	Short
Nitroglycerin, lingual (spray)	Nitrolingual Pumpspray, Nitromist	Short
Nitroglycerin, sublingual	Nitrostat	Short
Nitroglycerin, topical ointment	Nitro-Bid	Short
Nitroglycerin, transdermal	Minitran, Nitro-Dur, Nitrek, Deponit	Short
Nitroglycerin, transmucosal (buccal)	Nitrogard	Short

Source: Adapted from American College of Sports Medicine. *ACSM's Guidelines for Exercise Testing and Prescription.* 10th ed. Baltimore (MD): Lippincott Williams & Wilkins; 2017.

There are both long and short-acting nitrates and nitrites (see Table 7.9). Long-acting nitrates (*e.g.*, Isordil) begin to take effect within an hour of consumption and help maintain the oxygen demand balance for an extended period. Short-acting nitrites (*e.g.*, Nitrogard) take effect within minutes and can help quickly restore blood flow for a short period when symptoms arise (12). Long-acting nitrates have a longer half-life than short-acting nitrites, a fact that explains their extended period of action.

Side Effects

Two of the most common side effects of nitrates/nitrites are flushing of the face and headaches. These are common because nitrites dilate all blood vessels and increase blood flow to all areas of the body. Other side effects include dizziness, excessive hypotension, pale skin color, and weakness. Overconsumption of nitrates could potentially aggravate angina, especially in a patient who is unstable (12).

Related Drug Interactions

Nitrates and alcohol do not mix well together, especially in patients who have a severe hypotensive response to nitrates. Severe hypotension can also result from concurrent use of nitrates and sildenafil (Viagra) or other phosphodiesterase-5 inhibitors, because these medications increase smooth muscle relaxation, acting in a similar fashion to nitrates (12).

Effects on HR, BP, ECG, and Exercise

Both nitrates and nitrites decrease BP while they are active in the bloodstream. Nitrates increase the patient's ability to exercise (33), with higher doses being more effective. The myocardial O_2 consumption level is the same after nitrate consumption as before; that is, the triple product level is the same. The triple product level is equivalent to the aortic pressure times the HR times the ejection time. This effect is because of a decreased cardiac O_2 demand and beneficial distribution of blood flow to the ischemic myocardium (12). Resting HR is reduced, and exercise HR could be the same or increased, whereas the ischemic threshold is realized at a higher HR.

α-Blockers

α-Blockers are medications that block α_1 adrenergic receptors (Table 7.10). They are selective to inhibition of epinephrine and norepinephrine and work similar to β-blockers; however, they have different mechanisms of action.

Table 7.10	α-Blockers
Drug (Generic) Name	**Brand (Trade) Name**
Doxazosin	Cardura, Cardura XL
Prazosin	Minipress
Tamsulosin	Flomax
Terazosin	Hytrin

Source: American College of Sports Medicine. *ACSM's Guidelines for Exercise Testing and Prescription.* 10th ed. Baltimore (MD): Lippincott Williams & Wilkins; 2017.

Therapeutic Use

α-Blockers are used to treat patients with benign prostatic hyperplasia (BPH) as well as HTN. They are not first-line HTN medications but help decrease urinary symptoms in those with BPH. α-Blockers are often used in conjunction with β-blockers, diuretics, and other HTN medications; β-blockers improve the effectiveness of α-blockers.

Mechanism of Action

α-Blockers block α_1 adrenergic receptors at the postsynaptic level, producing decreased arteriolar resistance and increased venous capacity through decreased vasoconstriction. Vasodilation occurs in the cardiovascular and prostate areas. This decreased peripheral resistance and decreased venous return to the heart results in a reduced BP.

Depending on the level of receptor selectivity (prazosin having one of the highest), different α-blockers have different effects on BP and BPH. All α-blockers increase urine flow and allow smooth muscle relaxation in the prostate and urinary tract. Less mechanical pressure from the smooth muscle and less vasoconstriction allow urine to flow with less restriction and decreased symptoms. Terazosin has been found to have less prostate smooth muscle cell proliferation than other α-blockers, thus less mechanical pressure (34). A potential benefit of α-blockers is a reduction in LDL and TRIG concentrations with an increase in HDL concentration. The long-term benefits of these lipid changes in patients using α-blockers are not well understood (11).

Side Effects

Common side effects of α-blockers include constipation, diarrhea, fatigue, headache, nausea, and vomiting. These effects are usually seen initially until a patient becomes accustomed to taking the medication. A more serious side effect includes HF exacerbated by doxazosin (20). α-Blockers can also produce the "first dose phenomenon" (marked symptomatic orthostatic HTN up to 90 min after the first dose or a subsequent increase in dosage). Up to 50% of patients taking α-blockers will see no ill effects after a few doses (12).

Related Drug Interactions

α-Blockers can negatively interact with selected β-blockers (*e.g.*, atenolol, metoprolol, propranolol), increasing their effects and creating extreme hypotension. They can also negate the effects of verapamil, sildenafil, and tadalafil, increasing pulmonary HTN.

Effects on HR, BP, ECG, and Exercise

α-Blockers can increase or fail to reduce HR and cardiac output with exercise. Prazosin has little impact on HR or cardiac output, whereas doxazosin and tamsulosin increase HR and cardiac output with exercise. The decrease seen with total peripheral resistance may result in a lower systolic BP with exercise. There should be changes to the ECG (less ischemia seen with exercise); exercise tolerance is not significantly affected (12).

Central α-Agonists

Central α-agonists are similar to α-blockers; however, they act on the α_2 receptors in the central nervous system (CNS; Table 7.11).

Therapeutic Use

Although prescribed to treat HTN, central α-agonists are not usually first-line medications for BP control. They

Table 7.11	Central α-Agonists
Drug (Generic) Name	Brand (Trade) Name
Clonidine	Catapres, Catapres-TTS (patch), Duraclon (injection form), Kapvay
Guanabenz	Wytensin
Guanfacine	Intuniv, Tenex
Methyldopa	Aldoril

Source: American College of Sports Medicine. *ACSM's Guidelines for Exercise Testing and Prescription.* 10th ed. Baltimore (MD): Lippincott Williams & Wilkins; 2017.

are typically administered by mouth in the form of pills, and clonidine can also be administered using a patch or injection. Clonidine is sometimes given intravenously after an MI as adjunctive therapy. They have also been used to treat glaucoma but are not first-line medications for glaucoma.

Central α-agonists, especially clonidine, can be used during addiction recovery to help prepare addicted persons for withdrawal from alcohol, narcotics, or tobacco. The drugs are used because they help reduce sympathetic nervous system effects of withdrawal. Clonidine in particular may also help decrease the addict's longing for the drug. Other off-label uses for central α-agonists include treatment of atrial fibrillation, attention-deficit hyperactivity disorder, psychosis, and menopausal symptoms (35).

Mechanism of Action

Central α-agonists work at the level of the presynaptic α_2 receptors in the CNS to inhibit the release of norepinephrine at the neurosynapse. This leads to less norepinephrine being received at the postsynapse, resulting in decreased arteriolar resistance and increased venous capacity through decreased vasoconstriction; Grassi first reported this finding in patients with HF who were also taking β-blockers and ACE-I. They also act in the brainstem to provide antihypertensive benefits — a reduced increase in HR resulting in a lower systolic BP (35).

Side Effects

Severe bradycardia and dry mouth are the most common serious side effects of central α-agonists, especially clonidine. Sympathetic nervous system responses are also reduced — dizziness, drowsiness, and potential sedation can occur. Erectile dysfunction has also been shown to occur. Many of the side effects are dose dependent, and use of the skin patch helps reduce side effects; however, dermatitis can occur with use of the patch (35).

Related Drug Interactions

Patients taking pain medications (acetaminophen and derived medications) need to be aware of the central α-agonists' effects on blunting norepinephrine release — can result in lower HR and BP response to exercise. Other medications that affect the norepinephrine release or reception also need to be considered when prescribing central α-agonists. Too much blunting of the release or reception of norepinephrine can result in greater sedative effects than normally seen with central α-agonists — for example, dizziness and drowsiness.

Effects on HR, BP, ECG, and Exercise

There should be no appreciable change in cardiac output with central α-agonist use, and patients should realize lower HRs and BPs with exercise (28). Exercise capacity has not been shown to be diminished with central α-agonist use (36).

Direct Vasodilators

Direct vasodilators are medications that relax and dilate arterial smooth muscle.

Therapeutic Use

Direct vasodilators, either used on their own or combined with other cardiac medications, are used to treat HTN and HF (Table 7.12). Hydralazine, prior to being combined with other antihypertensive agents, was one of the first oral antihypertensive agents used in the U.S. Bidil (hydralazine plus isosorbide dinitrate) has been shown to reduce all-cause and cardiovascular mortality in patients who are African American (37) and those with a reduced EF (38). Sodium nitroprusside is effective in patients with advanced HF who have elevated systemic BP or mitral valve regurgitation or other mechanical insults after an MI (39). Minoxidil is typically used to treat hair loss, but it can also reduce BP in those resistant to other HTN medications.

Mechanism of Action

Vasodilation occurs because of blood vessel smooth muscle relaxation. This leads to a decreased systemic vascular resistance and a decreased afterload and preload; this is beneficial for HF and HTN treatment. BP is reduced through fluid reduction and vascular resistance reduction resulting in a reduced afterload. Direct vasodilators reduce afterload and assist with augmenting the stroke volume. They act at the arterial level to vasodilate, reduce ventricular filling pressure, and reduce pulmonary and systemic resistance. This allows stroke volume to remain as normal as possible in patients with HF and can help increase cardiac output because there is less stress on the ventricular walls. Maintenance of cardiac output in turn helps to improve renal function, making direct vasodilators helpful in promoting diuresis (39).

Some vasodilators have unique actions. Sodium nitroprusside's mechanism of action is through the NO-mediated vasodilation pathway discussed earlier in this chapter. Minoxidil decreases systemic vascular resistance by polarizing the K^+ channels in the vascular smooth muscle cells, resulting in dilation of blood vessels and a reduced afterload (39). Hydralazine has a combination effect from the HCTZ and isosorbide dinitrate. Each of these medications was discussed previously in this chapter.

Side Effects

Although minoxidil can exacerbate HF (24), all direct vasodilators can worsen hypotension. Excessive afterload reduction can also lead to reduced renal blood flow. Abdominal pain, convulsion/seizures, and mental status changes can occur with sodium nitroprusside and are signs of cyanide toxicity. Typical side effects of hydralazine include dizziness, fatigue, flushing, headache, hypotension, nausea, palpitations, tachycardia, and others depending on the formulation prescribed (+HCTZ or + isosorbide dinitrate); the other side effects are the same as those seen with HCTZ or isosorbide dinitrate individually as discussed previously in this chapter. Hydralazine and minoxidil can also produce angina pectoris from myocardial ischemia; this is because of the tachycardia and increased myocardial contractility side effect and can cause an MI. Hydralazine is not recommended for the treatment of HTN in patients with coronary artery

Table 7.12	Direct Vasodilators	
Drug (Generic) Name	Brand Name	Dosage Frequency
Hydralazine	Apresoline, (+HCTZ) Hydrazide, (+isosorbide dinitrate) Bidil	3–4 times daily
Minoxidil	Loniten Topical: Rogaine, Theroxidil	Once daily
Sodium nitroprusside	Nipride, Nitropress	Once daily
Verquvo	Vericiguat	Once daily

Source: Modified from American College of Sports Medicine. *ACSM's Guidelines for Exercise Testing and Prescription.* 10th ed. Baltimore (MD): Lippincott Williams & Wilkins; 2017.

disease (CAD) or those with multiple CAD risk factors, or in the elderly (39). Hydralazine can also induce immunological reactions that are similar to those of systemic lupus erythematosus (SLE). Because hydralazine is rarely prescribed on its own anymore, cases of lupus-like side effects are rare as well. Signs of this include excessive fatigue, arthralgia, arthritis, and fever (35). Minoxidil is used to treat male pattern baldness (topical Rogaine is an example), and excessive hair growth (hypertrichosis) is a side effect seen in both men and women when used for HTN treatment, typically for extended time periods (39). Alternatively, Rogaine can cause cardiovascular effects usually seen with minoxidil use for HTN.

Related Drug Interactions

Direct vasodilators taken along with ACE-I can result in an excessive afterload reduction and cause decreased renal blood flow. Hydralazine can increase the absorption of metoprolol and propranolol. Minoxidil should be taken with a diuretic as to not exacerbate HF (39).

Effects on HR, BP, ECG, and Exercise

Many of the effects seen with diuretics and nitrates are also seen with the use of direct vasodilating agents. The effects on HR, BP, and ECG, along with benefits or hindrances to exercise, are discussed in the sections on diuretics and nitrates. One key ECG change that can occur with minoxidil is a flattened or inverted T wave (see Chapter 6). This will resolve over time after cessation of the medication but is something CEPs need to be aware of when exercise testing or training individuals using minoxidil for male pattern baldness or HTN.

Peripheral Adrenergic Inhibitors

Peripheral adrenergic inhibitors act in the brain to restrict signals telling blood vessels to constrict. They are used when other BP medications fail to work for individuals or in those with severe HTN needing another BP agent to reach recommended BP levels. The best known is reserpine.

Therapeutic Use

Reserpine was the first pharmacological agent found to reduce BP by reducing the sympathetic nervous system effects — for example, reduce vasoconstriction. Because it is associated with severe adverse effects on the CNS, discussed shortly, it is now rarely prescribed and will not be discussed at length here. However, low-dose combination

Table 7.13	Peripheral Adrenergic Inhibitors
Drug (Generic) Name	Brand (Trade) Name
Reserpine	Raudixin, Serpalan, Serpasil

Source: American College of Sports Medicine. *ACSM's Guidelines for Exercise Testing and Prescription.* 10th ed. Baltimore (MD): Lippincott Williams & Wilkins; 2017.

therapy with thiazide has been shown to be effective with fewer side effects (see Table 7.13) (35, 40).

Mechanism of Action

Reserpine acts in the presynaptic vesicle to decrease the availability of norepinephrine. Secretion of norepinephrine results in increased HR and systolic BP. Blocking norepinephrine release therefore suppresses the increased HR and systolic BP seen with stress (35). Thus, HR, stroke volume, and peripheral arterial resistance are reduced with reserpine use.

Side Effects

Reserpine has been used to treat psychosis, as an overdose can sedate a patient; however, reserpine can cause depression and suicidal thoughts. It can also cause migraine headaches, nasal congestion, fatigue, and difficulty concentrating. These side effects cannot be reversed with other medications and tend to be long-lasting (35).

Related Drug Interactions

Reserpine decreases the effectiveness of CNS stimulants by decreasing catecholamine availability in the brain and at sympathetic nerve endings (35). There are also reports of interactions between reserpine and analgesics, anesthetics, and antidepressants. With these drugs, cardiac dysrhythmias (*e.g.*, premature ventricular contractions, ventricular tachycardia, and idioventricular rhythm) have occurred; further decreases in HR and BP are expected as well. Reserpine should be discontinued prior to administration of these medications (41).

Effects on HR, BP, ECG, and Exercise

Reserpine decreases both the resting and exercise HR and BP; however, there should be no change in ECG or exercise capacity (40). Reserpine is no longer routinely prescribed, so CEPs should not see many patients taking it.

Cardiac Glycosides

Cardiac glycosides are medications that increase the force of cardiac contraction and regulate cardiac rhythm.

Therapeutic Use

Cardiac glycosides were one of the first classes of medications used to treat HF and control arrhythmia (Table 7.14). The best-known cardiac glycoside is digoxin, extracted from the digitalis plant (foxglove). It was first discovered to be useful in the treatment of HF by Sir William Withering in 1785. Cardiac glycosides are used to support patients with dilated cardiomyopathy and acute decompensating HF. They are effective in relieving symptoms; however, they have not been shown to decrease mortality from HF (42).

Mechanism of Action

Cardiac glycosides help increase a patient's stroke volume by increasing contractility — a positive inotropic effect —

Table 7.14	Cardiac Glycosides
Drug (Generic) Name	Brand (Trade) Name
Amrinone (inamrinone)	Inocor
Digoxin	Lanoxin (pill form), Lanoxicaps (capsules form), Digitek (pill form)
Milrinone (intravenously or by mouth)	Primacor

Source: Bottle image reprinted from Kronenberger J, Ledbetter J. Lippincott Williams & *Wilkins' Comprehensive Medical Assisting.* 5th ed. Philadelphia (PA): Wolters Kluwer; 2016.

through an increase in myocardial cytosolic Ca^{2+} concentration (39). They assist with rhythm control by elevating vagal tone and inhibiting sympathetic nervous system activity and increasing the resting membrane potential in the atrial and AV node.

Side Effects

Side effects of cardiac glycosides include arrhythmias, nausea, vomiting, disorientation, and visual disturbances. Digoxin should be avoided in patients with AV nodal block without a pacemaker and in patients with Wolff–Parkinson–White syndrome — see Chapter 6 for more on these conditions. Patients having hypertrophic cardiomyopathy with a left ventricular outflow tract obstruction should not take digoxin (42). Digoxin toxicity can result in excessive sinus bradycardia; sinus arrest; first-, second-, or third-degree heart block; and lethal arrhythmias. Excessive dosages of digoxin can cause end-organ failure, hyperkalemia, and lethal ventricular arrhythmias if the action potential threshold is reduced too far (39, 43).

Related Drug Interactions

Elimination of cardiac glycosides is affected by renal function. Decreased renal function increases the risk of drug toxicity, especially digoxin toxicity (see the side effects above), because the serum concentration is increased. Cardiac glycoside serum concentrations are also affected by other medications — either increased by amiodarone, quinidine, verapamil, tetracycline, and erythromycin, or decreased by dexamethasone, phenytoin, and rifampicin. Patients taking cholestyramine or antacids should be instructed to take digoxin at least 2 hours before these drugs (43). CEPs need to be aware of potential toxicity and can alert providers if toxicity is suspected.

Effects on HR, BP, ECG, and Exercise

As discussed above, digoxin will decrease the HR in patients with atrial fibrillation; it may also do this in patients with CHF. Digoxin can produce nonspecific ST–T-wave changes on resting ECGs in addition to sinus bradycardia, sinus arrest, and first-, second-, and third-degree heart block, especially with digitalis toxicity. ST-segment depression can be seen on exercise ECGs. CEPs may be the first one to notice ECG changes in a patient taking cardiac glycosides and can communicate to the patient's provider as needed (see Chapter 6, for more information on these ECG findings).

Cardiac glycosides support exercise training and can be beneficial in increasing workloads achieved during exercise testing or training, especially in patients with atrial fibrillation or CHF. Exercise testing should be symptom-limited and event-limited. It has been done safely in small cohorts with few or no side effects (44, 45).

Symptom-limited exercise testing can be performed with patients taking milrinone or on a "milrinone drip" with caution; hypotension and significant cardiac arrhythmias are two side effects to be aware of. Milrinone provides inotropic support and can increase exercise test results (*e.g.*, 6-min walk, peak metabolic equivalents [METS], or $\dot{V}O_{2peak}$ (46)). Exercise training has been done on both adult and pediatric patients taking milrinone awaiting heart transplantation without significant side effects (44, 45).

Cardiotonic Agents

Cardiotonic agents are prescribed to help bolster the heart's cardiac output. This favorable effect is usually from an increased cardiac contractility.

Therapeutic Use

Cardiotonic agents are used to decrease the risk of hospitalization in symptomatic stable (New York Heart Association [NYHA] class II–III) patients with HF (Table 7.15). These patients can have symptomatic stable angina and worsening symptoms (*e.g.*, dyspnea with exertion, pitting edema). These agents are specific for those patients who have a reduced EF (EF < 35%), are in sinus rhythm, have a resting HR ≥ 70 beats per minute (bpm), and are either on a maximal β-blocker therapy or have contraindications for β-blocker usage. Ivabradine has been shown to decrease morbidity and mortality in these patients as well as decrease hospital admissions and cardiac death rates (47).

Mechanism of Action

Ivabradine, an SA node blocker, decreases the rate of atrial depolarization. It acts through blockage of cyclic nucleotide-gated channels responsible for the spontaneous cardiac pacemaker activity. This results in an HR reduction without affecting ventricular depolarization or

Table 7.15	Cardiotonic Agent
Drug (Generic) Name	Brand (Trade) Name
Ivabradine	Corlanor, Procoralan

Source: American College of Sports Medicine. *ACSM's Guidelines for Exercise Testing and Prescription.* 10th ed. Baltimore (MD): Lippincott Williams & Wilkins; 2017.

myocardial contractility. HR reduction is dose dependent, with a larger decrease in HR occurring with a higher dose and in those with a higher resting HR pre-ivabradine administration. Because ivabradine works at the SA node, it has no effect on the QRS complex or QT interval at the AV node (48). Greater time between beats can result in an increased end-diastolic volume, increased myocardial "stretch," and increased myocardial contractility — thus supporting an increased cardiac output.

Side Effects

Side effects of ivabradine include atrial fibrillation, BP increases, bradycardia, sinus arrest, heart block, and visual brightness. Those with second-degree heart block should not use ivabradine unless they already have a demand pacemaker (49).

Related Drug Interactions

Ivabradine should not be taken concurrently with verapamil or diltiazem as they can further lower a patient's HR. Patients should avoid ingesting grapefruit or grapefruit juice or St. John's wort while taking ivabradine as they increase and decrease the effects of ivabradine, respectively (49).

Effects on HR, BP, ECG, and Exercise

Ivabradine decreases HR and usually has little to no effect on BP. In some patients, however, it can cause heart block. CEPs need to be aware of this potential effect and should report any ECG changes seen for patients taking ivabradine.

Antiarrhythmic Agents

Antiarrhythmic agents are found in a variety of cardiac medications, many of which have already been discussed in this chapter (Table 7.16). This section will focus on those medications not already discussed previously.

Therapeutic Use

Antiarrhythmic agents are used to control irregular atrial (*e.g.*, atrial fibrillation, atrial flutter, supraventricular tachycardia) and ventricular (*e.g.*, premature ventricular contractions, ventricular fibrillation [VF], ventricular tachycardia) cardiac rhythms with the goal of maintaining normal sinus rhythm. The goal is to stop arrhythmias from progressing or prevent future arrhythmias. Many of these agents have other effects because they are used to treat other diseases (*e.g.*, BP control for HTN) (50).

Table 7.16	Antiarrhythmic Agents
Drug (Generic) Name	**Brand (Trade) Name**
Class I	
IA	
Disopyramide	Norpace (CR)
Procainamide	Procanbid
Moricizine	Ethmozine
Quinidine	Quinora, Quinidex, Quinaglute, Quinalan, Carioquin
IB	
Lidocaine	Xylocaine
Mexiletine	Mexitil
Phenytoin	Dilantin, Phenytek
IC	
Flecainide	Tambocor
Propafenone	Rythmol (SR)
Class II	
β-Blockers	
Acebutolol	Sectral
Atenolol	Tenormin
Bisoprolol	Zebeta
Esmolol	Brevibloc
Metoprolol	Lopressor, Lopressor SR, Toprol XL
Propranolol	Inderal, Inderal LA
Timolol	Blocadren
Class III	
Amiodarone	Cordarone, Nexterone (intravenous), Pacerone
Dofetilide	Tikosyn
Dronedarone	Multaq
Ibutilide	Covert (intravenous)
Sotalol	Betapace, Betapace AF, Sorine
Class IV	
Diltiazem	Cardizem CD or LA, Cartia XT, Dilacor XR, Dilt CD or XR, Diltia XT, Diltzac, Tiazac, Taztia XT
Verapamil	Calan, Calan SR, Covera HS, Verelan, Verelan PM

Source: Modified from American College of Sports Medicine. *ACSM's Guidelines for Exercise Testing and Prescription*. 10th ed. Baltimore (MD): Lippincott Williams & Wilkins; 2017.

Mechanism of Action

Class I medications block the Na^+ channel resulting in an increase in AV nodal block to slow the ventricular response in atrial fibrillation, atrial flutter, atrial tachycardia, AV nodal reentrant tachycardia (paroxysmal supraventricular tachycardia), ventricular tachycardia, and VF depending on the medication. Disopyramide, procainamide, lidocaine, and mexiletine are medications used in acute therapy, whereas quinidine, phenytoin, flecainide, and propafenone are used for chronic treatment of arrhythmia. Blocking the Na^+ channel long term is necessary to control the ventricular response and help maintain normal sinus rhythm (50).

Class II medications (β-blockers) slow AV nodal conduction and increase AV nodal refractory periods (for more information, see β-Blockers section).

Class III medications prolong the action potential required for stimulation and resultant ventricular contraction and block the K^+ channels. This results in a decreased energy threshold required for defibrillation, decreased VF burden from myocardial ischemia, and increased myocardial contractility. Amiodarone, dofetilide, and sotalol are common class III medications and control both atrial and ventricular arrhythmias (*e.g.*, atrial fibrillation, atrial flutter, ventricular tachycardia, VF; 50).

Class IV medications (diltiazem and verapamil) slow AV nodal conduction and increase AV nodal refractory periods through Ca^{2+} channel blockade. Please see the discussion of CCBs, specifically nondihydropyridines, previously in this chapter.

Side Effects

Many of the same side effects of other cardiac medications are seen with antiarrhythmic agents. Class II and Class IV medications have already been described in previous sections. Some class I and III medications (flecainide, disopyramide, dronedarone, and sotalol) can exacerbate HF (21). Class III medications lengthen cardiac action potentials and can result in torsades de pointes. Diltiazem and verapamil can prompt hypotension, especially with intravenous bolus administration. The same side effects of β-blockers and CCBs described in those sections of this chapter apply here as well. Noncardiac side effects of antiarrhythmic agents include neuromuscular paralysis as a result of procainamide or quinidine use, antithyroid actions from amiodarone, and muscle cramping from adenosine (50). Chronic amiodarone use can affect a patient's lung diffusing capacity (measured by diffusion capacity of the lung for carbon monoxide [DLCO]) and should not be taken by someone with identified lung disease, especially pulmonary fibrosis. Those with arthritis should not use procainamide long term, as it can exacerbate the symptoms and disease process.

It is important for CEPs to realize the potential side effects antiarrhythmic agents can have. Control of a patient's heart rhythm can require constant monitoring and medication adjustment, especially early in the treatment process. CEPs are vital to this and can identify cardiac and noncardiac issues as they arise, helping to improve patient care.

Related Drug Interactions

Adenosine and class I medication effects are reduced by dipyridamole and in patients with cardiac transplant. Caffeine and similar drugs require larger doses to create an antiarrhythmic effect. Class IC medication and digoxin dosages should be reduced with concomitant amiodarone use. Dofetilide should not be used in patients with renal function impairment, whereas dronedarone should not be taken at the same time as antifungal agents and macrolide antibiotics (50).

Effects on HR, BP, ECG, and Exercise

Many cardiac arrhythmia agents decrease resting HR and resting BP. The ECG effects are described above. Exercise tolerance has already been described for β-blockers and CCBs. Other antiarrhythmic agents have little effect on exercise tolerance.

Antianginal Agents
Therapeutic Use

Ranolazine, an antianginal agent, is primarily used to decrease anginal symptoms in patients with refractory symptomatic stable angina (Table 7.17). It is not a first-line medication for the treatment of angina but is usually prescribed together with other cardiac medications described previously (*e.g.*, ACE-I, ARBs, β-blockers, CCBs, and/or nitrates). Although research is ongoing, recent studies have used ranolazine for secondary purposes with

Table 7.17	Antianginal Agents
Drug (Generic) Name	Brand (Trade) Name
Ranolazine	Ranexa

Source: American College of Sports Medicine. *ACSM's Guidelines for Exercise Testing and Prescription.* 10th ed. Baltimore (MD): Lippincott Williams & Wilkins; 2017.

some success, including for control of atrial fibrillation and blood glucose, and for treatment of chemotherapy-induced cardiotoxicity, diastolic dysfunction, pulmonary arterial HTN, and refractory neuropathy pain (51). A number of randomized clinical trials have shown that ranolazine decreases the occurrence of atrial fibrillation, either new-onset or recurrent postcardioversion (52). CEPs should begin to see ranolazine use increase for these secondary purposes, either as off-label or after U.S. Food and Drug Administration (FDA) approval, especially in patients with refractory symptomatic stable angina and these secondary conditions (53).

Mechanism of Action

Ischemia occurs when an imbalance of oxygen availability and demand causes an ion imbalance in the myocytes. When there is an ion imbalance, the channels take longer to close with more Ca^{2+} flowing into the cell. This causes decreased left ventricular relaxation and increased diastolic left ventricular wall tension, resulting in impaired blood flow to the impacted myocardium and further ischemia. The patient is also at greater risk for arrhythmias with increases in Ca^{2+} flowing into the myocytes because the myocytes are more excitable. Ranolazine has direct effects on the Na^+ channels of cardiac myocytes (54) inhibiting the fast and late Na^+ channel currents slowing flow in and out of the myocytes. Cytosolic Ca^{2+} levels are then reduced with less calcium flowing into the cell. This reduces potential ischemia, resultant angina, and arrhythmias. The effects are seen in both the left and right ventricles. In the right ventricle, ranolazine results in decreased pulmonary artery HTN and arrhythmia control. QTc intervals (rate-corrected QT intervals) on the ECG are also increased by ranolazine from prolonged ventricular action potentials (51). In addition to the effects of ranolazine in cardiac myocytes, there have been reported effects in pancreatic islet α cells. The glycemic effects of ranolazine are not well understood at this time; however, improved blood glucose control has been seen with ranolazine use in patients with DM (51).

Side Effects

Ranolazine has similar side effects to other antianginal medications, with dizziness as one of the most commonly reported. Fatigue, headache, nausea, and weakness have also been commonly reported (55).

Related Drug Interactions

Ranolazine may be effective in increasing the effect of amiodarone to convert and control atrial fibrillation as it acts at the Na$^+$ channels of the cardiac myocytes. It has also been shown to work in concert with anticoagulants to help control atrial fibrillation in patients with refractory symptomatic stable angina. This is for both new-onset atrial fibrillation and the recurrence of atrial fibrillation after electrical cardioversion (52). Metformin at high doses (700 mg qd or greater) has been shown to negatively interact with ranolazine at higher doses (1,000 mg bid); (51). Cases of slow junctional rhythm, excessive QTc lengthening, and torsades de pointes have been reported with ranolazine use combined with ivabradine and verapamil (56). Neurological issues have also been reported with ranolazine use alongside clarithromycin (57), along with interactions in kidney transplant patients taking ranolazine and sirolimus (58).

Effects on HR, BP, ECG, and Exercise

With its effects on the Na$^+$ channels in cardiac myocytes, ranolazine helps to decrease the HR and BP at rest and with exercise. It also lengthens the QTc interval and can create T-wave inversions seen on ECG, along with decreasing episodes of ventricular tachycardia and supraventricular tachycardia. Recent studies have shown benefit in those with refractory symptomatic stable angina and in the secondary conditions listed above. Over time, these improvements could increase one's exercise capacity (51). Finch and colleagues realized increases in 6-minute walk distance in a small cohort of patients with HFpEF with pulmonary HTN (59).

Antilipemic Agents

Patients with dyslipidemia — abnormal levels of total cholesterol (CHOL), LDL, TRIG, and HDL — and patients with metabolic syndrome are commonly prescribed antilipemic agents, commonly known as lipid-lowering therapy (Table 7.18). They are used in primary and secondary prevention of CVD and to reduce the risk of cardiovascular events and mortality, especially in patients with DM, for whom CVD is the leading cause of death. Statins have been shown to decrease the risk of major vascular events by 10% (60).

Table 7.18	Antilipemic Agents	
Drug (Generic) Name	**Brand (Trade) Name**	**How Administered**
Bile Acid Sequestrants		
Cholestyramine	Locholest, Prevalite, Questran	Powder dissolved in liquid
Colesevelam	Welchol	Powder dissolved in liquid
Colestipol	Colestid	Powder dissolved in liquid
Fibric Acid Sequestrants		
Fenofibrate	Antara, Fenoglide, Lipofen, Lofibra, Tricor, Triglide, Trilipix	Tablet
Gemfibrozil	Lopid	Tablet
HMG-CoA Reductase Inhibitors (Statins)		
Atorvastatin	Lipitor	Tablet
Fluvastatin	Lescol (XL)	Tablet
Lovastatin	Mevacor, Altocor, Altoprev	Tablet
Lovastatin + Niacin	Advicor	Tablet
Pitavastatin	Livalo	Tablet
Pravastatin	Pravachol	Tablet
Rosuvastatin	Crestor, Ezallor	Tablet
Simvastatin	Zocor	Tablet

(continued)

Table 7.18	Antilipemic Agents (*continued*)	
Drug (Generic) Name	**Brand (Trade) Name**	**How Administered**
Simvastatin + Niacin	Simcor	Tablet
Statin 1 CCB		
Atorvastatin + Amlodipine	Caduet	Tablet
Nicotinic Acid		
Niacin (vitamin B$_6$)	Niaspan, Nicobid, Slo-Niacin	Tablet
Omega-3 Fatty Acid Ethyl Esters		
Omega-3-carboxylic acids (EPA and DHA)	Epanova	Capsule
Icosapent Ethyl (EPA)	Vascepa	Capsule
Omega-3 fatty acid ethyl esters (EPA and DHA)	Lovaza	Capsule
Cholesterol Absorption Inhibitor		
Ezetimibe	Zetia, (+Simvastatin) Vytorin	Tablet
PCSK9 Inhibitors		
Alirocumab	Praluent	Injection
Evolocumab	Repatha	Injection

CCB, calcium channel blocker; DHA, docosahexaenoic acid; EPA, eicosapentaenoic acid.

Source: Modified from American College of Sports Medicine. *ACSM's Guidelines for Exercise Testing and Prescription*. 10th ed. Baltimore (MD): Lippincott Williams & Wilkins; 2017.

Therapeutic Use

Antilipemic agents modify lipid profiles. Their action is often described as helping to "stabilize" arteries, especially those with atherosclerotic plaque. They are all prescribed along with lifestyle changes, like diet and exercise, and are usually added after lifestyle changes have been unsuccessful in modifying lipid profiles.

Each classification of antilipemic agent modifies different components of the lipid profile. Statins help to decrease CHOL, LDL, and TRIG and improve the total CHOL:HDL ratio. Nicotinic acid helps increase HDL. Fibric acid sequestrants help to decrease CHOL, LDL, and TRIG. Proprotein convertase subtilisin/kexin type 9 (PCSK9) inhibitors are prescribed to help decrease LDL (61).

When used individually, antilipemic agents, especially statins, decrease cardiovascular events, vasculopathy, and mortality (25). Statin therapy has the most benefit as long as the patient can tolerate taking a statin (57, 62). Higher doses of statins result in better results and less progression of CVD. How antilipemic agents may work together is still being debated. Bile acid sequestrants and fibric acid sequestrants are commonly prescribed with statins in patients with complex dyslipidemias or severe hypertriglyceridemia. Nicotinic acid has not been shown to be of benefit when prescribed with statins (25). PCSK9 inhibitors are prescribed either together with statins or individually when statins have not lowered LDLs sufficiently (61).

Statins are also prescribed for patients with heart transplant. Statin therapy, which begins early after heart transplant, is typically continued for life. Decreased rejection from hemodynamic compromise, vasculopathy, and mortality is benefit realized in patients with heart transplant (25). There are also off-label uses of antilipemic agents — statins include Alzheimer disease and anti-inflammatories. Statins have anti-inflammatory effects and reduce serum levels of C-reactive protein (CRP), lipoprotein-associated phospholipase A$_2$ (Lp-PLA$_2$), and matrix metalloproteinase-9 (MMP-9), resulting in fewer cardiovascular events (63). Bile acid sequestrants are also used to reduce itching caused by excess oxalate in the urine, which could lead to urinary stones.

Mechanism of Action

There are multiple mechanisms depending on the medication type. Each will be discussed separately.

Bile acid sequestrants decrease the intestinal absorption of bile acid and its transportation back to the liver. Instead, the bile travels through the GI tract to be excreted in feces. The subsequent decrease in bile results in greater LDL receptor activity and lower LDL concentrations in the blood. In the liver, cholesterol transformation into bile acid is enhanced (62).

Fibric acid sequestrants reduce LDL and TRIG levels and increase HDL levels by increasing lipoprotein lipase activity. This results in less very-low-density lipoprotein (VLDL) and TRIG formation, along with increased HDL formation (62). Decreases in VLDL result in decreased LDL formation.

Statins inhibit the activity of an enzyme called 3-hydroxy-3-methyl-glutaryl-CoA (HMG-CoA) reductase, which is involved in the production of cholesterol. Statins decrease the transformation of HMG-CoA to mevalonic acid (one of the steps in the creation of cholesterol and other isoprenoids like heme and sterol), thus reducing the amount of cholesterol produced by the liver. They target cholesterol production in the liver and enhance LDL receptor activity, removing LDL from the bloodstream (64).

Nicotinic acid decreases diacylglycerol acyltransferase-2 activity. This action reduces TRIG formation, LDL levels, and HDL breakdown by the liver. This results in lowered LDL and TRIG levels alongside increased HDL levels. These results lead to a decreased cardiovascular mortality with nicotinic acid monotherapy (62).

Omega-3 fatty acid (FA) ethyl esters have a few mechanisms of action. They decrease TRIG synthesis through hepatic suppression, lower LDL production and secretion in the liver, and elevate VLDL degradation in the liver. Omega-3 FAs are not as widely researched at this time as other antilipemic agents; however, early studies have shown some benefits to these agents, especially a decrease in TRIGs (62). They also appear to have antiatherogenic effects and to decrease BP.

Vytorin (a combination of simvastatin and ezetimibe) acts in two different ways: HMG-CoA reductase inhibition and cholesterol absorption by the intestines. This results in reduced cholesterol formation by the liver and decreased absorption in the intestines from dietary intake. Ezetimibe on its own decreases absorption of cholesterol in the intestines (65).

PCSK9 inhibitors (FDA approved in 2015) are injected one to two times monthly. The PCSK9 gene influences the LDL receptor numbers (mutations decrease receptors leading to higher LDL levels), and PCSK9 inhibitors transform the gene protein's capability subsequently increasing LDL receptor numbers. This assists the liver in reducing LDL levels. They are usually prescribed after statins and/or ezetimibe are not lowering LDL level sufficiently. PCSK9 inhibitors have also been shown to produce atheroma plaque regression (61).

Side Effects

Lipid-lowering agents are usually well tolerated. Some common side effects include flushing especially with nicotinic acid; GI distress (*e.g.*, bloating, upset stomach) with bile acid sequestrants, nicotinic acid, and omega-3 FAs; and muscle weakness seen with statins and combination agents. Fibric acid sequestrants have few side effects.

As just mentioned, muscle fatigue is a commonly reported side effect of statins. This fatigue can result from muscle-related toxicity (rhabdomyolysis) and can be increased with drug–drug interactions. For example, statins and fibric acid sequestrants taken concurrently increase the risk of muscle-related toxicity 5.5-fold. The FDA does not recommend that gemfibrozil, in particular, be taken concurrently with most statins (25). Fibric acid sequestrants also increase the risk for muscle weakness when taken independently of statins. The risk is approximately 10 times higher with gemfibrozil than with fenofibrate.

Specific statins increase the risk of developing Type 2 diabetes mellitus (T2DM), with increasing doses increasing risk. The lowest risk of T2DM is seen with pravastatin 40 mg per day (7% risk), whereas rosuvastatin (20 mg per d) has the highest risk (25% risk). Atorvastatin and simvastatin have an intermediate risk (15% and 21% risk, respectively). The proposed mechanisms for this risk, all center around impaired insulin secretion (60).

Ezetimibe has few side effects, and many have been linked to statins when ezetimibe is combined with simvastatin. Muscle myopathy has been reported with cholesterol absorption inhibitor use and usually recedes when ezetimibe use is stopped. Liver enzymes have increased in some patients, but this has been reversed when the patients cease ezetimibe use. Gallbladder disease has also been reported rarely with ezetimibe use and reversed when use is stopped (66).

Related Drug Interactions

Drug–drug interactions have been reported for several medications in combination with select statins. Amiodarone, amlodipine, colchicine, digoxin, diltiazem, dronedarone, fenofibric acid, ranolazine, ticagrelor, verapamil, and warfarin are considered safe to take concurrently when dosed appropriately. Others, including conivaptan, cyclosporine, everolimus, gemfibrozil, sirolimus, and tacrolimus are not considered safe with specific statins. Newer medications (*e.g.*, ivabradine, sacubitril/valsartan) currently show no safety concerns with some statins; however, there are insufficient data to make a determination. The American Heart Association published a scientific statement detailing drug–drug interactions with statins — see their statement for more details and recommendations (25).

Fibric acid sequestrants have been shown to increase the effects of warfarin (25). Ezetimibe can also increase the patient's international normalized ratio (INR), which is a measure of the time it takes blood to clot, increasing the effects of the anticoagulant warfarin (66). It is not recommended to use fibric acid sequestrants along with ezetimibe (66).

Effects on HR, BP, ECG, and Exercise

Antilipemic agents do not have any effect on HR, BP, ECG, or exercise capacity (28). Patients taking Caduet, a combination statin/CCB, may experience a decreased exercise HR and BP but not have an effect on the exercise capacity; this is from the CCB. Patients experiencing muscle fatigue from statin administration may have reduced exercise tolerance.

Blood Modifiers

The blood modifiers include anticoagulants and antiplatelets.

Anticoagulants

Anticoagulants, commonly called "blood thinners," impair the clotting response. There are various types of anticoagulants and various administration routes (Table 7.19). Anticoagulants help prevent blood clots and coagulation but have inherent risks. The anticoagulants to be covered in this section include direct thrombin inhibitors, low-molecular-weight heparin (LMWH), selective inhibitors of factor Xa, and vitamin K antagonist.

Therapeutic Use

Anticoagulants are used to treat and prevent thromboembolic disorders. They help decrease the risk of blood clots,

Table 7.19	Anticoagulants	
Drug (Generic) Name	**Brand (Trade) Name**	**Administration Route**
Direct Thrombin Inhibitor		
Argatroban	Acova	Intravenous
Bivalirudin	Angiomax	Intravenous
Dabigatran	Pradaxa	Tablet by mouth
Desirudin	Iprivask	Intramuscular
Lepirudin	Refludan	Intravenous
Low-Molecular-Weight Heparin (LMWH)		
Dalteparin	Fragmin	
Enoxaparin	Lovenox	Intramuscular
Fondaparinux	Arixtra	
Selective Inhibitor of Factor Xa, Serine Endopeptidase (*e.g.*, Prothrombinase, Thrombokinase, or Thromboplastin)		
Apixaban	Eliquis	Tablet by mouth
Edoxaban	Savaysa	Tablet by mouth
Rivaroxaban	Xarelto	Tablet by mouth
Vitamin K Antagonist		
Warfarin	Coumadin, Jantoven	Tablet by mouth, intravenous

intermittent claudication, MI, and CVA. Anticoagulants also decrease the risk of vascular death in those with a history of atrial fibrillation, deep venous thrombosis, ST-elevation MI, pulmonary embolus (PE), or thrombocytopenia from heparin use. Warfarin and selective inhibitors of factor Xa are prescribed for those with atrial fibrillation to decrease the risk of thromboembolic events in those at risk for CVA (67). Direct oral anticoagulants (DOACs) are more effective than warfarin and safer for use by patients with atrial fibrillation (68). Direct thrombin inhibitors are given intravenously to patients prior to percutaneous transluminal coronary angioplasty or coronary artery bypass surgery, whereas LMWH is given to those at risk of developing emboli in various areas of the body (69).

Mechanism of Action

The mechanisms of action differ according to the type of anticoagulant (see Table 7.19).

Direct thrombin inhibitors (argatroban, bivalirudin, dabigatran) do just as their name says; they inhibit thrombin and decrease clotting (69). Thrombin inhibition decreases platelet activation and clot formation. Direct thrombin inhibitors act quickly and typically do not need routine INR monitoring, as blood levels can be predicted based on dosage. They are used to prevent thromboembolism after surgery, especially hip or knee.

LMWH, such as dalteparin, enoxaparin, and fondaparinux and its derivatives, upregulates coagulant protease inhibitors (69). They attach to antithrombin (an important substance in blood clotting control produced by the liver) and accelerate antithrombin slowing of coagulation protease activity. LMWH acts quickly and is used to treat PE and venous thrombosis, as well as unstable angina and MI. Often another anticoagulant is started at the same time and given concurrently until the second anticoagulant has reached threshold levels in the bloodstream (*i.e.*, sufficient INR levels). Warfarin has commonly been used in this role.

Selective inhibitor of factor Xa (apixaban, edoxaban, rivaroxaban) such as factor Xa along with reduced prothrombinase activity results in prolonged prothrombin time (PPT) and activated partial thromboplastin time (APTT) and an increased INR. This reduces thrombin creation and potential thrombus (clot) formation (70). A treatment threshold concentration needs to be reached in the bloodstream for optimal efficacy.

In therapeutic levels, warfarin, the only vitamin K antagonist, blocks many steps in the coagulation cascade (*e.g.*, it limits vitamin K epoxide reductase activity);

thus, its efficacy must be followed closely with routine APTT, INR, and prothrombin time (PT) monitoring. It usually takes several days after starting warfarin before levels are therapeutic. Dosages are then modified to meet therapeutic levels based on APTT, INR, and PT monitoring. Levels too high increase the risk of bleeding externally and internally. Levels too low increase the risk of thromboembolic events, which warfarin is trying to prevent (69).

Side Effects

Warfarin is commonly called "rat poison." Excessive bleeding, especially extracranial and intracranial that can potentially be fatal, is the most common and serious side effect of all anticoagulants. However, apixaban (and potentially other selective inhibitors of factor Xa) has a decreased risk of bleeding and of hemorrhagic stroke compared to warfarin (67). Patients with prosthetic heart valves should not take apixaban, edoxaban, or rivaroxaban, as they have not been proven to be safe yet. Thrombocytopenia is a serious side effect sometimes seen with LMWH (69).

Related Drug Interactions

Patients taking warfarin are advised to limit their foods high in vitamin K (*e.g.*, green leafy vegetables) because too much vitamin K ingestion can lower the PT time. Warfarin and selective inhibitors of factor Xa should not be taken concomitantly. Warfarin use is not indicated for use with amiodarone, cholestyramine, cimetidine, clopidogrel, fluoxetine, loop diuretics, barbiturates, carbamazepine, rifampin, and coagulation factors — lowered PT times result (69).

Other anticoagulants and antiplatelet agents as well as long-term NSAID use increase the risk of bleeding (67). Patients switching from one drug to another require INR monitoring and should begin to take the other drug only after stopping the previous medication. Alternatively, the efficacy of selective inhibitors of factor Xa is decreased by dual inhibitors of Cytochrome P450 Family 3 Subfamily A Member 4 (CYP3A4) and P-glycoprotein 1 (P-gp, also known as multidrug resistance protein 1 [MDR1]). These types of medications (*e.g.*, carbamazepine, clarithromycin, ketoconazole, itraconazole, phenytoin, rifampin, ritonavir, St. John's wort) should not be taken concomitantly with anticoagulants. Antibiotics can lengthen PT time beyond therapeutic levels (69).

Patients taking chemotherapy agents are at an increased risk of venous thromboembolism. Many patients receiving chemotherapy are given anticoagulants, especially LMWHs, as part of primary prevention for thromboembolic events (69). However, some chemotherapy agents increase the risk of bleeding complications when taken with anticoagulants. Likewise, antiretroviral agents can impact the effectiveness of anticoagulants. Dabigatran has a low interaction rate with antiretroviral agents. Side effects are also likely not to occur between newer anticoagulants and antiretroviral agents (71).

Effects on HR, BP, ECG, and Exercise

Anticoagulants have not been shown to have an effect on HR, BP, or exercise tolerance. Patients having a history of atrial fibrillation are given anticoagulants to help maintain sinus rhythm and decrease the likelihood of blood clots caused for multiple reasons including atrial fibrillation.

Antiplatelet Agents

Antiplatelet agents are medications that inhibit activation or aggregation of platelets in the bloodstream. All antiplatelet agents are prescribed except for ASA. There are many types of antiplatelet agents (Table 7.20).

Table 7.20	Antiplatelet Agents
Drug (Generic) Name	**Brand (Trade) Name**
Adenosine Reuptake Inhibitor	
Dipyridamole	Persantine, (+ASA) Aggrenox
Adenosine Diphosphate-Ribose (ADP-R) Inhibitor	
Clopidogrel	Plavix
Prasugrel	Effient
Ticagrelor	Brilinta
Ticlopidine	Ticlid
Cyclooxygenase (COX-I) Inhibitor	
Aspirin	None, (+omeprazole) Yosprala, (+Pravastatin) Pravigard Pac
Phosphodiesterase (PDE) Inhibitor	
Cilostazol	Pletal
Others	
Pentoxifylline	Trental
Vorapaxar	Zontivity

Therapeutic Use

Antiplatelet agents are used in primary and secondary prevention for those at risk for and to prevent thromboembolic events (69). These events could cause an MI, CVA, transient ischemic attack (TIA), PE, or blood clot in the extremities. Primary prevention reduces the chance of a first thromboembolic event, whereas secondary prevention reduces the risk that a patient who has suffered a MI, ischemic CVA, TIA, or unstable angina will have a subsequent thromboembolic event. Those who have had percutaneous transluminal coronary angioplasty with or without a stent or a coronary bypass procedure are usually prescribed antiplatelet therapy to reduce the reocclusion or restenosis of the treated vessels. Combination therapy with two antiplatelet agents (*e.g.*, ASA and clopidogrel) is common for their superior effects when combined versus alone (72). Newer medications such as prasugrel act more quickly and predictably than others in the same class while having better outcomes (69).

Mechanism of Action

Antiplatelet agents reduce platelet activation or aggregation after injury to a blood vessel wall (69). Insult to the wall allows platelets to encounter tissue factors that trigger their activation, causing them to aggregate at the site of the injury and start to form a blood clot. When this happens inside a blood vessel, there is a risk that the clot will break off and travel to a smaller area of the vessel or a smaller branch. The clot can then become lodged in the artery, stopping blood flow past that point and "starving" the area downstream of oxygen and nutrients. The resulting event can be a CVA, TIA, MI, PE, or blood clot in the extremities.

Side Effects

Antiplatelet medications produce side effects similar to anticoagulants. Bleeding occurs with higher doses. Other side effects include diarrhea, nausea, and vomiting, especially with clopidogrel and ticlopidine. Ticlopidine is no longer commonly prescribed because of its serious side effects and blood dyscrasias (*e.g.*, hemophilia, leukemia), high rates of thrombotic thrombocytopenic purpura (TTP), and severe neutropenia. These conditions are serious blood disorders. Clopidogrel is more commonly prescribed because of its lower rate of side effects. Newer medications like ticagrelor have side effects similar to clopidogrel (69).

Related Drug Interactions

The antiplatelet effect of ASA peaks at 75 mg. When used at doses greater than 75 mg, it also acts as an NSAID. In contrast, other NSAIDs can block the antithrombotic actions of ASA (69). Antiretroviral agents can impact the effectiveness of antiplatelets. Clopidogrel and prasugrel have a low interaction rate with antiretroviral agents. Side interactions are also unlikely between newer antiplatelets and antiretroviral agents (71).

Effects on HR, BP, ECG, and Exercise

Antiplatelets have no known effect on HR, BP, ECG, or exercise tolerance. Recent data suggests vorapaxar doesn't benefit walking distance in intermittent claudication patients (73) Platelet aggregation could cause unstable angina or a subsequent MI negatively affecting exercise ability and tolerance.

PULMONARY DRUGS

This section begins with medications used for the treatment of two common chronic lower respiratory diseases: asthma and/or chronic obstructive pulmonary disease (COPD). Subsequently, medications used to relieve symptoms of allergies and respiratory infections, such as colds and influenza, will be discussed.

Medications Used for Asthma and/ or Chronic Obstructive Pulmonary Disease

Chronic lower respiratory diseases, including asthma and COPD, are the sixth leading cause of death in the U.S. (74). Medications important in the treatment of these diseases include inhaled corticosteroids, bronchodilators, leukotriene modifiers, and mast cell stabilizers.

Inhaled Corticosteroids

Globally, asthma is one of the most common chronic diseases effecting both adults and children. Patients with asthma have an underlying chronic inflammation of the airways characterized by activated mast cells, eosinophils, and T-helper 2 lymphocytes (75). This results in an increased responsiveness of the airways to potential triggers such as exercise, allergens, and air pollutants. This chronic inflammation underlies the typical symptoms of asthma, which include intermittent wheezing, coughing, dyspnea (difficulty breathing), and chest tightness. With corticosteroids the most effective treatment for these symptoms, inhaled corticosteroids have become first-line treatment for children and adults with persistent symptoms (Table 7.21).

Table 7.21	Inhaled Corticosteroids
Drug (Generic) Name	Trade (Brand) Name
Beclomethasone	Beclovent, Qvar, Vanceril
Budesonide	Pulmicort
Ciclesonide	Alvesco
Flunisolide	AeroBid
Fluticasone	Flovent
Mometasone	Asmanex
Triamcinolone	Azmacort

Therapeutic Use

Inhaled corticosteroids are considered the most effective long-term medication for control and management of asthma with regular use. In addition, they can be used for nasal polyps and rhinitis.

Mechanism of Action

Inflammation in asthma is characterized by the increased expression of multiple inflammatory genes, including those encoding for cytokines, chemokines, adhesion molecules, and inflammatory enzymes and receptors (75). Inhaled corticosteroids suppress airway inflammation by activating anti-inflammatory genes, switching off inflammatory gene expression, and inhibiting inflammatory cells. In addition, they enhance β_2-adrenergic signaling by increasing β_2-receptor expression and function, thereby controlling asthmatic symptoms in most patients.

Side Effects

Inhaled corticosteroids are not anabolic steroids; thus, they do not promote muscular hypertrophy, nor have they been shown to cause weak bones, suppress growth, or produce weight gain, all of which are side effects of anabolic steroids. In fact, few side effects are evident with inhaled corticosteroids, especially at lower doses. At high doses with chronic use, corticosteroids are known to promote HTN, hyperlipidemia, and glucose intolerance, established risk factors for CVD. Because the effect of corticosteroids on the cardiovascular system is dose-related, the low doses have few, if any, cardiovascular side effects (76).

Related Drug Interactions

When taken simultaneously, corticosteroids can sometimes make anticoagulants less effective. Also, corticosteroids have been known to decrease the effectiveness of oral antihyperglycemic medications used to treat DM. If both medications are necessary, blood glucose levels should be checked more regularly, and medication dosage may need to be adjusted.

Effects on HR, BP, ECG, and Exercise

In patients with exercise-induced asthma (EIA), daily use of an inhaled corticosteroid is not recommended as monotherapy; however, it may be used in combination with a short-acting β-agonist to help better manage symptoms (77).

Bronchodilators: An Overview

Bronchodilators are used to treat chronic conditions in which the airways become constricted and inflamed, such as asthma and COPD. Generally, symptoms are relieved by relaxing the muscles in the walls of the bronchi, thereby allowing the bronchi to widen and airflow to increase. Short-acting bronchodilators are used for acute relief from sudden, unexpected attacks of breathlessness, whereas long-acting bronchodilators are used regularly, to help control breathlessness in chronic asthma and COPD (78).

Bronchodilators may be used in combination with corticosteroids. By helping to keep the airways open, they increase the effectiveness of corticosteroids in reducing inflammation. Long-acting bronchodilators should never be taken without corticosteroids. Corticosteroids and bronchodilators may be taken separately in individual inhalers or taken in a combination preparation (Figure 7.3). Three types of popular bronchodilators currently used for the treatment of chronic asthma and COPD are muscarinic receptor antagonists, β$_2$-agonists, and xanthine derivatives (Table 7.22).

Bronchodilators: Muscarinic Receptor Antagonists

Muscarinic receptor antagonists were formally called anticholinergics (ACs). However, because they only block the muscarinic effects of acetylcholine, and not the nicotinic effects, the term anticholinergic is not entirely accurate (79). Currently, there are two long-acting muscarinic antagonists (LAMAs), glycopyrronium and tiotropium, and one short-acting muscarinic antagonist (SAMA), ipratropium.

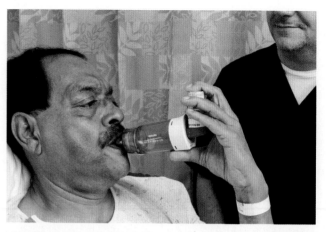

FIGURE 7.3 A small-volume nebulizer is commonly used to administer a medication combining a corticosteroid and bronchodilator. (From Rosdahl C. *Rosdahl's Textbook of Basic Nursing.* 12th ed. Philadelphia (PA): Wolters Kluwer; 2022.)

Therapeutic Use

Muscarinic receptor antagonists are primarily used for the management of bronchospasm related to COPD and are also indicated to reduce exacerbations in patients with COPD. They prevent wheezing, dyspnea, and difficult breathing caused by chronic bronchitis, emphysema, asthma, and other lung diseases.

Mechanism of Action

Muscarinic receptor antagonists block parasympathetic nerve reflexes that cause airway constriction. This dilation effect allows air passages to remain open. The LAMAs produce bronchodilation with a duration of action of over 24 hours; thus, they can be used once daily. Additionally, muscarinic receptor antagonists bind to muscarinic receptors and inhibit acetylcholine-mediated bronchospasm.

Side Effects

There are no serious side reactions associated with use of LAMAs and SAMAs.

Related Drug Interactions

No relevant drug interactions are evident with the use of muscarinic receptor antagonists.

Effects on HR, BP, ECG, and Exercise

Commonly, as with most atropinic agents, sinus tachycardia occurs with use. Cases of angina, supraventricular

Table 7.22	Bronchodilators	
Drug (Generic) Name	**Trade (Brand) Name**	**Combination Medications**
Muscarinic Receptor Antagonists		
Ipratropium (SAMA)	Atrovent	(+albuterol) Combivent
Glycopyrronium (LAMA)	Robinul	
Tiotropium (LAMA)	Spiriva	
β_2-Receptor Agonists		
Albuterol (SABA)	ProAir, Proventil, Ventolin	
Terbutaline (SABA)	Brethine, Brethaire, Bricanyl	
Levalbuterol (SABA)	Xopenex	
Metaproterenol (SABA)	Alupent, Metaprel	
Indacaterol (LABA)	Arcapta	
Salmeterol (LABA)	Serevent	(+fluticasone) Advair
Formoterol (LABA)	Foradil, Perforomist	(+budesonide) Symbicort (+mometasone) Dulera
Vilanterol (LABA)		(+fluticasone) Breo
Xanthine Derivatives		
Aminophylline	Phyllocontin, Truphylline	
Theophylline	Theo-24, Uniphyl	
Caffeine		

LABA, long-acting β_2-agonist; LAMA, long-acting muscarinic antagonist; SABA, short-acting β_2-agonist; SAMA, short-acting muscarinic antagonist.

tachycardia, and atrial fibrillation, while rare, have also been reported with the use of muscarinic antagonists (80).

Bronchodilators: β_2-Agonists

β_2-Agonists are medications used to relax smooth muscle. Both long-acting β_2-agonists (LABAs) and short-acting β_2-agonists (SABAs) are available.

Therapeutic Use

β_2-Agonists are used to relieve acute symptoms of asthma and manage all pulmonary disorders classified as COPD. SABAs help relieve acute symptoms of an asthmatic attack and can treat stable COPD in a patient with intermittent symptoms. LABAs are effective for treating COPD in a patient with persistent symptoms, and simultaneously to prevent exacerbations (81).

Mechanism of Action

β_2-Agonists are similar to muscarinic antagonists; however, instead of acting on the acetylcholine receptor pathway, they act on the β_2-adrenergic receptor pathway and possess sympathomimetic properties. Specifically, β_2-agonists work by stimulating β_2-receptors in the smooth muscles that line the bronchi, initiating relaxation and subsequent dilatation, and allowing greater airflow and easier breathing.

Side Effects

Common side effects include headache, anxiety, nausea, muscle tremors, hypokalemia, and nervousness; however, these are not pronounced when taken in low doses. One area of concern is for patients with COPD who also have DM; that is, β_2-receptor activation may lead to hepatic glycogenolysis and pancreatic release of glucagon, which increases plasma glucose concentrations (82).

Related Drug Interactions

Concurrent administration of β-adrenergic receptor antagonists (nonselective β-blockers) and $β_2$-agonists is contraindicated because the drugs inhibit each other's effect. β-Blockers not only block the therapeutic effects of β-agonists but may cause severe bronchospasm in patients with COPD (75, 83). Therefore, patients with COPD should not normally be treated with nonselective β-blockers.

Patients being treated concomitantly with a monoamine oxidase inhibitor (MAOI, a type of antidepressant), a tricyclic antidepressant, or a type 1A or 1C antiarrhythmic (drugs known to prolong the QTc interval on the ECG) should be closely monitored, because the effect of adrenergic agonists on the cardiovascular system may be potentiated by these agents (84). Drugs that are known to prolong the QTc interval confer an increased risk of ventricular arrhythmias, including torsades de pointes. Simultaneous treatment with xanthine derivatives, steroids, or diuretics may potentiate any hypokalemic effect of $β_2$-agonists.

Effects on HR, BP, ECG, and Exercise

Sinus tachycardia and palpitations may become apparent, especially in patients with existing CVD and irregular heart rhythms. Anginal symptoms may also become evident because of increased myocardial oxygen demand (82). $β_2$-Agonists taken prior to exercise provide significant protection against EIA in most patients. However, when taken daily, the duration of the protective effect of LABAs diminishes. Consequently, if an EIA attack occurs, recovery time is slower in response to their $β_2$-agonist than usual, and multiple doses may be required to achieve resting comfort (85). If a patient taking a $β_2$-agonist daily experiences problems with exercise, then the CEP should refer the patient back to their physician for potential modification of the treatment regimen to achieve better control of EIA.

Bronchodilators: Xanthine Derivatives (Methylxanthines)

The xanthine derivatives, also known as methylxanthines, are weak bronchodilators administered orally or by inhalation.

Therapeutic Use

Methylxanthines relax bronchial smooth muscle and help dilate constricted airways. Generally, a weak bronchodilator by themselves, methylxanthines are usually used in combination with other respiratory medications to treat asthma and COPD. In addition to being a weak bronchodilator, methylxanthines act as a respiratory stimulant, improving diaphragmatic contractility, and possess anti-inflammatory properties (86).

Mechanism of Action

The exact mechanism of action is not well understood, but it appears that methylxanthines inhibit the enzyme phosphodiesterase, which degrades cyclic adenosine monophosphate (AMP). Therefore, the concentration of cyclic AMP, a key component in the dilation of bronchial smooth muscle, is increased (87).

Side Effects

Common side effects of methylxanthines include heartburn, tremors, nausea, headache, nervousness, and tachycardia. Heartburn is a side effect of particular concern because, in patients with asthma, heartburn can actually increase dyspnea.

Related Drug Interactions

β-Blockers may decrease the efficacy of methylxanthines.

Effects on HR, BP, ECG, and Exercise

Methylxanthines have both ionotropic and chronotropic cardiac effects. The effects of caffeine on endurance exercise performance are well documented.

Leukotriene Modifiers

The leukotriene modifiers are divided into two classes (Table 7.23). Leukotriene-receptor antagonists (LTRAs) prevent leukotriene binding. Leukotriene-receptor inhibitors (LTRI) focus on synthesis inhibition.

Table 7.23	Leukotriene Modifiers
Drug (Generic) Name	Trade (Brand) Name
Montelukast (LTRA)	Singulair
Zafirlukast (LTRA)	Accolate
Zileuton (LTRI)	Zyflo

LTRA, leukotriene-receptor antagonist; LTRI, leukotriene-receptor inhibitor.

Therapeutic Use

Leukotriene modifiers are used to manage asthma (both treatment and prevention of acute asthmatic attacks), EIA, and allergic rhinitis. They are recommended as an alternative therapy to inhaled corticosteroids or in combination depending on the severity of symptoms. If a patient has been taking inhaled corticosteroids and their asthma still isn't well controlled, their physician may prescribe leukotriene modifiers concomitantly instead of increasing the dosage of the corticosteroid (88).

Mechanism of Action

In patients who are asthmatic, leukotriene-mediated effects include airway edema, smooth muscle contraction, and altered cellular activity associated with the inflammatory process (89). Leukotriene modifiers act by binding to cysteinyl leukotriene (CysLT) receptors and blocking their activation and the subsequent inflammatory cascade that causes the symptoms commonly associated with asthma and allergic rhinitis. More specifically, LTRAs prevent leukotrienes from binding to its receptors, whereas LTRIs prevent synthesis of leukotrienes by blocking the enzyme, 5-lipoxygenase, which is necessary for the formation of leukotrienes (90).

Side Effects

Leukotriene modifiers are well tolerated with few side effects. Headache, nausea, abdominal pain, cough, and rash are the most commonly reported. Hepatotoxicity linked to zafirlukast is rare, but occasionally severe cases have been reported (89).

Related Drug Interactions

Individuals on warfarin therapy should have close monitoring of their prothrombin time because leukotriene modifiers may significantly affect warfarin levels, resulting in PPTs (91).

Effects on HR, BP, ECG, and Exercise

Leukotriene modifiers have no effect on HR, BP, or ECG. Those leukotriene modifiers (*e.g.*, zafirlukast, montelukast, zileuton) prescribed for the prevention of asthma or EIA can increase one's exercise ability before an asthma attack occurs because there is less smooth muscle contraction of the bronchioles.

Mast Cell Stabilizers

Mast cell stabilizers are medications that stabilize the membrane of mast cells and thereby reduce the release of inflammatory mediators such as histamine (Table 7.24).

Therapeutic Use

Mast cell stabilizers are indicated in the management of patients with bronchial asthma and are used prophylactically to help prevent asthmatic attacks. In addition, they are used to prevent bronchospasm caused by exercise, exposure to cold, dry air, or environmental allergens. They are not used in emergency situations to alleviate exacerbated symptoms. At this time, cromolyn is the only available drug in the classification. Therefore, the rest of this review will refer to the drug cromolyn.

Mechanism of Action

Cromolyn acts by blocking calcium ions from entering mast cells, thereby inhibiting the release of inflammatory mediators. In response, both the immediate and non-immediate bronchoconstrictive reactions to inhaled antigens are inhibited.

Side Effects

The most frequently reported side reactions attributed to cromolyn are dry throat, cough, and nausea.

Related Drug Interactions

Using a rapid-acting inhaled insulin (Afrezza) concurrently with cromolyn may affect the absorption of insulin into the bloodstream. This may alter the effectiveness of the insulin.

Effects on HR, BP, ECG, and Exercise

Mast cell stabilizers have no effect on HR, BP, or ECG. They may increase one's ability to exercise because of the reduction in inflammation and potential asthma attack.

Table 7.24	Mast Cell Stabilizers
Drug (Generic) Name	**Trade (Brand) Name**
Cromolyn	Intal
Nedocromil	Tilade

Medications Used for Allergies and Respiratory Infections

Antihistamines

The inflammatory mediator histamine is responsible for many uncomfortable symptoms associated with inflammation, including a runny nose, watery eyes, and skin rash. Antihistamines counter these effects. They are sold both over-the-counter (OTC) and by prescription (Table 7.25).

Therapeutic Use

Antihistamines are commonly prescribed for allergy and cold and flu-like symptoms. Additionally, they treat allergic reactions, anaphylaxis (adjunctive), insomnia, motion sickness, skin pruritus (itching), rhinitis, sedation, and urticaria (hives). Whereas first-generation antihistamines are nonspecific for symptom management, second-generation antihistamines are specific for treating allergic reactions (*e.g.*, allergic rhinitis) and urticaria (hives).

Mechanism of Action

All antihistamines act not by preventing histamine release, but by blocking binding of circulating histamine to its receptor site. Antihistamines are reversible, competitive antagonists at histaminic (H1) receptors. Their action results in inhibition of respiratory, vascular, and GI smooth muscle constriction, a decrease in histamine-activated secretions from salivary and lacrimal glands, and anti-inflammatory effects. Antihistamines also decrease capillary permeability, which reduces the wheal and flare response to an allergen, as well as itching (92). Second-generation antihistamines are selective for peripheral H1 receptors. Consequently, they produce less sedation and AC effects than the nonselective first-generation antihistamines.

Side Effects

Common side effects of antihistamine use include dry mouth, drowsiness, dizziness, nausea, and vomiting. Rare but serious side effects include urinary retention, blurred vision, tinnitus, fast/irregular heartbeat, and confusion. Some antihistamines may include pseudoephedrine as part of its formulation and therefore may exhibit typical sympathomimetic effects.

Related Drug Interactions

Although several drugs have mild to moderate interactions with antihistamines, there are no major interactions seen in medications through the scope of practice of the CEP. Because of synergistic effects, patients simultaneously taking sleeping pills, sedatives, or muscle relaxants may experience considerable drowsiness.

Table 7.25	Antihistamines (Over the Counter and Prescription)	
	Drug (Generic) Name	Trade (Brand) Name
First-generation antihistamines	Brompheniramine	Dimetapp
	Carbinoxamine (prescription only)	Arbinoxa, Palgic
	Chlorpheniramine	Chlor-Trimeton
	Clemastine	Dayhist, Tavist
	Cyproheptadine	Periactin
	Diphenhydramine	Benadryl, Nytol
	Doxylamine	Vicks NyQuil, Alka-Seltzer Plus
Second-generation antihistamines	Acrivastine	Semprex-D
	Cetirizine	Zyrtec, Zyrtec-D
	Loratadine	Claritin, Claritin-D, Alavert, Alavert-D
	Fexofenadine	Allegra, Allegra-
	Levocetirizine (prescription only)	Xyzal
	Desloratadine (prescription only)	Clarinex, Clarinex-D

Effects on HR, BP, ECG, and Exercise

Second-generation antihistamines with pseudoephedrine may increase the HR and BP at rest and during exercise. Hypertensive individuals should avoid taking any product with pseudoephedrine.

Sympathomimetic/Adrenergic Agonists (Decongestants)

Sympathomimetic/adrenergic agonists are commonly known as decongestants. There are two preparations: phenylephrine and pseudoephedrine (Table 7.26).

Therapeutic Use

Sympathomimetic/adrenergic agonists are used to treat allergic rhinitis, nasal/sinus congestion, and congestion within the eustachian tubes. Preparations with phenylephrine are available OTC, whereas those with pseudoephedrine are now housed behind the counter where the consumer may have to sign for it or present a prescription depending upon the residing state.

Mechanism of Action

Sympathomimetic/adrenergic agonists act on α-adrenergic receptors in the mucosa of the respiratory tract, producing vasoconstriction, which in turn reduces swollen nasal membranes and nasal congestion. Also, sinus drainage may be enhanced.

Side Effects

Possible side effects include signs and symptoms of an allergic reaction: itching or hives, swelling in the face or hands, swelling or tingling in the mouth or throat, chest tightness, and dyspnea.

Related Drug Interactions

If an MAOI has been used within the past 2 weeks, phenylephrine and pseudoephedrine should not be used as they can intensify the sympathomimetic drug action.

Effects on HR, BP, ECG, and Exercise

Pseudoephedrine may increase the HR and BP at rest and during exercise. Hypertensive individuals should avoid taking any product with pseudoephedrine.

Guaifenesin (Expectorant)

Guaifenesin is a medication derived from guaiacum, a flowering plant native to North America. An expectorant, it helps the body clear mucus from the airways. It is available OTC.

Therapeutic Use

Guaifenesin is widely used to alleviate symptoms of excessive mucus accumulation in the chest and respiratory tract (Table 7.27).

Mechanism of Action

Guaifenesin helps loosen phlegm (mucus), thins bronchial secretions, and makes coughs more productive, thereby helping patients to clear their bronchial passageways of bothersome mucus. It is effective in patients with acute infections as well as in patients with stable chronic bronchitis (92). The mechanism by which its expectorant actions occur is poorly understood.

Side Effects

Guaifenesin is well tolerated and has a wide margin of safety.

Related Drug Interactions

No serious drug interactions within the scope of practice of the CEP have been reported.

Effects on HR, BP, ECG, and Exercise

There are no sympathomimetic effects exhibited by guaifenesin on cardiovascular measures or exercise.

Antitussives

Antitussives are medications that suppress or relieve coughs (*tussis* is Latin for cough).

Table 7.26	Sympathomimetic/Adrenergic Agonists
Drug (Generic) Name	Trade (Brand) Name
Phenylephrine	Sudafed PE
Pseudoephedrine	Sudafed; many combinations

Table 7.27	Expectorant
Drug (Generic) Name	Trade (Brand) Name
Guaifenesin	Robitussin, Mucinex, DayQuil

Therapeutic Use

Antitussives are indicated for the temporary symptomatic relief of a nonproductive cough because of minor throat and bronchial irritation, such as occurs with colds or inhaled irritants (93). They are available OTC and by prescription (Table 7.28). Codeine — a prescription antitussive — also possesses analgesic properties to help relieve pain.

Mechanism of Action

Antitussives suppress the cough reflex by a direct action on the cough center in the medulla of the brain (94).

Side Effects

Many antitussives, including codeine, are derived from opioids; therefore, they may cause drowsiness and constipation, and, additionally, may possess addictive properties.

Related Drug Interactions

In combination with an MAOI, dextromethorphan can cause severe serotogenic syndrome, HTN, and cardiac arrhythmias. This combination should be avoided if possible. There are no other serious drug interactions within the scope of practice of the CEP.

Effects on HR, BP, ECG, and Exercise

Antitussives may increase HR and BP.

DRUGS FOR METABOLIC DISORDERS

This section will review medications used in the treatment of DM, obesity, and renal disease.

Antidiabetic Medications

As discussed extensively in Chapter 10, DM is classified by etiology as either Type 1 (T1DM) or Type 2 (T2DM).

Table 7.28	Antitussives
Drug (Generic) Name	Trade (Brand) Name
Benzonatate	Tessalon
Codeine	Codeine
Dextromethorphan	Robitussin
Hydrocodone	

Briefly, when the pancreas has no viable β cells and can no longer produce insulin endogenously, T1DM is indicated. T2DM is diagnosed when insulin resistance is established and when insulin secretion is compromised. Treating DM requires not only managing blood glucose and hemoglobin A1C (HbA1C) levels, but alleviating symptoms of hyperglycemia (polyuria, polydipsia, polyphagia, fatigue), treating the associated comorbidities (dyslipidemia, HTN, obesity, and CVD), and preventing or reducing the microvascular and macrovascular complications associated with chronically mismanaged DM. This involves lifestyle modification (education, exercise, and nutrition) as well as pharmacological interventions.

The type of DM and level of glucose management (determined by HbA1C level) dictates the pharmacological treatment received. Individuals with T1DM are insulin-dependent (IDDM) and require administration of exogenous insulin to prevent ketoacidosis and sustain life. For individuals with T2DM, the level of glucose management determines the type of pharmacological treatment employed. Patients with T2DM under good control (HbA1C < 7%) are considered noninsulin dependent (NIDDM) and may require only diet and exercise management with perhaps one oral hypoglycemic agent (OHG). Patients with T2DM with fair control (HbA1C 7%–8%) or poor control (HbA1C > 8%) are typically either on mono or combination therapy with OHGs or become dependent on exogenous insulin. This section will discuss insulin preparations for IDDM as well as injectable and OHGs essential in the glycemic control of T2DM. An exhaustive list of drug interactions will not be provided. Only a list of common medications a CEP might notice in a cardiac or clinical environment will be presented.

Sulfonylureas

Sulfonylureas were one of the first oral medications developed to treat hyperglycemia in T2DM. There are two generations of sulfonylureas. Besides chemical structure, their primary differences are how they are eliminated from the body and their potency. First-generation sulfonylureas (Table 7.29) have been essentially replaced by the second-generation preparations (Table 7.30) because they are more potent and administered in lower doses, mainly on a once-a-day basis (95).

Therapeutic Use

Besides working acutely to lower elevated blood glucose levels, sulfonylureas have a significant effect on HbA1C levels, lowering them approximately 1.0%–2.0% (95).

Table 7.29	First-Generation Sulfonylureas
Drug (Generic) Name	Trade (Brand) Name
Chlorpropamide	Diabinese
Tolazamide	Tolinase
Tolbutamide	Orlinase

Table 7.30	Second-Generation Sulfonylureas	
Drug (Generic) Name	Trade (Brand) Name	Combination
Glimepiride	Amaryl	(+pioglitazone) Duetact (+rosiglitazone) Avandaryl
Glipizide	Glucotrol	(+metformin) Metaglip
Glyburide	DiaBeta, Glynase, Micronase	(+metformin) Glucovance

Sherifali et al. (96) and Hirst et al. (97) performed meta-analyses and reported on average a 1.5% and a 1.6% reduction in HbA1C levels, respectively, with sulfonylurea monotherapy. Consequently, the sulfonylureas remain a fundamental treatment of T2DM, especially when used in combination with metformin.

Mechanism of Action

Sulfonylureas are considered insulin secretagogues; in other words, they stimulate the pancreas to release insulin. Therefore, they only work in patients with T2DM who have viable β cells. Sulfonylureas bind to a specific site on the β cell, inhibiting the potassium adenosine triphosphate (ATP) channel complex, thereby allowing depolarization of the cell membrane and the subsequent reactions that produce insulin secretion (94). Conversely, they do not function to reduce insulin resistance. Unfortunately, the effects of sulfonylureas on insulin-producing β cells tend to diminish within approximately 2 years, resulting in a gradually less effective glucose reduction (95).

Side Effects

Although sulfonylureas appear to have no undesirable effects on cardiovascular function or ECG changes, there are two noteworthy side effects a CEP needs to acknowledge. Foremost, as a result of improved insulin secretion and its glucose-lowering effect, hypoglycemic episodes that may lead to syncope are a distinct possibility, especially when the patient is not eating properly. In addition, exercising during the medication's period of peak activity (within ~2–4 h of administration) may also lead to severe hypoglycemic events. Therefore, the patient should refrain from vigorous exercise 2–4 hours after taking a sulfonylurea. The second side effect is weight gain. Sulfonylureas may lead to increased body weight by limiting the amount of glucose excreted in the urine, thereby promoting reabsorption of glucose and storage as fat. This could potentially lead to a 1–4 kg (2–9 lb) gain in body weight. Ideally, with proper exercise and nutritional intake, weight gain may be counteracted. However, most individuals first diagnosed with DM do not embrace the necessary lifestyle modifications.

Related Drug Interactions

Because DM is a major risk factor for CAD, patients with DM may be on other medications, which could either enhance or interfere with the efficacy of their antidiabetic agent. The hypoglycemic effect of sulfonylureas may be heightened by sulfonamides, clofibrate, salicylates, alcohol, and anticoagulants. Conversely, the glucose-lowering effect may be weakened by β-blockers and CCBs (91). Ironically, β-blockers may also mask the symptoms of hypoglycemia; specifically, they may blunt the effects of epinephrine so patients may not experience the typical warning signs.

Meglitinides

Meglitinides are OHGs that act to help promote insulin release.

Therapeutic Use

Meglitinides are used to treat patients with T2DM whose blood glucose levels are not maintained in an optimal range, even though they are practicing prescribed lifestyle modifications, including exercising and following a healthy eating regimen (Table 7.31). Unlike sulfonylureas, which work most of the day, meglitinides work quickly; therefore, they should be taken just prior to the first bite of food. Because of the short half-life, they may be taken prior to each meal. Another advantage of their short half-life — and the primary indication for their use — is to prevent postprandial elevations of blood glucose (95). Increasing evidence suggests that postprandial excursions (glucose fluctuations) are a contributing factor to elevated

Table 7.31	Meglitinides	
Drug (Generic) Name	Trade (Brand) Name	Combination
Nateglinide	Starlix	
Repaglinide	Prandin	Prandimet (+metformin)

Table 7.32	Biguanides	
Drug (Generic) Name	Trade (Brand) Name	Combination
Metformin	Glucophage, Fortamet, Glumetza	Metaglip (+glipizide) Glucovance (+glyburide)

HbA1C levels in the development of the microvascular and macrovascular complications of T2DM (98). In addition to their postprandial effects, meglitinides lower HbA1C levels between 0.5% and 1.0% (99). A recent meta-analysis reported an average range of 0.5%–0.75% reduction in HbA1C levels (96).

Mechanism of Action

Like the sulfonylureas, meglitinides are considered insulin secretagogues. Insulin secretion is enhanced by blocking ATP-sensitive K^+ channels in pancreatic β cells, allowing the cascade of reactions producing insulin (95). Also like the sulfonylureas, the longer the medication is used, the greater the chance of secondary failure occurring.

Side Effects

As with sulfonylureas, the primary side effect of meglitinides is hypoglycemia. Considering the fact that meglitinides promote insulin release, this would make sense. However, meglitinides appear to trigger hypoglycemic events less commonly than sulfonylureas. This may be because of meglitinides' very short half-life and the fact that they are taken with food. Thus, meglitinides are advantageous for individuals with unpredictable schedules who cannot maintain consistent mealtimes. Repaglinide is more likely to cause hypoglycemia than nateglinide (95). Also, as in sulfonylureas, weight gain is a possibility, but is not as substantial.

Related Drug Interactions

Drugs that interact with sulfonylureas may also interact with meglitinides and potentiate the hypoglycemic response. Specifically, β-blockers, anticoagulants, NSAIDs, salicylates, and sulfonamides all promote enhanced glucose utilization (95).

Biguanides

A biguanide is an oral diabetes medication used to T2DM and produces its glucose-lowering effect by affecting the production of glucose that comes from digestion. Currently, metformin is the only available drug in the classification (Table 7.32). Therefore, the rest of this review will refer to the drug metformin.

Therapeutic Use

Metformin is considered a first-line treatment for T2DM and is the most widely prescribed antidiabetic medication. Usually taken twice a day, it is highly effective at lowering glucose levels as compared to other oral antidiabetes medications. Metformin is used as monotherapy as well as in combination with other oral agents for a synergistic effect. Metformin may also be used in combination with insulin in T2DM. It has also proved effective in delaying the progression of individuals with impaired glucose tolerance (IGT), also called prediabetes, to established T2DM (100). It is not effective in treating T1DM.

Like sulfonylureas, metformin has been shown to effectively lower HbA1C levels. Evidence suggests HbA1C levels are reduced by 1%–2% (101). Moreover, metformin may actually be associated with a reduction in cardiovascular outcomes (102, 103).

Mechanism of Action

Metformin primarily works by decreasing the rate of hepatic glucose output (HGO), resulting in lower blood glucose levels. Secondary actions include improving insulin sensitivity at the target tissue and increasing the amount of glucose stored in skeletal muscle. The hepatic effect is by far a more dominant role. Cellularly, AMP-dependent protein kinase activity is increased by metformin. The increase in AMP-protein kinase activity results in the stimulation of glucose uptake in muscle, FA oxidation in muscle and liver, lipogenesis, and the inhibition of hepatic glucose production (95).

Side Effects

GI issues such as nausea, vomiting, and diarrhea are the primary side effects triggered by metformin. However, with continued usage, these effects diminish over time. Titrating from a low dose to the prescribed dose may also diminish their severity and prevalence. Metformin therapy is contraindicated in patients with renal dysfunction, hypoxemic conditions (*e.g.*, severe anemia, MI, asphyxia, shock), dehydration (*e.g.*, severe diarrhea or vomiting), or sepsis. Patients with these conditions may be at increased risk for the development of lactic acidosis (LA), which is a rare but serious metabolic complication associated with elevated metformin accumulation in plasma (95). Although hypoglycemia is a common side effect in other oral agents, metformin does not cause hypoglycemic reactions. In addition, although weight gain occurs with other OHGs, metformin may actually lead to a slight reduction in body weight.

Related Drug Interactions

Two common medications produce a moderate interaction risk with metformin. Synthroid (levothyroxine), used for hypothyroidism, may reduce the effectiveness of metformin. Lasix (furosemide), a diuretic used for HTN, may lead to LA. Patients taking metformin should refrain from excessive alcohol use as it also may lead to LA (104).

Thiazolidinediones

Thiazolidinediones (TZDs) are a class of medications used to decrease insulin resistance (Table 7.33).

Therapeutic Use

TZDs are insulin sensitizers; therefore, endogenous insulin must be present. TZDs have no impact on T1DM.

TZDs are prescribed to manage blood glucose levels. Average reductions in HbA1C have been reported to be

Table 7.33	Thiazolidinediones	
Drug (Generic) Name	Trade (Brand) Name	Combination
Pioglitazone	Actos	Actoplus Met (XR) (+metformin)
		Duetact (+glimepiride)
Rosiglitazone	Avandia	Avandamet (+metformin)
		Avandaryl (+glimepiride)

between 0.5% and 1.5% (101). TZDs are effective both as monotherapy and in combination with sulfonylureas, metformin, or exogenous insulin. In addition to their effects on insulin receptors and glucose levels, TZDs have exhibited positive benefits on lipid metabolism by reducing plasma TRIGs and slightly raising HDL levels (94). However, use of TZDs is not indicated for abnormal lipid profiles. Although TZDs have elicited benefits in T2DM, they have also shown promise in reducing ($P < 0.0001$) progression from IGT to T2DM (105).

Mechanism of Action

As mentioned above, TZDs are insulin sensitizers. Specifically, they improve the sensitivity of insulin receptors, thereby increasing insulin action on skeletal muscle, adipose tissue, and the liver. These synergistic effects successfully work on glucose metabolism to achieve optimal glucose levels in T2DM. To accomplish this function, TZDs form a ligand with the peroxisome proliferator-activated receptor-γ (PPAR-γ). Ligands for this receptor have emerged as potent insulin sensitizers (106). In addition to stimulating glucose uptake into both muscle and adipose cells, TZDs reduce HGO and improve glucose uptake (95).

Side Effects

Although the pleiotropic effects of PPAR-γ ligands improve insulin sensitivity, the significance of side effects could potentially limit TZD use. The most common side effects are edema and weight gain. The potential for mild-to-moderate peripheral edema and a 2- to 4-kg (4–9 lb) gain in body weight with TZD is recognized. Patients in combination therapy with TZDs and insulin could potentially double the occurrence of edema and amount of weight gained. The greatest concern with TZD therapy is the increased prevalence of CHF and AMI (107). The FDA went so far as requesting manufacturers of the two TZD medications to place "black box" warnings on their labels on the high risk of CHF and potential AMI (108). Because of the high potential for edema and its latent effect for CHF, TZD use is contraindicated in patients currently diagnosed with CHF. Therefore, the CEP should always make a point of weighing patients prior to exercise sessions to assess for significant weight gain. Increases of 1.8 kg (4 lb) or more between sessions should be reported to the patient's physician.

Evidence reported from long-term treatment with TZDs includes the risk of hip and wrist fractures in women (109). Obviously, this may have implications for the CEP working with individuals with osteoporosis. Because both TZDs can be taken without regard to meals, hypoglycemia is not a major concern. However, when taken in combination with other oral agents, hypoglycemia may become apparent. Unlike troglitazone (Rezulin), the first TZD removed from the market for causing liver cancer, there is no evidence linking pioglitazone or rosiglitazone to drug-induced hepatotoxicity (110).

Related Drug Interactions

There are no reported drug interactions for TZDs that are of concern for the CEP.

α-Glucosidase Inhibitors

α-Glucosidase inhibitors (AGIs) are medications that help regulate blood glucose levels in patients with T2DM.

Therapeutic Use

AGIs have clear beneficial effects on glycemic control and postprandial glucose levels (Table 7.34). Specifically, fasting plasma glucose levels are reduced by approximately 1 mmol·L^{-1} (about 18 mg·dL^{-1}), HbA1C levels can be reduced on average between 0.5% and 0.8% (84), and postprandial glucose levels can be reduced by 2.0–2.5 mmol·L^{-1} (about 36–45 mg·dL^{-1}). In addition, AGIs lower resting and postload insulin levels (110). AGIs can be used as monotherapy, as well as combination therapy with other oral agents and insulin. Besides being used to treat T2DM, AGIs have established effectiveness in averting the progression of IGT to established T2DM.

Mechanism of Action

AGIs inhibit the enzyme α-glucosidase in the small intestine. Consequently, certain carbohydrates remain undigested, total absorption of carbohydrates from the GI tract is slowed, and postprandial glucose levels are reduced. Furthermore, AGIs stimulate the release of glucagon-like peptide-1 (GLP-1). GLP-1, a gut-derived hormone that possesses insulin-like effects, may contribute to the glucose-lowering effects of AGIs.

Side Effects

The most noticeable side effect with AGI use is GI distress, specifically, abdominal bloating, diarrhea, and hyperflatulence. AGIs do not promote weight gain or have noteworthy effects on plasma lipids. With monotherapy, hypoglycemia is not an issue. However, when taken with exogenous insulin or insulin secretagogues, hypoglycemia may be evident. When treating a hypoglycemic event with AGIs present, straight glucose should be used instead of sucrose or complex carbohydrates (95).

Related Drug Interactions

There are no major drug interactions for AGIs relative to the practice of the CEP.

Amylin Analogues

Amylin is a hormone produced in the β cells of the pancreas and naturally secreted with insulin following a meal. Pramlintide is a synthetic form of amylin approved for use in patients with T1DM and T2DM (Table 7.35).

Therapeutic Use

In patients with DM, pramlintide induces an HbA1C reduction of approximately 0.5%. Moreover, patients typically experience a 1.0- to 2.5-kg loss of weight over a 3- to 6-month period, and reduced insulin requirements (95).

Mechanism of Action

Pramlintide lowers blood glucose in three ways. By binding to amylin receptors in the brainstem, it triggers satiety (the feeling of fullness) during meals, and thereby reduces the amount of food consumed. It also delays gastric emptying (the rate at which food moves from the stomach to the small intestine), which keeps blood glucose from rising too quickly. Moreover, it blunts pancreatic glucagon release, thereby reducing the amount of glucose the liver produces.

Side Effects

The most common side effect of pramlintide is potentially severe hypoglycemia. Hypoglycemia is not a

Table 7.34	α-Glucosidase Inhibitors
Drug (Generic) Name	Trade (Brand) Name
Acarbose	Precose
Miglitol	Glyset

Table 7.35	Amylin Analogues
Drug (Generic) Name	Trade (Brand) Name
Pramlintide	Symlin

major concern during monotherapy. Conversely, when taken in conjunction with insulin, especially at mealtimes, an accelerated rate of hypoglycemia may occur. Consequently, a reduction in mealtime insulin doses by 30%–50% is recommended (95). With the GI effects produced by pramlintide, nausea and vomiting may also be evident.

Related Drug Interactions

There are no relevant interactions relative to the practice of the CEP. However, it is worth noting that pramlintide can slow digestion, and it may take longer for the body to absorb any medicines taken by mouth. Therefore, patients should avoid taking any oral medicines within 1 hour before or 2 hours after taking pramlintide.

Incretin-Based Therapies: An Overview

Before studying the two incretin-based therapies discussed ahead, it is essential to understand incretin physiology. Glucose homeostasis involves an intricate interaction of pancreatic hormones and incretins, insulinotropic hormones produced in the small intestine. Incretins are released after meals and stimulate β-cell insulin production. Glucagon-like peptide-1 (GLP-1) and glucose-dependent insulinotropic polypeptide (GIP) are the two primary incretin hormones. Their insulinotropic properties were identified more than 30 years ago. Once released, they exert their insulinotropic action through highly expressed receptors on pancreatic islet β cells. Although this appears to be an endogenous T2DM defense mechanism, unfortunately, soon after release, GLP-1 and GIP are acted upon by the enzyme dipeptidyl peptidase-4 (DPP-4), which inactivates them (their plasma half-life is 1–2 min), thereby terminating their insulinotropic action (Figure 7.4).

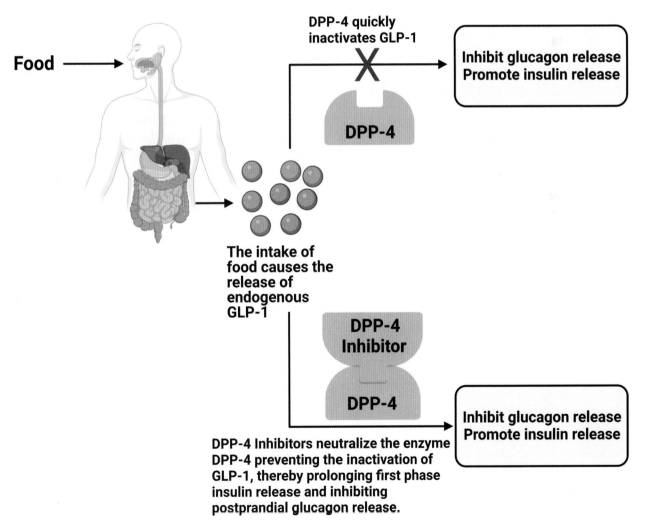

FIGURE 7.4 Interaction of GLP-1 and DPP-4. The naturally occurring "diabetes defense mechanism" of GLP-1 is short-lived because of the enzymatic action of DPP-4. DPP-4 inhibitors inactivate DPP-4 thus restoring the incretin actions of GLP-1. DPP-4, dipeptidyl peptidase-4; GLP-1, glucagon-like peptide-1. (Graphics program: Biorender.)

Given the insulinotropic actions of GLP-1 and its inactivation by DPP-4, two antidiabetic agents incorporating stimulation of insulin receptor signaling have been developed for treating T2DM. Both attempt to enhance levels of GLP-1 rather than GIP. Although the two incretins share certain qualities, GIP is not as effective for stimulating insulin release and lowering blood glucose levels in T2DM (111). Therefore, manufacturers have focused on GLP-1 for creating successful analogues to treat T2DM. The two incretin-based therapies are as follows:

■ Incretin mimetics are structurally similar to GLP-1; however, they are resistant to the actions of DPP-4. They are known as GLP-1 receptor agonists (or GLP-1 analogues).
■ Incretin enhancers act as DPP-4 inhibitors, preventing DPP-4 from inactivating GLP-1.

Incretin Mimetics: GLP-1 Receptor Agonists

Five glucagon-like peptide-1 receptor agonists (GLP-1RAs) are currently available (Table 7.36).

Therapeutic Uses

GLP-1RAs are the only hypoglycemic agent for the treatment of T2DM that is administered by injection. When originally released for use in 2005, they were approved only in combination therapy with metformin or sulfonylureas. In 2013, they received FDA approval to be used in monotherapy as a first-line treatment for T2DM.

GLP-1RAs mimic the actions of GLP-1, increasing the incretin effect and, as a result, promoting glucose-mediated insulin secretion in patients with T2DM. GLP-1RAs reduce HbA1C on average 1.1%–1.6% (112) while

Table 7.36	Glucagon-Like Peptide-1 Receptor Agonists
Drug (Generic) Name	Trade (Brand) Name
Exenatide (bid, qw)	Byetta
Liraglutide	Victoza
Albiglutide	Tanzeum
Dulaglutide	Trulicity
Semaglutide	Ozempic (injection)
	Rybelsus (oral)
	Wegovy (weight management)
Lixisenatide	Adlyxin

limiting hypoglycemia. Although previously not approved as a weight loss agent or in the treatment of obesity, GLP-1RAs have exhibited an average weight loss of 2.5–4 kg (5–9 lb (113)). Recently, the FDA-approved once-weekly semaglutide (Wegovy) for obesity management in adults with BMIs > 30 or >27 with weight-related comorbidities (114). A much lower dose is prescribed than for those taking semaglutide for DM. Researchers reported a 12.4% reduction of mean body weight versus placebo (115).

Because GLP-1 receptors are expressed on myocardial tissue, GLP-1RAs could possibly exert some cardiovascular benefits as well. Furthermore, liraglutide (116) and semaglutide (117) have been shown to reduce CVD risk in patients with established T2DM and/or high risk of CVD. The effects on CVD of the remaining GLP-1RAs in patients with established T2DM and/or high risk of CVD remain uncertain, but outcomes from ongoing clinical trials are forthcoming. Recently published results (116) from the liraglutide effect and action in diabetes: evaluation of cardiovascular outcome results (LEADER) trials indicate liraglutide significantly ($P = 0.01$) reduced the rates of major adverse cardiovascular events in patients with T2DM with elevated cardiovascular risk. In addition, there are reports of liraglutide improving systolic BP (118), modifying inflammatory markers of cardiovascular risk (119), reducing serum LDL-C (120), and improving postprandial lipemic excursions (121), an atherosclerotic risk factor. However, as of yet, GLP-1RAs are not indicated or approved for use in the treatment of CVD or its risk factors.

Mechanism of Action

All GLP-1RAs precipitate their action by activating the GLP-1 receptor, which is expressed not only by β cells, but by cells in the heart, kidney, and nervous systems. When activated, the GLP-1 receptor triggers the cyclic adenosine monophosphate–protein kinase A (cAMP-PKA) pathway, resulting in increased insulin production and release (95). Additionally, GLP-1RAs exert their action by inhibiting glucagon release, limiting HGO, delaying gastric emptying, reducing appetite, and decreasing postprandial glucose excursions.

Side Effects

No patterns of safety concerns exist for GLP-1RAs; however, common side effects include nausea and vomiting.

Related Drug Interactions

Because of delayed gastric emptying, GLP-1RAs should be used with caution when taking other medications, which also delay gastric emptying. Also, drugs that require rapid absorption through the GI system (*i.e.*, antibiotics and oral contraceptives) may not be absorbed quickly enough and may lose their effectiveness (95). When GLP-1RAs are used alone, hypoglycemic events are rare. However, when used in combination with sulfonylureas, bouts of hypoglycemia are more prevalent. There are no other relevant interactions relative to the practice of the CEP.

Incretin Enhancers: DPP-4 Inhibitors

Four DPP-4 inhibitors can be used as monotherapy or in combination with metformin, TZDs, sulfonylureas, or insulin (Table 7.37).

Therapeutic Use

Considered incretin enhancers, DPP-4 inhibitors are an OHG used to promote insulin secretion in response to a meal. In addition, they encourage a reduction in glucagon secretion and in both fasting and postprandial hyperglycemia. Specifically, they are used to support glycemic control: DPP-4 inhibitors reduce HbA1C levels by 0.6%–0.7% (122). They appear to have no effect on satiety; therefore, they are weight-neutral. There is no evidence of any cardiovascular benefits as noted with incretin mimetics.

Mechanism of Action

DPP-4 inhibitors inactivate the enzyme DPP-4, preventing the degradation of the endogenous incretin hormones (see Figure 7.4), thereby prolonging first-phase insulin release. Postprandial GLP-1 and GIP release inhibits glucagon release, which in turn increases insulin secretion, decreases gastric emptying, and decreases blood glucose levels.

Side Effects

DPP-4 inhibitors are well tolerated with no side effects reported or suggestions of cardiovascular risks (122). In contrast, some research findings (123) suggest that saxagliptin may reduce cardiovascular events (relative risk 0.44, 95% CI 0.24–0.82). Rare occurrences of hyperglycemia have been reported. Reports of hypoglycemia have only occurred when used in combination with sulfonylureas.

Related Drug Interactions

One reported drug interaction of interest to CEPs involves DPP-4 inhibitors with ACE-I. This combination is commonly prescribed for patients with T2DM to regulate HTN, preserve renal function, treat HF, or prevent MI (124). The interaction between sitagliptin and 10 mg of enalapril resulted in the possible blocking of the antihypertensive response of enalapril.

Sodium-Glucose Co-Transporter 2 Inhibitors

Sodium-glucose co-transporter 2 (SGLT2) inhibitors are the newest medications on the market for treating T2DM. Four SGLT2 inhibitors are used in monotherapy, and there are six combination drugs (Table 7.38).

Therapeutic Use

When used in conjunction with a healthy dietary plan and regular exercise, SGLT2 inhibitors improve glycemic

Table 7.37	Dipeptidylpeptidase-4 Inhibitors	
Drug (Generic) Name	Trade (Brand) Name	Combination
Alogliptin	Nesina	Kazano (+metformin)
Linagliptin	Trajenta	Oseni (+pioglitazone)
Saxagliptin	Onglyza	Kombiglyze (+metformin)
Sitagliptin Vildagliptin	Januvia Galvus	Janumet (+metformin)

Table 7.38	Sodium-Glucose Co-Transporter 2 Inhibitors	
Drug (Generic) Name	Trade (Brand) Name	Combination
Canagliflozin	Invokana	Invokamet (+metformin)
Dapagliflozin	Farxiga	Qtern (+saxagliptin)
Empagliflozin Ertugliflozin	Jardiance Steglatro	Glyxambi (+linagliptin) Synjardy (+metformin) Segluromet (+metformin) Steglujan (+sitagliptin)

control. A mean reduction in HbA1C ranging from 0.55% to 0.90% has been established (125) with no major episodes of hyperglycemia noted. In addition, weight loss and reductions in BP without increases in HR have been noted (126).

As with liraglutide, empagliflozin has shown promising effects on major side cardiovascular outcomes in patients with T2DM. Results from the landmark Empagliflozin, Cardiovascular Outcomes, and Mortality in Type 2 Diabetes study (EMPA-REG), a randomized, double-blind, placebo-controlled CV outcomes trial, indicated significantly ($P = 0.001$) lower rates of death from cardiovascular causes, which translated to a 38% relative risk reduction in cardiovascular mortality (127). Unlike the LEADER trials studying liraglutide, in which benefits were not noticed until about the 6-month mark, in the EMPA-REG trials, reduction of events occurred within the first few months. In addition to improved cardiovascular outcomes and lower mortality rates, results from a meta-analysis (128) suggested both dapagliflozin and empagliflozin reduced cardiovascular mortality ($P < 0.0001$) in patients with HFrEF. For patients with HFpEF, a multicenter randomized trial indicated significantly ($P < 0.001$) improved patient-reported symptoms, physical limitations and exercise function (128). Furthermore, empagliflozin significantly ($P < 0.001$) maintained renal function, preventing progression to renal failure in over 4,000 patients with T2DM (129, 130). Because of these momentous findings, empagliflozin could become a second-line treatment of T2DM behind metformin.

Mechanism of Action

SGLT2, a protein and a high-capacity glucose transporter, is located in the proximal tubule in the kidneys, where it facilitates glucose reabsorption from the renal filtrate. SGLT2 inhibitors prevent the reabsorption of glucose in the kidney, promote glucose excretion, and lower blood glucose levels. Additional glucose control is manifested by increasing insulin sensitivity, decreasing gluconeogenesis, and improving first-phase insulin release from the pancreas (131).

Side Effects

Vaginal yeast infections are the most common side effects in women, and urinary tract infections are common in women and uncircumcised men. In addition, an increased urge to urinate is evident. SGLT2 inhibitors are not indicated for patients with Type 1 diabetes (T1DM), frequent ketones in their blood or urine, or severe renal impairment, or in patients with ESRD receiving dialysis.

Related Drug Interactions

There are no relevant interactions relative to the practice of the CEP.

Exogenous Insulin

Insulin, a hormone produced in the pancreas, is primarily responsible for the uptake of glucose into muscle and fat cells. Additionally, it stimulates the synthesis of glycogen, lipids, and proteins. A great variety of exogenous insulin preparations are available (Table 7.39).

Therapeutic Use

Exogenous insulins are essential in the treatment of T1DM; however, they may also be used to treat T2DM when ideal glycemia cannot be maintained through lifestyle changes

Table 7.39	Insulin Preparations			
Rapid-Acting	Short-Acting	Intermediate-Acting	Intermediate- and Short-Acting Combination	Long-Acting
Lyumjev (ultra-rapid Lispro) Humalog (Lispro)	Humulin R	Humulin L	Humulin 70/30	Humulin U
Novolog (Aspart)	Novolin R	Humulin N	Novolin 70/30	Lantus (Insulin Glargine)
Apidra (Glulisine)		Novolin L	Novolog 70/30	Levemir (Insulin Detemir)
Afrezza (inhaled)		Novolin N	Humulin 50/50	
			Humalog 75/25	

and/or oral hypoglycemic therapy. All insulins used today are genetically engineered, so their structures are identical to that of human insulin. Multiple daily insulin injections or continuous subcutaneous infusions via a pump closely mimic pancreatic insulin secretion. Ultra-rapid-acting, rapid-acting, short-acting, intermediate-acting, combination, and long-acting insulins each have a specific purpose to help patients reach ideal glycemic control (132):

1. Ultra-rapid-acting: The newest approved endogenous insulin (Lyumjev) is a more rapid preparation of the rapid-acting Humalog (lispro). Researchers reported Lyumjev reached peak level at 13 min (compared to 19–27 for Humalog). In addition, the first effect on blood sugar lowering was observed at 15 minutes post injection and 2 to 3 hours post injection for its full effect. Although both Lyumjev and Humalog helped to reduce HbA1C levels, when compared to Humalog, Lyumjev manifested optimal reductions in blood sugar 1 to 2 hours postprandially (133).

2. Rapid-acting: Covers insulin needs for meals eaten at the same time as the injection. Usually is taken before a meal to prevent postprandial elevations in blood glucose. This type of insulin is usually used in combination with longer-acting insulins. Because Afrezza is inhaled, it is absorbed into the bloodstream through cells in the lungs. Therefore, it may have a faster onset of action than other types of rapid-acting insulins; and because it has a shorter duration of action, it may have less tendency to cause hypoglycemia. Additionally, it provides needle-free insulin for those who have trypanophobia (fear of needles).

3. Short-acting: Covers insulin needs for meals eaten within 30–60 minutes. Usually is taken approximately 30 minutes before a meal to cover the postprandial blood glucose elevations. This type of insulin is also generally used in combination with longer-acting insulin.

4. Intermediate-acting: Covers insulin needs for about half the day or overnight. More specifically, helps to control blood glucose elevations when rapid-acting insulins stop working. This type of insulin is often combined with rapid- or short-acting insulin and is usually taken twice a day, approximately 1 hour before a meal.

5. Combination (premixed): Generally taken two or three times a day before mealtime. Premixed insulins are more variable in peak and duration of action. Both peaks and durations of action have to be accounted for, especially when planning exercise sessions.

6. Long-acting: Usually covers insulin needs for about one full day. It lowers blood glucose levels when rapid-acting insulins stop working. This type of insulin is often combined with rapid- or short-acting insulin. It is taken once or twice a day.

Table 7.40 presents the pharmacokinetics of all types of insulin. Each type of insulin has its own unique therapeutic effect. The onset of action is how long it takes the hormone to start working at lowering blood glucose levels. The peak activity period is the point at which the dose is at the height of its therapeutic effectiveness, and the duration of action is how long the blood glucose-lowering effect of insulin lasts from injection to end. The key information from this table for the CEP is that the peak activity period should be accounted for when planning exercise sessions to prevent the incidence of hypoglycemia.

Mechanism of Action

Endogenous insulin is a hormone secreted by the pancreas. It regulates the uptake of glucose from blood into target tissues. Blood glucose is lowered by stimulating peripheral glucose uptake primarily by skeletal muscle and adipose cells, and by inhibiting gluconeogenesis in the

Table 7.40	Pharmacokinetics of Insulin		
Type of Insulin	Onset of Action	Peak Activity Period	Duration of Action
Afrezza (inhaled)	<15 min	Approx. 50 min	2–3 h
Ultra-rapid-acting	15-17 min	1-3 h	4-7 h
Rapid-acting	15–30 min	30 min–3 h	3–5 h
Short-acting	30 min–1 h	2–5 h	Up to 12 h
Intermediate-acting	1.5–4 h	4–12 h	Up to 24 h
Long-acting	1–4 h	Minimal peak	Up to 24 h

liver as well as HGO. Insulin also promotes conversion of excess glucose into fat. Exogenous insulin preparations replace insulin in patients with DM, increasing the uptake of glucose by cells and reducing the short- and long-term consequences of DM.

Side Effects

Common side effects from Afrezza may include acute bronchospasm, hypoglycemia, hypersensitivity, and decline in pulmonary function. Common side effects with traditional insulin preparations include hypoglycemia, weight gain because of the conversion of excess glucose into fat, and headaches.

Related Drug Interactions

The following drug interactions should be avoided if possible (134). β-Blockers may mask symptoms of hypoglycemia or prolong hypoglycemia and alter glucose metabolism. Repaglinide (Prandin) may increase the risk of hypoglycemia and/or MI. Rosiglitazone (Avandia) or rosiglitazone combination products increase the incidence of hypoglycemia, fluid retention, ischemia (manifested by angina symptoms), and CHF. Sulfonylureas may increase the risk of hypoglycemia; therefore, glucose levels should be monitored and adjusted accordingly.

Anti-Obesity Drugs (Anorectics)

Although several medications taken for other conditions exhibit the side effect of weight loss, currently, there are only four medications approved by the FDA for the long-term treatment of obesity (Table 7.41). There are also several drugs approved for short-term treatment; however, because obesity is a chronic condition and a high percentage of obese individuals do not adhere to lifestyle modifications (healthy eating and regular exercise), regain of the weight loss is common when patients cease using

these short-term medications. For this reason, this review focuses on the medications approved by the FDA for the long-term management of obesity.

GI Agents
Therapeutic Use

Orlistat is used for managing obesity in adults and adolescents 12 years old and older. Orlistat is indicated for patients who are obese with an initial body mass index (BMI) $\geq$30 kg·m^{-2} or $\geq$27 kg·m^{-2} in the presence of comorbidities (HTN, DM, dyslipidemia). It also helps to prevent relapse of weight gain after successful weight loss. Orlistat should be taken up to 1 hour after a meal containing fat. Subsequent digestion of fat does not enhance its effectiveness in producing weight loss (135).

Mechanism of Action

Normally after a meal containing fat, lipase enzymes hydrolyze TRIG into free FA, which are then absorbed in the small intestine. Orlistat is a GI lipase inhibitor. It promotes weight loss by inhibiting the breakdown of TRIG, which then precludes dietary fat absorption. Instead, the TRIG are excreted. The unabsorbed TRIGs provide a reduction in absorbed kilocalories, which may potentiate weight loss.

Side Effects

A common misunderstanding among patients taking orlistat is that, because fat absorption is being blocked, they can consume more fat. This is not the case. Increased dietary fat consumption causes GI side effects such as flatulence, oily stools, diarrhea, and stool incontinence. Therefore, it is important to remind patients to reduce their total fat intake while on orlistat to reduce the frequency and severity of these side effects. In addition, in patients with DM, taking orlistat may affect blood

Table 7.41	Anorectics	
Class	Drug (Generic) Name	Trade (Brand) Name
Gastrointestinal agent	Orlistat	Xenical (prescription — full dose) Alli (over the counter — half dose)
CNS stimulant	Lorcaserin	Belviq
CNS stimulant	Phentermine/topiramate	Qsymia
Opiate antagonist/antidepressant	Naltrexone/bupropion	Contrave

glucose levels (136). Therefore, their blood glucose levels should be monitored closely. It is suggested that patients check with their physician for possible adjustment of their DM medication. Because fat absorption is being inhibited, absorption of the fat-soluble vitamins may also be limited. A multivitamin should be taken at least 2 hours prior to or after orlistat to help promote optimal absorption (136).

Related Drug Interactions

For patients taking orlistat, no major interactions have been noted that are of concern for the CEP. However, patients concurrently taking an anticoagulant (*e.g.*, a patient with atrial fibrillation) may require more monitoring because of the potential for malabsorption of vitamin K (135).

CNS Stimulants

Therapeutic Use

Both lorcaserin and phentermine/topiramate are approved as an adjunct therapy to a well-balanced diet and regular physical activity for the treatment of obesity and the continued management of sustained weight loss. Both medications are indicated in patients 18 years of age and older with a BMI >30 kg·m^{-2} or >27 kg·m^{-2} in the presence of at least one comorbid condition such as HTN, T2DM, or hyperlipidemia. Lorcaserin is taken once a day in the morning, whereas phentermine/topiramate is taken twice a day.

Mechanism of Action

Although both medications are considered CNS stimulants, lorcaserin is more specifically a serotonin receptor agonist and phentermine/topiramate is a combination of a sympathomimetic amine and an anticonvulsant. Lorcaserin stimulates serotonin receptors in the CNS, particularly the hypothalamus, to reduce appetite. The mechanism of action of phentermine/topiramate has not been well established. It is speculated that the combination acts to suppress appetite and enhance satiety (137).

Side Effects

Some of the side effects of lorcaserin include hypoglycemia in patients with DM, bradycardic or irregular HR, and cognitive impairment. More common side effects are back pain, headache, and GI disturbances. For phentermine/topiramate, common side effects include depressed mood, anxiety, mild dizziness, insomnia, and constipation.

Related Drug Interactions

When lorcaserin or phentermine/topiramate are used with an MAOI (used to treat depression) in patients with HTN, the potential for a hypertensive emergency exists. BP should be monitored closely.

Opiate Antagonist/Antidepressant

Therapeutic Use

Naltrexone/bupropion is the most recent medication approved (in 2014) for use in the treatment of obesity. Like the other anorectics, naltrexone/bupropion is indicated for patients who are obese with an initial BMI ≥ 30 kg·m^{-2} or ≥ 27 kg·m^{-2} in the presence of comorbidities (HTN, DM, dyslipidemia).

Mechanism of Action

The mechanism by which the combination of naltrexone/bupropion induces weight loss is not entirely understood. Pathways that regulate food intake involve satiety and reward. It appears that naltrexone/bupropion targets both of these areas. It is speculated that bupropion could stimulate the hypothalamus to promote satiety, whereas naltrexone could block the reward feedback from eating. This combination is associated with a decline in body weight (138).

Side Effects

Common side effects include insomnia, dizziness, headache, and GI complications. The CEP should monitor the patient's BP, as elevations in BP sometimes occur. In addition, although rare, pain in the chest, arms, jaw, back, or neck mimicking angina symptoms may be exhibited (139).

Related Drug Interactions

As would be expected, individuals being treated for obesity may also be treated for HTN. Therefore, the CEP should take note when individuals are also taking amlodipine, lisinopril, or HCTZ as hypotensive responses may ensue.

ESRD Medications

Presently, there are no medications that cure or reverse ESRD. However, medications can treat the symptoms and complications, as well as prevent additional renal damage. A significant number of individuals with ESRD also experience HTN at various stages of the disease's progression. Therefore, medications that treat HTN are prescribed to patients with ESRD to help maintain their BP in an optimal range and prevent further kidney damage.

Commonly prescribed BP medications include ACE-I, ARBs, β-blockers, CCBs, diuretics, and vasodilators. All of these drug classes were discussed in the cardiovascular section of this chapter.

Furthermore, because DM is the leading cause of ESRD, a significant number of patients with ESRD will also be on one or more DM medications. In addition to managing HTN in patients with ESRD, medications are ordered to treat the symptoms and complications of ESRD. Two medications serve a dual purpose. Besides treating HTN, ACE-I and ARBs also work to control or reduce proteinuria. The mechanism by which this occurs is not fully understood.

Diuretics not only help reduce BP but also relieve fluid buildup caused by ESRD. Spironolactone, a diuretic and an aldosterone receptor agonist (ARA), is commonly used in combination with either ACE-I or ARBs. Eplerenone, a more selective ARA, can also be used. However, there may be a decrease in the GFR with either of these medications in conjunction with an ACE-I or ARB (10). A notable decrease in the GFR increases the risk of hyperkalemia; hence, ARAs are used with only stage 1 and 2 renal disease patients with sufficient GFR. The only medications for ESRD that are suggested to be prescribed concurrently are ARAs and ACE-I or ARBs. In addition, studies have shown patients with concomitant CHF realize morbidity and mortality benefits (10).

Recombinant human erythropoietin (rhEPO or EPO) is also employed to treat symptomatic anemia, a common component of ESRD. EPO stimulates the production of new red blood cells, reducing the need for blood transfusions. This therapy may be started prior to dialysis or used during dialysis treatments (140). When EPO therapy alone is not effective, iron therapy may help elevate iron levels in the body to help alleviate the anemia.

Continual dialysis treatments may eventually lead to soft, brittle bones. Therefore, vitamin D may be administered to help strengthen bones.

DRUGS FOR NEUROMUSCULAR AND AUTOIMMUNE DISORDERS

This section covers medications for Parkinson disease (PD), multiple sclerosis (MS), and SLE.

Drugs for PD

Most symptoms of PD are caused by insufficient levels of dopamine in the brain. Therefore, the pharmacological treatment of PD is designed to either temporarily replenish dopamine or mimic the action of dopamine. These dopaminergic medications generally help reduce the primary motor symptoms of PD, including resting tremor, muscle rigidity, bradykinesia, and postural imbalance.

Besides the brand name preparations of carbidopa/levodopa, dopamine agonists, MAOI, and ACs, there are multiple generic formulations. A patient taking a brand name Parkinson medication should be cautious about switching to a generic substitute. If a switch occurs, the CEP may need to monitor the patient more closely for changes in primary motor symptoms. Although the FDA requires that generic drugs show similar actions and results to the brand name drug prior to market approval, in some cases, this standard is not sufficient. A review supported by the National Parkinson's Foundation (141) reports convincing evidence that in the more advanced stages of the disease, switching from brand name to generic medications may prove ineffective.

Carbidopa/Levodopa

Carbidopa is a decarboxylase inhibitor. Levodopa is a synthetic dopamine precursor. Carbidopa/levodopa preparations are identified in Table 7.42.

Therapeutic Use

The combination of carbidopa and levodopa is manufactured as Sinemet and is the most effective drug for treating PD. Carbidopa/levodopa has a dramatic effect on the primary motor symptoms of PD. The beneficial effects are most significant in the early stages of the disease; therefore, it is imperative to start treatment as soon as PD is diagnosed.

The plasma half-life of levodopa is relatively short without carbidopa. When carbidopa and levodopa are administered together, the half-life of levodopa increases to about 1.5 hours. Therefore, CEPs working with patients

Table 7.42	Carbidopa/Levodopa Preparations
Trade (Brand) Name	Preparation
Sinemet	Oral
Parcopa	Orally disintegrating tablet
Sinemet CR	Oral (controlled-release)
Rytary	Oral (extended-release)
Duopa	Enteral suspension

with PD should encourage them to exercise approximately 1 hour after taking their medication to achieve their best possible motor responses. A limitation of the long-term use of carbidopa/levodopa may be a reduction in its efficacy; that is, a patient's motor state may fluctuate dramatically with each dose and may return to baseline more quickly than expected.

Mechanism of Action

Levodopa, the metabolic precursor of dopamine, crosses the blood–brain barrier, where dopamine cannot, and apparently is converted to dopamine in the brain. This is thought to be the mechanism whereby levodopa relieves symptoms of PD. However, if administered without carbidopa, levodopa is easily decarboxylated by the enzyme aromatic L-amino acid decarboxylase and very little of the drug reaches the brain (141). This is why levodopa is very rarely used alone in the treatment of PD. In addition, when administered together, carbidopa significantly reduces the amount of levodopa required to produce a given response; and increases both plasma levels and the plasma half-life of levodopa, while decreasing plasma and urinary dopamine levels (142).

Side Effects

Combining levodopa with carbidopa minimizes the nausea and vomiting that occurs when levodopa is taken alone. Although nausea and vomiting are still experienced by patients on carbidopa/levodopa, the severity is greatly reduced. Additional common side reactions when working with patients with PD include orthostatic hypotension, dyskinesia (sudden involuntary movements), and hallucinations and confusion, especially in elderly patients or patients with preexisting cognitive dysfunction (142).

Related Drug Interactions

For patients receiving antihypertensive drugs, symptomatic postural hypotension is evident when carbidopa/levodopa is taken concurrently. Therefore, check with the patient's physician to see if a dosage adjustment of the antihypertensive drug is possible. In addition, patients taking MAOI concomitantly with carbidopa/levodopa may experience severe orthostatic hypotension.

Dopamine Receptor Agonists

Dopamine receptor agonists (DRAs) are adjuncts to carbidopa/levodopa therapy that mimic the effects of dopamine (Table 7.43).

Table 7.43	Dopamine Agonists
Drug (Generic) Name	**Trade (Brand) Name**
Ropinirole	Requip, Requip XL
Pramipexole	Mirapex, Mirapex ER
Apomorphine (injection)	Apokyn
Rotigotine (transdermal patch)	Neupro

Therapeutic Use

DRAs stimulate sections of the brain influenced by dopamine. An adjunct to levodopa therapy, they are often used to manage dose-related fluctuations in the motor state while preventing motor complications (142). Addition of DRAs to patients' drug regimens allows a 20%–30% reduction in the dose of levodopa in practice and leads to improvement in disabling complications (143).

The two most commonly prescribed oral DRAs are ropinirole and pramipexole. Both also come in extended-release formulations. Apomorphine is a powerful fast-acting injectable that almost immediately relieves symptoms of PD; however, the effects are short-lived. Its primary use is for patients with PD who suddenly experience unexpected immobility when their medication wears off. Rotigotine uses a transdermal patch system, which has been shown in clinical trials to be as effective as ropinirole and pramipexole.

Mechanism of Action

The oxidative pathways by which levodopa is converted in the brain into dopamine can contribute to the formation of cytotoxic free radicals. In contrast, DRAs are not metabolized by oxidative pathways, and therefore do not lead to free radical formation (144). DRAs actually mimic the effects of dopamine without having to be converted; that is, they act directly on postsynaptic dopamine receptors, thus precluding the need for metabolic conversion, storage, and release.

Side Effects

Although well tolerated, DRAs are still associated with the usual dopaminergic side effects — nausea, hypotension, and exacerbation of dyskinesias. In addition, they can also cause confusion and hallucinations when used as an adjunct to levodopa (143).

Related Drug Interactions

The only interaction of note to the CEP is when DRAs are used in conjunction with antihypertensive medication. A hypotensive reaction is possible with this drug combination.

Anticholinergics

ACs are the oldest class of medications used to treat PD. Although there are several types on the market, two that are currently used in patients with PD are benztropine and trihexyphenidyl (Table 7.44).

Therapeutic Use

ACs block the action of the neurotransmitter acetylcholine in the brain; therefore, they are traditionally used to treat diseases like asthma, incontinence, GI cramps, muscular spasms, depression, and sleep disorders. However, because they balance the production of dopamine and acetylcholine in the body, and work to block involuntary movements of muscles, they may be helpful in treating tremor that is not adequately controlled with dopaminergic medications in patients with PD.

Mechanism of Action

The mechanism of action of ACs is not well understood. Researchers speculate that they work by inhibiting parasympathetic nerve impulses by blocking the binding of acetylcholine to its receptor present in nerve cells. Because the parasympathetic nervous system is responsible for the involuntary movement of muscles, blocking this action may control tremor (142).

Side Effects

The most acknowledged side effects are sedation and confusion. In addition, ACs may lead to hypohidrosis (reduction in sweat rate) or anhidrosis (absence of sweating (145)), which could lead to an increase in body temperature during exercise. Furthermore, if the patient also presents with DM, one of the key warning signs of hypoglycemia is lost.

Table 7.44	Anticholinergics
Drug (Generic) Name	Trade (Brand) Name
Benztropine	Cogentin
Trihexyphenidyl	Artane

Related Drug Interactions

No major interactions of concern for the CEP have been noted for patients taking ACs.

Monoamine Oxidase-B Inhibitors

Two isozymes of monoamine oxidase (MAO-A and MAO-B) exist. MAO-B is predominantly responsible for the oxidative metabolism of dopamine in the brain (142). Two specific MAO-B inhibitors selectively inactivate MAO-B through irreversible inhibition of the enzyme (Table 7.45).

Therapeutic Use

MAOIs are traditionally prescribed for depression. However, three selective MAO-B inhibitors are approved as adjunctive therapy to levodopa/carbidopa in patients whose symptoms of PD are not well-controlled on levodopa/carbidopa. They produce a modest suppression of symptoms of PD (142). Selegiline is well tolerated in younger patients in the early stages of PD, but not as well tolerated by elderly patients in the advanced stages.

Mechanism of Action

Selegiline elevates dopamine concentrations by inhibiting the enzyme that catabolizes dopamine MAO, and in so doing, extends the duration of action of each dose of levodopa. The precise mechanism of action of rasagiline is unknown; however, it is believed to be related to its MAO-B inhibitory activity.

Side Effects

No serious side effects in the scope of practice for the CEP have been noted.

Related Drug Interactions

No serious interactions in the scope of practice for the CEP have been noted.

Table 7.45	MAO-B Inhibitors (Adjunctive Parkinson Therapy)
Drug (Generic) Name	Trade (Brand) Name
Selegiline	Eldepryl, Carbex
Rasagiline	Azilect
Safinamide	Xadago

Catechol-O-Methyltransferase Inhibitors

Catechol-*O*-methyltransferase (COMT) inhibitors are PD medications that increase the availability of levodopa to the brain.

Therapeutic Use

COMT inhibitors have no direct effect on the primary motor symptoms of PD; however, they are used in conjunction with levodopa to prolong its effect (Table 7.46). In other words, they help to manage end-of-dose wearing-off with levodopa therapy. Because COMT inhibitors do not contain levodopa, they must be taken with levodopa in order to have any benefit (142). Additionally, COMT inhibitors may be prescribed when dopamine agonists are not tolerated.

Mechanism of Action

When levodopa is taken orally, an enzyme in the body called COMT converts a portion of the levodopa into a form (3-*O*-methyl dopa) that is useless. COMT inhibitors prevent the COMT enzyme from converting levodopa, thereby increasing the plasma half-life of levodopa. This effect increases the percentage of each dose that reaches the CNS, making more levodopa available in the brain to help reduce PD symptoms (142).

Side Effects

Patients taking tolcapone must have blood drawn periodically to monitor liver function and avoid liver toxicity (142). No other serious side effects in the scope of practice for the CEP have been noted.

Related Drug Interactions

No serious interactions in the scope of practice for the CEP have been noted.

Table 7.46	Catechol-*O*-Methyltransferase Inhibitors
Drug (Generic) Name	Trade (Brand) Name
Entacapone	Comtan
Tolcapone	Tasmar
Entacapone + levodopa/carbidopa	Stalevo
Opicapone	Ongentys

MS Drugs

MS is an autoimmune disease that causes progressive destruction of the myelin sheath covering nerve fibers in the CNS. The two types of MS are primary progressive MS (PPMS) and relapsing–remitting MS (RRMS). PPMS gets worse over time. There are no relapses or remissions. How quickly it progresses and the degree of disability it produces varies by individual. Ten to fifteen percent of people with MS have PPMS. They are usually diagnosed later in life. No pharmacological therapies have shown benefit for slowing the progression of PPMS, so treatment of PPMS revolves around treating symptoms to keep the patient comfortable.

RRMS, the most common form of the disease, has a variable course characterized by relapses that tend to become more frequent with age. Patients with RRMS are aggressively treated with medications to potentially lower the relapse rate and delay the formation of new CNS lesions. These disease-modifying medications are currently considered the best strategy available to delay the degenerating nature of RRMS (Table 7.47).

Table 7.47	Medications for RRMS
Drug (Generic) Name	Trade (Brand) Name
Injectable Medications	
Interferon-β	Avonex
	Betaseron
	Extavia
	Rebif
	Plegridy
Glatiramer acetate	Copaxone
	Glatopa
Daclizumab	Zinbryta
Oral Medications	
Teriflunomide	Aubagio
Fingolimod	Gilenya
Dimethyl fumarate	Tecfidera
Infused Medications	
Alemtuzumab	Lemtrade
Mitoxantrone	Novantrone
Natalizumab	Tysabri

Injectable Disease-Modifying Medications

β-Interferons are frequently prescribed as a first-line treatment for RRMS. They are injected subcutaneously or intramuscularly and work to reduce the frequency and severity of exacerbations (33%), as well as the appearance of new CNS lesions (67% (146)). However, the mechanism of action of these drugs in the treatment of MS has remained elusive. Their long-term safety profile is generally good. Common short-term side effects are headache, fatigue, and depression.

Glatiramer acetate injected subcutaneously also works to reduce the occurrence of exacerbations. Although the exact mechanism of action is unknown, it is intended to reduce the autoimmune attacks on myelin. The one side effect related to the work of CEPs is angina, which occurs at least once in approximately 13% of patients taking glatiramer acetate. The pain is usually transient, lacks characteristic symptomology, and appears to be deficient of clinical sequelae. Some patients experience more than one such episode, and episodes usually begin at least 1 month after the initiation of treatment (147). The pathogenesis of this symptom is unknown. Interactions between glatiramer acetate and other drugs have not been fully evaluated.

Daclizumab, the newest medication approved (in May 2016) for MS, is indicated for the treatment of adult patients with MS experiencing repeated exacerbations. Because of its safety profile, its use should largely be reserved for patients who have had a poor response to two or more other drugs indicated for the treatment of MS. The precise mechanism of action for daclizumab in MS is unknown but is presumed to involve modulation of IL-2–mediated activation of lymphocytes through binding to CD25 (148). Because it reduces immune function, the most common side effect is susceptibility to infections. Common types of infections manifested include upper respiratory tract infections, urinary tract infections, and viral infections (148).

Oral Disease-Modifying Medications for MS

Teriflunomide is indicated for the treatment of patients with RRMS. It works to reduce swelling and inflammation in the immune system. The mechanism of action by which teriflunomide exerts its therapeutic effect in MS is unknown but may involve a reduction in the number of activated lymphocytes in the CNS. Besides severe hepatotoxic and teratogenic effects, teriflunomide produces a slightly hypertensive response, so patients being treated for HTN need to be monitored on a regular basis (149).

Fingolimod, an immunosuppressant, is indicated for the treatment of patients with RRMS to reduce the frequency of clinical exacerbations and to delay established physical disability. Fingolimod blocks the capacity of lymphocytes to exit from lymph nodes, reducing the number of lymphocytes in peripheral blood. The mechanism of action by which fingolimod exerts therapeutic effects in MS is unknown, but it may reduce lymphocyte migration into the CNS (150). The primary side effect of interest to CEPs is the occurrence of bradycardia and all AV blocks. These conduction abnormalities are usually transient and asymptomatic, and resolve within the first 24 hours on treatment, but they occasionally require treatment with atropine or isoproterenol (150).

Dimethyl fumarate is indicated for the treatment of patients with RRMS to reduce the frequency of exacerbations. The mechanism by which dimethyl fumarate exerts its therapeutic effect in MS is unknown. Although there are several warnings and mild-to-moderate side effects, none are specific to the scope of practice for the CEP.

Infused Disease-Modifying Medications for MS

The infused disease-modifying medications are normally reserved for patients with advanced stages of MS. Because their mobility is severely limited, the CEP will rarely see them in practice.

Systemic Lupus Erythematosus

SLE is an autoimmune disease that causes chronic inflammation and a wide range of signs and symptoms, including fatigue, fever, swollen, painful joints, hair loss, and a characteristic skin rash, typically on the face. It can be difficult to diagnose because these signs and symptoms mimic those of other disorders. The pharmacological treatment for SLE varies according to the presentation. As signs and symptoms flare-up and subside, medications may need to be changed or dosages adjusted.

Traditionally, the standard therapy regimen for SLE has included only nonspecific agents, including analgesics, NSAIDs, and immunosuppressives and antimalarials, the latter of which suppress the entire immune system (Table 7.48). In contrast, belimumab (Benylsta), the first SLE medication approved by the FDA in over 50 years, is a monoclonal antibody; that is, an immune protein developed to find and attach to only one type of substance in the body. Belimumab specifically recognizes and blocks

Table 7.48	Standard Therapy for Systemic Lupus Erythematosus		
Drug Class	Drug (Generic) Name	Trade (Brand) Name	Symptoms Treated
Analgesic	Acetaminophen	Tylenol	Pain
Nonsteroidal anti-inflammatory drugs	Ibuprofen	Advil Motrin	Pain, inflammation, fever, arthritis
	Naproxen sodium	Aleve, Naprosyn, Anaprox	
	Acetylsalicylic acid	Ecotrin	
Corticosteroids	Prednisone	Rayos Prednisone Intensol	Decreases pain, swelling, warmth, tenderness associated with inflammation
Antimalarials	Hydroxychloroquine	Plaquenil	Decreases autoantibody production
	Chloroquine	Aralen	
Immunosuppressives	Cyclophosphamide	Cytoxan	Controls overactive immune system, inflammation
	Methotrexate	Rheumatrex	
	Azathioprine	Imuran	
Anticoagulants	Heparin	Calciparine	Helps prevent clotting
	Warfarin	Coumadin	

the biological activity of B-lymphocyte stimulator, a naturally occurring protein, which, when elevated, prolongs the survival of B-lymphocytes contributing to the production of autoantibodies. Belimumab reduces autoantibody levels and helps control autoimmune disease activity.

Belimumab is indicated to treat adults with active SLE who are receiving other medications. It is generally well tolerated. Typical side effects include nausea, diarrhea, fever, inflammation of the nose and throat, bronchitis, insomnia, pain in the extremities, depression, and migraine headache.

DRUGS FOR ORTHOPEDIC DISORDERS

This section covers drugs for osteoarthritis (OA), osteoporosis, and rheumatoid arthritis (RA).

Arthritis Drugs

OA is a chronic disease for which there is no cure. Treatments are available to manage symptoms such as stiffness, pain, and inflammation, as well as to improve joint mobility and flexibility. Pharmacologic therapy addresses the pain and inflammation, whereas appropriate physical activity designed by a CEP works to strengthen affected joints and improve joint mobility and flexibility. Common OA medications include analgesics, NSAIDs, and corticosteroids (Table 7.49).

Analgesics

Analgesics are drugs that relieve pain. Acetaminophen is a pain reliever and an antipyretic. It is available OTC as well as in prescription preparations. Its analgesic and antipyretic actions are similar to NSAIDs; however, it lacks the other typical actions of NSAIDs, such as anti-inflammatory activity, antiplatelet activity, and gastrotoxicity.

Although its mechanism of action is not fully understood, acetaminophen appears to be a weak inhibitor of prostaglandin (PG) synthesis. PGs are hormone-like lipid compounds that cause pain, fever, and inflammation. However, acetaminophen possesses only limited anti-inflammatory activity (151).

Acetaminophen is very well tolerated with minimal GI side effects. Chronic usage along with acute overdosing

Table 7.49	Common Osteoarthritis Medications		
Class	Drug (Generic) Name	Brand (Trade) Name	Selectivity
Analgesic	Acetaminophen	Tylenol (OTC)	
Nonsteroidal anti-inflammatory drugs	Acetylsalicylic acid (aspirin)	Ecotrin (OTC)	COX-1 selective
	Ibuprofen	Advil (OTC), Motrin (OTC and prescription strength)	COX nonselective
	Naproxen sodium	Aleve (OTC), Naprosyn, Anaprox	COX nonselective
	Celecoxib	Celebrex	COX-2 selective
	Diclofenac	Voltaren, Zorvolex, Zipsor	COX nonselective
Corticosteroids	Prednisone	Rayos, Prednisone Intensol	
	Cortisone	Cortone	

could lead to hepatotoxicity. Acute overdosing includes cases of excess doses within 24 hours, taking additional acetaminophen-containing products concurrently, or consuming alcohol while taking the drug (152). There are no related drug interactions of note for the CEP.

Nonsteroidal Anti-inflammatory Drugs

Therapeutic Use

NSAIDs are prescribed for the treatment of mild-to-moderate pain, fever, headache, and inflammation. In addition, they have proved effective in treating OA, RA, soft tissue inflammation that causes tendinitis and bursitis, and dysmenorrhea. Some are available OTC, whereas others are by prescription.

Mechanism of Action

NSAIDs work by reducing the production of PGs. PGs promote inflammation that is necessary for healing, support the blood clotting function of platelets, and protect the lining of the stomach from the damaging effects of gastric acid. Specifically, NSAIDs block the enzyme cyclooxygenase (COX) that leads to the production of PGs, thereby lowering PG synthesis and subsequently reducing inflammation, pain, and fever. Two COX enzymes, COX-1 and COX-2, support PG synthesis; however, only COX-1 is involved in the production of PGs that support platelets and protect the stomach. Certain NSAIDs have specific selectivity for COX-2 enzymes (see Table

7.49). These are potentially protective of platelets and the stomach lining.

Side Effects

NSAIDs that are not selective for COX-2 enzymes reduce PGs that protect the mucosal lining of the stomach, thereby increasing the risk for ulcers; in addition, they can promote excessive bleeding. Given the elevated risk for potential GI ulcers, the need for selective COX-2 inhibitors is clear. In addition to GI risks, well-controlled clinical trials have revealed an increase in the incidence of MI, stroke, and thrombosis in patients using all types of NSAIDs (152). In response to these concerns, the FDA has issued warnings about NSAIDs increasing the risk of MI or stroke in both patients with a risk of heart disease and patients without. The risk of an MI also appears to be dose dependent, with a higher risk at higher doses, and can develop within weeks of starting an NSAID. Additionally, that risk may increase the longer the NSAIDs are used (151).

Related Drug Interactions

Low-dose ASA is widely used as prevention for MI and other CVD; however, concurrent use with other NSAIDs may inhibit the antiplatelet effect of ASA (153, 154). Although the data are contradictory, it appears as if ibuprofen has the most consistent synergistic antiplatelet effect with ASA, whereas naproxen sodium, celecoxib, and diclofenac may have a possible effect. Acetaminophen has a minimal if any effect at all.

Corticosteroids/Glucocorticoids

Therapeutic Use

Corticosteroids have been among the most widely prescribed and effective treatments to manage inflammatory and autoimmune diseases (see Table 7.49). Specifically, corticosteroids are used to treat several types of arthritis, SLE, asthma, and bronchitis, as well as leukemias and lymphomas. Additionally, corticosteroids are commonly used as part of an antirejection regimen to suppress the immune system and prevent the body from rejecting transplanted organs.

Mechanism of Action

Corticosteroids mimic the effects of hormones the body produces naturally in the adrenal glands. When prescribed in doses that exceed normal levels, corticosteroids suppress inflammation. This can reduce the signs and symptoms of inflammatory conditions, such as arthritis and asthma. Corticosteroids also suppress the immune system, which can help control autoimmune conditions.

Side Effects

Corticosteroids can cause obesity and may lead to the development or worsening of T2DM. Corticosteroids are also referred to as glucocorticoids because of their effects on glucose metabolism. It is common for patients taking corticosteroids to experience increases in blood glucose levels. In addition, as just noted, corticosteroids suppress immune system function; therefore, an increased frequency or severity of infections is possible. Also, the effectiveness of vaccines and antibiotics may be compromised. Chronic corticosteroid use may also reduce bone mineral density (BMD), leading to the development of osteoporosis, which increases the risk for bone fractures (hip, wrist, vertebral). Patients taking long-term corticosteroids often receive supplements of calcium and vitamin D to counteract the effects on bones.

Related Drug Interactions

Corticosteroids can decrease the effectiveness of oral hypoglycemic medications used to treat DM. If both medications are necessary, blood glucose levels will usually be checked more regularly, and the dose of the DM medication may need to be adjusted. For patients on anticoagulant medications, adding corticosteroids may make the anticoagulants less effective, promoting the chances of clot formation. However, patients may experience excess bleeding resulting in bleeding from the gums, nosebleeds, unusual bruising, or dark stools.

Osteoporosis Drugs

Bone mineral homeostasis requires a balance between building and breakdown. With age, the rate of bone breakdown begins to increase. For women, menopause is the catalyst for this increased rate of breakdown, whereas men experience it from approximately age 70. At this point, the rebuilding process cannot keep pace; therefore, BMD decreases, and bones become fragile.

Osteoporosis medications help to slow down this process and thus to maintain bone density while decreasing the risk of an osteoporotic fracture. There are two types of osteoporosis medications. One type slows bone breakdown and builds bone mass, and the second builds new bone mass. Other complementary therapies available for bone health include vitamin D supplements, dietary calcium supplements, and weight-bearing exercise.

Bisphosphonates

Bisphosphonates are considered bone resorption inhibitors (Table 7.50). They have a strong affinity for bone targeting bone surfaces undergoing remodeling. Accordingly, they are extensively used in conditions characterized by osteoclast-mediated bone resorption, especially osteoporosis (155). Alendronic acid is one of the most widely prescribed medications for the prevention and treatment of osteoporosis.

Bisphosphonates show preferential localization to sites of bone resorption, specifically under osteoclasts. Although they do not interfere with osteoclast recruitment or attachment, they do inhibit osteoclast activity. Bisphosphonate treatment reduces bone turnover (*i.e.*,

Table 7.50	Bisphosphonates
Drug (Generic) Name	Brand (Trade) Name
Alendronic acid	Fosamax
Ibandronic acid	Boniva
Risedronic acid	Actonel
	Atelvia
Zoledronic acid	Reclast

the number of sites at which bone is remodeled). Consequently, bone formation exceeds bone resorption at these remodeling sites, leading to progressive gains in bone mass (156). Zoledronic acid, a third-generation bisphosphonate, generally has the same outcomes; however, instead of inhibiting osteoclast activity, zoledronic acid prevents calcium release from bone.

Side Effects

Although serious adverse reactions with chronic bisphosphonate use are rare, they include osteonecrosis of the jaw, atypical femur fracture, atrial fibrillation, and esophageal cancer. Typical side effects of rash and GI upset were minimal. For zoledronic acid, bone pain, back pain, muscle, joint pain, and edema in the feet or ankles are common side effects.

The incidence of upper GI side events was increased in patients receiving concomitant therapy with daily doses of NSAIDs.

Other Osteoporosis Medications

Although denosumab and teriparatide can be prescribed to anyone with osteoporosis, they are generally recommended for people with unique circumstances, such as severe osteoporosis with very low bone density, multiple fractures, and chronic steroid use. These drugs, which are injected, might also be given to people who can't tolerate an oral bisphosphonate. Denosumab has exhibited a reduction in the risk of osteoporotic fractures in women and men. It is also used in people with reduced kidney function who can't take a bisphosphonate (157). Teriparatide is usually reserved for men and postmenopausal women who have severely low bone density, have had osteoporotic fractures, have multiple risk factors for fracture, whose osteoporosis is caused by chronic steroid use, or who cannot tolerate other osteoporosis treatments. Currently, teriparatide is the only osteoporosis medication that has the potential to rebuild bone and actually somewhat reverse osteoporosis (157).

RA Drugs

RA is a chronic progressive inflammatory autoimmune disease characterized by pain, stiffness, inflammation, swelling, and sometimes destruction of joints. It gets worse over time unless the inflammation is stopped or slowed. There is no cure for RA; however, in extremely rare cases it goes into remission without treatment.

Traditional arthritis medications — NSAIDs, corticosteroids, and analgesics — play an essential role in controlling the symptoms of RA. These have been discussed earlier in this section. In the past, NSAIDs were also prescribed for RA treatment, before progressing to more potent RA drugs when signs of joint damage were manifested. Currently, however, a more aggressive approach using disease-modifying antirheumatic drugs (DMARDs) and biologic response modifiers (BRMs) is thought to be more effective. This more aggressive approach results in reduced symptoms, joint damage, and disability, and remission of symptoms is more likely (158, 159).

Disease-Modifying Antirheumatic Drugs

DMARDs are the most important drugs used in RA treatment (Table 7.51). Methotrexate is the drug of choice for treatment, but the complete arsenal also includes antimalarials and immunosuppressants. The primary function of DMARDs is to reduce pain and inflammation, slow the progression of RA, and protect the affected joints from permanent damage. Although very effective in the treatment of RA, these drugs may take several weeks before the benefits are exhibited.

The mechanism by which DMARDs work varies by drug; however, they ultimately slow or stop the progression of RA by suppressing immune system processes that promote inflammation (Table 7.52).

Common side reactions to DMARDs vary but may include hepatotoxicity, bone marrow suppression, and severe lung infections.

Although there are several serious drug interactions for methotrexate, the only one related to the scope of practice for the CEP is excessive bruising and bleeding when methotrexate is used with low-dose ASA. In addition, alcohol abuse increases the risk for hepatotoxicity. Methotrexate is safe to use in combination with other DMARDs and BRMs; in fact, it usually is combined with hydroxychloroquine and sulfasalazine for a more effective relief of several symptoms of RA.

Table 7.51	Disease-Modifying Antirheumatic Drugs
Drug (Generic) Name	Trade (Brand) Name
Methotrexate	Trexall, Otrexup, Rasuvo
Hydroxychloroquine	Plaquenil
Sulfasalazine	Azulfidine
Leflunomide	Arava

Table 7.52	Mechanism of Action of DMARDs
Drug	Mechanism of Action
Methotrexate	Anti-inflammatory effects because of interruption of adenosine; immunosuppressive effects due to inhibition of dihydrofolate reductase, the enzyme involved in the metabolism of folic acid.
Hydroxychloroquine	Alters antigen presentation.
Sulfasalazine	Promotes folate depletion.
Leflunomide	Not fully understood.

Source: Hopkinsarthritis.com. Rheumatoid arthritis treatment. 2016. Available from: http://www.hopkinsarthritis.org/arthritis-info/rheumatoid-arthritis/ra-treatment/.

Biologic Response Modifiers

BRMs are the newest class of medications approved to treat RA (Table 7.53). Although they do not cure RA, they target the part of the immune system response that leads to inflammation and joint damage. They thereby relieve symptoms and improve quality of life. In addition, they may slow the progression of RA or help induce remission (159). If the medication is stopped, symptoms may return.

Table 7.53	Biologic Response Modifiers	
Class	Drug (Generic) Name	Trade (Brand) Name
T-cell co-stimulatory blocker	Abatacept	Orencia
IL-1 receptor antagonist	Anakinra	Kineret
TNF-α inhibitors	Adalimumab	Humira
	Certolizumab	Cimzia
	Etanercept	Enbrel
	Golimumab	Simponi
	Infliximab	Remicade
B-cell depletion	Rituximab	Rituxan
IL-6 inhibitor	Tocilizumab	Actemra

TNF, tumor necrosis factor.

For the best possible response, BRMs are usually taken concomitantly with methotrexate.

The several subclasses of BRMs all work on the innate immune system; however, each has a specialized action (Table 7.54). As with most immunosuppressants, an

Table 7.54	Mechanism of Action of BRMs
Class of BRM	Mechanism of Action
TNF-α inhibitors	TNF-α inhibitors suppress the immune system by blocking the activity of TNF-α, a proinflammatory cytokine found in large quantities in the rheumatoid joint. TNF-α is one of the critical cytokines mediating joint damage and destruction.
T-cell costimulatory blocker	When abatacept binds to CD28 on the T-cell surface, it prevents the second signal from being delivered, thus turning down the T-cell response. It also decreases the production of T-cell–derived cytokines, including TNF.
IL-1 receptor antagonist	IL-1 is a proinflammatory cytokine implicated in the pathogenesis of RA. Tocilizumab is an endogenous blocker of IL-1.
IL-6 inhibitor	IL-6 is a pleiotropic proinflammatory cytokine produced by a variety of cell types. Tocilizumab binds specifically to both soluble and membrane-bound IL-6 receptors and has been shown to inhibit IL-6–mediated signaling through these receptors.
B-cell depletion	Rituximab binds to the CD20 molecule on the B-cell surface leading to the removal of B cells from the circulation. This leads to a rapid depletion of B-lymphocytes in the peripheral blood that is sustained for 6 mo–1 yr or possibly longer.

BRM, biologic response modifiers; RA, rheumatoid arthritis; TNF, tumor necrosis factor.

Source: Hopkinsarthritis.com. Rheumatoid arthritis treatment. 2016. Available from: http://www.hopkinsarthritis.org/arthritis-info/rheumatoid-arthritis/ra-treatment/.

increased risk of routine and opportunistic infections is prevalent. There appears to be a limited susceptibility to drug interactions with BRMs that would be related to the scope of practice for the CEP.

Oncology Treatments

Various treatments and medications are used to treat oncological diseases (cancers). Recent exercise research has focused on exercise programming effects. Little research has been done assessing the treatment and medication direct effects on HR and BP. Exercise capacity can be affected by the treatment and medication side effects, and this has been the focus of recent studies. New medications and treatments are constantly being developed, and it's difficult to ascertain the medication and/or treatment effects on HR, BP, and exercise capacity versus the disease process effects on exercise capacity.

This section will focus on selected treatments and their effects on the cardiovascular, pulmonary, and musculoskeletal systems — specifically as related to side effects and subsequently predicted changes in exercise capacity. Table 7.55 highlights treatments, drug classifications used to treat oncological diseases, and known deleterious effects on the cardiovascular, pulmonary, and musculoskeletal systems. Medications discussed earlier in this chapter can be used to treat the oncological treatment side effects.

Endocrine Treatment

Endocrine treatment (*e.g.*, hormone therapy) treats various types of cancers. Both men and women can receive endocrine treatment for various cancers (*e.g.*, breast, endometrial, prostate, and adrenal cancer). There are various types of endocrine treatment used for each cancer, including aromatase inhibitors and antiestrogens. Tamoxifen is an antiestrogen commonly used to treat some breast tumors. Endocrine treatments can have deleterious effects on the cardiovascular, pulmonary, and musculoskeletal systems (160–164), and the side effects can be reversed once treatment is stopped (165). Exercise capacity can be negatively affected during treatment (166).

Chemotherapy

Two chemotherapy drug classifications are anthracyclines and taxanes. Both have known deleterious effects on the cardiovascular, pulmonary, and musculoskeletal systems (167–172). Chemotherapy agents have been shown to decrease exercise capacity, while exercise training before and during treatment has been shown to

help alleviate cardiovascular (173) and musculoskeletal side effects (174).

Immunotherapy

Two immunotherapy drug classifications include PD-1 and PD ligand ½, and anti-CTLA-4 (Ipilimumab). These have known negative cardiovascular, pulmonary, and musculoskeletal system side effects (175–177). These side effects can negatively affect exercise capacity. Exercise training has been shown to positively influence outcomes (175).

Targeted Treatments

Targeted oncology treatments use drugs or other substances targeting certain cancer cell types. They are used either alone or in combination with standard chemotherapy, radiation therapy, or surgery. Targeted treatments have known deleterious effects on the cardiovascular, pulmonary, and musculoskeletal systems (178–180), potentially decreasing one's exercise capacity. Moderate-intensity exercise training has a protective effect on LVEF and exercise capacity after women received trastuzumab (181).

Monoclonal Antibody Therapy

Monoclonal antibodies are laboratory-developed immune system proteins. The antibodies target specific cancer cells. Rituximab is a monoclonal antibody used to identify cancer cells, helping to destroy them. These therapies have some cardiovascular, pulmonary, and musculoskeletal system side effects (182). These side effects could potentially decrease one's exercise capacity.

COVID-19 Medications

A recent health worldwide endemic has been the COVID-19 endemic. COVID-19 infection exacerbates other comorbidities. New drugs and treatments are being developed and released; however, there's insufficient data to warrant an extensive review of these medications. Studies have begun assessing pharmacologic efficacy, and minimal data are available regarding exercise considerations. It's too early to discern long-term effects of medications to treat acute COVID-19 infections. Further research needs to be done assessing the effect of medications (Table 7.56) taken during acute COVID-19 infection on long-term HR, BP, rating of perceived exertion (RPE), and exercise ability/tolerance among other variables.

Early research confirms the anecdotal reports regarding the deleterious effects of COVID-19 (183); however,

Table 7.55 Oncology Medications/Treatments

Treatment	Drug Classification	Cardiovascular System Effects Related to Exercise Capacity	Pulmonary System Effects Related to Exercise Capacity	Musculoskeletal System Effects Related to Exercise Capacity
Endocrine treatment (160–164)	Tamoxifen Aromatase inhibitors	CVD can increase in the long term. Tamoxifen for example included an approximately twofold to threefold increase relative risk of thromboembolic disease compared with placebo. People with cardiovascular risk factors are at even a higher risk of CVD.	Insufficient data exists.	Decrease in bone density because of estrogen deficiency. Increase in bone pain, joint pain, and arthralgias. Exercise as a benefit has been indicated to relieve some of the previously mentioned symptoms.
Chemotherapy (167–172)	Anthracyclines	Increase the risk of developing heart failure and significant associated morbidity and mortality. This can be caused by formation of reactive oxygen species, induction of apoptosis, DNA damage through interaction with topoisomerase II, and inhibition of protein synthesis. Myocyte damage can be a resultant factor with these types of medications. They can also be associated with left ventricular dysfunction and a decreased EF. There is a risk of developing chronotropic incompetence.	Drug-induced interstitial lung disease has been occasionally reported.	Greater increases of visceral fat have been associated with the use of anthracyclines.
	Taxanes	Chest discomfort/pain, tachycardia, and hypotension have been associated with the use of taxanes.	Associated with pulmonary toxicity such as pneumonitis and dyspnea. A syndrome of capillary leakage, resulting in peripheral edema, noncariogenic pulmonary edema, and pleural effusions.	Associated with both sensory and motor neuropathy. Myalgias and arthralgias can occur as well. The mechanisms of it remain unknown. The feelings would be described as numbness and tingling.
Immunotherapy (177)	Checkpoint inhibitor immunotherapy			

(continued)

Table 7.55 | **Oncology Medications/Treatments** *(continued)*

Treatment	Drug Classification	Cardiovascular System Effects Related to Exercise Capacity	Pulmonary System Effects Related to Exercise Capacity	Musculoskeletal System Effects Related to Exercise Capacity
	PD-1 and PD ligand 1/2	Kidney infections can be common. Heart palpitations have been associated with therapy. Inflammation in the heart and kidneys can occur. Venous thromboembolism has been seen. Myocarditis has been reported as well.	Can increase the risk of pneumonitis.	Fatigue specifically in the PD-1 agent. Muscle weakness can occur and nervous system issues such as numbness. Can cause inflammatory arthritis.
	Anti-CTLA-4 (Ipilimumab)	Chest pain and dizziness. In <1% arteritis, hypersensitivity angiitis, myocarditis, pericarditis, peripheral vascular disease, and vasculitis can occur. Nephrotoxicity can occur as well.	In <1% acute respiratory distress syndrome can occur. Pneumonitis can occur.	Muscle weakness is uncommon. Muscle weakness, muscle pain, and joint pain are rare. Arthralgia can occur as well. In <1% arthritis, myelitis, myositis (including orbital), polymyalgia rheumatica, polymyositis, rhabdomyolysis can occur.
Targeted treatment (178–180)	Herceptin	Cardiotoxicity such as reduction in LVEF and heart failure. Hypotension and angioedema. Swelling can occur in the ankles or legs and weight gain.	Dyspnea and bronchospasm. Herceptin may cause inflammation of the lungs. Symptoms include trouble breathing, cough, tiredness, and fluid in the lungs.	Insufficient information.
	Perjeta	Decreased left ventricular EF and anemia. Peripheral edema. Can be cardiotoxic.	Epistaxis and upper respiratory tract infection.	Fatigue and insomnia. Myalgia and arthralgia. Asthenia. Peripheral neuropathy.
	Enhurtu	Hypokalemia, Anemia, Decreased EF, peripheral edema, dizziness. Can be cardiotoxic. The drug even has concern for bone marrow suppression.	Upper respiratory tract infection, interstitial pulmonary disease, and pneumonia.	Fatigue and muscle weakness.
Monoclonal antibody therapy (182)	Rituximab	Hypotension and severe hypotension in <10% of the cases.	Bronchospasm and pneumonitis.	Back pain.

CVD, cardiovascular disease; EF, ejection fraction; LVEF, left ventricular ejection fraction; PD, Parkinson disease.

The authors would like to thank Chris Fitzmaurice, MS, CET, Carmen Calfa, MD, and Julio Rodriguiz, MS (University of Miami Medical Center Division of Oncology) for their insightful technical expertise in creating Table 7.55.

Table 7.56	COVID-19 Medications
Drug (Generic) Name	**Trade (Brand) Name**
Remdesivir	Veklury
Monoclonal antibody treatments: Bamlanivimab plus etesevimab Casirivimab plus imdevimab Sotrovimab	None
Convalescent plasma	None

little is known regarding lingering effects of medications used to treat acute COVID-19 infection. Current activity recommendations post-COVID-19 include no exercise until an individual is asymptomatic for 7 days (184). COVID-19 vaccination has reported myocarditis as a potential side effect (185), and medications discussed earlier in this chapter (*e.g.*, corticosteroids) are a medical treatment option.

The following section will discuss some COVID-19 treatment options (Table 7.56). COVID-19 treatments are rapidly changing in response to the disease.

Remdesivir (Veklury) is an FDA-approved antiviral for use in treating COVID-19. It has been shown to prevent disease progression in patients who are symptomatic COVID-19 positive and to improve outcomes in hospitalized patients with moderate-to-severe coronavirus disease (186, 187). Remdesivir has been tolerated well showing few adverse events (187).

Monoclonal antibody (mAb) treatments have been given emergency use authorizations (EUAs) by the FDA for the treatment and/or prevention of COVID-19. These infusion treatments are man-made in a laboratory and imitate antibodies. Three approved for EUA include bamlanivimab plus etesevimab, casirivimab plus imdevimab, and sotrovimab. They can stop the coronavirus causing COVID-19 from attaching to human cells. This limits the virus' ability to reproduce and cause further harm. mAbs have varying success against different COVID-19 variants (188).

Convalescent plasma (CCP) (*e.g.*, serum therapy) and other emerging treatment plans have also been used to treat COVID-19 with varying effectiveness. CCP — donated by previous patients with COVID-19 who have recovered from COVID-19 — is most effective when used early in the disease process (189). A recent randomized controlled trial on hospitalized patients who are nonvaccinated on supplemental noninvasive oxygen therapy showed no clinical status benefit using CCP within 7 days of symptom onset; these patients also received remdesivir and/or corticosteroids (190). Continued research is needed to assess current and emerging treatments. Published data analyzing these treatments and the interaction of treatments on clinical benefits are limited at the time of writing.

SUMMARY

Thousands of medications are available for the prevention and treatment of disease. This chapter focused only on the drugs of choice; that is, those that are either the most effective or the most utilized for the disease in question. HR and BP are the vital signs most commonly assessed to determine drug effects, but as discussed in this chapter, other assessments may be important for certain diseases. New drugs are being introduced into the clinical marketplace every year. The CEP should become knowledgeable about these new drugs and their effects on both the resting and exercising patient.

CHAPTER REVIEW QUESTIONS

1. Explain the therapeutic difference between cardioselective and noncardioselective β-blockers.
2. ACE-I and diuretics are well known for controlling BP. Discuss their combined role and mechanism of action in the prevention of HF.
3. Discuss the difference in mechanism of action between ACE-I and ARBs. Why are ARBs helpful in patients following an MI with an EF < 40%?
4. Loop diuretics interact with a long list of other medications in various ways. Discuss these interactions.
5. Discuss the mechanism of action of cardiac glycosides and relate it to the benefits seen during exercise testing and training.
6. Glucophage (metformin) is considered a first-line treatment for DM. Discuss its therapeutic benefit in terms of fasting blood glucose and HbA1C levels.

7. Compare the potential cardioprotective effects of GLP-1RAs and SGLT2 inhibitors.

8. Levodopa, the metabolic precursor of dopamine, is apparently converted to dopamine in the brain. This is thought to be the mechanism whereby levodopa relieves symptoms of PD. Discuss why levodopa is not administered alone and why the combination of carbidopa and levodopa is beneficial in the treatment of PD.

9. Discuss the mechanism of action of the two types of NSAIDs and the difference in potential for severe cardiovascular events with chronic use.

10. RA and SLE are considered chronic progressive inflammatory autoimmune diseases. Discuss similarities in their pharmacological treatment.

Case Study 7.1

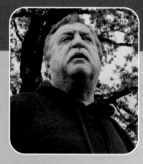

Bill is a 62-year-old Type-2 diabetic male on metformin (500 mg bid), atorvastatin (40 mg qd), and metoprolol (50 mg qd); he's 182 cm (71.62 inches) tall and weighs 145.5 kg (320 lbs). A new CPX showed his $\dot{V}O_{2Peak}$ was 18 mL·kg^{-1}·min^{-1} (89% predicted), and his max HR was 166 bpm; he stopped because of fatigue at RPE 18/20. His breathing reserve shows he's cardiovascularly limited. He had no arrhythmias during the test, and his systolic BP averaged a 12-mm Hg increase for each 1 MET increase reaching a max BP of 184/86. A resting echo showed an EF of 39%. A resting lipid profile revealed TC 284 mg·dL^{-1} (15.8 mmol·L^{-1}), LDL 148 mg·dL^{-1} (8.2 mmol·L^{-1}), HDL 37 mg·dL^{-1} (2.1 mmol·L^{-1}), and a fasting blood glucose level of 184 mg·dL^{-1} (10.2 mmol·L^{-1}). His resting BP is 124/82 and resting HR is 66 bpm.

He's a medical fitness center member and wants to "get better." Bill has not been exercising for the last 6 months and has been told to go back to the fitness center. You are assigned to guide him through an exercise program.

Case Study 7.1 Questions

1. What additional medication should Bill be prescribed? What would be the benefit?

2. How does Bill's medication regimen appear to be working for him?

3. What type of exercise program might you prescribe for Bill to assist him in improving his blood and lipid profile?

4. What are some medication side effects Bill should watch out for as he starts his exercise program? What should he do to monitor them?

Case Study 7.2

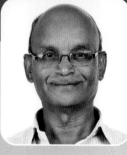

Steve, a 56-year-old male, comes to your cardiac rehabilitation program with a diagnosis of HF, nonischemic cardiomyopathy, sarcoidosis, pulmonary HTN, and T2DM. During his intake interview, he describes dyspnea with exertion (e.g., raking leaves, push mowing, and walking 1 mile in 20 min) and ranks it 5–7 of 10 (10-point scale). He also reports waking up at night with wheezing and shortness of breath; it goes away after sitting up for 5–10 minutes.

He recently had an automatic implantable cardioverter-defibrillator (AICD) implanted after a cardiac MRI showed an EF of 25% with no evidence of inducible myocardial ischemia and sarcoid infiltration into his right ventricle and lungs. During a cardiopulmonary exercise testing (CPET) test, Steve had premature ventricular couplets and a nonsustained 5 beat run of ventricular tachycardia at a rate of 135 bpm prior to the test being stopped. His resting ECG showed sinus rhythm with incomplete right bundle branch block; he had multifocal PVCs throughout exercise that did not decrease with exercise intensity. He was able to reach a maximal workload of 5 METs at a measured peak of 17 mg·kg^{-1}·min^{-1}.

Medication review shows he is on Toprol XL, sildenafil, flecainide, ASA, atorvastatin, methotrexate, torsemide, and glimepiride. His resting BP prior to exercise was 124/76 mm Hg with an HR of 84 bpm. His weight is 1.8 kg (4 lb) higher than what was measured 2 days ago during his intake interview/orientation. During Steve's first exercise session, he becomes dyspneic (5/10 on a 10-point scale) walking on the treadmill at 2.0 mph (3.2 kph)/0% grade; it is relieved by 5 minutes rest. The dyspnea reported is less than what he experiences at home and is "tolerable."

Case Study 7.2 Questions

1. In addition to the medications, Steve is currently prescribed, what other medications could be used to treat his HF?
2. What is a common indication for sildenafil (Viagra)? What effect on BP would you expect to see with exercise while taking sildenafil?
3. Flecainide is an antiarrhythmic medication. What is a class III antiarrhythmic that could be used to control the nonsustained ventricular tachycardia with exercise?
4. Steve reports his fasting blood sugar has been at least 180 mg·dL^{-1} for the past week. He states he has not changed his diet or activity pattern recently but has seen his fasting blood sugar increase from about 140 to at least 180 mg·dL^{-1}. In addition to the medications Steve is currently prescribed, what are some other medications that could help to control his blood sugar?

Case Study 7.3

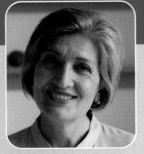

Janell, a 54-year-old female, was an accomplished triathlete through her 40s, often winning competitions in her age bracket. Over the past several years, she began to experience tremors, bradykinesia, and extremely stiff joints. Unable to compete and with her performance diminishing, she saw a neurologist specializing in movement disorders. She was diagnosed with PD and placed on Sinemet 200 mg PO q12 hr. Janell was instructed to continue her exercise routine and return to clinic in 3 months.

Case Study 7.3 Questions

1. Sinemet combines levodopa and carbidopa. What is the advantage of combining these two medications?
2. How should Janell coordinate her exercise regimen and her medication?
3. What should be monitored now that Janell has been prescribed Sinemet?

REFERENCES

1. McLaughlin M, Jacobs I. Exercise is medicine, but does it interfere with medicine? *Exerc Sport Sci Rev*. 2017;45(3):127–35.

2. Liguori G, Feito, Y, Fountaine, C, et al. *ACSM's Guidelines for Exercise Testing and Prescription*. 11th ed. Philadelphia (PA): Wolters Kluwer; 2022.

3. Riebe D, Ehrman JK, Liguori G, et al. *ACSM's Guidelines for Exercise Testing and Prescription*. 10th ed. Philadelphia (PA): Wolters Kluwer; 2018.

4. Priel E, Wahab M. Mondal T, et al. The impact of beta blockade on the cardio-respiratory system and symptoms during exercise. *Curr Res Physiol*. 2021;4:235–42.

5. Smith SC, Benjamin EJ, Bonow RO, et al; World Heart Federation and the Preventive Cardiovascular Nurses Association. AHA/ACCF secondary prevention and risk reduction therapy for patients with coronary and other atherosclerotic vascular disease: 2011 update: a guideline from the American Heart Association and American College of Cardiology Foundation [Erratum appears in *Circulation*. 2015;131(15):e408]. *Circulation*. 2011;124(22):2458–73.

6. January CT, Wann LS, Alpert JS, et al; ACC/AHA Task Force Members. 2014 AHA/ACC/HRS guideline for the management of patients with atrial fibrillation: a report of the American College of Cardiology/American Heart Association Task Force on practice guidelines and the Heart Rhythm Society [Erratum appears in *Circulation*. 2014;130(23):e272–4]. *Circulation*. 2014;130(23):2071–104.

7. Yancy CW, Jessup M, Bozkurt, B, et al. 2017 ACC/AHA/HFSA focused update of the 2013 ACCF/AHA guideline for the management of heart failure: a report of the American College of Cardiology/American Heart Association Task Force on Clinical Practice Guidelines and the Heart Failure Society of America. *Circulation*. 2017;136:e137–61.

8. Mason RP, Giles TD, Sowers JR. Evolving mechanisms of action of beta blockers: focus on nebivolol. *J Cardiovasc Pharmacol*. 2009;54(2):123–8.

9. Reed BN, Street SE, Jensen BC. Time and technology will tell: the pathophysiologic basis of neurohormonal modulation in heart failure. *Heart Fail Clin*. 2014;10(4):543–57.

10. Viazzi F, Bonino B, Cappadona F, Pontremoli R. Renin-angiotensin-aldosterone system blockade in chronic kidney disease: current strategies and a look ahead. *Intern Emerg Med*. 2016;11(5):627–35.

11. Chobanian AV, Bakris GL, Black HR, et al; Joint National Committee on Prevention, Detection, Evaluation, and Treatment of High Blood Pressure; National Heart, Lung, and Blood Institute; National High Blood Pressure Education Program Coordinating Committee. Seventh report of the Joint National Committee on prevention, detection, evaluation, and treatment of high blood pressure. *Hypertension*. 2003;42(6):1206–52.

12. Brunton LL, Hilal-Dandan R, Knollmann BC. *Goodman & Gilman's The Pharmacological Basis of Therapeutics*. 13th ed. New York (NY): McGraw-Hill Medical; 2018.

13. Drugs.com. Angiotensin converting enzyme inhibitors. 2022. Available from: https://www.drugs.com/drug-class/angiotensin-converting-enzyme-inhibitors.html.

14. Mignat C, Unger T. ACE inhibitors. Drug interactions of clinical significance. *Drug Saf*. 1995;12(5):334–47.

15. Boldt J, Muller M, Heesen M, Harter K, Hempelmann G. Cardiorespiratory effects of continuous i.v. administration of the ACE inhibitor enalaprilat in the critically ill. *Br J Clin Pharmacol*. 1995;40(5):415–22.

16. Vescovo G, Dalla Libera L, Serafini F, et al. Improved exercise tolerance after losartan and enalapril in heart failure: correlation with changes in skeletal muscle myosin heavy chain composition. *Circulation*. 1998;98(17):1742–9.

17. Li EC, Heran BS, Wright JM. Angiotensin converting enzyme (ACE) inhibitors versus angiotensin receptor blockers for primary hypertension. *Cochrane Database Syst Rev*. 2014;2014(8):CD009096.

18. Drugs.com. Ernesto. 2022. Available from: https://www.drugs.com/search.php?searchterm=entresto.

19. Nougué H, Pezel T, Picard F, et al. Effects of sacubitril/valsartan on neprilysin targets and the metabolism of natriuretic peptides in chronic heart failure: a mechanistic clinical study. *Eur J Heart Fail*. 2019;21(5):598–605.

20. Vitale G, Romano G, DiFranco A, et al. Early effects of sacubitril/Valsartan on exercise tolerance in patients with heart failure with reduced ejection fraction. *J Clin Med*. 2019;8(2):262. doi:10.3390/jcm8020262.

21. Esteras R, Perez-Gomez MV, Rodriguez-Osorio L, Ortiz A, Fernandez-Fernandez B. Combination use of medicines from two classes of renin-angiotensin system blocking agents: risk of hyperkalemia, hypotension, and impaired renal function. *Ther Adv Drug Saf*. 2015;6(4):166–76.

22. Zamponi GW, Striessnig J, Koschak A, Dolphin AC. The physiology, pathology, and pharmacology of voltage-gated calcium channels and their future therapeutic potential. *Pharmacol Rev*. 2015;67(4):821–70.

23. Russell RP. Side effects of calcium channel blockers. *Hypertension*. 1988;11(3 Pt 2):II42–4.

24. Page RL, O'Bryant CL, Cheng D, et al; On behalf of the American Heart Association Clinical Pharmacology and Heart Failure and Transplantation Committees of the Council on Clinical Cardiology; Council on Cardiovascular Surgery and Anesthesia; Council on Cardiovascular and Stroke Nursing; and Council on Quality of Care and Outcomes Research. Drugs that may cause or exacerbate heart failure: a scientific statement from the American Heart Association. *Circulation*. 2016;134(6):e32–69.

25. Wiggins BS, Saseen JJ, Page RL, et al; American Heart Association Clinical Pharmacology Committee of the Council on Clinical Cardiology; Council on Hypertension; Council on Quality of Care and Outcomes Research; and Council on Functional Genomics and Translational Biology. Recommendations for management of clinically significant drug-drug interactions with statins and select agents used in patients with cardiovascular disease: a scientific statement from the American Heart Association. *Circulation*. 2016;134(21):e468–95.

26. Xu G, Chen J, Jing G, Shaley A. Preventing beta-cell loss and diabetes with calcium channel blockers. *Diabetes*. 2012;61(4):848–56.

27. Uesawa Y, Takeuchi T, Mohri K. Integrated analysis on the physicochemical properties of dihydropyridine calcium channel blockers in grapefruit juice interactions. *Curr Pharm Biotechnol.* 2012;13(9):1705–17.

28. Reents S. *Sport and Exercise Pharmacology.* Champaign (IL): Human Kinetics; 2000.

29. Al-Makki A, DiPette D, Whelton PK, et al. Hypertension pharmacological treatment in adults: a world health organization guideline executive summary. *Hypertension.* 2022;79: 293–301.

30. Rabi DM, McBrien KA, Sapir-Pichhadze R et al. Hypertension Canada's 2020 comprehensive guidelines for the prevention, diagnosis, risk assessment, and treatment of hypertension in adults and children. *Can J Cardiol.* 2020;36:596–624.

31. Whelton PK, Carey RM, Aronow WS, et al. 2017 ACC/AHA/ AAPA/ABC/ACPM/AGS/APhA/ASH/ASPC/NMA/PCNA guideline for the prevention, detection, evaluation, and management of high blood pressure in adults: a report of the American College of Cardiology/American Heart Association Task Force on Clinical Practice Guidelines. *Hypertension.* 2018;71:e13–115. doi:10.1161/HYP.0000000000000065.

32. Kosmala W, Rojek A, Przewlocka-Kosmala M, Wright L, Mysiak A, Marwick TH. Effect of aldosterone antagonism on exercise tolerance in heart failure with preserved ejection fraction. *J Am Coll Cardiol.* 2016;68(17):1823–34.

33. Somani SM. *Pharmacology in Exercise and Sports.* Boca Raton (FL): CRC Press; 1996.

34. Lepor H, Williford WO, Barry MJ, et al. The efficacy of terazosin, finasteride, or both in benign prostatic hyperplasia. Veterans affairs cooperative studies benign prostatic hyperplasia study group. *N Engl J Med.* 1996;335(8):533–9.

35. Westfall JL, Westfall DP. Adrenergic agonists and antagonists. In: Brunton LL, Chabner B, Knollmann BC, editors. *Goodman & Gilman's The Pharmacological Basis of Therapeutics.* 12th ed. New York (NY): McGraw-Hill Medical; 2011. p. 277–333.

36. Grassi G, Turri C, Seravalle G, Bertinieri G, Pierini A, Mancia G. Effects of chronic clonidine administration on sympathetic nerve traffic and baroreflex function in heart failure. *Hypertension.* 2001;38(2):286–91.

37. Taylor AL, Ziesche S, Yancy CW, et al; African American Heart Failure Trial Investigators. Early and sustained benefit on event-free survival and heart failure hospitalization from fixed-dose combination of isosorbide dinitrate/hydralazine: consistency across subgroups in the African American Heart Failure Trial. *Circulation.* 2007;115(13):1747–53.

38. Cohn JN, Archibald DG, Ziesche S, et al. Effect of vasodilator therapy on mortality in chronic congestive heart failure. Results of a Veterans Administration Cooperative Study. *N Engl J Med.* 1986;314(24):1547–52.

39. Maron BA, Rocco TP. Pharmacotherapy of congestive heart failure. In: Brunton LL, Chabner B, Hilal-Dandan R, Knollmann BC, editors. *Goodman & Gilman's The Pharmacological Basis of Therapeutics.* 132th ed. New York (NY): McGraw-Hill Medical; 2018. p. 789–814.

40. Kronig B, Pittrow DB, Kirch W, Welzel D, Weidinger G. Different concepts in first-line treatment of essential hypertension. Comparison of a low-dose reserpine-thiazide combination with nitrendipine monotherapy. German Reserpine in Hypertension Study Group. *Hypertension.* 1997;29(2):651–8.

41. Jahr JS, Weber S. Ventricular dysrhythmias following an alfentanil anesthetic in a patient on reserpine for hypertension. *Acta Anaesthesiol Scand.* 1991;35(8):788–9.

42. Eichhorn EJ, Gheorghiade M. Digoxin—new perspective on an old drug. *N Engl J Med.* 2002;347(18):1394–5.

43. Ziff OJ, Kotecha D. Digoxin: the good and the bad. *Trends Cardiovasc Med.* 2016;26(7):585–95.

44. Arena R, Humphrey R, Peberdy MA. Safety and efficacy of exercise training in a patient awaiting heart transplantation while on positive intravenous inotropic support. *J Cardiopulm Rehabil.* 2000;20(4):259–61.

45. McBride MG, Binder TJ, Paridon SM. Safety and feasibility of inpatient exercise training in pediatric heart failure: a preliminary report. *J Cardiopulm Rehabil Prev.* 2007;27(4):219–22.

46. White M, Ducharme A, Ibrahim R, et al. Increased systemic inflammation and oxidative stress in patients with worsening congestive heart failure: improvement after short-term inotropic support. *Clin Sci (Lond).* 2006;110(4):483–9.

47. Yancy CW, Jessup M, Bozkurt B, et al. 2016 ACC/AHA/HFSA focused update on new pharmacological therapy for heart failure: an update of the 2013 ACCF/AHA guideline for the management of heart failure: a report of the American College of Cardiology/American Heart Association Task Force on Clinical Practice Guidelines and the Heart Failure Society of America. *J Am Coll Cardiol.* 2016;68(13):1476–88.

48. Borer JS, Tavazzi L. Update on ivabradine for heart failure. *Trends Cardiovasc Med.* 2016;26(5):444–9.

49. Cammarano C, Silva M, Comee M, Donovan JL, Malloy MJ. Meta-analysis of ivabradine in patients with stable coronary artery disease with and without left ventricular dysfunction. *Clin Ther.* 2016;38(2):387–95.

50. Sampson KJ, Kass RS. Anti-arrhythmic drugs. In: Brunton LL, Chabner B, Hilal-Dandan R, Knollmann BC, editors. *Goodman & Gilman's The Pharmacological Basis of Therapeutics.* 132th ed. New York (NY): McGraw-Hill Medical; 2018. p. 815–47.

51. Banerjee K, Ghosh RK, Kamatam S, Banerjee A, Gupta A. Role of ranolazine in cardiovascular disease and diabetes: exploring beyond angina. *Int J Cardiol.* 2017;227:556–64.

52. Gong M, Zhang Z, Fragakis N, et al. Role of ranolazine in the prevention and treatment of atrial fibrillation: a meta-analysis of randomized clinical trials. *Heart Rhythm.* 2017;14(1):3–11.

53. ClinCalc.com. Ranolazine: Drug usage statistics, United States, 2013–2020. 2022. Available from: http://clincalc.com/ DrugStats/Drugs/Ranolazine/.

54. Hasenfuss G, Maier LS. Mechanism of action of the new anti-ischemia drug ranolazine. *Clin Res Cardiol.* 2008;97(4): 222–6.

55. Zack J, Berg J, Juan A, et al. Pharmacokinetic drug-drug interaction study of ranolazine and metformin in subjects with type 2 diabetes mellitus. *Clin Pharmacol Drug Dev.* 2015;4(2):121–9.

56. Mittal SR. Slow junctional rhythm, QTc prolongation and transient torsades de-pointes following combined use of ivabradine, diltiazem and ranolazine. *J Assoc Physicians India.* 2014;62(5):426–7.

57. Mishra A, Pandya HV, Dave N, Mathew M, Sapre CM, Chaudhary S. A rare debilitating neurological adverse effect of ranolazine due to drug interaction with clarithromycin. *Indian J Pharmacol.* 2014;46(5):547–8.

58. Masters JC, Shah MM, Feist AA. Drug interaction between sirolimus and ranolazine in a kidney transplant patient. *Case Rep Transplant*. 2014;2014:548243.

59. Finch KT, Stratton EA, Farber HW. Ranolazine for the treatment of pulmonary hypertension associated with heart failure with preserved ejection fraction: a pilot study. *J Heart Lung Transplant*. 2016;35(11):1370–3.

60. Navarese EP, Buffon A, Andreotti F, et al. Meta-analysis of impact of different types and doses of statins on new-onset diabetes mellitus. *Am J Cardiol*. 2013;111(8):1123–30.

61. Rosenson RS, Hegele RA, Fazio S, Cannon CP. The evolving future of PCSK9 inhibitors. *J Am Coll Cardiol*. 2018;72(3):314–29.

62. Sando KR, Knight M. Nonstatin therapies for management of dyslipidemia: a review. *Clin Ther*. 2015;37(10):2153–79.

63. Nissen SE, Tuzcu EM, Schoenhagen P, et al; REVERSAL Investigators. Effect of intensive compared with moderate lipid-lowering therapy on progression of coronary atherosclerosis: a randomized controlled trial. *JAMA*. 2004;291(9):1071–80.

64. Giacomini KM, Sugiyama Y. Membrane transporters and drug response. In: Brunton LL, Chabner B, Hilal-Dandan R, Knollmann BC, editors. *Goodman & Gilman's The Pharmacological Basis of Therapeutics*. 132th ed. New York (NY): McGraw-Hill Medical; 2018. p. 89–121.

65. Kastelein JJ, Akdim F, Stroes ES, et al; ENHANCE Investigators. Simvastatin with or without ezetimibe in familial hypercholesterolemia [Erratum appears in *N Engl J Med*. 2008;358(18):1977]. *N Engl J Med*. 2008;358(14):1431–43.

66. Florentin M, Liberopoulos EN, Elisaf MS. Ezetimibe-associated adverse effects: what the clinician needs to know. *Int J Clin Pract*. 2008;62(1):88–96.

67. Carnicelli AP, Hong H, Connolly SJ, et al; COMBINE AF (A Collaboration Between Multiple Institutions to Better Investigate Non-Vitamin K Antagonist Oral Anticoagulant Use in Atrial Fibrillation) Investigators. Direct oral anticoagulants versus warfarin in patients with atrial fibrillation: patient-level network meta-analyses of randomized clinical trials with interaction testing by age and sex. *Circulation*. 2022;145(4):242–55.

68. Alexander JH, Lopes RD, Thomas L, et al. Apixaban vs. warfarin with concomitant aspirin in patients with atrial fibrillation: insights from the ARISTOTLE trial. *Eur Heart J*. 2014;35(4):224–32.

69. Johnston SC, Easton JD, Farrant M, et al; Clinical Research Collaboration, Neurological Emergencies Treatment Trials Network, and the POINT Investigators. Clopidogrel and aspirin in acute ischemic stroke and high-risk TIA. *N Engl J Med*. 2018;379(3):215–25.

70. Weitz JI. Blood coagulation and anticoagulant, fibrinolytic, and antiplatelet drugs. In: Brunton LL, Chabner B, Hilal-Dandan R, Knollmann BC, editors. *Goodman & Gilman's The Pharmacological Basis of Therapeutics*. 132th ed. New York (NY): McGraw-Hill Medical; 2018. p. 849–76.

71. Tripodi A, Padovan L, Veena C, Scalambrino E, Testa S, Peyvandi F. How the direct oral anticoagulant apixaban affects thrombin generation parameters. *Thromb Res*. 2015;135(6):1186–90.

72. Egan G, Hughes CA, Ackman ML. Drug interactions between antiplatelet or novel oral anticoagulant medications and antiretroviral medications. *Ann Pharmacother*. 2014;48(6):734–40.

73. Tsai S, Liu Y, Alaiti MA, Gutierrez JA, Brilakis ES, Banerjee S. No benefit of vorapaxar on walking performance in patients with intermittent claudication. *Vasc Med*. 2022;27(1):33–8.

74. Centers for Disease Control and Prevention. National Center for Health Statistics. Chronic Obstructive Pulmonary Disease (COPD) includes: chronic bronchitis and emphysema. 2020. Available from: http://cdc.gov/nchs/fastats/copd.htm/.

75. Barnes PJ, Adcock IM. How do corticosteroids work in asthma? *Ann Intern Med*. 2003;139(5 Pt 1):359–70.

76. Sholter DE, Armstrong PW. Adverse effects of corticosteroids on the cardiovascular system. *Can J Cardiol*. 2000;16(4):505–11.

77. Parsons JP, Hallstrand TS, Mastronarde JG, et al; American Thoracic Society Subcommittee on Exercise-induced Bronchoconstriction. An official American Thoracic Society clinical practice guideline: exercise-induced bronchoconstriction. *Am J Respir Crit Care Med*. 2013;187(9):1016–27.

78. National Health Service (UK). Bronchodilators. 2022. Available from: https://www.nhs.uk/conditions/bronchodilators/.

79. Montastruc JL, Durrieu G, Sommet A, Damase-Michel C, Lapeyre-Mestre M. Anticholinergics, antimuscarinics or atropinics? About the words in pharmacology. *Br J Clin Pharmacol*. 2010;69(5):561–2.

80. Ogale SS, Lee TA, Au DH, Boudreau DM, Sullivan SD. Cardiovascular events associated with ipratropium bromide in COPD. *Chest*. 2010;137(1):13–9.

81. MedlinePlus.gov. *COPD—Control Drugs*. Bethesda (MD): National Library of Medicine; 2022. Available from: https://medlineplus.gov/ency/patientinstructions/000025.htm.

82. Klabunde RE. Beta-adrenoceptor agonists: cardiovascular pharmacology concepts. 2022. Available from: https://www.cvpharmacology.com/cardiostimulatory/beta-agonist.

83. RxList.com. Performoist. 2022. Available from: https://www.rxlist.com/perforomist-side-effects-drug-center.htm.

84. MedicineNet. Which drugs or supplements interact with bronchodilators? 2022. Available from: https://www.medicinenet.com/bronchodilators_for_asthma/article.htm#which_drugs_or_supplements_interact_with_bronchodilators?.

85. Anderson SD, Caillaud C, Brannan JD. Beta$_2$-agonists and exercise-induced asthma. *Clin Rev Allergy Immunol*. 2006;31(2–3):163–80.

86. Barnes PJ. Theophylline in chronic obstructive pulmonary disease: new horizons. *Proc Am Thorac Soc*. 2005;2(4):334–9; discussion 340–1.

87. Drugs.com. Methylxanthines. 2022. Available from: https://www.drugs.com/drug-class/methylxanthines.html.

88. Banasiak NC, Meadows-Oliver M. Leukotrienes: their role in the treatment of asthma and seasonal allergic rhinitis. *Pediatr Nurs*. 2005;31(1):35–8.

89. National Library of Medicine, National Center for Biotechnology Information. LiverTox: Clinical and Research Information on Drug-Induced Liver Injury: Zafirlukast. Bethesda (MD): National Institute of Diabetes and Digestive and Kidney Diseases; 2012 [Updated 2019 Jun 4]. Available from: https://www.ncbi.nlm.nih.gov/books/NBK547915/.

90. Drugs.com. Leukotriene modifiers. 2022. Available from: https://www.drugs.com/drug-class/leukotriene-modifiers.html.

91. Krawiec ME, Wenzel SE. Use of leukotriene antagonists in childhood asthma. *Curr Opin Pediatr*. 1999;11(6):540–7.

92. Olin BR. *Antihistamines. Drug Facts and Comparisons.* 55th ed. St. Louis (MO): Facts and Comparisons; 2001. p. 698–707.

93. Drugs.com. Guaifenesin NR prescribing information. 2022. Available from: https://www.drugs.com/pro/guaifenesin-nr .html.

94. Irwin RS, Curley FJ, Pratter MR. The effects of drugs on cough. *Eur J Respir Dis Suppl.* 1987;153:173–81.

95. Powers AC, D'Alessio D. Endocrine pancreas and pharmacotherapy of diabetes. In: Brunton LL, Chabner B, Hilal-Dandan R, Knollmann BC, editors. *Goodman & Gilman's The Pharmacological Basis of Therapeutics.* 13th ed. New York (NY): McGraw-Hill Medical; 2018. p. 1237–73.

96. Sherifali D, Nerenberg K, Pullenayegum E, Cheng JE, Gerstein H. The effect of oral antidiabetic agents on A1C levels: a systematic review and meta-analysis. *Diabetes Care.* 2010;33(8):1859–64.

97. Hirst JA, Farmer AJ, Dyar A, Lung TWC, Stevens RJ. Estimating the effect of sulfonylurea on HbA1c in diabetes: a systematic review and meta-analysis. *Diabetologia.* 2013;56(5):973–84.

98. Ceriello A. Postprandial hyperglycemia and diabetes complications: is it time to treat? *Diabetes.* 2005;54(1):1–7.

99. Inzucchi SE, Bergenstal RM, Buse JB, et al; American Diabetes Association (ADA); European Association for the Study of Diabetes (EASD). Management of hyperglycemia in type 2 diabetes: a patient-centered approach: position statement of the American Diabetes Association (ADA) and the European Association for the Study of Diabetes (EASD). *Diabetes Care.* 2012;35(6):1364–79.

100. Knowler WC, Barrett-Connor E, Fowler SE, et al; Diabetes Prevention Program Research Group. Reduction in the incidence of type 2 diabetes with lifestyle intervention or metformin. *N Engl J Med.* 2002;346(6):393–403.

101. Nathan DM, Buse JB, Davidson MB, et al. Medical management of hyperglycemia in type 2 diabetes: a consensus algorithm for the initiation and adjustment of therapy: a consensus statement of the American Diabetes Association and the European Association for the Study of Diabetes. *Diabetes Care.* 2009;32(1):193–203.

102. Holman RR, Paul SK, Bethel MA, Matthews DR, Neil HA. 10-year follow-up of intensive glucose control in type 2 diabetes. *N Engl J Med.* 2008;359(15):1577–89.

103. Selvin E, Bolen S, Yeh HC, et al. Cardiovascular outcomes in trials of oral diabetes medications: a systematic review. *Arch Intern Med.* 2008;168(19):2070–80.

104. Drugs.com. Metformin interactions. 2022. Available from: https://www.drugs.com/drug-interactions/metformin.html.

105. DREAM (Diabetes REduction Assessment with ramipril and rosiglitazone Medication) Trial Investigators; Gerstein HC, Yusuf S, Bosch J, et al. Effect of rosiglitazone on the frequency of diabetes in patients with impaired glucose tolerance or impaired fasting glucose: a randomised controlled trial [Erratum appears in *Lancet.* 2006;368(9549):1770]. *Lancet.* 2006;368(9541):1096–105.

106. Rangwala SM, Lazar MA. Peroxisome proliferator-activated receptor gamma in diabetes and metabolism. *Trends Pharmacol Sci.* 2004;25(6):331–6.

107. Nissen SE, Wolski K. Effect of rosiglitazone on the risk of myocardial infarction and death from cardiovascular causes [Erratum appears in *N Engl J Med.* 2007;357(1):100]. *N Engl J Med.* 2007;356(24):2457–71.

108. Tanne JH. FDA places "black box" warning on antidiabetes drugs. *BMJ.* 2007;334(7606):1237.

109. Meier C, Kraenzlin ME, Bodmer M, Jick SS, Jick H, Meier CR. Use of thiazolidinediones and fracture risk. *Arch Int Med.* 2008;168(8):820–5.

110. Lebovitz HE, Kreider M, Freed MI. Evaluation of liver function in type 2 diabetic patients during clinical trials: evidence that rosiglitazone does not cause hepatic dysfunction. *Diabetes Care.* 2002;25(5):815–21.

111. van de Laar FA, Lucassen PL, Akkermans RP, van de Lisdonk EH, Rutten GE, van Weel C. Alpha-glucosidase inhibitors for patients with type 2 diabetes: results from a Cochrane systematic review and meta-analysis. *Diabetes Care.* 2005;28(1):154–63.

112. Aroda VR, Henry RR, Han J, et al. Efficacy of GLP-1 receptor agonists and DPP-4 inhibitors: meta-analysis and systematic review. *Clin Ther.* 2012;34(6):1247–58.e1222.

113. Amori RE, Lau J, Pittas AG. Efficacy and safety of incretin therapy in type 2 diabetes: systematic review and meta-analysis. *JAMA.* 2007;298:194–206.

114. Wilding JPH, Batterham RL, Calanna S, et al. Once weekly semaglutide in adults with overweight and obesity. *N Engl J Med.* 2021;384:989–1002. doi:10.1056/NEJMoa2032183.

115. Rubino DM, Greenway FL, Khalid, U, et.al; STEP 8 Investigators. Effect of weekly subcutaneous semaglutide vs daily liraglutide on body weight in adults with overweight or obesity without diabetes the step 8 randomized clinical trial. *JAMA.* 2022;327(2):138–50. doi:10.1001/jama.2021.23619.

116. Marso SP, Daniels GH, Brown-Frandsen K, et al; LEADER Steering Committee; LEADER Trial Investigators. Liraglutide and cardiovascular outcomes in type 2 diabetes. *N Engl J Med.* 2016;375(4):311–22.

117. Marso SP, Bain SC, Consoli A, et al; SUSTAIN-6 Investigators. Semaglutide and cardiovascular outcomes in patients with type 2 diabetes. *N Engl J Med.* 2016;375(19):1834–44.

118. Blonde L, Russell-Jones D. The safety and efficacy of liraglutide with or without oral antidiabetic drug therapy in type 2 diabetes: an overview of the LEAD 1-5 studies. *Diabetes Obes Metab.* 2009;11(Suppl 3):26–34.

119. Derosa G, Maffioli P, Salvadeo SA, et al. Exenatide versus glibenclamide in patients with diabetes. *Diabetes Technol Ther.* 2010;12(3):233–40.

120. Zinman B, Gerich J, Buse JB, et al; LEAD-4 Study Investigators. Efficacy and safety of the human glucagon-like peptide-1 analog liraglutide in combination with metformin and thiazolidinedione in patients with type 2 diabetes (LEAD-4 Met+TZD) [Erratum appears in *Diabetes Care.* 2010;33(3):692]. *Diabetes Care.* 2009;32(7):1224–30.

121. Meier JJ, Gethmann A, Gotze O, Gallwitz B, Holst JJ, Schmidt WE. Glucagon-like peptide 1 abolishes the postprandial rise in triglyceride concentrations and lowers levels of non-esterified fatty acids in humans. *Diabetologia.* 2006;49(3):452–8.

122. Monami M, Iacomelli I, Marchionni N, Mannucci E. Dipeptidyl peptidase 4 inhibitors in type 2 diabetes: a meta-analysis of randomized clinical trials. *Nutr Metab Cardiovasc Dis.* 2010;20(4):224–35.

123. Frederich R, Alexander JH, Fiedorek FT, et al. A systematic assessment of cardiovascular outcomes in the saxagliptin

drug development program for type 2 diabetes. *Postgrad Med.* 2010;122(3):16–27.

124. Brown NJ, Byiers S, Carr D, Maldonado M, Warner BA. Dipeptidyl peptidase-IV inhibitor use associated with increased risk of ACE inhibitor-associated angioedema. *Hypertension.* 2009;54(3):516–23.

125. Ferrannini E, Ramos SJ, Salsali A, Tang W, List JF. Dapagliflozin monotherapy in type 2 diabetic patients with inadequate glycemic control by diet and exercise: a randomized, double-blind, placebo-controlled, phase 3 trial. *Diabetes Care.* 2010;33(10):2217–24.

126. Liakos A, Karagiannis T, Athanasiadou E, et al. Efficacy and safety of empagliflozin for type 2 diabetes: a systematic review and meta-analysis. *Diabetes Obes Metab.* 2014;16(10):984–93.

127. Zinman B, Wanner C, Lachin JM, et al; EMPA-REG OUTCOME Investigators. Empagliflozin, cardiovascular outcomes, and mortality in type 2 diabetes. *N Engl J Med.* 2015;373(22):2117–28.

128. Zannad F, Ferreira, JP, Pocock SJ, et al. SGLT2 inhibitors in patients with heart failure with reduced ejection fraction: a meta-analysis of the EMPEROR-Reduced and DAPA-HF trials. *Lancet.* 2020;396:819–29.

129. Nassif ME, Windsor SL, Borlaug BA, et al. The SGLT2 inhibitor dapagliflozin in heart failure with preserved ejection fraction: a multicenter randomized trial. *Nat Med.* 2021;27(11):1954–60. doi:10.1038/s41591-021-01536-x.

130. Wanner C, Inzucchi SE, Lachin JM, et al; EMPA-REG OUTCOME Investigators. Empagliflozin and progression of kidney disease in type 2 diabetes. *N Engl J Med.* 2016;375(4):323–34.

131. Gallo LA, Wright EM, Vallon V. Probing SGLT2 as a therapeutic target for diabetes: basic physiology and consequences. *Diab Vasc Dis Res.* 2015;12(2):78–89.

132. Joslin Education Team. *Different Types of Insulin.* Boston (MA): Joslin Diabetes Center; 2022. Available from: https://www.joslin.org/patient-care/diabetes-education/diabetes-learning-center/different-types-insulin.

133. Leohr J, Dellva MA, LaBelle E, et al. Pharmacokinetic and glucodynamic responses of ultra-rapid lispro vs lispro across a clinically relevant range of subcutaneous doses in healthy subjects. *Clin Ther.* 2020;42(9):1762–77. doi:10.1016/J.Clinthera.2020.07.005.

134. Ogbru O. *Insulin for Diabetes Treatment (Types, Side Effects, and Preparations).* San Clemente (CA): MedicineNet, Inc; 2022. Available from: https://www.medicinenet.com/insulin_for_diabetes_treatment_types_side_effects/article.htm.

135. Hamdy O. *Obesity Medication.* New York (NY): Medscape; 2022. Available from: https://emedicine.medscape.com/article/123702-medication#showall.

136. Drugs.com. Orlistat. 2022. Available from: https://www.drugs.com/orlistat.html.

137. PDR.net. *Qsymia (phentermine/topiramate): Drug Summary.* Whippany (NJ): PDR, LLC; 2022. Available from: http://www.pdr.net/drug-summary/Qsymia-phentermine-topiramate-2564.2036.

138. Wadden TA, Foreyt JP, Foster GD, et al. Weight loss with naltrexone SR/bupropion SR combination therapy as an adjunct to behavior modification: the COR-BMOD trial. *Obesity (Silver Spring).* 2011;19(1):110–20.

139. Drugs.com. Contrave prescribing information. 2022. Available from: https://www.drugs.com/pro/contrave.html.

140. WebMD. What are the treatments for kidney disease? 2022. Available from: https://www.webmd.com/a-to-z-guides/understanding-kidney-disease-treatment#1.

141. Go CL, Rosales RL, Schmidt P, Lyons KE, Pahwa R, Okun MS. Generic versus branded pharmacotherapy in Parkinson's disease: does it matter? A review. *Parkinsonism Relat Disord.* 2011;17(5):308–12.

142. Standaert DG, Roberson ED. Treatment of central nervous system degenerative disorders. In: Brunton LL, Chabner B, Hilal-Dandan R, Knollmann BC, Editors. *Goodman & Gilman's The Pharmacological Basis of Therapeutics.* 132th ed. New York (NY): McGraw-Hill Medical; 2018. p. 609–28.

143. Brooks DJ. Dopamine agonists: their role in the treatment of Parkinson's disease. *J Neurol Neurosurg Psychiatry.* 2000;68(6):685–9.

144. Rascol O, Brooks DJ, Brunt ER, Korczyn AD, Poewe WH, Stocchi F. Ropinirole in the treatment of early Parkinson's disease: a 6-month interim report of a 5-year levodopa-controlled study. 056 Study Group. *Mov Disord.* 1998;13(1):39–45.

145. Lieberman JA. Managing anticholinergic side effects [Erratum appears in *Prim Care Companion J Clin Psychiatry.* 2012;14(1):PCC.12lcx01362]. *Prim Care Companion J Clin Psychiatry.* 2004;6(Suppl 2):20–3.

146. Rudick RA, Goelz SE. Beta-interferon for multiple sclerosis. *Exp Cell Res.* 2011;317(9):1301–11.

147. Drugs.com. Copaxone prescribing information. 2022. Available from: https://www.drugs.com/pro/copaxone.html.

148. Drugs.com. Zinbryta prescribing information. 2022. Available from: https://www.drugs.com/pro/zinbryta.html.

149. Drugs.com. Aubagio prescribing information. 2022. Available from: https://www.drugs.com/pro/aubagio.html.

150. Drugs.com. Gilenya prescribing information. 2022. Available from: https://www.drugs.com/pro/gilenya.html.

151. Grosser T, Smyth E, Fitzgerald GA. Anti-inflammatory, antipyretic and analgesic agents. In: Brunton LL, Chabner B, Hilal-Dandan R, Knollmann BC, editors. *Goodman & Gilman's The Pharmacological Basis of Therapeutics.* 13th ed. New York (NY): McGraw-Hill Medical; 2018. p. 959–1004.

152. Medline Plus. *Acetaminophen*; 2023. Available from: https://medlineplus.gov/druginfo/meds/a681004.html.

153. Coxib and traditional NSAID Trialists' (CNT) Collaboration; Bhala N, Emberson J, Merhi A, et al. Vascular and upper gastrointestinal effects of non-steroidal anti-inflammatory drugs: meta-analyses of individual participant data from randomised trials. *Lancet.* 2013;382(9894):769–79.

154. Hohlfeld T, Saxena A, Schror K. High on treatment platelet reactivity against aspirin by non-steroidal anti-inflammatory drugs—pharmacological mechanisms and clinical relevance. *Thromb Haemost.* 2013;109(5):825–33.

155. Friedman PA. Agents affecting mineral ion homeostasis and bone turnover. In: Brunton LL, Chabner B, Hilal-Dandan R, Knollmann BC, editors. *Goodman & Gilman's The Pharmacological Basis of Therapeutics.* 13th ed. New York (NY): McGraw-Hill Medical; 2018. p. 1275–306.

156. Drugs.com. Fosamax prescribing information. 2022. Available from: https://www.drugs.com/pro/fosamax.html.

157. Mayo Clinic. *Osteoporosis Treatment: Medications Can Help.* Rochester (MN): Mayo Foundation for Medical Education & Research; 2022. Available from: https://www

.mayoclinic.org/diseases-conditions/osteoporosis/in-depth/osteoporosis-treatment/art-20046869.

158. Mayo Clinic. *Rheumatoid Arthritis*. Rochester (MN): Mayo Foundation for Medical Education & Research; 2022. Available from: https://www.mayoclinic.org/diseases-conditions/rheumatoid-arthritis/symptoms-causes/syc-20353648.

159. WebMD. Rheumatoid arthritis drug guide. 2022. Available from: https://www.webmd.com/rheumatoid-arthritis/rheumatoid-arthritis-medications#1.

160. UpToDate. *Adjuvant Endocrine Therapy for Postmenopausal Women With Hormone Receptor Positive Breast Cancer*. Philadelphia (PA): Wolters Kluwer; 2022. Available from: https://www.uptodate.com/contents/adjuvant-endocrine-therapy-for-postmenopausal-women-with-hormone-receptor-positive-breast-cancer.

161. Condorelli R, Vaz-Luis I. Managing side effects in adjuvant endocrine therapy for breast cancer. *Expert Rev Anticancer Ther*. 2018;18(11):1101–12.

162. Khosrow-Khavar F, Filion KB, Al-Qurashi S, et al. Cardiotoxicity of aromatase inhibitors and tamoxifen in postmenopausal women with breast cancer: a systematic review and meta-analysis of random controlled trials. *Ann Oncol*. 2017;28:487–96.

163. Franzoi MA, Agostinetto E, Mastro LD, et al. Evidence-based approaches for the management of side-effects of adjuvant endocrine therapy in patients with breast cancer. *Lancet Oncol*. 2021;22:e303–13.

164. Yu Q, Xu Y, Yu E, Zheng Z. Risk of cardiovascular disease in breast cancer patients receiving aromatase inhibitors vs. tamoxifen: a systematic review and meta-analysis. *J Clin Pharm Ther*. 2022;47(5):575–87.

165. Cifra B, Chen CK, Fan CS, et al. Dynamic myocardial response to exercise in childhood cancer survivors treated with anthracyclines. *J Am Soc Echocardiogr*. 2018;31:933–42.

166. Bonsignore A, Marwick TH, Adams SC, et al. Clinical, echocardiographic, and biomarker associations with impaired cardiorespiratory fitness early after HER2-targeted breast cancer therapy. *JACC CardioOncol*. 2021;3(5):678–91.

167. UpToDate. *Clinical Manifestations Monitoring and Diagnosis of Anthracycline Induced Cardiotoxicity*. Philadelphia (PA): Wolters Kluwer; 2022. Available from: https://www.uptodate.com/contents/clinical-manifestations-monitoring-and-diagnosis-of-anthracycline-induced-cardiotoxicity?search=anthracycline&source=search_result&selectedTitle=1~150&usage_type=default&display_rank=1.

168. Jones LW, Haykowsky MJ, Swartz JJ, Douglas PS, Mackey JR. Early breast cancer therapy and cardiovascular injury. *J Am Coll Cardiol*. 2007;50(15):1435–41.

169. Hoshina H, Takei H. Drug-induced interstitial lung disease after anthracycline-combined chemotherapy for breast cancer: a case report and literature review. *Case Rep Oncol*. 2021;14:1671–6.

170. Kirkham AA, Haykowsky MJ, Beaudry RI, et al. Cardiac and skeletal muscle predictors of impaired cardiorespiratory fitness post-anthracycline chemotherapy for breast cancer. *Sci Rep*. 2021;11:14005.

171. UpToDate. *Acute Side Effects of Adjuvant Chemotherapy for Early-Stage Breast Cancer*. Philadelphia (PA): Wolters Kluwer; 2022. Available from: https://www.uptodate.com/contents/acute-side-effects-of-adjuvant-chemotherapy-for-early-stage-breast-cancer?search=taxanes%20side%20effects&source=search_result&selectedTitle=1~150&usage_type=default&display_rank=1#H4008994931.

172. Bertrand EM, Caru M, Lemay V, et al. Heart rate response and chronotropic incompetence during cardiopulmonary exercise testing in childhood acute lymphoblastic leukemia survivors. *Pediatr Hematol Oncol*. 2021;38(6):564–80 doi:10.1080/08880018.2021.1894279.

173. Gomes-Santos IL, Jordao CP, Passos CS, et al. Exercise training preserves myocardial strain and improves exercise tolerance in doxorubicin-induced cardiotoxicity. *Front Cardiovasc Med*. 2021;8:605993.

174. Gui Q, Li D, Zhuge Y, Xu C. Efficacy of exercise rehabilitation program in relieving oxaliplatin induced peripheral neurotoxicity. *Asian Pac J Cancer Prev*. 2021;22(3):705–9.

175. Gustafson MP, Wheatley-Guy CM, Rosenthal AC, et al. Exercise and the immune system: taking steps to improve responses to cancer immunotherapy. *J Immunother Cancer*. 2021;9:e001872.

176. Simsek NY, Demir A. Cold application and exercise on development of peripheral neuropathy during taxane chemotherapy in breast cancer patients: a randomized controlled trial. *Asia Pac J Oncol Nurs*. 2021;8:255–66.

177. UpToDate. *Toxicities Associated With Checkpoint Inhibitor Immunotherapy*. Philadelphia (PA): Wolters Kluwer; 2022. Available from: https://www.uptodate.com/contents/toxicities-associated-with-checkpoint-inhibitor-immunotherapy?search=Checkpoint%20inhibitor%20immunotherapy&source=search_result&selectedTitle=2~150&usage_type=default&display_rank=2.

178. Sodergren SC, Copson E, White A, et al. Systematic review of the side effects associated with anti-HER2-targeted therapies used in the treatment of breast cancer, on behalf of the EORTC quality of life group. *Target Oncol*. 2016;11:277–92.

179. Medline Plus. *Pertuzumab injection*. 2023. Available from: https://medlineplus.gov/druginfo/meds/a612027.html.

180. Medline Plus. *Fam-trastuzumab deruxtecan-nxki Injection*; 2023. Available from: https://medlineplus.gov/druginfo/meds/a620006.html.

181. Hojan K, Procyk D, Horynksa-Kestowicz D, Leporowska E, Litwiniuk M. The preventive role of regular physical training in ventricular remodeling, serum cardiac markers, and exercise performance changes in breast cancer in women undergoing trastuzumab therapy—an REH-HER study. *J Clin Med*. 2020;9:1379–94.

182. UpToDate. *Infusion Related Reactions to Therapeutic Monoclonal Antibodies Used for Cancer Therapy*. Philadelphia (PA): Wolters Kluwer; 2022. Available from: https://www.uptodate.com/contents/infusion-related-reactions-to-therapeutic-monoclonal-antibodies-used-for-cancer-therapy?search=herceptin%20and%20muscle%20spasms&anchor=H19&language=en-US&source=preview#H19.

183. Vonbank K, Lehmann A, Bernitzky D, et al. Predictors of prolonged cardiopulmonary exercise impairment after COVID-19 infection. a prospective observational study *Front Med*. 2021;8:773788.

184. Salman D, Vishnubala D, LeFeuvre P, et al. Returning to physical activity after COVID-19. *BMJ*. 2021;372:m4721.

185. Oster ME, Shay DK, Su JR, et al. Myocarditis cases reported after mRNA-based COVID-19 vaccination in the US from December 2020 to August 2021. *JAMA*. 2022;327(4):331–40.

186. Gottlieb RL, Vaca CE, Paredes R, et al; GS-US-540-9012 (PINETREE) Investigators. Early remdesivir to prevent progression to severe COVID-19 in outpatients. *N Engl J Med*. 2022;386:305–15.

187. Lai C, Chen CH, Wang CY, Chen KH, Wang YH, Hsueh PR. Clinical efficacy and safety of remdesivir in patients with COVID-19: a systematic review and network meta-analysis of randomized clinical trials. *J Antimicrob Chemother*. 2021;76:1962–8.

188. Casadevall A, Dragotakes Q, Johnson PW, et al. Convalescent plasma use in the USA was inversely correlated with COVID-19 mortality. *ELife*. 2021;10:e69866.

189. Takashita E, Kinoshita N, Yamayoshi S, et al. Efficacy of antibodies and antiviral drugs against COVID-19 omicron variant. *N Engl J Med*. 2022;386(10):995–8. doi:10.1056/NEJMc2119407.

190. Ortigoza MB, Yoon H, Goldfield KS, et al. Efficacy and safety of COVID-19 convalescent plasma in hospitalized patients: a random controlled trial. *JAMA Intern Med*. 2022;182(2):115–26.

CHAPTER 8

Respiratory Diseases

INTRODUCTION

Breathing is a vital process that sustains life through provision of oxygen and removal of carbon dioxide. By breathing 12 or more times per minute, every minute of every day, the average human being takes more than 500 million breaths during an average lifespan. Although we have a degree of conscious control over our breathing, the process is typically unnoticed. This is not to say that breathing occurs in a haphazard manner; in fact, a myriad of sensory and regulatory mechanisms ensure that the air ventilated by the lungs is sufficient to maintain oxygen and carbon dioxide at levels within a normal homeostatic range. This regulatory control is sensitive and dynamic enough to control oxygen and carbon dioxide levels even when the metabolic rate is increased 10-fold or more in healthy adults during exercise.

Unfortunately, things can and do go wrong within the respiratory system. Respiratory diseases affect airflow in and out of the lungs, they can cause areas within the lungs to be disproportionately ventilated with respect to the amount of blood flow they receive, and they can alter the structure of the lung parenchyma, thereby diminishing the efficiency of oxygen and carbon dioxide transport (gas exchange) across the alveolar–capillary interface. Moreover, the impact of respiratory disease extends beyond the lungs to contribute to skeletal muscle dysfunction altering the perception of physical effort, making physical activity feel disproportionately difficult for the actual intensity (Figure 8.1). Chronic respiratory disease burdens the sufferer with dyspnea and fatigue, anxiety, activity avoidance, and physical deconditioning. For those affected, physical capacity and productivity are lost, and quality of life is diminished.

EPIDEMIOLOGY OF RESPIRATORY DISEASE

Respiratory disease is an immense health burden, with five respiratory diseases (chronic obstructive pulmonary disease [COPD], asthma, acute lower respiratory infections, tuberculosis, and lung cancer) being among the most common causes of severe illness and death worldwide (1, 2). Analysis of data from the Global Burden of Diseases, Injuries, and Risk Factors Study 2017 showed that nearly 545 million people worldwide had a chronic respiratory illness in 2017, representing a nearly 40% increase in incidence since 1990 (3).

Communicable respiratory diseases such as pneumonia and acute lower respiratory tract infections account for as many as 2.4 million deaths annually (1, 4) and are a leading cause of death in children and adults older than 65 years of age (5–7). In 2020, the WHO estimated that 9.8 million people were infected with tuberculosis and as many as 1.5 million died from the disease (8). At the time of writing, there have been nearly 540 million confirmed cases of severe acute respiratory syndrome coronavirus 2 (SARS-CoV-2) and 6.3 million deaths worldwide from the virus that continues to give rise to new variants and infections (9). With exception of the recent increase in deaths attributable to SARS-CoV-2, the overall death rate because of all infectious respiratory diseases has been trending downward owing to improved infection control and disease management (4).

Chronic noncommunicable respiratory diseases such as COPD, asthma, cystic fibrosis, and lung cancer are a growing global burden. COPD is estimated to affect more than 200 million people and is the third leading cause of death, killing approximately 3.2 million people per year (1).

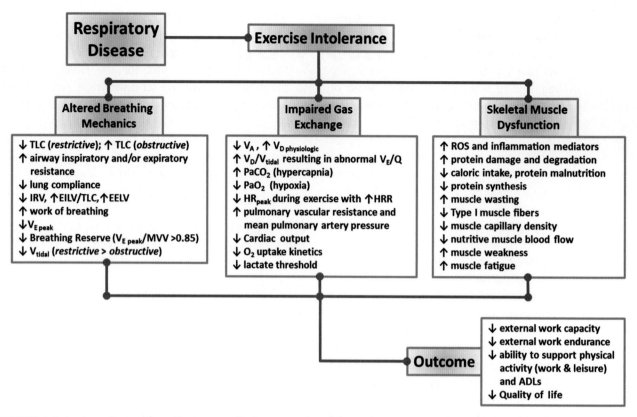

FIGURE 8.1 A schematic overview of factors contributing to exercise intolerance in those with respiratory disease. ADL, activities of daily living; EELV, end-expiratory lung volume; EILV, end-inspiratory lung volume; HRR, heart rate reserve; IRV, inspiratory reserve volume; MVV, maximum voluntary ventilation; ROS, reactive oxygen species; TLC, total lung capacity.

Asthma affects up to 350 million people worldwide, and it is the most common chronic disease in childhood (1). More than 250,000 deaths are attributed to asthma annually (10, 11). Lung cancer is the second most diagnosed cancer, and it is a leading cause of cancer-related death. In 2020, there were 2.2 million new lung cancer cases representing approximately one in 10 (11.4%) of all new cancers diagnosed; and 1.8 million lung cancer deaths representing one in 5 (18.0%) cancer deaths (12). In contrast, cystic fibrosis affects far fewer individuals. It is difficult to estimate accurately worldwide incidence rates for cystic fibrosis because many children die before diagnosis in countries lacking developed health care systems. Current estimates suggest that cystic fibrosis affects 70,000–160,000 people worldwide and, as with asthma, the burden of this disease is expected to grow (13). Approximately 1 in 20 Americans carries an abnormal cystic fibrosis transmembrane conductance regulator (*CFTR*) gene, and each heterozygous adult pair has a 25% chance of producing offspring with two abnormal *CFTR* genes and cystic fibrosis.

Altogether, it is clear that respiratory disease is a major public health burden, affecting people both acutely and chronically over their lifetime. Management strategies that ease the burden individually as well as from a public health perspective are needed to reduce the impact of respiratory disease.

Epidemiology of COPD

The Global Initiative for Chronic Obstructive Lung Disease (12) defines COPD as "... a common, preventable and treatable disease that is characterized by persistent respiratory symptoms and airflow limitation that is due to airway and/or alveolar abnormalities usually caused by significant exposure to noxious particles or gases." Frequent exposure to tobacco smoke, and environmental or occupational exposure to organic and inorganic dusts, chemical fumes, and pollution are recognized contributors to the development of COPD (7). Exposure to noxious substances provokes an enhanced inflammatory response that affects the large and small airways as well as the lung parenchyma (the acini or respiratory bronchioles, alveolar ducts, and alveoli). Hypersecretion of mucus from hypertrophied submucosal glands and goblet cells leads to the chronic cough and sputum production characteristic of chronic bronchitis. In emphysema, chronic inflammation increases small airway resistance through airway narrowing and loss, and it destroys the lung parenchyma, reducing both the lung's elastic recoil and the tethering between acini and small airways (13). The loss of structural support allows small airways to collapse during exhalation leading to lung hyperinflation and a sense of breathlessness. COPD is a chronic condition that worsens and becomes more debilitating over time.

As just noted, COPD is estimated to affect more than 200 million people worldwide and it is the third leading cause of death, killing approximately 3.2 million people per year (1). The true mortality rate may be much higher, as underdiagnosis and underreporting of COPD as the primary cause of death have been identified in many areas of the world (14). An increase in smoking in developing countries and an aging population in advanced nations is expected to increase the global prevalence of COPD further; in addition, by 2060, it is expected that there will be more than 5.4 million COPD-attributable deaths per year (14).

COPD is the third leading cause of death in the U.S., behind heart disease and cancer (15). An estimated 15.7 million Americans (6.4% of the population) have been diagnosed with COPD, and a similar number are likely to be living with undiagnosed COPD (15, 16). The age-adjusted mortality rate rose from 29.4 per 100,000 in 1968 to 67.0 per 100,000 in 1999 but has declined since then to 63.7 per 100,000 in 2011 (17). Similar mortality rates have been reported in the United Kingdom, Canada, and New Zealand (18–20). Prevalence is highest in smokers versus nonsmokers and in those over the age of 40 years (21). Males are more likely to be diagnosed with COPD, but the gender gap is narrowing (14, 17, 19).

The chronic and progressive nature of COPD makes the disease expensive to manage, and there is a direct relationship between disease severity and management cost. Exacerbations, which are periods of worsening symptoms requiring hospitalization or medication adjustments, account for the greatest proportion of direct health care spending for respiratory disease. An estimated 8 million outpatient visits and 1.5 million emergency department visits are made by patients with COPD per year in the U.S. As many as 726,000 hospitalizations annually are caused by COPD, with an average 6.3-day length of stay at a mean cost of USD$10,684 per stay (20, 22). The direct health care costs associated with COPD in the U.S. in 2010 were USD$32 billion with another USD$20.4 billion in indirect costs such as lost work productivity and disability (23). Similar total and proportional costs are incurred by the European Union (38.6 billion euros) and Canada ($1.7 billion) per year to manage COPD (16, 24).

The etiology of COPD is not completely understood but is thought to evolve from a complex interaction between genetics and the environment. The most well-established genetic link for the development of COPD is in those who are α1-antitrypsin deficient, but this deficiency accounts for only a small percentage of the world's COPD cases (25). Other single genes or polynucleotide polymorphisms and gene clusters may result in one or more COPD risk phenotypes but causal genes remain unidentified (26, 27). Aging is a risk factor for COPD and many age-related changes in the airways mimic those changes occurring as a result of COPD (28). Although men used to have greater prevalence and mortality from COPD, this is no longer the case as men and women now have similar COPD incidence and mortality rates; likely due to changes in smoking behavior (29, 30). Although not conclusive, emerging evidence suggests that women may incur greater harm from smoking (31). Tobacco and/ or marijuana smoking are directly related to the prevalence of COPD and are a common risk factor (32, 33). It must be noted, however, that up to 50% of heavy smokers do not develop COPD (21) and that COPD also occurs in nonsmokers (34). A study by McCloskey et al. (35) showed a strong familial risk for airflow limitation among parents and siblings of patients with severe COPD when compared to a sample population in Great Britain (35). Exposure to particles, organic and inorganic dusts, chemical agents and fumes, biomass combustion, and urban pollution is associated with a higher incidence of respiratory symptoms, airway obstruction, and COPD. Similarly, factors that affect lung growth and development, and having low socioeconomic status, asthma, airway hyperreactivity, frequent respiratory infections, and chronic bronchitis, are all established risk factors for developing COPD (14).

Epidemiology of Asthma

The Global Initiative for Asthma (GINA) defines asthma as ". . . a heterogeneous disease, usually characterized by chronic airway inflammation. It is defined by the history of respiratory symptoms such as wheeze, shortness of breath, chest tightness and cough that vary over time and in intensity, together with variable expiratory airflow limitation" (36). The Global Asthma Network estimates that more than 350 million men, women, and children of all ages and ethnic backgrounds have asthma (37). The burden of asthma is high causing nearly 500,000 deaths per year and it is a frequent cause of preventable hospital admission for children living in high-income countries. Asthma is the most common chronic disease in children and is often more severe in middle- and low-income countries with underdiagnosis and undertreatment common (1).

Asthma in the U.S.

About 8% of the U.S. population has asthma translating to approximately 25.5 million people, of which more than 5.9 million are children under the age of 17 years. The prevalence of asthma is 1.5 times greater for females than for males. The prevalence is higher among non-Hispanic Black people (10.4%) than among non-Hispanic Caucasians (8.0%) or Hispanics (6.4%), although Hispanics identifying as Puerto Rican are disproportionally affected (14.0%). The prevalence of asthma also varies with socioeconomic status, with higher rates among those with a household income below 100% of the poverty level as compared to those with a household income at 450% of the poverty level or higher (38).

Between 2016 and 2018, 11.7 million Americans reported having an asthma attack and 3.1 million were children under 17 years of age. There are 10.8 million physician office visits and 1.3 million hospital outpatient visits with 439,000 hospital discharges per year for which asthma was the primary reason or diagnosis. The age-adjusted death rate is 10.8 per million for all patients with asthma, and it is 2.7 per million for children under 18 years of age. Again, non-Hispanic Black people are affected more (29.5 per million) than other ethnic groups (38, 39). The economic burden of asthma is estimated at USD$56 billion per year when direct medical costs from hospital stays and indirect costs such as lost school and workdays are considered (40), and a recent probabilistic model estimates the total direct cost of asthma will be USD$300.6 billion with a total economic burden of USD$963.5 billion over the next 20 years (41).

Describing Asthma

Although a specific cause is unknown, asthma involves a complex interaction between host genetics and a wide range of environmental factors that result in the development of airflow obstruction, bronchial hyperresponsiveness, and inflammation. The dominant aspect of the disease that produces clinical symptoms is airway smooth muscle constriction and inflammation, both of which lead to airway narrowing and obstruction and make ventilation of the lungs more difficult. The disease is chronic with periods of acute flare-up during which the symptoms become exacerbated. Each flare-up is usually the result of exposure

to a triggering factor and/or poor disease control and management. Chronic inflammation leads to structural changes within the airways, including smooth muscle hyperplasia, subepithelial fibrosis, blood vessel proliferation, and infiltration of inflammatory cells (42, 43).

The view of asthma as a single disease or disease process is considered out of date. Asthma is now viewed as a collection of related diseases or disease phenotypes that result from multiple biologic mechanisms with discreet and overlapping elements. Researchers have described a variety of asthma phenotypes. (A *phenotype* is an observable manifestation of the interaction between an individual's genotype and their environment. A phenotype may change over time and with exposure to new environments.) These different asthma phenotypes may offer a mechanism by which different forms of asthma can be categorized. Further refinement of this concept has led some groups to propose that different asthma types can be arranged into different endotypes; that is, specific biologic pathways that explain the observable properties of the phenotype. Endotypes form distinct entities based on observable criteria such as symptoms, biomarkers, lung physiology, genetics, histopathology, immunology, and response to treatment. Although there is agreement that a classification system based on endotypes is necessary and could improve disease management and treatment selection, there is no widespread agreement on which endotype classification system should be used. Disagreement arises because a phenotype may fit into one or more endotypes and an endotype may contain more than one phenotype. A proposed endotype classification system is outlined in Table 8.1 (44).

Risk Factors Associated With Asthma

Although a family history is not necessary or sufficient for the development of asthma, several studies show that the offspring of affected parents have a much greater chance of developing asthma themselves (45, 46). Maternal inheritance appears stronger than paternal inheritance (47). Genetic studies illustrate that there is broad genetic heterogeneity in asthma with hundreds of genes potentially influencing asthma development. Genome-wide association studies to identify genetic differences in the population between those with and without asthma have found that the *17q21* locus differs between groups. Alteration of four genes within this locus (*ORMDL3, GSDMB, ZPBP2,* and *IKZF3*) interferes with protein folding in the endoplasmic reticulum, resulting in a proinflammatory effect that could contribute to the airway inflammation central to asthma pathology (48).

Table 8.1	Categorization of Asthma by Endotype		
Endotype	Phenotype	Clinical Characteristics	Natural History
T$_2$ High	Atopic or early-onset allergic asthma	• Well defined • Early onset • Steroid sensitive	• Mild to severe • *Identifiable and treatable* • Preserved lung function
	Late-onset eosinophilic asthma	• Older adults • Associated chronic rhinosinusitis with nasal polyps	• Severe from outset • More frequent exacerbations • Steroid resistant
	Aspirin-exacerbated respiratory disease	• Adult onset	• Severe from outset • More frequent exacerbations
Non-T$_2$ (T$_2$ Low)	Nonatopic	• Adult onset • Paucigranulocytic or neutrophilic	• Variable course and lung function
	Smokers	• Older adults • Steroid resistant	• More frequent exacerbations • Lower lung function
	Obesity related	• Often in female sex	• Severe symptoms • Preserved lung function
	Older adults	• Onset occurs at >50 to 65 years	• Steroid resistant

T$_2$ High, immune response driven (eosinophilic) asthma; Non-T$_2$ Low, non-eosinophilic, neutropenic asthma

Source: Data from Kuruvilla ME, Lee FE, Lee GB. Understanding asthma phenotypes, endotypes, and mechanisms of disease. *Clin Rev Allergy Immunol.* 2019;56(2):219–33. doi:10.1007/s12016-018-8712-1.

To complicate matters further, alteration of gene expression or transcription independent of the gene sequence (*i.e.*, epigenetic factors) is also implicated as potential cause of asthma. Differences in gene expression between those with and without asthma or in patients with asthma before and after steroid treatments have implicated hundreds of genes as possible contributors to the development of asthma (48). Despite having a clear role in the development of asthma, genetics cannot entirely explain the disease, as a study of Danish twins showed that the progress of asthma was not uniform in identical twins sharing presumably similar environmental exposure (39).

Probably the greatest difficulty in establishing clear genetic links to the development of asthma is the nearly impossible task of identifying and precisely quantifying a gene–environment interaction and exposure (49). There are numerous environmental risk factors that interact with an individual's genetic makeup and can lead to the expression of an asthma phenotype. Phenotype expression can also be influenced by the timing and/or the duration of exposure to a particular environmental risk factor or host of risk factors. Some known risk factors may

be encountered early in the prenatal period, and others during childhood or adulthood.

Prenatal maternal tobacco smoking is associated with early childhood wheezing, decreased airway caliber, and increased risk of food allergy. Prenatal consumption of foods rich in omega-3 fatty acids, vitamin E, and zinc are associated with a lower risk of childhood eczema and atopic wheezing. Excluding foods such as cow's milk and eggs have little protective effect against the development of atopic disease in offspring. There is a positive dose-response relationship between prenatal antibiotic use and an increased risk of the child developing persistent wheezing and asthma in early childhood. Finally, there is a two- to threefold increase in the development of atopic disease among infants delivered by an emergency but not elective C-section. This finding suggests that prenatal maternal stress may be a risk factor for the development of atopic disease in children (49).

Children are also exposed to a number of environmental risk factors for asthma. The role of breastfeeding in protecting the child against developing asthma is equivocal. There appears to be some risk reduction from exclusive breastfeeding for the first 3–6 months with late solid food introduction (*i.e.*, after 4–6 mo), especially in children with a parental history of atopic disease. Maternal dietary restriction (*i.e.*, avoidance of cow's milk and eggs) during breastfeeding has little effect on the subsequent development of asthma (50).

Reduced airway size during infancy, which is possibly due to prenatal maternal smoking and postnatal second-hand smoke exposure, predisposes children to reduced airway function, hyperresponsiveness, wheezing, and later development of asthma. Abnormal lung function can be detected as early as 3 years of age, and a fixed decrement in lung function can be observed in 7- to 9-year-olds with a history of wheezing and asthma that persists into adulthood.

Large family size (*i.e.*, >four children) may protect against asthma by increasing the child's exposure to a variety of microbial organisms that help the immune system develop into nonatopic phenotypes. This view must be balanced against the increased early wheezing and asthma risk associated with antibiotic use or the possibility that infection of the lower respiratory tract may promote aeroallergen sensitization (49).

Allergic sensitization during maturation of the immature immune system is a critical element in the development of asthma. The presence of high levels of immunoglobulin E (IgE) at birth is associated with greater aeroallergen sensitivity and incidence of atopic disease (45). Sensitization to the house dust mite, cat, and cockroach allergens is strongly associated with asthma; however, a number of studies have also shown that early-life exposure to dogs, cats, and farm animals can reduce the risk of developing asthma. Exposure to dogs may reduce sensitization to dog allergens as well as other allergens such as the house dust mite (51).

Adult-onset asthma may be new in origin or relapse or exacerbation of childhood asthma that was not diagnosed or recalled by the patient. New adult-onset asthma is often occupationally induced through exposure to various inhaled chemicals or pollutants. Example occupations and exposures include painters (isocyanates), hairdressers (various chemicals), firefighters (smoke and pollutants), commercial cleaners (cleaning solutions), health care workers (latex), and bakers (flour dust). Smoking tobacco or marijuana can also increase the risk of developing asthma as can the use of medicinal agents such as β-adrenergic antagonists, nonsteroidal anti-inflammatories, and hormone replacement drugs (49, 52). Being female and becoming obese along with stress exposure also appear to increase the risk of developing adult-onset asthma (52).

Again, asthma is a multifactorial disease. The etiology is difficult to pinpoint because there are so many potential genetic–environmental interactions to consider, in addition to the variable individual responses that occur among those exposed to similar triggers. Regardless of the underlying genetic–environmental interactions that predispose an individual to the development of asthma, the exaggerated immune response to specific antigens and the resulting inflammation "cause" the symptoms and chronic pathology. This may explain in part why treatment is currently focused on optimal management of asthma symptoms (36).

Epidemiology of Cystic Fibrosis

Cystic fibrosis is a life-threatening recessively inherited genetic disease that arises from defects in a single gene on the long arm of chromosome 7 (53). This gene, the *CFTR* gene, encodes for a protein that functions mainly as a chloride channel. The *CFTR* protein is widely distributed in epithelial surfaces of the paranasal sinus, airways, pancreas, gut, biliary tree, and vas deferens, as well as in skin sweat glands. More than 1,800 specific mutations have been identified in the *CFTR* gene (54–56). Defects result in the production of excessively salty sweat and thick, overly viscid mucous that blocks mucous ducts and epithelial-lined passages. Patients with cystic fibrosis suffer lung, liver, pancreas, gastrointestinal (GI), and reproductive dysfunction.

The incidence rate of cystic fibrosis varies by country and ethnicity. In the U.S., the incidence rate among Caucasians of northern European descent is approximately 1 in 3,000 births and represents 91.6% of all cases (54). The rate is lower among Latin Americans (1 in 4,000–10,000 births) and African Americans (1 in 15,000–20,000 births). Cystic fibrosis is uncommon in Africa and Asia, with Japan reporting an incidence rate of just one in 350,000 births (57). In the U.S., there were 31,411 individuals with cystic fibrosis listed on the 2020 Cystic Fibrosis Registry, and there are an estimated 70,000 patients with cystic fibrosis registered worldwide (54, 56). The number of children (<18 yr of age) living with cystic fibrosis in the U.S. remained steady at just over 10,000 since 1990. The number of adults living with cystic fibrosis continues to increase, and now adults with cystic fibrosis represent 57.2% (a 25% increase since 1990) of the total Registry (54).

It is expected that the adult patient population with cystic fibrosis will continue growing. In 1938, 70% of babies born with cystic fibrosis died within the first year of life. By the mid-1990s, cystic fibrosis infant mortality had dropped to less than 1 in 50 (58). The current age range of individuals listed on the 2020 Cystic Fibrosis Registry extends from birth to 89.7 years, with a median age of 20.3 years highlighting that the age distribution curve is heavily skewed toward younger individuals. Patient mortality rates continue to decline and now stand at 0.8 deaths per 100 patients with cystic fibrosis. This has increased the median predicted survival age, which now stands at 59 years of age (54).

Epidemiology of Lung Transplant

Because of advances in immunosuppressive therapies during the last 30 years, pulmonary (lung) transplantation has become an established treatment option for a carefully selected group of patients with end-stage lung disease, including cystic fibrosis, bronchiectasis, pulmonary hypertension, COPD, and pulmonary fibrosis. Worldwide, around 4,600 adult lung transplants are carried out each year, with 55% of all transplant operations performed in North America and 35% in Europe (59, 60).

The types of pulmonary transplant surgeries are discussed shortly. Approximately 85% of surgeries are bilateral (double) lung transplantation (59). Single lung transplantation is typically reserved for older patients with pulmonary fibrosis or nonsuppurative airway disease. Heart–lung transplantation is rare and is largely reserved for patients with complex congenital heart disease and irreversibly damaged pulmonary circulation. Worldwide, in 2015, there were only 58 such operations reported to the International Registry (60). Lung transplant is typically for patients with advanced lung disease and projected shortened life expectancy with compromised quality of life. Median posttransplant survival is estimated at 6.2 years, increasing to 8.3 for patients that survive the first year after surgery. Although pulmonary transplantation outcomes are improving, the median survival remains only 6.5 years. A shortage of donor organs is the major limitation to increasing accessibility to this potentially lifesaving therapy, which also vastly improves the quality of life in most recipients (59, 60).

Pathway to Transplantation

Patients are very carefully assessed following referral to a pulmonary transplant program. The aim is to identify individuals who are reasonably likely to have a good outcome from transplantation, achieving not just extension of life expectancy but improved quality of life. Some patients are referred with such advanced disease and poor functional status, and their chances of surviving the perioperative period are so low that transplantation is likely to be futile; moreover, it would deprive another individual of the opportunity to receive lungs and achieve a good outcome (61). Thus, such patients are deemed unsuitable for transplant.

Several factors are assessed in determining suitability for this physically and psychologically demanding treatment. These include the patient's social circumstances and support, and their ability to adhere to the postoperative rehabilitation program and report symptoms appropriately (61). Comorbidities that can affect longevity or the ability to rehabilitate following transplantation are also taken into account. Significant organ dysfunction (*e.g.*, cardiac failure or renal dysfunction) will usually result in a patient being deemed unsuitable. However, as pulmonary transplantation has evolved over the last 30 years, older patients with more comorbidities have increasingly been accepted onto waiting lists. Although patients over 70 years old can do well with pulmonary transplantation, they are at higher risk of significant disease of other organs and of having a limited functional reserve. These factors significantly reduce survival further out from transplantation; thus, transplantation in this population remains an area of controversy (62, 63). However, setting a rigid upper limit for pulmonary transplantation is also controversial.

For those deemed suitable candidates, functional status at the time of assessment, rate of deterioration in functional capacity, and the underlying disease determine the timing of transplantation. The aim is to monitor patients who are still reasonably functional and identify when they are deteriorating to the point at which life expectancy is becoming limited and the benefits of transplantation begin to outweigh the attendant risks of both surgery and its early complications, which lead to approximately 15% mortality by 1 year (60, 61). Initially, most patients will be put on an inactive waiting list; that is, they are suitable candidates, but not yet sick enough to require pulmonary transplantation. Some patients are referred with such advanced diseases that they are immediately placed on the active waiting list. A variety of scoring systems have been used to determine when patients should go on the list and their priority. The U.S. and Canada have adopted the Lung Allocation Scoring (LAS) system, which has proven reasonably accurate and acceptable in ensuring a cohesive national approach. Once on the active waiting list, the time to transplantation is highly variable and can be very prolonged if the recipient has a rare blood group, a very small or very large thoracic cavity, or multiple cross-reactive antibodies, which often result from previous blood transfusions (59, 64).

Lung Transplant Surgery

The most common surgery is bilateral single sequential lung transplantation. In this procedure, one lung is excised by dividing the main bronchus to that lung and the pulmonary artery and vein. Then the donor lung's main bronchus is sewn onto the remaining portion of the recipient's main bronchus and, similarly, the pulmonary artery and vein are anastomosed. Once the first donor lung is placed in the thorax, perfused, and inflated, the procedure is repeated on the other side. In approximately 50% of patients, the surgery is carried out with cardiopulmonary bypass (heart–lung machine) or extracorporeal membrane oxygenation. In the remaining patients, native lung function is adequate to sustain respiration while the first donor lung is being implanted. Then the newly implanted lung supports the patient during the implantation of the other new lung. The latter method avoids the need for heart–lung bypass with its attendant risks (65).

The classical surgical approach has been a clamshell incision; that is, the lower thorax is opened horizontally like a clam, cutting the lower sternum. Some surgeons prefer to do a median sternotomy (*i.e.*, a vertical incision down the middle of the sternum), as used in many heart surgeries. Finally, a bilateral posterior thoracotomy, dividing between two ribs and opening the chest from the back, is an alternative approach. Each approach has advantages and disadvantages in terms of ease of access to certain structures. Single lung transplantation is usually conducted through a posterior thoracotomy. Heart–lung transplantation is conducted through a median sternotomy, in which the trachea may be divided, and the donor trachea anastomosed to the recipient trachea (66).

GENERAL PATHOLOGY AND PATHOPHYSIOLOGY IN RESPIRATORY DISEASE

Normal Function and Age-Related Decline

The primary role of the respiratory system is to facilitate an exchange of oxygen and carbon dioxide between external environmental air and the body's interior. At rest, a healthy adult consumes approximately 300 mL·min^{-1} of oxygen while exhaling 250 mL·min^{-1} of carbon dioxide. During exercise, oxygen consumption and carbon dioxide production rates can increase 10- to 20-fold depending on the exercise intensity and the individual's level of fitness. Beginning around 25 years of age, the respiratory reserve capacity as measured by

forced expiratory volume in 1 second (FEV$_1$) and forced vital capacity (FVC) decreases by approximately 30 mL per year in men and 23 mL per year in women. This decline continues until about age 65 years, at which point it tends to accelerate for both sexes (67, 68). The age-associated loss of respiratory capacity is proportional to the decline in maximum aerobic capacity; however, respiratory reserve remains sufficiently high to support increased physical activity in all but perhaps older adult patients who are capable of undertaking intense physical activity (69, 70).

Figure 8.2 shows the ventilatory response to graded exercise in a healthy recreationally active young male. To support the increased metabolic rate of exercise, minute ventilation ($\dot{V}_E$) can increase from 10 L·min^{-1} at rest to nearly 200 L·min^{-1} at maximum effort, depending on the individual's age and training status. Breathing reserve, which is the difference between maximal voluntary ventilation (MVV) rate and the during peak exercise, is more or less preserved at greater than or equal to 20% in healthy aging as peak exercise and MVV tend to decrease proportionally.

To increase $\dot{V}_E$, tidal volume expands from approximately 0.5 to 2.5 L or more depending on body size. Breathing frequency also increases from 10 to 12 breaths·min^{-1} at rest to 40 breaths·min^{-1} or more at peak exercise (71). Tidal volume expansion and breathing frequency increase in a controlled manner to balance the work of breathing and dead space ventilation with the need to regulate blood pH, partial pressure of carbon dioxide in the arterial blood (PaCO$_2$), and partial pressure of oxygen in the arterial blood (PaO$_2$; see Figure 8.2). In young adults, tidal volume is increased through utilization of the inspiratory reserve volume (IRV) and to a lesser extent the expiratory reserve volume (ERV). This allows the tidal volume to range over the more linear portion of the lung–chest wall pressure–volume relationship. Beginning inspiration at a lower end-expiratory lung volume (EELV) allows for passive recoil of the chest wall to assist the respiratory muscles during inhalation. Both of these factors decrease the overall work of breathing during exercise.

This increase in tidal volume with exercise is reduced with aging. Moreover, the pattern of expansion favors utilization of the IRV with little or no expansion into the ERV at higher ventilation rates (28, 72–74). The emergence of this pattern in older adults is likely due to calcification of the costal cartilage and structural changes in the thorax, including spinal kyphosis or other osteoporosis-associated changes in the spine, as well as obesity, as these changes increase chest wall stiffness and limit expansion of thoracic volume (70). An age-related reduction in lung elasticity due to alveolar and distal duct enlargement without alveolar wall destruction (*i.e.*, in contrast to the

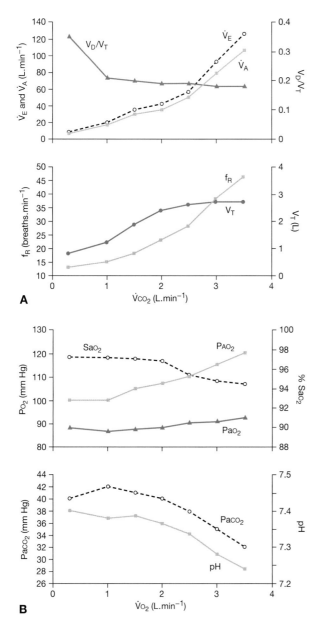

FIGURE 8.2 A. Ventilatory responses to progressively increasing steady-state exercise in a recreationally active young male ($\dot{V}O_{2max}$ = 45 mL·kg^{-1}·min^{-1}); total minute ventilation; V_A, alveolar ventilation; V_D/V_A, dead space to tidal volume ratio; f_R, respiratory frequency; carbon dioxide production. **B.** Arterial blood gases and acid–base status during progressive steady-state increases in work rate. SaO_2, percent arterial oxyhemoglobin saturation; P_AO_2, alveolar PO_2; PaO_2, arterial PO_2; $PaCO_2$, arterial PCO_2; pH, arterial pH. The fall in pH at the two highest work rates was caused by a rise in the concentration of lactic acid and a reduction in plasma bicarbonate in arterial blood. $PaCO_2$ is fairly constant over the first four work rates but falls commensurately with the metabolic acidosis at the two heaviest work rates. Thus, the arterial blood acid–base status at the two work rates is primarily metabolic acidosis partially compensated by hyperventilation (and hypocapnia). (Figure reproduced with permission from Farrell PA, Joyner MJ, Caiozzo VJ. *ACSM's Advanced Exercise Physiology.* 2nd ed. Philadelphia (PA): Wolters Kluwer; 2011.)

changes associated with emphysema), coupled with airway narrowing and inherent respiratory muscle weakness, which limits expiratory airflow, also shift the tidal volume range to higher end-inspiratory lung volume (EILV) and EELV when compared to younger adults (70, 73, 75, 76).

Minute ventilation is adjusted moment by moment to limit changes in PaO_2, $PaCO_2$, and pH over a wide range in metabolic rate by a respiratory control system consisting of a central controller (pons, medulla, and other parts of the brain), sensors (chemoreceptors and mechanoreceptors), and effectors (respiratory muscles) (77). Although the precise mechanisms by which the central controller matches exercise-induced hyperpnea to metabolic demand are still debated (78); changes in $\dot{V}_E$ appear coupled to $PaCO_2$ and arterial pH. During moderate-intensity exercise (*i.e.*, below the lactate threshold), $\dot{V}_E$ increases in proportion to carbon dioxide produced from aerobic metabolism. As exercise intensity increases above the lactate threshold, $\dot{V}_E$ also increases in proportion to CO_2 produced by aerobic metabolism and bicarbonate buffering of H^+ arising from increasing rates of glycolysis (*i.e.*, isocapnic buffering). At vigorous and very vigorous exercise intensities, $\dot{V}_E$ is further increased as a response to counter both high rates of CO_2 production and falling arterial pH caused by increasing metabolic acidosis (*i.e.*, the respiratory compensation point) (71, 79). PaO_2 is not believed to be a primary stimulus for increasing $\dot{V}_E$ unless PaO_2 drops below 50 mm Hg (77).

Oxygen and carbon dioxide sensitivity is diminished with aging, at rest, and during exercise (80, 81). During exercise, $\dot{V}_E$ tends to be greater for a given $\dot{V}CO_2$, and the $\dot{V}_E$ versus $\dot{V}CO_2$ slope during graded exercise is steeper for older versus younger adults (82, 83). This suggests older adults either maintain a lower $PaCO_2$ during exercise or there is an increase in the dead space to tidal volume ratio (V_D/V_T). Evidence suggests that both young and older adults remain isocapnic during moderate-intensity exercise and that $PaCO_2$ declines via respiratory compensation for metabolic acidosis during heavy exercise (80). Thus, an increased V_D/V_T is most likely driving a higher $\dot{V}_E$ during exercise in older adults.

Dead space in the respiratory system is made up of an anatomical component corresponding to the volume of the conducting airways plus a physiologic component due to poor diffusion across the alveolar membrane and ventilation of alveoli that are poorly perfused with blood. The physiologic dead space is approximately equal to the anatomical dead space and accounts for 25%–30% of the resting tidal volume, which decreases to approximately 15% during exercise. There is a small increase in anatomical dead space of approximately 10 mL per decade (84), presumably as a result of the age-related expansion of the terminal alveolar ducts and alveoli (85). This can increase the V_D/V_T by as much as 15%–20% in the older adults (86).

Physiologic dead space increases through an age-related decline in diffusion capacity of the lung at rest and during exercise. This decline is thought to reflect a gradual reduction in the alveolar–capillary density to alveolar diameter, a reduction in pulmonary blood volume, and increased alveolar ventilation-perfusion (V_A/Q) mismatching (75, 87). The age-associated V_A/Q mismatch appears to be due to increased heterogeneity in alveolar ventilation and pulmonary perfusion. That is, nonuniform loss of lung elastic recoil and connective support between alveoli and small airways causes some regions of the lung to be better ventilated than others, whereas age-related remodeling and vascular stiffness reduce vascular extensibility and recruitment potential to create a more heterogeneous perfusion of the lung (88, 89). In spite of the age-related increase in V_T/V_D and V_A/Q, older adults appear to maintain adequate alveolar ventilation and a near-normal alveolar–capillary diffusion rate that together maintain arterial blood gases within normal ranges even during heavy exercise. Although there is a general decline in external work capacity with aging, it does not appear that this decline is the direct result of a diminished respiratory capacity, as the ability to perform external work declines in parallel to the decline in respiratory capacity (76, 85, 90).

Pathology and Pathophysiology in COPD

COPD is primarily a disease of the large and small airways and the lung parenchyma that is characterized by inflammation, airway narrowing, and poorly reversible airflow obstruction (91). COPD itself or some aspect associated with COPD such as disuse, causes variable changes in skeletal muscle leading to dysfunction (92, 93). For the individual, COPD manifests as dyspnea, skeletal muscle weakness, and exercise intolerance.

Pathology

The central pathology of COPD is an exaggerated inflammatory response due to chronic exposure to noxious gases and particulate (*i.e.*, tobacco and biomass fuel smoke; see Figure 8.3). Depending on the interplay between different inflammatory and repair mechanisms, chronic bronchitis, emphysematous, mixed, or asthma–COPD overlap phenotype of the disease can emerge (94).

In large airways, overproduction of mucus from hypertrophied submucosal glands and enlarged goblet cells leads to the productive cough typically present in COPD.

An inability to clear excess mucus provides an environment that promotes microbial infection and inflammation. The clinical exercise physiologist (CEP) can instruct and assist the patient in some manual and active cycle of breathing techniques to promote removal of airway mucus (95).

The characteristic airflow limitation of COPD arises primarily from small airways less than 2 mm in diameter. In these small airways, goblet cells undergo metaplasia and the mucus produced can displace surfactant. This in turn can increase acini surface tension and predispose them to collapse. Epithelial cells injured by exposure to noxious stimuli instigate recruitment of neutrophils, macrophages, and cytotoxic T lymphocytes. Cytokines, chemokines, reactive oxygen species, elastases, proteinases, and myeloperoxidases form an inflammatory milieu that directly damages the extracellular matrix of the acini connective tissue. Excessive growth factor production leads to airway smooth muscle growth and fibrosis, which narrows the airway lumen and increases airway resistance. Emphysema results when the alveoli, alveolar ducts, and respiratory bronchioles become irreversibly damaged (14, 94, 96, 97).

Pathological changes to the large airways in COPD have relatively little impact on airflow. Instead, airflow resistance is increased in the small (<2 mm diameter) airways. Increased mucus production plugs these airways and chronic inflammation stimulates airway smooth muscle growth and reactivity that effectively reduces the total airway cross-sectional area and increases airway resistance (98). Inflammatory-driven destruction of the lung parenchyma results in the loss of structural interdependence of the alveolar units and alveolar attachment to small airways. The tethering effect of the alveoli on each other and on smaller airways to hold them open during exhalation is lost. Collapsed airways are more difficult to reinflate and offer increased resistance to expiratory airflow; therefore, greater expiratory muscle effort is required to empty the lung. This only serves to exacerbate the problem because increased transmural airway pressure causes further narrowing and collapse of the airways (99). Destruction of the lung parenchyma also reduces elastic recoil of the lung tissue, resulting in a loss of passive force to help empty the lungs of air during exhalation. This shifts the operating lung volume higher on the lung pressure–volume relationship curve, increasing the muscular effort required to ventilate the lung. This is especially true during exercise, when volume expansion may be limited by inspiratory capacity (IC) and breathing frequency (77, 100, 101).

Pathophysiology

The hallmark expiratory airflow limitation characteristic of COPD develops gradually over many years. Although

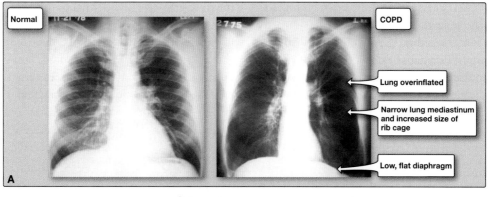

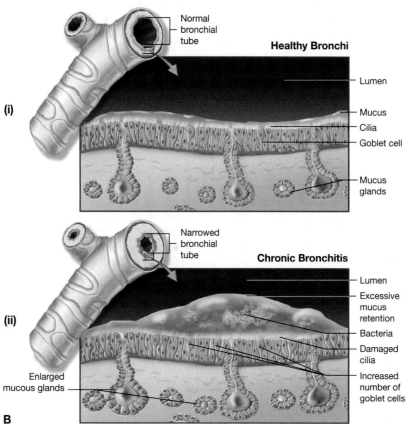

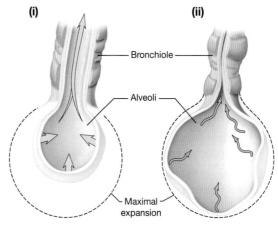

FIGURE 8.3 A. Radiographs of the normal lung (left) and the lung of a patient with chronic obstructive pulmonary disease (COPD). **B.** The upper panel **(i)** depicts a normal healthy bronchial tube, whereas the lower panel **(ii)** depicts a bronchial tube of a patient with chronic bronchitis. Irritant-induced inflammation leads to mucus production that over time becomes excessive due to goblet cell hypertrophy and hyperplasia. Reduced mucociliary clearance leads to blocked airways that have been narrowed by inflammation-induced airway remodeling. **C.** The left panel **(i)** depicts normal elastic recoil in a healthy alveolus. The end inspiration volume is shown by the dotted line and alveolar volume decreases with exhalation. Panel **(ii)** shows how the loss of alveolar elastic recoil due to emphysema leads to a larger end expiratory alveolar volume and air trapping. (Panel A from Looper-Woodford SK, Adkison LR. *Lippincott Illustrated Reviews: Integrated Systems*. 1st ed. Philadelphia (PA): Wolters Kluwer; 2015. Panels B and C from Braun C, Anderson C. *Applied Pathophysiology*. 3rd ed. Philadelphia (PA): Wolters Kluwer; 2016.)

a diagnosis of COPD is typically given when spirometry testing reveals the ratio of FEV_1 to forced vital capacity (FEV_1/FVC) becomes less than or equal to 0.7, the disease process is already well established by this point. When the postbronchodilator administration FEV_1 is less than 80% of the predicted value, there is a tendency toward air trapping and lung hyperinflation (21). However, patients with COPD seldom describe their dyspnea as an inability to exhale. Instead, they describe their dyspnea as an "inability to get their air" or the result of "muscular weakness" during exercise (76, 102). Figure 8.4 compares normal and pathological lung volumes and capacities. During the later

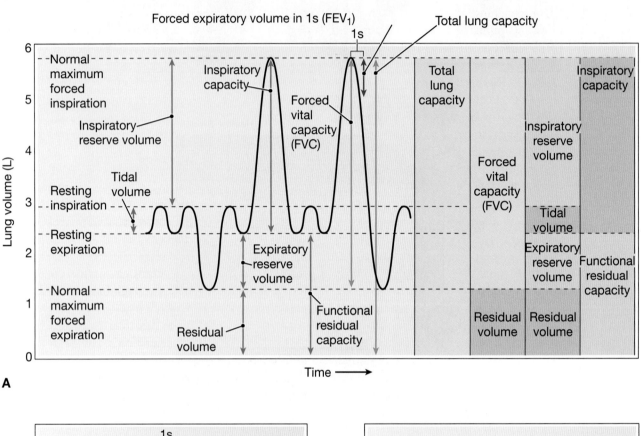

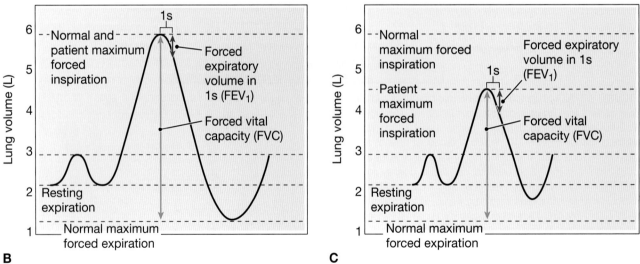

FIGURE 8.4 A. A normal spirogram tracing with lung volumes and capacities identified. **B.** A spirogram tracing of a forced vital capacity (FVC) maneuver performed by someone with obstructive lung disease: One-second forced expiratory volume (FEV_1) is low; FVC is normal. **C.** A spirogram tracing of an FVC maneuver performed by someone with restrictive lung disease: Both FEV_1 and FVC are low. (From McConell TH. *Nature of Disease.* 2nd ed. Philadelphia (PA): Wolters Kluwer; 2013.)

stages of COPD, the total lung capacity (TLC) is typically increased to more than 120% of the predicted value. The residual volume (RV) also increases above normal, and an RV/TLC% greater than 35% is indicative of air trapping. Lung hyperinflation is present when both the TLC and RV/TLC% are elevated above normal. The pattern of change in RV results in the vital capacity (VC) either decreasing (TLC unchanged) or remaining the same (TLC increasing). The IC (defined as TLC minus FRC) is typically reduced in COPD because the functional residual capacity (FRC) is increased due to less lung elastic recoil force opposing chest wall expansion (87, 103, 104). The IC represents the operational volume limit for tidal volume expansion through inhalation. When resting IC values are less than 80% of the predicted value can suggest an expiratory flow limitation. Worsening of the airflow limitation will increase FRC causing further decline in the IC. The IC/TLC% can be used as an indirect measure of lung hyperinflation if TLC is stable. Mortality is increased in patients with COPD who have an IC/TLC% that is less than 25% (105–107).

A consequence of lung hyperinflation is that the lung operating volume shifts higher on the lung's pressure–volume curve. During hyperinflation, the diaphragm is flattened and has less force-generating potential because it is operating over a shorter overall range within the muscle length–tension relationship (108). Several lines of evidence from both animal models and from human specimens suggest that over time the diaphragm muscle adapts and shortens the optimal length of the muscle fibers through sarcomere deletion, thereby improving the ability of the diaphragm to generate force during hyperinflation (109). Even with this adaptation, patients with COPD and lung hyperinflation have a reduced capacity for generating diaphragmatic pressure (110). It is generally accepted that the diaphragm of patients with COPD produces less force than in their healthy counterparts. Central to lost force-generating capacity is a shift toward predominantly more type I fibers with an overall reduction in the fiber diameter and myosin content in type I and remaining type II fibers. The reduction in myosin content leads to a lower cross-bridge density and reduced force-generating capacity. The shift toward a greater proportion of type I fibers improves the overall metabolic capacity of the diaphragm by increasing the capacity for aerobic adenosine triphosphate (ATP) production, which compensates to some extent the loss in mechanical efficiency (109, 111).

The EELV, defined as the volume of air in the lung at the end of a tidal breath, can be variable depending on the tidal volume, airway resistance, and rate of airflow. With normal "quite" breathing at rest, EELV approximates FRC in that the respiratory musculature relaxes and the tidal breath is fully exhaled. In COPD, airway narrowing or collapse during exhalation of a tidal breath can add airway resistance reducing air flow and increasing the time needed to fully exhale the tidal breath. If inspiration takes place before the first breath is fully exhaled, the new inspired volume will be added to what remained from the previous breath. If this continues over several breaths, the EELV will progressively increase as a portion of air is "trapped" with each breath and the lung begins to hyperinflate (76). As the EELV increases, there is a rightward shift along the lung's pressure–volume curve increasing the respiratory muscle force needed to inflate the lung while at the same time shifting the diaphragm, intercostal muscles, and accessory muscles of respiration to shorter, less optimal muscle lengths for force development. A lung volume of 70% of the predicted TLC approximates the balance point for chest wall compliance. For patients with severe or dynamic hyperinflation, at least a portion of the tidal volume will use lung volumes in excess of 70% predicted TLC (107). The net effect of these shifts is to greatly increase the work and oxygen cost of breathing because the respiratory muscles must generate enough force to overcome a positive inspiratory threshold load or a positive end-expiratory pressure (PEEPi) resulting from EELV being greater than FRC when inspiration begins prior to complete evacuation of the preceding breath (103, 112, 113). In a historical study by Levison and Cherniack (114), the respiratory muscle oxygen cost of breathing during cycling was measured to be 1.96 and 6.3 mL of oxygen per 1 L of ventilation at rest in healthy adults and patients with COPD, respectively. The increase in respiratory muscle oxygen cost in patients with COPD was more than double that of the healthy adults (4.2 vs. 9.3 mL of oxygen per L of ventilation) when the $\dot{V}_E$ was raised to 20 L·min^{-1}. The total oxygen cost was not different between the patients with COPD and healthy adults for an equivalent external workload, meaning that a greater proportion of the oxygen uptake during the exercise was needed to support ventilation and was not available to support locomotor muscles. Not surprisingly, the external work capacity of patients with COPD was severely reduced (114).

To increase $\dot{V}_E$ during exercise, both the tidal volume and breathing frequency increase. The typical pattern for tidal volume expansion in healthy adults is for the EILV to increase up to 70%–80% of the TLC. At the same time, active recruitment of expiratory muscles lowers the EELV below FRC to allow further expansion of the tidal volume within the linear portion of the pressure–volume curve. However, the capacity to lower EELV in older adults is limited (73, 86, 103, 115, 116). In healthy patients, expiratory flow rates are sufficiently high enough that EELV only increases slightly even with a peak breathing frequency of 30–40 breaths·min^{-1}. In COPD, however, a dynamic lung hyperinflation develops because the expiratory airflow limitation slows the emptying of the lungs and the shortened expiratory time invariably leads to a progressive increase in air trapping and EELV. On average, EELV increases by 0.3–0.6 L above resting volumes in 85% of patients with moderate to severe COPD during cycling exercise (101). Dynamic hyperventilation could be seen as a positive compensatory mechanism as there is greater pulmonary stretching and radial traction, reduced airway collapse, and higher expiratory flow rates at larger lung volumes; however, the progressive increase in EELV that occurs with exercise is superimposed on the existing lung hyperventilation of COPD. Those with the highest EELVs are the most limited when it comes to tidal volume expansion and must rely on increased ventilatory frequency to raise the $\dot{V}_E$. This only serves to hasten the time required to reach their critical minimal IRV and exercise is terminated (100). The typical scenario is that during exercise, tidal volume expansion

represents greater and greater proportions of the IC until the tidal volume accounts for 70% of the IC or the remaining IRV is roughly 90% of the age-predicted TLC. At this point, further expansion of the tidal volume is limited and $\dot{V}_E$ increases primarily through the ventilatory rate. This places greater load on already weakened respiratory muscles that must increase their shortening velocity in the face of reduced dynamic lung compliance. Respiratory neural drive approaches near-maximum levels as does the sense of dyspnea, and a greater proportion of the exercise oxygen consumption is used to support respiratory muscle. This series of events can lead to hypoxia, hypercapnia, muscular fatigue, and termination of exercise at relatively low intensity compared to age- and gender-matched peers (107).

Dyspnea is perhaps the most distressing symptom of COPD, and it is often the primary reason for seeking treatment (Figure 8.5). In general, dyspnea is a multidimensional sensation described as air hunger, increased effort, or chest tightness. Dissociation between respiratory motor output and the mechanical/muscular response of the respiratory system, especially during lung hyperinflation, is believed to be central to the increased perception of unsatisfied inspiration (117). Patients with COPD must develop greater neural activation to compensate for inherent respiratory muscle weakness, fatigue, and mechanical loading. In addition, increased corollary discharge to the sensory cortex is perceived as increased respiratory muscle effort. This is reflected reasonably well by the relationship between the effort displacement ratio and the perceived intensity of inspiratory difficulty. Effort displacement ratio is equal to tidal esophageal pressure relative to maximum inspiratory pressure divided by the tidal volume displacement as a proportion of age-predicted VC. This ratio crudely reflects the operating tidal volume in relation to the lung pressure–volume curve (76, 118). Afferent discharge from intercostal and accessory muscles of ventilation may also contribute to the sensations of dyspnea (118).

Lung hyperinflation also affects cardiovascular function. High intrathoracic pressure (ITP), similar to a Valsalva maneuver, during hyperinflation can exceed right atrial pressure reducing right-side venous return and right ventricular preload. Compression of alveolar blood vessels and increased wall thickening in pulmonary vessels causes pulmonary vascular resistance to increase. In combination with a compromised left ventricle, pulmonary wedge pressure and right ventricular afterload are elevated (*i.e.*, pulmonary hypertension). In COPD,

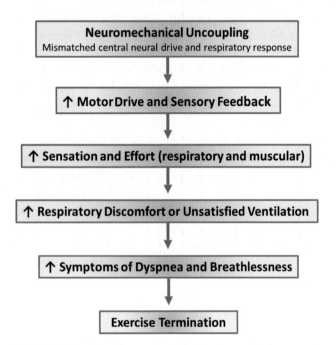

FIGURE 8.5 A schematic overview of the development of dyspnea and breathlessness leading to exercise termination in respiratory disease.

elevated pulmonary vascular resistance is typical at rest and becomes more severe during exercise in response to exercise-induced vasoconstrictor signals (*i.e.*, hypoxemia, acidosis, and increased sympathetic tone) and worsening lung hyperinflation (119–122). As a result of reduced right ventricular filling and increased resistance, right ventricular output does not rise sufficiently during exercise (123, 124). On the heart's left side, lung hyperinflation limits end-diastolic left ventricular volume, and reduced right ventricular ejection volumes limit left ventricular filling. A high ITP decreases left ventricular compliance and further limits left ventricular volume expansion (*i.e.*, pneumonic cardiac tamponade). Volume expansion can also be limited by a leftward shift of the intraventricular septum due to enlargement of the right ventricle in the face of rising afterload pressures (121, 125). Ultimately, limited left ventricular volume expansion reduces stroke volume. Cardiac output increases as expected during exercise but remains lower for individuals with COPD at peak and submaximal exercise intensities. The heart rate is usually higher in patients with COPD for a given exercise intensity to preserve cardiac output in the face of reduced stroke volume (107, 126, 127). Competition for a smaller cardiac output contributes to the limited exercise capacity in patients with COPD as overworked respiratory muscles siphon a greater proportion of the cardiac output away from locomotor muscles. An insufficient blood supply to locomotor muscles would lower oxygen delivery, promoting early metabolic acidosis and sensations of muscular fatigue and breathlessness (76, 118, 128, 129).

COPD compromises both ventilation and perfusion of the lung to cause regional $\dot{V}_A/\dot{Q}$ mismatching that can result in hypoxia, hypercapnia, or both at rest and during exercise. This is most likely due to an increased ventilatory dead space (V_D) volume. In lung areas where emphysema is the dominant pathology, the alveolar–capillary bed is destroyed, and ventilation of the area fails to support gas exchange. In areas of the lung where chronic bronchitis is the dominant pathology, perfusion is preserved to the alveolar units but airway narrowing reduces ventilation of the alveolus and gas exchange is compromised. Pulmonary venous blood gas values represent the sum of all alveolar units and, in the case of severe COPD, blood returning to the left ventricle may be somewhat hypoxic and hypercapnic, especially during exercise (130). In those with mild to moderate COPD, an increase in $\dot{V}_E$ relative to healthy adults is sufficient to minimize the impact of an increased V_D and allow arterial blood gases to be maintained within normal ranges

at rest and during exercise. Over time, however, maintaining an increased $\dot{V}_E$ will hasten lung hyperinflation, increase dyspnea relative to exercise intensity, and limit exercise performance compared to healthy adults (131, 132). In those with severe COPD, a constrained ability to expand the tidal volume prevents $\dot{V}_E$ from increasing enough to compensate for the increased physiologic dead space volume. Any existing V_A/Q mismatch worsens exacerbating arterial hypoxia and hypercapnia. Although hypoxia itself is a weak stimulus for ventilation, hypercapnia is a potent stimulus that can drive high ventilation rates (133). As $\dot{V}_E$ is driven higher in response to hypercapnia, lung hyperinflation worsens and V_A/Q mismatching becomes even more pronounced, physiologic dead space expands, and blood gases are deranged even further, leading to greater respiratory distress, dyspnea, and exercise intolerance.

Although dyspnea is the most commonly reported reason for terminating exercise involving endurance walking or cycling among patients with COPD, leg fatigue is also cited in up to 25% and 70% of cases for walking and graded maximal effort cycling, respectively (134, 135). Skeletal muscle dysfunction is the most common extrapulmonary manifestation of COPD. The dysfunction results from a complex combination of functional, metabolic, and anatomical changes (*e.g.*, atrophy, altered fiber type, metabolism) to both ventilatory and nonventilatory skeletal muscle groups. The dysfunction tends to worsen with symptom severity, and it reduces patient function (93). Skeletal muscle function in COPD is characterized by weakness that manifests as a reduction in muscular strength or endurance, or both. Quadriceps strength may be 20%–30% lower in patients with COPD compared to healthy age-matched adults. Muscle dysfunction appears to be greater in the lower limb compared to the upper limb muscles (93, 136–139). The overall severity of muscular weakness is prognostic in COPD, with increased mortality associated with greater levels of muscular weakness (140, 141).

The respiratory muscles (*i.e.*, the diaphragm, intercostal, and accessory muscles) and peripheral muscles are all striated skeletal muscles that can adapt positively or negatively to various stressors. As discussed earlier, in COPD, the respiratory muscles are exposed to excess lengthening and mechanical loading and undergo positive adaptation to these stimuli. They respond by shortening their overall length and undergoing adaptations that improve their aerobic capacity. These adaptations include an increase in the percentage of oxidative fibers, capillarization, mitochondrial density, and aerobic enzyme content that helps the muscle to meet the high metabolic demand of ventilating a lung with airflow limitation and hyperinflation (93, 109–111, 142).

Numerous studies have shown that patients with COPD have diminished peripheral muscular strength (140, 141, 143–145), muscle cross-sectional area or mass (143, 146, 147), and whole-body fat-free mass (148) when compared to healthy counterparts. Unlike the respiratory muscle, peripheral muscles undergo a number of negative adaptations that contribute to muscular weakness. There is a reduction in the proportion of type I oxidative skeletal muscle fibers in both moderate (149, 150) and severe COPD (151) with a corresponding increase in the proportion of type IIb fibers (152). Type II fibers typically atrophy, however, with prolonged corticosteroid use, further weakening the muscle (153, 154). Consistent with a reduction in aerobic capacity are diminished capillarization (152, 155), mitochondrial derangement (156), and diminished levels of aerobic enzymes (157), all of which are observed in the peripheral muscle of patients with COPD.

Although the pathology of muscle weakness associated with COPD is reasonably well established, the cause is not well understood and is most likely multifactorial (93). Systemic inflammation, oxidative stress, and malnutrition appear central to muscle degradation and wasting. Many of the negative structural and biochemical skeletal muscle adaptations that take place in COPD are similar to those that occur with deconditioning and disuse. Physical deconditioning and a sedentary lifestyle are common in those with COPD, and exercise training can improve skeletal muscle function. It should be noted, however, that not all of the skeletal muscle dysfunction results from deconditioning because muscle dysfunction persists in the hand despite the fact that hand muscles are continually used even by patients with very severe COPD (138) and because exercise training does not fully reverse muscle abnormality (158–160).

Pathology and Pathophysiology in Asthma

Pathology

The term *asthma* has evolved into an umbrella term that describes a cluster of clinical symptoms that include wheezing, breathlessness, chest tightness, and cough. The modern asthma diagnosis should be followed by an investigation into what type of asthma someone has so

that the specific molecular underpinnings of the asthma type can be identified and treatment targeted according to disease endotype (44, 161–163). An overview of asthma pathology is shown in Figure 8.6. Historically, asthma was viewed to be an exaggerated inflammatory response following exposure of the airway to triggering stimuli such as dust or pollen, viral infection, or airway drying. Inflammation affected the trachea, bronchi, and/or bronchioles, leading to airway hyperreactivity and narrowing. Chronic inflammation cycles resulted in extensive airway remodeling that over time caused irreversible airway obstruction or development of an asthma–COPD hybrid form of respiratory disease (164). From these historic foundational views, the pathology underpinning asthma is being actively expanded according to fundamental inflammatory endotypes (Table 8.1) and delineation of the molecular pathways driving different types of the disease (44).

The eosinophilic or type 2 immune response-driven (T_2-high) endotype encompasses several asthma phenotypes (*e.g.*, atopic, late-onset, and aspirin-exacerbated respiratory disease) found in children and adults. The general paradigm of the T_2-high endotype involves a dysregulated epithelial barrier that facilitates translocation of allergens, air pollution, and viruses that stimulate airway epithelial cells to release cytokine alarmins to initiate an adaptive type 2 immune response. The alarmin thymic stromal lymphopoietin primes dendritic cells to induce differentiation of naive T cells into Th2 cells. Th2 cells release IL-4 to activate B cells that differentiate into plasma cells. The alarmins IL-25 and IL-33 activate eosinophils, basophils, and mast cells along with group 2 innate lymphoid cells highlighting the current view that immune processes outside the classic allergen-specific pathways are also involved in asthma pathology. Activated cells produce a variety of inflammatory mediators (*e.g.*, IL-3, IL-4, IL-5, IgE, cysteinyl leukotrienes, eosinophil cationic protein and peroxidase, eosinophil-derived neurotoxin, and prostaglandin D2) that affect airway hyperresponsiveness, and ultimately result in smooth muscle hypertrophy and airway remodeling (44).

The non-eosinophilic or T2-low asthma endotype is less well characterized but includes the paucigranulocytic or neutrophilic, smoking-related, obesity-related, and older adult asthma phenotypes. It is more the absence of T2-high biomarkers rather than the presence of specific biomarkers that characterize the T2-low endotype. The endotype is generally characterized by neutrophilic (sputum neutrophils >40% to 60%) or

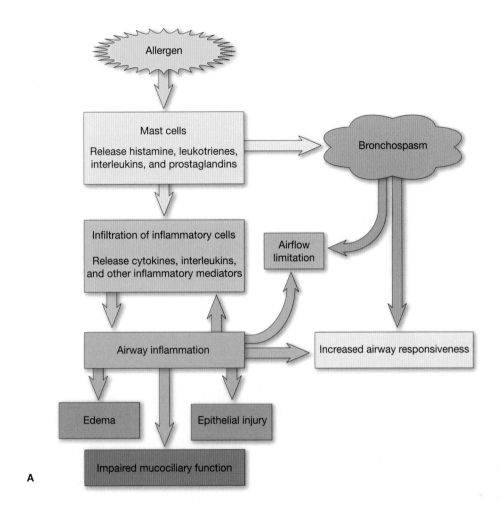

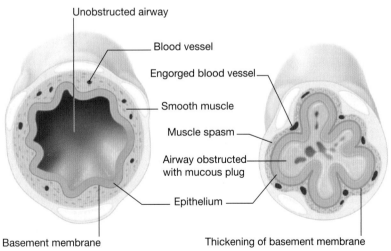

FIGURE 8.6 The pathology of asthma. **A.** A schematic overview of the steps leading from allergen exposure to development of bronchial obstruction. **B.** Morphological changes in the bronchial tubes due to asthma. (From Braun C, Anderson C. *Applied Pathophysiology.* 3rd ed. Philadelphia (PA): Wolters Kluwer; 2016.)

paucigranulocytic (*i.e.*, normal sputum levels of eosinophils and neutrophils) inflammation and a lack of response to corticosteroid therapy. T2-low asthma is linked to TH1 and/or Th17 cell activation with pathogenesis linked to activation of NLRP3 inflammasome and elevated IL-1β, IL-8, IL-17A, IL-17F, IL-22, and interferon-gamma (IFN-γ) (44, 165).

As proinflammatory environments associated with both the T2-high and T2-low endotypes become chronic, components such as vascular endothelial growth factor (VEGF) promote angiogenesis leading to vascular leakage and airway edema. Production of transforming growth factor-β, IL-9, and IL-13 induces fibroblast and airway smooth muscle proliferation as well as extracellular matrix deposition. Over time, this chronic inflammatory response results in airway remodeling that is characteristic of asthma (42, 44, 165–167).

Pathophysiology

During an acute asthma attack, contraction of airway smooth muscle and swelling of the airway epithelium cause airway narrowing that obstructs airflow, making it more difficult to ventilate the lungs. Patients may wheeze, gasp, or be short of breath; or in extreme circumstances, suffocate to death.

Chronic asthma is linked to significant airway remodeling over time. Although airway remodeling is commonly attributed to chronic inflammation, other mechanisms are also thought to be involved because the use of anti-inflammatory medications to treat asthma has had limited success (44, 168). Asthmatic airway remodeling is characterized by epithelial sloughing, mucous gland and smooth muscle hyperplasia, basement membrane thickening, and airway edema. These changes narrow the airway lumen and increase airway resistance. Goblet cell hyperplasia in the airway epithelium results in excessive mucus production that can accumulate in the small airways, causing airway obstruction. Airway remodeling and development of an airflow obstruction leads to the development of lung hyperinflation. As in COPD, static and dynamic lung hyperinflation can have a significant impact on dyspnea symptoms, exercise capacity, and quality of life.

Exercise-induced asthma (EIA) and exercise-induced bronchoconstriction (EIB) are terms often used interchangeably to describe wheezing or difficulty breathing during or after exercise. However, there are distinctions. The vast majority of diagnosed asthma patients will experience bronchoconstriction during exercise because exercise is one of many possible triggers of their existing asthma. The term *EIA* most appropriately describes this condition. For other individuals, exercising at a high intensity or in a cold environment is the trigger for an inflammatory response that induces airway constriction and difficulty breathing. EIB most appropriately describes this form of asthma, which is believed to be caused by evaporative airway epithelial water loss and cooling in response to high ventilation rates. Drying the epithelium initiates an IgE-mediated inflammatory response and contracture of the airway smooth muscle (169).

Pathology and Pathophysiology in Cystic Fibrosis

Pathology

The basic defect in cystic fibrosis is loss of function and/or expression of the CFTR protein; however, the exact role of diminished transepithelial transport in the pathogenesis of cystic fibrosis is not completely understood. The CFTR protein functions mainly as a cyclic AMP–regulated chloride channel that also plays a role in the inhibition of sodium transport through epithelial sodium channels as well as the inhibition of calcium-activated chloride channels. It regulates outwardly flowing chloride channels and ATP channels; intracellular vesicle transport; and intracellular acidification; in addition, it is involved in transepithelial bicarbonate–chloride exchange (53, 57). The majority of *CFTR* mutations involve three or fewer nucleotides that result in amino acid substitutions, frameshifts, splice site, or nonsense mutations. The most common mutation involves a three-base pair deletion coding for phenylalanine at position 508 (F508del) of the CFTR protein (53).

CFTR gene mutations produce six different phenotype categories that are identified in Table 8.2. Class I, II, and III mutations result in the synthesis of reduced or nonfunctional CFTR proteins. This is a severe disease phenotype generally associated with low pulmonary and pancreatic function. Class IV and V mutations result in the synthesis of CFTR proteins with some residual function; therefore, the resulting disease phenotype is milder than for classes I, II, III, and VI. Patients with class VI mutations have not been widely studied, but their disease phenotype tends to be severe (53, 55–57, 170).

It should be noted that the above description is a generalization and that disease severity can vary between patients with the same *CFTR* gene mutation. This variation is likely due to polymorphism in genes other than the *CFTR* gene (*i.e.*, transforming growth factor-β (171)).

Table 8.2	*CFTR* Gene Mutation Classification and Description	
Class	Functional CFTR Protein	Description of Dysfunction
Severe Disease Phenotype		
I	No	Stop codon or splicing defects; CFTR is not synthesized.
II	No or substantially reduced amount	CFTR synthesized in an immature form; defective trafficking or increased degradation prevents CFTR from inserting in apical membrane.
III	Nonfunctioning CFTR protein inserted into membrane	CFTR protein synthesized and inserted into apical membrane; however, activation and regulation by ATP or cAMP dysfunctional
Moderate Disease Phenotype		
IV	Yes	CFTR synthesized and inserted into apical membrane, but chloride conductance is reduced.
V	Yes	Reduced CFTR synthesis rate
Severe Disease Phenotype		
VI	Yes	CFTR is synthesized and inserted into the apical membrane but is rapidly turned over; reduced ion conductance for ions other than Cl⁻

Source: Adapted from Strausbaugh SD, Davis PB. Cystic fibrosis: a review of epidemiology and pathobiology. *Clin Chest Med.* 2007; 28:279–88; O'Sullivan BP, Freedman SD. Cystic fibrosis. *Lancet.* 2009;373:1891–904; Lubamba B, Dhooghe B, Noel S, Leal T. Cystic fibrosis: insight into CFTR pathophysiology and pharmacology. *Clin Biochem.* 2012;45:1132–44.

Pathophysiology

An overview of cystic fibrosis pathophysiology is presented in Figure 8.7. Mucus is a viscoelastic substance composed of mucins (*e.g.*, glycoproteins), water, electrolytes, epithelial cells, and leukocytes. A layer of mucus a few tens of micrometers thick covers epithelial surfaces of airways, the GI tract, and ducts within the biliary, pancreatic, and reproductive systems. It is produced by specialized epithelial cells (*e.g.*, goblet cells) and small submucosal glands. It keeps the epithelial surface moist and serves as a barrier to bacteria and other foreign particles that become trapped in the sticky material. In the lungs, cilia on epithelial cells move mucus and any trapped particles out of the lung toward the pharynx at a rate of approximately 1 cm·min⁻¹. Evacuated mucus is either swallowed or coughed out. In the GI tract, mucus provides a barrier to protect the epithelium from mechanical and chemical trauma and acts as a lubricant to facilitate food moving through the digestive system (172).

Cystic fibrosis has long been associated with the formation of abnormally thick, sticky mucus that blocks ducts and passages in the lungs, liver, pancreas, GI tract, and reproductive tract. Despite this association, there is little evidence directly connecting CFTR to mucus hypersecretion or abnormal mucin production. CFTR is not expressed by mucin-secreting cells (*i.e.*, goblet cells), and mucin secretion is normal in the mucosal cells of patients with cystic fibrosis; moreover, some mucus-producing glands (*i.e.*, salivary and lacrimal glands) are unaffected by CFTR defects (173). Together, these observations suggest that CFTR is not likely involved in mucin production or secretion and that there is an indirect relationship between CFTR expression/function and mucus quantity, quality, and consistency. Hypotheses connecting abnormal CFTR with mucus hypersecretion and abnormally thick mucus production generally fall into one of two central themes:

1. According to the dehydration hypothesis, the CFTR defect leads to a loss of the ionic gradients necessary to prevent the mucus layer from drying out and becoming thick and sticky. When this happens in the lung, there is a loss of lubrication and the mucus compresses the cilia, reducing normal mucus clearance from the lung. Mucus plugs then block smaller passages and harbor bacteria such as *Pseudomonas aeruginosa* that maintain and sustain cycles of chronic infection and inflammation.

2. According to the innate immune response hypothesis, defective CFTR results in the production of mucus that has reduced antimicrobial activity. High chloride levels in the periciliary layer diminish the effectiveness of innate antibiotic molecules (*i.e.*, β-defensin-1), allowing bacteria that would normally be cleared to persist in the airways. *P. aeruginosa* fails to bind to nonfunctional CFTR. Normally, this binding would initiate a rapid self-limiting innate immune response. Finally,

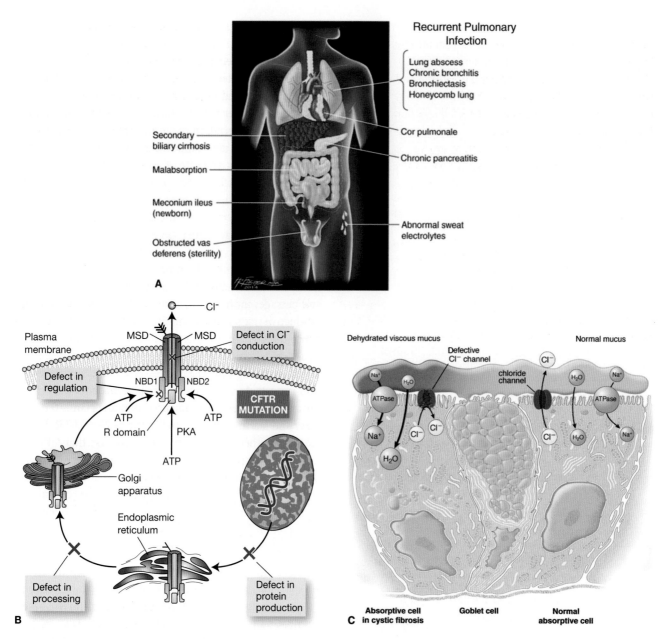

FIGURE 8.7 The pathology of cystic fibrosis. **A.** Organs affected by defective cystic fibrosis transmembrane conductance regulator (CFTR) function. **B.** Cellular sites of disruption in the synthesis of CFTR in cystic fibrosis. ATP, adenosine triphosphate; Cl$^-$, chloride ion; MSD, membrane spanning domain; NBD, nucleotide-binding domain; PKA, protein kinase A. **C.** A schematic depiction of how dysfunctional Cl$^-$ transport alters mucus quality in cystic fibrosis. A defect in the CFTR protein reduces Cl$^-$ transport into the lumen of a bronchial tube or organ duct. Sodium ion resorption from the luminal surface is then increased, and water moves into the cell along the resulting osmotic gradient. As a result, the mucus layer becomes dehydrated and viscous. It is difficult for the mucociliary escalator to convey this thickened mucus out of the respiratory tract, and it therefore clogs the lumen. Na, sodium ion; H$_2$O, water.

lung lavage studies show an imbalance in pro- and anti-inflammatory mediators that favor inflammation in patients with cystic fibrosis (57, 173).

Pulmonary Manifestations

Infants carrying the defective *CFTR* gene have normal lungs at birth (again highlighting that defective *CFTR* likely does not directly affect the quality or quantity of mucus production), but a cycle of repeated infection, inflammation, and impaired mucus clearance soon begins. The lungs are quickly colonized by *P. aeruginosa* and *Staphylococcus aureus*, and other bacterial species can also be present (174, 175). Chronic airway infection and inflammation leads to lung infiltrates (areas of denser than normal lung on a radiograph), bronchiectasis (irreversibly irregular and dilated airways), or hyperlucency (areas of the lung that are less dense than normal on a radiograph). Lower respiratory tract disease is the usual predominant clinical finding, although some patients also develop nasal polyps and chronic rhinitis that can limit nasal breathing and serve as a source of bacterial colonization that may contribute to lung infection. Bronchiectasis can be detected in infants, and the incidence increases with age (176). There is often detectable airway obstruction in children at or over 5 years old, and typical findings include reduced FEV_1, forced expiratory flow between 25% and 75% of FVC (FEF_{25-75}), and evidence of hyperinflation such as an increased RV and RV/TLC%. FEF_{25-75} is affected by disorders of the small bronchi and larger bronchioles (175).

In Children and adults with cystic fibrosis, disease severity becomes worse as the FEV1 declines (*e.g.*, FEV1 ≥ 90% normal; 70%–89% mild; 40%–60% moderate, <40% severe). For many patients with cystic fibrosis, the progressive loss of lung tissue and increasingly severe obstruction leads to respiratory failure and death (22). The speed with which the disease progresses is variable and likely influenced by gene polymorphism of other traits (171). Children displaying the classic symptoms of cystic fibrosis in infancy usually have the poorest prognosis, while those with atypical or episodic milder symptoms that present in adolescence or adulthood have a better prognosis (177).

Other pulmonary manifestations of cystic fibrosis include a barrel chest deformity, which is indicative of lung hyperinflation, use of accessory muscles of respiration to assist ventilation, hypertrophic pulmonary osteoarthropathy (enlargement of the phalanges and the ends of long bones of the forearm or lower leg), pneumothorax, hemoptysis (coughing up blood or bloody sputum from the lung), and exercise intolerance. Near the end stage of lung disease, there may be pulmonary hypertension, cor pulmonale, and respiratory failure with cyanosis (53).

Gastrointestinal Manifestations

Between 85% and 90% of infants born with cystic fibrosis develop pancreatic insufficiency, leading to low digestive enzyme availability. Combined with biliary insufficiency, this results in poor digestion and malabsorption of nutrients, especially fats. Fats that are poorly broken down and absorbed cause abdominal distension and malodorous stool. Chronic malnutrition leads to a failure to thrive when young, and many adults struggle to maintain an age-appropriate body mass. Male and female adults who can maintain their body mass index (BMI) above 23 and 22 $kg \cdot m^{-2}$, respectively, usually have better pulmonary outcomes (175, 178). Malnutrition is also associated with an increased incidence of bone disease in cystic fibrosis, especially in the second decade of

life (56, 178). There is a reduced bone mineral accrual in late childhood and early adulthood, leading to reduced bone mineral density. Inactivity, malnutrition, chronic airway inflammation, and chronic steroid use promote greater bone resorption while suppressing bone formation (179, 180). In a systemic review, the prevalence of osteoporosis in adult patients with cystic fibrosis was estimated at 23.5%, with radiologically confirmed vertebral and nonvertebral fractures occurring in 14% and 19.7% of patients, respectively (181).

Pancreatic dysfunction is caused by obstruction of the pancreatic ducts with thickened secretions. Over time, autolysis and scarring of pancreatic tissue destroy islet cells, reducing insulin secretion and resulting in glucose dysregulation. By early adolescence, 15%–20% of patients with cystic fibrosis have impaired glucose tolerance, and 10%–15% have cystic fibrosis–related diabetes. The prevalence of impaired glucose tolerance decreases slightly between 15 and 65 years of age, whereas the prevalence of cystic fibrosis–related diabetes increases from 15% to 45% over the same age range (175, 178).

Most patients with cystic fibrosis develop some form of liver disease. Nonalcoholic fatty liver disease is present in 20%–60% of patients, with a small number progressing to cirrhosis (55). Liver disease accounted for 15 of 448 (3.3%) deaths in patients with cystic fibrosis in 2015 (178). Biliary tract disease with formation of gallstones is also prevalent.

Reduced Exercise Tolerance

Compared to healthy individuals, those with cystic fibrosis have reduced exercise tolerance, lower $\dot{V}O_{2peak}$, and lower peak work capacity (182–185). Pulmonary dysfunction is a key contributor to exercise intolerance in those with severe disease and ventilatory inefficiency limits exercise tolerance in those with mild to moderate disease (186); however, it may not be the primary limiting factor in those with mild to moderate disease (187, 188). The reduced exercise capacity in early or mild stable disease does not always correlate well with spirometry and may reflect nonpulmonary disease processes such as malnutrition. Over time, lung function generally deteriorates (189, 190) and the reduced exercise capacity appears as the result of a decreased lung function (183, 191). For those who develop pulmonary-based exercise intolerance, there is generally a progressive increase in dead space. To preserve V_A, tidal volume and breathing frequency are increased to compensate for the increased dead space volume. Eventually, tidal volume expansion becomes limited by the IC and remaining IRV. Increased breathing frequency can partially compensate; however, the compensation becomes insufficient to sustain adequate $\dot{V}_E$ as patients often reach or even exceed their breathing reserve during exercise (192,

193). In addition, air trapping can lead to lung hyperinflation as it does in COPD, and limit ventilation and exercise by similar mechanisms (184). In a study of adolescents 12–18 years of age with mild to moderately severe disease, the presence of static hyperventilation (defined as an RV/TLC > 30%) resulted in early exercise termination due to inspiratory muscle fatigue resulting from dynamic lung hyperinflation and the increased work of breathing, as is seen in COPD (194).

Gas exchange can also become compromised in patients with cystic fibrosis. Oxygen desaturation and carbon dioxide retention occur during exercise in those with exercise limitation and moderate to severe disease. Those with resting oxygen saturation levels below 90% or an FEV_1 below 50% predicted are more likely to have oxygen desaturation during exercise (195). Also, patients with cystic fibrosis with lower FEV_1 are more likely to retain carbon dioxide. During maximal exercise, children (11–15 yr) who retained carbon dioxide (defined as a rise ≥5 mm Hg from rest to peak followed by a ≥3 mm Hg decrease after the peak work rate) had lower FEV_1 values. Carbon dioxide retention is reported to correlate with a faster rate of decline in FEV_1 among patients with cystic fibrosis (186, 196).

Recent evidence suggests skeletal muscle in patients with cystic fibrosis may have a reduced ability to use oxygen (197). Specifically, the phase II component of the $\dot{V}O_2$ kinetic response during exercise appears to be slowed. This slowing could reflect cardiopulmonary limitations, but it is also believed to reflect the kinetics of muscle oxygen uptake. Patients with cystic fibrosis tend to have slower $\dot{V}O_2$ kinetics when breathing normoxic air (21% oxygen). Switching from normoxic to hyperoxic air (40% oxygen) does not change $\dot{V}O_2$ kinetics even though oxygen saturation levels are increased by hyperoxia (198). The expression of CFTR by skeletal muscle raises the possibility that defective CFTR alters skeletal muscle contractile or metabolic function (199, 200). Consistent with a skeletal muscle mechanism driving exercise intolerance in cystic fibrosis is the finding that dyspnea scores are often poorly correlated with resting pulmonary function (201). In a study of 104 patients with cystic fibrosis, reported leg fatigue scores at peak exercise were higher than breathlessness scores in those with mild to moderate disease, whereas breathlessness scores were higher than leg fatigue scores in those with more severe disease. Supporting physiologic data showed normal lactate, $\dot{V}_E$, and attainment of the predicted heart rate maximum in those with less severe disease, all of which suggest a nonpulmonary limitation to exercise. In contrast, in those with more severe disease, lower lactate levels and the presence of heart

rate reserve but little breathing reserve underscore a pulmonary limitation to exercise. Thus, even though exercise capacity is reduced in those with cystic fibrosis compared to healthy individuals, the mechanism responsible for reduced capacity appears to be nonpulmonary in origin initially with pulmonary mechanisms contributing more with increasing disease severity (202).

The cardiovascular response to exercise appears normal in patients with mild to moderate cystic fibrosis, as does cardiac output and the oxygen cost of cycling (*i.e.*, 10 mL $O_2 \cdot W^{-1}$) (183, 203). Peak heart rates meet age-predicted norms, but the slope of a heart rate versus $\dot{V}O_2$ relationship is steep, reflecting reduced activity and deconditioning. In those with severe disease, peak heart rates are lower than predicted because of the pulmonary limitation to exercise, and there is evidence of a smaller stroke volume (204, 205). This is likely due to the influence of hyperinflation on ventricular filling. Those with the most severe disease and malnutrition typically have the most significant cardiac limitation to exercise (192).

Pathology and Pathophysiology in Lung Transplant

Following lung transplant, five major pathophysiologies may degrade lung function. They include loss of bronchial arterial supply, loss of airway receptors, loss of feedback from stretch receptors, airway hyperresponsiveness, and chronic lung allograft dysfunction (CLAD).

Loss of Bronchial Arterial Supply

Although a few transplant surgeons around the world anastomose the donor bronchial arteries to the recipient arteries, the great majority of transplant surgeons sacrifice the bronchial circulation at the level of the bronchial anastomoses. The viability of the bronchial system (bronchial wall and mucosa) relies on blood supply from the pulmonary circulation from distal anastomoses between the two circulations, bronchial and pulmonary. The ability of the pulmonary circulation to pick up the load is variable, and 10%–15% of patients experience extensive bronchial wall ischemia leading to necrosis of bronchial cartilage and the development of either bronchial stenosis from scarring or bronchomalacia from loss of cartilage, with airway collapse during inspiration. Shortening the donor airway to only one cartilage ring above the first division of the airways decreases but does not abolish the risk of these serious and potentially crippling complications. In the initial postoperative period, there is a profound loss of mucociliary function, which improves slowly over the initial weeks unless there has been extensive mucosal destruction by ischemia distal to the anastomosis.

Loss of Airway Receptors

From the anastomosis onward, the airways are deinnervated following transplantation. This results in the patient being unaware of distal airway secretions. In the immediate postoperative period when mucociliary function is reduced, patients are at high risk for retained secretions leading to infection or mucous plugging and deteriorating respiratory function. Immediately on weaning from mechanical ventilation, patients require vigorous and frequent chest physiotherapy concentrating on pulmonary clearance techniques to improve bronchial patency. As they recover and become increasingly mobile, secretion clearance as a rule is less of an issue. However, they require teaching that their permanent lack of awareness of peripheral secretions means they have to be more vigilant for other signs and symptoms of lower respiratory tract infections and to reinstitute pulmonary clearance measures.

Loss of Feedback From Stretch Receptors

Loss of the feedback from stretch receptors in the lung and central airways results in the loss of the Hering–Breuer reflex, which turns off inflation at high tidal volumes during exercise. Although altered breathing patterns have been reported in lung transplant recipients, they tend to be minor, and there is no convincing evidence that this loss of feedback significantly alters exercise capacity. This may be because feedback to the respiratory control centers from the chest wall continues, monitoring chest wall expansion and thus lung volume on inspiration.

Airway Hyperresponsiveness

An increase in bronchial hyperresponsiveness on inhalational bronchial challenge is recognized. This increase possibly reflects the loss of cholinergic innervation of the allograft lung below the bronchial anastomoses. This is rarely of any clinical significance to the individual recipient.

Chronic Lung Allograft Dysfunction

CLAD is a late complication of pulmonary transplantation that all recipients and their transplant team fear. At least 50% of transplant recipients will develop this complication, which is the principal cause of suboptimal outcomes of pulmonary transplantation (206). CLAD is a poorly understood phenomenon. Although often referred to as a chronic rejection, this remains unproven.

CLAD can occur at any time from 3 months to more than 10 years posttransplantation, after a period of stable lung function. Patients who have had several episodes of acute rejection or episodes of cytomegalovirus (CMV) pneumonitis are at increased risk. It may appear to be triggered by a simple intercurrent infection, such as an adenovirus infection. Although its impact on lung function and rate of progression is variable, within a few months, it can lead to death from respiratory failure or from a variety of patterns of very slow progressive falls in lung function or episodes of abrupt deterioration interspersed with periods of reduced but stable lung function (207, 208).

CLAD manifests in two distinct forms. The most common form is bronchiolitis obliterans (BO), in which an inflammatory process first narrows and then obliterates small airways. BO leads to wheezing, exertional dyspnea, and difficulties with pulmonary clearance. The rarer form is a chronic restrictive interstitial process, characterized by fibrosis of the lung parenchyma, often starting in the upper lobes and progressing through the lung. This is called restrictive CLAD as the lung function tests show a restrictive pattern as seen in pulmonary fibrotic diseases (207, 208).

Again, although its rate of progression is variable, CLAD is usually rapidly progressive and almost always leads to death from respiratory failure within the year. Altering immunosuppressive therapy has not been demonstrated to improve the clinical course of either type of CLAD. In addition, increasing immunosuppression in a patient with failing lungs and increasing difficulty maintaining pulmonary clearance of secretions is not without risk (207, 208).

Posttransplant, pulmonary function is largely influenced by patient factors existing prior to surgery (*e.g.*, underlying disease in the case of a single lung transplant), operative factors (*e.g.*, pleural or diaphragm injury), and posttransplant complications (*e.g.*, bronchial strictures). In the first few weeks after surgery, pain and early graft dysfunction hamper pulmonary function; however, peak pulmonary function is typically reached within 3–12 months after surgery. Average function tends to decline thereafter due to a 50% prevalence in CLAD within 5 years of surgery (209). Most patients undergoing bilateral lung transplant will eventually produce normal pulmonary function values for FEV_1, FVC, and TLC, but those undergoing single lung transplant often remain below normal due to the initial underlying disease (*e.g.*, COPD, pulmonary arterial hypertension, or idiopathic pulmonary fibrosis) (209). In bilateral lung transplant patients, exercise tolerance and peak aerobic capacity are often below normal despite having normal FEV_1, FVC, and TLC values. Peripheral factors including skeletal muscle dysfunction are suspected to cause diminished exercise capacity (210–212).

DIAGNOSIS OF RESPIRATORY DISEASE

As with any diagnosis, the diagnosis of respiratory disease begins with the patient history and physical examination. The findings from these assessments guide the choice of the precise diagnostic tests that follow, including for COPD, asthma, and cystic fibrosis.

COPD-Specific Considerations in Diagnostic Testing

The diagnosis of COPD is made based on patient history, physical examination, laboratory testing, and a chest x-ray. COPD should be suspected in anyone presenting with increased or chronic cough, purulent sputum production, wheezing, dyspnea, and occasional fever. In the early stages of the disease, a slowed expiration phase and wheezing may be observed. Breath sounds are typically diminished, heart sounds may be distant, and crackles may be heard at the base of the lung. In the later stages of the disease, fatigue, weight loss, and anorexia become more common. Patients may have a barrel-shaped chest, and their use of accessory muscles may be visible during breathing. Coughing spells may become violent or prolonged enough to fracture ribs or cause syncope. Ankle swelling could be present, indicating cor pulmonale or right-side heart failure. Depression and/or anxiety are also common in those with COPD and are associated with increased risk for exacerbation and poor health status (21, 213).

Tobacco smoking is a key risk factor for the development of COPD, so the patient's history in terms of pack-years (the number of cigarette packs smoked per day multiplied by the number of years smoked) should be established. A smoking history of 40–70 pack-years has been cited as indicative of the presence of COPD (14, 94). Other occupational and/or environmental exposure to dust, vapors, and particulates should also be considered because as many as 20% of COPD cases result from such exposure. A history of asthma, allergy, sinusitis or nasal polyps, frequent respiratory infections, or a family history of COPD also increases the risk for COPD (14).

Spirometry Testing

Spirometry testing, consisting primarily of an FVC maneuver after administration of a short-acting inhaled bronchodilator, is necessary to confirm the presence of an airflow limitation, which is required to establish a diagnosis of COPD. A postbronchodilator FEV_1/FVC ratio of less than or equal to 0.70 confirms an airflow limitation that is not fully reversible (14). Spirometry testing equipment is commercially available and suitable for use in hospital, laboratory, or clinic environments. Most manufacturers have adopted reasonably consistent specifications that meet current American Thoracic Society (ATS) and European Respiratory Society (ERS) guidelines (214).

The FVC maneuver requires the patient to perform a maximal inspiration followed by a forceful exhalation of air that continues until the end of the test. The technician should demonstrate this maneuver for the patient. To begin the maneuver, the patient should have the spirometry mouthpiece in place, with the lips forming a good seal to prevent air escaping. The patient should inhale quickly to their maximum inspiratory lung volume (*e.g.*, inflate to TLC) and without pausing, exhale with maximum effort. Patients should be informed "to inhale as deeply as possible" rather than simply "take a deep breath" and that inhaling to TLC is unnatural and may feel uncomfortable. They should be instructed to "blast" not just "blow" the air from their lungs. Exhalation should continue until the volume-versus-time curve plateaus (*i.e.*, <0.025 L change over ≥1 s) and the subject has tried to exhale for greater than or equal to 6 seconds for those 10 years of age or older or greater than or equal to 3 seconds for children less than 10 years of age. The technician should provide verbal encouragement to elicit the patient's best effort, but the test should be terminated if the subject cannot or should not continue because of symptoms such as light-headedness or syncope. Allowing the patient to see the flow versus volume trace or digital data in real time may provide additional encouragement or cueing to continue the exhalation effort. Note that some patients with COPD may require more than 6 seconds to reach their EELV; however, it should also be noted that exhalation times greater than 15 seconds rarely change the clinical diagnosis or treatment decisions and place the patient at greater risk for discomfort or syncope. Upon completing the forced exhalation, the patient should be instructed to inhale as deeply and quickly as possible with maximal effort to their maximal inspiratory volume. This provides a measure of the patient's forced inspiratory capacity (FIVC). If the FVC is less than the PIVC, it suggests that the patient began the expiratory maneuver before reaching maximal inspiratory volume that in turn reduces the test accuracy. A maneuver with an FIVC − FVC difference of more than 0.100 L or 5% of FVC is considered unacceptable. The exhalation and inhalation phases of the FVC maneuver should be consistent and even because coughing, hesitation, pausing, or consciously slowing the exhalation rate reduces the accuracy of the test (214).

Overall, an acceptable FVC maneuver meets the following criteria: There should be a plateauing of the volume-versus-time curve; a satisfactory start to the test with no hesitation or cough; sufficient exhalation duration; no Valsalva maneuver; no air leak from around the mouthpiece; no obstruction from the tongue or from biting of the mouthpiece; and no variable effort or evidence of the patient taking a breath during prolonged exhalation. Examples of acceptable and unacceptable quality FVC maneuver traces are shown in Figure 8.8. At least three traces meeting these criteria should be obtained for analysis, with the two largest FVC and FEV_1 values within 0.150 L of each other when testing over 6 years of age. Testing should continue until these criteria are met or the subject has performed a total of eight tests (214).

Additional pulmonary function testing includes measurement of lung volumes (*i.e.*, TCL, RV, IC, and EC), dead space ventilation, and diffusion limitations (*i.e.*, D_LCO). These can be undertaken to support a COPD diagnosis and determine disease severity (214).

Spirometry testing is generally safe; however, it can be risky for certain patients, especially when maximal or forced maneuvers are performed in outpatient settings. The high pressure generated by the thorax or abdomen could precipitate a pneumothorax or aneurysm rupture, or cause separation of tissues healing from recent surgery. There is also the potential for a significant rise and fall in blood pressure that could affect the heart and brain, causing syncope, dizziness, or light-headedness. Moreover, spirometry requires maximal expansion of the lungs and chest wall, which may cause pain or discomfort or incite paroxysmal coughing and bronchial constriction. Even with fastidious infection control, there is a risk of communicable disease transmission between patients and/or staff.

To prevent rupture of healing surgical wounds, most medical organizations recommend delaying pulmonary function testing by 4–6 weeks following surgery. This delay may be reduced to 1 or 2 weeks following laparoscopic procedures. Spirometry testing recommendations are

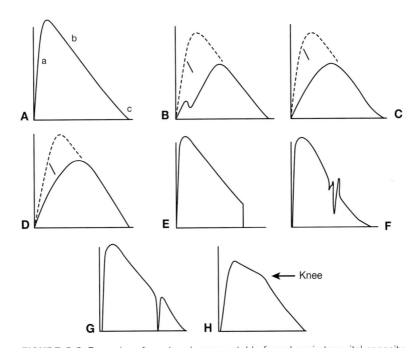

FIGURE 8.8 Examples of good and unacceptable forced expiratory vital capacity maneuvers. **A.** Excellent effort. (*a*) Rapid climb to peak flow; (*b*) continuous decrease in flow; (*c*) termination at 0–0.05 L·s^{-1} of zero flow. **B.** Hesitating start makes curve unacceptable. **C.** Subject did not exert maximal effort at the start of expiration: test needs to be repeated. **D.** Such a curve almost always indicates failure to exert maximal effort initially, but occasionally, it is reproducible and valid, especially in young nonsmoking females. This is called a rainbow curve. This curve may be found in children, patients with neuromuscular disease, or subjects who perform the maneuver poorly. In **B**, **C**, and **D**, the dashed line indicates the expected curve, and the arrow indicates the reduction in flow caused by the performance error. **E.** Curve shows a good start, but the subject quit too soon; test needs to be repeated. Occasionally, this is reproducible, and this curve can be normal for some young nonsmokers. **F.** Coughing during the first second will decrease the forced expiratory volume in 1 second. The maneuver should be repeated. **G.** Subject stopped exhaling momentarily; test needs to be repeated. **H.** This curve with a "knee" is a normal variant that often is seen in nonsmokers, especially young women. (Figure reproduced with permission from Hyatt RE, Scanlon PD, Masao N. *Interpretation of Pulmonary Function Tests.* 4th ed. Philadelphia (PA): Wolters Kluwer; 2014.)

generally conservative with respect to eye surgery because peak changes in intraocular pressure are thought to be damaging postoperatively. During spirometry, ITP is increased, but the increase is typically less than the amount generated when producing maximal expiratory pressure or during a cough (215). It is difficult to know exactly how

much ITP transfers to intraocular pressure during spirometry, but it appears to be less than 1:1. Conservatively, spirometry testing 2–3 weeks after eye surgery is considered to be a relative contraindication and classified as a moderate risk (215). Absolute and relative contraindications to spirometry testing are outlined in Table 8.3 (214, 215).

Table 8.3	Absolute and Relative Contraindications to Spirometry Testing		
Contraindication	Type	Reason to Avoid Testing	Wait Time
Recent myocardial infarction	Absolute	Risk further infarction and cardiac arrest	1 wk post event
Unstable angina	Absolute	May precipitate cardiac arrest	Perform only if necessary
Ascending aortic aneurysm	Absolute	Risk of rupture leading to catastrophic or fatal event; especially high if >6 cm or rapid growth	1 wk post repair
Pulmonary embolism	Absolute	Risk of hypoxia, respiratory failure, and death	Perform only if necessary
Brain, thorax, and abdominal surgery	Relative	Risk of rupture to repaired tissues, pain, and discomfort	4–6 wk post
Eye surgery	Relative	Risk of rupture to repaired tissues, pain, and discomfort	2–3 wk post
Pacemaker implant	Relative	Insertion site healing time	2–3 wk
Pneumothorax	Relative	Pain, discomfort, worsening of pneumothorax	2-wk post resealing
Hemoptysis	Relative	Increased bleeding and aspiration to noninfected regions of lung; suspected pulmonary emboli or myocardial infarction	Perform only if necessary
Severe hypertension	Relative	For >200 mm Hg systolic and/or 120 mm Hg diastolic, risk of syncope; cerebrovascular or aneurysm rupture; measure BP prior to testing	Variable depending on pressure and time to effective intervention
Mental confusion or instability	Relative	Patient may not understand or comply with testing procedures; consider test validity; usefulness may be compromised	Perform only if necessary
Diarrhea	Relative	Patient discomfort and embarrassment	Wait until symptoms abate
Respiratory infection	Relative	Patient discomfort, cross-contamination risks	Wait until symptoms abate

Absolute: Lung function testing should be avoided in most cases; specialist medical consultation advised to establish risks versus benefits; Relative: the risk versus benefit of testing should be considered on a case-by-case basis before proceeding with testing.

Source: Data from Cooper BG. An update on contraindications for lung function testing. *Thorax*. 2010;66(8):714–23. doi:10.1136/thx.2010.139881 with permission from BMJ Publishing Group Ltd.

Table 8.4	Combined ATS/ERS and GOLD Airflow Limitation Ranking Scheme for Chronic Obstructive Pulmonary Disease Using Postbronchodilator Spirometry	
Severity Classification	**Postbronchodilator FEV$_1$/FVC**	**FEV$_1$ as a Percentage of the Predicted Value**
At risk[a]	>0.7	≥80
Mild (GOLD 1)	≤0.7	≥80
Moderate (GOLD 2)	≤0.7	50–79
Severe (GOLD 3)	≤0.7	30–49
Very severe (GOLD 4)	≤0.7	<30

[a]Based on patients who smoke or are exposed to occupational and environmental risk factors and present with cough and/or sputum and dyspnea.

ATS, American Thoracic Society; ERS, European Respiratory Society; FEV$_1$, forced expired volume in 1 second; FVC, forced vital capacity; GOLD. Global Initiative for Chronic Obstructive Lung Disease.

Source: Adapted with permission of the © ERS 2018: Celli BR, MacNee W, Agusti A, et al. Standards for the diagnosis and treatment of patients with COPD: a summary of the ATS/ERS position paper. *Eur Respir J.* 2004;23(6):932–46. doi:10.1183/09031936.04.00014304; GOLD. Global strategy for the diagnosis, management, and prevention of COPD: 2022 Report, Global Initiative for Chronic Obstructive Lung Disease (GOLD). 2022: Available from: http://goldcopd.org.

Staging

Staging criteria to classify the severity of COPD have been proposed by the Global Initiative for Chronic Obstructive Lung Disease (GOLD) and the ATS and ERS. These are outlined in Table 8.4. Although this is useful for predicting health status, utilization of health care resources, development of exacerbations, and mortality, FEV$_1$ has been shown to correlate poorly with an individual patient's symptoms and health status (34, 216, 217). To capture the true patient COPD burden and inform clinical decision-making, COPD symptom severity and impact on functionality should be assessed and graded to identify those at high risk for exacerbation requiring medication adjustment, medical intervention, or hospitalization. Two classification systems have emerged for this purpose: the BMI, airflow obstruction, dyspnea, and exercise capacity (BODE) index and the GOLD ABE Tool (218).

The BODE index is a composite score that reflects the sum of component scores assigned to four factors that were shown to predict death in a cohort of patients with COPD (Table 8.5). To calculate the BODE index, BMI is measured by standard methodology. The FEV$_1$ is

Table 8.5	Guide for Calculating the BODE Index				
	Points Awarded Based on Measured Value				
Variable	**0**	**1**	**2**	**3**	**Score**
FEV$_1$ (% of predicted)	≥65	50–64	36–49	≤35	
Distance (m) walked in 6 min	≥350	250–349	150–249	≤149	
MMRC dyspnea scale score	0–1	2	3	4	
Body mass index (kg·m^{-2})	>21	≤21			
Sum for composite score					

The composite score sums to between 0 and 10 with higher scores indicative of increased mortality and disease severity.

BODE, BMI, airflow obstruction, dyspnea, and exercise capacity; FEV$_1$, forced expired air volume in 1 second; MMRC, the Modified Medical Research Council dyspnea scale.

Source: Adapted from Celli BR, Cote CG, Marin JM, et al. The body-mass index, airflow obstruction, dyspnea, and exercise capacity index in chronic obstructive pulmonary disease. *N Engl J Med.* 2004;350(10):1005–12. Reprinted with permission from Massachusetts Medical Society.

measured by spirometry and expressed as a percentage of the patient's age-predicted value. Dyspnea is measured using the Modified Medical Research Council (MMRC) dyspnea scale. The patient's exercise capacity is scored based on the outcome of a 6-minute walk test (6MWT) (219). The BODE index has been modified to include a measured value expressed as a percentage of the age-predicted value in place of the 6MWT (220). Both the BODE and modified BODE indexes have similar capacities for predicting mortality (221); however, a graded maximal exercise test provides a more robust assessment of exercise limitation than the 6MWT.

The GOLD ABE Tool is similar to the BODE index but emphasizes the impact of symptoms and disease burden on daily living over airflow limitation (see Figure 8.9).

FEV_1 is still measured by spirometry and ranked according to the patient's predicted value to guide prognostic and therapeutic decision-making. To overcome the poor correlation between FEV_1 and an individual's symptoms or health status, the patient's exacerbation history with and without hospitalization, as well as the symptomatic burden of COPD, are measured by questionnaire. Although the MMRC dyspnea scale can be used, the most recent GOLD recommendations suggest using the COPD Assessment Test (CAT) due to its simplicity, good correlation with more complicated tools (*i.e.*, St Georges Respiratory Questionnaire), and its assessment of symptoms beyond breathlessness (*i.e.*, MMRC dyspnea scale). The new GOLD ABE Tool forgoes a composite score in favor of categorizing patients according to exacerbation history,

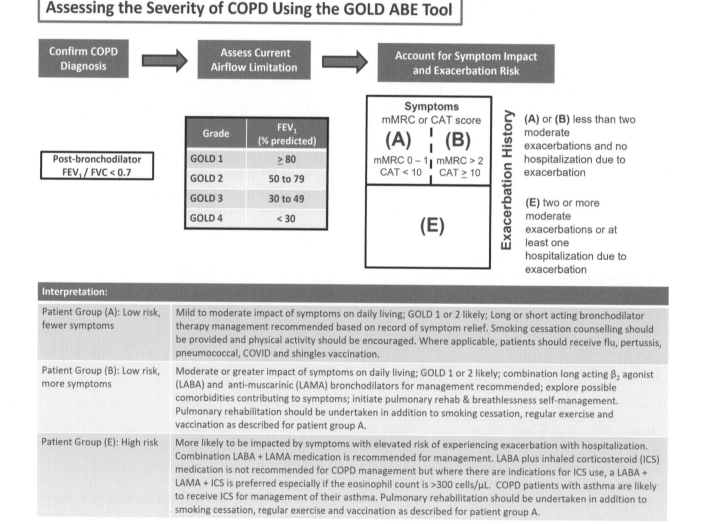

Assessing the Severity of COPD Using the GOLD ABE Tool

Confirm COPD Diagnosis → Assess Current Airflow Limitation → Account for Symptom Impact and Exacerbation Risk

Post-bronchodilator $FEV_1 / FVC < 0.7$

Grade	FEV_1 (% predicted)
GOLD 1	≥ 80
GOLD 2	50 to 79
GOLD 3	30 to 49
GOLD 4	< 30

Symptoms mMRC or CAT score

(A)	(B)
mMRC 0 – 1 CAT < 10	mMRC > 2 CAT ≥ 10

(E)

Exacerbation History

(A) or (B) less than two moderate exacerbations and no hospitalization due to exacerbation

(E) two or more moderate exacerbations or at least one hospitalization due to exacerbation

Interpretation:

Patient Group (A): Low risk, fewer symptoms	Mild to moderate impact of symptoms on daily living; GOLD 1 or 2 likely; Long or short acting bronchodilator therapy management recommended based on record of symptom relief. Smoking cessation counselling should be provided and physical activity should be encouraged. Where applicable, patients should receive flu, pertussis, pneumococcal, COVID and shingles vaccination.
Patient Group (B): Low risk, more symptoms	Moderate or greater impact of symptoms on daily living; GOLD 1 or 2 likely; combination long acting β₂ agonist (LABA) and anti-muscarinic (LAMA) bronchodilators for management recommended; explore possible comorbidities contributing to symptoms; initiate pulmonary rehab & breathlessness self-management. Pulmonary rehabilitation should be undertaken in addition to smoking cessation, regular exercise and vaccination as described for patient group A.
Patient Group (E): High risk	More likely to be impacted by symptoms with elevated risk of experiencing exacerbation with hospitalization. Combination LABA + LAMA medication is recommended for management. LABA plus inhaled corticosteroid (ICS) medication is not recommended for COPD management but where there are indications for ICS use, a LABA + LAMA + ICS is preferred especially if the eosinophil count is >300 cells/µL. COPD patients with asthma are likely to receive ICS for management of their asthma. Pulmonary rehabilitation should be undertaken in addition to smoking cessation, regular exercise and vaccination as described for patient group A.

FIGURE 8.9 The Global Initiative for Obstructive Lung Disease (GOLD) ABE Assessment Tool for categorization of patients with obstructive pulmonary disease. (Adapted from GOLD. Global strategy for the diagnosis, management and prevention of COPD: 2023 Report, Global Initiative for Chronic Obstructive Lung Disease (GOLD). 2023. Available from: http://goldcopd.org.)

exacerbation-induced hospitalization, and symptom burden (218). The GOLD ABE Tool builds on the earlier 2017 GOLD Index that was argued to better identify the cause(s) of current symptoms, thereby facilitating more precise treatment compared to other approaches (21). Both the BODE and GOLD indexes appear useful for predicting morbidity and mortality (21, 219); however, at least one study suggests that neither instrument assesses factors that seem to be the main predictors of acute exacerbations (222). The new GOLD ABE Tool still requires validation with clinical research (218).

Asthma-Specific Considerations in Diagnostic Testing

Diagnosis of asthma requires clinical experience and judgment because the presenting signs and symptoms can vary between patients and even within a patient at different times. A diagnosis of asthma is based on identifying a characteristic pattern of several respiratory symptoms that are usually present simultaneously (especially in adults) and include wheezing, shortness of breath, chest tightness, cough, and a variable or reversible airflow limitation. As the symptoms themselves can be present in many different respiratory diseases, the key to diagnosis is the respiratory symptom pattern. Symptoms are often triggered by viral infection (*e.g.*, colds) exercise, allergen exposure changes in weather, laughter, or irritants such as car exhaust fumes, smoke, or strong smells. Symptoms are worse at night or during early morning, and they vary over time and in intensity. The symptoms are less likely to be asthma-related if cough is the only symptom, there is chronic production of sputum, there is shortness of breath with dizziness, paresthesia, or chest pain, or there is noisy inspiration during exercise-induced dyspnea (*i.e.*, vocal cord dysfunction) (36).

Medical history should highlight the time frame of symptom onset, history of allergic rhinitis or eczema, and familial history of asthma or atopic disease. Family and social history may identify potential causal factors and allergen triggers. Current medications should be considered, as nonsteroidal anti-inflammatories and β-adrenergic antagonists can worsen asthma symptoms and angiotensin-converting enzyme inhibitors can cause a chronic cough that imitates asthma. Physical examination is often normal, but respiratory wheezing (rhonchi) can sometimes be detected by auscultation, especially when exhalation is forced. Crackles and inspiratory wheezing are not typically present in asthma. Examination of the nasal sinus may reveal polyps or signs of allergic rhinitis (36).

Spirometry Testing

A key feature of asthma is the presence of a variable airflow limitation. Spirometry conducted by trained individuals using well-maintained and calibrated equipment is the recommended method for detecting and measuring an airflow limitation. A forced expiratory maneuver with measurement of FVC, FEV_1, FEV_1/FVC%, and PEFR (*i.e.*, peak expiratory flow rate) is used to document the severity of the limitation. Because asthmatic airflow limitations are variable, the presence or absence of a flow limitation is not diagnostic for asthma. It is the pattern of variability or reversibility of the airflow limitation that supports an asthma diagnosis.

An airflow limitation is established when the FEV_1 is reduced and the measured FEV_1/FVC% is less than 75% to 80% in adults or less than 90% in children and there is additional evidence of excessive variability in lung function. Excessive variability in lung function can manifest as a reversible airflow limitation where FEV_1 improves by more than 12% (or 200 mL above baseline) 10–15 minutes after administration of 200–400 μg of albuterol or equivalent. A 12% variance from baseline in FEV_1 in adults and children on successive follow-up appointments can indicate excessive variability of lung function. It may also be evident if FEV_1 decreases by more than 10% or 200 mL from baseline in adults or more than 12% in children during exercise or when average PEFR varies by more than 10% in adults or 13% in children when measured twice daily over 2 weeks.

Airway hyperresponsiveness is a feature of asthma, and it can be identified through inhalation of standard dosages of methacholine, mannitol, or hypertonic saline, or by hyperventilation. In patients with asthma, these challenges produce a typical decrease in FEV_1 of greater than or equal to 20% (methacholine) and more than 15% for the other challenges. Serial testing is important. Finally, an improvement in FEV_1 by 12% or PEFR greater than 20% following 4 weeks of anti-inflammatory treatment is suggestive of asthma (36, 223, 224).

Other Testing

Other tests may be used to support an asthma diagnosis or rule out other causes of the patient's symptoms. A chest x-ray may show hyperinflation or other abnormalities associated with pneumonia, pneumothorax, malignancy, or heart failure. Sputum may be examined for evidence of increased eosinophil and neutrophil counts. The fractional concentration of exhaled nitric oxide (FENO) may be measured as a noninvasive marker of airway inflammation, but its usefulness in establishing an asthma diagnosis is debated. Finally, allergy testing by skin prick testing can be used to identify atopic status; however, a skin reaction to a specific allergen does not mean that the allergen causes the patient's symptoms, nor does it confirm the presence of asthma (36).

Most patients with asthma will experience bronchoconstriction in response to exercise. In order to identify individuals with EIB, exercise-based testing or eucapnic voluntary hyperpnea testing can be used. Exercise is undertaken to increase $\dot{V}_E$ approximately 20-fold for 8–10 minutes. FEV_1 is then measured at 5, 10, 15, and 30 minutes, postexercise. Using a baseline FEV_1 obtained before exercise for comparison, a decrease in FEV_1 of greater than or equal to 10% on two consecutive postexercise time points is considered positive evidence for the presence of EIB (225). Eucapnic voluntary hyperpnea can also be used in place of, or in tandem with, exercise testing to identify the presence of EIB. Eucapnic voluntary hyperpnea requires the patient to hyperventilate through a system that monitors and maintains end-tidal carbon dioxide at a constant level. Patients may be asked to perform graded (*e.g.*, 30%, 60%, and 90% of MVV for 3 min each) or single-stage (*e.g.*, 85% MVV for 6 min) hyperventilation tests. Multistage tests are usually performed in those with severe uncontrolled disease, and the test is terminated if evidence for EIB is found. In both test types, FEV_1 is measured at 1, 5, 10, 15, and 20 minutes after the patient has hyperventilated for the required duration (*e.g.*, 3 or 6 min) and intensity (*e.g.*, %MVV). The test is considered positive if the FEV_1 decreases by greater than or equal to 10% of the baseline value obtained prior to hyperventilation (226).

Cystic Fibrosis–Specific Considerations in Diagnostic Testing

The Cystic Fibrosis Foundation guidelines state that diagnosis should be based on the presence of one or more clinical features of cystic fibrosis, history of cystic fibrosis in a sibling, or a positive newborn screen, and laboratory findings of abnormal *CFTR* gene or protein function (178).

Broad implementation of newborn screening programs in North America, Europe, and Australasia identifies a significant proportion of new patients with cystic fibrosis, which improves outcomes later in life. Newborn screening requires the measurement of immunoreactive trypsinogen (IRT) from a blood spot (heel prick) test. Very high IRT levels are indicative of pancreatic injury but are not specific for cystic fibrosis. The IRT test is repeated at 3 weeks, and the sample is also screened for the presence of one of the 40 most frequent *CFTR* mutations (57).

The gold standard test for confirming a cystic fibrosis diagnosis is the sweat chloride test with genetic testing to identify the specific *CFTR* mutation that in turn directs (54, 227). It is recommended that all newborns with a positive screen undergo diagnostic sweat testing even when the presence of two cystic fibrosis genetic mutations has been identified. Sweat chloride testing involves iontophoresis of pilocarpine on skin patches of the arms or legs. Using standardized procedures, sweat is collected in gauze and analyzed. Normal mean sweat chloride levels are typically around 10 $mmol \cdot L^{-1}$. Generally speaking, sweat chloride levels greater than 60 $mmol \cdot L^{-1}$ are consistent with a diagnosis of cystic fibrosis, and sweat test chloride levels between 30 and 59 $mmol \cdot L^{-1}$ are considered borderline or indeterminate, and test values less than 30 $mmol \cdot L^{-1}$ are considered negative (227).

Additional laboratory testing can be undertaken to support a diagnosis of cystic fibrosis, especially in older individuals or those with mild symptoms or to monitor disease progression. Testing should include sputum culture, chest radiograph, blood sampling for complete cell counts, liver and renal function testing, nutritional status assessment (total protein and albumin levels, fat-soluble vitamin status), blood glucose monitoring (cystic fibrosis–related diabetes), spirometry, and aerobic capacity testing. Most patients with cystic fibrosis have mild lung disease and variable levels of airway obstruction and hyperinflation. Regular spirometry testing can identify acute or declining FEV_1 or FEF_{25-75} that highlight worsening lung function (54, 178). A single measure of aerobic capacity is correlated with long-term survival in that those with higher $\dot{V}_E$ values have longer life expectancy. Regular exercise testing is also important for monitoring disease progression as those who maintain aerobic capacity have a better long-term prognosis (228).

MEDICAL MANAGEMENT OF RESPIRATORY DISEASE

Respiratory diseases are often chronic and progressive, and in many cases cannot be cured. Management is therefore aimed primarily at reducing disease symptoms, improving exercise tolerance, limiting disease progression, and preventing disease exacerbations and premature mortality. Comprehensive disease management includes pharmacological therapy, influenza and pneumococcal vaccination, oxygen therapy, exercise and psychosocial assessment and management, and lung volume reduction or transplant surgery. These interventions typically address lung dysfunction, inflammation, and dynamic hyperinflation. Pulmonary rehabilitation programming includes exercise, smoking cessation, and other behavioral support. These interventions address systemic extrapulmonary consequences of the disease, such as physical deconditioning and exercise intolerance or behaviors such as smoking that predispose to disease progression. Psychosocial components of pulmonary rehabilitation are vital for improving patients' overall health and well-being, as depression is common in this patient population.

In addition, secondary disease prevention (*e.g.*, prevention of cardiovascular disease) is important. Medical management should also aim to preserve functionality, enabling patients to continue working and participating in recreational activities, as well as to maintain activities of daily living. These efforts will help patients maintain a higher quality of life.

Pulmonary Rehabilitation

The ATS and ERS define pulmonary rehabilitation as ". . . a comprehensive intervention based on a thorough patient assessment followed by patient-tailored therapies, which include, but are not limited to, exercise training, education and behavior change, designed to improve the physical and emotional condition of people with chronic respiratory disease and to promote the long-term adherence of health-enhancing behaviors" (229–231). Pulmonary rehabilitation is an integrated multidisciplinary strategy of disease management that involves active collaboration between patients and family and the health care providers, including CEPs, involved in their care. It actively promotes patient self-efficacy and provides an opportunity to coordinate patient care throughout the clinical course of an individual's disease.

Pulmonary rehabilitation can be beneficial for patients with any chronic respiratory disease that reduces pulmonary function to cause exercise intolerance in spite of optimal pharmacologic management (232). It can be effective when initiated at any stage of a patient's disease, including during or immediately following acute disease exacerbation (233). Although patients with severe disease are typically referred to pulmonary rehabilitation programs, those with mild disease also appear to benefit significantly from attendance (234). The American College of Physicians, American College of Chest Physicians, ATS, and ERS recommend that patients with an FEV_1 less than 50% of the predicted value be referred to a pulmonary rehabilitation program. It is acknowledged that patient disease burden is not always reflected by the degree

of airflow limitation; therefore, an individual with FEV_1 greater than 50% predicted who is symptomatic or has exercise intolerance should also be referred to pulmonary rehabilitation. Other reasons for program referral include reduced functional status, reduced occupational performance, inability to maintain activities of daily living, difficulty following medical regimen, nutritional concerns, depression or behavioral health concerns, gas exchange abnormalities, or an increase in medical resource consumption (229).

Development of patient self-efficacy and exercise training are central components of pulmonary rehabilitation. Programs are holistic and intensive, and include individualized patient assessment, individualized exercise prescription, supervised exercise training, self-management education, psychosocial support, breathing retraining, and nutritional counseling. The majority of insurance providers will cover up to 36 sessions if medically necessary. Typically, patients attend program sessions two to three times per week for 12 weeks, with attendance in at least 20 sessions being the threshold for obtaining benefit. Any achieved benefits are usually lost within 1 year unless some form of maintenance programming is adopted (229).

There is no consensus on ideal program length, but longer programs appear better, especially for those with severe COPD (235–237). It is likely that all chronic respiratory diseases benefit from longer interventions, because these conditions are incurable and most often progressive. It is unreasonable to expect an intervention lasting only a few weeks to provide adequate treatment for a condition that could persist for a decade or more. It is often necessary to repeat pulmonary rehabilitation one or more times and/or supplement formal pulmonary rehabilitation with maintenance-style programming to reinforce patient self-efficacy throughout the course of the patient's disease.

Pulmonary rehabilitation can be offered in a hospital-, community-, or home-based setting. The safety and efficacy of community-based programs can equal hospital-based programs if they are supported by appropriate medical and allied health professionals and they are staffed by CEPs specifically trained to assess exercise capacity and prescribe exercise to individuals with chronic health conditions (238). Home-based pulmonary rehabilitation programs are typically limited to exercise training with periodic tele-monitoring or telephone support and are thus more suited to patients who are highly motivated and self-directed rather than those with severe disease. For some, home-based programs are economical and convenient, especially for improving or maintaining exercise tolerance and quality of life. It should be noted, however, that home-based programs lack group support and the opportunity to develop social support networks, which are also important to well-being and disease self-management. This can be alleviated to an extent if the home-based program includes periodic group sessions in a community or hospital-based setting. Additionally, the cost of home-based programs may not be covered by the patient's insurance provider, causing an increased financial responsibility for the patient.

Pulmonary rehabilitation is more than just exercise training. In hospital- and community-based programs, patients are likely to receive education around pharmacotherapy and learn how to manage exacerbations, including how to better identify when they should seek hospital care. Patients receive nutritional counseling to manage cachexia or obesity. Psychological and behavior change support are provided to manage depression and anxiety, as well as facilitate smoking cessation and adoption of regular physical activity. Breathing (*i.e.*, pursed-lip, diagrammatic, and paced) and mucus-clearing techniques (*i.e.*, postural drainage or forced expiration) are taught to patients for better management of dyspnea. Patients may also receive other specialized interventions such as respiratory muscle training through inspiratory resistive training, threshold loading, or normocapnic hyperpnea training. Some programs include hospice care and end-of-life planning, as many patients are unaware of the severity of their disease. In a study that interviewed patients in pulmonary rehabilitation in the month before they died, approximately 70% reported that they believed they would survive for at least 1 year (229–231, 239).

COPD-Specific Medical Management

In addition to pulmonary rehabilitation, pharmacological therapy is used in COPD to induce bronchodilation, reduce inflammation, and manage or prevent respiratory infection. Bronchodilators act to relax airway smooth muscle and reduce airway resistance to improve FEV_1 and symptoms. They reduce airway hyperinflation at rest and during exercise, and they improve exercise capacity (14).

Use of long- or short-acting β_2-adrenergic agonists and anticholinergic drugs that block M_3 muscarinic receptors achieve bronchodilation through cell signaling pathways that increase intracellular cyclic AMP in the airway smooth muscle (240, 241). Cyclic AMP–mediated signaling pathways cause airway smooth muscle relaxation that widens the airways. Common bronchodilator medications are listed in Table 8.6. Short-acting bronchodilators are usually the first line of drugs used for airway

management, or they are prescribed as rescue medications for periods of acute worsening of symptoms because they have a rapid onset of action and can be used on an as-needed basis. There is little difference in efficacy or symptom relief between the two different drug classes, but each has its own side-effect profile and cost, which may direct preference. Long-acting β_2-adrenergic agonists and anticholinergic drugs prescribed alone or in combination improve FEV_1 and symptoms and reduce exacerbation risk without affecting mortality. They are often used to treat moderate to severe COPD and have a prolonged but slow onset of action. A short-acting bronchodilator is typically coprescribed to manage acute symptoms of airflow worsening. Long-acting anticholinergics may be better for preventing exacerbations than long-acting β_2-adrenergic agonists (21); however, combination therapy using long-acting β_2-adrenergic and anticholinergic medications appears to be most effective (14). Methylxanthines are also prescribed for bronchodilation and work through a generalized inhibition of phosphodiesterases to increase airway smooth muscle cyclic AMP in a "shot gun"–type approach. The therapeutic dose window is small, and methylxanthines have a side-effect profile that limits their usefulness in COPD. Other specific cyclic AMP phosphodiesterase inhibitors such as roflumilast have been developed that are much more effective and have fewer side effects (242).

Inhaled corticosteroids and oral glucocorticoids are used to reduce airway inflammation. Evidence suggests that inhaled cortical steroids maybe useful for preserving lung function and reducing exacerbations in current and ex-smokers. Efficacy of inhaled corticosteroids is much greater when used in combination with long-acting β_2-adrenergic and anticholinergic medications. The benefit of long-term corticosteroid use as a means to treat COPD remains equivocal. Patients experiencing frequent exacerbations, with blood eosinophil counts less than 300 cells·μL^{-1}, and a history of asthma appear to derive the greatest benefit from inhaled corticosteroids. Oral glucocorticoid therapy is mainly used to treat acute exacerbation of COPD because of the negative side-effect profile associated with long-term oral glucocorticoid use (14). Antibiotics (*i.e.*, azithromycin), vaccinations, and mucolytics (*i.e.*, acetylcysteine) are also used to prevent and manage respiratory infections to reduce the frequency and severity of exacerbations. Antitussives to reduce cough are not recommended despite the potential for symptom relief because coughing is essential for clearing the airways and improving airflow (94).

Table 8.6	Common Drugs Used to Treat Respiratory Disease
Drug	**Main Action and Exercise Considerations**
β2-Adrenergic Agonists (Short Acting)	
Fenoterol, levalbuterol, pirbuterol, salbutamol/albuterol, terbutaline	• Bronchodilation achieved through activation of β_2-adrenergic receptor pathway. Increased intracellular cAMP that promotes airway smooth muscle relaxation • Improves exercise capacity by reducing bronchoconstriction and improving airflow; timing of administration effects impacts exercise performance and ability to prevent bronchospasm • May ↑ HR and BP at rest or during exercise
β2-Adrenergic Agonists (Long Acting)	
Arformoterol, formoterol, indacaterol, olodaterol, salmeterol	• Similar in action and effect as short-acting β_2 agonist drugs • Salmeterol may cause skeletal muscle tremor and hypokalemia.
cAMP Agonists	
Aminophylline, theophylline, caffeine, roflumilast (PDE-4 inhibitor)	• Bronchodilation achieved through inhibition of PDE that reduce intracellular cAMP • Inhibition of histamine-induced airway smooth muscle constriction; anti-inflammatory activity in COPD • Improve exercise capacity by relieving bronchoconstriction and improving airflow • At therapeutic doses may have cardiac effects; ↑HR and may increase PVC incidence
Anticholinergics (Short Acting)	
Ipratropium bromide, oxitropium bromide	• Bronchodilation achieved through inhibition of muscarinic receptors, resulting in airway smooth muscle relaxation • Improves exercise capacity by relieving bronchoconstriction and improving airflow • May ↑HR • Preferred rescue medication for those using β-blocking medications with action on β_2 receptors • Side-effect profile includes dry mouth and bitter metallic aftertaste; may increase cardiovascular events in patients with COPD.
Combination β2-Adrenergic Agonists and Anticholinergic Drugs	
Short acting: Fenoterol/ipratropium, salbutamol/ipratropium **Long acting:** Formoterol/aclidinium, formoterol/glycopyrronium, vilanterol/umeclidinium, olodaterol/tiotropium	• Combined medications have similar effect and side-effect profile as individual medications.

(continued)

Table 8.6	Common Drugs Used to Treat Respiratory Disease *(continued)*

Anti-inflammatories

| **Systemic steroids:**
Prednisone, prednisolone, methylprednisolone
Inhaled steroids:
Budesonide, beclomethasone flunisolide, fluticasone, triamcinolone
Leukotriene modifiers:
Zafirlukast, zileuton, montelukast
Miscellaneous:
Cromolyn/nedocromil (mast cell stabilizers), omalizumab (anti-IgE), ibuprofen | • Various mechanisms exploited to reduce immune system activity and heightened inflammatory responses
• No direct effect on exercise or exercise capacity identified but can indirectly improve exercise capacity through reduction in inflammatory symptoms and improvement in lung function
• Although risk is greatest with systemic steroid use, side effects include increased risk of osteoporosis, muscle atrophy, hypertension, diabetes, cataracts, oral thrush, and cough |

Antibiotics

| Ciprofloxacin, co-trimoxazole, tobramycin, cephalexin, colistin, dicloxacillin, azithromycin | • Both oral and inhaled antibiotics used to prevent, treat, or reduce bacterial load to reduce airway inflammation
• No direct effect on exercise, indirectly may improve function through reduction in airway inflammation |

Antihistamines

| Loratadine, cetirizine, fexofenadine | • Improvement in exercise
• May ↑HR at rest
• Timing of administration should be considered to obtain benefit during exercise. |

Mucolytics

| Guaifenesin, DNase, nebulized hypertonic saline, *N*-acetylcysteine | • Reduce mucus viscosity, aid in mucus removal
• No direct effect on exercise, indirectly may increase exercise capacity by improving airflow and lung function |

Nasal Sprays

| Beconase, Flonase, Nasel, Nasacort, Rhinocort, Vancenase | • Symptom relief for rhinitis and sinusitis; no known direct effect on exercise capacity |

Gastrointestinal Support Medications

| Pancrelipase (pancreatic enzyme supplement), omeprazole, ranitidine (for gastroesophageal reflux relief), docusate, casanthranol (stool softener) | • Symptom relief, no known direct effect on exercise capacity |

Nutritional Supplements

| ADEK, Fer-in-Sol, poly-vi-flor drops, aquasol A, aquasol E, drisdol | • Nutrition support, no known direct effect on exercise capacity |

↑, increase; ↓, decrease; ↔, variable effect; BP, blood pressure; cyclic AMP, cyclic 3′5′-adenosine monophosphate; HR, heart rate; PDE, phosphodiesterase; PVC, premature ventricular contraction.

There is a long-standing history supporting the use of supplementary oxygen therapy in patients with COPD and arterial hypoxemia (*i.e.*, $PaO_2 = 55$ mm Hg or 8 kPa or $SaO_2 < 88\%$). Breathing air enriched with oxygen increases the oxygen partial pressure of alveolar air that in turn facilitates greater diffusion of oxygen into the blood. The goal of oxygen therapy is to prevent arterial hypoxemia and improve tissue oxygen delivery by maintaining SaO$_2$ at greater than or equal to 90% at rest and during exercise. Early studies showed that long-term oxygen therapy significantly reduces hospital admissions and mortality (243, 244), improves polycythemia (245), reduces pulmonary hypertension (246), and supports neuropsychiatric function (247). Supplemental oxygen also improves exercise capacity and may improve exercise training results for both conventional and high-intensity interval training (HIIT) by improving peripheral muscle oxygenation and reducing dyspnea (248–251).

Although the benefits of oxygen supplementation in those with severe or acute hypoxemia are clear, long-term oxygen therapy may not be suitable for all patients with COPD. A recent parallel group randomized clinical trial conducted by the Long-term Oxygen Treatment Trial Research Group found that stable patients with COPD with moderate resting or exercising arterial desaturation (*i.e.*, SaO$_2$ 89%–93%) who were prescribed long-term oxygen therapy (*n* = 368) fared no better than patients who were not prescribed long-term oxygen therapy (*n* = 370) in terms of time to death and time to first hospital admission. In fact, both groups had similar rates for all hospitalizations, COPD-related hospitalizations, and other secondary outcome measures such as quality of life, lung function, and distance walked in 6 minutes (252). Given that there are some side effects associated with long-term oxygen therapy (*i.e.*, nasal dryness and bleeding, reduced ventilatory drive leading to CO$_2$ retention, and fire hazard risk), more research is necessary to determine which patients can benefit most from long-term oxygen therapy.

Asthma-Specific Medical Management

Asthma is one of the world's most common chronic illnesses, and it cannot be cured. Medical treatment of asthma is therefore aimed toward management of symptoms and prevention of disease exacerbations. The cycle for achieving good asthma control includes three key steps:

1. Thorough assessment of symptoms, lung function, risk factors, and therapeutic adherence,
2. Adjustment of medications and nonpharmacologic treatments to match disease status and treatment of modifiable risk factors, and
3. Regular review of symptoms, exacerbations, treatment side effects, lung function, and patient satisfaction (28).

Pharmacologic therapy for asthma (Table 8.6) follows a step-up or step-down algorithm so that therapy can be adjusted to match changing symptom severity. The gold

standard therapy is to initiate therapy consisting of a low-dose inhaled corticosteroid with a long-acting β$_2$-adrenergic agonist (*e.g.*, formoterol). In some patients, it is necessary to include an on-demand short-acting β$_2$-adrenergic agonist. From the initial treatment, dosages can be titrated up or down based on symptoms. In all cases, the medication, device, and dose for controller and reliever should be individualized (36). A leukotriene receptor inhibitor or theophylline may be prescribed in place of a corticosteroid. When symptoms are severe, therapy may be stepped up by adding a long-acting inhaled β-adrenergic agonist to progressively increasing doses of inhaled corticosteroids. Other preventer medications such as a long-lasting anticholinergic (*i.e.*, tiotropium bromide) or anti-IgE (*i.e.*, omalizumab) can be added as needed. Therapy should be monitored so that medications can also be stepped down when they are no longer required. The goal should be to use the lowest inhaled corticosteroid dosage possible while still maintaining optimal symptom management. Although inhaled corticosteroid use poses less risk than systemic steroid use, prolonged daily use of high-dose inhaled corticosteroids does increase the risk of developing clinically significant adverse side effects. Daily use of low-dose corticosteroids is not associated with significant adverse side effects (36). EIB can usually be managed with the use of a short-acting β-adrenergic agonist, but some cases may require the addition of one or more controllers to achieve effective symptom control (169, 253). To improve pharmacologic therapy, appropriate inhaler devices should be prescribed, and the patient should be taught how to use the device to ensure that each medication dose is delivered to the lungs and not deposited on the oropharynx (254).

Addressing certain comorbidities is also useful for achieving optimal symptom control. The presence of rhinitis and rhinosinusitis increases the risk of exacerbation and may increase the use of rescue medication. Treatment of any underlying rhinopathy will likely improve overall asthma symptom control. Obesity increases the risk for developing asthma and the presence of obstructive sleep apnea. Obesity-related asthma is often refractory to inhaled corticosteroids, whereas a 5%–10% reduction in body weight generally improves symptoms and quality of life (255). Gastroesophageal reflux disease (GERD) and reduced lung volumes make asthma harder to manage. The presence of GERD even among normal-weight individuals may induce coughing and precipitate asthma attacks. Avoidance of asthma triggers (*e.g.*, aspirin, indoor and outdoor allergens, first- and secondhand tobacco smoke, environmental pollutants, and some foods or chemicals) is encouraged as a means of preventing exacerbation of asthma symptoms (36).

Cystic Fibrosis–Specific Medical Management

Although their life expectancy has improved dramatically, most patients with cystic fibrosis will still die from respiratory failure. A major emphasis of medical management is aimed at preventing lung infection and preserving lung function (256). Improvement in disease management is increasing life expectancy for those with cystic fibrosis. Between 2000 and 2010, the median age for patients with cystic fibrosis increased by 2.4 years. Median survival for male and female children born in 2010 is projected to be 40 and 37 years, respectively, based on current mortality rates. Median survival could reach 50 years if the mortality rate continues to decline as it has from 2000 to 2010 (257). Development and U.S. Food and Drug approval of more CFTR modulator drugs like the new triple-combination therapy (*e.g.*, Trikafta; elexacaftor/tezacaftor/ivacaftor) for individuals aged 12 years and older and have at least one allele with the F508del variant is expected to significantly improve morbidity and mortality from CF (258).

Preventing Infection and Inflammation

Considerable emphasis is placed on the prevention and management of recurrent and chronic infection to mitigate the damaging effects of inflammation. Mucociliary clearance is compromised in cystic fibrosis. The thick, sticky mucus not only obstructs small airways but also harbors microorganisms that produce infection (Table 8.6). Thus, central to prevention of infection are various nonpharmacologic airway clearance techniques. Percussive or rhythmic clapping on the exterior chest wall or chest wall vibration can loosen secretions or prompt an airway-clearing cough, especially when the chest wall is vibrated during exhalation. In some cases, an inflatable vest can be worn for percussive and vibration therapy. The vest is connected to an air pump that produces oscillatory chest compressions at various frequencies. Other airway-clearing techniques include active cycle breathing, autogenic drainage, positive expiratory pressure therapies, Huff coughing technique, and exercise. Patients are also encouraged to put themselves into positions that promote postural drainage. Chest physiotherapy sessions typically require 20–30 minutes, and they are performed at least twice per day (259). Clearing mucus from the airways can be enhanced through inhalation of aerosolized hypertonic saline (7%) or mannitol powder to rehydrate the airways, or through inhalation of dornase alfa, a human deoxyribonuclease 1 enzyme that cleaves DNA and reduces viscoelasticity of mucus, making it easier to clear. Regular collection of airway cultures and aggressive antibiotic therapy following positive cultures is part of the strategy to minimize cycles of infection and inflammation. Long-term antibiotic therapy is recommended to manage chronic infections as the treatment benefits outweigh the risk of developing antibiotic resistance (256).

Chronic airway inflammation is ever present in cystic fibrosis, and it is likely the major contributor to airway destruction and development of bronchiectasis and obstruction. Inhaled and oral corticosteroids have often been used to manage airway inflammation in cystic fibrosis; however, several reviews have concluded that they provide limited benefit for improving lung function in children and adults. In children, oral corticosteroids are associated with glucose metabolism abnormalities, cataract formation, and retarded linear growth. In adults, oral corticosteroids are associated with abnormal glucose metabolism, osteoporosis, and skeletal muscle myopathy. The limited evidence for benefit of inhaled corticosteroids and the increased adverse risk profile of oral corticosteroids led the Cystic Fibrosis Foundation to recommend against the use of inhaled and oral corticosteroids to manage airway inflammation in those with cystic fibrosis in the absence of asthma or allergic bronchopulmonary *aspergillosis* (36, 260). Other oral anti-inflammatories such as leukotriene modifiers and cromolyn (sodium cromoglycate) are of limited use as evidence showing benefit is lacking. Daily ibuprofen 15–31.6 mg·kg^{-1} per day has been shown to slow the decline in FEV_1 among patients aged 5–39 years, but there is insufficient evidence to support recommended usage as chronic therapy (36). Inhaled macrolide antibiotics (*e.g.*, azithromycin) effectively improve lung function, probably because of their antibiotic and anti-inflammatory properties, even though they are not particularly effective against *P. aeruginosa*. Maintenance therapy reduces pulmonary exacerbations in young patients; however, there is some concern that prolonged use will lead to the development of resistant strains. Newer inhaled antibiotics such as colistin, tobramycin, aztreonam lysine, and levofloxacin appear effective for managing *P. aeruginosa* infection (261).

Improving Lung Function

Bronchodilators are often prescribed to patients with cystic fibrosis. Inhaled β_2-adrenergic agonists consistently improve FEV_1 and peak expiratory flow. Long-acting agonists (*i.e.*, salmeterol) improve lung function better than short-acting agonist (*i.e.*, salbutamol or albuterol), but both are well tolerated. Two recent studies of inhaled β_2-adrenergic agonist use produced equivocal results, prompting the Cystic Fibrosis Foundation to alter earlier recommendations concerning chronic use of these drugs.

Current recommendations recognize that β_2-adrenergic agonists can benefit those with airway hyperresponsiveness (*i.e.*, increased sensitivity to bronchoconstrictors) and can relieve acute bronchospasm; however, daily chronic use is no longer recommended (54, 260, 262). Inhaled anticholinergic agents are not recommended because the level of evidence supporting their use in patients with cystic fibrosis is lacking or of poor quality. Trials of the short-acting anticholinergic medication ipratropium bromide showed that it can improve FEV_1 for most patients, but a small number of patients showed decreases in FEV_1. There have been no studies of long-term use, and none of the long-acting medications have been sufficiently studied to recommend their use (260).

Medications and practices that improve airway function should generally increase exercise capacity. Long-term use of systemic glucocorticosteroids is associated with the development of osteoporosis and skeletal muscle myopathy, which can result in reduced muscular strength and increased injury risk. Load-bearing exercise can be used to offset these effects (263, 264), but they must be considered by the exercise practitioner when interpreting functional test scores and designing the exercise prescription. It should be noted that inhaled β_2-agonist bronchodilators may cause tachycardia or cough or worsen bronchoconstriction in some patients. Oral bronchodilators such as theophylline may cause tachycardia, ventricular dysrhythmia, and/or tachypnea.

Improving Nutrition and Metabolism

In addition to preventing infection and preserving pulmonary function, medical management aims to improve nutritional status and metabolic health. Maintaining good nutrition and a BMI close to the target range is critical to long-term survival in cystic fibrosis and for supporting and maintaining physical activity, which also contributes to long-term survival. The target BMI for children and adolescents is the 50th percentile for their age and gender; female and male patients should aim to achieve and maintain a BMI of 22 and 23 $kg \cdot m^{-2}$, respectively (256).

Nutritional management includes anticipatory guidance consisting of behavioral modification and motivational interviewing to reinforce adherence to diet and to sodium and enzyme supplementation recommendations. During moderate malnutrition, oral supplements and meal replacements may be introduced to increase caloric and nutrient intake. Temporary nasogastric or nasal jejunal feeding may be used. During severe malnutrition, a gastric tube may be used for long-term enteral feeding.

Many patients develop pancreatic insufficiency; thus, pancreatic enzymes (*i.e.*, lipase, amylase, and protease) are taken as an oral supplement to improve fat, carbohydrate, and protein digestion (265). Fat digestion is often compromised because cystic fibrosis affects the liver's ability to secrete bile, which aids in the digestion and absorption of fats and fat-soluble vitamins. Supplementation of the diet with fat-soluble vitamins is somewhat standard (266).

Precision Medicine Using Gene Therapy

CFTR modulator drugs enhance or even restore the expression, function, and stability of a defective CFTR. Each modulator acts distinctively, and they are classified into five main groups depending on their effects on *CFTR* mutations: potentiators, correctors, stabilizers, readthrough agents, and amplifiers. For example, ivacaftor targets class III and IV *CFTR* mutations (*i.e.*, channels that reach the plasmalemma membrane but fail to open) and increases the likelihood that the channel will open to facilitate chloride transport. To target the more prevalent Phe508del mutation that causes CFTR misfolding (class II mutation), ivacaftor has been combined with lumacaftor, which improves trafficking of the CFTR protein to the plasmalemmal surface. The combined drug approach improves the likelihood of channels inserting into the plasmalemma and opening to function as chloride transporters. This approach has been shown to improve FEV_1 and reduce sweat chloride levels in patients homozygous for Phe508del. Trials using the trade name drug Orkambi (a combination of ivacaftor and lumacaftor) showed modest improvement after use in lung function and quality of life (267). The newly approved elexacaftor-tezacaftor-ivacaftor triple-combination CFTR-modulating therapy contains two correctors and a potentiator of the CFTR channel. Clinical trials have demonstrated superior efficacy against other therapies with respect to improving lung function, sweat chloride reduction, and decreasing exacerbation frequency with minimal side effects (268). Although CFTR modulators are proven to significantly improve CF treatment, use of the modulating drugs to improve exercise tolerance remains understudied. In a small case study, it was reported that Trikafta/Kaftrio (*i.e.*, elexacaftor/tezacaftor/ivacaftor) improved $\dot{V}O_{2max}$ by 18%, 52%, and 33% for the three adolescent participants following 6 weeks of treatment (269). In contrast, a similar study showed that three of four adolescent participants receiving the tezacaftor/ivacaftor combination failed to improve $\dot{V}O_{2max}$ after 8 months of treatment (270). Future studies are needed to evaluate the impact of CFTR-modulating therapies on exercise function.

Lung Transplant Medical Management

Immunosuppressive Therapies

The lung is an active organ of innate immune function, responding to exposure to damaging particles and microorganisms in every breath. Thus, despite receiving significantly higher doses of immunosuppressant drugs, lung transplant recipients have a more acute rejection than patients with other solid organ transplants (*e.g.*, heart transplantation). Inevitably, this higher level of immunosuppression, which is primarily directed at cell-mediated immunity rather than antibody-mediated immunity, increases the risk of complicating infections, particularly atypical infections: atypical bacteria, parasites, and fungi. Episodes of acute rejection are common in the first year and are treated with augmented immunosuppression using short bursts of high doses of corticosteroids often combined with alterations in the patient's background immunosuppressive regimen. The target concentrations of immunosuppressive drugs are gradually reduced over the first 6–24 months as the risk of acute rejection decreases. A standard regimen consists of a corticosteroid, prednisone, combined with a calcineurin antagonist, tacrolimus or cyclosporine, and either azathioprine or mycophenolate mofetil as an immunosuppressant.

Long-term Risks of Immunosuppressive Therapies

For long-term survivors (more than 8–10 yr), there are major adverse effects of taking these therapies for life. Lung transplant recipients receive more immunosuppression than other single organ transplant populations, and this contributes to a greater risk for the development of cancer posttransplant. The most common cancers in lung transplant recipients are non-melanoma skin cancers, followed by lung cancer and posttransplant lymphoproliferative disorder (PTLD) (271). Renal dysfunction caused by calcineurin inhibitors (tacrolimus and cyclosporine) can lead to renal failure and the need for either long-term hemodialysis or a renal transplant. About 20% of patients who survive for 10 years posttransplant will have chronic renal failure, and 3%–7% will require renal replacement therapy (272). Posttransplant immunotherapy also increases the risk for developing diabetes primarily due to the side effect of calcineurin inhibitors and glucocorticoids. There are increased risks for developing cardiovascular disease (*e.g.*, hypertension and hyperlipidemia), cytopenia, thromboembolic disease, avascular necrosis of the femoral head, gastrointestinal complications, and neurologic complications (273).

Osteopenia is almost universal in patients with advanced respiratory failure, and many develop overt osteoporosis. Following transplant, there can be improvement in bone density with the combination of increased activity and medication. However, with long-term corticosteroid therapy, there is a high risk of progressive osteoporosis (273).

EXERCISE TESTING AND TRAINING IN RESPIRATORY DISEASE MANAGEMENT

Exercise intolerance is defined as an inability to perform exercise or physical activity at an intensity that would be expected of others of the same age and gender. Exercise intolerance and exertional dyspnea are the primary symptoms that prompt many patients to consult with their physician. Evaluation of exercise capacity is a key element of respiratory disease management and pulmonary rehabilitation programming, as it provides the information needed to develop a safe and individualized exercise prescription that, when combined with optimized pharmacotherapy, is the most effective way to treat exercise intolerance (229, 274, 275).

Most diagnostic and treatment optimization testing is done while the patient is at rest. The results of such testing (*i.e.*, FEV_1) often correlate poorly with exertional symptoms (134). It is only when the system is stressed by exercise that the true extent of the disease impact and factors contributing to exercise intolerance can be identified. Lung function is often clearly the central limiting factor to exercise capacity in those with severe respiratory disease, but for those with mild to moderate respiratory disease, exercise capacity may be limited more by skeletal muscle dysfunction, poor physical conditioning, and/or comorbidities such as heart disease. Exercise testing that combines physiologic and subjective measurements (*i.e.*, dyspnea scale or rating of perceived exertion [RPE] scales) is the most accurate method for assessing and identifying specific factors limiting a patient's exercise capacity.

Cardiopulmonary Exercise Testing

Cardiopulmonary exercise testing is recognized as the best method for evaluating the physiologic response to exercise. The test is well characterized, and it provides a comprehensive assessment of cardiac, respiratory, and skeletal muscle physiology under load up to failure. It is a laboratory-based test involving treadmill or cycle ergometer exercise that becomes progressively more difficult over time until the patient elects to stop (*i.e.*, volitional exhaustion) or an abnormal physiologic response occurs (*e.g.*, cardiac pain), and the test is terminated by the supervising clinician (Table 8.7).

Testing Modality

The decision to use a treadmill or cycle ergometer for testing should be dictated by the modality of exercise best suited to the patient and by the availability of equipment. An important advantage of treadmill testing is that walking is an activity of daily living, and the patient will be accustomed to it. It is a suitable modality of exercise for all but the most severely deconditioned or those with compromised balance and coordination. Peak oxygen consumption rates ($\dot{V}O_2$) are typically 5%–10% higher when a treadmill is used instead of cycle ergometry (276), and treadmill testing results in greater arterial oxygen desaturation than cycling, which may be advantageous for measuring exercise-induced arterial desaturation in patients with COPD (135, 277, 278). Treadmill testing is necessary for patients with pacemakers that rely on accelerometry to match heart rate to an increased cardiac output demand (71). The central disadvantage of treadmill exercise is that it can present a falls risk for some patients especially when being stabilized for blood pressure measurement and because the external work rate varies due to body mass, gait dynamics, and by the patient holding onto the handrails for balance. Cycle ergometers offer the advantage of a well-established energetic cost (*i.e.*, 10 mL·min^{-1} of oxygen per watt) that is minimally affected by body mass or technique. In addition, cycle ergometry negates issues associated with balance while exercising or the need to stabilize the patient while measuring blood pressure and drawing arterial blood samples. Perhaps the greatest advantage offered by cycle ergometry is that the patient can stop exercise safely when needed by ceasing to pedal. During treadmill exercise, the patient must signal the desire to stop and the clinician must decrease the treadmill speed and inclination gradually because abruptly ceasing to continue walking or stopping the belt will likely result in loss of balance and potential injury (71, 279).

Testing Protocol

Two types of exercise testing protocols are used for patients with respiratory diseases:

1. Incremental work protocols and
2. Continuous or endurance work protocols

Incremental Protocols

During incremental protocols, the exercise intensity is gradually increased over time in steps, or it is ramped at a constant rate. For cycling, the patient warms up for 2–3 minutes with unloaded pedaling before the resistance is increased by 5–30 W every 1–3 minutes depending on the fitness level. It is recommended that a test should last

Table 8.7	Contraindications to Continuing Exercise
Absolute	**Relative**
1. Patient requests to stop 2. Drop in systolic BP of >10 mm Hg from baseline despite an increase in workload when accompanied by other evidence of ischemia 3. Moderately severe angina > 2 on the 4-point angina scale 4. Increasing nervous system symptoms 5. Signs of poor perfusion 6. Technical difficulties 7. Sustained ventricular tachycardia 8. ECG ST-segment elevation (>1.0 mm) in leads without a diagnostic Q-wave	1. Drop in systolic BP of >10 mm Hg from baseline despite an increase in workload in the absence of other evidence of ischemia 2. ECG ST-segment or QRS changes such as excessive ST depression (>2 mm horizontal or downsloping ST-segment depression) or a marked axis shift 3. Arrhythmias other than sustained VT, including multifocal PVCs, triplets of PVCs, supraventricular tachycardia, heart block, or bradyarrhythmias 4. Fatigue, shortness of breath, wheezing, leg cramps, or claudication 5. Development of bundle branch block or interventricular conduction delay 6. Increasing chest pain 7. Hypertensive response (systolic BP > 250 mm Hg and or diastolic BP > 115 mm Hg)

Source: Fletcher GF, Balady GJ, Froelicher VF, Hartley LH, Haskell WL, Pollock ML. Exercise standards: a statement for healthcare professionals from the American Heart Association. *Circulation*. 1995;91(2):580–615. ©1995 American Heart Association, Inc.

between 8 and 12 minutes; however, those with severe disease may not be able to exercise continuously for this long. A test duration of 5 minutes is likely sufficient for analysis in severely deconditioned patients (71). Benzo et al. (280) compared 4, 8, and 16 $W \cdot min^{-1}$ continuous ramp cycle protocols to an 8 $W \cdot min^{-1}$ step cycle protocol in patients with severe COPD (*i.e.*, $FEV_1 < 38\%$ predicted), and found that $\dot{V}O_{2peak}$, maximal $\dot{V}_E$, peak heart rate, and peak RPE were not different between protocols in spite of the test duration being significantly shorter and the maximal work rate being higher in the 16 $W \cdot min^{-1}$ ramp protocol.

A routine for estimating 1-minute step workload increases needed to achieve a cycle ergometer test that is approximately 10 minutes long is outlined below (71):

1. Estimate the oxygen cost of unloaded cycling:
   unloaded cycling $(mL \cdot min^{-1}) = 150 + (6 \times$ body weight in kilograms)
2. Estimate the maximal oxygen uptake rate:
   Peak $(mL \cdot min^{-1}) = $ (height in centimeters $-$ age in yr) $\times 20$ for sedentary men or $\times 14$ for sedentary women

   For those with an FEV_1 or D_{LCO} approximately 80% of age-predicted norms, $\dot{V}O_{2peak}$ will be slightly overestimated so the test may be less than 10 minutes long.

   For those with an FEV_1 or D_{LCO} between 80% and 50% of age-predicted norms, actual $\dot{V}O_{2peak}$ will be 60%–70% of the predicted value.

   For those with an FEV_1 or D_{LCO} between 50% and 30% of age-predicted norms, actual $\dot{V}O_{2peak}$ will be 30%–50% of the predicted value.
3. Calculate work rate increment:
   Work rate increment $(W \cdot min^{-1}) = $ (Peak $\dot{V}O_{2peak} - \dot{V}O_{2peak}$ unloaded cycling)/10 minutes.

Incremental treadmill protocols for exercise testing individuals with respiratory diseases alter workload by increasing the treadmill belt speed and inclination. Standard exercise testing protocols such as the Bruce protocol are generally criticized for being too demanding for patients with significant respiratory disease. The modified Balke-Ware or Naughton protocols may be suitable alternatives (281). Cooper et al. (282) developed a treadmill-based protocol for use in patients with moderate to severe COPD that is outlined in Table 8.8. The protocol has an approximately linear increase in work rate over time, and in a sample population of 519 patients with COPD, the average test duration was approximately 9 minutes.

Continuous or Endurance Protocols

Continuous or endurance work rate protocols require the patient to warm up by cycling or walking at a very low

Table 8.8	Speed and Grade Adjustments for Treadmill Testing in Patients With Moderate to Severe COPD		
Test Phase	Elapsed Time (min)	Speed mph (kph)	Grade (%)
Warm-up	1	1.0 (1.6)	0
	2	1.0 (1.6)	0
	3	1.0 (1.6)	0
Exercise	4	1.0 (1.6)	1
	5	1.0 (1.6)	2
	6	1.0 (1.6)	3
	7	1.0 (1.6)	5
	8	1.5 (2.4)	5
	9	1.5 (2.4)	7
	10	2.0 (3.2)	7
	11	2.0 (3.2)	8
	12	2.5 (4.0)	8
	13	2.5 (4.0)	9
	14	3.0 (4.8)	9
	15	3.5 (5.6)	9
	16	4.0 (6.4)	9
	17	4.5 (7.2)	9
	18	5.0 (8.0)	9
Recovery	19	1.0 (1.6)	0
	20	1.0 (1.6)	0

kph, kilometers per hour; mph, miles per hour.

Source: Adapted from Cooper CB, Abrazzado M, Legg D, Kesten S. Development and implementation of treadmill exercise testing protocols in COPD. *Int J Chron Obstruc Pulmon Dis.* 2010;5:375–85. Originally published by and used with permission from Dove Medical Press Ltd.

workload for 2–3 minutes. The workload is then abruptly increased above critical power (*i.e.*, <75% or more of the patient's peak $\dot{V}O_2$) and the patient continues until volitional fatigue, or the test is terminated by the supervising technician (259). A limitation of this approach is the requirement of a prior incremental test to establish the workload; however, there is emerging evidence that constant load tests are superior to incremental tests for evaluating pulmonary rehabilitation or drug interventions to improve exercise capacity (283). The decision to use an incremental or constant load test protocol should be based on the test objective (*i.e.*, characterizing the response to exercise vs. measuring improvement to an intervention).

Test Components

At a minimum, incremental and continuous tests should include collection of expired air for volume and gas analysis; a 12-lead electrocardiogram; regular hemodynamic monitoring by auscultation; an RPE measure; a dyspnea measure; and pulse oximetry. It should be noted that the measurement reliability of pulse oximeters may become questionable for saturation levels below 90% (284). In addition to the standard measures, arterial blood gas and lactate concentrations can be measured if the patient is fitted with a brachial artery catheter. Key physiologic parameters derived from the measured data include peak oxygen consumption rate ($\dot{V}O_{2peak}$); the ventilatory equivalents for oxygen and carbon dioxide ($\dot{V}O_2/\dot{V}_E$ and $\dot{V}CO_2/\dot{V}_E$); the anaerobic threshold (AT); the dead space to tidal volume ratio (V_D/V_T); the respiratory exchange ratio (RER); the alveolar minus arterial oxygen and carbon dioxide difference ($P(A-a)O_2$); the arterial minus end-tidal carbon dioxide difference ($P(a-ET)CO_2$); the oxygen pulse (O_2-pulse); and the breathing and heart rate reserve.

Responses

Cardiopulmonary exercise testing in those with respiratory disease typically shows a lower-than-expected peak work rate and a $\dot{V}O_{2peak}$ that is below age-predicted norms. The $\dot{V}O_2$ versus work relationship is usually normal during the initial exercise stages (*i.e.*, 10 mL·min^{-1} O_2·W^{-1}) but may be reduced as the test progresses depending on disease severity. The relationship between $\dot{V}CO_2$ and $\dot{V}_E$ is linear, and the line has a slope between 23 and 28 in healthy subjects. The slope increases in proportion to disease severity in those with respiratory disease. The RER is typically less than 1.0 at rest and increases above 1.0 during progressive exercise. In those with severe respiratory disease, the RER may exceed 1.0 at rest, identifying patients who are hyperventilating with respect to oxygen demand. In some patients, the RER may not increase above 1.0 during exercise because exercise is terminated prior to reaching the AT. The AT is usually at the lower end of normal due to physical deconditioning but may be absent in those with very severe airflow limitations because peak exercise occurs before the AT is reached. In these instances, the patient is unable to increase $\dot{V}_E$ in response to increasing arterial carbon dioxide and continues to exercise. The v-slope method is thought to be more sensitive than the ventilatory equivalent method for detecting the AT (71, 279, 285).

As would be expected, ventilatory responses are abnormal in those with respiratory disease. Peak $\dot{V}_E$ is less than the expected value, as is the maximum voluntary ventilation (MVV) rate. As exercise progresses, breathing reserve is typically exhausted because of plateauing of tidal volume expansion combined with an expiratory flow limitation that prevents the breathing rate from exceeding 40 breaths·min^{-1} (although it may reach 50 breaths·min^{-1} in restrictive disorders). The cardiovascular response is mostly normal unless cardiac or pulmonary vascular disease is also present. O_2-pulse and heart rate should increase normally, although heart rate may increase somewhat steeply (due to deconditioning). The heart rate should maintain a linear relationship with $\dot{V}O_2$, and the heart rate maximum should be unchanged; however, heart rate reserve is often more than 20% at peak exercise because exercise is limited by noncardiac factors before the cardiovascular system is maximally stressed (71, 279, 285).

During exercise testing in someone with respiratory disease, V_A/Q and gas exchange abnormalities are often observed. The V_D/V_T is a useful measure because it provides an estimate of the degree of mismatching between ventilation and perfusion of the lung. The lower the V_D/V_T, the better ventilation and perfusion are matched. In healthy individuals, the V_D/V_T falls from roughly 0.33 at rest to 0.20 during exercise. In those with respiratory disease, the V_D/V_T may be normal or slightly elevated at rest and will fail to decrease during exercise. The high proportion of "wasted" ventilation means a higher $\dot{V}_E$ is required to maintain normal $PaCO_2$ and PaO_2. As a result, both the $\dot{V}O_2/\dot{V}_E$ and $\dot{V}CO_{2peak}/\dot{V}_E$ tend to be higher and fail to decrease below 28 and 32 at their respective nadirs. The degree of elevation is proportional to the severity of the disease. As a result of overventilation of poorly perfused areas of the lung, $P(a-ET)CO_2$ is typically increased and remains constant, whereas it would typically decrease and become negative in healthy individuals. This often distinguishes uneven ventilation from uneven perfusion as the cause of V_A/Q inequality (71). $P(A-a)O_2$ is also elevated above normal due to ventilation of poorly ventilated airspaces. Despite an increased $\dot{V}_E$ to maintain $PaCO_2$, PaO_2 often falls during exercise (71, 279, 285).

Safety

Maximal cardiopulmonary exercise testing has been shown to be extremely safe even in high-risk populations. The risk of experiencing an acute myocardial infarction, ventricular fibrillation, hospitalization, or death ranges from 2 to 5 per 100,000 tests to approximately 6 per 10,000 tests. Testing risks can be minimized by using proper pretest screening procedures and patient risk stratification; adherence to recognized contraindications to exercise testing and exercise test termination criteria (see Tables 8.7 and 8.9); adequate monitoring during testing; use of adequately trained staff (*e.g.*, training in clinical exercise testing and advanced cardiac life support); and rapid access to an automated external defibrillator (AED), oxygen, and airway support (286, 287).

Field-Based Walking Tests of Cardiopulmonary Fitness

Although exercise testing is the recommended method for assessing exercise intolerance and dyspnea in respiratory disease, it is limited to use in laboratory and clinical settings. Several field-based walking tests that are less reliant on expensive equipment can be used to measure the impact of disease on functional capacity and efficacy of treatment. A technical standard was recently developed by the ERS and ATS to provide clinicians, therapists, and exercise specialists with standardized procedures for using walking-based field tests (288). Absolute and relative

contraindications to field-based walking tests are identified in Table 8.10.

The 6-Minute Walk Test

The 6MWT is perhaps the most widely used field test in clinical and research settings and is required for the calculation of a BODE score (see Table 8.5). During the test, the patient walks at a self-selected pace as far as possible in 6 minutes on a 30-m (98 feet) linear course. The self-selected pace means that the patient typically exercises at a submaximal effort. Testing should not be undertaken on a treadmill, as this reduces 6MWT distance (289). Some patients may need to slow down or pause during the test, but the timing is not interrupted. The track should be indoors with a firm flat surface that is clearly marked in 3-m (9.8 feet) intervals (290). Patients may need to use supplemental oxygen or wheeled walkers to complete the test. Serial testing should be undertaken at the same time of day using the same support devices, and the patients should follow their usual medication routine to ensure test consistency. In addition to the distance completed, heart rate, blood pressure, and dyspnea should be measured before and at the completion of the test. Oxygen saturation should be measured continuously during the test and the lowest value achieved recorded. Encouragement

Table 8.9	Contraindications for Initiating a Cardiopulmonary Exercise Test
Absolute	**Relative**
1. Recent change in the resting ECG, suggesting significant ischemia, recent myocardial infarction (within 2 d), or other acute cardiac event 2. Unstable angina 3. Uncontrolled cardiac dysrhythmia causing symptoms or hemodynamic compromise 4. Symptomatic severe aortic stenosis 5. Uncontrolled symptomatic heart failure 6. Acute pulmonary embolus or pulmonary infarction 7. Suspected or known dissecting aneurysm 8. Acute systematic infection, accompanied by fever, body aches, or swollen lymph glands	1. Left main coronary stenosis 2. Moderate stenotic valvular heart disease 3. Electrolyte abnormalities (e.g., hypokalemia, hypomagnesemia) 4. Severe arterial hypertension (*i.e.*, SBP > 200 mm Hg and/or DBP > 110 mm Hg) at rest 5. Tachydysrhythmia or bradydysrhythmia 6. Hypertrophic cardiomyopathy and other forms of outflow tract obstruction 7. Neuromuscular, musculoskeletal, or rheumatoid disorders that are exacerbated during exercise 8. High-degree atrioventricular block 9. Ventricular aneurysm 10. Uncontrolled metabolic disease (*e.g.*, diabetes, thyrotoxicosis, or myxedema) 11. Chronic infectious disease (*e.g.*, mononucleosis, hepatitis, AIDS) 12. Mental or physical impairment leading to inability to exercise adequately

Source: Data from Fletcher GF, Ades PA, Kligfield P, et al. Exercise standards for testing and training: a scientific statement from the American Heart Association. *Circulation*. 2013;128(8):873–934. ©2013 American Heart Association, Inc.

Table 8.10	Absolute and Relative Contraindications for Field Walking Tests

Absolute	Relative
1. Acute (3–5 d) postmyocardial infarction 2. Unstable angina 3. Symptomatic uncontrolled arrhythmias 4. Syncope 5. Active endocarditis 6. Acute myocarditis or pericarditis 7. Symptomatic severe aortic stenosis 8. Uncontrolled heart failure 9. Acute pulmonary embolism or infarction 10. Lower extremity thrombosis 11. Suspected dissecting aneurysm 12. Uncontrolled asthma 13. Pulmonary edema 14. Room air oxygen Sat ≤ 85% unless ambulatory supplemental oxygen provided 15. Acute respiratory failure 16. Acute noncardiopulmonary disorder that could be aggravated by exercise (*i.e.*, infection, renal failure, thyrotoxicosis) 17. Mental impairment leading to an inability to follow test instructions	1. Left main coronary artery stenosis or its equivalent 2. Moderate stenotic valvular heart disease 3. Severe untreated arterial hypertension at rest (*i.e.*, ≥200 mm Hg systolic and/or 120 mm Hg diastolic) 4. Tachyarrhythmias or bradyarrhythmias 5. High-degree atrioventricular block 6. Hypertrophic cardiomyopathy 7. Significant pulmonary hypertension 8. Advanced complicated pregnancy 9. Electrolyte abnormalities 10. Orthopedic impairments that prevent or are made worse by walking

Source: Adapted with permission of the © ERS 2018: Holland AE, Spruit MA, Troosters T, et al. An official European Respiratory Society/American Thoracic Society technical standard: field walking tests in chronic respiratory disease. *Eur Respir J.* 2014;44(6):1428–46. doi:10.1183/09031936.00150314.

and updates can be given to the patient during testing, but only standardized phrases (Table 8.11) should be used periodically to avoid influencing the patient's self-selected pacing strategy (291). Repeatability studies show that the

Table 8.11	Standardized Feedback for the 6-Minute Walk Test

1 min: "You are doing well. You have 5 minutes to go."
2 min: "Keep up the good work. You have 4 minutes to go."
3 min: "You are doing well. You are halfway."
4 min: "Keep up the good work. You only have 2 minutes left."
5 min: "You are doing well. You have only 1 minute to go."
6 min: "Please stop where you are."

Note: If a patient stops during the test, say, "Please resume walking whenever you feel able" every 30 seconds once their oxygen saturation is >85%.

Source: Adapted with permission of the © ERS 2018: Holland AE, Spruit MA, Troosters T, et al. An official European Respiratory Society/American Thoracic Society technical standard: field walking tests in chronic respiratory disease. *Eur Respir J.* 2014;44(6):1428–46. doi:10.1183/09031936.00150314.

distance walked during the first trial is shorter than it is in subsequent trials so at least two trials with up to 1 hour of rest in between should be performed to overcome the learning effect of repeat testing (288, 291).

The primary outcome measure of the 6MWT is the total distance walked, which is correlated with functional capacity, disease severity, and prognosis (291, 292). It is thought that the 6MWT distance better reflects limitations in activities of daily living than peak $\dot{V}O_2$ values measured during exercise testing (291). In addition to the total distance walked, the average walking speed over 6 minutes and the number of times and total duration that the subject had to stop walking should be recorded. These may provide alternate metrics for pre- and postintervention assessment in patients who cannot walk continuously for 6 minutes. Exercise-induced arterial desaturation is an important finding during a 6MWT as this is associated with low daily physical activity, lower FEV_1, and a declining prognosis if it worsens over time (288).

The average distance walked by 40- to 80-year-old healthy subjects is estimated to be 571 ± 90 m (624.5 ± 31.7 yards) with males walking on average 30 m (32.81 yards) farther than females. The 6MWT distance is reduced with normal aging, and age-specific reference standards for males and females are available (293). The 6MWT distance is reduced in those with respiratory disease, and many reference equations are available for predicting walking distance. Unfortunately, a wide range of predicted values can be generated from the available reference equations. Although there is moderately good correlation ($r = 0.73$) between 6MWT distance and $\dot{V}O_{2peak}$ for groups of patients with COPD, it should be highlighted that there can be significant individual variability between distance walked and the calculated $\dot{V}O_{2peak}$ for these equations (294). A prediction equation can be used to derive the peak cycle ergometer work rate from the 6MWT distance (295):

$$\text{Peak work rate} = (0.122 \times \text{6MWT distance [m]}) + (72.683 \times \text{height [m]}) - 117.109$$

This equation could be useful for estimating cycle ergometer workloads used in exercise rehabilitation training, but it should not be viewed as a surrogate for exercise testing, as the 6MWT provides little information to identify factors responsible for exercise intolerance and dyspnea.

The 6MWT is most often used as an outcome measure to evaluate the effect of treatment or rehabilitation in patients with pulmonary disease. There is considerable controversy, however, regarding the minimal clinically important difference (MCID) that should be used to compare pre- to postintervention outcomes. The MCID is reported to be as low as 20 m (21.87 yards) and as high as 54 m (59.06 yards). Alternatively, an increase in 6MWT distance of 10%–14% of the preintervention could be used (296, 297).

The Incremental and Endurance Shuttle-Walk Tests

In addition to the 6MWT, the incremental shuttle-walk test (ISWT) and the endurance shuttle-walk test (ESWT) can be used to evaluate functional capacity in a field-based setting. The ISWT is an incremental maximal exercise test and should follow similar contraindications as exercise testing (see Tables 8.7, 8.9, and 8.10). Subjects travel between two traffic pylons spaced 10 m (10.94 yards) apart and should reach each cone in time with a series of "beeps" which could be played electronically. The interval between beeps shortens as the test progresses to the increased walking speed by 10 m·min^{-1}. The 12-stage test continues until the patient can no longer continue or keep the required pace. The ESWT is completed on the same course as the ISWT. After a 2-minute warm-up of walking at a low to moderate pace, the patient is required to walk between the traffic pylons at 85% of the maximum

sustainable walking speed using audible beeps to ensure proper speed is maintained. The patient walks until severe breathlessness or fatigue develops or 20 minutes of test time has elapsed. Supplemental oxygen can be used during the ISWT and ESWT (288, 292).

The primary outcome measure for both the ISWT and ESWT is the total distance walked, which reflects peak $\dot{V}O_{2peak}$ in patients with mild to severe COPD (298). Dyspnea, RPE, and oxygen saturation are also important outcome measures that may be useful for evaluating the degree of impairment. Both the ISWT and ESWT distances are sensitive to therapeutic intervention, but the MCID is not yet established. A 50–200 m (54.68–218.72 yard) of improvement has been reported for ISWT and 150–300 m (164.04–328.08 yard) of improvement to various interventions have been reported with some suggestion that the ESWT is more sensitive than the 6MWT (296). To date, there has been only limited development of reference values and predictive equations for the ISWT and ESWT. The ISWT for healthy adult males and females was reported to be 606 ± 167 m (662.67 ± 182.63 yard) and 443 ± 117 m (484.43 ± 127.95 yard), respectively (299). In a second study (300), the mean ISWT was 810 m (885.83 yards), with a large degree of variability (IQR$_{25\%-27\%}$ = 572–1,030 m or 625.55–1126.42 yards). In both studies, age, height, weight, gender, and BMI explained most of the variability. The ISWT distance is further reduced in populations that are chronically ill; for example, male and female patients entering cardiac rehabilitation walked 395 ± 165 m (431.98 ± 180.45 yards) and 269 ± 118 m (294.18 ± 129.05 yards), respectively (276). There is a paucity of information regarding reference values or predictive equations for ESWT distances.

Musculoskeletal Testing

In addition to cardiopulmonary function, musculoskeletal function is negatively affected by respiratory disease. Loss of skeletal muscle mass and a shift toward a less oxidative metabolic profile contribute to exercise intolerance, low physical activity levels, and reduced ability to complete tasks of daily living. Musculoskeletal testing is an objective way to monitor disease progression, treatment efficacy, and the impact of rehabilitation for the patient.

Isometric strength is important in daily activities such as carrying groceries, sitting down, and standing up from a chair, and pushing and pulling open doors (301). Static maximal isometric strength is easily measured by isometric dynamometry in clinical and rehabilitation environments. The patient performs a maximal voluntary contraction (MVC), and the muscle force produced is measured by a strain gauge, cable tensiometer, force platform, or force transducer. The tests are reproducible and sensitive if the measurement procedure is standardized. MVC force varies with joint angle and the angle of muscle pull, so it is important to use a goniometer to record the joint angle to improve the accuracy of retesting. There are a range of reference values for upper and lower limb muscles.

Handheld, spring, or computerized dynamometers and strain gauges can be used to measure muscle force–generating capacity. Handheld dynamometers are affordable and portable measurement devices that allow the assessment of muscle strength over a range of joint angles and actions. The weaknesses are the difficulty in standardizing measurement and a lack of widespread acceptance of reference values. Computerized dynamometers measure similar single joint actions but often use a mechanical platform to isolate joint and limb movement, thereby increasing the repeatability of measurement. They produce valid, reliable, and reproducible measurements of muscular strength, but their use is often limited by their high cost and complexity of operation (302). Grip strength is an inexpensive, easy, and reliable method to estimate overall muscle strength from childhood to old age, and its decline is associated with an increased risk of all-cause mortality in healthy adults (303) and in patients with COPD (304). Grip strength may not correlate well with COPD severity or functional impairment, but it does correlate with health-related quality of life and higher exacerbation risk (305, 306). Thus, additional strength testing should be undertaken in COPD, including testing that evaluates quadriceps strength, as it is more clinically relevant (307).

Isometric movements and strength may not be relevant to movements made during activities of daily living or rehabilitative exercise training because the measured strength is specific to joint/muscle pull angle and muscle fiber length. Dynamic testing allows strength to be measured over the whole range of motion (ROM) while the external load remains fixed, but the velocity of movement may vary. This better reflects natural movement. The one repetition maximum (1RM) test is widely used, and it assesses the maximum load that can be lifted through the whole ROM with proper form for one repetition. 1RM testing can be used to assess muscle isolation exercises (*e.g.*, leg extension for quadriceps strength) or multi-joint and complex exercises (*e.g.*, bench press for pectoral, triceps, and anterior deltoid muscles) in healthy adults, athletes, older adults, and those with chronic disease (281). Both machine and free weights can be used to provide the appropriate resistance. Testing is generally contraindicated in those meeting the contraindication criteria for exercise testing (see Table 8.9) in addition to those with musculoskeletal conditions or injuries that may be made worse by exerting maximal effort.

Prior to testing, the patient engages in a warm-up of the exercise being assessed using light loads for 5–10 repetitions. The weight is increased to approximately 80% of the 1RM load, which is lifted three to five times. After 3–5 minutes of rest, the weight is further increased, and the lift is attempted. If successful, the weight is increased, and the lift is attempted after 3–5 minutes of rest (281). It can be difficult and time consuming to identify the 1RM, especially for patients with COPD who are susceptible to muscle fatigue. As an alternative, the 1RM can be estimated from the 2RM to 10RM (*i.e.*, the maximum load lifted for 2–10 repetitions) because a relationship exists between muscular strength, endurance, and the number of repetitions to fatigue (308). Measurement or estimate of the 1RM may not be feasible in some patients, and in these cases, measurement of muscle force by handheld dynamometry may be a better option. With handheld dynamometry, the tester identifies the muscle or muscle group to be tested. The patient then pushes or pulls against a handheld dynamometer (*e.g.*, micro-FET®; Hogan Scientific), and the force developed is recorded. Forces developed for most muscle groups can be compared to population norms (309, 310). Assessment of muscular endurance may be more relevant and sensitive for detecting change in physical function, especially for those with COPD (237, 311). Unfortunately, there are no standardized tests of muscular endurance available nor are there reference data available for comparison in patients with chronic respiratory disease (312).

Flexibility is often overlooked, yet it is important to possess and maintain an appropriate ROM across all joints to facilitate activities of daily living that require bending, reaching, squatting, and rotating. ROM is most often assessed using a two-armed goniometer. One arm of the goniometer is positioned to align with the fixed proximal segment whereas the other arm is adjusted to align with the distal segment. The center of the device is fixed at the joint's axis of rotation, and the joint angle is read from the device's protractor. Other flexibility tests such as the forward trunk flexion test and back-scratch test may also be used, as there are normative data sets for comparison (281). Flexibility tests are common components of fitness test batteries such as the Seniors Fitness Test, which may also be useful for evaluating the functional capacity of patients with respiratory disease (313).

Asthma-Specific Considerations in Exercise Testing

Cardiopulmonary exercise testing is not routinely required in patients diagnosed with asthma unless there is a decline in exercise tolerance that is disproportionate to the patient's symptoms and degree of airflow restriction. When testing is undertaken for diagnostic or prescriptive purposes, individuals diagnosed with controlled asthma have the same contraindications for exercise or exercise testing as the general population. It is prudent to forgo graded maximal exercise testing or training when a patient is experiencing an acute bronchospasm or unusual chest tightness, shortness of breath, or pain. All patients should have access to their rescue medications in case they are required to counteract symptoms that develop during or following testing. Exercise professionals conducting testing should be aware that some asthma medications may increase resting and/or exercise heart rate or blood pressure (*e.g.*, β_2-adrenergic agonists) or increase the risk of premature ventricular contractions occurring (*e.g.*, theophylline). In patients with poorly controlled asthma, severe deconditioning, or disease comorbidity, the increased risks associated with maximal exercise testing should be balanced against the usefulness of the information to patients' medical management and exercise prescription development. In older adult patients or those with significant disease or comorbidity, field-based walking or submaximal testing may provide sufficient information to guide exercise prescription design. There are no asthma-specific concerns related to musculoskeletal assessment except for the possible impact of long-term high-dose corticosteroid use. Specific exercise testing for diagnosis of EIB is presented in the section on Other Testing for Asthma-specific Diagnostic Considerations.

Cystic Fibrosis–Specific Considerations in Exercise Testing

Standardized cardiopulmonary exercise testing is a recommended part of the annual assessment of patients with cystic fibrosis (314, 315). Cystic fibrosis is a complex disease affecting multiple body systems, and exercise places stress on these systems in a way that provides useful insight for evaluating physical limitations, symptoms, and possible abnormal responses to exercise. Exercise testing provides the most accurate information on which to base an exercise prescription, and it may provide useful adjunct information to guide decision-making concerning lung transplant decisions (316). In patients with cystic fibrosis, aerobic capacity may be a better predictor of mortality and quality of life than pulmonary function testing (*i.e.*, FEV_1), especially when serial testing highlights a decline in $\dot{V}O_{2peak}$ (228, 317).

It is recommended that all patients with cystic fibrosis greater than or equal to 10 years of age undergo cardiopulmonary exercise testing. Younger children can be tested to familiarize them with the test and motivate them for regular exercise participation. All able newly diagnosed patients should also be tested unless there are contraindications or clear explanations for any symptoms (315).

To standardize cardiopulmonary exercise testing in patients with cystic fibrosis, clinicians should use the Godfrey cycle ergometer protocol (183), which is a continuous incremental test protocol for volitional fatigue with pulse oximetry, ventilatory gas analysis, and heart rate measurement. Use of the Godfrey cycle ergometer protocol without ventilatory gas analysis is considered the second-best option. The Bruce or modified Bruce treadmill protocols are options that may be useful for patient evaluation if cycle exercise is not possible for some reason. Field tests can be utilized for assessment in cystic fibrosis, but these tests provide limited information.

The Godfrey protocol is easy to administer relative to treadmill testing even among children as young as 6 years of age. A specialized pediatric cycle ergometer with adjustable crank arms will be required for testing patients less than 130 cm (51 inches) tall. The Godfrey protocol should require 8–12 minutes of cycling against a resistance load. The test begins with the patient seated on the ergometer for 3 minutes, followed by 3 minutes of unloaded cycling to warm up. The initial and incremental workloads are determined by patient height: 10 W for those less than 120 cm (48 inches), 15 W for those between 120 and 150 cm (48–60 inches), and 20 W for those greater than 150 cm (60 inches). For patients with severe disease (*i.e.*, $FEV_1 < 30\%$ of the predicted value), smaller initial and incremental workloads may be required. Each test stage is 1-minute long, with heart rate and oxygen saturation measured during the last 15 seconds of each stage. The test can be completed by patients requiring supplemental oxygen; however, expired gas analysis may not be possible depending on the gas analysis equipment used. In cases where expired gas analysis was not undertaken, peak work rate can be recorded and $\dot{V}O_{2peak}$ estimated using predictive equations accepting that the true values may be over- or underestimated (315).

For example, to estimate peak work rate (W_{peak}) in healthy adolescent children (183):

$$W_{peak\,(males)} = 2.87 \times \text{height (cm)} - 291$$

$$W_{peak\,(females)} = 2.38 \times \text{height (cm)} - 238$$

To estimate $\dot{V}O_{2peak}$ in healthy adolescent children (318):

$$\dot{V}O_{2peak}\ (\text{L·min}^{-1}) = (216.3 - 138.7 \times \text{gender}) + (11.5 \times W_{peak}); \text{ where male} = 0 \text{ and female} = 1$$

Other predictive equations and normative cardiopulmonary test values for children, adolescents, and adults with cystic fibrosis can be found in Hebestreit et al. (315), and special guidelines and recommendations for exercise testing in pediatric populations should be reviewed prior to testing pediatric patients (319).

Assessment of muscular strength, power, and endurance can provide insight into factors other than cardiopulmonary dysfunction that limit exercise tolerance or the ability of a patient with cystic fibrosis to perform activities of daily living. Patients with mild to moderate disease may be limited more by reduced mitochondrial efficiency and muscular strength than by reduced aerobic capacity (185, 320, 321). In addition, anaerobic fitness is important to many activities of daily living, especially in children (322), and it has been shown to be reduced in those with cystic fibrosis (323). An anaerobic cycling test called the Wingate test is useful for assessing anaerobic muscle power and endurance in patients with cystic fibrosis. The Wingate test involves cycling at maximal speed and effort for 30 seconds against a fixed resistance that is traditionally set at 0.075 kp·kg^{-1} of body weight. Note that a kilopond (kp) is equal to the standard gravitational force (*i.e.*, 9.80665 m·s^{-2}) acting on 1 kg of mass or 9.8 N. In practical terms, a 1-kg weight added to the braking pan of a Monarch cycle ergometer produces 1 kp of resistance. The test is believed to assess anaerobic power because approximately 85% of the energy required to complete the test is derived from ATP-PC (28% of total) and glycolytic metabolic pathways (56% of total). The ATP-PC system is thought to be the dominant energy supply system during the first 3–5 seconds of the test, with the glycolytic system reaching its peak contribution between 10 and 15 seconds. Despite this being an anaerobic test, the aerobic system contributes about 15% of the total energy required to complete the test (324).

A typical Wingate test begins with a 3- to 5-minute low-load warm-up on the cycle ergometer. At the end of the warm-up, the patient is instructed to begin cycling as fast as possible. Within 3–5 seconds, the patient will reach a peak pedaling rate and the resistance load can be applied to the ergometer. In healthy nonathletic adults and children, the resistance load is typically 7.5% of the body mass, but this can be lowered in patients with severe disease. For example, in a protocol used by Klijn et al. (325), resistance was set relative to age, gender, and body weight (*i.e.*, boys 9–14 yr 5.5% of body weight; boys 15–19 yr, 7% of body weight; girls 9–14 yr, 5.3% of body weight; girls 15–19 yr, 6.7% of body weight) (299). The patient cycled as fast as possible for 30 seconds, after which a cool-down of low-resistance load cycling was initiated to facilitate recovery. Verbal encouragement and progress updates (*i.e.*, 10 s to go) are helpful as this is a maximal effort test, and encouragement is useful for eliciting a maximal effort. Use of toe straps will increase both peak and mean power. The test is relatively insensitive to differences in environmental temperature and hydration status (326). Useful metrics obtained from the test include peak anaerobic power (*i.e.*, power produced during the first 5 s), mean anaerobic power (*i.e.*, the average power produced over the 30-s test), and the fatigue index (*i.e.*, proportion of power lost during the test) (327).

Studies using the Wingate test have demonstrated that individuals with cystic fibrosis have lower anaerobic power when compared to those who are healthy. In a study of 41 male adolescents with cystic fibrosis, peak power was lower when compared to healthy individuals. A subgroup analysis of the patients with cystic fibrosis suggested that nutritional status and sexual maturity rather than pulmonary function per se were the main determinants of peak anaerobic power in this group; however, it has also been shown that anaerobic performance in patients with cystic fibrosis is determined by fat-free mass and FEV$_1$ (325, 328). Either way, it appears that anaerobic performance on a Wingate test is diminished by the severity of the disease when measured by FEV$_1$ and nutritional status (323).

Lung Transplant-Specific Considerations in Exercise Testing and the Exercise Response

Cardiopulmonary exercise testing is useful for assessing exercise function, and it can reveal causes of exercise intolerance in patients post lung transplant. The denervation of the lung during transplant surgery, in addition to the loss of the cough receptors, could affect the control of ventilation as stretch and irritant receptors below the bilateral bronchial anastomoses are lost. In both heart transplant recipients and heart–lung transplant recipients, there is a loss of the chronotropic response of the heart to exercise. This condition, also referred to as chronotropic incompetence, has been demonstrated to contribute to exercise limitation (329). Pulmonary transplant recipients have a permanent reduced exercise capacity despite adequate graft function in the majority of cases. Following any type of lung transplant (heart–lung, single lung, or bilateral lung transplant), peak $\dot{V}O_{2peak}$ is reduced very significantly to 40%–60% predicted with only rare cases achieving a normal peak (330, 331).

The cause for this reduced exercise capacity is multifactorial, with the exact contribution of each component varying in each recipient. The first factor relates to the period prior to transplantation, when the underlying lung disease leading to transplantation causes exercise limitation and varying degrees of deconditioning, including reduction in peripheral skeletal muscle mass. This has been most extensively studied in patients with COPD. Type I muscle fiber proportion increases in the diaphragm, which improves fatigue resistance; however, the loss of type II fibers can negatively impact force development by the diaphragm. At the same time, there is a loss of type I fibers in skeletal muscle and an increase in type IIb fibers and reduced activity of aerobic enzymes. The reduction in skeletal muscle type I fibers has been correlated with the degree of impairment in peak $\dot{V}O_{2peak}$ (332).

The second factor involves the perioperative and the early postoperative periods, when primary allograft dysfunction, prolonged intensive care unit (ICU) or hospital stay, acute rejection, or infective episodes may damage graft function or limit potential functional recovery. Critical illness myopathy and polyneuropathy can be particularly devastating and lead to poor long-term recovery.

Exercise capacity will plateau at 6–24 months and will be suboptimal in virtually all recipients. One contributing factor may be anemia, although most patients on medication will have a hemoglobin concentration either in the lower part of the normal range or mildly reduced. Whereas anemia could affect oxygen delivery during high-intensity exercise, it is not able to explain very significant long-term limitations on exercise capacity.

Following bilateral lung transplantation, a mild restrictive defect is normal. This may reflect altered chest wall compliance from the surgical incision. Gas transfer is often mildly reduced, suggesting altered V_A/Q matching. However, the arterial–alveolar oxygen gradient is normal, and desaturation does not occur during exercise, suggesting there is no limitation of gas exchange during exercise and no evidence of a ventilatory limitation to exercise. In a recent study of patients post lung transplant, patients had lower than average $\dot{V}O_{2peak}$ and those with lower $\dot{V}O_{2peak}$ report greater muscle pain at peak exercise. Greater muscle pain was associated with elevated acidosis at rest and early onset of the lactate threshold and faster increase in RER during exercise. Greater muscle pain was also associated with less breathing reserve at $\dot{V}O_{2peak}$ and for some patients in the study, higher $\dot{V}_E$ was associated with higher dyspnea ratings (211). Studies demonstrate that in many lung transplant patients the dominant limitation is poor peripheral muscle oxygen utilization (331). What is unclear is the cause: myopathy, loss of muscle mass pretransplant, and deconditioning have all been proposed. In a group of patients who had undergone a lung transplant for COPD, it has been reported that the arterial-mixed venous oxygen content difference rises during exercise rather than falls, suggesting that muscle oxygen extraction is reduced (333).

Exercise Training

Exercise training is a fundamental component of pulmonary rehabilitation and the most effective method for reducing exercise intolerance and dyspnea symptoms when combined with optimal pharmacotherapy (229). The exercise prescription in chronic respiratory disease should be comprehensive, including cardiorespiratory training, resistance exercise to improve muscular function, and flexibility training to maintain or improve mobility. Inspiratory muscle training may be of benefit to some, but not all, patients (22). Neuromotor or balance training may be beneficial for some patients as well, especially if they are at high risk for falls. The current pulmonary rehabilitation exercise prescription guidelines and recommendations endorsed by the American College of Sports Medicine (ACSM), the American Association of Cardiovascular and Pulmonary Rehabilitation (AACVPR), the ATS, the British Thoracic Society, and the ERS are summarized in Table 8.12.

The purpose of exercise training is to improve an individual's capacity to perform external work. This is accomplished by repeatedly requiring multiple body systems to operate at levels exceeding those usually required during normal daily activity. The repeated overloading of body systems causes a positive adaptive stress response, or training effect, which increases operational capacity and allows the trained system to operate at a higher level than before. Training responses are achieved using the well-established FITT-VP (frequency, intensity, time, type, volume, and progression) principle to apply a progressively increasing overload stimulus. Although use of the FITT-VP principle establishes a somewhat formulaic approach to developing

Table 8.12	Recommendations to Guide Development of Exercise Prescriptions in Pulmonary Rehabilitation					
Training Type	Frequency	Intensity	Time (Duration)	Type	Progression	Special Considerations
Aerobic	3–5 d per wk	30%–80% of peak work rate; RPE 11–13/20 or 4–6/10	20–60 min total; 4- to 12-wk program length	Target large muscle groups, especially quadriceps, i.e., walking and cycling, dancing, swimming, rowing	Emphasize continuous duration over intensity; consider client preferences to support compliance.	Use of interval training may increase exercise duration, intensity, or both; may require multiple daily sessions to meet duration requirement
Resistance (no non-COPD respiratory disease-specific recommendations available)	≥2 d per wk	Low resistance, high repetition; 8–15RM or 40%–70% of the 1RM for 10–15 reps	1–4 sets; 2–3 min rest between sets	Machine or free weights, resistance bands, or body mass to add resistance	No specific guidance: increase resistance when all reps and sets can be completed or exceeded	Emphasis on exercises that target the quadriceps and muscles of the upper back, shoulders, and arms
Flexibility and balance	1–3 d or more	Extend end ROM to feeling of tightness or slight discomfort.	10–60 s hold; 2–4 reps	Static stretching; one exercise per major muscle group	Extend hold duration to 30–60 s; increase reps up to 4	Avoid ballistic stretching or bouncing at the end of the ROM; longer programs (>8 wk) may confer more benefit

Source: From Compiled from American Association of Cardiovascular and Pulmonary Rehabilitation. *American Association of Cardiovascular and Pulmonary Rehabilitation Guidelines for Pulmonary Rehabilitation Programs.* Champaign (IL): Human Kinetics; 2011; American College of Sports Medicine. *ACSM's Guidelines for Exercise Testing and Prescription.* Philadelphia (PA): Lippincott Williams and Wilkins; 2013; Bolton CE, Bevan-Smith EF, Blakey JD, et al. British Thoracic Society Pulmonary Rehabilitation Working Group; British Thoracic Society Standards of Care Committee. BTS guidelines on pulmonary rehabilitation in adults. *Thorax.* 2013;68(Suppl 2):ii1–30; Ehrman JK, ed. *Clinical Exercise Physiology.* 3rd ed. Champaign (IL): Human Kinetics; 2013; Spruit MA, Singh SJ, Garvey C, et al. An official American Thoracic Society/European Respiratory Society Statement: key concepts and advances in pulmonary rehabilitation. *Am J Respir Crit Care Med.* 2013;188(8):e13–64; Heyward VH. *Advanced Fitness Assessment and Exercise Prescription.* Champaign (IL): Human Kinetics; 2014.

an exercise prescription, each exercise prescription should be individualized and developed from objective assessment of the patient's functional capacity. The default emphasis of clinical exercise prescription is often to focus on general whole-body conditioning; however, the patient may be better served by a prescription that focuses more on one aspect of a patient's physical capacity over another at different times (i.e., alternating mesocycles of strength, power, and endurance training or emphasizing muscular strength development over aerobic conditioning). In the end, each

exercise prescription developed must be accepted by the patient and compatible with the patient's physical capability, medical condition, and prescribed medical management to be both safe and effective. With effective training, it is expected that the patient's maximal aerobic, muscular, and functional capacities will be improved. Submaximal exercise endurance will also improve as evidenced by a longer work time and reduced exercise heart rate, blood lactate, $\dot{V}CO_2$, and $\dot{V}_E$ for the same level of external work. As a result of becoming trained, patients typically report less severe dyspnea and breathlessness, reduced anxiety, and improved quality of life.

The general principles involved in training individuals with chronic respiratory diseases are not different from those used to train healthy or athletic populations. Prescriptions typically contain a warm-up routine, focused exercise training, and cool-down activities. The framework established by ACSM for development and maintenance of cardiorespiratory, musculoskeletal, and neuromotor fitness in apparently healthy adults (334) can be used in addition to the current pulmonary rehabilitation exercise prescription guidelines and recommendations (see Table 8.12) to develop training programs for individuals with chronic respiratory diseases outlined in *ACSM's Guidelines for Exercise Testing and Prescription* (287). Considerable research effort has focused on optimizing exercise training for patients with COPD, and many of these findings are relevant for individuals with other chronic respiratory diseases. This work is summarized in the following sections with disease-specific considerations outlined at the end of the section.

Aerobic Exercise Training

Typical aerobic exercise training sessions are structured to include a warm-up, a conditioning, and a cool-down phase. To warm up, patients should undertake 5–10 minutes of whole-body exercise beginning at low activity intensity ($<40\%$ of the $\dot{V}O_2$ reserve; $\dot{V}O_2R = \dot{V}O_{2rest}$ + (Intensity percentage)/100 [$\dot{V}O_{2max} - \dot{V}O_{2rest}$]) and gradually increase this to a level that does not exceed the training intensity. Heart rate reserve (*i.e.*, $HRR = HR_{max} - HR_{rest}$) can be used in place of the $\dot{V}O_2$ reserve. The patient should warm up with activities similar to those used during the conditioning phase of the training session. Mobility, ROM, and flexibility exercises should have purpose and thus need to be structured into the warm-up session appropriately. The warm-up should prepare the cardiac and muscular systems for conditioning exercise by improving blood flow, speeding up neural impulse transmission, increasing internal body temperature, and promoting joint readiness.

A cool-down period of gradually decreasing whole-body aerobic exercise intensity ($<40\%$ R) is recommended after completing the conditioning phase of a training session. The cool-down phase should continue for 5–10 minutes to allow the body to return toward resting state. Rhythmic contraction of muscle prevents venous pooling in the lower extremities that can precipitate cardiac arrhythmia, hypotension, dizziness, and syncope. Gradual cool-down may also prevent bronchospasm.

Static stretching and other flexibility exercises can be performed after the patient has sufficiently recovered from the conditioning exercises, but these activities should not be used as the primary cool-down activity (281, 335).

Frequency

In most cases, patients should engage in aerobic endurance exercise 3–5 days per week. For patients who are obese, exercise training of up to 7 days per week (300 min per wk) may be necessary to achieve the required caloric deficit that will promote and maintain weight loss (336). Individuals with poor cardiorespiratory fitness may need to undertake multiple short exercise bouts per day to accumulate a sufficient total volume of exercise. There is typically no difference in training effect between those who exercise on three consecutive days versus those who exercise every other day (337). It is recommended that at least one exercise session per week be supervised by a CEP as the efficacy of home-based exercise is not yet established for pulmonary disease. Recent meta-analyses show that home-based pulmonary rehabilitation provides therapeutic benefit in the short term; however, large-scale randomized controlled trials are still needed to identify an optimal standard for short-and long-term home-based pulmonary rehabilitation programming (338, 339).

Intensity

The aerobic training intensity is typically prescribed as a percentage of the patient's peak or maximal $\dot{V}O_2$, heart rate, or work rate; or as a percentage of the patient's reserve capacity (*i.e.*, $\dot{V}O_2R$ or HRR). Peak $\dot{V}O_2$ and heart rate should be measured by exercise testing rather than estimated from predictive equations. Many of the standard predictive equations were developed for use in healthy populations. These equations fail to consider the impact of medications with chronotropic action (340, 341), or that the estimate variability is often too high to be useful on an individual level even when the predictive equations are specifically developed for the patient population with COPD (294, 342).

When exercise testing is not possible or practical, exertion scales such as the RPE scale (6–20) or the BORG CR10 scale (1–10) can be useful for prescribing exercise intensity. In chronic respiratory disease, these subjective scales, along with dyspnea and breathlessness scales, are useful for setting and adjusting the training intensity as needed to match symptom variability or fitness level improvement (335).

Exercise training intensity is usually described using the terms *low*, *moderate*, or *vigorous*. In a rehabilitation setting, low-intensity exercise requires 20%–39% of the $\dot{V}O_2R$, moderate-intensity training generally describes any training activity requiring 40%–59% of the $\dot{V}O_2R$ to complete, and vigorous-intensity training requires greater than or equal to 60% of the $\dot{V}O_2R$ (287). Many studies and guidelines recommend *high-intensity training*. This can often be misunderstood to mean only exercise that requires near-maximal effort and high training loads. High-intensity exercise generally applies to any exercise intensity that is greater than or equal to 60% of the $\dot{V}O_{2peak}$ or HR_{peak}. High-intensity exercise is typically used in interval training where periods of high-intensity exercise are separated by periods of low-intensity exercise. The term *sprint interval* or *high-intensity low-volume training* should be reserved for training programs that require near maximal or supramaximal (*i.e.*, $\geq 100\%$ of the $\dot{V}O_{2peak}$) to complete (343–345).

Training below 50% $\dot{V}O_{2peak}$ can produce health benefits without necessarily improving aerobic capacity. In healthy adults, aerobic capacity is generally increased when training intensities of 50%–100% of the $\dot{V}O_{2peak}$ are used. Training at 90%–100% $\dot{V}O_{2peak}$ results in the largest increases in aerobic capacity. Training above $\dot{V}O_{2peak}$ (*i.e.*, supramaximal intensities) improves $\dot{V}O_{2peak}$, but the increase may be lower than what it would be if training were undertaken below 100% $\dot{V}O_{2peak}$ (346). Supramaximal training quickly leads to muscle fatigue and limits the amount of training that can be completed during a session. Use of recovery intervals between successive bouts of supramaximal exercise alleviates this problem even in clinical populations by allowing the muscle to recover between work intervals (343, 345, 347).

It is difficult to identify an appropriate or optimal exercise intensity target or range for aerobic training of individuals with chronic respiratory disease. The chronic and progressive nature of the disease and periods of disease exacerbation create a wide variance with respect to airflow limitation, dyspnea severity, skeletal muscle weakness, exercise intolerance, comorbidity development, pharmacotherapy, patient safety, and motivation that all influence a patient's ability and willingness to exercise. The recommended aerobic training intensity for those with COPD ranges from 50% to 80% of the peak work rate (see Table 8.12). The astute CEP will recognize that training intensity may need to be adjusted upward or downward to match the patient's changing health status. The exercise intensity recommendations presented in Table 8.12 are suitable for patients living with other chronic respiratory conditions.

Regardless of the exercise intensity used, oxygen saturation should be maintained at greater than or equal to 88%. This can be achieved through use of an ambulatory supplemental oxygen supply (348). Those who are on long-term oxygen will need to continue therapy during exercise. The oxygen flow rate will likely need to be increased to maintain oxygen saturation levels in the required range. Although oxygen supplementation improves exercise capacity for patients with COPD in a laboratory environment, widespread use of oxygen supplementation to support increased training levels is not recommended because research has produced equivocal findings with regard to efficacy (229, 349).

Time

Ideally, patients will complete 20–60 minutes of cardiorespiratory exercise during each training session. Patients who are severely deconditioned or have moderate to severe disease may not be able to sustain 20 minutes or more of continuous exercise. For these individuals, interval training is a most useful approach to help them meet training duration recommendations. Varying the work interval intensity and duration as well as altering the type (active vs. passive) and length of the recovery interval can delay exercise-limiting fatigue, dyspnea, and breathlessness. Progression toward the goal of 30 minutes of continuous activity can be accomplished by a combination of lengthening each work interval and reducing the recovery interval duration. This approach is recommended in principle by current pulmonary rehabilitation exercise guidelines (229, 287, 348, 350); however, there is insufficient research evidence at this time to support specific guidelines for application in patients with respiratory disease. A recent review of HIIT studies conducted in patients with COPD concluded that a prescription consisting of 30-second exercise intervals at 80% of the workload peak separated by 20–40 second rest intervals for 30–40 minutes effectively increases exercise capacity when performed three to four times per week (351). In summary, it is recommended that the work and/or recovery intervals used during training of individuals with respiratory diseases be guided by use of the patient's RPE and dyspnea scale scores obtained during exercise, as well as the level of fatigue during and after the training session. The use of HIIT in patients living with respiratory disease is discussed further below.

Type

For patients with chronic respiratory disease, arm and leg fatigue often limit exercise tolerance and the ability to perform leisure and daily living activities (352, 353). The most commonly employed exercise modalities involve walking or cycling to engage the lower limb. Arm cycling is sometimes prescribed to improve unsupported arm capacity; however, it can produce significant dyspnea and patient distress if the accessory muscles of inspiration in patients who rely on them to assist ventilation become fatigued (354, 355). Other modes of endurance exercise can be used successfully, including rowing, aerobic dance, stepping, swimming, and ice-skating. Outdoor exercise in cold temperatures may cause bronchoconstriction and exacerbate symptoms. Patients should consider wearing a scarf over the mouth and nose to warm the air when ice-skating or outdoors in cold weather (335, 356). The type of exercise used should be varied and be accepted by the patient to promote uptake and sustain long-term interest.

There has been significant research interest in the use of HIIT in clinical populations. Higher training intensities produce greater improvement in aerobic capacity (345, 346); however, patients with respiratory disease are often unable to perform high-intensity aerobic activity for very long because their low AT leads to early lactate acidosis and carbon dioxide loading. This in turn stimulates increased ventilation, exacerbating lung hyperventilation and exhausting the ventilatory reserve (76). The intermittent application of high-intensity workloads imposes high muscular load while reducing the overall physiologic response when compared to continuous training. This moderates the ventilatory increase and minimizes lung hyperinflation to enable patients to spend greater proportions of their training time exercising at higher intensities than would be possible using a continuous mode (357, 358).

The general consensus at this time is that both continuous and interval training protocols improve exercise capacity and quality of life in patients with COPD, and there are few if any clinically important differences between approaches. This is likely due to the practice of matching total work between protocols in research studies. Early studies indicated that interval training reduced exercise dyspnea compared to continuous training, but more recent studies have found little difference. This may be due to longer work interval lengths used in the later studies ($\geq$1 min vs. $\leq$30 s), and it highlights the fact that the optimal work and recovery interval characteristics have not been established. A recent meta-analysis of eight randomized controlled trials that compared continuous to interval training outcomes in patients with moderate to severe COPD concluded that both approaches improved exercise capacity and health-related quality of life (359). One such training study showed that continuous and interval training favorably improved the capillary-to-fiber ratio and the fiber-type distribution within vastus lateralis. In addition, both training modalities increased the muscle oxidative capacity and cross-sectional area of type I and

type IIa fibers while the number of type IIb fibers was reduced (358). A follow-up study by this group showed similar levels of expression of genes regulating muscle fiber hypertrophy (*i.e.*, insulin-like growth factor 1 [IGF-1] and mechano-growth factor [MGF]) and regeneration (*i.e.*, myoblast determination protein [MyoD]) (130).

There are no evidence-based recommendations available to guide decision-making with respect to choosing a continuous or interval-based training program. The decision should be guided by client preference, symptoms, and willingness to adhere to the program as well as by the therapeutic goals that have been established. In practical application, an interval program may allow patients to complete a greater total volume of work per training session. Patients with very severe COPD take fewer unintended breaks when performing interval versus continuous exercise (360). Some additional practical recommendations that may lead the practitioner to consider using interval training include:

1. A severe air flow obstruction (*i.e.*, $FEV_1 < 40\%$ predicted),
2. A low exercise capacity (*i.e.*, peak work rate $< 60\%$ predicted),
3. A limited capacity for continuous exercise (*i.e.*, <10 min), or
4. An exercise oxygen saturation that decreases to less than 85% or intolerable dyspnea during continuous exercise.

Interval training is best completed in a supervised environment using an exercise bike, treadmill, or recumbent stepper to control workload and pace. Self-paced HIIT can be effective; however, it has been shown that self-paced interval training undershoots the target intensity levels (361). A possible strategy for prescribing self-supervised interval exercise may be to encourage the patient to walk through their neighborhood, speeding up between two successive streetlights, fire hydrants, or other repeating landmarks, while slowing to recover over the distance to the next landmark.

Resistance Training

Skeletal muscle atrophy and weakness in the upper and lower limbs are common among those with chronic respiratory disease. Possible causes include systemic inflammation- and oxidative stress-induced myopathy, chronic hypercapnia, malnutrition, corticosteroid use, and physical inactivity (76, 362). Quadriceps muscle strength is correlated with both 6MWT distance and $\dot{V}O_{2peak}$ (138, 363). For many patients, muscle dysfunction contributes to exercise intolerance, and it is a significant contributor to the severity of symptoms experienced by those with COPD

(138, 362). It creates a vicious downward cycle in which ventilatory limitation leads to shortness of breath during exercise, which leads to the patient avoiding exercise and physical activity, which in turn leads to greater skeletal muscle detraining and amplification of dyspnea symptoms during activity (93). The loss of muscular strength is proportional to the degree of muscle wasting experienced, and there is a preferential muscle loss in the lower limbs of patients with COPD (143). Reduced skeletal muscle strength in COPD is associated with an increased use of health care resources, poor prognosis, and increased mortality (141, 364).

Resistance training is an effective way to increase muscle size and strength in healthy adults (365, 366) and in patients living with COPD (367). In fact, resistance training appears to be more effective than aerobic endurance training for increasing muscle size and strength (144, 367-370). Even older patients with COPD appear to improve muscle size and strength after engaging in a program of heavy resistance skeletal muscle training. In a small-scale study, patients aged 65 years or older with moderate to severe COPD undertook a resistance training program consisting of two 60-minute training sessions per week over 12 weeks. Patients completed four sets of eight repetitions at 80% of the patient's 1RM for leg press, knee extension, and knee flexion exercises. The patients were instructed to complete the concentric phase of each lift with an explosive tempo and rest for 2-3 minutes between each set. The study included a patient control group that completed unsupervised resistance exercises over the 12 weeks. Those patients who undertook the prescribed resistance training showed a 4% increase in quadriceps cross-sectional area and a 15%-20% increase in knee extension and leg press strength, maximum gait speed, stair-climbing ability, and self-reported health (371). The study is significant not only because it highlighted a hypertrophic response in patients with COPD but also because it revealed that intense high-load resistance training can be safely undertaken by patients with COPD even when they are older and have moderate to severe disease.

Some research suggests that muscle strength is increased more by a combined aerobic resistance training program than by programs consisting of either aerobic or resistance training alone. Vonbank et al. (372) allocated 36 patients with COPD ($n = 30$ GOLD stage 2 and 3) into a resistance-only, aerobic-only, or combined resistance and aerobic training groups. The 3-month resistance training program consisted of 2 weekly sessions of eight weightlifting exercises that targeted major muscle groups. Patients performed 8-15 repetitions per exercise for two sets. Progression of the program was achieved by increasing the number of sets completed and increasing the resistance once the patient could complete 15 repetitions of the assigned resistance. The endurance-only group completed two endurance-cycling exercise sessions per week at 60% of their measured heart rate reserve. The aerobic training sessions were 20 minutes long and progressed by 5 minutes every 4 weeks. The combined training group completed both training programs simultaneously. Peak work rate was increased by approximately 10% in all three groups; however, $\dot{V}O_{2peak}$ was higher in the endurance and combined training groups only. Posttraining program muscle strength was higher in all three groups for leg press, bench press, and bench pull exercises. The resistance and combined training program group strength increase were approximately 20% greater than it was for the aerobic training group.

Consistent with these findings are the conclusions of a recent systematic review that concluded resistance training consistently improves strength in patients with COPD despite wide variation in training program characteristics such as repetition number, resistance load intensity, set number, and type of exercise (*i.e.*, machine or free weight or resistance bands). The meta-analysis conducted by the authors showed that resistance training typically improved maximal knee extensor strength by 25% compared to only 10% for aerobic endurance exercise training. It did not significantly improve maximal aerobic capacity or respiratory function, however (373). Similar conclusions were also reached by Liao et al. in their recent review (374). They reviewed 18 trials totaling 750 patients with COPD and found that resistance training consistently improved muscle strength and reduced dyspnea symptoms during exercise. Also noted was a small improvement in FEV_1 when compared to a nonexercise control group. Muscle strength and health-related quality of life were higher in patients who completed a combined resistance and aerobic endurance training program compared to an aerobic program alone, despite both programs achieving similar improvement in 6MWT distance, $\dot{V}O_{2peak}$, and peak exercise workload. These findings are supported by those of a second systematic review of 14 randomized control trials involving 592 patients that found a similar improvement in health-related quality of life, dyspnea, activities of daily living, walking distance, lean body mass, muscle strength, and exercise capacity between resistance and endurance training programs (375).

Overall, these studies suggest that patients may receive similar benefit from aerobic, resistance, and combined aerobic resistance training programs. In practice, patients who are severely limited in their ability to undertake continuous or interval aerobic training may be better served initially by completing resistance training due to its lower demand for oxygen and lower dyspnea scores. In contrast, a higher-functioning patient would benefit from a combined program that could potentially improve strength and aerobic capacity to a greater degree than a unimodal program. Current pulmonary rehabilitation exercise programming recommendations support the use of combined aerobic and resistance training with no specific recommendations to guide when it might be appropriate to emphasize one modality over another (see Table 8.12).

The current pulmonary rehabilitation recommendations with respect to resistance training describe a program that includes 8–10 whole-body exercises that involve the major muscle groups (*i.e.*, arms, shoulders, chest, abdomen, back, and legs). Patients should perform 1–3 sets of 8–12 repetitions on 2–3 days each week. The recommended resistance intensity for beginners is 60%–70% of the 1RM. This intensity increases to 80% for experienced patients, who should complete 2–4 sets of 8–12 RM (*i.e.*, the patient can perform no more than 8–12 repetitions without loss of proper form). For those unable to undergo 1RM or 1RM predictive testing, resistance training intensity can be guided using an RPE scale score of 5–6 of 10 for moderate or 7–8 of 10 for high-intensity training (376).

Using 2–3 minutes of recovery time between sets, most resistance programs can likely be completed within 30–40 minutes. The CEP should remain aware of the total time commitment required by the patient. A training program containing aerobic and strength conditioning and flexibility training could easily require 60–90 minutes or more to complete when a warm-up and cool-down are also factored in. A frequently identified barrier to undertaking exercise training is that it requires too much time.

Resistance exercise can be prescribed using almost any type of resistance element, such as machine or free weights, elastic resistance bands, weighted grocery bags or other common items, or the patient's own body mass. Complex multi-joint exercises such as a squat are more appropriately prescribed in a patient population as a sit-to-stand exercise from a chair or as a seated leg press rather than as a free-weight exercise. The CEP should also consider that in some cases even the lowest setting on a machine may provide more resistance than the patient can overcome.

As noted earlier, unsupported arm exercise can produce significant levels of dyspnea in patients with COPD, presumably because the accessory muscles of inspiration (*i.e.*, scalene, sternocleidomastoid, and serratus anterior) are active during the exercise, become fatigued, and are thus less able to assist ventilation. This may also explain why patients with COPD often complain of dyspnea when performing activities of daily living that are dependent on upper body musculature (354, 355). Several studies and reviews show that patients with COPD tolerate and benefit from upper arm extremity exercise, but there is no conclusive evidence showing that upper arm training alone improves activities of daily living or physical functioning (229). Therefore, upper limb training should be combined with other types of training with an awareness that exercise involving the upper arms may contribute to dyspnea if the accessory muscles of inspiration become fatigued.

There are no clear recommendations concerning specific exercises to improve the function of the accessory muscles of ventilation, but general training principles for muscular improvement should be effective (21). In patients with severe disease who rely on accessory muscles of ventilation to meet the ventilatory requirements of exertion, caution is required so as to not fatigue these muscles with training and cause the patient undue discomfort and breathlessness. In the past, inspiratory muscle training was undertaken to improve inspiratory muscle strength and reduce symptoms of breathlessness and dyspnea. Typically, the patient breathes through a handheld device that provides airflow resistance to inspiration (~30% of the maximum inspiratory pressure must be generated to induce flow). Inspiratory muscle training improves inspiratory muscle strength and endurance; however, it is unlikely that the gains achieved are greater than that achieved through aerobic training. Current guidelines state that while inspiratory muscle training is effective, it should be considered an adjunct therapy to other forms of exercise training. Scientific evidence does not support routine use in pulmonary rehabilitation, and it should only be considered for select patients with reduced inspiratory muscle weakness and breathlessness despite optimal pharmacological therapy (229, 377).

There are no specific recommendations concerning resistance training progression or program-variable manipulation for chronic respiratory disease (see Table 8.12). As in the cardiopulmonary system, a training response is created in skeletal muscle by repeatedly contracting the muscle against a load or resistance that is not typically experienced in daily living. Because the muscle adapts to the overload stimulus that is applied, the resistance load should be progressively increased to promote continued adaptation. Adaptation of skeletal muscle is specific, meaning that it is shaped by the demands of the training program. Thus, training the leg produces very little gain in arm strength, and minimal explosive power is gained from static isometric training.

Periodization should be considered for any resistance training program as it is superior to standard progression programs (281, 378). Periodization systematically varies the intensity and volume of resistance training to prioritize strength, power, hypertrophy, and endurance gains by altering the applied training stimulus. It tends to reduce the negative effects of overtraining and boredom that can discourage patients from continuing their training. In a classic linear periodization model, a macrocycle (*i.e.*, 12 months) is divided into three or four mesocycles. The volume of exercise (*i.e.*, the number of repetitions × number of sets) is gradually reduced as the intensity of the exercise is increased during each successive mesocycle. In a linear model, the three to four microcycles within each mesocycle are used to make progressive adjustments in intensity, repetitions, and sets of exercises. Nonlinear or undulating periodization programs may prioritize strength, power, hypertrophy, or endurance within a mesocycle and as a result, the microcycles within the mesocycle change frequently and variably to achieve the desired training goal.

Flexibility Training

Flexibility is recognized as important in the current pulmonary rehabilitation guidelines (see Table 8.12). Specifically, impaired posture can affect ventilation and increase the work of breathing (379). Common postural impairment in COPD includes thoracic kyphosis, increased anterior–posterior diameter, shoulder elevation, and trunk flexion (380). Nevertheless, no clinical trials demonstrating the effectiveness of flexibility training on respiratory disease symptom management have been undertaken to date. Thus, there are no specific flexibility guidelines for pulmonary rehabilitation at this time. ACSM advocates for applying the general flexibility exercise recommendations for healthy individuals and older adults. Stretching programs can be undertaken every day, but a minimum frequency of 2–3 days per week is recommended. The flexibility program should contain a regimen of exercises that stretch each major muscle–tendon group (*i.e.*, neck, chest, shoulders, upper and lower back, abdomen, hips, thigh, and lower leg). During each exercise, the patient should move gently to the end of the joint ROM until they feel a slightly uncomfortable stretching sensation and then hold the position for 10–30 seconds. Progression can be added by holding the end ROM position for up to 60 seconds. Each stretching exercise should be repeated two to four times (287).

Asthma-Specific Considerations in Exercise Training

The etiology and pathophysiology of asthma can be vastly different from one individual to another. Some patients with asthma are severely limited in their capacity to undertake physical activity and exercise whereas others can compete at the Olympic level in events heavily dependent on cardiorespiratory function and capacity such as cross-country skiing. Complicating matters is the fact that the symptom severity and the limitations imposed by the symptoms may be variable day to day, week to week, or year to year. Any exercise prescription developed will require periodic adjustment to remain effective and compatible with changes in disease symptoms or progression, medical management (*i.e.*, medication changes), and patient preferences and capabilities.

Prior to undertaking exercise training, therapeutic control of the patient's asthma should be maximized by their medical practitioner, and the patient's symptoms are well controlled. Exercise training should be avoided during periods of acute exacerbation or severe symptoms. Exercising with a severe airflow restriction (*i.e.*, <75% predicted FEV_1) can result in lung hyperventilation, increased work of breathing, and possible respiratory muscle fatigue, as well as arterial oxygen desaturation and hypercapnia. Exercise can lead to severe shortness of breath and could ultimately culminate in death, although fortunately, this outcome is rare (381). Despite these risks, moderate and vigorous exercise is well tolerated and safe for patients whose asthma is well controlled (382).

Prophylactic use of medications prior to exercise may reduce the incidence of EIA and EIB and prevent development of significant or severe dyspnea. Long- and short-acting β_2-adrenergic agonists may provide protection for up to 12 and 3 hours, respectively, postexercise; however, prolonged regular use may induce medication tolerance and reduced effectiveness. Current asthma management is likely to include an anti-inflammatory management medication (*e.g.*, corticosteroid) and short-acting β_2-adrenergic agonist rescue medication for better control of symptoms.

Once therapy is optimized and symptoms are well controlled, exercise recommendations and guidelines are the same for individuals with asthma as they are for healthy individuals across the age groups. In fact, those with asthma can participate in the same high-level training that is required to achieve maximal athletic performance at an Olympic level.

As discussed earlier, each training session should include a warm-up, conditioning section, and cool-down. For moderately trained athletes with asthma, a warm-up consisting of 15 minutes of continuous exercise at 60% of $\dot{V}O_{2peak}$ significantly reduces the incidence of post-EIB. Interval-based warm-up routines (*i.e.*, short maximal sprints) may be helpful but appear less effective than continuous exercise (383, 384).

The conditioning portion of the training session should be developed based on objective assessment of the patient's exercise capacity and individualized according to specific needs and goals. As is recommended for healthy individuals, the conditioning portion of the training session should begin at a lower intensity and gradually progress as the fitness level improves. Ideally, the exercise intensity will require at least 40%–60% of the $\dot{V}O_{2peak}$ to promote aerobic conditioning. Dyspnea and Borg scales can be useful for setting the exercise intensity in patients who are severely deconditioned or are symptom limited. Level walking on a treadmill is suitably intense for severely deconditioned and symptom-limited individuals. Sprint interval training is suitable for those who are highly conditioned and have optimally controlled asthma.

Most exercise modalities are suitable for patients with asthma; however, participation in scuba diving is actively discouraged. In countries where licensing is required, those with asthma may not meet the medical requirement because there is an increased risk of precipitating an asthma attack by breathing cold, dry, compressed air during the heavy exertion associated with diving (169). Swimming is often recommended as a training modality for those with asthma because humidified air is less drying to the epithelium. There is some concern that chloramines that form in the air present at indoor pools could act as an airway irritant that provokes or worsens existing asthma symptoms (385). Exercise in cold environments, such as ice-skating, cross-country skiing, and snowshoeing, should be limited to avoid triggering bronchoconstriction. Other activities such as road cycling, mountain biking, and hiking may also expose individuals to a host of possible asthma triggers. Reactivity to air humidity, air temperature, pollutant exposure, allergens, and other environmental exposures should be considered on an individual basis to minimize possible negative influences on asthma control and overall health and safety of the individual.

Physical activity and exercise should be encouraged for all patients with asthma to improve functional capacity and quality of life and to reduce the risk of developing comorbid conditions such as obesity, Type 2 diabetes, and cardiovascular disease. Children with asthma appear to have physical activity levels that are similar to their peers without asthma so long as barriers such as disease severity and parental concerns are not present (386). Adults, however, are less active than their age-matched healthy peers and place more self-imposed limits on physical activity (387). The decision to exercise is often weighed against concerns about experiencing symptoms. Harmful anticipation was shown to significantly increase the perception of visceral changes during exercise, creating wide variability between the degree of airway obstruction, exercise tolerance, and dyspnea severity ratings. Patient attitudes toward exercise and how they perceive both their symptoms and their body's response to exercise need to be considered when constructing and implementing an exercise prescription (388).

Given the complexity of asthma pathology and pathophysiology, it is expected that exercise and training responses can be quite variable for and between patients with asthma. Overall, there are the expected training-related improvements in $\dot{V}O_{2peak}$, O_2 pulse, lactate threshold, muscular strength, power and endurance, flexibility, balance, and emotional outlook (389). Aside from the normal responses expected, it has been reported that patients with asthma show blunted sympathoadrenal responses to exercise (390), altered potassium homeostasis, and excessive growth hormone secretion (22). The impact of these observations in the face of such varied pathophysiology is not well understood at this time.

Exercise training and regular physical activity reduce the risk of asthma exacerbations and can attenuate lung function decline, but it does not appear to reduce airway inflammation (391, 392). In a study of adults with mild to moderate asthma undertaking 10 weeks of supervised high-intensity exercise on various modalities (i.e., 80%–90% of age-predicted heart rate max or 7–8 out of 10 using the Borg RPE Scale), improved aerobic capacity, walking distance, and a reduction in asthma symptoms and anxiety were reported postprogram (393). Patients participating in the study were followed for 3 years postprogram, and it was found that asthma symptom reduction was limited to those patients who continued exercising one to two times per week after the original intervention was complete (394). Several systematic reviews have concluded that exercise training will lead to an improvement in cardiorespiratory fitness without increasing asthma symptoms, but there is little evidence that exercise training improves lung function or reduces lung inflammation (389, 391, 395, 396). A Cochrane Review that examined 21 randomized studies that included 772 patients over 8 years of age who completed at least 20 minutes of exercise two times per week for a period of at least 4 weeks found that $\dot{V}O_{2peak}$ increased on average by 4.92 mL·kg^{-1}·min^{-1} (95% confidence interval 3.98–5.87 mL·kg^{-1}·min^{-1}); however, no statistically significant changes in FEV$_1$, FVC, PEFR, or maximal were observed. Additionally, the study found some evidence to support an improvement in health-related quality of life that was both statistically and clinically significant (395).

Physical activity and exercise training are generally safe and well tolerated by patients with well-controlled asthma. The benefits of undertaking exercise training include improved fitness, fewer exacerbations, and risk reduction of comorbid conditions. Unfortunately, exercise itself does not appear to improve lung function compromised by asthma.

Cystic Fibrosis–Specific Considerations in Exercise Training

Habitual physical activity and exercise have been shown to slow declining lung function and reduce pulmonary exacerbations and hospitalization among patients with cystic fibrosis (397, 398). Patients who are active typically enjoy greater aerobic and anaerobic capacity, mobility, and quality of life when compared to patients who are less active (399–401); however, a recent Cochrane Review found that there is only low-quality evidence to support that exercise training improves aerobic capacity, pulmonary function, and health-related quality of life (402). Perhaps the more important finding is that patients who increase their current physical activity levels often improve several aspects of health-related quality of life (399). Thus, the inclusion of regular exercise into the routine care of patients with cystic fibrosis has become an important component of overall disease management despite the lack of widely endorsed recommendations and guidelines to direct CEPs in applying exercise prescriptions for this patient population. Recently, a group of international experts in exercise and cystic fibrosis put forward a series of evidence-based recommendations to guide clinicians and exercise practitioners on the application of exercise and physical activity for all patients with cystic fibrosis (403). The recommendations are consistent with other general physical activity and exercise recommendations made regarding children and adolescents as well as those presented in Table 8.12.

The exercise prescription for patients with cystic fibrosis should be focused on achieving several goals, including improvement in aerobic capacity and muscular strength; slowing of physiologic decline; improvement of disease symptoms; reduction in frequency of exacerbations; improvement in quality of life; and promotion of lifelong physical activity. Because the exercise prescription will only be successful if the patient is willing to engage in

the proposed activities, the CEP should consider patient preferences and goals when designing the program.

Considerations for Children

Because the cystic fibrosis disease process begins essentially at birth and continues into middle adulthood, an additional challenge for the CEP is to develop age-appropriate intervention strategies. Adults can often accept traditional exercise or rehabilitation training programs, but children and adolescents may not find these programs engaging. They may be more motivated by active play and athletic activities that include their peers, such as team-based sports and games. Formal resistance training can begin as early as 7–8 years of age (403); however, children and youth do well when their program matches their level of muscular development, strength, coordination, and skill levels. The use of active play, including real-life activities and video games that require running, jumping, dancing, bending, and reaching, can engage children while providing a sufficient training load to help them meet current physical activity guidelines (404–406). Including parents in the exercise prescription design is often critical to the overall success of the program because parents may feel exercise will negatively affect their child and because the parent will most likely be required to facilitate travel to and from program activity sites.

Children with mild to moderate cystic fibrosis can be physically active but often are not. Inactivity among children with cystic fibrosis is sometimes encouraged by parents, other caregivers, teachers, and various health care professionals because of a lack of understanding of disease–exercise interactions. Other reasons for inactivity include a patient's fear of provoking symptoms or disease exacerbation, self- or peer-imposed social isolation, and a perceived lack of time due to the time required to complete other tasks associated with disease management (407). It is important that children with cystic fibrosis overcome these barriers because limited participation in physical activity in turn leads to deconditioning that leads to further worsening of the disease. Although exercise will not change the pathophysiologic process of the disease, maintenance of aerobic and muscular capacity reduces the rate of physiologic decline and overall mortality (193, 407–409).

Considerations for Adults

Adult patients with cystic fibrosis have many of the same compliance issues as their healthy counterparts. More and more adult patients with cystic fibrosis secure employment and begin careers as well as start families. Treatment may become more and more complex and time consuming as the disease progresses, limiting the time available for participating in exercise training. Facilitating the uptake of regular physical activity and helping the patient with cystic fibrosis overcome barriers to exercise may be more important than the actual elements of the exercise training program.

Precautions

Because of the nature of cystic fibrosis pathology, some precautions should be observed by patients and CEPs when undertaking exercise training. Patients with cystic fibrosis are at increased risk for developing dehydration. They should be taught the symptoms (*i.e.*, light-headedness, heat intolerance, flushed skin, production of a small volume of dark yellow urine, nausea, headache, and muscle cramping) and the prevention (*i.e.*, consume 120 mL or 4 oz of water every 20 minutes; for children, it is often easier to advise them to take eight gulps of water every 20 minutes) (410). Patients with cystic fibrosis also risk sodium loss with excessive sweating because of the concentrated nature of their sweat, so including electrolytes (*i.e.*, 50 mmol·L^{-1} sodium chloride) can be helpful (411). Cystic fibrosis–related diabetes can result in episodes of hypoglycemia. These episodes can be prevented by monitoring blood glucose levels before and after exercise; adjusting the dose of insulin and where it is administered to avoid areas of active muscle such as the legs; consuming supplemental carbohydrates (*e.g.*, 15 g if blood glucose is <100 mg·dL^{-1} or 5.5 mmol·L^{-1}); and timing exercise earlier in the day because late afternoon or evening training sessions could lead to hypoglycemia during sleeping hours (412).

Moderate exercise can induce coughing. Severe coughing can increase the risk of hemoptysis (*i.e.*, coughing up blood) and pneumothorax. Exercise should be discontinued if hemoptysis is moderate (5–250 mL) to severe (>250 mL) and should not be resumed until there has been a period of 24–48 hours with no new bleeding (403). Coughing during exercise also presents a risk to other patients in that respiratory droplets of patients infected with *P. aeruginosa* and *Burkholderia cepacia* can become airborne and spread to other patients. The microorganisms can survive on dry surfaces for several days, so fastidious cleaning of equipment (*i.e.*, ergometers, stethoscopes, etc.) and hands is required, but at this time there are no recommendations suggesting the use of masks, gloves, and/or gowns is necessary. It has been shown that contamination of respiratory droplets from coughing can occur over 1–2 meters (413), so many centers instruct patients to maintain a 2-meter distance from one another and often schedule patients with similar microbial infections to use their clinic facilities at common times.

Pneumothorax is more likely to occur in patients with poor lung function. To protect against pneumothorax, patients should perform airway-clearing exercises prior to exercise. Patients with a pneumothorax should not lift weights greater than 2.5 kg (~5.5 lb) or perform activities that precipitate a Valsalva maneuver for 2 weeks after the pneumothorax has resolved. High-altitude training and scuba diving are also contraindicated during this time (403).

Some patients may suffer from bronchoconstriction during exercise. This should be easily managed with the use of prescribed short-term β-adrenergic agonist inhalers. Some patients are at risk of arterial oxygen desaturation and should be monitored regularly. For patients with significant desaturation of less than 89%, supplemental oxygen should be used.

Participation in team-based sports is not contraindicated in cystic fibrosis. However, patients with feeding tubes, liver disease–related coagulation disorders, and swollen visceral organs (*i.e.*, spleen and liver) should avoid contact sports because of the risk of injury to these organs and internal bleeding.

Patients with cystic fibrosis should be encouraged to perform resistance exercises to offset malnutrition-induced osteopenia and osteoporosis. They should be instructed to avoid ballistic movements and motions that involve vigorous flexion and/or rotation of the trunk to avoid injury. Stretching the upper torso and neck while strengthening muscles that retract the scapula can alleviate some of the discomfort associated with thoracic kyphosis and altered breathing mechanics (380).

Finally, the CEP should be aware that there is a high prevalence of depression in patients with cystic fibrosis. The prevalence of depression is estimated to range between 8% and 29% among children and adolescents and between 13% and 33% among adults. Depression is associated with decreased lung function, lower BMI, low treatment program adherence, lower quality of life, and more frequent hospitalizations. The Patient Health Questionnaire 9-item scale (PHQ-9), Generalized Anxiety Disorder 7-item scale (GAD-7), or the Children's Depression Inventory (CDI) may be useful for identifying individuals who would benefit from referral to appropriate mental health professionals (414).

Lung Transplant–Specific Considerations in Exercise Training

There are three distinct and clearly separate phases in which exercise training is important for lung transplant patients: during the waiting period prior to transplantation; in recovery during the postoperative period; and during long-term maintenance beginning approximately 6 months posttransplant.

Prospective Transplantation

The first phase is prior to transplantation when the patient is on the inactive or active waiting list. To maximize the chances of surviving what is a major surgical procedure with a high postoperative complication rate, it is essential to ensure that the patient remains as fit as possible up to the time of surgery. Once on the active transplant waiting list, the patient will often have to wait a considerable period for a suitable donor who matches their blood group and is of a similar size. During the waiting period, the patient's condition progressively deteriorates, and exercise training has the ability to slow down this progression to an extent. This is often referred to as "prolonging the window of opportunity" for transplantation. Patients whose condition deteriorates to the point at which they are very wasted and have very poor function are unlikely to survive the perioperative period and are typically removed from the transplant waiting list permanently.

There is clear evidence that the poorer the patient's pretransplant functional capacity, the poorer their outcomes postoperatively (415). Research has shown that quadriceps function is significantly reduced in pulmonary transplant candidates, and lower limb muscle strength is affected more than upper limb strength (393). There is evidence that pulmonary rehabilitation can help patients maintain their general condition, as measured by the 6-minute walk distance (6MWD), during their period on the active waiting list despite their progressive deterioration in lung function (394). Recent systematic reviews have demonstrated that prerehabilitation programs including at least moderate intense aerobic exercise prior to surgery can improve exercise capacity and reduce postoperative complications by nearly 50%, and it can reduce hospital length of stay in high-risk lung cancer surgery populations (210, 416)

Patterns of exercise are similar in prerehabilitation exercise programs to those used in pulmonary rehabilitation programs, although the severity of the transplant candidate's disease may require some modification to standard protocols. Traditionally, patients with pulmonary hypertension were excluded from exercise training, but recent studies have shown that exercise training has clear benefits. Nevertheless, high-intensity exercise, resistance training, and Valsalva maneuvers are generally avoided. As the aim of the exercise program at the preoperative stage is to maintain functional status, patients should be advised to undertake both outpatient and home-based exercise regimens, use of oxygen on exertion, and how to conserve their energy to maximize their ability to complete their exercise training sessions, irrespective of whether they are at home or in an institutional setting.

The patient's exercise program and functional status can be affected by complications during the waiting period by exacerbations or intercurrent infections and hospitalization. During such events, patients and health care providers need to focus on early mobilization, and measures to control breathlessness and use pharmacological interventions, to protect their exercise capacity. Following such events, interventions to recover lost ground are essential.

A recent publication from an experienced transplant center reviews the evidence and offers guidance on functional assessment and pretransplant exercise prescription for transplant candidates (212). It is recommended as an excellent resource.

Aiding Recovery of Function in the Postoperative Period

By the time patients undergo lung transplantation, they have had advanced respiratory failure and/or chronic infection for a prolonged period. This impacts directly on functionality, muscle mass, and strength. In addition, there is associated comorbidity ranging from osteoporosis to loss of physiologic reserve in other organs (*e.g.*, cardiac damage from persistent hypoxia). During the hospital admission at the time of transplantation, there is a 15%–32% further fall in quadriceps strength (212), proving there is further deconditioning in a patient who already had very limited functional ability preoperatively. Although even within diagnostic groups there is considerable heterogeneity, and some patients have a very straightforward recovery from this major surgical procedure, perioperative complications are common and prolonged ICU admissions and primary graft dysfunction are relatively frequent. Physical rehabilitation of these patients is both challenging and essential to ensure a positive outcome from the procedure. A personalized approach for each individual is critical.

Exercise has to commence as early as possible, including in the ICU in the conscious patient even if still on a ventilator. Sitting, upper arm exercise, and standing should be encouraged. Although no evidence specific to pulmonary transplant recipients supports this recommendation, it has been demonstrated to be effective and improve survival in other populations who are critically ill in whom muscle wasting has been shown to occur early. Recipients who have a complicated postoperative course and prolonged ICU admission on a background of reduced muscle strength and mass are very vulnerable to the development of ICU-acquired myopathy and polyneuropathy, with their resultant threats to both survival and long-term recovery.

Most transplant units encourage a vigorous rehabilitation program in the first few weeks after discharge from the ICU to help the recovery of muscle strength. The exercise program often includes supplemental oxygen in the first days or even weeks posttransplant. Numerous complications may occur in this particularly vulnerable period, including inadequate pain control, infections, acute rejection, or mental health issues such as depression and anxiety. During such events, the aim should be to modify and adapt the exercise program, not discontinue it, as exercise is essential to achieve the best possible functional outcome. In the initial postoperative period, 6MWD deteriorates but then progressively improves as the patient recovers from the operative procedure. Following discharge from the hospital, an outpatient rehabilitation program should be completed for a period of between 4 and 12 weeks. Again, the exact duration and content of the program has to be tailored to the individual patient. There is evidence that this approach improves outcomes (210, 416).

Quadriceps muscle strength takes 3–4 months to recover to the level of strength present in the immediate preoperative period. Many services use 6MWD to monitor progress. Current evidence suggests that the slow recovery of exercise capacity is not due to the lung graft, which usually has adequate function relatively early in the posttransplant period but is due to slow recovery of muscle strength (417).

During any readmission to the hospital due to complications, exercise may have to be modified to accommodate changes in the patient's physical condition; however, it must be continued, and its importance emphasized. Again, a recent review of the role of pulmonary rehabilitation in lung transplant programs offers guidance regarding the continuum of pulmonary rehabilitation from ICU to discharge and suggestions for rehabilitation therapy in the early posttransplant outpatient period (212).

Maintaining Long-term Functional Success

Most patients will achieve their maximal posttransplant 6MWD within 6–12 months. From 6 months onward, patients who are doing well will often be back in employment and leading a near-normal life. Unfortunately, recipients are at significant lifelong risk of major complications in the posttransplant period; therefore, the better their functional status, the more likely they are to have a good clinical outcome and recover from any step-down in their functional ability. Six-minute walk testing suggests that those patients who achieve greater percentages of their predicted walking distance have better long-term outcomes (418). Even if they are unfortunate enough to develop chronic allograft dysfunction with resultant reduced respiratory function, if they have maintained muscle condition through activity, then they will have less dyspnea at any given workload compared to a deconditioned recipient.

Another potential threat to recipients is weight gain, commonly seen from 2 to 18 months posttransplant (419). Some weight gain reflects recovery from the malnutrition seen in some patients with advanced lung disease. Medications, particularly long-term corticosteroid therapy, also contribute. Patients should be warned about the dangers of excessive weight gain, including its implications for general health and for exercise ability. Key tasks for the exercise team are educating the patient about the value of incorporating exercise into their daily routine and encouraging and advising on how best to maintain their posttransplantation fitness and a healthy weight. Increasing numbers of modern devices offer the ability to monitor activity levels and setting a mutually agreed target level of exercise long term can help to motivate recipients to maintain muscle strength and functional ability.

Rather than arbitrarily imposing a specific exercise regimen, the transplant team should explore with patients their preferred exercise pursuits and counsel them on recommended duration and intensity. By taking up activities that they enjoy, patients are more likely to be motivated to persist with the activity long term. The aim is long-term adherence to a pattern of exercise activity that allows patients to achieve maximal function and maintain that level of function (403).

SUMMARY

Respiratory diseases impose a significant health burden worldwide. Those suffering from these diseases endure a significant loss of health that reduces their well-being, productivity, and quality of life. Respiratory disease is expensive to manage, costing world health care systems billions of dollars. Although the causes may be different for COPD (*i.e.*, pollutant/irritant inhalation), asthma (*i.e.*, allergic immune response), and cystic fibrosis (*i.e.*, *CFTR* mutation), all three diseases have a common pathology in that inflammation is central to disease symptoms and severity. All three diseases often share a final "last ditch" effort for medical treatment in the form of a lung transplant. Although this is often a successful treatment, it is neither optimal nor is it cost effective for routine disease management.

Engagement in regular physical activity and/or prescriptive exercise unfortunately will not cure respiratory disease, but it will enable patients to better manage their symptoms, reduce disease exacerbations, and slow the decline in lung function. In addition, regular physical activity and exercise reduce the risk of developing secondary comorbid health conditions such as obesity, Type 2 diabetes, and cardiovascular disease, thereby reducing the overall disease burden. Thus, the CEP plays an important role in helping patients manage their disease. When the initial exercise prescription and adjustments over time are compatible with the patient's disease status and medical management, exercise training can have a major impact on the overall success of each patient's treatment.

CHAPTER REVIEW QUESTIONS

1. What is the primary etiology common to COPD, asthma, cystic fibrosis, and post lung transplant loss of function?
2. What pathological mechanisms result in airflow limitation in patients with COPD?
3. Why is exercise ventilation limited in patients with obstructive respiratory disease?
4. What is the difference between exercise-induced asthma and exercise-induced bronchoconstriction?
5. Of the six different *CFTR* gene mutation phenotypes, which manifests as the most severe?
6. Following lung transplant, what are the five major pathologies that degrade lung function?
7. How is the BODE index different from the GOLD index when it comes to classifying disease severity among patients with COPD?
8. What are the key objectives of pulmonary rehabilitation programs?
9. What are the potential causes of muscle atrophy and weakness in patients with chronic respiratory disease?
10. Describe nonpharmacologic airway clearance techniques in patients with cystic fibrosis.

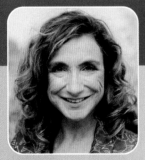

Case Study 8.1

Heather was born in March 1981. At the age of 18 months, she was diagnosed with the autosomal recessive, life-limiting disease, cystic fibrosis. Her older brother also had cystic fibrosis. She had a relatively normal childhood and engaged in plenty of exercise, although she was often kept out of school to prevent her from getting ill when other children were not well. Heather had nasal polyps removed at age 11, and her appendix removed at age 17

years. She was diagnosed with hyperglycemia at age 19. Up until this time, she was moderately active, primarily engaged in surfing and dancing.

Timeline and Medical History

At Age 21 Years:
Heather was first hospitalized because of a cystic fibrosis complication. She was treated for infections caused by *Staphylococcus aureus* and *Pseudomonas aeruginosa*, two common pathogens that result in severe pneumonia. After recovering, she was able to trek in Nepal.

(*continued*)

Case Study 8.1 (*continued*)

At Age 22 Years:

Heather began injecting insulin because of cystic fibrosis–related Type 1 diabetes. At age 23 years, she was again hospitalized, this time for 2 weeks with *S. aureus* and *P. aeruginosa* pneumonia. Despite these severe infections, she recovered sufficiently well to go on a second trek in Nepal.

At Age 24 Years:

Heather was diagnosed with thrombophilia, a tendency for the blood to clot, found in approximately 20% of people with cystic fibrosis. A few months later, Heather was again hospitalized for 2 weeks with *S. aureus* and *P. aeruginosa* pneumonia. She was finding her ability to exercise was diminishing rapidly.

At Age 27 Years:

Heather's FEV_1 was down to 42%. She was suffering from the effects of cystic fibrosis, loss of weight, chest infections, and low respiratory function. Six months after her last severe bout of bacterial pneumonia, Heather was hospitalized again for the same condition.

At Age 29 Years:

Heather had a feeding tube inserted to try to slow down her weight loss. By now she weighed 36 kg (80 lb), approximately the weight of an 11-year-old child. At this time, her FEV_1 was only 17% and she could barely walk or breathe. She was also diagnosed with osteopenia and over the subsequent several years broke six ribs through coughing and was given a zoledronate infusion, a powerful bisphosphonate to prevent her ribs from fracturing.

At Age 30–34 Years:

Heather continued to have severe bouts of pneumonia. Her FEV_1 got down to 23%, and she needed home help. Her life was predominantly engaged in a regimen of feeding, using nebulizers, and very limited attempts to exercise.

Age 35 Years:

In 2015 and through June 2016, Heather was diagnosed with and treated for pneumonia, pleurisy, osteoporosis, iron deficiency anemia, and collapsed veins from clots and intravenous lines and lures. She was in significant pain all the time and was given a wheelchair. Her FEV_1 was 24%, and she was placed on night-time oxygen.

Age 36 Years:

In June 2016, Heather was placed on the waiting list for a double lung transplant. Two months later, she received a bilateral sequential lung transplant. Although pleural effusion drainage was required postoperatively, 2 months after the transplant, Heather was back at work. Her night-time feeds and nebulizer were stopped, and she no longer suffered bouts of coughing or dyspnea. Her 6MWD was 613 m, and FEV_1 was 54%. By November, her FEV_1 was 71%.

Exercise Capacity:

Heather conducted the following exercise over the 12 months prior to becoming eligible for the transplant waiting list:

- Daily 5 km (3.2 miles) on an Exercycle with no resistance (took ~15–20 min to complete).
- Shoulder and chest stretches to "open up" her shoulders to increase chest capacity and prevent "hunching over."
- Upper body strengthening exercises. Heather found this was too difficult to manage due to very low energy, and it caused too much coughing. The priority remained the Exercycle.

After surgery:

Commencing 18 days posttransplant and while Heather was in the rehabilitation unit for 3 weeks, she conducted a mixture of the following daily for an hour at least:

- Exercycle
- Treadmill
- Three types of arm weights
- Walking stairs
- Standing up from the sitting position
- Leg weights
- Leg presses
- Squats
- Walks and being generally active

After being discharged from the rehabilitation unit, Heather continued at home with an Exercycle, treadmill, arm weights, and general walking.

Seven Months After Her Transplant:

Heather rides her bicycle easily for 14.5 km (9 miles) and uses her Exercycle most days for 15 km (9 miles). She uses arm weights of 3 kg (7 lb) on each arm for an hour and stretches for an hour. She can now do most forms of exercise without hesitation. Heather is still working hard to regain thigh muscle strength, her only limiting factor.

Case Study 8.1 Questions

1. *Staphylococcus aureus* and *Pseudomonas aeruginosa* are two common pathogens that result in severe pneumonia. Heather was first diagnosed with these at the age of 23 years. Is there a connection between these common pathogens and her resulting double lung transplant?

2. What are the possible patient outcomes of a double lung transplant?

3. Worldwide, around 4,000 adult lung transplants are carried out each year. What five groups of patients with end-stage lung disease can benefit from lung transplantation?

Case Study 8.2

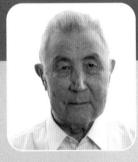

Chris, a 66-year-old male patient, was referred to the exercise rehabilitation clinic by his primary care physician for improvement of exercise intolerance and secondary prevention of cardiovascular disease. At the time of referral, Chris was becoming increasingly sedentary because he experienced shortness of breath when walking continuously for more than 10 minutes. Chris had diagnoses of recurrent supraventricular tachycardia that was managed with diltiazem (180 mg OD) and moderate to severe COPD for which Chris had been prescribed a Duolin inhaler (salbutamol 100 μg and ipratropium bromide 20 μg). Chris was recovering from a recent inguinal hernia operation 3 weeks prior and was advised to limit heavy lifting activity for 4–6 weeks. Finally, Chris had a 20-year history of depression managed with the 5-hydroxytryptamine (5-HT, serotonin) uptake inhibitor, paroxetine (20 mg OD). Anthropometric, pulmonary function testing, and a graded maximal effort cardiopulmonary exercise test were undertaken by the clinician to assess the extent to which Chris's cardiovascular and pulmonary diseases were contributing to his reduced functional capacity.

Patient Assessment Data

A staged cycle ergometry protocol was used to assess Chris's maximal aerobic capacity. Chris cycled at 35 W for 5 minutes to warm up after which the resistance was increased in 10 W increments every 2 minutes. The results of testing are shown in panels A–I in Figure 1. Chris reached a peak workload of 75 W and voluntarily terminated the test due to leg fatigue (RPE = 9 of 10) and shortness of breath (score = 3 out of 4). Chris did not report any chest pain or lightheadedness. Chris's oxygen consumption rate ($\dot{V}O_{2\,peak}$) increased predictably with power output. The slope of this relationship was 12.3 mL $O_2 \cdot W^{-1}$, which suggests a slightly increased O_2 cost during cycling exercise (normal slope = 10 mL $O_2 \cdot W^{-1}$) perhaps due to an increased work of breathing. The peak $\dot{V}O_{2peak}$ achieved was 72% of the predicted value for similarly aged males, indicating a moderate reduction in aerobic capacity (Figure 1A).

Table 1		Patient Assessment Data				
Anthropometry		**Spirometry**			**Cardiopulmonary**	
Height (m)	1.77	FEV$_1$ (L)	1.39	41% of predicted	HR$_{rest}$ (bpm)	108
Weight (kg)	70.3	FVC (L)	3.21	71% of predicted	HR$_{max}$ (bpm)	140
BMI (kg·m^{-2})	22.4	FEV$_1$/FVC	0.43	58% of predicted	BP$_{rest}$ (mm Hg)	112/70
WC (cm)	95	PEFR (L·min^{-1})	188	36% of predicted	BP$_{max}$ (mm Hg)	190/72
		MVV (L·min^{-1})	48.6	41% of predicted	O$_2$ saturation$_{rest}$ (%)	95
					O$_2$ saturation$_{max}$ (%)	92
					RPE$_{max}$	9/10
					Dyspnea scale$_{max}$	9/10

(continued)

Case Study 8.2 (*continued*)

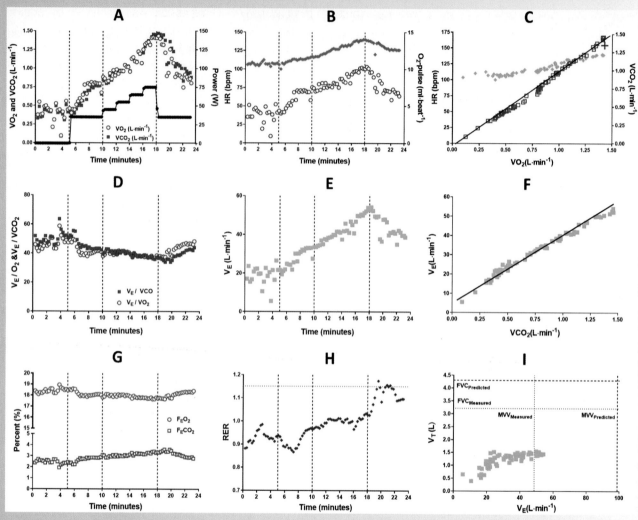

FIGURE 1. A nine-panel plot of data from Chris's maximal cardiopulmonary exercise test is presented in panels A–I. A detailed explanation of the data can be found in the text. The vertical dotted lines identify from right to left the end of rest, the end of warm-up exercise, and the start of active recovery. Abbreviations used are as follows: the rate of oxygen consumption ($\dot{V}O_2$), heart rate (HR), the carbon dioxide production rate ($\dot{V}CO_2$), the ventilatory equivalent for oxygen ($\dot{V}O_2/\dot{V}_E$) and carbon dioxide ($\dot{V}CO_2/\dot{V}_E$), minute ventilation ($\dot{V}_E$), mixed expired fraction of oxygen (F_EO_2) and carbon dioxide (F_ECO_2), tidal volume (V_{Tidal}), respiratory exchange ratio (RER), forced vital capacity (FVC), maximal voluntary ventilation (MVV) rate.

Chris was tachycardic at rest (108 bpm), and his peak exercise heart rate reached 90% of his age-predicted maximum. Chris's exercise ECG showed occasional premature ventricular contractions but was otherwise normal. The O_2 pulse increased to a peak during incremental exercise. The peak O_2 pulse was slightly lower than expected, given a $\dot{V}O_2$ of 1.4 L·min^{-1}. Overall, Chris's tachycardia continued during exercise. As a result, Chris appeared to have limited cardiac reserve at peak exercise, and it is likely his tachycardia contributes to his reported shortness of breath symptoms (Figure 1B).

A clear ventilatory threshold (VT_1) was not detected by either the v-slope or ventilatory equivalent methods (Figure 1C and D), suggesting that volitional fatigue occurred before the onset of significant metabolic acidosis or the need for respiratory compensation (*i.e.*, absent respiratory compensation point or VT_2; Figure 1D and F). This is suggestive of a ventilatory-based exercise limitation. Chris's spirometry measures are consistent with those expected in a patient diagnosed with moderate COPD. The manifestation of Chris's expiratory flow limitation is reflected by an excessive minute ventilation in relation to a given oxygen consumption and carbon dioxide elimination rate (Figure 1D) and in his lack of ventilatory reserve at peak exercise (Figure 1I). Clearly, Chris is limited in his ability to expand his V_{Tidal} (likely because of exercise-induced hyperinflation), which limits his ability to increase minute ventilation.

Exercise Prescription

Chris struggles to sustain continuous moderate-intensity exercise, and this is affecting his quality of life and placing him at increased risk for sedentarism. COPD is a chronic and progressive disease that cannot be cured with exercise. Exercise training can however improve patient exercise capacity and symptom management.

The decision was made to include a mix of continuous moderate-intensity training (CMIT) and high-intensity interval training (HIIT) aerobic exercise training sessions into Chris's exercise prescription. Using a stationary cycle or programmable treadmill, Chris performed 2 HIIT and 1 CMIT session each week. Following an adequate warm-up, the HIIT session included one set of 4 × 1-minute work intervals (*e.g.*, 100% peak workload) separated by 2-minute recovery intervals (*e.g.*, 30% peak workload). Progression was achieved by adding repetitions and/or by increasing the work interval duration in 15-second increments. CMIT sessions consisted of 10 minutes of cycling or treadmill walking at 50% of the peak workload. These sessions were progressed by increasing the exercise duration and intensity. Flexibility training with static and dynamic balance exercises were included to complete Chris's program. At week 4, resistance exercises that targeted large muscle groups were also introduced into Chris's program.

After 12 weeks of exercise rehabilitation, Chris increased his peak cycling workload to 85 W and his 6MWD improved by 68 m. Chris reported improvement in his symptoms and was able to resume his favorite recreational activity, golf, without being unduly short of breath.

Case Study 8.2 Questions

1. What is the primary reason that patients with chronic obstructive pulmonary disease are referred to rehabilitation programs?
2. Why was the decision made to include a mix of continuous moderate-intensity training (CMIT) and high-intensity interval training (HIIT) aerobic exercise training sessions into Chris's exercise prescription?
3. For Chris, was the outcome expected, and can all patients with COPD expect the same outcome?

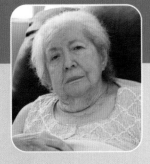

Case Study 8.3

Martha is a 72-year-old pleasant female with a history of severe COPD, hypertension, hyperlipidemia, and diabetes. She reports increased difficulty with completing activities of daily living due to exertional dyspnea and not having the strength to lift items comfortably. Martha also stated that she experienced a fall last month in her apartment when she tripped on the edge of her rug. She was referred to pulmonary rehabilitation to help improve her fitness and regain her physical independence. A 6-minute walk test, timed up and go, and 30-second chair stand test were performed during her pulmonary rehabilitation orientation visit.

Patient Assessment Data

During the 6-minute walk test, Martha stopped periodically due to dyspnea (rating 3 out of 4) with her oxygen saturation staying above 90% at all times. She was only able to walk a total of 197 meters. The results of her timed up and go test and 30-second chair stand test were also poor (27 s and 2 stands, respectively).

(*continued*)

Case Study 8.3 (*continued*)

Exercise Prescription

Martha's results indicate that she is frail and would benefit from performing an exercise program that is designed to increase strength and improve. Accordingly, resistance exercise was primarily performed to include 8–10 whole-body exercises. The first week consisted of 1 set of 12 repetitions, which then progressed to two sets by the third week of the program. Because Martha was hesitant to perform a one repetition max test, and RPE of five to six of 10 was used to guide the intensity of activity. Flexibility, static, and dynamic balance exercises were also incorporated into the remaining time left in the exercise sessions. Both continuous and interval aerobic exercise training were increasingly incorporated as Martha demonstrated greater exercise tolerance.

At the end of the 12-week program, Martha was able to complete the 6-minute walk test with only taking one short break and improved her walking distance by 52 m. Although Martha still experienced physical limitations, she reported noticeable improvements in her ability to carry on activities of daily living.

Case Study 8.3 Questions

1. Why did the initial exercise prescription predominantly focus on resistance exercise?
2. Why was aerobic exercise incorporated into the exercise regimen?
3. Although Martha's follow-up 6-minute walk distance was not associated with physical independence, was her improvement clinically meaningful?

REFERENCES

1. Forum of International Respiratory Societies. *The Global Impact of Respiratory Disease.* 3rd ed. European Respiratory Society; 2021. [cited 2021 Sept 22]. Available from: https://www.firsnet.org/images/publications/FIRS_Master_09202021.pdf.

2. World Health Organization [Internet]. The top 10 causes of death. World Health Organization; [cited 2020 Dec 20]. Available from: https://www.who.int/newsroom/fact-sheets/detail/the-top-10-causes-of-death.

3. Labaki WW, Han MK. Chronic respiratory diseases: a global view. *Lancet Respir Med.* 2020;8(6):531–3.

4. Ferkol T, Schraufnugal D. The global burden of respiratory disease. *Ann Am Thorac Soc.* 2014;11(3):404–6.

5. Wardlaw TM, Johansson EW, Hodge M. Pneumonia: the forgotten killer of children. World Health Organization. 2006. Available from: https://apps.who.int/iris/bitstream/handle/10665/43640/9280640489_eng.pdf?sequence=1&isAllowed=y.

6. Walker CL, Rudan I, Lui L, et al. Global burden of childhood pneumonia and diarrhoea. *Lancet.* 2013;381:1405–16.

7. Lim SS, Vos T, Flaxman AD, et al. A comparative risk assessment of burden of disease and injury attributable to 67 risk factors and risk factor clusters in 21 regions, 1990–2010: a systematic analysis for the Global Burden of Disease Study 2010. *Lancet.* 2012;380:2224–60.

8. World Health Organization. *Global Tuberculosis Report 2013.* Geneva (IL): World Health Organization; 2013.

9. World Health Organization [Internet]. WHO Coronavirus (COVID-19) dashboard. Available from: https://covid19.who.int/.

10. Kudo M, Ishigatsubo Y, Aoki I. Pathology of asthma. *Front Mircobiol.* 2013;4:263.

11. Masoli M, Fabian D, Holt S, Beasley R; Global Initiative for Asthma (GINA) Program. The global burden of asthma: executive summary of the GINA Dissemination Committee report. *Allergy.* 2004;59:469–78.

12. Sung H, Ferlay J, Siegel RL, et al. Global Cancer Statistics 2020: GLOBOCAN estimates of incidence and mortality worldwide for 36 cancers in 185 countries. *CA Cancer J Clin.* 2021;71(3):209–49.

13. Guo J, Garratt A, Hill A. Worldwide rates of diagnosis and effective treatment for cystic fibrosis. *J Cyst Fibros.* 2022; 21(3):456–62.

14. Global Initiative for Chronic Obstructive Lung Disease. Global strategy for the diagnosis, management and prevention of COPD: 2022 report. 2021. Available from: https://goldcopd.org/2022-gold-reports.

15. National Center for Health Statistics. *Health, United States, 2015 With Special Feature on Racial and Ethnic Health Disparities.* Hyattsville (MD): National Center for Health Statistics; 2016.

16. American Lung Association. Trends in COPD (chronic bronchitis and emphysema): morbidity and mortality. 2013. Available from: http://www.lungusa.org/finding-cures/our-research/trend-reports/copd-trend-report.pdf.

17. Ford ES. Trends in mortality from COPD among adults in the United States. *Chest.* 2015;148(4):962–70.

18. Levack WMM, Weatherall M, Reeve JC, Mans C, Mauro A. Uptake of pulmonary rehabilitation in New Zealand by people with chronic obstructive pulmonary disease in 2009. *N Z Med J.* 2012;125(1348):23–33.

19. Lopez-Campos JL, Ruiz-Ramos M, Soriano JB. Mortality trends in chronic obstructive pulmonary disease in Europe, 1994–2010: a joinpoint regression analysis. *Lancet Respir Med.* 2014;2(1):54–62.

20. Ehrman JK. *Clinical Exercise Physiology.* 3rd ed. Champaign (IL): Human Kinetics; 2013.

21. Global Initiative for Chronic Obstructive Lung Disease. Global strategy for the diagnosis, management and prevention of COPD: 2017 report. Global Initiative for Chronic Obstructive Lung Disease (GOLD) 2017. 2016. Available from: https://goldcopd.org/archived-reports/.

22. Mannino DM, Buist AS. Global burden of COPD: risk factors, prevalence and future trends. *Lancet.* 2007;370(9589):765–73.

23. Guarascio AJ, Ray SM, Finch CK, Self TH. The clinical and economic burden of chronic obstructive pulmonary disease in the USA. *Clinicoecon Outcomes Res.* 2013;5:235–45.

24. Public Health Agency of Canada. *Life and Breath: Respiratory Disease in Canada, 2007.* Ottawa: Public Health Agency of Canada; 2007. Available from: https://www.canada.ca/en/public-health/services/reports-publications/2007/life-breath-respiratory-disease-canada-2007.html.

25. Stoller JK, Aboussouan LS. Alpha1-antitrypsin deficiency. *Lancet.* 2005;365(9478):2225–36.

26. Le Rouzic O, Roche N, Cortot AB, et al. Defining the "Frequent Exacerbator" phenotype in COPD: a hypothesis-free approach. *Chest.* 2018;153(5):1106–15.

27. Lee YJ, Choi S, Kwon SY, et al. A Genome-Wide Association Study in early COPD: identification of one major susceptibility loci. *Int J Chron Obstruct Pulmon Dis.* 2020;15:2967–75.

28. MacNee W. Is chronic obstructive pulmonary disease an accelerated aging disease? *Ann Am Thorac Soc.* 2016;13(Suppl 5):S429–37.

29. Ntritsos G, Franek J, Belbasis L, et al. Gender-specific estimates of COPD prevalence: a systematic review and meta-analysis. *Int J Chron Obstruct Pulmon Dis.* 2018;13:1507–14.

30. Montserrat-Capdevila J, Marsal JR, Ortega M, et al. Clinico-epidemiological characteristics of men and women with a new diagnosis of chronic obstructive pulmonary disease: a database (SIDIAP) study. *BMC Pulm Med.* 2021;21(1):44.

31. Sørheim I-C, Johannessen A, Gulsvik A, Bakke PS, Silverman EK, DeMeo DL. Gender differences in COPD: are women more susceptible to smoking effects than men? *Thorax.* 2010;65(6):480–5.

32. Vestbo J, Hurd S, Agusti AG, et al. Global strategy for the diagnosis, management and prevention of chronic obstructive pulmonary disease: GOLD executive summary. *Am J Respir Crit Care Med.* 2013;187(4):347–65.

33. Tan WC, Lo C, Jong A, et al. Marijuana and chronic obstructive lung disease: a population-based study. *CMAJ.* 2009;180:814–20.

34. Celli BR, MacNee W, Agusti A, et al; American Thoracic Society (ATC)/European Respiratory Society (ERS)Task Force. Standards for the diagnosis and treatment of patients with COPD: a summary of the ATS/ERS position paper. *Eur Respir J.* 2004;23:932–46.

35. McCloskey SC, Patel BD, Hinchliffe SJ, Reid ED, Wareham NJ, Lomas DA. Siblings of patients with severe chronic obstructive pulmonary disease have a significant risk of airflow obstruction. *Am J Respir Crit Care Med.* 2001;164(8 Pt 1):1419–24.

36. Global Initiative for Asthma. Global strategy for asthma management and prevention. 2022. Available from: www.ginasthma.org/gina-reports/.

37. Global Asthma Network. The global asthma report 2018. 2018. Available from: http://globalasthmareport.org/2018/index.html.

38. Pate CA, Zahran HS, Qin X, Johnson C, Hummelman E, Malilay J. Asthma surveillance — United States, 2006–2018. *MMWR Surveill Summ.* 2021;70(5):1–32.

39. Skadhauge LR, Christensen K, Kyvik KO, Sissgaard T. Genetic and environmental influence on asthma: a population-based study of 11,688 Danish twin pairs. *Eur Respir J.* 1999;13:8–14.

40. United States Environmental Protection Agency. Asthma facts. 2016. Available from: https://19january2017snapshot.epa.gov/asthma/2016-asthma-factsheet_.html.

41. Yaghoubi M, Adibi A, Safari A, FitzGerald JM, Sadatsafavi M. The projected economic and health burden of uncontrolled asthma in the United States. *Am J Respir Crit Care Med.* 2019;200(9):1102–12.

42. Barnes PJ. Immunology of asthma and chronic obstructive pulmonary disease. *Nat Rev Immunol.* 2008;8(3):183–92.

43. Holgate ST. Pathogenesis of asthma. *Clin Exp Allergy.* 2008;38(6):872–97.

44. Kuruvilla ME, Lee FE, Lee GB. Understanding asthma phenotypes, endotypes, and mechanisms of disease. *Clin Rev Allergy Immunol.* 2019;56(2):219–33.

45. Diamant Z, Diderik Boot JD, Virchow JC. Summing up 100 years of asthma. *Respir Med.* 2007;101(3):378–88.

46. Ober C, Yao TC. The genetics of asthma and allergic disease. *Immunol Rev.* 2011;242:10–30.

47. Lim RH, Kobzik L, Dahl M. Risk for asthma in offspring of asthmatic mothers verses fathers: a meta analysis. *PLoS One.* 2010;5:e10134.

48. Mims JW. Asthma: definitions and pathology. *Int Forum Allergy Rhinol.* 2015;5(Suppl 1):S2–6.

49. Subbarao P, Mandhane PJ, Sears MR. Asthma: epidemiology, etiology and risk factors. *CMAJ.* 2009;181(9):E181–90. doi:10.1503/cmaj.080612.

50. Muraro A, Dreborg S, Halken S, et al. Dietary prevention of allergic diseases in infants and small children. Part III: critical review of published peer-reviewed observational and interventional studies and final recommendations. *Pediatr Allergy Immunol.* 2004;15:291–307.

51. Almqvist C, Egmar AC, Hedlin G, et al. Direct and indirect exposure to pets — risk of sensitization and asthma at 4 years in a birth cohort. *Clin Exp Allergy.* 2003;33(9):1190–7.

52. Kuruvilla ME, Vanijcharoenkarn K, Shih JA, Lee FE. Epidemiology and risk factors for asthma. *Respir Med.* 2019;149:16–22.

53. Lubamba B, Dhooghe B, Noel S, Leal T. Cystic fibrosis: insight into CFTR pathophysiology and pharmacology. *Clin Biochem.* 2012;45:1132–44.

54. Cystic Fibrosis Foundation. *Cystic Fibrosis Patient Registry 2020. Annual Data Report.* Bethesda (MD): Cystic Fibrosis Foundation; 2021. Available from: https://www.cff.org/sites/default/files/2021-10/2019-Patient-Registry-Annual-Data-Report.pdf.

55. Strausbaugh SD, Davis PB. Cystic fibrosis: a review of epidemiology and pathobiology. *Clin Chest Med.* 2007;28:279–88.

56. Chen Q, Shen Y, Zheng J. A review of cystic fibrosis: basic and clinical aspects. *Animal Model Exp Med.* 2021;4(3):220–32.

57. O'Sullivan BP, Freedman SD. Cystic fibrosis. *Lancet.* 2009;373:1891–904.

58. Dodge JA, Morison S, Lewis PA, et al. Incidence, population, and survival of cystic fibrosis in the UK, 1968–95. UK Cystic Fibrosis Survey Management Committee. *Arch Dis Child.* 1997;77(6):493–6.

59. van der Mark SC, Hoek RAS, Hellemons ME. Developments in lung transplantation over the past decade. *Eur Respir Rev.* 2020;29(157):190132.

60. Yusen RD, Edwards LB, Dipchand AI, et al; International Society for Heart and Lung Transplantation. The Registry of the International Society for Heart and Lung Transplantation: thirty-third adult lung and heart–lung transplant report-2016; focus theme: primary diagnostic indications for transplant. *J Heart Lung Transplant.* 2016;35(10):1170–84.

61. Leard LE, Holm AM, Valapour M, et al. Consensus document for the selection of lung transplant candidates: an update from the International Society for Heart and Lung Transplantation. *J Heart Lung Transplant.* 2021;40(11):1349–79.

62. Hayanga AJ, Aboagye JK, Hayanga HE, et al. Contemporary analysis of early outcomes after lung transplantation in the elderly using a national registry. *J Heart Lung Transplant.* 2015;34(2):182–8.

63. Olson MT, Elnahas S, Biswas Roy S, et al. Outcomes after lung transplantation in recipients aged 70 years or older. *Clin Transplant.* 2022;36(1):e14505.

64. Maxwell BG, Levitt JE, Goldstein BA, et al. Impact of the lung allocation score on survival beyond 1 year. *Am J Transplant.* 2014;14(10):2288–94.

65. Hayanga JW, D'Cunha J. The surgical technique of bilateral sequential lung transplantation. *J Thorac Dis.* 2014;6(8):1063–9.

66. Yeung JC, Keshavjee S. Overview of clinical lung transplantation. *Cold Spring Harb Perspect Med.* 2014;4(1):a015628.

67. Hankinson JL, Odencrantz JR, Fedan KB. Spirometric reference values from a sample of the general U.S. population. *Am J Respir Crit Care Med.* 1999;159:179–87.

68. Kerstjens HA, Rijcken B, Schouten JP, Postma DS. Decline of FEV1 by age and smoking status: facts, figures, and fallacies. *Thorax.* 1997;52(9):820–7.

69. Kasch FW, Boyer JL, Van Camp SP, Verity LS, Wallace JP. Effect of exercise on cardiovascular aging. *Age Aging.* 1993;22:5–10.

70. Roman MA, Rossiter HB, Casaburi R. Exercise, aging and the lung. *Eur Respir J.* 2016;48:1471–86.

71. Wasserman K, Hansen JE, Sue DY, et al. *Principles of Exercise Testing and Interpretation Including Pathophysiology and Clinical Applications.* 5th ed. Philadelphia (PA): Lippincott Williams & Wilkins, a Wolters Kluwer business; 2012.

72. Henke KG, Sharratt M, Pegelow D, Dempsey JA. Regulation of end-expiratory lung volume during exercise. *J Appl Physiol.* 1988;64:135–46.

73. Johnson BD, Reddan WG, Seow KC, Dempsey JA. Mechanical constraints on exercise hyperpnea in a fit aging population. *Am Rev Respir Dis.* 1991;143:968–77.

74. Johnson BD, Saupe KW, Dempsey JA. Mechanical constraints on exercise hyperpnea in endurance athletes. *J Appl Physiol.* 1992;73:874–86.

75. Taylor BJ, Johnson BD. The pulmonary circulation and exercise responses in the elderly. *Semin Respir Crit Care Med.* 2010;31:528–38.

76. Vogiatzis I, Zakynthinos S. Factors limiting exercise tolerance in chronic lung diseases. *Compr Physiol.* 2012;2:1779–817.

77. West JB. *Respiratory Physiology. The Essentials.* 6th ed. Baltimore (MD): Lippincott Williams & Wilkins; 2000.

78. Ward SA. Exercise physiology: exercise hyperpnea. *Curr Opin Physiol.* 2019;10:166–72.

79. Ward SA. Ventilation/carbon dioxide output relationships during exercise in health. *Eur Respir Rev.* 2021;30(160):200160.

80. Brischetto MJ, Millman RP, Peterson DD, Silage DA, Pack AI. Effect of aging on the ventilatory response to exercise and CO_2. *J Appl Physiol Respir Environ Exerc Physiol.* 1984;56:1143–50.

81. Garcia-Rio F, Vilamor A, Gomez-Mendieta A, et al. The progressive effects of aging on chemosensitivity in healthy subjects. *Respir Med.* 2007;101:2192–8.

82. Inbar O, Oren A, Scheinowitz M, Rotstein A, Dlin R, Casaburi R. Normal cardiorespiratory responses during incremental exercise in 20 to 70 year old men. *Med Sci Sports Exerc.* 1994;26:538–46.

83. Poulin MJ, Cunningham DA, Paterson DH, Rechnitzer PA, Ecclestone NA, Koval JJ. Ventilatory response to exercise in men and women 55 to 86 years of age. *Am J Respir Crit Care Med.* 1994;149:408–15.

84. Cotes JE. *Lung Function. Assessment and Application in Medicine.* Oxford: Blackwell Scientific; 1979.

85. Shephard RJ. Aging, respiratory function, and exercise. *J Aging Phys Act.* 1993;1:59–83.

86. Johnson BD, Dempsey JA. Demand vs. capacity in the aging pulmonary system. *Exerc Sport Sci Rev.* 1991;19:171–210.

87. Madama VC. *Pulmonary Function Testing and Cardiopulmonary Stress Testing.* Albany (NY): Delmar Publishers; 1998.

88. Cardus J, Burgos F, Diaz O, et al. Increase in pulmonary ventilation-perfusion inequality with age in healthy individuals. *Am J Respir Crit Care Med.* 1997;156((2 Pt 1)):648–53.

89. Levin DL, Buxton RB, Spiess JP, Arai T, Balouch J, Hopkins SR. Effects of age on pulmonary perfusion heterogeneity measured by magnetic resonance imaging. *J Appl Physiol.* 2007;102(5):2064–70.

90. Burtscher J, Millet GP, Gatterer H, Vonbank K, Burtscher M. Does regular physical activity mitigate the age-associated decline in pulmonary function? *Sports Med.* 2022;52(5):963–70.

91. Grundy S. COPD 1: pathophysiology, diagnosis and prognosis. *Nursing Times.* 2019;116(4):27–30.

92. Jeffery Mador M, Bozkanat E. Skeletal muscle dysfunction in chronic obstructive pulmonary disease. *Respir Res.* 2001;2(4):216–24.

93. Jaitovich A, Barreiro E. Skeletal muscle dysfunction in chronic obstructive pulmonary disease. What we know and can do for our patients. *Am J Respir Crit Care Med.* 2018;198(2):175–86.

94. Mehta GR, Mohammed R, Sarfraz S, et al. Chronic obstructive pulmonary disease: a guide for the primary care physician. *Dis Mon.* 2016;62:164–87.

95. Belli S, Prince I, Savio G, et al. Airway clearance techniques: the right choice for the right patient. *Front Med (Lausanne).* 2021;8:544826.

96. Barnes PJ, Shapiro SD, Pauwels RA. Chronic obstructive pulmonary disease: molecular and cellular mechanisms. *Eur Respir J.* 2003;22(4):672–88.

97. Alfahad AJ, Alzaydi MM, Aldossary AM, et al. Current views in chronic obstructive pulmonary disease pathogenesis and management. *Saudi Pharm J.* 2021;29(12):1361–73.

98. MacNee W. ABC of chronic obstructive pulmonary disease pathology, pathogenesis and pathophysiology. *BMJ.* 2006;332:1202–4.

99. Hyatt RE. Expiratory flow limitation. *J Appl Physiol.* 1983;55:1–8.

100. Milne KM, Domnik NJ, Phillips DB, et al. Evaluation of dynamic respiratory mechanical abnormalities during conventional CPET. *Front Med (Lausanne).* 2020;7:548.

101. O'Donnell DE, Revill S, Webb KA. Dynamic hyperinflation and exercise intolerance in chronic obstructive pulmonary disease. *Am J Respir Crit Care Med.* 2001;164:770–7.

102. Casaburi R, Rennard SI. Exercise limitation in chronic obstructive pulmonary disease. The O'Donnell threshold. *Am J Respir Crit Care Med.* 2015;191(8):873–5.

103. Levitzky MG. *Pulmonary Physiology.* 5th ed. New York (NY): McGraw-Hill Health Professions Division; 1999.

104. Ruppel G. What is the clinical value of lung volumes? *Respir Care.* 2012;57(1):26–35.

105. Casanova C, Cote C, de Torres JP, et al. Inspiratory-to-total lung capacity ratio predicts mortality in patients with chronic obstructive pulmonary disease. *Am J Respir Crit Care Med.* 2005;171(6):591–7.

106. O'Donnell DE, Guenette JA, Maltais F, Webb KA. Decline of resting inspiratory capacity in COPD: the impact on breathing pattern, dyspnea and ventilatory capacity during exercise. *Chest.* 2012;141:753–62.

107. O'Donnell DE, Webb KA, Neder JA. Lung hyperinflation in COPD: applying physiology to clinical practice. *COPD Res Pract.* 2015;1:4 doi:10.1186/s40749-015-0008-8.

108. Polkey MI, Kyroussis D, Hamnegard CH, Mills GH, Green M, Moxham J. Diaphragm strength in chronic obstructive pulmonary disease. *Am J Respir Crit Care Med.* 1996;154:1310–7.

109. Clanton TL, Levine S. Respiratory muscle fiber remodeling in chronic hyperinflation: dysfunction or adaptation? *J Appl Physiol(1985).* 2009;107:324–35.

110. Bellemare F, Grassino A. Force reserve of the diaphragm in patients with chronic obstructive pulmonary disease. *J Appl Physiol.* 1983;55:8–15.

111. Ottenheijm CAC, Heunks LMA, Dekhuijzen RPN. Diaphragm adaptations in patients with COPD. *Respir Res.* 2008;9(12):12.

112. Dodd DS, Yarom J, Loring SH, Engel LA. O$_2$ cost of inspiratory and expiratory resistive breathing in humans. *J Appl Physiol(1985).* 1988;65(6):2518–23.

113. Stubbing DG, Pengelly LD, Morse JL, Jones NL. Pulmonary mechanics during exercise in subjects with chronic airflow obstruction. *J Appl Physiol Respir Environ Exerc Physiol.* 1980;49:511–5.

114. Levison H, Cherniack M. Ventilatory cost of exercise in chronic obstructive pulmonary disease. *J Appl Physiol.* 1968;25(1):21–7.

115. Sharratt MT, Henke KG, Aaron EA, Pegelow DF, Dempsey JA. Exercise-induced changes in functional residual capacity. *Respir Physiol.* 1987;70:313–26.

116. Vogiatzis I, Aliverti A, Golemati S, et al. Respiratory kinematics by optoelectric plethysmography during exercise in men and women. *Eur J Appl Physiol.* 2005;93:581–7.

117. O'Donnell DE, Webb KA. Exertional breathlessness in patients with chronic airflow limitation. The role of lung hyperinflation. *Am Rev Respir Dis.* 1993;148:1351–7.

118. Stendardi L, Binazzi B, Scano G. Exercise dyspnea in patients with COPD. *Int J Chron Obstruct Pulmon Dis.* 2007;2(4):429–39.

119. Luecke T, Pelosi P. Clinical review: positive end-expiratory pressure and cardiac output. *Crit Care.* 2005;9:607–21.

120. Matthay RA, Berger HJ, Davies RA, et al. Right and left ventricular exercise performance in chronic obstructive pulmonary disease: radionucleotide assessment. *Ann Intern Med.* 1980;93:234–9.

121. Panagiotou M, Kastanakis E, Vogiatzis I. Exercise limitation in COPD. *Pneumon.* 2013;26(3):245–56.

122. Pinsky MR. Cardiovascular issues in respiratory care. *Chest.* 2005;128(5 Suppl 2):592S–7S.

123. Mahler DA, Brent BN, Loke J, Zaret BL, Matthay RA. Right ventricular performance and central hemodynamics during upright exercise in patients with chronic obstructive pulmonary disease. *Am Rev Respir Dis.* 1984;130:722–9.

124. Matthay RA, Arroliga AC, Weidemann HP, Schulman DS, Mahler DA. Right ventricular function at rest and during exercise in chronic obstructive pulmonary disease. *Chest.* 1992;101:255S–62S.

125. Slutsky R, Hooper W, Ackerman W, et al. Evaluation of left ventricular function in chronic pulmonary disease by exercise gated equilibrium radionucleotide angiography. *Am Heart J.* 1981;101:414–20.

126. Hilde JM, Skjørten I, Hansteen V, et al. Haemodynamic responses to exercise in patients with COPD. *Eur Respir J.* 2013;41:1031–41.

127. Holverda S, Bogaard HJ, Groepenhoff H, Postmus PE, Boonstra A, Vonk-Noordegraaf A. Cardiopulmonary exercise test characteristics in patients with chronic obstructive pulmonary disease and associated pulmonary hypertension. *Respiration.* 2008;76:160–7.

128. Aliverti A, Macklem PT. The major limitation to exercise performance in COPD is inadequate energy supply to the respiratory and locomotor muscles. *J Appl Physiol (1985).* 2008;105:749–51.

129. Borghi-Silva A, Oliveira CC, Carrascosa C, et al. Respiratory muscle unloading improves leg muscle oxygenation during exercise in patients with COPD. *Thorax.* 2008;63:910–5.

130. Vogiatzis I, Stratakos G, Simoes D, et al. Effects of rehabilitative exercise on peripheral muscle TNFalpha, IL-6, IGF-I and MyoD expression in patients with COPD. *Thorax.* 2007;62:950–6.

131. Elbehairy AF, Ciavaglia CE, Webb KA, et al. Pulmonary gas exchange abnormalities in mild chronic obstructive pulmonary disease. Implications for Dyspnea and Exercise Intolerance. *Am J Respir Crit Care Med.* 2015;191(12):1384–94.

132. O'Donnell DE, Neder JA, Elbehairy AF. Physiological impairment in mild COPD. *Respirology.* 2016;21:211–23.

133. Nishino T. Dyspnea: underlying mechanisms and treatment. *Br J Anaesth.* 2011;106(4):463–74.

134. Killian KJ, Leblanc P, Martin DH, Summers E, Jones NL, Campbell EJ. Exercise capacity and ventilatory, circulatory, and symptom limitation in patients with chronic airflow limitation. *Am Rev Respir Dis.* 1992;146:935–40.

135. Man WD, Soliman MG, Gearing J, et al. Symptoms and quadriceps fatiguability after walking and cycling in chronic obstructive pulmonary disease. *Am J Respir Crit Care Med.* 2003;168:562–7.

136. Castagana O, Boussuges A, Vallier JM, Prefaut C, Brisswalter J. Is impairment similar between arm and leg cranking exercise in COPD patients? *Respir Med.* 2007;101:547–53.

137. Gosselink R, Troosters T, Decramer M. Distribution of muscle weakness in patients with stable chronic obstructive pulmonary disease. *J Cardiopulm Rehabil.* 2000;20:353–60.

138. Gosselink R, Troosters T, Decramer M. Peripheral muscle weakness contributes to muscle weakness in COPD. *Am J Respir Crit Care Med.* 1996;153:976–80.

139. Hamilton AL, Killian KJ, Summers E, Jones NL. Muscle strength, symptom intensity, and exercise capacity in patients with cardio-respiratory disorders. *Am J Respir Crit Care Med.* 1995;152:2021–31.

140. Burtin C, Ter Riet G, Puhan MA, et al. Handgrip weakness and mortality risk in COPD: a multicentre analysis. *Thorax.* 2016;71(1):86–7.

141. Swallow EB, Reyes D, Hopkinson NS, et al. Quadriceps strength predicts mortality in patients with moderate to severe chronic obstructive pulmonary disease. *Thorax.* 2007;62(2):115–20.

142. Gea J, Pascual S, Casadevall C, Orozco-Levi M, Barreiro E. Muscle dysfunction in chronic obstructive pulmonary disease: update on causes and biological findings. *J Thorac Dis.* 2015;7(10):E418–38.

143. Bernard S, LeBlanc P, Whittom F, et al. Peripheral muscle weakness in patients with chronic obstructive pulmonary disease. *Am J Respir Crit Care Med.* 1998;158(2):629–34.

144. Clark CJ, Cochrane LM, Mackay E, Paton B. Skeletal muscle strength and endurance in patients with mild COPD and the effects of weight training. *Eur Respir J.* 2000;15:92–7.

145. Maltais F, Decramer M, Casaburi R, et al; ATS/ERS Ad Hoc Committee on Limb Muscle Dysfunction in COPD. An official American Thoracic Society/European Respiratory Society statement: update on limb muscle dysfunction in chronic obstructive pulmonary disease. *Am J Respir Crit Care Med.* 2014;189:e15–62.

146. Engelen MP, Schols AM, Does JD, Wouters EF. Skeletal muscle weakness is associated with wasting of extremity fat-free mass but not with airflow obstruction in patients with chronic obstructive pulmonary disease. *Am J Clin Nutr.* 2000;71:733–8.

147. Marquis K, Debigare R, Lacasse Y, et al. Midthigh cross-sectional area is a better predictor of mortality than body mass index in patients with chronic obstructive pulmonary disease. *Am J Respir Crit Care Med.* 2002;166(6):809–13.

148. Schols AM, Broekhuizen R, Weling-Scheepers CA, Wouters EF. Body composition and mortality in chronic obstructive pulmonary disease. *Am J Clin Nutr.* 2005;82(1):53–9.

149. Barreiro E, Gea J. Molecular and biological pathways of skeletal muscle dysfunction in chronic obstructive pulmonary disease. *Chron Respir Dis.* 2016;13(3):297–311.

150. Gosker HR, van Mameren H, van Dijk PJ, et al. Skeletal muscle fibre-type shifting and metabolic profile in patients with chronic obstructive pulmonary disease. *Eur Respir J.* 2002;19:617–25.

151. Jakobsson P, Jorfeldt L, Brundin A. Skeletal muscle metabolites and fibre types in patients with advanced chronic obstructive pulmonary disease (COPD), with and without chronic respiratory failure. *Eur Respir J.* 1990;3:192–6.

152. Whittom F, Jobin J, Simard PM, et al. Histochemical and morphological characteristics of the vastus lateralis muscle in patients with chronic obstructive pulmonary disease. *Med Sci Sports Exerc.* 1998;30(10):1467–74.

153. Decramer M, Lacquet LM, Fagard R, Rogiers P. Corticosteroids contribute to muscle weakness in chronic airflow obstruction. *Am J Respir Crit Care Med.* 1994;150:11–6.

154. Dekhuijzen PN, Decramer M. Steroid-induced myopathy and its significance to respiratory disease: a known disease rediscovered. *Eur Respir J.* 1992;5(8):997–1003.

155. Jobin J, Maltais F, Doyon JF, et al. Chronic obstructive pulmonary disease: capillarity and fiber-type characteristics of skeletal muscle. *J Cardiopulm Rehabil.* 1998;18(6):432–7.

156. Puente-Maestu L, Lazaro A, Humanes B. Metabolic derangements in COPD muscle dysfunction. *J Appl Physiol.* 2013;114(9):1282–90.

157. Maltais F, LeBlanc P, Whittom F, et al. Oxidative enzyme activities of the vastus lateralis muscle and the functional status in patients with COPD. *Thorax.* 2000;55:848–53.

158. Bloomfield SA. Changes in musculoskeletal structure and function with prolonged bed rest. *Med Sci Sports Exerc.* 1997;29:197–206.

159. Maltais F, LeBlanc P, Simard C, et al. Skeletal muscle adaptations to endurance training in patients with chronic obstructive pulmonary disease. *Am J Respir Crit Care Med.* 1996;154:442–7.

160. Sala E, Roca J, Marrades RM, et al. Effects of endurance training on skeletal muscle bioenergetics in chronic obstructive pulmonary disease. *Am J Respir Crit Care Med.* 1999;159:1726–34.

161. Ray A, Camiolo M, Fitzpatrick A, Gauthier M, Wenzel SE. Are we meeting the promise of endotypes and precision medicine in asthma? *Physiol Rev.* 2020;100(3):983–1017.

162. Pavord ID, Beasley R, Agusti A, et al. After asthma: redefining airways diseases. *Lancet.* 2018;391(10118):350–400.

163. Bush A. Pathophysiological mechanisms of asthma. *Front Pediatr.* 2019;7:68.

164. Kim S-R, Rhee YK. Overlap between asthma and COPD: where the two diseases converge. *Allergy Asthma Immunol Res.* 2010;2(4):209–14.

165. Papi A, Brightling C, Pedersen SE, Reddel HK. Asthma. *Lancet.* 2018;391(10122):783–800.

166. National Asthma Education and Prevention Program. *Third Expert Panel on the Diagnosis and Management of Asthma.* Bethesda (MD): National Heart, Lung and Blood Institute (US); 2007. Available from: https://www.epa.gov/sites/default/files/2014-09/documents/asthgdln.pdf.

167. Ishmael FT. The inflammatory response in the pathogenesis of asthma. *J Am Osteopath Assoc.* 2011;111(11 Suppl 7):S11–7.

168. Killeen K, Skora E. Pathophysiology, diagnosis and clinical assessment of asthma in the adult. *Nurs Clin North Am.* 2013;48:11–23.

169. Morton AR, Fitch KD. Australian association for exercise and sports science position statement on exercise and asthma. *J Sci Med Sport.* 2011;14:312–6.

170. Zielenski J. Genotype and phenotype in cystic fibrosis. *Respiration.* 2000;67:117–33.

171. Drumm ML, Konstan MW, Schluchter MD, et al. Genetic modifiers of lung disease in cystic fibrosis. *N Engl J Med.* 2005;353(14):1443–53.

172. Guyton AC, Hall JE. *Textbook of Medical Physiology.* 10th ed. Philadelphia (PA): W.B. Saunders Company; 2000.

173. Kreda SM, Davis CW, Rose MC. CFTR, mucins, and mucus obstruction in cystic fibrosis. *Cold Spring Harb Perspect Med.* 2012;2:a009589.

174. Rosenfeld M, Gibson RL, McNamara, et al. Early pulmonary infection, inflammation, and clinical outcomes in infants with cystic fibrosis. *Pediatr Pulmonol.* 2001;32(5):356–66.

175. Lee AJ, Huffmyer JL, Thiele EL, Zeitlin PL, Chatterjee D. The changing face of cystic fibrosis: an update for anesthesiologists. *Anesth Analg.* 2022;134(6):1245–59.

176. Stick SM, Brennan S, Murry C, et al; Australian Respiratory Early Surveillance Team for Cystic Fibrosis (AREST CF). Bronchiectasis in infants and preschool children diagnosed with cystic fibrosis after newborn screening. *J Pediatr.* 2009;155(5):623–8.e1.

177. De Boeck K, Wilschanski M, Castellani C, et al. Cystic fibrosis: terminology and diagnostic algorithms. *Thorax.* 2006;61:627–35.

178. Cystic Fibrosis Foundation. *Cystic Fibrosis Foundation Patient Registry, 2015. Annual Data Report.* Bethesda (MD): Cystic Fibrosis Foundation; 2016. Available from: https://www.cisztasfibrozis.hu/wpcontent/files/registry/int/CF%20Foundation%20-%20USA/2015-CFFPatient-Registry-Annual-Data-Report.pdf.

179. Aris RM, Merkel PA, Bachrach LK, et al. Guide to bone health and disease in cystic fibrosis. *J Clin Endocrinol Metab.* 2005;90(3):1888–96.

180. Putman MS, Anabtawi A, Le T, Tangpricha V, Sermet-Gaudelus I. Cystic fibrosis bone disease treatment: current knowledge and future directions. *J Cyst Fibros.* 2019;18(Suppl 2):S56–65.

181. Haworth CS. Impact of cystic fibrosis on bone health. *Curr Opin Pulm Med.* 2010;16(6):616–22.

182. Freeman W, Stableforth DE, Cayton RM, Morgan MDL. Endurance exercise capacity in adults with cystic fibrosis. *Respir Med.* 1993;87:541–9.

183. Godfrey S, Mearns M. Pulmonary function and response to exercise in cystic fibrosis. *Arch Dis Child.* 1971;46:144–50.

184. Pastré J, Prévotat A, Tardif C, Langlois C, Duhamel A, Wallaert B. Determinates of exercise capacity in cystic fibrosis patients with mild to moderate lung disease. *BMC Pulm Med.* 2014;14:74. Available from: http://www.biomedcentral.com/1471-2466/14/74.

185. Shei R-J, Mackintosh KA, Peabody Lever JE, McNarry MA, Krick S. Exercise physiology across the lifespan in cystic fibrosis. *Front Physiol.* 2019;10:1382.

186. Paolo MD, Teopompi E, Savi D, et al. Reduced exercise ventilatory efficiency in adults with cystic fibrosis and normal to moderately impaired lung function. *J Appl Physiol (1985).* 2019;127(2):501–12.

187. Dodd JD, Barry SC, Gallagher CG. Respiratory factors do not limit maximal symptom-limited exercise in patients with mild cystic fibrosis lung disease. *Respir Physiol Neurobiol.* 2006;152(2):176–85.

188. Stevens D, Oades PJ, Armstrong N, Williams CA. Early oxygen uptake recovery following exercise testing in children with chronic chest diseases. *Pediatr Pulmonol.* 2009;44(5):480–8.

189. Dodd JD, Barry SC, Barry RB, Gallagher CG, Skehan SJ, Masterson JB. Thin-section CT in patients with cystic fibrosis: correlation with peak exercise capacity and body mass index. *Radiology.* 2006;240(1):236–45.

190. Klijn PH, van der Net J, Kimpen JL, Helfers PJ, van der Ent CK. Longitudinal determinants of peak aerobic exercise performance in children with cystic fibrosis. *Chest.* 2003;124(6):2215–9.

191. Cropp GJ, Pullano TP, Cerny F, Nathanson IT. Exercise tolerance and cardiorespiratory adjustments at peak work capacity in cystic fibrosis. *Am Rev Respir Dis.* 1982;126:211–6.

192. Moorcroft AJ, Dodd ME, Webb AK. Exercise limitations and training for patients with cystic fibrosis. *Disabil Rehabil.* 1998;20(6–7):247–53.

193. Rand S, Prasad SA. Exercise as part of a cystic fibrosis therapeutic routine. *Expert Rev Respir Med.* 2012;6(3):341–51.

194. Werkman MS, Hulzebos HJ, Arets HGM, van der Net J, Helders PJM, Takken T. Is static hyperinflation a limiting factor during exercise in adolescents with cystic fibrosis? *Pediatr Pulmonol.* 2011;46:119–24.

195. Henke KG, Orenstein DM. Oxygen saturation during exercise in cystic fibrosis. *Am Rev Respir Dis.* 1984;129:708–11.

196. Javadpour SM, Selvadurai H, Wilkes DL, Schneiderman-Walker J, Coates AL. Does carbon dioxide retention during exercise predict a more rapid decline in FEV_1 in cystic fibrosis? *Arch Dis Child.* 2005;90(8):792–5.

197. Williams CA, Saynor ZL, Tomlinson OW, Barker AR. Cystic fibrosis and physiological responses to exercise. *Expert Rev Respir Med.* 2014;8(6):751–62.

198. Kusenbach G, Wieching R, Barker M, Hoffmann U, Essfeld D. Effects of hyperoxia on oxygen uptake kinetics in cystic fibrosis patients as determined by pseudo-random binary sequence exercise. *Eur J Appl Physiol Occup Physiol.* 1999;79(2):192–6.

199. Lamhonwah AM, Bear CE, Haun LJ, Kim Chiaw P, Tein I. Cystic fibrosis transmembrane conductance regulator in human muscle: dysfunction causes abnormal metabolic recovery in exercise. *Ann Neurol.* 2010;67(6):802–8.

200. Wells GD, Wilkes DL, Schneiderman JE, et al. Skeletal muscle metabolism in cystic fibrosis and primary ciliary dyskinesia. *Pediatr Res.* 2011;69(1):40–5.

201. de Jong W, van de Schans CP, Mannes GPM, van Alderen WM, Grevink RG, Köeter GH. Relationship between dyspnea, pulmonary function and exercise capacity in patients with cystic fibrosis. *Respir Med.* 1997;91:41–6.

202. Moorcroft AJ, Dodd ME, Morris J, Webb AK. Symptoms, lactate and exercise limitation at peak cycle ergometry in adults with cystic fibrosis. *Eur Respir J.* 2005;25(6):1050–6.

203. Lands LC, Heigenhauser JF, Jones NL. Analysis of factors limiting maximal exercise performance in cystic fibrosis. *Clin Sci.* 1992;83:391–7.

204. Favoriti A, Lanbiase C, Cimino G, et al. What's the role of stroke volume and cardiac output during exercise in cystic fibrosis? *Eur Respir J.* 2015;46:PA2062.

205. Pianosi P, Pelech J. Stroke volume during exercise in cystic fibrosis. *Am J Respir Crit Care Med.* 1996;153:1105–9.

206. Meyer KC, Raghu G, Verleden GM, et al; ISHLT/ATS/ERS BOS Task Force Committee; ISHLT/ATS/ERS BOS Task Force Committee. An international ISHLT/ATS/ERS clinical practice guideline: diagnosis and management of bronchiolitis obliterans syndrome. *Eur Respir J.* 2014;44(6):1479–503.

207. Verleden GM, Glanville AR, Lease ED, et al. Chronic lung allograft dysfunction: Definition, diagnostic criteria, and approaches to

treatment–a consensus report from the Pulmonary Council of the ISHLT. *J Heart Lung Transplant.* 2019;38(5):493–503.

208. Gauthier JM, Hachem RR, Kreisel D. Update on chronic lung allograft dysfunction. *Curr Transplant Rep.* 2016;3(3):185–91.

209. Thabut G, Mal H. Outcomes after lung transplantation. *J Thorac Dis.* 2017;9(8):2684–91.

210. Hume E, Ward L, Wilkinson M, Manifield J, Clark S, Vogiatzis I. Exercise training for lung transplant candidates and recipients: a systematic review. *Eur Respir Rev.* 2020;29(158):200053.

211. Braccioni F, Bottigliengo D, Ermolao A, et al. Dyspnea, effort and muscle pain during exercise in lung transplant recipients: an analysis of their association with cardiopulmonary function parameters using machine learning. *Respir Res.* 2020;21(1):267.

212. Wickerson L, Rozenberg D, Janaudis-Ferreira T, et al. Physical rehabilitation for lung transplant candidates and recipients: an evidence-informed clinical approach. *World J Transplant.* 2016;6(3):517–31.

213. Standards for the diagnosis and care of patients with chronic obstructive pulmonary disease. American Thoracic Society. *Am J Respir Crit Care Med.* 1995;152:S77–S121.

214. Graham BL, Steenbruggen I, Miller MR, et al. Standardization of spirometry 2019 update. An Official American Thoracic Society and European Respiratory Society Technical Statement. *Am J Respir Crit Care Med.* 2019;200(8):e70–88.

215. Cooper BG. An update on contraindications for lung function testing. *Thorax.* 2011;66:714–23.

216. Han MK, Muellerova H, Curran-Everett D, et al. GOLD 2011 disease severity classification in COPDGene: a prospective cohort study. *Lancet Respir Med.* 2013;1(1):43–50.

217. Jones PW. Health status and spiral of decline. *COPD.* 2009;6(1):59–63.

218. Global Initiative for Chronic Obstructive Lung Disease. Global strategy for the diagnosis, management, and prevention of chronic obstructive pulmonary disease (2023 report). 2022. Available from: https://goldcopd.org/2023-goldreport-2/

219. Celli BR, Cote C, Marin JM, et al. The body-mass index, airflow obstruction, dyspnea, and exercise capacity index in chronic obstructive pulmonary disease. *N Engl J Med.* 2004; 350:1005–12.

220. Cardoso F, Tufanin AT, Colucci M, Nascimento O, Jardim JR. Replacement of the 6 minute walk test with maximal oxygen consumption in the BODE index applied to patients with COPD: an equivalency study. *Chest.* 2007;132:477–82.

221. Cote C, Pinto Plata V, Marin JM, Nekach H, Dordelly LJ, Celli BR. The modified BODE index: validation with mortality in COPD. *Eur Respir J.* 2008;32:1269–74.

222. Faganello MM, Tanni SE, Sanchez FF, Pellegrino NR, Lucheta PA, Godoy I. BODE index and GOLD staging as predictors of 1-year exacerbation risk in chronic obstructive pulmonary disease. *Am J Med Sci.* 2010;339(1):10–4.

223. Larsson K, Kankaanranta H, Janson C, et al. Bringing asthma care into the twenty-first century. *NPJ Primary Care Respir Med.* 2020;30(1):25.

224. Papi A, Blasi F, Canonica GW, Morandi L, Richeldi L, Rossi A. Treatment strategies for asthma: reshaping the concept of asthma management. *Allergy Asthma Clin Immunol.* 2020;16(1):75.

225. Parsons JP, Hallstrand TS, Mastronarde JG, et al; American Thoracic Society Subcommittee on Exercise-induced Bronchoconstriction. An official American Thoracic Society clinical practice guideline: exercise-induced bronchoconstriction. *Am J Respir Crit Care Med.* 2013;187(9):1016–27.

226. Hull JH, Ansley L, Price OJ, Dickinson JW, Bonini M. Eucapnic voluntary hyperpnea: gold standard for diagnosing exercise-induced bronchoconstriction in athletes? *Sports Med.* 2016;46:1083–93.

227. Farrell PM, White TB, Ren CL, et al. Diagnosis of cystic fibrosis: consensus guidelines from the Cystic Fibrosis Foundation. *J Pediatr.* 2017;181S:S4–15.e1.

228. Pianosi P, LeBlanc J, Almudevar A. Relationship between FEV$_1$ and peak oxygen uptake in children with cystic fibrosis. *Pediatr Pulmonol.* 2005;40(4):324–9.

229. Spruit MA, Singh SJ, Garvey C, et al; ATS/ERS Task Force on Pulmonary Rehabilitation. An official American Thoracic Society/European Respiratory Society Statement: key concepts and advances in pulmonary rehabilitation. *Am J Respir Crit Care Med.* 2013;188(8):e13–64.

230. Troosters T, Blondeel A, Janssens W, Demeyer H. The past, present and future of pulmonary rehabilitation. *Respirology.* 2019;24(9):830–7.

231. Holland AE, Cox NS, Houchen-Wolloff L, et al. Defining modern pulmonary rehabilitation. An official American Thoracic Society workshop report. *Ann Am Thorac Soc.* 2021;18(5):e12–29.

232. Corhay J-L, Nguyen Dang D, Van Cauwenberge H, Louis R. Pulmonary rehabilitation and COPD: providing patients a good environment for optimizing therapy. *Int J Chron Obstruct Pulmon Dis.* 2014;9:27–39.

233. Burtin C, Decramer M, Gosselink R, Janssens W, Troosters T. Rehabilitation and acute exacerbations. *Eur Respir J.* 2011;38:702–12.

234. Berry MJ, Rejeski WJ, Adair NE, Zaccaro D. Exercise rehabilitation and chronic obstructive pulmonary disease stage. *Am J Respir Crit Care Med.* 1999;160:1248–53.

235. Beauchamp MK, Janaudis-Ferreira T, Goldstein RS, Brooks D.. Optimal duration of pulmonary rehabilitation for individuals with chronic obstructive pulmonary disease — a systematic review. *Chron Respir Dis.* 2011;8(2):129–40.

236. Rossi G, Florini F, Romagnoli M, et al. Length and clinical effectiveness of pulmonary rehabilitation in outpatients with chronic airway obstruction. *Chest.* 2005;127(1):105–9.

237. Salman GF, Mosier MC, Beasley BW, Calkins DR. Rehabilitation for patients with chronic obstructive pulmonary disease: meta analysis of randomized controlled trials. *J Gen Intern Med.* 2003;18(3):213–21.

238. Collins EG, Bauldoff G, Carlin B, et al; American Association of Cardiovascular and Pulmonary Rehabilitation. Clinical competency guidelines for pulmonary rehabilitation professionals. position statement of the American Association of Cardiovascular and Pulmonary Rehabilitation. *J Cardiopulm Rehabil Prev.* 2014;34:291–302.

239. Bernard S, Ribeiro F, Maltais F, Saey D. Prescribing exercise training in pulmonary rehabilitation: a clinical experience. *Rev Port Pneumol.* 2014;20(2):92–100.

240. Williams DM, Rubin BK. Clinical pharmacology of bronchodilator medications. *Respir Care.* 2018;63(6):641–54.

241. Melani AS. Long-acting muscarinic antagonists. *Expert Rev Clin Pharmacol.* 2015;8(4):479–501.

242. Rabe KF. Update on roflumilast, a phosphodiesterase 4 inhibitor for the treatment of chronic obstructive pulmonary disease. *Br J Pharmacol.* 2011;163(1):53–67.

243. Long term domiciliary oxygen therapy in chronic hypoxic cor pulmonale complicating chronic bronchitis and emphysema. Report of the Medical Research Council Working Party. *Lancet.* 1981;1:681–6.

244. Continuous or nocturnal oxygen therapy in hypoxemic chronic obstructive lung disease: a clinical trial. Nocturnal Oxygen Therapy Trial Group. *Ann Intern Med.* 1980;93:391–8.

245. Levine BE, Biglow DB, Hamstra RD, et al. The role of long-term continuous oxygen administration in patients with chronic airway obstruction with hypoxemia. *Ann Intern Med.* 1967;66:639–50.

246. Abraham AS, Cole RB, Bishop JM. Reversal of pulmonary hypertension by prolonged oxygen administration to patients with chronic bronchitis. *Circ Res.* 1968;23:147–57.

247. Heaton RK, Grant I, McSweeny AJ, Adams KM, Petty TL. Psychologic effects of continuous and nocturnal oxygen therapy in hypoxemic chronic obstructive pulmonary disease. *Arch Intern Med.* 1983;143:1941–7.

248. Bradely BL, Garner AE, Billiu D, Mestas JM, Forman J. Oxygen-assisted exercise in chronic obstructive lung disease. The effect on exercise capacity and arterial blood gas tensions. *Am Rev Respir Dis.* 1978;118:239–43.

249. Neunhäuserer D, Steidle-Kloc E, Weiss G, et al. Supplemental oxygen during high-intensity exercise training in nonhypoxemic chronic obstructive pulmonary disease. *Am J Med.* 2016;129(11):1185–93.

250. Pierce AK, Paez PN, Miller WF. Exercise training with the aid of a portable oxygen supply in patients with emphysema. *Am Rev Respir Dis.* 1965;91:653–9.

251. Wadell K, Henriksson-Larsen K, Lundgren R. Physical training with and without oxygen in patients with chronic obstructive pulmonary disease and exercise-induced hypoxemia. *J Rehabil Med.* 2001;33:200–5.

252. Albert RK, Au DH, Blackford AL, et al. A randomized trial of long-term oxygen for COPD with moderate desaturation. *N Engl J Med.* 2016;375(17):1617–27.

253. Del Giacco SR, Firinu D, Bjermer L, Carlsen K-H. Exercise and asthma: an overview. *Eur Clin Respir J.* 2015;2:27984.

254. Crapo RO, Casaburi R, Coates A, et al. Guidelines for methacholine and exercise challenge testing — 1999. This official statement of the American Thoracic Society was adopted by the ATS Board of Directors, July 1999. *Am J Respir Crit Care Med.* 2000;161(1):309–29.

255. Baff CW, Winnica DE, Holguin F. Asthma and obesity: mechanisms and clinical implications. *Asthma Res Pract.* 2015;1:1.

256. Smyth AR, Bell SC, Bojcin S, et al; European Cystic Fibrosis Society. European Cystic Fibrosis Society standards of care: best practice guidelines.. *J Cyst Fibros.* 2014;13(Suppl 1):S23–42.

257. MacKenzie T, Gifford AH, Sabadosa KA, et al. Longevity of patients with cystic fibrosis in 2000 to 2010 and beyond: survival analysis of the Cystic Fibrosis Foundation patient registry. *Ann Intern Med.* 2014;161(4):233–41.

258. Lopes-Pacheco M. CFTR modulators: the changing face of cystic fibrosis in the era of precision medicine. *Front Pharmacol.* 2020;10:1662.

259. Lester MK, Flume PA. Airway-clearance therapy guidelines and implementation. *Respir Care.* 2009;54(6):733–50.

260. Flume PA, O'Sullivan BP, Robinson KA, et al; Cystic Fibrosis Foundation, Pulmonary Therapies Committee. Cystic fibrosis pulmonary guidelines: chronic medications for maintenance of lung health. *Am J Respir Crit Care Med.* 2007;176:957–69.

261. Taccetti G, Francalanci M, Pizzamiglio G, et al. Cystic fibrosis: recent insights into inhaled antibiotic treatment and future perspectives. *Antibiotics (Basel).* 2021;10(3):338.

262. Mogayzel PJ, Naureckas ET, Robinson KA, et al; Pulmonary Clinical Practice Guidelines Committee. Cystic fibrosis pulmonary guidelines: chronic medications for maintenance of lung health. *Am J Respir Crit Care Med.* 2013;187(7):680–9.

263. LaPier TK. Glucocorticoid-induced muscle atrophy. The role of exercise in treatment and prevention. *J Cardiopulm Rehabil.* 1997;17:76–84.

264. Moghadam-Kia S, Werth VP. Prevention and treatment of systemic glucocorticoid side effects. *Int J Dermatol.* 2010;49(3):239–48.

265. Wier H, Kuhn RJ. Pancreatic enzyme supplementation. *Curr Opin Pediatr.* 2011;23(5):541–4.

266. Grammatikopoulou MG, Vassilakou T, Goulis DG, et al. Standards of nutritional care for patients with cystic fibrosis: a methodological primer and AGREE II analysis of guidelines. *Children (Basel).* 2021;8(12):1180.

267. Spoonhower KA, Davis PB. Epidemiology of cystic fibrosis. *Clin Chest Med.* 2016;37:1–8.

268. Ridley K, Condren M. Elexacaftor-Tezacaftor-Ivacaftor: the first triple-combination cystic fibrosis transmembrane conductance regulator modulating therapy. *J Pediatr Pharmacol Ther.* 2020;25(3):192–7.

269. Causer AJ, Shute JK, Cummings MH, et al. Elexacaftor-Tezacaftor-Ivacaftor improves exercise capacity in adolescents with cystic fibrosis. *Pediatr Pulmonol.* 2022;57(11):2652–8.

270. Ahmed M, Dayman N, Madge J, Gaillard E. P91 Cardiopulmonary exercise testing in CF adolescents after starting Tezacaftor/Ivacaftor. *Thorax.* 2021;76(Suppl 1):A136.1–A136.

271. Shtraichman O, Ahya VN. Malignancy after lung transplantation. *Ann Transl Med.* 2020;8(6):416.

272. Ojo AO, Held PJ, Port FK, et al. Chronic renal failure after transplantation of a nonrenal organ. *N Engl J Med.* 2003;349(10):931–40.

273. Lyu DM, Zamora MR. Medical complications of lung transplantation. *Proc Am Thorac Soc.* 2009;6(1):101–7.

274. McCarthy B, Casey D, Devane D, Murphy K, Murphy E, Lacasse Y. Pulmonary rehabilitation for chronic obstructive pulmonary disease. *Cochrane Database Syst Rev.* 2015;2015(2):CD003793.

275. Pritchard A, Burns P, Correia J, et al. ARTP statement on cardiopulmonary exercise testing 2021. *BMJ Open Respir Res.* 2021;8(1):e001121.

276. McArdle WD, Katch FI, Pechar GS. Comparison of continuous and discontinuous treadmill and bicycle tests for max VO$_2$. *Med Sci Sports.* 1973;5:156–60.

277. Hsia D, Casaburi R, Pradham A, Torres E, Porszasz J. Physiologic responses to linear treadmill and cycle ergometer exercise in COPD. *Eur Respir J.* 2009;34:605–15.

278. Turner SE, Eastwood PR, Cecins NM, Hillman DR, Jenkins SC. Physiologic responses to incremental and self-paced exercise in COPD: a comparison of three tests. *Chest.* 2004;126:766–73.

279. Datta D, Normandin E, ZuWallack R. Cardiopulmonary exercise testing in the assessment of exertional dyspnea. *Ann Thorac Med.* 2015;10(2):77–86.

280. Benzo RP, Parmesh S, Patel SA, Slivka WA, Sciurba F. Optimal protocol selection for cardiopulmonary testing in severe COPD. *Chest.* 2007;132(5):1500–5.

281. Heyward VH. *Advanced Fitness Assessment and Exercise Prescription.* 7th ed. Champaign (IL): Human Kinetics; 2014.

282. Cooper CB, Abrazzado M, Legg D, Kesten S. Development and implementation of treadmill exercise testing protocols in COPD. *Int J Chron Obstruct Pulmon Dis.* 2010;5:375–85.

283. Palange P, Ward SA, Carlsen K-H, et al. Recommendations on the use of exercise testing in clinical practice. *Eur Respir J.* 2007;29:185–209.

284. Nickerson BG, Sarkisian C, Tremper K. Bias and precision of pulse oximeters and arterial oximeters. *Chest.* 1988;93:515–7.

285. Stickland MK, Butcher SJ, Marciniuk DD, Bhutani M. Assessing exercise limitation using cardiopulmonary exercise testing. *Pulm Med.* 2012;2012:824091. doi:10.1155/2012/824091.

286. Myers J, Forman DE, Balady GJ, et al; American Heart Association Subcommittee on Exercise, Cardiac Rehabilitation, and Prevention of the Council on Clinical Cardiology, Council on Lifestyle and Cardiometabolic Health, Council on Epidemiology and Prevention, and Council on Cardiovascular and Stroke Nursing. Supervision of exercise testing by non-physicians: a scientific statement from the American Heart Association. *Circulation.* 2014;130:1014–27.

287. Riebe D, Ehrman JK, Liguori G, Magal M. *ACSM's Guidelines for Exercise Testing and Prescription.* 10th ed. Baltimore (MD): Lippincott Williams & Wilkins; 2018.

288. Holland AE, Spruit MA, Troosters T, et al. An official European Respiratory Society/American Thoracic Society technical standard: field walking tests in chronic respiratory disease. *Eur Respir J.* 2014;44:1428–46.

289. de Almeida FG, Victor EG, Rizzo JA. Hallway vs. treadmill 6 minute walk tests in patients with chronic obstructive pulmonary disease. *Respir Care.* 2009;54:1712–6.

290. Butland RJ, Pang J, Gross ER, Woodcock AA, Geddes DM. Two-, six-, and 12 minute walking tests in respiratory disease. *B Med J (Clin Res Ed).* 1982;284(6329):1607–8.

291. ATS Committee on Proficiency Standards for Clinical Pulmonary Function Laboratories. ATS statement: guidelines for the six minute walk test. *Am J Respir Crit Care Med.* 2002;166(1):111–7.

292. Pichurko BM. Exercising your patient: which test(s) and when? *Respir Care.* 2012;57(1):100–10.

293. Casanova C, Celli BR, Barria P, et al; Six Minute Walk Distance Project (ALAT). The 6-min walk distance in healthy subjects: reference standards from seven countries. *Eur Respir J.* 2011;37(1):150–6.

294. Ross RM, Murthy JN, Wollak ID, Jackson AS. The six minute walk test accurately estimates mean peak oxygen uptake. *BMC Pulm Med.* 2010;10:31.

295. Hill K, Jenkins SC, Cecins N, Phillippe DL, Hillman DR, Eastwood PR. Estimating maximum work rate during incremental cycle ergometry testing from six-minute walk distance in patients with chronic obstructive pulmonary disease. *Arch Phys Med Rehabil.* 2008;89(9):1782–7.

296. Borel B, Provencher S, Saey D, Maltais F. Responsiveness of various exercise-testing protocols to therapeutic interventions in COPD. *Pulm Med.* 2013;2013:410748. doi:10.1155/2013/410748.

297. Huang L-H, Chen Y-J. The 6-minute walk test to assess exercise capacity of patients with chronic obstructive pulmonary disease. *Eur Respir J.* 2016;48(Suppl 60):PA1385.

298. Benzo RP, Sciurba FC. Oxygen consumption, shuttle walking test and the evaluation of lung resection. *Respiration.* 2010;80(1):19–23.

299. Jurgensen SP, Antunes LCDO, Tanni SE, et al. The incremental shuttle walk test in older Brazilian adults. *Respiration.* 2011;81:223–8.

300. Probst VS, Hernandes NA, Teixeira DC, et al. Reference values for the incremental shuttle walking test. *Respir Med.* 2012;106:243–8.

301. Butcher SJ, Pikaluk BJ, Chura RL, Walkner MJ, Farthing JP, Marciniuk DD. Associations between isokinetic muscle strength, high-level functional performance, and physiological parameters in patients with chronic obstructive pulmonary disease. *Int J Chron Obstruct Pulmon Dis.* 2012;7:537–42.

302. Robles PG, Mathur S, Janaudis-Ferreira T, Dolmage TE, Goldstein RS, Brooks D. Measurement of peripheral muscle strength in individuals with chronic obstructive pulmonary disease: a systematic review. *J Cardiopulm Rehabil Prev.* 2011;31:11–24.

303. Strand BH, Cooper R, Bergland A, et al. The association of grip strength from midlife onwards with all-cause and cause-specific mortality over 17 years of follow up in the Tromosø Study. *J Epidemiol Community Health.* 2016;70:1214–21.

304. Fonseca J, Machado FVC, Santin LC, et al. Handgrip strength as a reflection of general muscle strength in chronic obstructive pulmonary disease. *COPD.* 2021;18(3):299–306.

305. Jeong M, Kang HK, Song P, et al. Hand grip strength in patients with chronic obstructive pulmonary disease. *Int J Chron Obstruct Pulmon Dis.* 2017;12:2385–90.

306. Martinez CH, Diaz AA, Meldrum CA, et al; COPDGene Investigators. Handgrip strength in chronic obstructive pulmonary disease. Associations with acute exacerbations and body composition. *Ann Am Thorac Soc.* 2017;14(11):1638–45.

307. Nyberg A, Saey D, Maltais F. Why and how limb muscle mass and function should be measured in patients with chronic obstructive pulmonary disease. *Ann Am Thorac Soc.* 2015;12(9):1269–77.

308. Brzycki M. Strength testing — predicting a one repetition max from reps-to-fatigue. *J Phys Ed Rec Dance.* 1993;64(1):88–90.

309. Kolber MJ, Cleland JA. Strength testing using hand-held dynamometry. *Phys Ther Rev.* 2005;10(2):99–112.

310. Andrews AW, Thomas MW, Bohannon RW. Normative values for isometric muscle force measurements obtained with hand-held dynamometers. *Phys Ther.* 1996;76(3):248–59.

311. Coronell C, Orozco-Levi M, Mendez R, Ramirez-Sarmiento A, Galditz JB, Gea J. Relevance of assessing quadriceps endurance in patients with COPD. *Eur Respir J.* 2004;24:129–36.

312. Holland AE, Spruit MA, Singh SJ. How to carry out a field walking test in chronic respiratory disease. *Breathe (Sheff).* 2015;11(2):128–39.

313. Rikli R, Jones CJ. *Senior Fitness Test Manual.* Champaign (IL): Human Kinetics; 2001.

314. Urquhart DS, Saynor ZL. Exercise testing in cystic fibrosis: who and why? *Paediatr Respir Rev.* 2018;27:28–32.

315. Hebestreit H, Arets HGM, Aurora P, et al; European Cystic Fibrosis Exercise Working Group. Statement on exercise testing in cystic fibrosis. *Respiration*. 2015;90:332–51.

316. Radtke T, Faro A, Wong J, Boehler A, Bendon C. Exercise testing in pediatric lung transplant candidates with cystic fibrosis. *Pediatr Transplant*. 2011;15:294–9.

317. Orenstein DM, Nixon PA, Ross EA, Kaplan RM. The quality of well-being in cystic fibrosis. *Chest*. 1989;95(2):344–7.

318. Werkman MS, Hulzebos EH, Helders PJ, Arets BG, Takken T. Estimating peak oxygen uptake in adolescents with cystic fibrosis. *Arch Dis Child*. 2014;99:21–5.

319. Washington RL, Bricker T, Alpert BS, et al. AHA Medical/Scientific Statement Special Report. Guidelines for exercise testing in the pediatric age group. From the Committee on Atherosclerosis and Hypertension in Children, Council on Cardiovascular Disease in the Young, the American Heart Association. *Circulation*. 1994;90(4):2166–79.

320. Darbee J, Watkins M. Isokinetic evaluation of muscle performance in individuals with cystic fibrosis. *Pediatr Pulmonol*. 1987;3(Suppl):140–1.

321. deMeer K, Jeneson JAL, Gulmans VAM, van der Laag J, Berger R. Efficiency of oxidative work performance of skeletal muscle in patients with cystic fibrosis. *Thorax*. 1995;50:980–3.

322. Bailey RC, Olson J, Pepper SL, Porszasz J, Barstow TJ, Cooper DM. The level and tempo of children's physical activities: an observational study. *Med Sci Sports Exerc*. 1995;27:1033–41.

323. Cabrera ME, Lough MD, Doershuk CF, De Rivera GA. Anaerobic performance — assessed by the Wingate Test — in patients with cystic fibrosis. *Pediatr Exerc Sci*. 1993;5:78–87.

324. Smith JC, Hill DW. Contribution of energy systems during a Wingate power test. *Br J Sports Med*. 1991;25(4):196–9.

325. Klijn PH, Terheggen-Lagro SW, van der Ent CK, van der Net J, Kimpen JL, Helders PJ. Anaerobic exercise in pediatric cystic fibrosis. *Pediatr Pulmonol*. 2003;36:223–9.

326. Bar-Or O. The Wingate Anaerobic Test: an update on methodology, reliability and validity. *Sports Med*. 1987;4:381–94.

327. Haff GG, Dumke C. *Laboratory Manual for Exercise Physiology*. Champaign (IL): Human Kinetics; 2012.

328. Boas SR, Joswiak ML, Nixon PA, Fulton JA, Orenstein DM. Factors limiting anaerobic performance in adolescent males with cystic fibrosis. *Med Sci Sports Exerc*. 1996;28(3):291–8.

329. Savin WM, Haskell WL, Schroeder JS, Stinson EB. Cardiorespiratory responses of cardiac transplant patients to graded, symptom-limited exercise. *Circulation*. 1980;62(1):55–60.

330. Ulvestad M, Durheim MT, Kongerud JS, Hansen BH, Lund MB, Edvardsen E. Cardiorespiratory fitness and physical activity following lung transplantation: a National Cohort Study. *Respiration*. 2020;99(4):316–24.

331. Williams TJ, McKenna MJ. Exercise limitation following transplantation. *Compr Physiol*. 2012;2(3):1937–79.

332. Guerrero K, Wuyam B, Mezin P, et al. Functional coupling of adenine nucleotide translocase and mitochondrial creatine kinase is enhanced after exercise training in lung transplant skeletal muscle. *Am J Physiol Regul Integr Comp Physiol*. 2005;289(4):R1144–54.

333. Systrom DM, Pappagianopoulos P, Fishman RS, Wain JC, Ginns LC. Determinants of abnormal maximum oxygen uptake after lung transplantation for chronic obstructive pulmonary disease. *J Heart Lung Transplant*. 1998;17(12):1220–30.

334. Garber CE, Blissmer B, Deschenes MR, et al; American College of Sports Medicine. American College of Sports Medicine position stand: quantity and quality of exercise for developing and maintaining cardiorespiratory, musculoskeletal, and neuromotor fitness in apparently healthy adults: guidance for prescribing exercise. *Med Sci Sports Exerc*. 2011;43:1334–59.

335. American College of Sports Medicine. *ACSM's Resource Manual for Guidelines for Exercise Testing and Exercise Prescription*. 7th ed. Baltimore (MD): Wolters Kluwer Lippincott Williams & Wilkins; 2014.

336. Donnelly JE, Blair SN, Jakicic JM, Manore MM, Rankin JW, Smith BK. Appropriate physical activity intervention strategies for weight loss and prevention of weight regain for adults. *Med Sci Sports Exerc*. 2009;41(2):459–71.

337. Moffatt RJ, Stamford BA, Neill RD. Placement of tri-weekly training sessions: Importance regarding enhancement of aerobic capacity. *Res Q Exerc Sport*. 1977;48:583–91.

338. Lui XL, Tan JY, Wang T, et al. Effectiveness of home-based pulmonary rehabilitation for patients with chronic obstructive pulmonary disease: a meta-analysis of randomized controlled trials. *Rehabil Nurs*. 2014;39(1):36–59.

339. Stafinski T, Nagase FI, Avdagovska M, Stickland MK, Menon D. Effectiveness of home-based pulmonary rehabilitation programs for patients with chronic obstructive pulmonary disease (COPD): systematic review. *BMC Health Serv Res*. 2022;22(1):557.

340. Brawner CA, Ehrman JK, Schairer JR, Cao JJ, Keteyian SJ. Predicting maximum heart rate among patients with coronary heart disease receiving beta-adrenergic blockade therapy. *Am Heart J*. 2004;148(5):910–4.

341. Hulo S, Inamo J, Dehon A, Le Rouzic O, Edme J-L, Neviere R. Chronotropic incompetence can limit exercise tolerance in COPD patients with lung hyperinflation. *Int J Chron Obstruct Pulmon Dis*. 2016;11:2553–61.

342. Chuang M-L, Lin I-F, Vintch JRE. Comparison of estimated and measured maximal oxygen uptake during exercise testing in patients with chronic obstructive pulmonary disease. *Intern Med J*. 2004;34:469–74.

343. Burgomaster KA, Hughes SC, Heigenhauser GJ, Bradwell SN, Gibala MJ. Six sessions of sprint interval training increases muscle oxidative potential and cycle endurance capacity in humans. *J Appl Physiol*. 2005;98:1985–90.

344. Gibala MJ, Little JP, MacDonald MJ, Hawley JA. Physiologic adaptations to low-volume, high intensity interval training in health and disease. *J Physiol*. 2012;590(5):1077–84.

345. Ross LM, Ryan R, Porter J, Durstine L. High-intensity interval training (HIIT) for patients with chronic diseases. *J Sport Health Sci*. 2016;5:139–44.

346. Wenger HA, Bell GJ. The interactions of intensity, frequency and duration of exercise training in altering cardiorespiratory fitness. *Sports Med*. 1986;3(5):346–56.

347. Warburton DER, McKenzie DC, Haykowsky MJ, et al. Effectiveness of high-intensity interval training for the rehabilitation of patients with coronary artery disease. *Am J Cardiol*. 2005;95:1080–4.

348. American Association of Cardiovascular and Pulmonary Rehabilitation. *American Association of Cardiovascular and Pulmonary Rehabilitation Guidelines for Pulmonary Rehabilitation Programs*. 4th ed. Champaign (IL): Human Kinetics; 2011.

349. Alison JA, McKeough ZJ, Leung RWM, et al. Oxygen compared to air during exercise training in COPD with exercise-induced desaturation. *Eur Respir J.* 2019;53(5):1802429.

350. Bolton CE, Bevan-Smith EF, Blakey JD, et al; British Thoracic Society Pulmonary Rehabilitation Guideline Development Group; British Thoracic Society Standards of Care Committee. British Thoracic Society guideline on pulmonary rehabilitation in adults. *Thorax.* 2013;68(Suppl 2):ii1–30.

351. Kortianou EA, Nasis IG, Spetsioti ST, Daskalakis AM, Vogiatzis I. Effectiveness of interval exercise training in patients with COPD. *Cardiopulm Phys Ther J.* 2010;21(3):12–9.

352. Killian KJ, Summers E, Jones NL, Campbell EJ. Dyspnea and leg effort during incremental cycle ergometry. *Am Rev Respir Dis.* 1992;145:1339–45.

353. Lahaije AJMC, van Helvoort HAC, Dekhuijzen PN, Heijdra YF. Physiologic limitations during daily life activities in COPD patients. *Respir Med.* 2010;104(8):1152–9.

354. Celli BR, Rassulo J, Make BJ. Dyssynchronous breathing during arm but not leg exercise in patients with chronic airflow obstruction. *N Engl J Med.* 1986;314:1485–90.

355. Tangri S, Woolf CR. The breathing pattern in chronic obstructive lung disease during the performance of some common daily activities. *Chest.* 1973;63:126–7.

356. Pelham TW, Holt LE, Moss MA. Exposure to carbon monoxide and nitrogen dioxide in enclosed ice arenas. *Occup Environ Med.* 2002;59:224–33.

357. Sabapathy S, Kingsley RA, Schneider DA, Adams L, Morris NR. Continuous and intermittent exercise responses in individuals with chronic obstructive pulmonary disease. *Thorax.* 2004;59:1026–31.

358. Vogiatzis I, Nanas S, Kastanakis E, Georgiadou O, Papazahou O, Roussos C. Dynamic hyperinflation and tolerance to interval exercise in patients with advanced COPD. *Eur Respir J.* 2004;24:385–90.

359. Beauchamp MK, Nonoyama M, Goldstein RS, et al. Interval versus continuous training in individuals with chronic obstructive pulmonary disease — a systematic review. *Thorax.* 2010;65:157–64.

360. Gloeckl R, Marinov B, Pitta F. Practical recommendations for exercise training in patients with COPD. *Eur Respir J.* 2013;22(128):178–86.

361. Varga J, Porszasz J, Boda K, Casaburi R, Somfay A. Supervised high intensity continuous and interval training vs. self-paced training in COPD. *Respir Med.* 2007;101:2297–304.

362. Storer TW. Exercise in chronic pulmonary disease: resistance exercise prescription. *Med Sci Sports Exerc.* 2001;33(7 Suppl):S680–92.

363. Probst VS, Troosters T, Pitta F, Decramer M, Gosselink R. Cardiopulmonary stress during exercise training in patients with COPD. *Eur Respir J.* 2006;27:1110–18.

364. Decramer M, Gosselink R, Troosters T, Verschueren M, Evers G. Muscle weakness is related to utilization of health care resources in COPD patients. *Eur Respir J.* 1997;10(2):417–23.

365. Charette SL, McEvoy L, Pyka G, et al. Muscle hypertrophy response to resistance training in older women. *J Appl Physiol.* 1991;70(5):1912–6.

366. Frontera WR, Meridith CN, O'Reilly KP, Knuttgen HG, Evans WJ. Strength conditioning in older men: skeletal muscle hypertrophy and improved function. *J Appl Physiol.* 1988;64:1038–44.

367. Ortega F, Toral J, Cejudo P, et al. Comparison of the effects of strength and endurance training in patients with chronic obstructive pulmonary disease. *Am J Respir Crit Care Med.* 2002;166:669–74.

368. Spruit MA, Gosselink R, Troosters T, De Paepe K, Decramer M. Resistance verses training in patients with COPD and peripheral muscle weakness. *Eur Respir J.* 2002;19:1072–8.

369. Bernard S, Whittom F, Leblanc P, et al. Aerobic and strength training in patients with chronic obstructive pulmonary disease. *Am J Respir Crit Care Med.* 1999;159:896–901.

370. Clark CJ, Cochrane LM, Mackay E. Low intensity peripheral muscle conditioning improves exercise intolerance and breathlessness in COPD. *Eur Respir J.* 1996;9:2590–6.

371. Kongsgaard M, Backer V, Jørgensen K, Kjaer M, Beyar N. Heavy resistance training increased muscle size, strength and physical function in elderly male COPD patients — a pilot study. *Respir Med.* 2004;98:1000–7.

372. Vonbank K, Strasser B, Mondrzyk J, et al. Strength training increases maximum working capacity in patients with COPD — randomized clinical trial comparing three training modalities. *Respir Med.* 2012;106:557–63.

373. O'Shea SD, Taylor NF, Paratz JD. Progressive resistance exercise improves muscle strength and may improve elements of performance of daily activities for people with COPD: a systematic review. *Chest.* 2009;136:1269–83.

374. Liao W-h, Chen J-W, Chen X, et al. Impact of resistance training in subjects with COPD: a systematic review and meta-analysis. *Respir Care.* 2015;60(8):1130–45.

375. Iepsen UW, Jørgensen K, Ringback T, Hansen H, Skrubbeltrang C, Lange P. A systematic review of resistance training verses endurance training in COPD. *J Cardiopulm Rehabil Prev.* 2015;33(3):163–72.

376. Nelson ME, Rejeski WJ, Blair SN, et al. Physical activity and public health in older adults: recommendations from the American College of Sports Medicine and the American Heart Association. *Med Sci Sports Exerc.* 2007;39(8):1435–45.

377. Figueiredo RIN, Azambuja AM, Cureau FV, Sbruzzi G. Inspiratory muscle training in COPD. *Respir Care.* 2020;65(8):1189–201.

378. Bird SP, Tarpenning KM, Marino FE. Designing resistance training programmes to enhance muscular fitness: a review of the acute programme variables. *Sports Med.* 2005;35(10):841–51.

379. Massery M. Musculoskeletal and neuromuscular interventions: a physical approach to cystic fibrosis. *J R Soc Med.* 2005;98(Suppl 45):55–66.

380. Tattersall R, Walshaw MJ. Posture and cystic fibrosis. *J R Soc Med.* 2003;96(Suppl 43):18–22.

381. Becker JM, Rogers J, Rossini G, Mirchandani H, D'Alonzo GE Jr. Asthma deaths during sports: report of a 7-year experience. *J Allergy Clin Immunol.* 2006;113(2):264–7.

382. Weisgerber M, Webber K, Meurer J, Danduran M, Berger S, Flores G. Moderate and vigorous exercise programs in children with asthma: safety, parental satisfaction, and asthma outcomes. *Pediatr Pulmonol.* 2008;43(12):1175–82.

383. Cypcar D, Lemanske DF. Asthma and exercise. *Clin Chest Med.* 1994;15:351–68.

384. McKenzie DC, McLuckie SL, Stirling DR. The protective effects of continuous and interval exercise in athletes with exercise-induced asthma. *Med Sci Sports Exerc.* 1994;26(8):951–6.

385. Thickett KM, McCoach JS, Gerber JM, Sadhra S, Burge PS. Occupational asthma caused by chloramines in indoor swimming-pool air. *Eur Respir J*. 2002;19(5):827–32.

386. Nystad W. The physical activity level in children with asthma based on a survey among 7–16 year old school children. *Scand J Med Sci Sports*. 1997;7:331–5.

387. Mancuso CA, Sayles W, Robbins R, et al. Barriers and facilitators the healthy physical activity in asthma patients. *J Asthma*. 2006;43:137–43.

388. Meyer R, Froner-Herwig B, Sporkel H. The effect of exercise and induced expectations on visceral perception in asthmatic patients. *J Psychosom Res*. 1990;34:454–60.

389. Heikkinen SAM, Quansah R, Jaakkola JJK, Jaakkola MS. Effects of regular exercise on adult asthma. *Eur J Epidemiol*. 2012;27:397–407.

390. Warren JB, Keynes RJ, Brown MJ, Jenner DA, McNicol MW. Blunted sympathoadrenal response to exercise in asthmatic subjects. *Br J Dis Chest*. 1982;76:147–50.

391. Hansen ESH, Pitzner-Fabricius A, Toennesen LL, et al. Effect of aerobic exercise training on asthma in adults: a systematic review and meta-analysis. *Eur Respir J*. 2020;56(1):2000146.

392. Garcia-Aymerich J, Varraso R, Anto JM, Camargo CA Jr. Prospective study of physical activity and risk of asthma exacerbations in older women. *Am J Respir Crit Care Med*. 2009;179:999–1003.

393. Emtner M, Herela M, Stalenheim G. High intensity physical training in adults with asthma. *Chest*. 1998;109:323–30.

394. Emtner M, Finne M, Stalenheim G. A 3-year follow-up of asthmatic patients participating in a 10-week rehabilitation program with emphasis on physical training. *Arch Phys Med Rehabil*. 1998;79:539–44.

395. Carson KV, Chandratilleke MG, Picot J, Brinn MP, Esterman AJ, Smith BJ. Physical training for asthma. *Cochrane Database Syst Rev*. 2013;30(9):CD00116.

396. Ram FS, Robinson SM, Black PN, Picol J. Physical training for asthma. *Cochrane Database Syst Rev*. 2005;(4):CD001116.

397. Pérez M, Groeneveld IF, Santana-Sosa E, et al. Aerobic fitness is associated with lower risk of hospitalization in children with cystic fibrosis. *Pediatr Pulmonol*. 2014;49(7):641–9.

398. Schneiderman JE, Wilkes DL, Atenafu EG, et al. Longitudinal relationship between physical activity and lung health in patients with cystic fibrosis. *Eur Respir J*. 2014;43:817–23.

399. Hebestreit H, Scmid K, Kieser S, et al. Quality of life is associated with physical activity and fitness in cystic fibrosis. *BMC Pulm Med*. 2014;14:26. Available from: http://Biomedcentral.com/1471-2466/14/26.

400. Selvaduria HC, Blimkie CJ, Cooper PJ, Mellis CM, Van Asperen PP. Gender differences in habitual activity in children with cystic fibrosis. *Arch Dis Child*. 2004;89:928–33.

401. Thobani A, Alverez JA, Blair S, et al. Higher mobility scores in patients with cystic fibrosis are associated with better lung function. *Pulm Med*. 2015;2015:423219. doi:10.1155/2015/423219.

402. Radtke T, Nevitt SJ, Hebestreit H, Kriemler S. Physical exercise training for cystic fibrosis. *Cochrane Database Syst Rev*. 2017;11(11):CD002768.

403. Swisher AK, Hebestreit H, Mejia-Downs A, et al. Exercise and habitual physical activity for people with cystic fibrosis:

404. Belcastro AN, Morrison KS, Hicks E, Matta H. Cardiorespiratory and metabolic responses associated with children's physical activity during self-paced games. *Can J Physiol Pharmacol*. 2012;90(9):1269–76.

405. Prickett K, Reading SA. The energy expenditure of guided active play games in a feild setting. *Appl Physiol Nutr Metab*. 2012;37:S30.

406. Reading SA, Prickett K. Evaluation of children playing a new-generation motion-sensitive active videogame by accelerometry and indirect calorimetry. *Games Health J*. 2013;2(3):166–73.

407. Williams CA, Stevens D. Physical activity and exercise training in young people with cystic fibrosis: current recommendations and evidence. *J Sport Health Sci*. 2013;2:39–46.

408. Lannefors L. Physical training: vital for survival and quality of life in cystic fibrosis. *Breathe*. 2012;8(4):309–13.

409. Shoemaker MJ, Hurt H, Arndt L. The evidence regarding exercise training in the management of cystic fibrosis: a systematic review. *Cardiopulm Phys Ther J*. 2008;19(3):75–83.

410. Kriemler S, Wilk B, Schurer W, Wilson WM, Bar-Or O. Preventing dehydration in children with cystic fibrosis who exercise in the heat. *Med Sci Sports Exerc*. 1999;31(6):774–9.

411. Williams CA, Benden C, Stevens D, Radtke T. Exercise training in children and adolescents with cystic fibrosis: theory and practice. *Int J Pediatr*. 2010;2010:670640.

412. Younk LM, Mikeladze M, Tate D, Davis SN. Exercise-related hypoglycemia in diabetes mellitus. *Expert Rev Endocrinol Metab*. 2011;6(1):93–108.

413. Festini F, Taccetti G, Galici V, et al. A 1-m distance is not safe for children with cystic fibrosis at risk for cross-infection with Pseudomonas aeruginosa. *Am J Infect Control*. 2010;38:244–5.

414. Quittner AL, Abbott J, Georgiopoulos AM, et al; International Committee on Mental Health; EPOS Trial Study Group. International Committee on Mental Health in Cystic Fibrosis: Cystic Fibrosis Foundation and European Cystic Fibrosis Society consensus statements for screening and treating depression and anxiety. *Thorax*. 2016;71:26–34.

415. Martinu T, Babyak MA, O'Connell CF, et al; INSPIRE Investigators. Baseline 6-min walk distance predicts survival in lung transplant candidates. *Am J Transplant*. 2008;8(7):1498–505.

416. Langer D. Rehabilitation in patients before and after lung transplantation. *Respiration*. 2015;89(5):353–62.

417. Walsh JR, Chambers DC, Davis RJ, et al. Impaired exercise capacity after lung transplantation is related to delayed recovery of muscle strength. *Clini Transplant*. 2013;27(4):E504–11.

418. Mejia-Downs A, DiPerna C, Shank C, Johnson R, Rice D, Hage C. Predictors of long-term exercise capacity in patients who have had lung transplantation. *Prog Transplant*. 2018;28(3):198–205.

419. Singer LG, Brazelton TR, Doyle RL, Morris RE, Theodore J; International Lung Transplant Database Study Group. Weight gain after lung transplantation. *J Heart Lung Transplant*. 2003;22(8):894–902.

expert consensus, evidence-based guide for advising patients. *Cardiopulm Phys Ther J*. 2015;26:85–98.

Clinical Exercise Testing

INTRODUCTION

Clinical exercise testing has been part of the diagnostic and exercise prescription paradigm for patients with known or suspected cardiopulmonary disease for at least 50 years (1), since the pioneering work of Drs. Bruno Balke, Robert Bruce, John Naughton, and other founders in preventive cardiology (2–4). This early work was the historic legacy of Dr. Arthur Master, who used electrocardiographic (ECG) responses following stepping exercise (5). It also incorporated the recognition of maximal oxygen consumption ($\dot{V}O_2max$) (6) and anaerobic threshold (7) as fundamental markers of exercise tolerance. Together, this research formed the scientific background for clinical exercise testing as it is known today. The purpose of this chapter is to briefly summarize the critical issues and practical steps required to successfully perform clinical exercise testing, primarily as a diagnostic tool for patients with cardiopulmonary disease.

USE OF CLINICAL EXERCISE TESTING

Exercise testing is a valuable noninvasive diagnostic test commonly used in clinical practice to evaluate and assess cardiorespiratory fitness (CRF), severity of coronary ischemia, and clinical decision-making. There are many ways an exercise test may be referred to in the literature, a graded exercise test (GXT), cardiac stress test, clinical exercise test, exercise tolerance test (ETT), or when using metabolic or ventilatory gas exchange analysis during exercise, termed a cardiopulmonary exercise test (CPX or CPET). A clinical exercise test can be used for diagnostic (identify abnormal responses), prognostic (identify the outcomes with a given pathology), or therapeutic (identify the impact of intervention) purposes (1). Evidence-based consensus statements regarding the use of clinical exercise testing are available from several sources (8–14).

General Guidelines for Performing a Clinical Exercise Test

Indications for clinical exercise testing are determined by the physician using an algorithmic approach, as recommended by the American College of Cardiology (ACC) and the American Heart Association (AHA) (11). Exercise stress testing is beneficial in assessing ischemia, arrhythmia, conduction abnormality, and chronotropic incompetence. This test is most often used for older adults to evaluate symptoms related to exertion. Specifically, a clinical exercise test can be used for:

- Evaluating the cause of symptoms in patients who present to the physician with complaints (angina pectoris, dyspnea, leg pain) suggestive of cardiopulmonary diseases
- Identifying coronary artery disease (CAD) before it presents clinically in individuals who are at elevated risk (see Figure 3.1). In a substantial percentage of patients (more than 30% in males, more than 10% in females), the first presentation of cardiovascular disease (CVD) may be fatal
- Risk stratification of patients with postmyocardial infarction, designed to help physicians determine the nature of follow-up therapy and intervention
- Risk stratification in patients considered for coronary revascularization
- Risk stratification before noncardiac surgery in patients with known/suspected CAD or those at high risk for CAD
- Evaluating patients for advanced cardiac intervention candidacy
- Evaluating effectiveness of therapeutic interventions
- Developing an exercise prescription

■ Evaluating individuals prior to returning to work for those whose jobs require physically demanding labor

Exercise stress testing is part of medical diagnostics and is intimately linked to the history and physical examination performed by the physician or other qualified health care provider. Historically, physicians have conducted exercise testing with the help of nonphysician allied health professionals. Over the past several decades, transition to nonphysician staff conducting tests has occurred such as clinical exercise physiologists (CEPs), nurses, physical therapists, and physician assistants. According to the ACC and AHA, nonphysician staff such as the CEPs should have the appropriate training and practical skills to conduct the exercise test (15). Standing protocols still require physician oversight to provide for emergencies and test interpretation. Physicians may be available for direct supervision (*i.e.*, patients at high risk), on premises for immediate assistance, or available by phone (healthy, asymptomatic low risk). Appropriately trained nonphysician staff can safely administer maximal clinical exercise tests as outlined by the AHA (16).

If the patient is ambulatory, able to exercise, and has a normal resting ECG, a basic clinical exercise test may be indicated as a safe, cost-effective, and reliable first option for diagnosis, prognosis, or evaluation. The sensitivity or specificity of ECG exercise testing to identify CAD varies. Pooled results suggest a sensitivity (likelihood of a person with disease to have an abnormal result) of 68% and a specificity (likelihood of a person without disease to have a normal result) of 77%. When workup bias is eliminated (*e.g.*, only testing individuals with a high likelihood of having disease), the sensitivity is slightly lower, and the specificity is somewhat higher. Ischemic heart disease (IHD) is the most common indication for testing. The probability of detecting disease with a clinical exercise test depends on age, gender, severity of symptoms, and the cohort of patients undergoing the test (1). The ACC and the AHA have developed a logistic approach for evaluating someone presenting with stable chest pain (11). The clinical exercise test provides valuable cardiorespiratory data predictive of health and disease as highlighted by professional agencies as well as findings from the Fitness Registry and the Importance of Exercise National Database (FRIEND) (12, 13, 17).

Contraindications

Prior to administering clinical exercise tests, it is important for overall patient safety to avoid unstable ischemic, rhythm, or hemodynamic conditions that may increase

Box 9.1 Absolute and Relative Contraindications to Exercise Testing

Absolute

- A recent significant change in the resting electrocardiogram [ECG] suggesting significant ischemia, recent myocardial infarction (within 2 d), or other acute cardiac event
- Unstable angina
- Uncontrolled cardiac dysrhythmias causing symptoms or hemodynamic compromise
- Symptomatic severe aortic stenosis
- Uncontrolled symptomatic heart failure
- Acute pulmonary embolus or pulmonary infarction
- Acute myocarditis or pericarditis
- Suspected or known dissecting aneurysm
- Acute systemic infection, accompanied by fever, body aches, or swollen lymph glands

Relative

- Left main coronary stenosis
- Moderate stenotic valvular heart disease

- Electrolyte abnormalities (*e.g.*, hypokalemia or hypomagnesemia)
- Severe arterial hypertension (*i.e.*, systolic blood pressure of >200 mm Hg and/or a DBP of >110 mm Hg) at rest
- Tachyarrhythmia or bradyarrhythmia
- Hypertrophic cardiomyopathy and other forms of outflow tract obstruction
- Neuromotor, musculoskeletal, or rheumatoid disorders that are exacerbated by exercise
- High-degree atrioventricular block
- Ventricular aneurysm
- Uncontrolled metabolic disease (*e.g.*, diabetes, thyrotoxicosis, or myxedema)
- Chronic infectious disease (*e.g.*, human immunodeficiency virus [HIV])
- Mental or physical impairment leading to inability to exercise adequately

the risk associated with testing. Box 9.1 outlines the absolute and relative contraindications to exercise stress testing. Except in extraordinary cases, which must be actively decided by both the referring and the supervising physician on a case-by-case basis, the patient should not perform the exercise test if an absolute contraindication is present. However, for patients with relative contraindications to exercise, stress testing should be considered if the benefits gained, in terms of better physician management of the patient, outweigh the risks. Given the low absolute risk of exercise stress testing, about 1.5/10,000 tests for fatal or life-threatening events (15), and the observation that a substantial percentage of abnormal findings are made only near peak exercise capacity (18, 19), the risk to benefit ratio often favors performing the exercise test. However, the reduced risk of clinical exercise testing compared to reports from a generation ago reflects growth in recognition of the value of identifying and respecting contraindications to exercise testing (10). The utility of evaluating CRF has proved to be very useful in the detection and quantification of cardiovascular abnormalities as exercise tolerance has become an important outcome measure in patients with chronic obstructive pulmonary disease (COPD), chronic heart failure (CHF), and other chronic diseases (13).

EXERCISE MODALITIES AND PROTOCOLS

The clinical exercise test commonly assesses functional capacity using treadmill walk time and ECG response measuring hemodynamics and ischemic response to evaluate exercise tolerance. Two popular modalities for clinical exercise tests are the treadmill and the cycle ergometer as the means to stress physiological response while using ECG acquisition to evaluate oxygen perfusion with cardiac demand. Depending on referral and rationale for clinical exercise testing by the physician, the objective of the test can vary. Testing protocols may be designed to reach maximal workloads, submaximal thresholds, or symptom-limited tolerance. It is paramount for CEP to monitor physiological response throughout the test assessing for exercise intolerance or abnormal response.

Treadmill

Treadmills are thought to be especially useful as walking is a more common and familiar mode of exercise than cycling. Because of this, most exercise stress tests in the

U.S. are performed using a treadmill. Walking or running uses a larger muscle mass compared to cycling and typically elicits about a 9% greater max metabolic equivalent (MET) level (18). Additionally, treadmill tests usually result in a higher maximal heart rate (HR) and rate pressure product (RPP; discussed shortly) than cycling (20, 21).

It can be more difficult using a treadmill to obtain accurate blood pressure (BP) and ECG readings because of body motion during walking compared to cycling. Assessing manual BP during exercise, the arm must be released from the handrail and relaxed. The CEP should support the patient's arm in a fully extended elbow position to enhance access of the brachial artery for auscultation of Korotkoff sounds. Additionally, adequate skin prep for electrode placement and stabilization of ECG wires are especially helpful to minimize motion artifact. Moreover, although walking is a normal form of exercise to most people, a substantial percentage of patients are initially uncomfortable on the treadmill and, therefore, reach for handrail support. Gripping the handrail can cause a substantial and highly unpredictable overestimation of exercise capacity (22, 23). Because exercise capacity is strongly linked with prognosis in all classes of patients, ranging from healthy individuals to patients with CHF (12, 24–26; see Figure 9.1), allowing handrail support results in an overestimate of exercise capacity, and thus to an erroneously favorable prognosis, and to "undertreating" the patient. Even exercise capacity prediction equations that

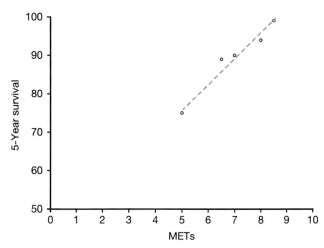

FIGURE 9.1 Anticipated 5-year survival in middle-aged individuals in relation to exercise capacity, regardless of the presence or absence of known cardiovascular disease. When the exercise capacity is more than 9 metabolic equivalents (METs), the 5-year survival approximates 100%. (Data from Myers J, Prakash M, Froelicher V, Do D, Partington S, Atwood JE. Exercise capacity and mortality among men referred for exercise testing. *N Engl J Med.* 2002;346(11):793–801.)

specifically account for the presence of handrail support (20, 21, 23, 27) have larger prediction errors than seen in equations based on nonhandrail-supported exercise performance.

The Bruce treadmill protocol is the most widely used protocol in the U.S. (15) likely because of physician familiarity. Dr. Bruce's original criteria for conducting an exercise test includes beginning at a distinctly submaximal level, progress in stages long enough to allow physiologic accommodation to the stage, and have increments between stages that are reasonable relative to the patient's exercise capacity. However, now that exercise tests are often performed in older and more debilitated individuals, the original Bruce treadmill protocol often does not meet Dr. Bruce's own criteria, particularly with reference to the initial workload and the magnitude of increments between stages. Aerobic requirements associated with the first stage of the Bruce protocol (~5 METs) combined

with large increases between stages (~3 METs) make the protocol less than optimal for patients with cardiovascular or pulmonary disease who may have low functional capacity. The CEP should consider the individual's medical and physical activity history and symptomology with protocol selection.

Testing protocols are dependent on the rationale for the exercise test, and with the wide variety of protocols available, appropriateness is based on pathophysiology suitability of each individual patient. Typically, an incremental protocol using progressive increase in work rate or continuous ramp workloads are used to evaluate symptom-limited response or volitional fatigue. A variety of tables have been created to enable clinicians to estimate exercise capacity when not performing metabolic testing during a GXT (see Tables 9.1–9.4). These tables are based either on observations of the specific protocol duration or maximal measured MET response in a wide variety of

Table 9.1	Bruce Treadmill Protocol				
Stage	Time (min)	Speed (mph)	Grade (%)	METs No HRS	METs With HRS
1	1	1.7	10	3.2	3.0
	2			3.9	3.7
	3			4.6	4.4
2	4	2.5	12	5.2	5.0
	5			5.9	5.7
	6			6.6	6.4
3	7	3.4	14	7.2	7.0
	8			7.9	7.7
	9			8.6	8.3
4	10	4.2	16	9.7	9.0
	11			10.9	9.6
	12			12.1	10.3
5	13	5.0	18	13.3	10.9
	14			14.6	11.6
	15			15.7	12.2
6	16	5.5	20	16.9	12.9
	17			17.9	13.5
	18			18.9	14.2

HRS, handrail support; METs, metabolic equivalents.

Table 9.2	Modified Bruce Protocol				
Stage	Time (min)	Speed (mph)	Grade (%)	METs No HRS	METs With HRS
1	1	1.4	0	1.8	1.6
2	2	1.7	5	3.0	2.9
3	3	1.7	10	4.6	4.4
4	4	2.0	11	5.2	5.0
5	5	2.4	11	6.0	5.6
6	6	2.5	12	6.6	6.4
7	7	2.8	13	7.3	6.9
8	8	3.2	14	8.2	7.5
9	9	3.4	14	8.6	8.3
10	10	3.6	15	9.7	9.0
11	11	3.8	16	11.0	9.6
12	12	4.2	16	12.1	10.3
13	13	4.2	17	13.3	11.0
14	14	4.6	18	14.5	11.6
15	15	5.0	18	15.7	12.2
16	16	5.0	19	16.8	12.9
17	17	5.3	20	17.9	13.6
18	18	5.5	20	18.9	14.2

HRS, handrail support; METs, metabolic equivalents.

Table 9.3	Modified Balke Protocol				
Stage	Time (min)	Speed (mph)	Grade (%)	METs No HRS	METs With HRS
1	2	2.0/2.5/3.0/3.5	0	2.2/2.5/2.8/3.2	2.1/2.4/2.7/3.0
2	4	2.0/2.5/3.0/3.5	2.5	2.8/3.3/3.7/4.2	2.7/3.2/3.6/4.1
3	6	2.0/2.5/3.0/3.5	5	3.4/4.0/4.6/5.3	3.3/3.9/4.5/5.1
4	8	2.0/2.5/3.0/3.5	7.5	4.0/4.8/5.5/5.3	3.9/4.6/5.3/6.1
5	10	2.0/2.5/3.0/3.5	10.0	4.6/5.5/6.4/7.4	4.4/5.3/6.2/7.1
6	12	2.0/2.5/3.0/3.5	12.5	5.2/6.3/7.3/8.4	5.0/5.0/6.8/7.7
7	14	2.0/2.5/3.0/3.5	15.0	5.8/7.0/8.2/9.5	5.6/6.6/7.5/8.5
8	16	2.0/2.5/3.0/3.5	17.5	6.4/7.8/8.1/10.5	6.1/7.2/8.3/9.4
9	18	2.0/2.5/3.0/3.5	20.0	7.0/8.5/10.0/11.6	6.5/7.9/9.0/10.2
10	20	2.0/2.5/3.0/3.5	22.5	7.6/9.3/10.9/12.6	7.0/8.4/9.7/11.0
11	22	2.0/2.5/3.0/3.5	25.0	8.2/10.0/11.8/13.7	7.5/9.0/10.4/11.9
12	24	2.0/2.5/3.0/3.5	27.5	8.8/10.7/12.7/14.7	8.0/9.6/11.1/12.8
13	26	2.0/2.5/3.0/3.5	30.0	9.4/11.4/13.6/15.7	8.5/10.2/11.8/13.7

During the first stage, the fastest walking speed that is comfortable for the patient should be established, usually the fastest that doesn't require handrail support. Thereafter, workload increases should be accomplished by elevations of the grade. If the test is terminated when a stage has not been completed, the METs are calculated by interpolation based on the proportional time completed in the last stage.

HRS, handrail support; METs, metabolic equivalents.

Table 9.4	Modified Naughton Treadmill Protocol				
Stage	Time (min)	Speed (mph)	Grade (%)	METs No HRS	METs With HRS
1	2	2.0	0	1.9	1.7
2	4	2.0	3.5	2.9	2.8
3	6	2.0	7.0	3.8	3.6
4	8	2.0	10.5	4.7	4.5
5	10	2.0	14.0	5.6	5.3
6	12	2.0	17.5	6.5	6.1
7	14	3.0	12.5	7.4	6.9
8	16	3.0	15.0	8.4	7.7
9	18	3.0	17.5	9.3	8.4
10	20	3.0	20.2	10.2	9.2
11	22	3.0	22.5	11.1	9.9
12	24	3.4	20.0	12.1	10.7
13	26	3.4	22.0	13.0	11.4
14	28	3.4	24.0	13.9	12.2
15	30	3.4	26.0	14.8	13.0

HRS, handrail support; METs, metabolic equivalents.

people (10, 12, 21, 27, 28). The Bruce and Balke treadmill protocols are commonly used with the aim to reach volitional fatigue. Figure 9.2 displays variation in workload across different protocols; note, the modified Bruce protocol is designed to avoid large changes in workload that occur during the widely used Bruce protocol.

The option to conduct an independent treadmill protocol (Table 9.5) provides flexibility for the CEP to custom design the exercise protocol to fit individual needs of the patient. The independent protocol aims to conclude the test in 8–12 minutes with the CEP adjusting workloads each minute in speed or incline based on patients' comfort. This patient-friendly format should be considered when the CEP predicts the initial workload may be too high or the increments between stages are too large to conduct an orderly test. During the last minute of the test, the maximal speed grade achieved during protocol-independent treadmill exercise test is used to estimate functional exercise capacity (20).

The selected test should require little skill on the part of the patient. Given that some patients have difficulty with treadmill walking, it may be advisable to allow a brief (1–2 min) period of habituation to help the patient ambulate comfortably with or without minimal handrail support. This habituation period should include ambulation at a very slow speed, with progressive reductions in the amount of handrail support, and with the chosen protocol beginning only when the patient is able to ambulate comfortably without handrail support. The additional time required to perform this habituation will increase the likelihood of conducting a high-quality test.

The testing modality should use large muscle groups, unless the patient has orthopedic or peripheral limitations, in which case arm ergometry is indicated. As a general principle, the greater the total muscle mass used, the more likely the test will reveal pathologic conditions if present.

FIGURE 9.2 Common treadmill and stationary cycle ergometry protocols used in symptom-limited maximal exercise testing with exercise workload and metabolic demand. METs reflect the estimated value for each stage. CHF, chronic heart failure; kg, kilogram; KPM, kilopond meter; METs, metabolic equivalents of task; MPH, miles per hour; %GR, percent grade. *Source:* From Liguori G. *ACSM's Guidelines for Exercise Testing and Prescription.* 11th ed. Philadelphia (PA): Wolters Kluwer; 2021. (Adapted from Fletcher GF, Ades PA, Kligfield P, et al. Exercise standards for testing and training: a scientific statement from the American Heart Association. *Circulation.* 2013;128(8):873–934.)

The following table reproduces the data shown in Figure 9.2.

METS	CYCLE ERGOMETER (for 70 kg body weight)	RAMP (per 30 sec) MPH / %GR	MOD. BRUCE 3 min MPH	MOD. BRUCE 3 min %GR	BRUCE 3 min MPH	BRUCE 3 min %GR	NAUGHTON 2 min MPH	NAUGHTON 2 min %GR	MOD. NAUGHTON (CHF) 2 min MPH	MOD. NAUGHTON (CHF) 2 min %GR
21	FOR 70 KG BODY WEIGHT									
20			6.0	22	6.0	22				
19	1 WATT = 6.1 Kpm/min									
18			5.5	20	5.5	20				
17										
16	Kpm/min									
15			5.0	18	5.0	18				
14	1,500								3.0	25
13		3.0 / 25.0; 3.0 / 24.0	4.2	16	4.2	16			3.0	22.5
12	1,350	3.0 / 23.0; 3.0 / 22.0							3.0	20
11	1,200	3.0 / 21.0; 3.0 / 20.0							3.0	17.5
10	1,050	3.0 / 19.0; 3.0 / 18.0; 3.0 / 17.0	3.4	14	3.4	14			3.0	15
9	900	3.0 / 16.0; 3.0 / 15.0					2	17.5	3.0	12.5
8		3.0 / 14.0; 3.0 / 13.0					2	14.0		
7	750	3.0 / 12.0; 3.0 / 11.0; 3.0 / 10.0	2.5	12	2.5	12			3.0	10
6	600	3.0 / 9.0; 3.0 / 8.0; 3.0 / 7.0					2	10.5	3.0	7.5
5	450	3.0 / 6.0; 3.0 / 5.0	1.7	10	1.7	10	2	7.0	2.0	10.5
4	300	3.0 / 4.0; 3.0 / 3.0; 3.0 / 2.0					2	3.5	2.0	7.0
3	150	3.0 / 1.0; 3.0 / 0; 2.5 / 0	1.7	5			2	0	2.0	3.5
2		2.0 / 0; 1.5 / 0	1.7	0			1	0	1.5	0
1		1.0 / 0; 0.5 / 0							1.0	0

Cycle Ergometer

Cycle ergometry provides another modality for patients who have ambulatory, orthopedic, or peripheral vascular limitations. In general, they are less expensive than treadmills, more portable, and permit easier BP and ECG readings. Additionally, cycle ergometers may be less intimidating than treadmills for people with balance instabilities.

However, patients not familiar with cycling may experience localized leg fatigue before the cardiovascular system is maximally challenged. Electrically braked cycle ergometers, which automatically accommodate changes in pedaling rate to allow exercise at a predetermined power output, are easier to use than mechanically braked ergometers. In clinical practice, many patients have difficulty maintaining a desired pedaling rate, which means control of power output is less than optimal.

Cycle ergometer exercise elicits approximately 9% lower maximal MET values than treadmill tests, a difference attributable to both a reduced muscle mass used and local muscle fatigue during cycling (29). The HR response is usually lower on the cycle, but the systolic blood pressure (SBP) is typically higher. The diagnostic accuracy of ECG stress testing may be slightly better on the treadmill, but not so much as to dictate one manner of testing over another (30–32).

Table 9.5	Protocol-Independent Treadmill Protocol				
Speed (mph)% Grade	2.0	2.5	3.0	3.5	4.0
0	2.2/2.0	2.5/2.3	2.8/2.6	3.2/3.0	3.5/3.2
1	2.4/2.2	2.8/2.6	3.2/3.0	3.6/3.4	4.0/3.8
2	2.7/2.5	3.1/2.9	3.6/3.3	4.0/3.7	4.5/4.2
3	2.9/2.7	3.4/3.1	3.9/3.7	4.4/4.2	4.9/4.7
4	3.1/2.9	3.7/3.5	4.3/4.1	4.9/4.7	5.4/5.2
5	3.4/3.2	4.0/3.8	4.6/4.4	5.3/5.1	5.9/5.7
6	3.6/3.4	4.3/4.1	5.0/4.8	5.7/5.5	6.4/6.1
7	3.9/3.7	4.6/4.3	5.4/5.2	6.1/5.9	6.9/6.5
8	4.1/3.9	4.9/4.7	5.7/5.5	6.5/6.2	7.3/6.8
9	4.3/4.1	5.2/5.0	5.1/5.8	7.0/6.5	7.8/7.2
10	4.6/4.2	5.5/5.3	6.4/6.1	7.4/6.9	8.3/7.6
11	4.8/4.5	5.8/5.6	6.8/6.4	7.8/7.2	8.8/8.0
12	5.1/4.9	6.1/5.8	7.2/6.7	8.2/7.5	9.3/8.4
13	5.3/5.1	6.4/6.1	7.5/7.0	8.6/7.9	9.7/8.8
14	5.5/5.3	6.7/6.3	7.9/7.3	9.0/8.2	10.2/9.1
15	5.8/5.6	7.0/6.6	8.2/7.5	9.5/8.5	10.7/9.5
16	6.0/5.8	7.3/6.8	8.6/7.8	9.9/8.9	11.2/9.9
17	6.3/6.0	7.6/7.0	9.0/8.1	10.3/9.2	11.7/10.3
18	6.5/6.2	7.9/7.3	9.3/8.4	10.7/9.5	12.1/10.7
19	6.7/6.3	8.2/7.5	9.7/8.7	11.1/9.9	12.6/11.0
20	7.0/6.5	8.5/7.8	10.0/9.0	11.6/10.2	13.1/11.4
21	7.2/6.7	8.8/8.0	10.4/9.3	12.0/10.5	13.6/11.8
22	7.5/6.9	9.1/8.2	10.8/9.6	12.4/10.9	14.1/12.2

Begin with the patient walking slowly on the treadmill at 0% grade. Every minute, ask the patient if they want to go faster or steeper, and adjust the treadmill accordingly. Metabolic equivalents (METs) are calculated based on no/with handrail support. Use the highest speed and grade completed (no credit for partial stages).

Historically, cycle protocols are common in exercise labs that evaluate pediatric patients and adults with congenital heart disorders (Table 9.6). Cycle protocols are easier for children to perform, which commonly include metabolic testing. Multistage incremental protocols permit feasibility of obtaining estimation or measurement of functional capacity and conducted within the duration of 8- to 12-minutes test. Cycle ergometer protocols are either staged (*e.g.*, James, McMaster, Godfrey) or continuous ramping (progressive incremental). Ramp-type cycle protocols permit the CEP to choose the appropriate incremental workload tailored for each patient's fitness ability (10, 33).

Arm Ergometry

If the patient cannot perform lower body exercises, arm ergometry may be an appropriate exercise testing

Table 9.6		Cycle Ergometer Pediatric Protocols			
Protocol	Rate (rpm)	Body Measure	Initial Load	Increment	Stage Duration (min)
McMaster	50	Height (cm)	(Watts)	(Watts)	
		<120	12.5	12.5	2
		120–140	12.5	25	2
		140–160	25	25	2
		>160	25	50 (male)	2
				25 (female)	2
James	60–70	Body surface area (BSA) (m^2)	(Kg m/min)	(Kg m/min)	
		<1.0	200	100	3
		1.0–1.2	200	200	3
		>1.2	200	300	3
Godfrey	60	Height (cm)	(Watts)	(Watts)	
		<120	10	10	1
		120–150	15	15	1
		>150	20	20	1

rpm, revolutions per minute.

BSA = 1/6(WH)0.5, where W is body weight in kg and H is body height in m.

Adopted from Chung EK, Tighe DA. *Pocket Guide to Stress Testing*. Malden (MA): Blackwell Publishing Inc; 1997.

modality. However, because there is less muscle mass involved using only upper extremity, peak exercise can be about 5%–20% lower than treadmill values (1, 34). Obtaining BP and ECG may be more difficult during arm ergometry because it requires brief interruptions of the exercise load. Additionally, the test endpoint will most likely be because of arm fatigue rather than reaching maximal cardiorespiratory challenge.

Previous data suggest that arm exercise capacity, like whole-body exercise capacity, is a strong indicator of prognosis (35). Protocols for the arm cycle ergometer are similar to those for the upright cycle ergometer, as the intensity can either be increased in a graded fashion or ramping. Arm cycle ergometry is typically used in a testing setting when the subject is unable to perform a standard treadmill or cycle test secondary to a physical limitation such as being wheelchair bound. Arm ergometers are more commonly used in a cardiac or pulmonary rehabilitation setting. Because of the difficulties involved in performing arm ergometry testing, this modality has largely been replaced with pharmacologic stress testing rather than physical exercise, discussed later in this chapter.

After choosing the appropriate protocol, the clinical exercise test should last approximately 8–12 minutes, permitting adequate time for warm-up and a gradual increase in the hemodynamic response. As a general principle, each stage of the exercise test should last 2–3 minutes granting hemodynamic and ECG response to stabilize and be evaluated. The test should start well below maximal workload levels for the patient. If an error is made at this stage of the test (*e.g.*, starting too easy), it is comparatively simple to increase the rate of progression of intensity. But it is hard to "go back" from too high an initial exercise intensity. This principle is particularly important when testing older or more debilitated patients. For example, the starting point for the Bruce treadmill protocol is approximately 5 METs, which may represent a near-maximal exercise level in deconditioned patients. This can be a major drawback for this protocol and highlights the importance of the CEP evaluating suitability of the testing protocol based on patients' needs (36, 37). There should be a gradual and regular increase in the workload, averaging about 1 MET per minute in most situations, but with faster or slower progression in individuals with predicted high or low exercise capacities, respectively. In this regard, it is sometimes of value to use a nonexercise estimate of the exercise capacity, based on age, sex, body weight, and activity tolerance. There are excellent questionnaire models for estimating exercise capacity before beginning the exercise test (38, 39). The Duke Activity Status Index is a self-administered questionnaire to evaluate functional capacity of patients with CVD (Figure 9.3).

General Exercise Testing Preparation

Prior to commencing the test, adequate preparticipation health screening and informed consent must be completed (see Chapter 3). Review the patient's medical history, including the reason for the current test (especially recent symptoms) and medications that the patient is currently taking, including those that have been temporarily discontinued before the test. The CEP should review with the patient the reason for testing, medical history, current symptoms, medications, and consent before initiating the test.

The exercise laboratory should contain appropriate exercise modalities (treadmill, cycle ergometer, arm ergometer), monitoring (ECG, BP) equipment, and necessary emergency items (defibrillator, drug cart). Appropriately trained personnel (physicians, nurse practitioners, physician assistants, CEPs) should either be present or rapidly available (in less than 1 min) to assure patient safety.

	Yes	No
1. Can you take care of yourself (eating, dressing, bathing, or using the toilet)?	2.75	0
2. Can you walk indoors, such as around your house?	1.75	0
3. Can you walk a block or two on level ground?	2.75	0
4. Can you climb a flight of stairs or walk up a hill?	5.50	0
5. Can you run a short distance?	8.00	0
6. Can you do light work around the house, such as dusting or washing dishes?	2.70	0
7. Can you do moderate work around the house, such as vacuuming, sweeping floors, or carrying in groceries?	3.50	0
8. Can you do heavy work around the house, such as scrubbing floors or lifting and moving heavy furniture?	8.00	0
9. Can you do yard work, such as raking leaves, weeding, or pushing a power mower?	4.50	0
10. Can you have sexual relations?	5.25	0
11. Can you participate in moderate recreational activities, such as golf, bowling, dancing, doubles tennis, or throwing a baseball or football?	6.00	0
12. Can you participate in strenuous sports, such as swimming, singles tennis, football, basketball, or skiing?	7.50	0

Positive responses are summed for total score, range 0 to 58.2.

The higher score indicates higher functional capacity.

Duke Activity Status Index (DASI) = sum of "Yes" replies ——————

$\dot{V}O_2$ peak = (0.43 × DASI) + 9.6

$\dot{V}O_2$ peak = —————— mL/kg/min ÷ 3.5 mL/kg/min = —————— METS

FIGURE 9.3 The self-administered 12-Item scale, Duke Activity Status Index (DASI), provides assessment of functional capacity and an objective measure of maximal exercise capacity. (Adapted from Hlatky MA, Boineau RE, Higginbotham MB, et al. A brief self-administered questionnaire to determine functional capacity (The Duke Activity Status Index). *Am J Cardiol.* 1989;64(10):651–4.)

Proper electrode preparation, including cleaning the skin surface, is critical for achieving a clear ECG with minimal artifact. Mason–Likar electrode placement provides the best option for exercise (see Chapter 6, Box 6.5). Preparing equipment prior to beginning the test is essential for the CEP to multitask and conduct the test. Depending on the patient's hemodynamic needs during the exercise test, equipment required to measure and monitor variables consist of the following:

- Manual BP cuff and stethoscope to acquire resting and exercise measurements, although some laboratories may use automatic cuffs
- Pulse oximeter to assess oxygen saturation
- Subjective rating scales for perceived exertion, dyspnea, angina, claudication

The room temperature should be approximately 20°C (72°F) with less than 60% relative humidity. It is ideal if there is a general movement of air over the patient to optimize thermoregulation, as the microclimate next to the patient's body can rapidly become warm and humid during exercise in a room with little air movement even if the room temperature is quite low.

During the test, it is important for the CEP to monitor the patient for isometric contractions (including gripping treadmill handrails or cycle handlebars). The pressor response should be avoided to decrease the likelihood of disproportionate increases in HR, BP, and ECG artifact. Table 9.7 identifies the recommended monitoring intervals associated with maximal graded exercise testing.

FLOW OF THE TEST

Pretest

Before beginning the test, clearly explain testing instructions to the patient including what the test will involve and physical expectations. Ascertain that the patient understands that the test requires physical exertion and may be uncomfortable. If the patient presents with symptoms (chest discomfort, dyspnea, claudication), the primary goal of exercise testing will be to reproduce the presenting symptoms and then use the available technology to determine the nature of the pathology/pathologies causing the symptoms. Patients should understand that they are likely to become symptomatic, or at least very tired, during the

Table 9.7	Recommended Monitoring Intervals Associated With a Symptom-Limited Maximal Exercise Test		
Variable	**Before Exercise Test**	**During Exercise Test**	**After Exercise Test**
Electrocardiogram	Monitored continuously; recorded supine position and posture of exercise	Monitored continuously; recorded during the last 5–10 s of each stage (interval protocol) or every 2 min (ramp protocols)	Monitored continuously; recorded immediately postexercise, during the last 15 s of first minute of recovery, and then every 2 min thereafter
Heart rate[a]	Monitored continuously; recorded supine position and posture of exercise	Monitored continuously; recorded during the last 5–10 s of each minute	Monitored continuously; recorded during the last 5 s of each minute
Blood pressure[b]	Measured and recorded in supine position and posture of exercise	Measured and recorded during the last 30–60 s of each stage (interval protocol) or every 2-min period (ramp protocols)	Measured and recorded immediately postexercise and then every 2 min thereafter
Signs and symptoms	Monitored continuously; recorded as observed	Monitored continuously; recorded as observed	Monitored continuously; recorded as observed
Rating of perceived exertion	Explain scale	Recorded during the last 5–10 s of each exercise stage or every 2 min with ramping protocol	Obtain peak exercise value; then not measured in recovery

[a]In addition, BP and HR should be assessed and recorded whenever adverse symptoms or abnormal ECG changes occur.

[b]An unchanged or decreasing systolic blood pressure with increasing workloads should be retaken (*i.e.*, verified immediately).
Source: Liguori G. *ACSM's Guidelines for Exercise Testing and Prescription.* 11th ed. Philadelphia (PA): Wolters Kluwer; 2021.

stress test. In the absence of signs or symptoms, the CEPs should encourage the patient to continue exercising until reaching volitional fatigue.

The most accurate diagnosis of CAD will be made at or near maximal HR. A test should not be terminated simply because the patient achieved a predetermined threshold based on age-predicted maximal HR (or 85% of age-predicted maximal HR). Cumming (18) and Jain et al. (19) have demonstrated that about 60% of ECG abnormalities will occur by the time 85% of the age-predicted maximal HR has been reached. These findings have led to a tendency to terminate tests at this point. However, these findings also mean that about 40% of ischemic/hemodynamic abnormalities are not going to be seen until after 85% of age-predicted maximal HR has been achieved. Given the modest sensitivity of exercise ECG for detecting CAD, the practice of stopping clinical exercise tests arbitrarily at 85% of the age-predicted maximal HR (itself a value of limited accuracy) has little plausible defense. Exerting physical demands of the body in the controlled exercise testing laboratory environment provides the opportunity to uncover possible pathology or abnormal responses, especially with patients pursing vigorous exercise. Given that patients who "pass" an exercise test might be encouraged to participate in more vigorous activities, it is critical that an adequate diagnosis be made in the laboratory (rather than during unsupervised strenuous activity).

Prior to beginning a clinical exercise test, the CEP should obtain the patient's resting vital signs and ECG tracings including supine and standing BP to check for orthostatic hypotension. Physiological variables assessed during the test include HR, ECG, BP, oxygen saturation, rating of perceived exertion (RPE), and signs and symptoms (*i.e.*, dyspnea, angina, and claudication). In this regard, it is important to remember that dyspnea (*e.g.*, "running out of air") is an angina equivalent in older individuals (more than 60 years old; Table 9.7).

Exercise Test

Monitoring exercise tolerance using a protocol consisting of 2- to 3-minute stages is recommended for physiologic accommodation to allow the patient to reach steady-state prior to collecting hemodynamic measurements. Although it is possible to ramp exercise tests (36, 37), so the workload is constantly changing, more often tests are conducted using definite stages. The CEP should focus on progressively guiding the patient through continuous exercise to reach elevated physiological demands. If a diagnosis can be made at low-level exercise, pushing the test

until a cardiopulmonary event occurs has little logic. On the other hand, a test that remains normal, in a patient who was referred for testing by the physician to rule out pathology, should be encouraged to continue exercising at least until the patient is volitionally fatigued.

The physiological responses monitored during the test include the following: HR, SBP, diastolic blood pressure (DBP), and RPP, as described in Table 9.7.

Heart Rate

In general, HR should increase 10 ± 2 beats per minute (bpm) with each 1 MET increase during the test (1). If the patient is on a β-blocker or other medication that changes the chronotropic response, the HR will usually be blunted (it will fail to rise normally with incrementally harder work). If the HR fails to increase linearly with an increasing workload or the peak HR is more than 20 bpm below predicted maximal levels without drug therapy that influences HR, the patient may be experiencing chronotropic incompetence, which has unfavorable prognostic implications (40). An additional HR marker that is useful as a prognostic indicator is the failure of the HR to decrease appropriately (more than 12 bpm in the first minute) during recovery, whether sitting or performing very low-level exercise (41).

Systolic Blood Pressure

Like HR, SBP should exhibit a linear increase with increasing work. In general, there should be a 10 ± 2 mm Hg increase in SBP with each 1 MET level increase (1). If the patient is on medications that influence the BP response, the increase in SBP will be slower, but should still exhibit a generally linear increasing pattern. At maximal exercise, the BP response for men will typically be 20 ± 5 mm Hg higher than women (1).

Some recommendations suggest stopping the test if the patient's SBP rises above 250 mm Hg. However, given the profound BP response during lifting and carrying (42), stopping the test at a SBP above 250 mm Hg may not be necessary unless symptoms are also present.

A flat or hypotensive response in SBP to an increased workload often indicates ischemia or pump failure (1). Indications of a hypotensive response include less than 20 mm Hg increase in SBP from rest, maximal SBP less than 140 mm Hg (if the patient is not on medications that blunt the SBP response to exercise), a decrease below resting SBP values, or a 10 mm Hg decrease in SBP with an increase in workload. A decrease in SBP in the presence of other evidence of myocardial ischemia (angina and ECG changes) is adequate criteria for immediate termination of an exercise test. Following exercise, SBP should decrease in an orderly way. Because true peak exercise SBP is not always able to be measured accurately, it is probably best to make sure that the 3-minute postexercise SBP is less than the 1-minute postexercise SBP as an index of normal recovery (43).

Diastolic Blood Pressure

During the exercise stress test, DBP should stay the same or decrease slightly because of vasodilation in the vessels of the exercising muscles. An increase of less than 10 mm Hg in DBP from resting values is considered normal if the resting values are within the normal range of 50–90 mm Hg at rest (1). An isolated 15 mm Hg increase in DBP may indicate that the patient has stiff vessels, meaning that the arterioles are not dilating appropriately. The test should be stopped if DBP reaches 115 mm Hg. It is important to recognize that the measurement of DBP during exercise can be difficult and changes in DBP are, at best, secondary criteria for stopping an exercise test.

Rate Pressure Product

The RPP, or *double product*, provides an indirect measure of myocardial oxygen consumption. RPP is calculated by multiplying HR by SBP. The RPP at which angina (ischemia) occurs is very reproducible and one goal of most therapies is to shift this value upward. More importantly, in the absence of abnormal findings during the exercise test, the physician is obliged to ascertain whether the patient's cardiac function is truly normal or if something has been missed in the diagnosis. An RPP at or above 25,000 can be thought of as a "security blanket" that a normal test accurately represents a patient without pathology. The normal range for RPP is 25,000–40,000 (1).

Subjective Ratings

In addition to monitoring the ECG tracing, HR and BP during the test, symptoms suggestive of myocardial ischemia must also be monitored. It can be helpful to ask the patient to gauge exertion during each stage of the test. RPE is a standardized scale used to assess how hard the patient feels while they are working. The RPE scale is highly correlated with physiologic responses during progressive exercise. The most common scale is the Borg scale; either 15-point (6–20) or the 10-point scale (0–10) (Figure 9.4). Assessing physiological symptoms during the test and throughout recovery include signs of light-headedness,

Borg CR10 Scale®

0	Nothing at all	
0.3		
0.5	Extremely weak	Just noticeable
0.7		
1	Very weak	
1.5		
2	Weak	Light
2.5		
3	Moderate	
4		
5	Strong	Heavy
6		
7	Very strong	
8		
9		
10	Extremely strong	"Maximal"
11		
∫		
•	Absolute maximum	Highest possible

FIGURE 9.4 The Borg category-ratio scale. *Source:* From Liguori G. *ACSM's Guidelines for Exercise Testing and Prescription.* 11th ed. Philadelphia (PA): Wolters Kluwer; 2021. (Reprinted from Borg G, Borg E. *The Borg CR Scales Folder.* Hässelby (Sweden): Borg Perception; 2010.)

angina, dyspnea, claudication, and fatigue. Standardized scales for angina, dyspnea, and claudication (Figure 9.5) are helpful in evaluating specific symptoms. Each scale is assessed using a 0–4 scale, and a rating of 3 out of 4 is an indication to stop exercising. Careful documentation should be noted regarding timing, character, magnitude of symptoms, or if symptoms resolve.

Indications for Stopping the Test

While watching for appropriate physiologic responses to exercise, the CEP monitors the patient for additional indications for stopping the clinical exercise test. Box 9.2 outlines the absolute and relative indications for stopping the test. Any occurrence of an absolute indication should lead to immediate termination of the test. However, if relative indications occur, how the patient looks and feels should be part of the decision-making process to terminate the test. Terminating exercise for symptomatic indications, relative or absolute, the CEP should initiate inactive recovery (stop exercising), assist to the supine position, and continue to monitor BP, HR/ECG, and signs of appropriate

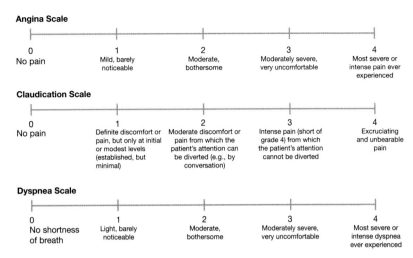

Angina Scale

0	1	2	3	4
No pain	Mild, barely noticeable	Moderate, bothersome	Moderately severe, very uncomfortable	Most severe or intense pain ever experienced

Claudication Scale

0	1	2	3	4
No pain	Definite discomfort or pain, but only at initial or modest levels (established, but minimal)	Moderate discomfort or pain from which the patient's attention can be diverted (e.g., by conversation)	Intense pain (short of grade 4) from which the patient's attention cannot be diverted	Excruciating and unbearable pain

Dyspnea Scale

0	1	2	3	4
No shortness of breath	Light, barely noticeable	Moderate, bothersome	Moderately severe, very uncomfortable	Most severe or intense dyspnea ever experienced

FIGURE 9.5 Frequently used scales for assessing the individual's level of angina (top), claudication (middle), and dyspnea (bottom). (Reprinted from Liguori G. *ACSM's Guidelines for Exercise Testing and Prescription.* 11th ed. Philadelphia (PA): Wolters Kluwer; 2021.)

Box 9.2   Indications for Terminating Exercise Testing

Absolute

- Drop in systolic blood pressure (SBP) of more than 10 mm Hg with an increase in work rate, or if SBP decreases below the value obtained in the same position prior to testing when accompanied by other evidence of ischemia
- Moderately severe angina (defined as 3 on standard scale)
- Increasing nervous system symptoms (*e.g.*, ataxia, dizziness, or near syncope)
- Signs of poor perfusion (cyanosis or pallor)
- Technical difficulties monitoring the electrocardiogram (ECG) or SBP
- Subject's desire to stop
- Sustained ventricular tachycardia
- ST elevation (+1.0 mm) in leads without diagnostic Q waves (other than V_1 or aVR)

Relative

- Drop in SBP of more than 10 mm Hg with an increase in work rate, or if SBP below the value obtained in the same position prior to testing
- ST or QRS changes such as excessive ST depression (>2 mm horizontal or downsloping ST-segment depression) or marked axis shift
- Arrhythmias other than sustained ventricular tachycardia, including multifocal premature ventricular contractions (PVCs), supraventricular tachycardia, heart block, or bradydysrhythmias
- Fatigue, shortness of breath, wheezing, leg cramps, or claudication
- Development of bundle branch block or intraventricular conduction delay that cannot be distinguished from ventricular tachycardia
- Increasing chest pain
- Hypertensive response (SBP of >250 mm Hg and/or a DBP of >115 mm Hg)

Source: Fletcher GF, Balady GJ, Froelicher VF, Hartley LH, Haskell WL, Pollock ML. Exercise standards: a statement for healthcare professionals from the American Heart Association. *Circulation.* 1995;91(2):580–615.

---

perfusion, and symptoms in the recovery stage for at least 6 minutes. The purpose of conducting the test (*e.g.*, evaluating presenting symptoms, screening for occult CAD, and obtaining maximum MET level for returning to work) should always be a primary consideration. Obviously, if the clinical question that prompted the test has been answered (*e.g.*, ST-segment depression correlated with angina-type chest discomfort or dyspnea, particularly if linked to abnormal BP responses), then the test should be terminated. In this context, it is useful to remember that the concept of "clinical correlation" is high on the list of important findings when physicians are trying to make diagnoses. However, in the absence of a clear sign to stop, the test should be continued until there is a clear reason to stop (*e.g.*, fatigue).

Posttest

Postexercise recovery is an essential component of the clinical exercise test and continued monitoring of vital signs for abnormal response to exercise is imperative. Once the decision has been made to terminate the test, obtain maximal BP, HR, RPE, and ECG readings at peak exercise. For most commercial equipment, once initiated, the recovery protocol will commence automatically, and workloads will be reduced. Each laboratory should develop standardized procedures for postexercise recovery (active vs. inactive recovery and monitoring duration). Tests terminated for absolute or relative symptomatic responses use inactive recovery immediately following exercise with the patient placed supine and continue observing hemodynamics and signs of myocardial ischemia. Active recovery provides low-intensity exercise helping to support venous return and hemodynamic stability. If the treadmill does not automatically initiate reduce workloads, manually lower the speed and grade promptly, instruct the patient to continue walking at a slow pace (*e.g.*, 1 mph or 1.6 kph, 0% grade), to prevent postexercise hypotension. If using a cycle ergometer, lower the resistance (10–20 W) and have the patient continue pedaling. Once the workload is reduced, continuous ECG, BP, and HR should be obtained every 2 minutes monitoring the pattern of recovery. This recovery stage should continue until near resting values have been obtained during cooldown.

Normally, HR will decrease more than 12 bpm in the first minute (41). BP should recover steadily, such that the 3-minute postexercise SBP should be less than the 1-minute postexercise SBP (43). Failures of HR and BP to recover adequately are unfavorable prognostic signs. In most cases, the postient should not be taken off ECG and hemodynamic monitoring until symptoms have resolved, the ECG has fully normalized, and the HR is less than 100 bpm.

Testing Data and Prognosis

Exercise test scoring is a powerful prognostic indicator for patients with CAD. The most widely used tool is the Duke Treadmill Score (44), a nomogram using prognostic markers of exercise capacity and exercise-induced ischemia (angina and ST-segment changes on the ECG). The Duke Score awards points for the number of minutes of exercise — conveniently, the standard Bruce protocol increments at about 1 MET per minute so the CEP can substitute METs achieved for exercise time. Points are subtracted for angina (more if the angina was limiting vs. just being present) and the magnitude of ST-segment depression. The weighted index is a prognostic score related to annual and the 5-year survival probability.

Using the calculated score to categorize patients into low-, moderate-, and high-risk subgroups has several distinct advantages as physicians may use the data to choose between more conservative or aggressive therapies. If the physician believes the patient is unlikely to survive with the disease, then a more aggressive approach to therapy (revascularization such as bypass surgery, angioplasty, and/or stent placement) may be indicated. If, on the other hand, the patient's prognosis is relatively good, then less aggressive medical/behavioral therapies may be given a reasonable chance as the first line of therapy.

An example of the computation and prognostic estimates from the Duke Treadmill Score is presented in Figure 9.6. Exercise capacity provides powerful assessment for clinical decision-making when applied to this scoring method as a predictor of survival rates (24–26).

Interpreting ECG tracings from the test requires evaluation of ischemia, presence of arrhythmia, conduction disturbances, axis, and evidence of prior infarction, as described in Chapter 6.

METABOLIC TESTING

When a clinical exercise test includes analysis of expired gases during exercise, it is termed "cardiopulmonary exercise test" (CPX or CPET) or a metabolic exercise test. CPET provides an ideal modality for evaluating exertional dyspnea, fatigue, circulatory impairment, pulmonary limitations, functional capacity, and differential diagnosis with suspected cardiovascular or respiratory diseases. Direct measurement of expired gases uses a metabolic cart to analyze, in real time, open circuit spirometry and oxygen saturation of blood through pulse oximetry, during the exercise test. The analysis of expired gas overcomes errors associated with estimating exercise capacity from peak workload and is the most accurate measure of exercise capacity and useful index of overall cardiopulmonary health (1).

The CPET provides additional data that are not available in stress testing conducted without expired gas analysis, such as the respiratory exchange ratio (RER), ventilatory anaerobic threshold (VAT), and the rate of change of minute ventilation (volume of expired air per unit time [$\dot{V}_E$]) to change in volume of carbon dioxide exhaled ($\dot{V}CO_2$) during exercise (*i.e.*, $\dot{V}_E/\dot{V}CO_2$ slope, an indicator of ventilatory efficiency) (11). Maximal $\dot{V}O_2$ consumption is used to assess fitness and functional capacity measured both in absolute (mL/min) and indexed to patient weight (mL/kg/min). Heart rate reserve is an important indicator, determined by age, to assess physiological response to increasing workloads (refer to Chapter 4, Table 4.1).

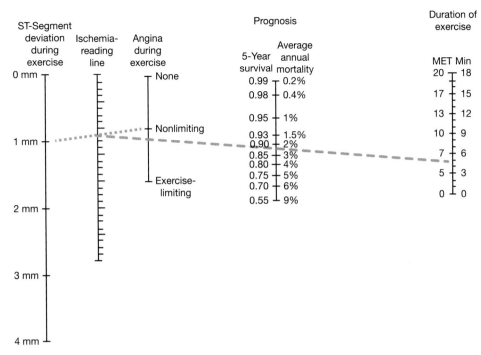

FIGURE 9.6 The Duke Index. An ischemic score is created by drawing a line between the maximal degree of ST depression and the presence and character of angina during exercise. This ischemic score is balanced with either the duration of exercise on the Bruce treadmill protocol or the number of metabolic equivalents (METs) achieved. By drawing a line between the ischemic score and the exercise score, either the 5-year survival or the average annual mortality can be computed. Depending on the judgment of the physician, 5-year survival predictions more than 95% may indicate that medical/behavioral therapy should be given a chance as first-line therapy. In contrast, 5-year survival predictions less than 70% may indicate that invasive therapy should be the first line of therapy. A higher exercise duration or MET capacity inherently suggests less invasive therapy. Because handrail support spuriously elevates the exercise capacity, the presence of even minimal handrail support will confound the findings of the Duke Index. In the example patient, a 1-mm ST-segment depression, nonlimiting angina, and a 6-MET exercise capacity predict a 5-year survival of about 89%. (Adapted from Mark DB, Shaw L, Harrell F, et al. Prognostic value of a treadmill exercise score in outpatients with suspected coronary disease. *N Engl J Med.* 1991;325(12):849–53. Reprinted with permission from Massachusetts Medical Society.)

Prior to performing CPET, resting spirometry measurements, including forced expiratory volume (FEV_1), forced vital capacity (FVC) and maximum voluntary ventilation (MVV), are conducted to help gauge lung function and calculate breathing reserve for maximal CPET data. Separate trials of spirometry need to be repeatable and reproducible to be valid and deemed a maximal effort (refer to Chapter 8 on respiratory diseases).

Testing Variables

CPET is typically performed with the intent of exercising the patient to volitional fatigue to reach maximal effort. Interpreting maximal effort achieved includes the following criteria:

- Plateau in HR despite increases in workload
- RER value greater than ≥1.1
- Plateau in VO_2 with increased workload
- RPE greater than 17 on the 6–20 scale or greater than 7 on the 0–10 scale

- Postexercise venous lactate concentration greater than 8.0 mM

Reaching three of the above-mentioned criteria has commonly been used to characterize an exercise test effort as "maximal". However, due to limited validity, there is no consensus within the literature on the number of criteria that needs to be met. Additionally, failure to obtain 85% or more peak HR, when evaluated as a maximal exercise test, indicates chronotropic incompetence. This abnormal response is independently associated with increased risk of morbidity and mortality.

Testing Findings

Impaired physiologic response obtained by exercise gas exchange analysis with CPET may be indicative of cardiopulmonary disorders. Numerous common conditions may reveal impaired responses to CPET demonstrating cardiac, ventilatory, or gas exchange abnormalities (45). CPET permits the CEP to differentiate cardiac from pulmonary disorders optimizing decision-making for designing exercise prescriptions. Assessing exercise capacity provides enhanced understanding of the efficacy of therapy for patients with CVD or the need for intervention. The benefits for using CPET provides integrative multiorgan physiological evaluation which is helpful to optimize health-related outcomes (46).

A wealth of scientific evidence has consistently demonstrated the prognostic utility of peak $\dot{V}O_2$. This is not surprising considering that this noninvasive measure assesses the integrated response of multiple organ systems to a graded exercise challenge. Although peak $\dot{V}O_2$ maintains a high level of clinical utility, additional measures acquired during a CPET can help reveal cardiopulmonary abnormalities and/or refine the decision-making process to pursue advanced therapies. For instance, the slope of the change in ventilation to change in carbon dioxide (CO_2) production (termed the $\dot{V}_E/\dot{V}CO_2$ slope) strongly predicts clinical events and mortality in patients with heart failure (1). This measure only requires a submaximal effort; a clear advantage when considering that individuals with diagnosed or suspected heart failure may hesitate to fully exert themselves during a CPET. A ventilatory classification scheme (Figure 9.7) help practitioners stratify a patient's level of risk for adverse events. The slope increases in proportion to disease severity in those with diagnosed or suspected cardiopulmonary disorders.

Exercise oscillatory ventilation (EOV) is an additional clinically meaningful parameter that is revealed with gas exchange analysis during exercise testing. Rather than observing a gradual increase in ventilation with graded exercise, EOV is an oscillatory ventilatory pattern that persists for at least 60% of the exercise test at amplitude 15% or more of the average resting value (10). Although the mechanisms explaining this observation have not been fully elucidated, it has been associated with pulmonary

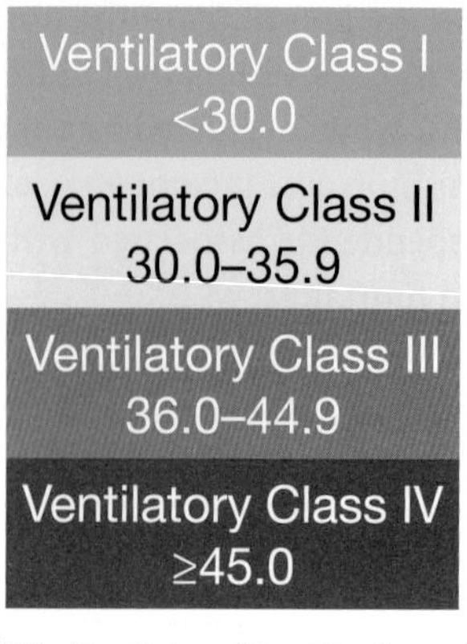

| Ventilatory Class I
<30.0 |
| Ventilatory Class II
30.0–35.9 |
| Ventilatory Class III
36.0–44.9 |
| Ventilatory Class IV
≥45.0 |

FIGURE 9.7 $\dot{V}_E/\dot{V}CO_2$ Ventilatory Classifications. (Information from Guazzi M, Bndera F, Ozemek C, et al. Cardiopulmonary exercise testing: what is its value? *J Am Coll Cardiol*. 2017;70(13):1618–36.)

interstitial congestion and a delayed circulatory transit time. End-tidal CO_2 pressure ($P_{ET}CO_2$) measured at rest and in response to exercise is another measure that adds prognostic value to CPET interpretation as it may help reveal impaired cardiac output. The attenuated increase in cardiac output with exercise translates to reduced $P_{ET}CO_2$ because of a reduction in the delivery of CO_2 to the lung and mismatching of ventilation and perfusion caused by impaired cardiac output. It is important to note, however, that this measure requires expired gases to be quantified by a metabolic cart capable of performing breath-by-breath analyses. Normal resting values are considered to be 33.0 mm Hg and more with values increasing by 3–8 mm Hg during the CPET.

Lastly, practitioners should take a multidimensional approach to interpreting CPET outcomes. Although peak $\dot{V}O_2$, $\dot{V}_E/\dot{V}CO_2$, EOV, and $P_{ET}CO_2$ are independent markers of poor prognosis, the presence of multiple abnormal responses indicates poorer clinical outcomes compared to one on its own.

DECIDING ON APPROPRIATE ALTERNATIVE TESTS

If the patient cannot exercise or does not have a normal resting ECG, the following information may help the health care team decide which alternative test may be the best option. There are two specific considerations to keep in mind when an alternative test is used:

1. Patients with COPD or other pulmonary diseases should be considered for nuclear testing because the enlarged lung area may interfere with echocardiographic images.
2. Patients with left bundle branch block (LBBB) should be considered for vasodilator pharmacologic testing with a myocardial perfusion agent, because the abnormal wall motion induced by exercise or dobutamine can result in a reduced septal uptake of the tracer, resulting in a false-positive test result.

Testing for Patients Who Can Exercise

If the patient has an abnormal resting ECG (*i.e.*, nonspecific ST-T changes, left ventricular hypertrophy, prescription digitalis therapy, Wolff–Parkinson–White syndrome), but can still exercise, perfusion imaging or stress echocardiography with exercise as the stressor should be the first consideration. In this regard, it is important to recognize that the information obtained from the exercise capacity and the HR and BP response retain their value, even if ECG changes are not central to the diagnosis.

With perfusion testing, a regular exercise test in conjunction with myocardial perfusion scanning using either thallium or cardiolite (sestamibi/technetium 99m) is useful. These images should be compared to resting images. Normally, cardiolite is preferred over thallium because it is a brighter photon and has a shorter half-life, leading to better images and a smaller radiation exposure. Cardiac gaiting can also be conducted with cardiolite because of the better visibility of myocardial segments. Several protocols exist for administration of radioactive tracers, depending on the patient's availability to return to the hospital on two consecutive days and what type of stressor is used in conjunction with the tracer. Refer to Henzlova et al., for more information on nuclear protocols (47).

If the patient is functionally able to exercise, a normal exercise test combined with the use of echocardiographic imaging, called "stress echocardiography," may be conducted. This test requires imaging of the heart before and immediately after maximum exercise. To image the heart as near to peak stress as possible, the cooldown period will be omitted to permit echocardiography in the supine position.

If leg exercise, such as treadmill walking or cycle ergometry, is not possible or difficult (*i.e.*, poor balance, orthopedic limitations, peripheral arterial disease [PAD]), arm exercise should be considered before resorting to pharmacologic testing, as arm exercise can provide increased physiological demand to the coronary circulation and can provide independent prognostic information (35). The beginning level and rate of progression of workload may need to be reduced (from approximately 20 W per stage to approximately 10 W per stage). Hemodynamic monitoring may require the patient to drop one arm while BP is recorded, and there may need to be brief interruptions of the workload at the end of each stage to allow an artifact-free ECG recording, but otherwise the principles of exercise testing are the same.

Testing for Patients Who Cannot Exercise

If the patient cannot exercise, pharmacologic stress testing using a vasodilator may be conducted with perfusion scanning (thallium or cardiolite) and compared to normal resting images. Alternatively, if the patient cannot exercise

and has contraindications to vasodilators, dobutamine may be used as the stressor. Normal diagnostic criteria including reversible reductions in myocardial perfusion at peak stress or new wall-motion abnormalities during stress are the same as when the stress is provided by exercise.

Vasodilators

Three commonly prescribed vasodilator stressors, with the ability to stimulate adenosine A2A receptors, are used with pharmacologic testing. Understanding considerations and major contraindications can be helpful for the CEP to understand when working with patients and providing patient education.

Adenosine works by directly vasodilating the coronary arteries, resulting in a 3.5- to 4-fold increase in myocardial blood flow in nonstenosed arterial segments. Because of the large increase in vessel diameter, the nondiseased segments essentially "steal" blood flow from the diseased segments, resulting in less blood flow and imaging uptake. Adenosine may cause activation of the A2b and A3 receptors, resulting in bronchospasm; therefore, it should not be used in patients who are asthmatic. A slight increase in HR and a slight decrease in BP should be expected with adenosine. If the patient has second- or third-degree atrioventricular block without a pacemaker or has SBP less than 90 mm Hg, adenosine should not be used. Adenosine has the unique advantage of a very short (approximately 10 s) half-life, so even in the case where it causes problems, the short duration of action is favorable.

The blood thinner and vasodilator dipyridamole (*e.g.*, persantine) indirectly results in coronary artery vasodilation by preventing the intracellular reuptake of adenosine during a nuclear stress test. Contraindications and hemodynamic responses are similar to adenosine. However, dipyridamole may result in a higher frequency of side effects (flushing, chest pain, headache, dizziness, and hypotension) than adenosine (1). Low-level exercise after the administration of dipyridamole and adenosine may attenuate the side effects and may increase uptake of the radiotracer. Persistent side effects with dipyridamole and its relatively long half-life (approximately 30 min) may require reversal with aminophylline.

Diagnostic imaging agent regadenoson (*e.g.*, Lexiscan) works by specifically activating the adenosine A2A receptor and results in coronary vasodilation, increasing coronary blood flow. An increase in HR and decrease in BP should be expected within 45 minutes after administration (1). Because regadenoson typically causes less bronchospasm than adenosine, it is becoming the vasodilator of choice in most situations.

Dobutamine

When there are contraindications to vasodilators, a dobutamine test may be used. Dobutamine causes direct stimulation of the β_1 and β_2 receptors, resulting in an increase in HR and myocardial contractility producing similar physiological responses occurring with exercise.

Blood flow will increase to the subepicardium and subendocardium, except where blood flow is impeded by stenotic arteries. Approximately 75% of patients will experience side effects, which may include palpitation, chest pain, headache, flushing, dyspnea, or supraventricular arrhythmias. For a more thorough discussion, with extensive reference to the literature, the reader is referred to the AHA Scientific Statement "Exercise Standards for Testing and Training" (11).

SUMMARY

Clinical exercise testing is part of the history and physical examination that physicians use in the diagnosis of cardiopulmonary disease. It may also be used to evaluate the effects of therapy, to evaluate patients for the safety of other surgical procedures, for defining prognosis in the case of known disease, and baseline data for exercise prescription. In most cases, the diagnostic value of clinical exercise testing depends on evaluating the clinical correlation between the patients' history, the symptoms they experience during incremental exercise, and either the ECG or hemodynamic findings. Classically, clinical exercise testing is based on progressive graded exercise intensities, performed either on the treadmill or on the cycle ergometer. A variety of protocols are in wide use, but all operate on the premise of starting at submaximal intensity, having gradual increases in the workload approximately 1 MET per minute, and with the target of either provoking signs and symptoms or causing fatigue within 8–12 minutes of exercise. Alternative ways of providing stress, using either arm ergometry or various pharmacologic stressors, are important adjuncts, particularly when combined with methods to augment information obtained from ECG findings (*e.g.*, myocardial perfusion or left ventricular function).

Clinical exercise testing should be performed based on well-established indications and contraindications, which define the likely value and likely risk of the procedure. When ECG criteria are central to the diagnostic scheme, it is important to recognize that changes from rest are the primary diagnostic criteria and that the presence of resting abnormalities indicates the need for adjunctive procedures.

Clinical exercise testing is a diagnostic procedure. As such, medical practitioners are the specific end user and must make the final interpretation of results. However, as a practical matter, it is common to have the procedure performed and sometimes the preliminary diagnosis by appropriately trained nonphysicians, including CEPs.

CHAPTER REVIEW QUESTIONS

1. Describe how typical hemodynamics should respond with increasing workload. What is the corresponding terminology for failure of the HR to increase during the exercise stress test?
2. How can the Duke Treadmill Score be helpful with interpreting testing data?
3. When is using handrail support during a treadmill stress test appropriate?
4. Describe the importance of calculating RPP during the stress test.
5. List the five criteria commonly used to interpret maximal effort when administering a CPET.
6. In preparation to conduct an exercise test with a new patient, briefly outline important instructions to discuss with the patient prior to starting the protocol.
7. List absolute contraindications when stress testing would not be permitted.
8. In general, when should a stress test be terminated? Also, identify absolute indications for stopping a test.
9. Compare similarities and differences in hemodynamic responses during stress tests using treadmill versus cycle ergometers. Are there benefits to using a cycle ergometer over a treadmill during a stress test?
10. List alternative tests that may be used instead of the exercise stress test and provide reasoning why certain tests would be more appropriate.

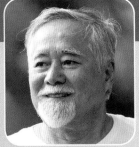

Shutterstock

Case Study 9.1

Bob is a 65-year-old active runner who was referred to exercise stress testing because he was experiencing chest pain while jogging. He is relatively healthy other than a 10-year history of controlled hypertension. He reports that his father died of a myocardial infarction (MI) at 70 years old. He also has known LBBB on his resting ECG.

Case Study 9.1 Questions

1. Identify Bob's risk factors for chronic disease.

2. What would be the appropriate exercise stress test for Bob? Explain your reasoning.

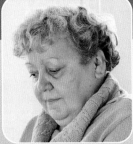

Shutterstock

Case Study 9.2

Laurie is an 80-year-old female referred to stress testing before she undergoes an abdominal aortic aneurysm repair next month. Her surgeon wants to make sure her heart can take the stress of undergoing this complicated surgery. Laurie has a history of hypertension, dyslipidemia, and a 60-year history of smoking. She was diagnosed with ischemic heart disease 5 years ago and is also obese. She reports she has difficulty walking and uses a walker for stability.

Case Study 9.2 Questions

1. Identify Laurie's risk factors for chronic disease and for complications during surgery.

2. What would be the appropriate exercise stress test for Laurie? Explain your reasoning.

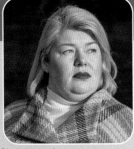

Shutterstock

Case Study 9.3

Jennifer is a 39-year-old female complaining of dyspnea and unusual fatigue during activities of daily life (such as walking up steps, carrying groceries). Her physical assessment includes body mass index (BMI) 36 kg/m^2, resting BP 136/88, fasting glucose 132 mg/dL, waist circumference 38 inches, low-density lipoprotein (LDL) 140 mg/dL, high-density lipoprotein (HDL) 38 mg/dL, triglycerides 160 mg/dL; she is sedentary and reports no family history for heart disease. Her physician requires health screening prior to obtaining clearance to join a fitness facility.

Case Study 9.3 Questions

1. Evaluate Jennifer's risk factors and determine if she meets the criteria for metabolic syndrome. List each criterion and describe your justification.

2. Which would be the appropriate exercise test for Jennifer? Explain your reasoning.

REFERENCES

1. Liguori G. *ACSM's Guidelines for Exercise Testing and Prescription*. 11th ed. Philadelphia (PA): Wolters Kluwer; 2021.
2. Balke B. The effect of physical exercise on the metabolic potential, a crucial measure of physical fitness. In: *Exercise and Fitness: A Collection of Papers Presented at the Colloquium on Exercise and Fitness*. Urbana (IL): Athletic Institute; 1960.
3. Bruce RA. Exercise testing of patients with coronary heart disease. Principles and normal standards for evaluation. *Ann Clin Res*. 1971;3(6):323–32.
4. Patterson JA, Naughton J, Pietras RJ, Gunnar RM. Treadmill exercise in assessment of the functional capacity of patients with cardiac disease. *Am J Cardiol*. 1972;30(7):757–62.
5. Master AM, Rosenfeld I. The "two-step" exercise test brought up to date. *N Y State J Med*. 1961;61:1850–8.
6. Shephard RJ, Allen C, Benade AJ, et al. The maximum oxygen intake. An international reference standard of cardiorespiratory fitness. *Bull World Health Organ*. 1968;38(5):757–64.
7. Wasserman K, Mcilroy MB. Detecting the threshold of anaerobic metabolism in cardiac patients during exercise. *Am J Cardiol*. 1964;14(6):844–52.
8. American Thoracic Society, American College of Chest Physicians. ATS/ACCP statement on cardiopulmonary exercise testing. *Am J Respir Crit Care Med*. 2003;167(2):211–77.
9. Arena R, Myers J, Williams MA, et al; American Heart Association Committee on Exercise, Rehabilitation, and Prevention of the Council on Clinical Cardiology; American Heart Association Council on Cardiovascular Nursing. Assessment of functional capacity in clinical and research settings: a scientific statement from the American Heart Association Committee on Exercise, Rehabilitation, and Prevention of the Council on Clinical Cardiology and the Council on Cardiovascular Nursing. *Circulation*. 2007;116(3):329–43.
10. Balady GJ, Arena R, Sietsema K, et al; American Heart Association Exercise, Cardiac Rehabilitation, and Prevention Committee of the Council on Clinical Cardiology; Council on Epidemiology and Prevention; Council on Peripheral Vascular Disease; Interdisciplinary Council on Quality of Care and Outcomes Research. Clinician's guide to cardiopulmonary exercise testing in adults: a scientific statement from the American Heart Association. *Circulation*. 2010;122(2):191–225.
11. Fletcher GF, Ades PA, Kligfield P, et al; American Heart Association Exercise, Cardiac Rehabilitation, and Prevention Committee of the Council on Clinical Cardiology; Council on Nutrition, Physical Activity and Metabolism; Council on Cardiovascular and Stroke Nursing; Council on Epidemiology and Prevention. Exercise standards for testing and training: a scientific statement from the American Heart Association. *Circulation*. 2013;128(8):873–934.
12. Mezzani A, Agostoni P, Cohen-Solal A, et al. Standards for the use of cardiopulmonary exercise testing for the functional evaluation of cardiac patients: a report from the Exercise Physiology Section of the European Association for Cardiovascular Prevention and Rehabilitation. *Eur J Cardiovasc Prev Rehabil*. 2009;16(3):249–67.
13. Palange P, Ward SA, Carlsen KH, et al. Recommendations on the use of exercise testing in clinical practice. *Eur Respir J*. 2007;29(1):185–209.
14. Rodgers GP, Ayanian JZ, Balady G, et al. American College of Cardiology/American Heart Association Clinical Competence Statement on Stress Testing. A report of the American College of Cardiology/American Heart Association/American College of Physicians–American Society of Internal Medicine Task Force on Clinical Competence. *Circulation*. 2000;102(14):1726–38.
15. Myers J, Forman DE, Balady GJ, et al; American Heart Association Subcommittee on Exercise, Cardiac Rehabilitation, and Prevention of the Council on Clinical Cardiology; Council on Lifestyle and Cardiometabolic Health; Council on Epidemiology and Prevention; Council on Cardiovascular and Stroke Nursing. Supervision of exercise testing by nonphysicians: a scientific statement from the American Heart Association. *Circulation*. 2014;130(12):1014–27.
16. Myers J, Voodi L, Umann T, Froelicher VF. A survey of exercise testing: methods, utilization, interpretation, and safety in the VAHCS. *J Cardiopulm Rehabil*. 2000;20(4):251–8.
17. Peterman JE, Arena R, Myers J, et al. Reference standards for cardiorespiratory fitness by cardiovascular disease category and testing modality: data from FRIEND. *J Am Heart Assoc*. 2021;10(22):e022336.
18. Cumming GR. Yield of ischaemic exercise electrocardiograms in relation to exercise intensity in a normal population. *Br Heart J*. 1972;34(9):919–23.
19. Jain M, Nkonde C, Lin BA, Walker A, Wackers FJ. 85% of maximal age-predicted heart rate is not a valid endpoint for exercise treadmill testing. *J Nucl Cardiol*. 2011;18(6):1026–35.
20. Foster C, Crowe AJ, Daines E, et al. Predicting functional capacity during treadmill testing independent of exercise protocol. *Med Sci Sports Exerc*. 1996;28(6):752–6.
21. Foster C, Jackson AS, Pollock ML, et al. Generalized equations for predicting functional capacity from treadmill performance. *Am Heart J*. 1984;107(6):1229–34.
22. Haskell WL, Savin W, Oldridge N, DeBusk R. Factors influencing estimated oxygen uptake during exercise testing soon after myocardial infarction. *Am J Cardiol*. 1982;50(2):299–304.
23. McConnell TR, Foster C, Conlin N, Thompson NN. Prediction of functional capacity during treadmill testing: effect of handrail support. *J Cardiopulm Rehabil*. 1991;11(4):255–60.
24. Mancini DM, Eisen H, Kussmaul W, Mull R, Edmunds LH Jr, Wilson JR. Value of peak exercise oxygen consumption for optimal timing of cardiac transplantation in ambulatory patients with heart failure. *Circulation*. 1991;83(3):778–86.
25. Myers J, Prakash M, Froelicher V, Do D, Partington S, Atwood JE. Exercise capacity and mortality among men referred for exercise testing. *N Engl J Med*. 2002;346(11):793–801.
26. Ross R, Blair SN, Arena R, et al; American Heart Association Physical Activity Committee of the Council on Lifestyle and Cardiometabolic Health; Council on Clinical Cardiology; Council on Epidemiology and Prevention; Council on Cardiovascular and Stroke Nursing; Council on Functional Genomics and Translational Biology; Stroke Council. Importance of assessing cardiorespiratory fitness in clinical practice: a case for fitness as a clinical vital sign: a scientific statement from the American Heart Association. *Circulation*. 2016;134(24):e653–99.

27. Foster C, Pollock ML, Rod JL, Dymond DS, Wible G, Schmidt DH. Evaluation of functional capacity during exercise radionuclide angiography. *Cardiology*. 1983;70(2):85–93.

28. Myers J, Arena R, Franklin B, et al; American Heart Association Committee on Exercise, Cardiac Rehabilitation, and Prevention of the Council on Clinical Cardiology; the Council on Nutrition, Physical Activity, and Metabolism; the Council on Cardiovascular Nursing. Recommendations for clinical exercise laboratories: a scientific statement from the American Heart Association. *Circulation*. 2009:119(24):3144–61.

29. Shephard RJ. Tests of maximum oxygen intake. A critical review. *Sports Med*. 1984;1(2):99–124.

30. Hambrecht RP, Schuler GC, Muth T, et al. Greater diagnostic sensitivity of treadmill versus cycle exercise testing of asymptomatic men with coronary artery disease. *Am J Cardiol*. 1992;70(2):141–6.

31. Wicks JR, Sutton JR, Oldridge NB, Jones NL. Comparison of the electrocardiographic changes induced by maximum exercise testing with treadmill and cycle ergometer. *Circulation*. 1978;57(6):1066–70.

32. Niederberger M, Bruce RA, Kusumi F, Whitkanack S. Disparities in ventilatory and circulatory responses to bicycle and treadmill exercise. *Br Heart J*. 1974;36(4):377–82.

33. Paridon SM, Alpert BS, Boas SR, et al; American Heart Association Council on Cardiovascular Disease in the Young, Committee on Atherosclerosis, Hypertension, and Obesity in Youth. Clinical stress testing in the pediatric age group: a statement from the American Heart Association Council on Cardiovascular Disease in the Young, Committee on Atherosclerosis, Hypertension, and Obesity in Youth. *Circulation*. 2006;113(15):1905–20.

34. Franklin BA. Exercise testing, training and arm ergometry. *Sports Med*. 1985;2(2):100–19.

35. Ilias NA, Xian H, Inman C, Martin WH 3rd. Arm exercise testing predicts clinical outcome. *Am Heart J*. 2009;157(1):69–76.

36. Myers J, Buchanan N, Walsh D, et al. Comparison of the ramp versus standard exercise protocols. *J Am Coll Cardiol*. 1991;17(6):1334–42.

37. Whipp BJ, Davis JA, Torres F, Wasserman K. A test to determine parameters of aerobic function during exercise. *J Appl Physiol Respir Environ Exerc Physiol*. 1981;50(1):217–21.

38. Hlatky MA, Boineau RE, Higginbotham MB, et al. A brief self-administered questionnaire to determine functional capacity (the Duke Activity Status Index). *Am J Cardiol*. 1989; 64(10):651–4.

39. Jackson AS, Blair SN, Mahar MT, Wier LT, Ross RM, Stuteville JE. Prediction of functional aerobic capacity without exercise testing. *Med Sci Sports Exerc*. 1990;22(6):863–70.

40. Brubaker PH, Kitzman DW. Chronotropic incompetence: causes, consequences, and management. *Circulation*. 2011;123(9):1010–20.

41. Cole CR, Blackstone EH, Pashkow FJ, Snader CE, Lauer MS. Heart-rate recovery immediately after exercise as a predictor of mortality. *N Engl J Med*. 1999;341(18):1351–7.

42. Williams MA, Haskell WL, Ades PA, et al; American Heart Association Council on Clinical Cardiology; American Heart Association Council on Nutrition, Physical Activity, and Metabolism. Resistance exercise in individuals with and without cardiovascular disease: 2007 update: a scientific statement from the American Heart Association Council on Clinical Cardiology and Council on Nutrition, Physical Activity, and Metabolism. *Circulation*. 2007;116(5):572–84.

43. McHam SA, Marwick TH, Pashkow FJ, Lauer MS. Delayed systolic blood pressure recovery after graded exercise: an independent correlate of angiographic coronary disease. *J Am Coll Cardiol*. 1999;34(3):754–9.

44. Mark DB, Shaw L, Harrell FE Jr, et al. Prognostic value of a treadmill exercise score in outpatients with suspected coronary artery disease. *N Engl J Med*. 1991;325(12):849–53.

45. Sietsema KE, Sue DY, Stringer WW, Ward SA. *Wasserman & Whipp's Principles of Exercise Testing and Interpretation*. 6th ed. Baltimore (MD): Lippincott, Williams & Wilkins; 2021.

46. Guazzi M, Bandera F, Ozemek C, et al. Cardiopulmonary exercise testing: what is its value? *J Am Coll Cardiol*. 2017;70(13):1618–36.

47. Henzlova MJ, Duvall WL, Einstein AJ, Travin MI, Verberne HJ. ASNC imaging guidelines for SPECT nuclear cardiology procedures: stress, protocols, and tracers. *J Nucl Cardiol*. 2016;23(3):606–39.Table 9.5

Obesity and Endocrine Conditions

INTRODUCTION

This chapter discusses three chronic conditions that the clinical exercise physiologist (CEP) is likely to encounter in practice: overweight/obesity, diabetes mellitus, and polycystic ovary syndrome (PCOS). In the U.S., more than 50% of adults aged 20 and older are obese. Rates of both Type 1 diabetes mellitus (T1DM) and Type 2 diabetes mellitus (T2DM) are increasing, and overweight/ obesity has been shown to be a risk factor for both. PCOS is also rising in incidence and may affect 20% of women with overweight/obesity. Insulin resistance is a key factor in both diabetes and PCOS and develops during weight gain. Physical activity/exercise is important in the prevention and treatment of overweight/obesity and insulin resistance, and therefore of both diabetes mellitus (DM) and PCOS. Thus, the CEP has a unique opportunity to design interventions to reduce morbidity and mortality in a majority of patients.

DEFINING OVERWEIGHT AND OBESITY

The term "overweight" refers to a weight that exceeds a defined standard. The term "obesity" specifically refers to excess adiposity. Body mass index (BMI) is the accepted clinical surrogate of adiposity for children ages 2 years and older. BMI is a ratio of body weight measured in kilograms to height measured in square meters ($kg \cdot m^{-2}$ or in scientific notation, $kg \cdot m^{-2}$). It is inexpensive and convenient to measure, but provides no information about body fat distribution, is limited by reduced sensitivity and specificity for estimating body adiposity in the overweight category in youth (1), and its predictive value for body composition and health outcomes differs by race and ethnicity. For example, for a given amount of adiposity by age and sex, Asian Americans compared to Whites have lower

BMIs by approximately 2–3 $kg \cdot m^{-2}$ and develop T2DM and cardiovascular disease (CVD) at these lower BMI values (2). Several more direct measures of body composition and body fat distribution are commonly used in research, including dual-energy x-ray absorptiometry (DEXA), air displacement plethysmography (e.g., Bod-Pod), bioimpedance analysis, magnetic resonance imaging (MRI), magnetic resonance spectroscopy (to assess intra-organ lipids), and computed tomography (CT).

Contemporary clinical and public health guidelines for obesity treatment recommend the use of BMI to define categories of healthy weight, overweight, and degrees of obesity (3), and the U.S. Preventive Services Task Force recommends the use of BMI to screen for obesity in youth starting at 6 years of age (4). Absolute BMI cutoffs are used to define weight categories for adults. By contrast, in children, BMI percentile (%ile) values should be used based on the age- and sex-specific Centers for Disease Control and Prevention's (CDC) BMI Growth Charts. BMI z-scores have been a widely reported as a research outcome in pediatrics. However, clinically, the meaning of a BMI z-score is less intuitive. Additionally, current BMI z-scores are a statistically invalid measure of adiposity for children and adolescents with severe obesity (4). For these reasons, BMI for youth with obesity are most often expressed relative to the age- and sex-specific CDC growth chart's 95th percentile, as a percent above the 95th percentile (Table 10.1) (4). More recently, it has been noted that a lower BMI is related to the development of metabolic disease in individuals in and from Southeast Asia (reviewed in (5)).

In the U.S., a primary source of obesity prevalence data comes from the National Health and Nutrition Examination Survey (NHANES), which has combined interview with physical examination data since the 1960s. Among adults aged 20 years or older in the 2017–2018 cycle, the NHANES age-adjusted prevalence rate for a BMI 30.0 $kg \cdot m^{-2}$ and more (class 1 obesity or higher) was 42.4%

Table 10.1	Criteria for Classifying Overweight and Obesity in Children (4) and Adults (3, 5)	
	Adults (≥18 yr)	Children (≤17 yr)
BMI Category	Absolute BMI Values	BMI %iles or % Above the 95th %ile for Age and Sex
Healthy	18.5 to <25 kg·m^{-2}	5th through the 84th %ile
Overweight	25 to <30 kg·m^{-2}	85th through the 94th %ile
Class 1 obesity	30 to <35 kg·m^{-2}	95th %ile through 119% of the 95th %ile
Class 2 obesity	35 to <40 kg·m^{-2}	120% through 139% of the 95th %ile OR 35 kg·m^{-2} (whichever is lower)
Class 3 obesity	≥40 kg·m^{-2}	≥140% of the 95th %ile OR 40 kg·m^{-2} (whichever is lower)
Asian and South Asian Population		
Overweight	23–24.9 kg·m^{-2}	
Obesity	≥25 kg·m^{-2}	

and for a BMI 40.0 kg·m^{-2} and more (class 3 severe obesity) was 9.2% (6). Class 3 severe obesity affects women more than men (11.5% vs. 6.9%) and non-Hispanic Black adults more than other racial and ethnic groups (13.8% vs. 9.3% in non-Hispanic White, 7.9% in Hispanic, and 2% in non-Hispanic Asian adults). Among youth aged 2 through 19 years in 2015–2016 cycle, 18.5% had class 1 obesity or higher and 1.9% had class 3 severe obesity (1.8% in girls and 2% in boys) (7). Non-Hispanic African American and Hispanic children had higher prevalence rates of overweight and all classes of obesity compared with other race and ethnicity groups. According to the World Health Organization (8), worldwide obesity has nearly tripled since 1975, and 13% of the world's population now has obesity.

ROLE OF PHYSICAL ACTIVITY IN WEIGHT REGULATION

Physical activity is a critically important contributor to regulation of body weight and composition. Because adherence to physical activity and inactivity guidelines is generally low, lack of sufficient physical activity is inarguably part of the causal pathway for increasing prevalence in overweight and obesity worldwide (9, 10). The most obvious benefit is the direct energy expenditure achieved during physical activity. While resting, energy expenditure averages about 1–1.5 kcal·min^{-1}, even relatively easy exercise raises that by three to fivefold, and during high-intensity

exercise, energy expenditure can reach 20 kcal·min^{-1}. It is clear that achieving just the minimum physical activity recommendation of 150 minutes of moderate exercise per week results in many hundreds of expended kcals relative to a sedentary lifestyle (10–12). But the role for physical activity is far more complex than just the direct energy expenditure as potential compensatory behavior in the form of greater food consumption and/or increased sedentary time can conspire to limit the "expected" weight loss from a simple calculation of energy balance (13, 14). Age, sex, genetics/epigenetics, shifts in body composition, and other factors are also contributors to the effects of increasing activity on body weight (10, 15, 16).

Weight Loss With Endurance Modes of Physical Activity

It is basically impossible to make blanket statements about the magnitude of weight loss in response to initiating a physical activity training program without intentional restriction of energy intake. In general, the overwhelming consensus has been that the addition of physical activity causes some weight loss, but, on average, it is not dramatic (17, 18), without a concurrent reduction in energy intake.

As shown in Figure 10.1, although mean body mass change after 12 weeks of supervised exercise training was −3.3 kg (−7.3 lb), changes spanned the gamut from large reductions to small increases. These studies revealed that the effect of exercise on appetite regulation involves at least two processes: an increase in the overall (orexigenic)

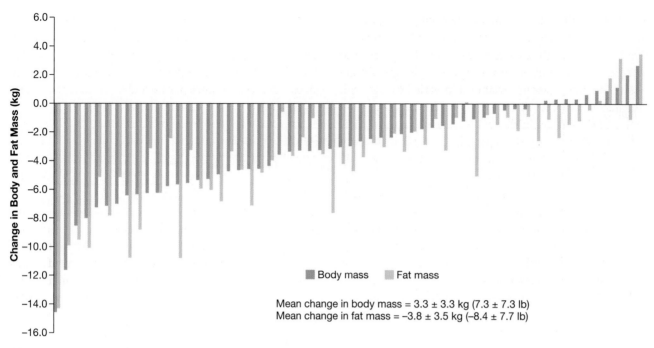

FIGURE 10.1 Individual variability in the response to supervised exercise. (Data from McLean et al. (18) redrawn from King et al. (19, 20).)

drive to eat and a concomitant increase in the satiating efficiency of a fixed meal. The individual variability in the overall response is likely rooted, at least in part, in how exercise differentially affects these two processes between individuals (13, 19).

Strictly focusing on body weight misses an important component; however, increasing physical activity can cause desirable changes in lean body mass, which can at least partly offset losses in body fat and blunt the magnitude of total weight loss. Accounting for changes in body composition is important as health benefits are far more dependent on loss of body fat than total weight. In fact, the mean change in fat mass noted above was -3.8 kg (-8.4 lb), exceeding the loss of body weight, implying a small gain of lean mass. But again, as Figure 10.1 shows, even accounting for lean mass changes, there were still 25% of participants who lost less than 2.0 kg (4.4 lb) of fat mass and some who actually gained. This wide variation in body weight and fat changes is consistent across other well-designed and controlled studies (17, 18, 20).

The Physical Activity Guidelines for Americans (PAG) Advisory Committees' original publication (Physical Activity Guidelines Advisory Committee. Physical Activity Guidelines Advisory Report, 2008. Washington D.C.: U.S. Department of Health and Human Services 2008) reviewed the literature to examine the effect of physical activity on weight loss. Intervention studies that were reviewed and included in this report ranged from about 8 to 16 months

in duration. The dose of physical activity across the studies ranged from 180 to 360 minutes per week at a moderate-to-vigorous intensity. Weight loss typically ranged from 1 to 3 kg (2.2–6.6 lb). The American College of Sports Medicine (ACSM) Position Stand on "Appropriate Physical Activity Strategies for Weight Loss and Prevention of Weight Regain for Adults" (10) concluded that there was no significant change in weight in studies in which physical activity was less than 150 minutes per week. The consensus was that physical activity more than 150 minutes per week resulted in significant weight loss, with a dose–response relationship observed. It was suggested that approximately 2-3 kg (4.4–6.6 lb) of weight loss occurs with more than 150 minutes per week of physical activity, whereas increasing that dose to 225–420 minutes per week increased the efficacy from 5 to 7.5 kg (11.0–16.5 lb). More recently, the 2018 PAG Advisory Committee reviewed literature that included studies done after ACSM Position Stand was published in 2009 (21). The updated report did not directly address the role of physical activity in weight loss, but instead focused on the role of physical activity in the prevention of weight gain and development of obesity. That report reinforced the 2009 ACSM report by concluding that there was strong evidence that the relationship between physical activity and blunted weight gain is most apparent when physical activity exceeds 150 minutes per week (21). They found that the evidence for the reported dose–response relationship between physical activity and weight was limited, and there was strong evidence that time spent in moderate-to-vigorous physical activity was positively associated with weight maintenance as opposed to weight gain. Evidence was not sufficient to determine whether the same was true for light intensity activity. The dose–response relationship varied by age with the report concluding that the relationship was strongest in young adults and diminished with increasing age. In addition, the relationship did not appear to vary by sex. There was insufficient evidence to determine if the relationship was mediated by socioeconomic status, race, or ethnicity.

Several well-designed studies initially suggested that weight loss achieved through exercise without prescribed energy restriction differs between men and women, and this perception is still widely held. An example of this is the first Midwest Exercise Trial (MET) (17). Young adults (17–35 years of age) were randomized to supervised exercise or no treatment control for a period of 16 months. The exercise consisted of the duration progressing from 20 to 45 minutes per day and intensity progressing from 60% to 75% of heart rate reserve by 6 months, for 5 days per week. Among men, the exercise resulted in a decrease of 5.2 kg (11.46 lb) compared to controls. The women in the exercise condition gained 0.6 kg (1.3 lb), which was less than the 2.9 kg (6.4 lb) weight gain observed in women in the control condition.

However, the same group of investigators postulated that the difference in pattern of weight change between men and women may have been a result of differences in energy expenditure generated by the structured exercise, as energy expenditure (EE) was 667 kcal per exercise session in men and 438 kcal per exercise session in women. A second study was conducted that compared weight loss effects between men and women when assigned to exercise that elicited 400 kcal per session or 600 kcal per session across 10 months (18, 20). Weight loss with 400 kcal per session was 3.9 kg (8.6 lb) and with 600 kcal per session was 5.2 kg (11.46 lb), with no difference between men and women at either threshold of exercise. A very well-designed study by Caudwell et al., in which the energy expenditure for structured exercise was held strictly constant for men and women, indicated exactly the same thing (22). Overall, these studies suggest that men and women can achieve similar weight change in response to exercise when energy expenditure is similar. It will be important to better disseminate this message to practitioners and the general public.

Magnitude of Weight Loss With Type of Exercise

Most studies have examined the effect of endurance modes of physical activity (*e.g.,* walking, cycling) on weight loss, but resistance exercise has been studied as well. A general consensus is exercise training alone (usually walking, jogging, and cycling) without enforced diet restriction generally results in only modest weight loss (10, 11, 15, 23). Doses of endurance exercise at 50% VO_2peak varying from 70 to 190 minutes per week did not cause appreciable weight loss in adults with obesity (24).

Even the highest volume group in the Studies of a Targeted Risk Reduction Intervention through Defined Exercise (STRRIDE) trial who averaged 17 miles of walking per week (estimated 1,600–1,800 kcal of expenditure only lost about 3.5% of initial body weight) (25). But it is critical to note that there was loss of both subcutaneous and visceral (which is strongly associated with insulin resistance and prediabetes/T2DM) fat and improvement in other key health factors (*e.g.,* insulin sensitivity) after this intervention (26). Higher doses of moderate-intensity exercise seem to be required to manifest weight loss greater than 5% of initial body weight, as evidenced by the Midwest exercise trials 1 and 2, in which participants exercised more frequently than the typical three to four times per week of most trials, expended more kcals/session (400 kcal in MET 1 and 400 or 600 in MET 2). Total kilocalories expended in those two trials exceeded 2,000 kcal per week, even with the lower dose. Taken together, there is good reason to suspect that the recommendation from the 2009 ACSM paper that it likely takes 225–420 minutes per week of moderate exercise to induce clinically relevant (*i.e.,* more than 5%–10% of initial body weight) is reasonable (10).

Fewer trials have been conducted to independently evaluate resistance training-only as a means to induce weight loss (*e.g.,* see the STRRIDE-AT/RT trial) (27), and there is a theoretical foundation to project how resistance exercise could be effective in this regard (10, 11). Resistance training expends energy during the activity itself and also can enhance muscle mass and strength, potentially raising resting metabolic rate (RMR). Early studies and literature reviews by Donnelly and others concluded that resistance exercise probably has minimal effects on weight loss because the overall energy expended during training is not sufficient (10, 11, 28, 29). Public health guidelines and position stands of professional organizations also suggest that resistance training may have only modest effects on weight loss. For example, the 2008 PAG Advisory Report concluded that resistance exercise may result in a modest reduction in body weight, typically less than 1 kg (2.2 lb), or no change in body weight, reinforced by a 2016 review by Swift et al. (11) and ACSM Position Stand on "Appropriate Physical Activity Strategies for Weight Loss and Prevention of Weight Regain for Adults" (10). However, as noted with endurance training, regular resistance training provides body composition and skeletal, muscular, metabolic, and other health benefits even in the absence of clinically relevant weight loss. To date, there has been little direct testing of weight loss in response to contemporary workout regimens like high-intensity interval training (*e.g.*, spring interval training, functional training like CrossFit). These workouts are often of relatively short duration (sometimes very short — several minutes a day), they are often done at exceptionally high intensity. There is good evidence showing that these workouts can provide fitness and even health benefits that rival those gained from exercise regiments requiring vastly longer durations. Whether those benefits include weight/fat loss remains to be directly tested in rigorous clinical trials. Further research is needed to determine if those results are germane to inducing or maintaining reduced body weight over the longer term.

COMBINING PHYSICAL ACTIVITY WITH A REDUCTION IN ENERGY INTAKE FOR WEIGHT LOSS

Although physical activity alone, either in the form of endurance modes (walking, cycling, etc.) or resistance modes (weight training), may have only a modest impact on weight loss, a more common strategy to treat overweight and obesity is through the combination of physical activity to increase energy expenditure and dietary change to decrease energy intake. Numerous studies have demonstrated that these two behaviors when used in combination are more effective for weight loss than when either behavior (diet or physical activity) is used in isolation (10). As noted, the volume of exercise defined as total energy expended, which incorporates intensity, duration, and frequency, is the most critical driver of weight loss. Therefore, at any given intensity, longer duration of exercise (and greater frequency) will have a larger effect on energy expenditure. It is worth repeating that favorable health benefits (*e.g.*, insulin sensitivity, lipids) occur even in the absence of substantial weight loss.

Short-Term Effects of Combining Physical Activity and Diet for Weight Loss

Most recommendations for weight loss encourage the combination of an energy-restricted diet plus physical activity (11, 15). There have been numerous studies comparing the short-term (defined as ≤6 months) effects of restricting energy intake alone to an energy-restricted diet plus increased energy expenditure via physical activity. Note that in studies comparing the same amount of energy deficit generated in different ways (most notably the Comprehensive Assessment of Long-term Effects of Reducing Intake of Energy [CALERIE] study in which a 25% deficit in energy balance was achieved either by reducing energy intake 25% or by combining a 12.5% decrease in energy intake with a 12% increase in energy output for 6 months), weight loss appears to be roughly the same regardless of how the energy deficit was generated (30, 31). The general consensus is that the reduced energy intake is the primary driving force in weight loss, both in the laboratory and in "real-world" situations. As described in Chapter 10 of the first volume of this book, adding physical activity in the range of the common guidelines (*e.g.*, 150 minutes/week), typically increases average weight loss by only a couple of kilograms(1–3 kg [2.2–6.6 lb]), accounting for about 10%–20% of overall weight loss. This is also consistent with the conclusions of ACSM based on the literature review conducted by Donnelly et al. for the 2009 Position Stand (10) — note that the position stand is being updated for release in 2023.

When physical activity is sufficiently high, the added benefit to energy restriction is more marked. Following a 6-month intervention in which participants with class 2 or 3 obesity consumed a prescribed diet of 1,200–2,100 kcal per day (based on initial body weight of the participant), weight loss averaged 8.2 kg (18.1 lb) compared to 10.9 kg (24.0 lb) when the same diet was combined with physical activity that progressed to 300 minutes per week. Participants in the added physical activity group also had larger changes in BMI, waist circumference, and total body fat (32). When physical activity is ramped up to extreme levels, much more weight loss is possible, as best exemplified by the popular television show "The Biggest Loser." Contestants performed prodigious amounts of both endurance and resistance exercise, often exceeding 2–3 hours per day while also consuming a somewhat energy-restricted (but not very low calorie) diet. Contestants lost as much as 230 pounds over the course of 30 weeks. Clearly in these cases, the majority of weight loss was ascribable to the massive dose of physical activity, but these methods are not generally applicable to the general population. Whether this kind of massive weight loss would even be sustainable will be discussed in the next section.

In summary, adding physical activity to an energy-restricted diet can enhance weight loss compared to the weight loss achieved with a similar energy-restricted diet that does not include physical activity. However, the additional weight loss is relatively small, on the order of a couple of kilogram, unless the physical activity input is extremely high.

Long-Term Effects of Physical Activity and Diet for Prevention of Weight Regain

Although many people focus on short-term weight loss, the goal for individuals with overweight and obesity is clearly to maintain a lower weight in the longer term. This outcome has proven elusive for the majority of people who have lost weight in the first 6 months. Weight regain has been reported to average 25%–50% of initial weight loss within 1–3 years of achieving weight loss (31, 33). Even intensive long-term lifestyle interventions, such as the Diabetes Prevention Program (DPP) Study and the Look AHEAD (Action for Health in Diabetes) Study, observe significant weight regain following initial weight loss (34, 35).

There is a general understanding among leading research scientists and, increasingly, clinical practitioners, that physical activity is far more critical to successful maintenance of lower body weight and fat than for initial weight loss. Further, there is broad consensus that the dose of physical activity required to maintain weight loss is greater than the 150 minutes per week dose found to be effective for other health benefits, for example, reducing risk for T2DM, CVD, or certain cancers. As noted in reviews, position stands and the prior version of this chapter (10, 11, 16, 23, 36), the public health recommendation is 150 minutes per week of moderate-to-vigorous intensity physical activity, but the dose required to maintain long-term weight loss is likely 1.5- to 2-fold higher. Although it is a challenge for much of the general public to adopt and sustain this level of physical activity (given that the 150-minutes/week threshold is already only met by a minority of the population), the current evidence strongly this as an important clinical recommendation.

Importantly, there is objective evidence to support this higher dose of physical activity. Schoeller et al. (37) used doubly labeled water to quantify energy expenditure 1 year after weight loss in women who were categorized as highly active, moderately active, or sedentary. Weight regain averaged 2.5 kg (5.5 lb) in the highly active category, 9.9 kg (21.8 lb) in the moderately active category, and 7.0 kg (15.4 lb) in the sedentary category. The investigators concluded that energy expenditure equivalent to 80 minutes per day of moderate-intensity activity or 35 minutes

per day of vigorous-intensity activity will significantly limit weight regain following initial weight loss. Note that this dose of activity is more than four times the 150 minute per week blanket recommendation.

High-quality data are also available from the National Weight Control Registry. The National Weight Control Registry was designed to identify individuals who were able to successfully lose 13.6 kg and more (~30 lb) and sustain that magnitude of weight loss for at least 1 year. A key finding from this registry is that individuals who are successful at achieving and maintaining this magnitude of weight loss self-report engaging in expending approximately 2,500 kcal per week in leisure-time physical activity (roughly translatable to 25 miles of walking — or just over an hour of physical activity per day at a 3-mile per hour walking pace) (33, 38). Jakicic et al. (39) assessed the level of physical activity associated with considerable 18-month weight loss, with physical activity measured using a wearable monitor. Participants were categorized based on the magnitude of weight change at 18 months (weight gain, <5% weight loss, 5% to <10% weight loss, ≥10% weight loss). Participants who achieved 10% and more weight loss were engaging in significantly more moderate-to-vigorous intensity physical activity as compared to participants in the other categories of weight change. A secondary analysis (40) observed that participants who best maintained weight loss averaged about 10,000 steps per day, with 3,500 of those steps coming from moderate-to-vigorous physical activity.

As noted earlier, Hall and colleagues have used the show "The Biggest Loser" as a seminatural experiment to understand the metabolic adaptations to weight loss and weight regain in people who have undergone prodigious weight loss with energy restriction and considerable physical activity. RMR went down by a considerable amount in the active weight loss period, despite participants generally maintaining their muscle mass (for those interested, this may be an example of the "constrained total energy expenditure" hypothesis proposed by Pontzer et al.) (41). Somewhat surprisingly, metabolic rate remained considerably depressed after the intervention, even at 6 years of follow-up (42). Even more surprisingly, the people with the most sustained reduction in RMR was NOT the people who had regained the most weight, quite the opposite — there was a negative association between depressed metabolic rate and weight regain (42). Defying common wisdom, but potentially consistent with the idea of a constraint on total daily energy expenditure, the people with the most sustained reduction in RMR were also the individuals who had best maintained high levels of physical activity (43). One of the conclusions from this longitudinal study over a 6-year time frame was that variation in weight regain among former participants was mainly explained by how effectively they had maintained a high level of physical activity.

DIETARY APPROACHES FOR WEIGHT LOSS

Obesity is an epidemic that affects 41.9% of the American adult population. When coupled with data that include overweight individuals, excess body weight affects over 73.6% of the American people (CDC, https://www.cdc.gov/nchs/fastats/obesity-overweight.htm). The abundance of obesity-related diseases such as T2DM hypertension (HTN), CVD, sleep apnea, and several types of cancers confers a tremendous burden on the health care system. Weight loss reduces many of these comorbidities, improves health span, and thus can be an important objective for many overweight individuals. The biology of weight loss is predicated on the notion that energy intake is less than energy expenditure, and prolonged energy deficit will result in a measurable reduction in body weight. There are many types of diets that are effective at reducing energy intake. These include but are not limited to diets that allow all food types but encourage caloric restriction (*e.g.*, calorie counting), diets that encourage ad labium eating but eliminate certain foods/food groups (*e.g.*, keto, high protein low fat, low fat, Paleo, Mediterranean), and diets that alter the timing of food consumption (*e.g.*, intermittent fasting and time-restricted eating).

Reducing body weight (through decreased adiposity) can be an important goal for many exercising individuals because weight loss improves health span and reduces many of the comorbidities associated with obesity. The biology of weight loss is predicated on the notion that energy intake is less than energy expenditure, and prolonged energy deficit will result in a measurable reduction in body weight. When energy intake (through diet) is equivalent to energy expenditure (primarily through basal metabolism and physical activity), an individual should remain in weight maintenance. In contrast, when energy intake exceeds energy expenditure, weight gain will occur, whereas when energy intake is less than energy expenditure, weight loss will occur. What reads as a seemingly simply concept is complicated by the fact that energy intake and expenditure are influenced by multiple factors such as hormones, psychology, and metabolism,

thus creating a challenge for both scientists studying diet and clients wishing to achieve weight loss.

Caloric Restriction

Reducing calories to cause weight loss is often the first line of defense when trying to combat obesity, but the task can be daunting for some. Sometimes, it is helpful to be able to prescribe a goal for calorie deficit (*e.g.*, 500 kcals/day) or an optimal amount of body weight that needs to be lost in order to see health benefits. Long-term studies have shown that reductions in body weight between 5% and 10% prevent the progression to T2DM in insulin-resistant individuals and greatly improves many clinically important metabolic parameters including blood glucose, systolic and diastolic blood pressure (BP), and high-density lipoprotein (HDL) cholesterol (44). In endocrine disorders that are highly associated with insulin resistance such as PCOS, improvements in fertility have been noted with lower reductions (2%–5%) in body weight (45). A study by Lean et al. found that T2DM was revered most in individuals who were able to achieve a 15% decrease in body weight through low-calorie diet compared to those who lost less weight (46). The general take-home message for those wondering how much weight to lose depends on the outcome desired but can be summarized to say that some weight loss is beneficial, and more is often better.

Some studies have found that significant weight loss occurs when calories are lowered, but a mix of carbohydrates, fats, and proteins are eaten, a diet that more typically reflects a "balanced" diet (*i.e.*, 45%–55% carbohydrate, 15%–25% protein, and 25%–30% fat). For example, Dansinger et al. compared weight loss in individuals with obesity who were randomized to the Atkins, Ornish, Weight Watchers, or Zone diets and found similar (~3%) decreases across the four diets at the end of 1 year (43). This study points to the idea that caloric deficit drives weight reduction, and diet composition is secondary when one is concerned with long-term weight loss. Other review papers have also reported successful weight loss with popular commercial diets as well with phone and computer app-based tracking programs that help individuals quantify food intake (47–49).

Very Low-Calorie Diets

Very low-calorie diets (VLCD) are a subset of caloric restriction. These diets restrict caloric intake to 500–800 kcals per day and are often overseen by a physician or dietitian for safety. VLCD results in rapid weight loss, sometimes as much as 3–5 lbs a week with the goal being 20% reduction in body weight in 6 months' time. This study points to the idea that caloric deficit drives weight reduction, and diet composition is secondary when one is concerned with long-term weight loss. These types of diets are incredibly successful, but failure to maintain weight loss in the long term is a criticism (50).

Although most individuals who are trying to lose weight would prefer to do so rapidly, such as with what can be achieved with a VLCD, there may be advantages to a slower rate of weight loss. A study reported on the effects of both rapid and slow weight loss on the body composition and metabolic risk factors following energy restriction in postmenopausal women with obesity (51). The findings demonstrated that although both the slow and rapid weight loss groups significantly lost weight, the rapid weight loss group also lost significantly more lean body mass. In addition, decreases in fasting triglyceride (TG) concentrations and diastolic BP were only observed in the slow weight loss group. This may suggest that within the context of weight loss, to maximize retention of lean body mass and to improve certain cardiometabolic risk factors, a more modest rate of weight loss may be preferred to a rapid weight loss such as that achieved with a VLCD.

Macronutrient Composition Manipulation and Weight Loss

Counting calories can be difficult for some. Moreover, many popular diet books have called into question the notion that energy-in must be less than energy-out to induce weight loss. Some popular diets hypothesize that not all calories are created equal and metabolic advantages may be achieved by eating diets that eliminate major macronutrient groups (Atkins, others).

These authors tend to promote a carbohydrate–insulin model of weight loss over an energy balance model promoting the connections that low-carbohydrate intake results in lower insulin secretion, less fat storage, greater fat oxidation, and less hunger, all factors that work in concert to aid in weight loss (52), In addition, if carbohydrate intake is low enough (generally between 20 and 50 g/day of carbohydrate), the liver produces ketones that provide body and brain with sufficient fuel. Low-carbohydrate ketogenic diets like these have been prescribed to treat epilepsy since the 1920s (53), and the notion that these diets can enhance weight loss and or be used to treat T2DM has been more extensively studied over the last 50 years. Conversely, low-fat

proponents argue that by eliminating fat and increasing protein, foods with lower energy density are consumed, better satiety is achieved, and weight loss ensues. On the whole, the data indicate that eliminating foods or food groups can result in successful weight loss and no one diet stands out as a clear champion.

There are many low-carbohydrate diet studies that have assessed the effectiveness of restricting carbohydrates. Although there is no standard definition of a low-carbohydrate diet, generally it is accepted that 20–50 g of carbohydrates constitutes a low-carb ketogenic diet, whereas 20–120 g is a low-carbohydrate diet.

Almost always carbohydrate restriction results in energy restriction that results in weight loss. This is true in men, women, obese, and overweight individuals with T2DM. Meta-analysis and review papers generally conclude that greater short-term weight loss occurs with low-carb diets compared to other interventions, but this difference disappears when studies are carried out for more than 12 months (54–56), although not always (57). To highlight this effect, consider data from a large, randomized control study that found in individuals who are obese, a low-carbohydrate diet resulted in an 11% decrease in body weight at year 1 and a 7% reduction at year 2. The successful weight loss at year 2 could have been explained by the intense behavior training and weekly and monthly meetings the subjects had access to during the study (58). Regardless, this study is one of the only of a few that shows the effects of a 2-year low-carbohydrate diet intervention in humans.

Just as there are data that support the effectiveness of low-carbohydrate diets, the same can be found for low-fat diets. These diets gained popularity after data suggested an association between high saturated fat intake, circulating cholesterol, and coronary heart disease (59, 60). What followed was decades of research aimed at understanding the effectiveness of lowering fat to reduce weight. Well-controlled clinical research studies using metabolic chambers to measure energy expenditure have shown that low-fat diets result in greater fat loss in individuals with obesity, at least in the short term (61). Clinical trials in men and women with overweight and obesity have documented weight loss ranging from 1 to 9 kg (2.2–19.8 lb) depending on the design of the study (62, 63). In addition, data from the National Weight Control Registry supports the idea that individuals who maintain weight loss for 5 years or more tend to eat a lower fat diet. Overall, it seems fair to conclude that low-fat diets cause weight loss in individuals with overweight and obesity.

INTERMITTENT ENERGY RESTRICTION AND FASTING DIETS

Fasting is a concept that most individuals are familiar with whether it be the natural daily fasts that occur during the overnight interval between the last meal of the day and breakfast or the more prolonged fasts often associated with religious practices (*e.g.*, Ramadan, Lent, Yom Kippur). Fasting is not a new concept, but using fasting or fasting mimetic diets to aid in weight loss is a more recent area of research.

There are several fasting regimens that can be used to achieve weight loss. These include intermittent fasting, alternate-day fasting, and time-restricted eating. Intermittent fasting is when no food is consumed for a certain length of time, but the duration and frequency of the fast can vary. Alternate-day fasting (fast 1 day, eat the next, repeat) and a 5:2 protocol (5 days of ad libitum eating and 2 consecutive days of fasting) are two prime examples. Time-restricted eating, where food is only consumed between a defined time period of the day (say between 10 AM and 6 PM) is another popular option. Catenacci et al. found that in men and women who are obese, 8 weeks of alternate-day fasting resulted in a 9% decrease in weight loss and decreases in low-density lipoprotein (LDL), fasting TGs, and insulin sensitivity (64). Interestingly, although the daily caloric deficit was higher with alternate-day fasting, the weight loss in this group was not different compared to the group that followed moderate daily caloric restriction (64). To determine the effects of a year of alternate-day fasting, Trepanowski et al. studied 100 men and women who were obese and found that weight was reduced by 6% at the 1-year mark with alternate-day fasting. Again though, this decrease was not different than those who participated with daily caloric restriction (65). Time-restricted feeding limits caloric intake to a specific window of time, most typically 8 hours. This intervention has been shown to decrease weight and BP in individuals who were obese (66). Liu et al. recently published data (67) indicating that although intermittent fasting results in weight loss, there does not seem to be a scientific advantage promoting use of this strategy over daily caloric restriction. Of important note, one concern with implementing intermittent fasting for long-term weight loss is the loss of lean muscle mass that happens unless resistance training is coupled with the diet. More data are needed to understand if the loss in lean muscle mass can be offset with every other day eating and exercise.

ANTI-OBESITY MEDICATIONS AND PHYSICAL ACTIVITY

When lifestyle-based modifications are insufficient to adequately treat physical and/or mental health complications associated with obesity, adjunct biologically based tools including pharmacotherapy should be considered. The U.S. guidelines for the pharmacologic management of obesity in adults were most recently published in 2015 (68), and a foundational expert opinion statement for the use of anti-obesity medications in pediatrics was published in 2019 (69). Anti-obesity medications are recommended as an adjunct to behaviorally based multicomponent interventions (*e.g.*, nutrition, physical activity, sleep) for adults with a BMI of 27 kg·m^{-2} or more plus a comorbidity or BMI of 30 kg·m^{-2} or more, and for adolescents with a BMI of 95th %ile or more plus a comorbidity or BMI of 120% or more of the 95th %ile. The most commonly prescribed medications include sympathomimetic amines (*e.g.*, phentermine, diethylpropion), topiramate, bupropion/naltrexone, orlistat, and glucagon-like peptide-1 receptor agonists (GLP-1 RAs) (*e.g.*, semaglutide). Additionally, tirzepatide, a GLP-1R/gastric inhibitory peptide (GIP) co-agonist, is a promising agent with unprecedented weight loss efficacy reported in adults (70).

Exercise physiologists may benefit from understanding the mechanism of action and side-effect profile of anti-obesity medications to the extent that they affect exercise performance and tolerance. However, the specific interaction between anti-obesity medications and physical activity has not been well studied to date. Most anti-obesity medications act primarily on the hypothalamus to suppress appetite and promote fullness, which can impact nutrient intake and meal schedule/routine. Ideally, these medications facilitate caloric reduction without oversuppressing appetite or promoting meal skipping. However, if hunger is too potently suppressed, this can lead to increased fasting periods, which has been associated with decreased prolonged aerobic performance (71). Additionally, if carbohydrate intake decreases compared to pre-medication baseline, this can decrease plasma glucose and lower glycogen stores, which may lead to early fatigue (72). Further, if hydration typically occurs during mealtimes and mealtimes are less frequent, symptoms of dehydration including dizziness or nausea may be present, which can decrease overall exercise tolerance. Finally, side effects associated with individual medications, as detailed below, vary by person, but may include increased heart rate and BP, increased risk of overheating, dizziness, gastrointestinal upset, nausea, vomiting, sleep disturbance and mood changes.

Phentermine

Sympathomimetic amines like phentermine act on the central nervous system including through modulation of norepinephrine to reduce hunger and increase satiation. The mean weight loss response above the effect of lifestyle changes is approximately 3.58 kg (7.9 lb) over 2–24 weeks (68). Like other stimulants, these medications may increase heart rate and BP and are not recommended for individuals with uncontrolled HTN, arrhythmias, coronary artery disease, or heart failure. Side effects can include increased energy, restlessness, irritability, anxiety, insomnia, dizziness, and dry mouth. Phentermine can be taken with or without food, and should be taken in the morning to prevent sleep disturbance.

Phentermine + Topiramate

The combination of phentermine and topiramate has been studied in large clinical intervention trials in adults (73, 74) and adolescents [https://doi.org/10.1056/EVIDoa2200014 — Kelly et al. NEJM Evidence, April 30, 2022. This study is not yet indexed in PubMed]. The precise mechanism by which topiramate potentiates appetite suppression and early fullness is unknown but is thought to be related to enhancing central gamma-aminobutyric acid (GABA) activity. This medication combination results in a placebo-subtracted mean weight loss of 14.5–18.9 lb at 1 year on low and high doses, respectively. The side-effect profile reflects each medication individually. Topiramate's side effects include paresthesias, fatigue, dizziness, difficulty with concentration, memory, and/or word finding, and rarely decreased sweating (oligohydrosis) and overheating, particularly in children. The combination is taken with or without food in the morning.

Bupropion Sustained Release + Naltrexone Sustained Release

The combination of bupropion (a dopamine and norepinephrine reuptake inhibitor) and naltrexone (an opioid antagonist) has only been rigorously studied in adults to date (75, 76). It results in a placebo-subtracted mean weight loss of 7.7–10.4 lb at 1 year on low and high doses, respectively. Side effects can include nausea, vomiting, constipation, headaches, and dizziness. It is taken twice daily (morning and evening) and not with a high-fat meal.

Orlistat

Orlistat is the only noncentrally acting anti-obesity medication in current use and has been well studied in adults and adolescents (77, 78). It is a pancreatic and gastric lipase inhibitor that blocks the absorption of approximately 30% of ingested fat. The placebo-subtracted mean weight loss is 6.5–7.5 lb in adults at 1 year. In participants 12–16 years old, there was a 1.1 lb weight gain seen (vs. 6.9 lb gain in the placebo group) but with a 0.86-kg·m^{-2} placebo-subtracted BMI reduction. Side effects primarily impact the gastrointestinal system and include abdominal pain, bowel urgency, oily stools, and fat-soluble vitamin deficiencies. It is taken three times daily with meals.

Glucagon-Like Peptide-1 Receptor Agonists

GLP-1 RAs, which were originally studied and have been extensively used for the treatment of T2DM, have now also been rigorously evaluated for the treatment of obesity without T2DM in adults and adolescents (79-81). GLP-1 RAs enhance glucose-dependent insulin secretion, reduce glucagon secretion, and decrease gastric emptying (82) to reduce food intake and body weight. Mean placebo-subtracted weight loss at 1 year varies by agent ranging from 9.9 lb in adolescents/12.3 lb in adults with the daily 3 mg liraglutide injection to 28 lb in adults/39 lb in adolescents with the weekly 2.4 mg semaglutide injection. Side effects commonly include nausea/vomiting, abdominal pain, headache, and increased heart rate. This subcutaneous injection is administered at the same time of day/same day of the week with or without food.

GLP-1 RAs/Gastric Inhibitory Peptide

Tirzepatide is a combination GLP-1 RA/GIP co-agonist used for the treatment of T2DM with recently published results for adults with obesity without T2DM (70). After a year at goal dose, mean placebo-subtracted weight loss was 30.2 lb at the lowest (5 mg) dose and 46.7 lb at the highest (15 mg) dose. Side effects include nausea, diarrhea, constipation, and increased heart rate. This is a once-weekly subcutaneous injection administered on the same day of the week with or without food.

METABOLIC AND BARIATRIC SURGERY

Lifestyle interventions with or without pharmacotherapy will not achieve optimal risk reduction for all individuals, particularly those with severe obesity. Metabolic and bariatric surgery (MBS) is the most effective and durable treatment for severe obesity and associated complications in adolescents and adults (83–86). Health care providers should discuss MBS alongside all other indicated treatment options in a standardized way for those who medically qualify. Such a uniform approach would help to combat the damaging bias and stigma still strongly associated with treating obesity (87, 88). Given the chronic, relapsing nature of obesity, MBS is increasingly recognized as one of a combination of tools that can be used to minimize health risks and maximize quality of life over the course of the lifespan. Indications for MBS in the U.S. for adults are a BMI of 35 kg·m^{-2} or more or of 30 kg·m^{-2} or more with metabolic disease ($\geq$30 kg·m^{-2} with metabolic disease for Asian individuals) (89). For adolescents, indications are a BMI of 35 kg·m^{-2} or more (or BMI $\geq$ 120% of the 95th %ile in youth) with a comorbidity or BMI of 40 kg·m^{-2} or more (or BMI $\geq$ 140% of the 95th %ile in youth) (90). The most common MBS procedures are sleeve gastrectomy and Roux-en-Y gastric bypass, which result in an estimated long-term average weight loss of approximately 25%. Gastric banding procedures have fallen out of favor because of high complication rates.

In adults, MBS has been associated with major cardiometabolic improvements, including T2DM remission, reduced T2DM-associated micro- and macrovascular complications, and death; lower risk of progression from nonalcoholic steatohepatitis to cirrhosis, hepatocellular carcinoma, or liver transplantation; and lower risks of myocardial infarction, stroke, and mortality among those with preexisting heart disease (91–93). In adolescents, MBS has been associated with high remission rates of T2DM, prediabetes, elevated BP, dyslipidemia, abnormal alanine aminotransferase, and abnormal kidney function 3 to 5 years postoperatively (94–96). Further, MBS has shown consistent superiority versus medical therapy in improving glycemic control for adolescents and adults with T2DM (85, 97). Interestingly, remission rates of T2DM and HTN are higher in adolescents versus adults 5 years after gastric bypass, despite similar weight loss (98).

In addition to associations with numerous adverse cardiometabolic health outcomes, obesity is a risk factor for osteoarthritis, chronic musculoskeletal pain, decreased functional mobility, and subsequent joint arthroplasty, which have significant individual health and broader economic consequences (99). MBS is associated with improved joint pain, physical function, quality of life, and decreased disability in adolescents and adults (96, 100, 101).

The mechanisms through which MBS mediates weight loss and improves cardiometabolic and musculoskeletal health have not yet been fully elucidated and extend well beyond the simple restriction of energy intake and nutrient malabsorption. Additional mechanisms include accelerated gastric emptying, changes in gastrointestinal peptides (e.g., increased cholecystokinin, GIP, GLP-1, peptide YY, and neurotensin) that result in decreased energy intake and increased satiation/satiety, alterations in the gut microbiota and bile acid signaling (including increased circulating fibroblast growth factor 19), and decreased systemic inflammation (102).

For sleeve gastrectomy and gastric bypass, short-term risks include bleeding, infection, leak, and venous thromboembolism, and long-term risks include micronutrient deficiencies, cholelithiasis, and the need for abdominal reoperations. Procedure-specific long-term risks for sleeve gastrectomy include sleeve stricture, gastroesophageal reflux disease (GERD), and incisional hernia and for gastric bypass include dumping syndrome, marginal ulceration, internal hernia, and anastomotic stricture (103).

For the musculoskeletal system, clear benefits of MBS are balanced against increased fracture risk in adults, which is highest after malabsorptive bariatric procedures (104, 105) along with bone loss and changes in bone microarchitecture after both bypass and sleeve gastrectomy. Limited adolescent studies primarily 1–2 years after sleeve gastrectomy have demonstrated decreased volumetric bone mineral density of the lumbar spine but increased cortical volumetric bone mineral density peripherally with no decline in measures of bone strength (106), which suggest potentially important differences compared to adults. Notably, the 2019 MBS guidelines from the American Academy of Pediatrics do not require a minimum age or pubertal stage for consideration of MBS and instead recommend that surgical timing be driven by medical necessity (90). Prepubertal youth with obesity experience accelerated linear growth and advanced bone age, then lose this height velocity advantage with earlier growth plate closure during puberty, resulting in a similar final adult height compared to peers with healthy BMI (107). Longer-term bone health/metabolism data are still needed for youth who undergo MBS earlier in life.

Changes in bone metabolism after MBS are thought to be multifactorial and related to decreased absorption of calcium and vitamin D with associated secondary hyperparathyroidism, decreased insulin, changes in body composition, and decreased mechanical load after weight loss (106, 108). Current adult and pediatric MBS guidelines recommend postoperative calcium and vitamin D supplementation, and adult guidelines additionally recommend DEXA of the proximal femur and lumbar spine preoperatively and at 2 years postoperatively (109).

It is worth noting that although the mean weight loss response to MBS is significant, the individual response is highly variable (110–112), similar to all obesity interventions. Further, for a subset with very high starting BMI, even after expected weight loss, obesity or severe obesity may persist with associated mechanical and psychological health risks related to a larger body size/shape. Thus, many will require adjunctive postoperative multicomponent interventions, including physical activity, to achieve optimal long-term risk reduction and health promotion over their lifetime.

The impact of physical activity before and after MBS on weight loss, prevention and treatment of weight regain, body composition, and reduction of bone mass loss have been studied primarily in adults. Only approximately 10% of adults who present for bariatric surgery meet national physical activity recommendations preoperatively, and this proportion does not increase postoperatively when measured objectively (113, 114). It is important to note that increased activity, even if it does not meet standard recommendations, may still confer meaningful metabolic improvements in this population. In one of few adolescent studies, Teen–Longitudinal Assessment of Bariatric Surgery (Teen-LABS) participants followed one of two distinct trajectories postoperatively: more active (>9,000 steps/day) or less active (<4,000 steps/day). Despite both groups being significantly below moderate-to-vigorous physical activity goals for age, the more active group had superior improvements in fasting insulin and insulin resistance independent of changes in BMI and adiposity at 6 months, which persisted to 36 months postoperatively (115).

Barriers to preoperative activity may include cardiorespiratory limitations (*e.g.*, angina, asthma), musculoskeletal pain, and low body esteem. A small study of unsupervised aerobic physical activity for 30 days before MBS demonstrated increased VO_2max, decreased inflammation, and shorter hospital stay (116). Postoperatively, the 2022 ACSM consensus statement for adults with T2DM summarizes the potential benefits of aerobic exercise training, which include improved weight maintenance, glycemic control, insulin sensitivity, endothelial function (independent of weight and adipose loss), and cardiac autonomic function (117). Postoperative resistance training may reverse muscle strength deficits seen in adults after MBS (118). A 2015 systematic review of four pre- and four postoperative activity interventions noted significant heterogeneity in intervention structure/timing, but concluded that beneficial programs (in terms of cardiometabolic, fitness, and functional capacity outcomes) were 3 months or more in duration, targeted 65% peak heart rate/VO_2max for intensity, and were at least partially supervised (119). Finally, a 2022 systematic review and meta-analysis of any supervised or unsupervised

structured exercise training programs 3 months or more in duration postoperatively in adults was associated with improved bone mineral density at the total hip, femoral neck, lumbar spine, and radius (120).

From a practical standpoint, physical activity pre- or postoperatively may be most successful when tailored to the individual's physical abilities and within a framework that identifies, and addresses barriers related to social determinants of health (*e.g.*, access to a gym/safe space to exercise) and psychosocial barriers (*e.g.*, concerns about body image/fear of judgment/stigma).

DIABETES MELLITUS

Diabetes is a complex heterogeneous disease characterized by hyperglycemia (high blood glucose levels) resulting from defects in insulin secretion, insulin action, or both. T2DM is classified by hyperglycemia per the American Diabetes Associations (ADA) cutoffs on 2 separate days and the absence of anti-pancreatic antibodies, and is the most common, accounting for 90%–95% of diabetes (121, 122). Type 1 diabetes mellitus (T1DM) is an immune-mediated disease, is characterized by pancreatic β-cell destruction that usually leads to absolute insulin deficiency (121). The four most common antibodies are islet cell autoantibodies, insulin autoantibodies, glutamic acid decarboxylase (GAD_{65}), and zinc antibodies. The rate of β-cell destruction varies widely (121). T1DM accounts for only 5%–10% of all cases of diabetes. Other forms of diabetes that are rarer have no known etiology (idiopathic diabetes), and there are numerous types of mature-onset diabetes of youth (MODY), which are defined by a single genetic mutation affecting glucose sensing or insulin secretion (121).

Because hyperglycemia appears to play a significant role in the pathophysiology of diabetes complications, medical treatment of all types of diabetes focuses on achieving near-normal blood glucose and HbA1C concentrations as safely as possible without inducing hypoglycemia (123). The landmark study informing the glucose targets for T1DM and T2DM and insulin dosing goals in T1DM was the Diabetes Control and Complication Trial (DCCT) that was designed to assess whether intensive insulin therapy was better than conventional therapy in those with T1DM (124). At the end of the 6.5 years of the DCCT, the mean HbA1C was 7.2% in the intensive therapy group versus 9% in the conventional therapy group. Subsequently, intensive insulin therapy reduced the risk of development and progression of microvascular and neuropathic complications by 35% and 76%, respectively, and decreased the progression of intima-media thickness, a sensitive marker for coronary and cerebral vascular disease in patients with diabetes (125, 126). Glucose targets include an HbA1C of less than 7.0% (53 mmol·mol^{-1}), fasting glucose of 80–130 mg·dL^{-1} (4.4–7.2 mmol·L^{-1}), and postprandial glucose of less than 180 mg·dL^{-1} (10.0 mmol·L^{-1}), although goals should be adjusted for individuals based on factors such as hypoglycemic unawareness, known comorbidities, and age/life expectancy (123). The ADA recommendations for youth with diabetes are separate from those for adults and also distinct for older adults (123, 127, 128).

Defining Normal Glucose Metabolism and Diabetes

The ADA recommends screening for T2DM in asymptomatic people at any age who have overweight or obesity and have at least one additional risk factor for T2DM (121). Some of these risk factors include lack of physical activity, first-degree relative with T2DM, high risk because of race or ethnicity (African American, Latino, and Native American), HTN, and history of CVD (129). The ADA further recommends that individuals without these additional risk factors should be tested for diabetes beginning at 45 years of age and at least every 3 years thereafter if results are normal. In pediatrics, screening should be performed in youth with a BMI of more than 85th percentile.

The ADA uses four criteria for the diagnosis of diabetes (126), with nonfasted HbA1C of 6.5% or more the most common test. Other tests include a fasting glucose, or the glucose 2 hours after the ingestion of a standard 75 g glucose drink (oral glucose tolerance test [OGTT]) (121).

Type 1 Diabetes Mellitus

T1DM is diagnosed more commonly in children and adolescents, but onset can occur at all ages, even among the elderly (121). Children and adolescents may present with ketoacidosis, which occurs when a high level of ketones (β-hydroxybutyrate, acetoacetate) are produced as a byproduct of incomplete fatty acid metabolism (130). In T1DM, the combination of deficient insulin and increased counter-regulatory hormones (*e.g.*, catecholamines, cortisol, glucagon) results in excessive ketone production and metabolic acidosis. Recently it has been described that those with T1DM also have significant insulin resistance, perhaps related to the subcutaneous delivery on insulin (131–133). Adults with T1DM may not present with

ketoacidosis for many years because they maintain some β-cell function. Instead, they may have modest fasting hyperglycemia that can quickly change to severe hyperglycemia and/or ketoacidosis.

Both genetics and environmental factors, such as viral infection or infant exposure to antibiotics, are thought to influence development of T1DM; however, precise risk factors are unknown (132). Patients' BMI patterns reflect that of the general population, and when individuals have obesity, it can be difficult to determine the type of diabetes until antibody results are reviewed.

Patients with T1DM are at increased risk for other autoimmune disorders as part of the spectrum of autoimmune polyglandular syndrome. Related autoimmune disease include Graves disease, Hashimoto thyroiditis, Addison disease, vitiligo, celiac, autoimmune hepatitis, myasthenia gravis, and pernicious anemia. Women with T1DM are also at an increased risk for PCOS, perhaps related to increased ovary exposure to insulin, because of the subcutaneous dosing of insulin and lack of primary portal clearance of insulin (134).

Type 2 Diabetes Mellitus

T2DM is characterized predominantly by insulin resistance with relative insulin deficiency from decreased β-cell pancreatic secretion (121). Insulin resistance is defined as a reduction in the bodily tissue responses elicited by a given insulin concentration. Insulin resistance manifests in a failure in suppression of hepatic glucose release, glucose disposal in skeletal muscle, and suppression of free fatty acid release from adipose tissue over time to name a few (135). Most patients with T2DM have obesity and/or have abdominal adiposity (121). Risk factors for T2DM include (121):

- Age 35 years or older
- BMI of 25 kg·m^{-2} or more or central adiposity (defined by waist circumference)
- Having a first-degree relative with T2DM
- African American, Latino, Native American, Asian American, or Pacific Islander race/ethnicity
- Past diagnosis of Gestational type 2 diabetes mellitus (GT2DM)
- PCOS
- HTN (≥140/90 mm Hg or on therapy for HTN)
- Presence of a low level of HDL cholesterol
- Prediabetes (HbA1C of 5.7%–6.4%, fasting glucose of 100–125 mg·dL^{-1}, and 2-hour OGTT glucose of 140–199 mg·dL^{-1})

■ Other clinical conditions associated with insulin resistance such as HIV medications, certain atypical antipsychotics, or chronic steroids

Screening for diabetes should start at age 35 years for lower risk individuals and those with a history of gestational diabetes mellitus (GDM), and then performed every 3 years. Individuals with prediabetes should undergo screening annually. Many adults with T2DM go undiagnosed because hyperglycemia often develops gradually and there are no classic symptoms; hence, regular screening is needed.

Prospective studies indicate an association between low physical fitness and the development of T2DM (136–139). In a population-based prospective study that directly measured fitness by a maximal exercise test, men in the low-fitness group had a 1.9-fold higher risk for prediabetes and a 3.7-fold higher risk for the development of T2DM compared to men in the high-fitness group (140). These associations persist even after adjustment for age, parental history of diabetes, alcohol consumption, and cigarette smoking. Higher levels of fitness are also associated with a reduced risk of developing T2DM in women (141). In another study, middle-aged Finnish men in the lowest quartile of cardiorespiratory fitness (<25.8 mL·kg^{-1}·min^{-1}) were more than four times as likely to develop T2DM as men in the highest two quartiles of fitness (>31.1 mL·kg^{-1}·min^{-1}) (142). A 6-year longitudinal study demonstrated that men in the lowest fitness group (the least fit 20% of the cohort) at the time of enrollment had a greater risk for prediabetes and T2DM compared with those in the highest fitness groups (the most fit 40% of the cohort) (140). Consistent with these data, in individuals at high risk for T2DM, the ADA recommends at least 150 minutes per week to prevent conversion to T2DM (129). Thus, it appears that physical fitness may be a major factor to prevent or reduce the development of T2DM.

T2DM can occur in children and adolescents after the onset of puberty. Risks for T2DM in youth include obesity, reduced physical activity, and the transient influence of pubertal hormones on increasing insulin resistance (143). The restoring insulin secretion (RISE) study demonstrated that insulin resistance in youth is at least twofold increased over results in similar adults (144). Glycemia does relate to insulin resistance (145). The treatment options for T2DM in adolescents and youth (TODAY) study demonstrate that those of Black race, Hispanic ethnicity, and female sex are at higher risk for developing T2DM and that socioeconomic status is lower (146, 147). Rates of prediabetes in youth are also increasing portending a higher T2DM incidence in youth (148).

Gestational Diabetes Mellitus

GDM has been defined for many years as any degree of carbohydrate intolerance with onset or first recognition during pregnancy (149). Hyperglycemia in the first 10 weeks of gestation leads majority of physical birth defects, and hyperglycemia through the pregnancy can lead to small or large for gestational age infants and an increased risk of delivery complications such as preeclampsia and preterm birth. Preconception counseling is suggested for all women and highly recommended for women with existing diabetes or a history of GDM in a previous pregnancy (150). Women with a high risk (central obesity, prior GDM, strong family history of T2DM, PCOS, Black race, and Hispanic ethnicity) for GDM should be screened at the first prenatal visit. Women who do not have known diabetes get screened for GDM at 24–28 weeks of gestation by undergoing a 75-g OGTT. Glycemic targets in pregnancy are lower, with a goal HbA1C of less than 6%, fasting glucose of 70–95 mg·dL^{-1} (3.9–5.3 mmol·L^{-1}), 1-hour postprandial glucose of 110–140 mg·dL^{-1} (6.1–7.8 mmol·L^{-1}), and 2-hour postprandial glucose of 100–120 mg·dL^{-1} (5.6–6.7 mmol·L^{-1}) (149). Treatment for GDM consists of a low glycemic diet, increased physical activity, and insulin therapy (149).

Complications of Diabetes

Complications from diabetes are secondary to hyperglycemia and insulin resistance. Macrovascular complications may include HTN and hyperlipidemia, which contribute to coronary artery disease, stroke, and peripheral artery disease (129). Microvascular complications often include renal disease, diabetic retinopathy, and diabetic neuropathy (125). In individuals with T2DM, there is a higher rate of nonalcoholic fatty liver disease, depression, and obstructive sleep apnea (151, 152). Patients with diabetes should be regularly assessed for early risk markers for disease including a urine microalbumin, fasting lipid panels, alanine aminotransferase, annual eye examinations, and sensory foot examinations (153). It is recommended that patients are seen every 3 months, but a minimum of two times a year. There are sex-related difference in the risk for CVD in T2DM (154). Weight control and normoglycemia are very important for preventing comorbidities (155).

LIFESTYLE APPROACHES FOR PREVENTION OF T2DM

The DPP was a multicenter randomized clinical trial that examined whether a pharmacological approach using medication (metformin) or a lifestyle approach focused on weight loss through diet and physical activity would reduce the onset of developing T2DM (156). Participants initially identified with prediabetes, but not T2DM, were followed up for an average duration of 2.8 years (range 1.8–4.6 years). Results showed that lifestyle intervention resulted in weight loss across the observation period of 5.6 kg (12.35 lb) in the lifestyle group compared to 2.1 kg (4.63 lb) in the group receiving metformin and 0.1 kg (0.22 lb) in the control group receiving placebo. Moreover, the lifestyle approach was the most effective approach to reducing the incidence of T2DM in this cohort of participants ($N = 3,234$). The estimated cumulative incidence of diabetes was 14.4% in the lifestyle group, 21.7% in the metformin group, and 28.9% in the placebo control group. Thus, the incidence of diabetes was 58% and 39% lower in the lifestyle group compared to the placebo control group and the metformin group, respectively. The incidence of diabetes was 31% lower in the metformin group compared to the placebo control group. In an earlier study, Gregg et al. also demonstrated that weight loss of 4.5 kg (9.92 lb), whether achieved through diet, physical activity, or the combination of diet and physical activity, significantly reduced the relative risk of developing T2DM in adults with either normal or prediabetes prior to treatment (157).

Effect of Exercise/Physical Activity in Patients With T1DM

As with healthy individuals and those with T2DM, patients with T1DM should be encouraged to perform regular exercise because of its ability to improve known risk factors for atherosclerosis and CVD. In prospective epidemiological studies, physical activity has been linked to reduced CVD mortality in patients with T1DM (158). During a 6-year follow-up period, patients with T1DM in the lowest quintile of reported baseline physical activity had a sixfold and fourfold all-cause mortality rate in men and women, respectively, compared to the quintile with the highest physical activity level even after controlling for potential confounding variables such as age, BMI, insulin dose, cigarette smoking, and alcohol consumption (158). Many types of exercise are beneficial for those with T1DM (159).

Children and adolescents with T1DM may show signs of atherosclerosis, but those who exercise more than 60 min/d have higher arterial flow-mediated dilation(160), suggesting benefits of physical activity on endothelial function. A randomized controlled clinical trial in patients with T1DM showed that 12–16 weeks of aerobic exercise training at 60%–80% of maximal effort produced favorable changes in lipid, lipoprotein, and apolipoprotein levels. The amount of aerobic activity was inversely associated with TG levels and directly associated with the apolipoprotein AI (APOA1)/apolipoprotein B (APOB) ratio even after controlling for adiposity and glycemic control (161). Six months of exercise training improved HbA1C levels and reduced insulin requirements in children, adolescents, and young adults with T1DM (162). In a meta-analysis of exercise interventions of adults with T1DM, HbA1C levels were reduced by 0.33% units between treatment and controls (163). In summary, the benefits of exercise training in individuals with T1DM include a reduction in CVD risk factors and reduced HbA1C levels; thus, patients are encouraged to perform regular aerobic exercise.

Exercise can affect glucose concentrations, because of exercise-induced muscle glucose uptake (164). Many patients experience overnight hypoglycemia when exercise is performed in the latter half of that day. Some patients have a higher glucose immediately following exercise, but insulin dosing for that may further exacerbate later hypoglycemia. Hypoglycemia is best managed with the use of a pump and continuous glucose monitor, where the system stops insulin delivery when blood sugars decline (165). There are also challenges when a patient uses a pump but is in a sport such as swimming where a pump can be used. Careful coordination between the endocrinologist and exercises specialist is needed.

Effects of Exercise/Physical Activity on Risk for T2DM

The clinical importance of physical activity in T2DM is underscored by studies that indicate that a low level of physical fitness is associated with increased risk of all-cause and CVD mortality (166–168). Men who improve their physical fitness reduce their all-cause mortality risk by approximately 44% (169). Significant progress has been made toward an understanding of the molecular basis underlying the beneficial effects of exercise training in stimulating the entry of glucose into tissue responsive to insulin action (170, 171). Accordingly, it is well accepted that regular physical exercise offers an effective therapeutic intervention to improve insulin action in skeletal muscle and adipose tissue in insulin-resistant individuals. Chronic exercise results in numerous physiologic and cellular adaptations that favor sustained improvement in insulin action (168, 170). The link between physical inactivity and insulin resistance was first noted in migrant populations who experienced dramatic increases in the incidence of T2DM after exposure to a more westernized environment that was quite different from their traditional lifestyles. Japanese migrants living in Hawaii had an elevated risk of T2DM compared to their counterparts living in Hiroshima (172). Likewise, Pima Indians in rural Mexico living a traditional Pima Indian lifestyle have markedly lower rates of T2DM compared to the Arizona Pima's consuming a westernized diet and maintaining a sedentary lifestyle (173). The difference in the prevalence of T2DM in these populations despite the similarity in genetic background can directly be attributed to changes in lifestyle behavior, in particular the level of habitual physical activity.

Additional evidence to support the hypothesis that physical inactivity plays a significant role in the increased incidence of T2DM is provided by observational and retrospective studies (174). Data from the University of Pennsylvania Alumni study document a 6% lower risk of T2DM for each 500 kcal per week of self-reported leisure-time physical activity (175). In the Physician Health Studies, the risk of T2DM was approximately 35% lower for females who reported vigorous exercise at least once per week, whereas men who exercised vigorously five or more times per week showed a 42% reduction in the age-adjusted risk of T2DM compared to those who exercised less than once per week, suggesting a dose–response relationship between increased physical activity and T2DM risk (176).

Prospective studies also document the beneficial effects that physical activity and fitness (44, 129) play in reducing the incidence of T2DM. The Nurses' Health Study showed that brisk walking for at least 2.5 hours per week was associated with a 25% reduction in T2DM over an 8-year follow-up period (176). Data from the Women's Health Study demonstrated that participants who reported walking 2–3 hours per week were 34% less likely to develop T2DM than women who reported no exercise (177). Furthermore, in the Women's Health Initiative Observational Study, participants in the lowest quartile of total energy and walking energy expenditure had, respectively, a 22% and 18% higher risk of developing T2DM compared to women in the highest quartiles (178). These studies support the hypothesis that a sedentary lifestyle

and low cardiorespiratory fitness play a significant role in the progression from normal glucose tolerance to T2DM. In a small sample of individuals with T2DM, aerobic training alone and a combined exercise program of aerobic and resistive training reduced HbA1C after only 16 weeks (179). In a randomized clinical trial of 39- to 70-year-old men and women with T2DM, 6-month community-based programs of aerobic, resistive, and aerobic plus resistive training also reduced HbA1C, with the greatest effect observed in the combined group (180). A meta-analysis of 14 randomized clinical trials indicates a 0.74 percentage point reduction in HbA1C after moderate-intensity exercise training in patients with T2DM compared to no change in a control group (181). High-intensity resistance training interventions were also very effective in reducing HbA1C in patients with T2DM with an absolute change of up to 1.2% (182, 183). A review of the literature of yoga-based programs indicated that yoga may improve risk profiles of individuals with T2DM, but considering the limitations of many of the 25 studies that were reviewed, no firm conclusions can be drawn about the effectiveness of this type of physical activity (184).

Exercise also reduces comorbidities in T2DM. In a randomized clinical trial, an exercise program consisting of 2 days per week aerobic and resistive training improved physical fitness and reduced HbA1C levels, systolic and diastolic BP, LDL, and waist circumference compared to a counseling control group (185). Maintaining a healthy body weight, not smoking, exercising moderately or vigorously 30 minutes per day, and eating a lower calorie and saturated fat diet results in more than an 80% reduction in the incidence of coronary events (44, 168, 186). Therefore, increased physical activity, along with a heart-healthy diet, is an effective treatment that yields significant health benefits in patients with T2DM.

MEDICAL TREATMENT OF T1DM

Insulin therapy is required in T1DM to control hyperglycemia (187). There are two primary insulin delivery methods: multiday injections with a long-acting insulin to control hepatic glucose release and a rapid-acting insulin administered at the time of meals. However, there are four types of insulin to allow for precise dosing: rapid-acting (peak action: 0.5–1.0 hours), short-acting (peak action: 2–3 hours), intermediate-acting (peak action: 4–10 hours), or long-acting (peak action: sustained for 20–24 hours). The other option that is becoming more popular is an insulin pump, which is loaded with a short-acting insulin which is given at different rates at all-time (187). Glucose control is generally better with the pumps. Further, current pumps can coordinate with a continuous glucose monitor and can decrease insulin delivery in the setting of hypoglycemia (188). Medications for insulin sensitivity such as metformin have been demonstrated to induce improvements in metabolic health in those with T1DM (189, 190).

MEDICAL TREATMENT OF T2DM

T2DM is a complex chronic disease that requires adequate management of hyperglycemia, its microvascular and macrovascular complications, and other comorbid physiologic dysfunctions such as dyslipidemia, HTN, and elevated thrombotic factors, which are highly associated with insulin resistance and increase the risk for CVD (129, 153, 168). Therefore, achieving metabolic control via tight monitoring of fasting and postprandial glucose and HbA1C is essential. Approaches for managing dysglycemia and weight need to include shared decision-making to set therapeutic goals, Specific Measurable Achievable Responsive Timely — SMART goals, continued patient engagement, and a culturally sensitive approach (153). Because of the beneficial effects of improved insulin sensitivity, improved glucose tolerance, and reduction in the risk of cardiovascular complications, the first line of therapy for patients newly diagnosed with T2DM is the implementation of an intensive lifestyle modification of increased physical activity and adoption of a heart-healthy diet (44, 129). A common recommendation is to reduce body weight by 5%–10%. Weight loss up to 10% improves insulin sensitivity and, in overweight individuals with T2DM, has been shown to reduce fasting blood glucose (FBG) by 2–3 mmol·L^{-1} and HbA1C by 1 or more percentage points (191). However, the United Kingdom Prospective Diabetes Study demonstrated that only 25% of the patients were able to maintain the optimal HbA1C levels of less than 7% after 9 years without an oral agent or insulin (192). The Look AHEAD Study in patients with T2DM and obesity found that the lifestyle intervention was effective at eliciting weight loss, improving diabetes control, and improving many cardiometabolic risk factors after the initial year of treatment (193); however, weight regain and regression in the cardiometabolic improvements occurred in subsequent years (194, 195). The researchers proposed that this regain and regression reflected the inability of study participants to maintain the

recommended dietary patterns and physical activity. Although there was no decrease in comorbidity risk after 9.6 years, there was a relationship between greater weight loss and decrease in CVD comorbidities, with a threshold of 10% weight loss (196). These data suggest that long-term compliance with lifestyle programs is important but tends to be less than optimal and that mediations are required for most. Other nonpharmacologic treatments include screening for and treating obstructive sleep apnea that is common in individuals with T2DM and can contribute to hyperglycemia (152).

Metformin

Upon failure of glycemic or weight goals, the primary pharmaceutical recommendation is to start metformin, with a target dose of 2,000 mg per day (187, 197, 198). The most common side effects are nausea, vomiting, and diarrhea, and thus patients work up to the full dose over the course of a month. There is also a rare risk of lactic acidosis, which can be prevented by adequate hydration. Metformin typically reduces fasting glucose by 2–4 mmol·L^{-1} with corresponding decreases in HbA1C of 1–2 percentage points (187). Metformin works improving insulin action in hepatic tissue, adipose tissue (199), and, to a lesser extent, in skeletal muscle (187, 189, 200, 201).

Glucagon-Like Peptide-1 Receptor Agonists

GLP-1 RAs reduce hyperglycemia and weight (187, 198). Exenatide treatment typically result in a 0.5- to 1.0-percentage point decrease in HbA1C, 1.4 mmol·L^{-1} decrease in fasting plasma glucose (FPG), and a 2- to 3-kg (4.4–6.6 lb) decline in body mass, whereas liraglutide results in a 1% decline in HbA1C and a 1- to 3-kg (2.2–3.3 lb) body mass loss (187, 202, 203). Most recently, there is a trend for using semaglutide, as it has superior reductions in glycemia and weight loss compared to other available medications in this class (204). After treatment of 2.0 injectable semaglutide for 40 weeks, adults with a mean HbA1C of 8.9% at baseline had a 2.1% reduction in HbA1C compared with a 1.9% reduction for those assigned 1 mg semaglutide (205). GLP-1 RAs are not currently considered first line and are often added to metformin with impressive effects (206). Treatment with GLP-1 RAs has also been shown to reduce progression of CVD, making them a good choice for those with existing or at high risk for CVD (207).

Sodium Glucose Transporter

Sodium glucose transporter 2 (SGLT-2) medications work by reducing the renal threshold for glucose excretion from 200 mg·dL^{-1} to approximately 140–160 mg·dL^{-1} (198). They have been shown to reduce HbA1C by 2.1%–2.3% as compared to placebo (187, 208). In addition to improving dysglycemia, they have impressive effects on not only preventing CVD progression, but actually reducing the severity of existing CVD, in particular heart failure (207, 209). They are now recommended for CVD indications and are included in American Heart Association guidelines (210, 211). Concomitant with improved cardiac outcomes, exercise tolerance is improved with SGLT-2 (212). SGLT-2 should not be used in those with severe renal impairment, and they increase the risk of normoglycemic ketoacidosis (187).

Thiazolidinediones

Thiazolidinediones (TZDs), such as pioglitazone, are also insulin sensitizers that improve whole-body insulin sensitivity via multiple actions on gene regulation (198). TZD treatment effectively control glycemia by altering cellular mechanisms in tissues such as muscle, adipose tissue, and liver, thereby improving insulin action (200). The metabolic effects observed in skeletal muscle tissue include increases in glucose uptake, glycolysis, glucose oxidation, and inconsistent changes in glycogenesis. The metabolic effects observed in adipose tissue include an increase in glucose uptake, fatty acid uptake, lipogenesis, and preadipocyte differentiation. The metabolic effects observed in the liver include a decrease in gluconeogenesis, glycogenolysis, and an increase in lipogenesis and glucose uptake. TZD agents reduce HbA1C by 0.5–1.5 percentage points (187). Their use has decreased secondary to weight gain and after concerns for heart disease were published (187, 213).

GLP-1 RAs/Glucagon Inhibiting Protein

The mechanisms of this class of medications and the only current drug tirzepatide are discussed above. In addition to impressive weight loss, the medications have a remarkable effect in lowering HbA1C (range of 2.1%–2.3% decrease in HbA1C) (214, 215). Additionally, a recent study revealed that tirzepatide is more effective than semaglutide for weight loss and reductions in HbA1C (216). Tirzepatide also reduces hepatic fat in individuals with T2DM and nonalcoholic fatty liver disease (217).

Dipeptidylpeptidase-4 Inhibitors

Dipeptidylpeptidase-4 (DPP-4) work as inhibitors and prolong and enhance the activity of the insulin secretagogue, incretin. The main two molecules that fulfill the criteria for being an incretin, GLP-1 and GIP, are intestinal hormones that amplify the postprandial secretion of insulin but are rapidly degraded by the enzyme DPP-4. DPP-4 inhibitors decrease HbA1C by 0.5–1.0 percentage points (218). They also improve fasting and postprandial glucose, with low risk of hypoglycemia (219–221). Because of improved efficacy of GLP-1 RAs and SGLTs, these are no longer commonly used, except in patients with contradictions to the prior medication classes (187, 198).

Amylinomimetic Agents

Amylinomimetic agents, such as pramlintide, are synthetic versions of the human hormone called "amylin," which modulates gastric emptying, prevents the postprandial rise in plasma glucagon, and causes early satiety (222). Provided through subcutaneous injections, amylinomimetic agents decrease HbA1C by 0.5%–1.0% points and body mass by approximately 2 kg (4.4 lb).

Insulin Secretagogues

Insulin secretagogues, such as sulfonylureas and glinides, lower circulating blood glucose by enhancing pancreatic insulin secretion (187, 223). However, because the hypoglycemic effect of this class of drugs is attributable to increased insulin secretion, its effectiveness is highly dependent on adequate β-cell function. Fasting glucose levels decrease with these drugs by 2–4 mmol·L^{-1} with an accompanying decrease in HbA1C of 1–2 percentage points (223). Enthusiasm for these medication has decreased, as it has been demonstrated that they accelerate the need for use of exogenous insulin (187).

Bromocriptine, a dopamine agonist, when dosed with the quick release formulation "Cycloset" has been shown to have limited efficacy in glucose control in T2DM (187, 224). The benefits are an oral preparation, but side effects and limited efficacy have precluded widespread use of this medication.

Insulin

Insulin is usually the last line of treatment and is reserved for those patients who fail to respond adequately to a combination of orals and injectable antidiabetic agents, whose glycemic control continues to deteriorate despite adequate drug combinations, and for whom safety and efficacy considerations favor its use as the drug of choice, such as in cases of pregnancy or severe hepatic and renal impairments (149, 187). In patients who present with a very high HbA1C, insulin can be used briefly for immediate glucose control, whereas oral or injectable medications are titrated to an effective dose. Insulin is typically constrained to long-acting formations, with postprandial dosing either by short-acting insulin or an insulin pump reserved for individuals with more extreme β-cell failure (187).

Treatments for Youth

ADA recommendations for treatment of dysglycemia in youth with diabetes are distinct from those for adults (127). The primary therapy for T2DM in youth is lifestyle modification and metformin, based on evidence that these can reduce hyperglycemia and diabetes complications (197). In youth with T2DM, the TODAY demonstrated that failure of oral medications metformin or thiazolidinediones or lifestyle occurred more rapidly than in adults and related to race and ethnicity (225, 226). Aggressive control of HbA1C is recommended, often requiring off-label use of new medication, as the rate of related morbidity and mortality in youth-onset T2DM is greatly accelerated (227). MBS is also highly recommended, as it can promote remission of T2DM in youth, especially compared to medical and lifestyle therapy (85).

POLYCYSTIC OVARY SYNDROME

PCOS is a condition of elevated testosterone and menstrual irregularities. It is a leading cause of female infertility and is closely associated with obesity and metabolic disease (228). PCOS often manifests in adolescence with persistently irregular menses and symptoms of excess testosterone such a hirsutism, acne, and androgenic alopecia, although many women are not diagnosed until adulthood when they seek care for difficulty with conception, or presentation for endometrial hyperplasia or carcinoma (229–232). The diagnosis for PCOS was defined most recently in the 2018 international guidelines, which merged previous contradictory definitions. Women with PCOS have irregular menses, clinical and laboratory evidence of elevated testosterone, and in women more than 8 years postmenarche, ultrasound of the ovary is also used (228). The cause of PCOS is not known (233). There are

three popular theories for the cause of hyperandrogenism: (i) functional ovarian dysfunction, (ii) insulin resistance and hyperinsulinism inducing theca cell hypertrophy, and (iii) hypothalamic/pituitary dysfunction causing an increased luteinizing hormone (LH) production (234–236). All of these pathways have been shown to be abnormal in PCOS, although which one is primary is unclear.

Metabolic Disease Related to PCOS

Women with PCOS are more likely to have overweight or obesity, although the exact prevalence is unknown, because of many patients not having a formal diagnosis (228). Women with PCOS have very high rates of metabolic syndrome, which may vary by race and ethnicity (237–240). Related to the increase in metabolic syndrome are very high rates of insulin resistance, which can be measured in women without obesity as well (241–245). The relative risk of developing T2DM is almost eight times higher in women with PCOS and obesity and two times in women without obesity, and is 18-fold higher in adolescents with PCOS (228, 246, 247). It is not clear if there is an increase in primary outcomes of myocardial infarction, stroke, or CVD-related death in women with PCOS, although risk factors for CVD including HTN, hyperlipidemia, early atherosclerosis deposition, and endothelial dysfunction is present in women with PCOS (248). Rates of nonalcoholic fatty liver disease are higher in PCOS, even in adolescents (244, 249).

Treatment for PCOS

The primary treatment for all women with PCOS, regardless of BMI, is lifestyle modification. Similar to diabetes, SMART goals should be created with patient involvement, and providers should "use a respectful and considerate approach" (228). For lean women, this includes 60 minutes vigorous activity three times a week. In women who have overweight or obesity, there is more than 5% weight loss goal, as weight loss has been associated with improvement in menstrual frequency in up to 60% of women. Activity recommendations include 250 minutes of moderate or 150 vigorous activities. However, the data supporting these guidelines are a little controversial (250). In terms of diet, the recommended energy deficit is 30% (1,200–1,500 kcal/day) (228). Because of these more ambitious goals, the use of weight loss medications is encouraged (228). Other strategies for weight loss from women with PCOS, including different types of exercise and diet recommendations, have recently been reviewed (253). Briefly, there are similar results to high-intensity exercise compared to aerobic exercise, and a lower glycemic diet is favored, but the best diet is the one that the patient prefers and induces weight loss (251–253).

Medications for PCOS are primarily estrogen-containing contraceptives and metformin (228, 254, 255). Other therapies such as long-acting progestins, which help with endometrial protection are also used (256). In terms of cosmetic treatment, antiandrogens such as spironolactone can be used, although these can cause a lower BP at higher dose (200 mg/day), so care should be taken in initiating an exercise protocol in these women (228). Thioglitazones are very effect for restoring menstrual cycles and treatment metabolic syndrome; however, their use is limited because of associated weight gain (228, 257). Weight loss medications including topiramate, phentermine, and GLP-1 RAs are also used (as previously described) (228, 251). Limited data on bariatric surgery are also very promising (258).

There are several other related comorbidities that may need to be addressed prior to being able to enact lifestyle changes. Women with PCOS have a twofold to threefold risk for obstructive sleep apnea, and treatment of this can lead to metabolic improvements, independent of weight loss (228, 259–262). Rates of depression, anxiety, and sexual dysfunction are also higher in women with PCOS (228, 263–265). Often, starting treatment for psychological conditions is required prior to patients being able to enact lifestyle changes (266). In summary, the potential treatment options for PCOS are varied and should be tailored to the individual patients' preferences and metabolic need.

OTHER ENDOCRINE CONDITIONS WITH EXERCISE IMPLICATIONS

There are several other endocrine conditions that can be accompanied by obesity or have exercise limitations. Once treated, exercise guidelines for the general population can be applied, although responses may vary.

Thyroid

Significant hyperthyroidism is often accompanied by HTN and tachycardia at rest, and cardiovascular and metabolic changes during exercise are abnormal (267, 268). Exercise that elevates the heart rate further should be avoided in these patients, until their hyperthyroidism has been controlled. However, once thyroid concentrations are normalized, even 3 weeks of walking and strength training exercises are beneficial (269). In the hypothyroid state, the overall metabolic rate is decreased through multiple mechanisms, weight gain is often present as are cardiovascular abnormalities (270). Again, exercise should be avoided when bradycardia is present during inadequately treated hypothyroidism. However, once hypothyroidism is treated, patients can participate in the exercise program deemed best by the CEP.

Hypogonadism

In both males and females with hypogonadism, exercise performance can be lower than anticipated, and efforts to build muscle mass attenuated. However, exercise is important to both mediate CVD risk and increase loading on the bone to improve bone health (271). Testosterone replacement, when done at physiologic levels, improves exercise performance in men, but monitoring for signs of androgenic steroid abuse is critical (272).

Adrenal Insufficiency

Medical adrenal insufficiency is defined as inadequate cortisol release, either because of abnormalities in the adrenal gland or in the hypothalamus/pituitary and is confirmed with standardized medical testing (273, 274). Currently, nonmedically diagnosed adrenal insufficiency is blamed for fatigue, weight gain, difficultly sleeping, or exercising and a number of other health complaints. Findings from individuals with true disease, such as autoimmune Addison disease or genetic congenital adrenal hyperplasia are described here. Exercise in the setting of untreated adrenal disease can be dangerous, as the body cannot produce the required cortisol, and in the case of primary adrenal disease, epinephrine and leptin, for a normal exercise response and hypoglycemia and hypotension may ensue (275, 276). In individuals with treated Addison adrenal insufficiency cardiometabolic responses to 1 hour of intensive exercise were lower than healthy controls and did not improve when additional hydrocortisone was administered (277). Similar results were found in treated individuals with congenital adrenal hyperplasia performing short high-intensity exercise (275, 278). Treated adults with congenital adrenal hyperplasia also had abnormal exercise responses following 90-minutes of brisk walking (279). It is unknown if additional stress hydrocortisone should be given for prolonged intense races such as marathons or triathlons. Perhaps in part because of this attenuated response to exercise, individuals with congenital adrenal hyperplasia have increased central adiposity and higher risks for cardiometabolic disease (280,

281). This underscores the need for exercise in these individuals once they are adequately treated, even if the responses are less.

SUMMARY

Exercise is critical in the treatment and prevention of overweight/obesity, DM, and PCOS. It should be considered a critical part of a comprehensive patient plan, which may include dietary modification and medical or surgical management. Plans may need to be tailored for the needs and conditions of the patient.

CHAPTER REVIEW QUESTIONS

1. A patient presents with a BMI that meets the criteria for obesity. They are willing to engage in a treatment program for 3–6 months to determine if this can be effective for weight loss before considering more advanced medical treatments for her obesity such as pharmacotherapy or bariatric surgery. What is the most appropriate lifestyle approach to maximize weight loss during this 3- to 6-month period that will be both efficacious and safe?

2. A patient presents with obesity and is interested in making changes to their diet that will facilitate weight loss. What would you recommend as the most appropriate dietary approach that will be effective for weight loss in this patient?

3. A patient recently engaged in a weight loss program and lost 11.3 kg (25 lb) over 6 months. The patient has lost this much weight in the past, only to regain weight over the subsequent 6–12 months. What advice can be given to this patient to increase the likelihood that they will be successful in maintaining the weight loss?

4. An adult is concerned about age-related weight gain as they get older and has heard about the negative health outcomes associated with sitting. Thus, this individual has invested in a standing desk at their office. However, despite using this standing desk for about 2 hours of each working day, they continue to experience gradual weight gain. What might explain why this reduced sedentary behavior is not effective to prevent weight gain?

5. An adult who is overweight initiates a resistance training exercise program with the goal of losing 10% of their current body weight. After engaging in this program for a period of 6 months, they have not observed any change in weight. What factors might

explain this lack of weight loss with resistance exercise training?

6. An adult has a biological parent and at least one sibling who has been diagnosed with T2DM. Thus, they are concerned about developing T2DM and seeks the advice of a health fitness professional regarding approaches to reduce their risk. What approaches should the health fitness professional suggest to this individual to reduce their risk of developing T2DM?

7. There is likely a genetic and/or metabolic predisposition for some individuals to have a greater risk of developing T2DM compared to others. Knowing this may cause some patients to request medications to prevent or treat T2DM, what evidence suggests that modifiable lifestyle factors contribute to the development of T2DM and should be important lifestyle intervention targets for treatment?

8. What is the primary treatment for PCOS? How does it differ for lean women with PCOS and those with obesity? What other kinds of treatment are recommended?

9. There is a common perception that when men start an exercise training program they lose more weight than do women. Does the evidence support that viewpoint? If not, what explains early study results suggesting there was a difference between the sexes in the efficacy of exercise training for weight loss?

10. Based on relatively low total energy expended during exercise and the knowledge that a larger percentage of energy comes from fat during low-intensity exercise, it might seem unlikely that high-intensity interval training (HIIT) would be a big part of a training plan designed to drive weight loss. Do you agree? If not, what rationale would you have for incorporating HIIT into your recommendations for a client highly motivated to lose weight?

Case Study 10.1

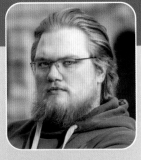

Jorge, a 35-year-old male patient, presents at a clinical visit for an annual physical examination. Prior to this visit, blood was drawn for a fasting blood panel. All values are within normal ranges. Clinical measurements during the visit include nonmedicated resting heart rate (68 beats per minute [bpm]), nonmedicated resting BP (systolic: 118 mm Hg; diastolic: 68 mm Hg), and BMI (32.5 kg·m^{-2}). The health history indicates that the patient reports engaging in structured physical activity in the form of walking on 3–4 days per week for approximately 30 minutes per session, and this has been ongoing for approximately 3 months. However, the patient reports disappointment in his weight loss, which has been a total of 1.8 kg (4 lb) during this period and says that he expected greater weight loss given his effort to regularly engage in physical activity. The physician seeks the advice of an exercise physiologist on this matter prior to counseling the patient. Consider the following when determining the appropriate advice that should be used to direct the care of this patient.

Case Study 10.1 Questions

1. What factors should be considered with regard to the patient's current physical activity that may elicit a greater weight loss response?

2. What dietary changes could elicit a greater weight loss response for this patient?

Case Study 10.2

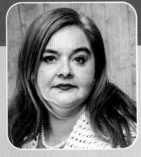

Chanda, a 45-year-old female patient, presents at a clinical visit for an annual physical examination. Prior to this visit, blood was drawn for a fasting blood panel that reveals high TG and FPG indicative of impaired glucose tolerance (IGT). Clinical measurements during the visit include nonmedicated resting heart rate (72 bpm), nonmedicated resting BP (systolic: 130 mm Hg; diastolic: 88 mm Hg), BMI (34.7 kg·m^{-2}), and waist circumference (38 inches, 96.5 cm). The health history also indicates that the patient gave birth to two children over the past 10 years and that both weighed more than 4.08 kg (9 lb), and the patient currently does not report engaging in regular periods of moderate-to-vigorous physical activity.

Case Study 10.2 Questions

1. The physician evaluating this patient is concerned that the patient is at risk for developing T2DM. What factors indicate that this concern is warranted?

2. What treatment plan should be considered for this patient to provide the greatest potential reduction in risk for developing T2DM?

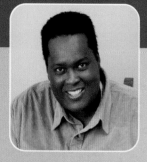

Case Study 10.3

Jeff, a 52-year-old male patient, presents at a clinical visit for an annual physical examination. Prior to this visit, blood was drawn for a fasting blood panel that reveals elevated fasting TG, a low level of HDL cholesterol, and elevated FPG. During the examination, it is determined that the patient has a BMI that meets the criteria for obesity, a waist circumference that meets the criteria for elevated abdominal adiposity, and elevated BP. The health history reveals that the patient engages in regular physical activity for 30 minutes per day on 5–6 days per week and reports eating a low-fat diet, which has been the patient's typical lifestyle pattern for the past 6 months.

Case Study 10.3 Questions

1. The physician evaluating this patient is concerned about the presence of metabolic syndrome and will begin to treat these numerous risk factors. However, both the physician and the patient are surprised that regular physical activity is not effective in impacting these risk factors, and a follow-up graded exercise test demonstrates that the cardiorespiratory fitness of the patient is low. What other interventions are potentially helpful for this patient?

2. The metabolic syndrome consists of numerous risk factors, and many are present in this patient. Given the presence of so many of these risk factors, how should the physician prioritize the treatment plan for this patient?

REFERENCES

1. Freedman DS, Sherry B. The validity of BMI as an indicator of body fatness and risk among children. *Pediatrics.* 2009;124(Suppl 1):S23–34.

2. Jih J, Mukherjea A, Vittinghoff E, et al. Using appropriate body mass index cut points for overweight and obesity among Asian Americans. *Prev Med.* 2014;65:1–6.

3. Jensen MD, Ryan DH, Apovian CM, et al; American College of Cardiology/American Heart Association Task Force on Practice Guidelines; Obesity Society. 2013 AHA/ACC/TOS guideline for the management of overweight and obesity in adults: a report of the American College of Cardiology/American Heart Association task force on practice guidelines and The Obesity Society. *Circulation.* 2014;129(25 Suppl 2): S102–38.

4. US Preventive Services Task Force; Grossman DC, Bibbins-Domingo K, Curry SJ, et al. Screening for obesity in children and adolescents: US Preventive Services Task Force recommendation statement. *JAMA.* 2017;317(23):2417–26.

5. Misra A. Ethnic-specific criteria for classification of body mass index: a perspective for Asian Indians and American Diabetes Association position statement. *Diabetes Technol Ther.* 2015;17(9):667–71.

6. Hales CM, Carroll MD, Fryar CD, Ogden CL. Prevalence of obesity and severe obesity among adults: United States, 2017–2018. *NCHS Data Brief.* 2020;(360):1–8.

7. Skinner AC, Ravanbakht SN, Skelton JA, Perrin EM, Armstrong SC. Prevalence of obesity and severe obesity in US children, 1999–2016. *Pediatrics.* 2018;141(3):e20173459.

8. World Health Organization. Obesity and overweight. 2017. Available from: http://www.who.int/en/news-room/fact-sheets/detail/obesity-and-overweight.

9. Benedetti L, Guiotto R. Atypical echographic image of hepatic miliary tuberculosis. *Radiol Med.* 1988;76(1–2):107–8.

10. Donnelly JE, Blair SN, Jakicic JM, Manore MM, Rankin JW, Smith BK; American College of Sports Medicine. American College of Sports Medicine position stand. Appropriate physical activity intervention strategies for weight loss and prevention of weight regain for adults. *Med Sci Sports Exerc.* 2009;41(2):459–71.

11. Swift DL, McGee JE, Earnest CP, Carlisle E, Nygard M, Johannsen NM. The effects of exercise and physical activity on weight loss and maintenance. *Prog Cardiovasc Dis.* 2018;61(2):206–13.

12. King AC, Whitt-Glover MC, Marquez DX, et al; 2018 Physical Activity Guidelines Advisory Committee. Physical activity promotion: highlights from the 2018 Physical Activity Guidelines Advisory Committee systematic review. *Med Sci Sports Exerc.* 2019;51(6):1340–53.

13. Hall KD, Guo J. Obesity energetics: body weight regulation and the effects of diet composition. *Gastroenterology.* 2017;152(7):1718–27.e3.

14. Gordon GD, Commerford PJ. Myocardial salvage—a perspective. *S Afr Med J.* 1988;73(9):509–10.

15. Bray GA, Heisel WE, Afshin A, et al. The science of obesity management: an Endocrine Society scientific statement. *Endocr Rev.* 2018;39(2):79–132.

16. Varkevisser RDM, van Stralen MM, Kroeze W, Ket JCF, Steenhuis IHM. Determinants of weight loss maintenance: a systematic review. *Obes Rev.* 2019;20(2):171–211.

17. Donnelly JE, Hill JO, Jacobsen DJ, et al. Effects of a 16-month randomized controlled exercise trial on body weight and composition in young, overweight men and women: the Midwest Exercise Trial. *Arch Intern Med.* 2003;163(11): 1343–50.

18. Donnelly JE, Washburn RA, Smith BK, et al. A randomized, controlled, supervised, exercise trial in young overweight men and women: the Midwest Exercise Trial II (MET2). *Contemp Clin Trials.* 2012;33(4):804–10.

19. King NA, Horner K, Hills AP, et al. Exercise, appetite and weight management: understanding the compensatory responses in eating behaviour and how they contribute to variability in exercise-induced weight loss. *Br J Sports Med.* 2012;46(5): 315–22.

20. Schubert MM, Washburn RA, Honas JJ, Lee J, Donnelly JE. Exercise volume and aerobic fitness in young adults: the Midwest Exercise Trial-2. *Springerplus.* 2016;5:183.

21. Piercy KL, Troiano RP, Ballard RM, et al. The Physical Activity Guidelines for Americans. *JAMA.* 2018;320(19):2020–8.

22. Caudwell P, Gibbons C, Hopkins M, King N, Finlayson G, Blundell J. No sex difference in body fat in response to supervised and measured exercise. *Med Sci Sports Exerc.* 2013;45(2):351–8.

23. Jakicic JM, Powell KE, Campbell WW, et al; 2018 Physical Activity Guidelines Advisory Committee. Physical activity and the prevention of weight gain in adults: a systematic review. *Med Sci Sports Exerc.* 2019;51(6):1262–9.

24. Morss GM, Jordan AN, Skinner JS, et al. Dose response to exercise in women aged 45–75 yr (DREW): design and rationale. *Med Sci Sports Exerc.* 2004;36(2):336–44.

25. Slentz CA, Duscha BD, Johnson JL, et al. Effects of the amount of exercise on body weight, body composition, and measures of central obesity: STRRIDE—a randomized controlled study. *Arch Intern Med.* 2004;164(1):31–9.

26. Houmard JA, Tanner CJ, Slentz CA, Duscha BD, McCartney JS, Kraus WE. Effect of the volume and intensity of exercise training on insulin sensitivity. *J Appl Physiol (1985).* 2004;96(1):101–6.

27. AbouAssi H, Slentz CA, Mikus CR, et al. The effects of aerobic, resistance, and combination training on insulin sensitivity and secretion in overweight adults from STRRIDE AT/RT: a randomized trial. *J Appl Physiol (1985).* 2015;118(12): 1474–82.

28. Wakamatsu Y, Obika M, Ozato K. Induction of xanthophores from non-pigmented dermal cells of xanthic goldfish in vitro. *Cell Differ.* 1987;20(2–3):161–70.

29. Yin F, He H, Zhang B, et al. Effect of deubiquitinase ovarian tumor domain-containing protein 5 (OTUD5) on radiosensitivity of cervical cancer by regulating the ubiquitination of Akt and its mechanism. *Med Sci Monit.* 2019;25:3469–75.

30. Redman LM, Heilbronn LK, Martin CK, et al; Pennington CALERIE Team. Metabolic and behavioral compensations in response to caloric restriction: implications for the maintenance of weight loss. *PLoS One.* 2009;4(2):e4377.

31. Catenacci VA, Ogden LG, Stuht J, et al. Physical activity patterns in the National Weight Control Registry. *Obesity (Silver Spring).* 2008;16(1):153–61.

32. Goodpaster BH, Delany JP, Otto AD, et al. Effects of diet and physical activity interventions on weight loss and cardiometabolic risk factors in severely obese adults: a randomized trial. *JAMA.* 2010;304(16):1795–802.

33. Catenacci VA, Grunwald GK, Ingebrigtsen JP, et al. Physical activity patterns using accelerometry in the National Weight Control Registry. *Obesity (Silver Spring).* 2011;19(6):1163–70.

34. Pi-Sunyer X. The Look AHEAD trial: a review and discussion of its outcomes. *Curr Nutr Rep.* 2014;3(4):387–91.

35. Looney SM, Raynor HA. Behavioral lifestyle intervention in the treatment of obesity. *Health Serv Insights.* 2013;6:15–31.

36. Jakicic JM, Rogers RJ, Donnelly JE. The health risks of obesity have not been exaggerated. *Med Sci Sports Exerc.* 2019;51(1):222–5.

37. Schoeller DA, Shay K, Kushner RF. How much physical activity is needed to minimize weight gain in previously obese women? *Am J Clin Nutr.* 1997;66(3):551–6.

38. Vos NJ, Pollock PJ, Harty M, Brennan T, de Blaauw S, McAllister H. Fractures of the cervical vertebral odontoid in four horses and one pony. *Vet Rec.* 2008;162(4):116–9.

39. Jakicic JM, Tate DF, Lang W, et al. Objective physical activity and weight loss in adults: the step-up randomized clinical trial. *Obesity (Silver Spring).* 2014;22(11):2284–92.

40. Creasy SA, Lang W, Tate DF, Davis KK, Jakicic JM. Pattern of daily steps is associated with weight loss: secondary analysis from the step-up randomized trial. *Obesity (Silver Spring).* 2018;26(6):977–84.

41. Pontzer H, Durazo-Arvizu R, Dugas LR, et al. Constrained total energy expenditure and metabolic adaptation to physical activity in adult humans. *Curr Biol.* 2016;26(3):410–7.

42. Fothergill E, Guo J, Howard L, et al. Persistent metabolic adaptation 6 years after "The Biggest Loser" competition. *Obesity (Silver Spring).* 2016;24(8):1612–9.

43. Kerns JC, Guo J, Fothergill E, et al. Increased physical activity associated with less weight regain six years after "The Biggest Loser" competition. *Obesity (Silver Spring).* 2017;25(11):1838–43.

44. American Diabetes Association Professional Practice Committee. 5. Facilitating behavior change and well-being to improve health outcomes: Standards of Medical Care in Diabetes—2022. *Diabetes Care.* 2022;45(Suppl 1):S60–82.

45. Ryan DH, Yockey SR. Weight loss and improvement in comorbidity: differences at 5%, 10%, 15%, and over. *Curr Obes Rep.* 2017; 6(2):187–94.

46. Lean ME, Leslie WS, Barnes AC, et al. Primary care-led weight management for remission of type 2 diabetes (DiRECT): an open-label, cluster-randomised trial. *Lancet.* 2018;391(10120):541–51.

47. Aguilar-Martínez A, Solé-Sedeño JM, Mancebo-Moreno G, Medina FX, Carreras-Collado R, Saigí-Rubió F. Use of mobile phones as a tool for weight loss: a systematic review. *J Telemed Telecare.* 2014;20(6):339–49.

48. Gudzune KA, Doshi RS, Mehta AK, et al. Efficacy of commercial weight-loss programs: an updated systematic review. *Ann Intern Med.* 2015;162(7):501–12.

49. Chin SO, Keum C, Woo J, et al. Successful weight reduction and maintenance by using a smartphone application in those with overweight and obesity. *Sci Rep*. 2016;6:34563.

50. Moreno B, Bellido D, Sajoux I, et al. Comparison of a very low-calorie-ketogenic diet with a standard low-calorie diet in the treatment of obesity. *Endocrine*. 2014;47(3):793–805.

51. Senechal M, Arguin H, Bouchard DR, et al. Effects of rapid or slow weight loss on body composition and metabolic risk factors in obese postmenopausal women. A pilot study. *Appetite*. 2012;58(3):831–4.

52. Ludwig DS, Ebbeling CB. The carbohydrate-insulin model of obesity: beyond "Calories In, Calories Out." *JAMA Intern Med*. 2018;178(8):1098–103.

53. Wheless JW, History of the ketogenic diet. *Epilepsia*. 2008; 49(Suppl 8):3–5.

54. Nordmann AJ, Nordmann A, Briel M, et al. Effects of low-carbohydrate vs low-fat diets on weight loss and cardiovascular risk factors: a meta-analysis of randomized controlled trials. *Arch Intern Med*. 2006;166(3):285–93.

55. Hession M, Rolland C, Kulkarni U, Wise A, Broom J. Systematic review of randomized controlled trials of low-carbohydrate vs. low-fat/low-calorie diets in the management of obesity and its comorbidities. *Obes Rev*. 2009;10(1):36–50.

56. Shai I, Schwarzfuchs D, Henkin Y, et al. Weight loss with a low-carbohydrate, Mediterranean, or low-fat diet. *N Engl J Med*. 2008;359(3):229–41.

57. Gardner CD, Kiazand A, Alhassan S, et al. Comparison of the Atkins, Zone, Ornish, and LEARN diets for change in weight and related risk factors among overweight premenopausal women: the A TO Z Weight Loss Study: a randomized trial. *JAMA*. 2007;297(9):969–77.

58. Foster GD, Wyatt HR, Hill JO, et al. Weight and metabolic outcomes after 2 years on a low-carbohydrate versus low-fat diet: a randomized trial. *Ann Intern Med*. 2010;153(3):147–57.

59. La Berge AF. How the ideology of low fat conquered America. *J Hist Med Allied Sci*. 2008;63(2):139–77.

60. Oppenheimer GM. Becoming the Framingham Study 1947–1950. *Am J Public Health*. 2005;95(4):602–10.

61. Hall KD, Bemis T, Brychta R, et al. Calorie for calorie, dietary fat restriction results in more body fat loss than carbohydrate restriction in people with obesity. *Cell Metab*. 2015;22(3):427–36.

62. Puska P, Iacono JM, Nissinen A, et al. Controlled, randomised trial of the effect of dietary fat on blood pressure. *Lancet*. 1983; 1(8314–5):1–5.

63. Hammer RL, Barrier CA, Roundy ES, Bradford JM, Fisher AG. Calorie-restricted low-fat diet and exercise in obese women. *Am J Clin Nutr*. 1989;49(1):77–85.

64. Catenacci VA, Pan Z, Ostendorf D, et al. A randomized pilot study comparing zero-calorie alternate-day fasting to daily caloric restriction in adults with obesity. *Obesity (Silver Spring)*. 2016;24(9):1874–83.

65. Trepanowski JF, Kroeger CM, Barnosky A, et al. Effect of alternate-day fasting on weight loss, weight maintenance, and cardioprotection among metabolically healthy obese adults: a randomized clinical trial. *JAMA Intern Med*. 2017;177(7):930–8.

66. Gabel K, Hoddy KK, Haggerty N, et al. Effects of 8-hour time restricted feeding on body weight and metabolic disease risk factors in obese adults: a pilot study. *Nutr Healthy Aging*. 2018;4(4):345–53.

67. Liu D, Huang Y, Huang C, et al. Calorie restriction with or without time-restricted eating in weight loss. *N Engl J Med*. 2022;386(16):1495–504.

68. Apovian CM, Aronne LJ, Bessesen DH, et al. Pharmacological management of obesity: an Endocrine Society clinical practice guideline. *J Clin Endocrinol Metab*. 2015;100(2):342–62.

69. Srivastava G, Fox CK, Kelly AS, et al. Clinical considerations regarding the use of obesity pharmacotherapy in adolescents with obesity. *Obesity (Silver Spring)*. 2019;27(2):190–204.

70. Jastreboff AM, Aronne LJ, Ahmed NN, et al; SURMOUNT-1 Investigators. Tirzepatide once weekly for the treatment of obesity. *N Engl J Med*. 2022;387(15):205–16.

71. Aird TP, Davies RW, Carson BP. Effects of fasted vs fed-state exercise on performance and post-exercise metabolism: a systematic review and meta-analysis. *Scand J Med Sci Sports*. 2018; 28(5):1476–93.

72. Coggan AR, Coyle EF. Carbohydrate ingestion during prolonged exercise: effects on metabolism and performance. *Exerc Sport Sci Rev*. 1991;19:1–40.

73. Gadde KM, Allison DB, Ryan DH, et al. Effects of low-dose, controlled-release, phentermine plus topiramate combination on weight and associated comorbidities in overweight and obese adults (CONQUER): a randomised, placebo-controlled, phase 3 trial. *Lancet*. 2011;377(9774):1341–52.

74. Garvey WT, Ryan DH, Look M, et al. Two-year sustained weight loss and metabolic benefits with controlled-release phentermine/topiramate in obese and overweight adults (SEQUEL): a randomized, placebo-controlled, phase 3 extension study. *Am J Clin Nutr*. 2012;95(2):297–308.

75. Greenway FL, Fujioka K, Plodkowski RA, et al; COR-I Study Group. Effect of naltrexone plus bupropion on weight loss in overweight and obese adults (COR-I): a multicentre, randomised, double-blind, placebo-controlled, phase 3 trial. *Lancet*. 2010;376(9741):595–605.

76. Apovian CM, Aronne L, Rubino D, et al. A randomized, phase 3 trial of naltrexone SR/bupropion SR on weight and obesity-related risk factors (COR-II). *Obesity (Silver Spring)*. 2013;21(5):935–43.

77. Finer N, James WP, Kopelman PG, Lean ME, Williams G. One-year treatment of obesity: a randomized, double-blind, placebo-controlled, multicentre study of orlistat, a gastrointestinal lipase inhibitor. *Int J Obes Relat Metab Disord*. 2000;24(3):306–13.

78. Chanoine JP, Hampl S, Jensen C, Boldrin M, Hauptman J. Effect of orlistat on weight and body composition in obese adolescents: a randomized controlled trial. *JAMA*. 2005; 293(23):2873–83.

79. Pi-Sunyer X, Astrup A, Fujioka K, et al; SCALE Obesity and Prediabetes NN8022-1839 Study Group. A Randomized, controlled trial of 3.0 mg of liraglutide in weight management. *N Engl J Med*. 2015;373(1):11–22.

80. Wilding JPH, Batterham RL, Calanna S, et al; STEP 1 Study Group. Once-weekly semaglutide in adults with overweight or obesity. *N Engl J Med*. 2021;384(11):989–1002.

81. Kelly AS, Auerbach P, Barrientos-Perez M. et al. A randomized, controlled trial of liraglutide for adolescents with obesity. *N Engl J Med*. 2020;382(22):2117–28.

82. Drucker DJ. GLP-1 physiology informs the pharmacotherapy of obesity. *Mol Metab*. 2022;57:101351.

83. Zhou X, Yu J, Li L, et al. Effects of bariatric surgery on mortality, cardiovascular events, and cancer outcomes in obese

patients: systematic review and meta-analysis. *Obes Surg.* 2016;26(11):2590–601.

84. Carlsson LMS, Sjöholm K, Jacobson P, et al. Life expectancy after bariatric surgery in the Swedish obese subjects study. *N Engl J Med.* 2020;383(16):1535–43.

85. Inge TH, Laffel LM, Jenkins TM, et al; Teen–Longitudinal Assessment of Bariatric Surgery (Teen-LABS) and Treatment Options of Type 2 Diabetes in Adolescents and Youth (TODAY) Consortia. Comparison of surgical and medical therapy for type 2 diabetes in severely obese adolescents. *JAMA Pediatr.* 2018;172(5):452–60.

86. Pedroso FE, Angriman F, Endo A, et al. Weight loss after bariatric surgery in obese adolescents: a systematic review and meta-analysis. *Surg Obes Relat Dis.* 2018;14(3):413–22.

87. Rubino F, Puhl RM, Cummings DE, et al. Joint international consensus statement for ending stigma of obesity. *Nat Med.* 2020;26(4):485–97.

88. Pont SJ, Puhl R, Cook SR, Slusser W; Section on Obesity; Obesity Society. Stigma experienced by children and adolescents with obesity. *Pediatrics.* 2017;140(6):e20173034.

89. Eisenberg D, Shikora SA, Aarts E, et al. 2022 American Society of Metabolic and Bariatric Surgery (ASMBS) and International Federation for the Surgery of Obesity and Metabolic Disorders (IFSO) indications for metabolic and bariatric surgery. *Obes Surg.* 2023;33(1):3–14.

90. Armstrong SC, Bolling CF, Michalsky MP, Reichard KW; Section On Obesity, Section On Surgery. Pediatric metabolic and bariatric surgery: evidence, barriers, and best practices. *Pediatrics.* 2019;144(6):e20193223.

91. Schauer PR, Mingrone G, Ikramuddin S, Wolfe B. Clinical outcomes of metabolic surgery: efficacy of glycemic control, weight loss, and remission of diabetes. *Diabetes Care.* 2016;39(6):902–11.

92. Aminian A, Al-Kurd A, Wilson R, et al. Association of bariatric surgery with major adverse liver and cardiovascular outcomes in patients with biopsy-proven nonalcoholic steatohepatitis. *JAMA.* 2021;326(20):2031–42.

93. Doumouras AG, Wong JA, Paterson JM, et al. Bariatric surgery and cardiovascular outcomes in patients with obesity and cardiovascular disease: a population-based retrospective cohort study. *Circulation.* 2021;143(15):1468–80.

94. Inge TH, Courcoulas AP, Jenkins TM, et al; Teen-LABS Consortium. Weight loss and health status 3 years after bariatric surgery in adolescents. *N Engl J Med.* 2016;374(2):113–23.

95. Olbers T, Beamish AJ, Gronowitz E, et al. Laparoscopic Roux-en-Y gastric bypass in adolescents with severe obesity (AMOS): a prospective, 5-year, Swedish nationwide study. *Lancet Diabetes Endocrinol.* 2017;5(3):174–83.

96. Bout-Tabaku S, Gupta R, Jenkins TM, et al; Teen-Labs Consortium. Musculoskeletal pain, physical function, and quality of life after bariatric surgery. *Pediatrics.* 2019;144(6):e20191399.

97. Schauer PR, Bhatt DL, Kirwan JP, et al; STAMPEDE Investigators. Bariatric surgery versus intensive medical therapy for diabetes—5-year outcomes. *N Engl J Med.* 2017;376(7):641–51.

98. Inge TH, Courcoulas AP, Jenkins TM, et al; Teen–LABS Consortium. Five-year outcomes of gastric bypass in adolescents as compared with adults. *N Engl J Med.* 2019;380(22):2136–45.

99. Callahan LF, Ambrose KR, Albright AL, et al. Public Health Interventions for Osteoarthritis—updates on the Osteoarthritis Action Alliance's efforts to address the 2010 OA Public Health Agenda Recommendations. *Clin Exp Rheumatol.* 2019;37 Suppl 120(5):31–9.

100. Koremans FW, Chen X, Das A, Diwan AD. Changes in back pain scores after bariatric surgery in obese patients: a systematic review and meta-analysis. *J Clin Med.* 2021;10(7):1443.

101. Heuts EAF, de Jong LD, Hazebroek EJ, Wagener M, Somford MP. The influence of bariatric surgery on hip and knee joint pain: a systematic review. *Surg Obes Relat Dis.* 2021;17(9):1637–53.

102. Xu G, Song M. Recent advances in the mechanisms underlying the beneficial effects of bariatric and metabolic surgery. *Surg Obes Relat Dis.* 2021;17(1):231–8.

103. Arterburn DE, Telem DA, Kushner RF, Courcoulas AP. Benefits and risks of bariatric surgery in adults: a review. *JAMA.* 2020;324(9):879–87.

104. Zhang Q, Chen Y, Li J, et al. A meta-analysis of the effects of bariatric surgery on fracture risk. *Obes Rev.* 2018;19(5):728–36.

105. Ahlin S, Peltonen M, Sjöholm K, et al. Fracture risk after three bariatric surgery procedures in Swedish obese subjects: up to 26 years follow-up of a controlled intervention study. *J Intern Med.* 2020;287(5):546–57.

106. Misra M, Bredella MA. Bone metabolism in adolescents undergoing bariatric surgery. *J Clin Endocrinol Metab.* 2021;106(2):326–36.

107. De Leonibus C, Marcovecchio ML, Chiavaroli V, de Giorgis T, Chiarelli F, Mohn A. Timing of puberty and physical growth in obese children: a longitudinal study in boys and girls. *Pediatr Obes.* 2014;9(4):292–9.

108. Gregory NS. The effects of bariatric surgery on bone metabolism. *Endocrinol Metab Clin North Am.* 2017;46(1):105–16.

109. Mechanick JI, Apovian C, Brethauer S, et al. Clinical practice guidelines for the perioperative nutrition, metabolic, and nonsurgical support of patients undergoing bariatric procedures—2019 update: cosponsored by American Association of Clinical Endocrinologists/American College of Endocrinology, The Obesity Society, American Society for Metabolic and Bariatric Surgery, Obesity Medicine Association, and American Society of Anesthesiologists. *Obesity (Silver Spring).* 2020;28(4):O1–58.

110. de Hollanda A, Ruiz T, Jiménez A, Flores L, Lacy A, Vidal J. Patterns of weight loss response following gastric bypass and sleeve gastrectomy. *Obes Surg.* 2015;25(7):1177–83.

111. Ryder JR, Kaizer AM, Jenkins TM, Kelly AS, Inge TH, Shaibi GQ. Heterogeneity in response to treatment of adolescents with severe obesity: the need for precision obesity medicine. *Obesity (Silver Spring).* 2019;27(2):288–94.

112. Courcoulas AP, King WC, Belle SH, et al. Seven-year weight trajectories and health outcomes in the Longitudinal Assessment of Bariatric Surgery (LABS) Study. *JAMA Surg.* 2018;153(5):427–34.

113. King WC, Hsu JY, Belle SH, et al. Pre- to postoperative changes in physical activity: report from the Longitudinal Assessment of Bariatric Surgery-2 (LABS-2). *Surg Obes Relat Dis.* 2012;8(5):522–32.

114. Bond DS, Jakicic JM, Unick JL, et al. Pre- to postoperative physical activity changes in bariatric surgery patients: self-report vs. objective measures. *Obesity (Silver Spring).* 2010;18(12):2395–7.

115. Price PH, Kaizer AM, Inge TH, Eckel RH. Physical activity impacts insulin sensitivity post metabolic bariatric surgery in adolescents with severe obesity. *Int J Obes (Lond)*. 2020;44(7):1479–86.

116. Gilbertson NM, Eichner NZM, Khurshid M, et al. Impact of pre-operative aerobic exercise on cardiometabolic health and quality of life in patients undergoing bariatric surgery. *Front Physiol*. 2020;11:1018.

117. Kanaley JA, Colberg SR, Corcoran MH, et al. Exercise/Physical activity in individuals with type 2 diabetes: a consensus statement from the American College of Sports Medicine. *Med Sci Sports Exerc*. 2022;54(2):353–68.

118. Oppert JM, Bellicha A, Roda C, et al. Resistance training and protein supplementation increase strength after bariatric surgery: a randomized controlled trial. *Obesity (Silver Spring)*. 2018;26(11):1709–20.

119. Pouwels S, Wit M, Teijink JA, Nienhuijs SW. Aspects of exercise before or after bariatric surgery: a systematic review. *Obes Facts*. 2015;8(2):132–46.

120. Diniz-Sousa F, Boppre G, Veras L, Hernández-Martínez A, Oliveira J, Fonseca H. The effect of exercise for the prevention of bone mass after bariatric surgery: a systematic review and meta-analysis. *Obes Surg*. 2022;32(3):912–23.

121. American Diabetes Association Professional Practice Committee. 2. Classification and diagnosis of diabetes: Standards of Medical Care in Diabetes—2022. *Diabetes Care*. 2022;45 (Suppl 1):S17–38.

122. Dabelea D, Pihoker C, Talton JW, et al; SEARCH for Diabetes in Youth Study. Etiological approach to characterization of diabetes type: the SEARCH for diabetes in youth study. *Diabetes Care*. 2011;34(7):1628–33.

123. American Diabetes Association Professional Practice Committee. 6. Glycemic targets: Standards of Medical Care in Diabetes—2022. *Diabetes Care*. 2022;45(Suppl 1):S83–96.

124. The Diabetes Control and Complications Trial Research Group. The effect of intensive treatment of diabetes on the development and progression of long-term complications in insulin-dependent diabetes mellitus. *N Engl J Med*. 1993;329(14):977–86.

125. Nathan DM, Cleary PA, Backlund JY, et al; Diabetes Control and Complications Trial/Epidemiology of Diabetes Interventions and Complications (DCCT/EDIC) Study Research Group. Intensive diabetes treatment and cardiovascular disease in patients with type 1 diabetes. *N Engl J Med*. 2005;353(25):2643–53.

126. Nathan DM, Lachin J, Cleary P, et al; Diabetes Control and Complications Trial; Epidemiology of Diabetes Interventions and Complications Research Group. Intensive diabetes therapy and carotid intima-media thickness in type 1 diabetes mellitus. *N Engl J Med*. 2003;348(23):2294–303.

127. American Diabetes Association. 13. Children and adolescents: Standards of Medical Care in Diabetes—2019. *Diabetes Care*. 2019;42(Suppl 1):S148–64.

128. American Diabetes Association Professional Practice Committee. 13. Older adults: Standards of Medical Care in Diabetes—2022. *Diabetes Care*. 2022;45(Suppl 1):S195–207.

129. American Diabetes Association Professional Practice Committee. 3. Prevention or delay of type 2 diabetes and associated comorbidities: Standards of Medical Care in Diabetes—2022. *Diabetes Care*. 2022;45(Suppl 1):S39–45.

130. Duca LM, Reboussin BA, Pihoker C, et al. Diabetic ketoacidosis at diagnosis of type 1 diabetes and glycemic control over time: the SEARCH for diabetes in youth study. *Pediatr Diabetes*. 2019;20(2):172–9.

131. Cree-Green M, Stuppy JJ, Thurston J, et al. Youth with type 1 diabetes have adipose, hepatic and peripheral insulin resistance. *J Clin Endocrinol Metab*. 2018;103(10):3647–57.

132. Nokoff NJ, Rewers M, Cree-Green M. The interplay of autoimmunity and insulin resistance in type 1 diabetes. *Discov Med*. 2012;13(69):115–22.

133. Nadeau KJ, Regensteiner JG, Bauer TA, et al. Insulin resistance in adolescents with type 1 diabetes and its relationship to cardiovascular function. *J Clin Endocrinol Metab*. 2010;95(2):513–21.

134. Thong EP, Milat F, Joham AE, Mishra GD, Teede H. Obesity, menstrual irregularity and polycystic ovary syndrome in young women with type 1 diabetes: a population-based study. *Clin Endocrinol (Oxf)*. 2020;93(5):564–71.

135. Cree-Green M, Gupta A, Coe GV, et al. Insulin resistance in type 2 diabetes youth relates to serum free fatty acids and muscle mitochondrial dysfunction. *J Diabetes Complications*. 2017;31(1):141–8.

136. Lipton RB, Liao Y, Cao G, Cooper RS, McGee D. Determinants of incident non-insulin-dependent diabetes mellitus among blacks and whites in a national sample. The NHANES I Epidemiologic Follow-up Study. *Am J Epidemiol*. 1993;138(10):826–39.

137. Manson JE, Rimm EB, Stampfer MJ, et al. Physical activity and incidence of non-insulin-dependent diabetes mellitus in women. *Lancet*. 1991;338(8770):774–8.

138. Momma H, Sawada SS, Lee IM, et al. Consistently high level of cardiorespiratory fitness and incidence of type 2 diabetes. *Med Sci Sports Exerc*. 2017;49(10):2048–55.

139. Kawakami R, Sawada SS, Lee IM, et al. Long-term impact of cardiorespiratory fitness on type 2 diabetes incidence: a cohort study of Japanese men. *J Epidemiol*. 2018;28(5): 266–73.

140. Lyerly GW, Sui X, Lavie CJ, Church TS, Hand GA, Blair SN. The association between cardiorespiratory fitness and risk of all-cause mortality among women with impaired fasting glucose or undiagnosed diabetes mellitus. *Mayo Clin Proc*. 2009;84(9):780–6.

141. Sui X, Hooker SP, Lee IM, et al. A prospective study of cardiorespiratory fitness and risk of type 2 diabetes in women. *Diabetes Care*. 2008;31(3):550–5.

142. Lynch J, Helmrich SP, Lakka TA, et al. Moderately intense physical activities and high levels of cardiorespiratory fitness reduce the risk of non-insulin-dependent diabetes mellitus in middle-aged men. *Arch Intern Med*. 1996;156(12):1307–14.

143. Cree-Green M, Triolo TM, Nadeau KJ. Etiology of insulin resistance in youth with type 2 diabetes. *Curr Diab Rep*. 2013;13(1):81–8.

144. Arslanian SA, El Ghormli L, Kim JY, et al. OGTT glucose response curves, insulin sensitivity, and β-cell function in RISE: comparison between youth and adults at randomization and in response to interventions to preserve β-cell function. *Diabetes Care*. 2021;44(3):817–25.

145. Chan CL, Pyle L, Morehead R, Baumgartner A, Cree-Green M, Nadeau KJ. The role of glycemia in insulin resistance

in youth with type 1 and type 2 diabetes. *Pediatr Diabetes.* 2017;18(6):470–7.

146. Zeitler P, Epstein L, Grey M, et al; Today Study Group. Treatment options for type 2 diabetes in adolescents and youth: a study of the comparative efficacy of metformin alone or in combination with rosiglitazone or lifestyle intervention in adolescents with type 2 diabetes. *Pediatr Diabetes.* 2007;8(2):74–87.

147. Copeland KC, Zeitler P, Geffner M, et al; TODAY Study Group. Characteristics of adolescents and youth with recent-onset type 2 diabetes: the TODAY cohort at baseline. *J Clin Endocrinol Metab.* 2011;96(1):159–67.

148. Andes LJ, Cheng YJ, Rolka DB, Gregg EW, Imperatore G. Prevalence of prediabetes among adolescents and young adults in the United States, 2005–2016. *JAMA Pediatr.* 2020;174(2):e194498.

149. American Diabetes Association Professional Practice Committee. 15. Management of diabetes in pregnancy: Standards of Medical Care in Diabetes—2022. *Diabetes Care.* 2022; 45(Suppl 1):S232–43.

150. ACOG Committee Opinion No. 762: prepregnancy counseling. *Obstet Gynecol.* 2019;133(1):e78–89.

151. Badescu SV, Tătaru C, Kobylinska L, et al. The association between diabetes mellitus and depression. *J Med Life.* 2016;9(2):120–5.

152. Bruyneel M, Kleynen P, Poppe K. Prevalence of undiagnosed glucose intolerance and type 2 diabetes in patients with moderate-to-severe obstructive sleep apnea syndrome. *Sleep Breath.* 2020;24(4):1389–95.

153. American Diabetes Association Professional Practice Committee. 4. Comprehensive medical evaluation and assessment of comorbidities: Standards of Medical Care in Diabetes—2022. *Diabetes Care.* 2022;45(Suppl 1):S46–59.

154. Huebschmann AG, Huxley RR, Kohrt WM, Zeitler P, Regensteiner JG, Reusch JEB. Sex differences in the burden of type 2 diabetes and cardiovascular risk across the life course. *Diabetologia.* 2019;62(10):1761–72.

155. Purnell JQ, Zinman B, Brunzell JD. The effect of excess weight gain with intensive diabetes mellitus treatment on cardiovascular disease risk factors and atherosclerosis in type 1 diabetes mellitus: results from the Diabetes Control and Complications Trial/Epidemiology of Diabetes Interventions and Complications Study (DCCT/EDIC) study. *Circulation.* 2013;127(2):180–7.

156. Knowler WC, Barrett-Connor E, Fowler SE, et al; Diabetes Prevention Program Research Group. Reduction in the incidence of type 2 diabetes with lifestyle intervention or metformin. *N Engl J Med.* 2002;346(6):393–403.

157. Gregg EW, et al; Association of an intensive lifestyle intervention with remission of type 2 diabetes. *JAMA,* 2012;308(23):2489-96.

158. Moy CS, Songer TJ, LaPorte RE, et al. Insulin-dependent diabetes mellitus, physical activity, and death. *Am J Epidemiol.* 1993;137(1):74–81.

159. Tavoian D, Russ DW, Law TD, et al. A randomized clinical trial comparing three different exercise strategies for optimizing aerobic capacity and skeletal muscle performance in older adults: protocol for the DART Study. *Front Med (Lausanne).* 2019;6:236.

160. Trigona B, Aggoun Y, Maggio A, et al. Preclinical noninvasive markers of atherosclerosis in children and adolescents with type 1 diabetes are influenced by physical activity. *J Pediatr.* 2010;157(4):533–9.

161. Laaksonen DE, Atalay M, Niskanen LK, et al. Aerobic exercise and the lipid profile in type 1 diabetic men: a randomized controlled trial. *Med Sci Sports Exerc.* 2000;32(9):1541–8.

162. Salem MA, AboElAsrar MA, Elbarbary NS, ElHilaly RA, Refaat YM. Is exercise a therapeutic tool for improvement of cardiovascular risk factors in adolescents with type 1 diabetes mellitus? A randomised controlled trial. *Diabetol Metab Syndr.* 2010;2(1):47.

163. Conn VS, Hafdahl AR, Lemaster JW, Ruppar TM, Cochran JE, Nielsen PJ. Meta-analysis of health behavior change interventions in type 1 diabetes. *Am J Health Behav.* 2008;32(3):315–29.

164. Paiement K, Frenette V, Wu Z, et al. Is better understanding of management strategies for type 1 diabetes associated with a lower risk of developing hypoglycemia during and after physical activity? *Can J Diabetes.* 2022;46(5):526–34.

165. Calhoun PM, Buckingham BA, Maahs DM, et al. Efficacy of an overnight predictive low-glucose suspend system in relation to hypoglycemia risk factors in youth and adults with type 1 diabetes. *J Diabetes Sci Technol.* 2016;10(6):1216–21.

166. Wei M, Gibbons LW, Mitchell TL, Kampert JB, Lee CD, Blair SN. The association between cardiorespiratory fitness and impaired fasting glucose and type 2 diabetes mellitus in men. *Ann Intern Med.* 1999;130(2):89–96.

167. Ekelund LG, Haskell WL, Johnson JL, Whaley FS, Criqui MH, Sheps DS. Physical fitness as a predictor of cardiovascular mortality in asymptomatic North American men. The Lipid Research Clinics Mortality Follow-up Study. *N Engl J Med.* 1988;319(21):1379–84.

168. American Diabetes Association. 10. Cardiovascular disease and risk management: Standards of Medical Care in Diabetes—2021. *Diabetes Care.* 2021;44(Suppl 1):S125–50.

169. Blair SN, Kohl HW 3rd, Barlow CE, Paffenbarger RS Jr, Gibbons LW, Macera CA. Changes in physical fitness and all-cause mortality. A prospective study of healthy and unhealthy men. *JAMA.* 1995;273(14):1093–8.

170. Ivy JL, Zderic TW, Fogt DL. Prevention and treatment of non-insulin-dependent diabetes mellitus. *Exerc Sport Sci Rev.* 1999;27:1–35.

171. Zierath JR. Invited review: exercise training-induced changes in insulin signaling in skeletal muscle. *J Appl Physiol (1985).* 2002;93(2):773–81.

172. Kawate R, Yamakido M, Nishimoto Y, Bennett PH, Hamman RF, Knowler WC. Diabetes mellitus and its vascular complications in Japanese migrants on the Island of Hawaii. *Diabetes Care.* 1979;2(2):161–70.

173. Ravussin E, Valencia ME, Esparza J, Bennett PH, Schulz LO. Effects of a traditional lifestyle on obesity in Pima Indians. *Diabetes Care.* 1994;17(9):1067–74.

174. Centers for Disease Control and Prevention. National Diabetes Statistics report. 2022. Available from: https://www.cdc.gov/diabetes/data/statistics-report/index.html.

175. Helmrich SP, Ragland DR, Leung RW, Paffenbarger RS Jr. Physical activity and reduced occurrence of non-insulin-dependent diabetes mellitus. *N Engl J Med.* 1991;325(3): 147–52.

176. Manson JE, Nathan DM, Krolewski AS, Stampfer MJ, Willett WC, Hennekens CH. A prospective study of exercise and

incidence of diabetes among US male physicians. *JAMA.* 1992;268(1):63–7.

177. Weinstein AR, Sesso HD, Lee IM, et al. Relationship of physical activity vs body mass index with type 2 diabetes in women. *JAMA.* 2004;292(10):1188–94.

178. Hsia J, Wu L, Allen C, et al; Women's Health Initiative Research Group. Physical activity and diabetes risk in postmenopausal women. *Am J Prev Med.* 2005;28(1):19–25.

179. Marcus RL, Smith S, Morrell G, et al. Comparison of combined aerobic and high-force eccentric resistance exercise with aerobic exercise only for people with type 2 diabetes mellitus. *Phys Ther.* 2008;88(11):1345–54.

180. Sigal RJ, Kenny GP, Boulé NG, et al. Effects of aerobic training, resistance training, or both on glycemic control in type 2 diabetes: a randomized trial. *Ann Intern Med.* 2007;147(6):357–69.

181. Liu JX, Zhu L, Li PJ, Li N, Xu YB. Effectiveness of high-intensity interval training on glycemic control and cardiorespiratory fitness in patients with type 2 diabetes: a systematic review and meta-analysis. *Aging Clin Exp Res.* 2019;31(5):575–93.

182. Castaneda C, Layne JE, Munoz-Orians L, et al. A randomized controlled trial of resistance exercise training to improve glycemic control in older adults with type 2 diabetes. *Diabetes Care.* 2002;25(12):2335–41.

183. Dunstan DW, Daly RM, Owen N, et al. High-intensity resistance training improves glycemic control in older patients with type 2 diabetes. *Diabetes Care.* 2002;25(10):1729–36.

184. Innes KE, Vincent HK. The influence of yoga-based programs on risk profiles in adults with type 2 diabetes mellitus: a systematic review. *Evid Based Complement Alternat Med.* 2007;4(4):469–86.

185. Balducci S, Zanuso S, Nicolucci A, et al. Effect of an intensive exercise intervention strategy on modifiable cardiovascular risk factors in subjects with type 2 diabetes mellitus: a randomized controlled trial: the Italian Diabetes and Exercise Study (IDES). *Arch Intern Med.* 2010;170(20):1794–803.

186. Shapiro JS. Primary prevention of coronary heart disease in women through diet and lifestyle. *N Engl J Med.* 2000;343(24):1814.

187. American Diabetes Association Professional Practice Committee. 9. Pharmacologic approaches to glycemic treatment: Standards of Medical Care in Diabetes—2022. *Diabetes Care.* 2022;45(Suppl 1):S125–43.

188. American Diabetes Association Professional Practice Committee. 7. Diabetes technology: Standards of Medical Care in Diabetes—2022. *Diabetes Care.* 2022;45(Suppl 1):S97–112.

189. Cree-Green M, Bergman BC, Cengiz E, et al. Metformin improves peripheral insulin sensitivity in youth with type 1 diabetes. *J Clin Endocrinol Metab.* 2019;104(8):3265–78.

190. Beysel S, Unsal IO, Kizilgul M, Caliskan M, Ucan B, Cakal E. The effects of metformin in type 1 diabetes mellitus. *BMC Endocr Disord.* 2018;18(1):1.

191. Petersen KF, Dufour S, Befroy D, Lehrke M, Hendler RE, Shulman GI. Reversal of nonalcoholic hepatic steatosis, hepatic insulin resistance, and hyperglycemia by moderate weight reduction in patients with type 2 diabetes. *Diabetes.* 2005;54(3):603–8.

192. Intensive blood-glucose control with sulphonylureas or insulin compared with conventional treatment and risk of complications in patients with type 2 diabetes (UKPDS 33). UK Prospective Diabetes Study (UKPDS) Group. *Lancet.* 1998;352(9131):837–53.

193. Wing RR, Bolin P, Brancati FL, et al; Look AHEAD Research Group. Cardiovascular effects of intensive lifestyle intervention in type 2 diabetes. *N Engl J Med.* 2013;369(2):145–54.

194. Pi-Sunyer X, Blackburn G, Brancati FL, et al; Look AHEAD Research Group. Reduction in weight and cardiovascular disease risk factors in individuals with type 2 diabetes: one-year results of the Look AHEAD trial. *Diabetes Care.* 2007;30(6):1374–83.

195. Wing RR; Look AHEAD Research Group. Long-term effects of a lifestyle intervention on weight and cardiovascular risk factors in individuals with type 2 diabetes mellitus: four-year results of the Look AHEAD trial. *Arch Intern Med.* 2010;170(17):1566–75.

196. Gregg EW, Jakicic JM, Blackburn G, et al; Look AHEAD Research Group. Association of the magnitude of weight loss and changes in physical fitness with long-term cardiovascular disease outcomes in overweight or obese people with type 2 diabetes: a post-hoc analysis of the Look AHEAD randomised clinical trial. *Lancet Diabetes Endocrinol.* 2016;4(11):913–21.

197. Effect of intensive blood-glucose control with metformin on complications in overweight patients with type 2 diabetes (UKPDS 34). UK Prospective Diabetes Study (UKPDS) Group. *Lancet.* 1998;352(9131):854–65.

198. Guo Z, Priefer R. Current progress in pharmacogenomics of type 2 diabetes: a systemic overview. *Diabetes Metab Syndr.* 2021;15(5):102239.

199. Fischer M, Timper K, Radimerski T, et al. Metformin induces glucose uptake in human preadipocyte-derived adipocytes from various fat depots. *Diabetes Obes Metab.* 2010;12(4):356–9.

200. Hallsten K, Virtanen KA, Lönnqvist F, et al. Rosiglitazone but not metformin enhances insulin- and exercise-stimulated skeletal muscle glucose uptake in patients with newly diagnosed type 2 diabetes. *Diabetes.* 2002;51(12):3479–85.

201. Johnson AB, Webster JM, Sum CF, et al. The impact of metformin therapy on hepatic glucose production and skeletal muscle glycogen synthase activity in overweight type II diabetic patients. *Metabolism.* 1993;42(9):1217–22.

202. Madsbad S. Exenatide and liraglutide: different approaches to develop GLP-1 receptor agonists (incretin mimetics)—preclinical and clinical results. *Best Pract Res Clin Endocrinol Metab.* 2009;23(4):463–77.

203. Tzefos M, Olin JL. Glucagon-like peptide-1 analog and insulin combination therapy in the management of adults with type 2 diabetes mellitus. *Ann Pharmacother.* 2010;44(7-8):1294–300.

204. Chan M, Dimitriou A, Lam S. Semaglutide: a novel oral glucagon-like peptide receptor agonist for the treatment of type 2 diabetes mellitus. *Cardiol Rev.* 2021;29(2):100–8.

205. Frias JP, Auerbach P, Bajaj HS, et al. Efficacy and safety of once-weekly semaglutide 2.0 mg versus 1.0 mg in patients with type 2 diabetes (SUSTAIN FORTE): a double-blind, randomised, phase 3B trial. *Lancet Diabetes Endocrinol.* 2021;9(9):563–74.

206. Rosenstock J, Allison D, Birkenfeld AL, et al; PIONEER 3 Investigators. Effect of additional oral semaglutide vs sitagliptin on glycated hemoglobin in adults with type 2 diabetes uncontrolled with metformin alone or with sulfonylurea:

the PIONEER 3 randomized clinical trial. *JAMA*. 2019; 321(15):1466–80.

207. Uneda K, Kawai Y, Yamada T, et al. Systematic review and meta-analysis for prevention of cardiovascular complications using GLP-1 receptor agonists and SGLT-2 inhibitors in obese diabetic patients. *Sci Rep*. 2021;11(1):10166.

208. Chipkin SR. Tirzepatide for patients with type 2 diabetes. *JAMA*. 2022;327(6):529–30.

209. Wei R, Wang W, Pan Q, Guo L. Effects of SGLT-2 inhibitors on vascular endothelial function and arterial stiffness in subjects with type 2 diabetes: a systematic review and meta-analysis of randomized controlled trials. *Front Endocrinol (Lausanne)*. 2022;13:826604.

210. Reid T. Cardiometabolic risk reduction: a review of clinical guidelines and the role of SGLT-2 inhibitors. *J Fam Pract*. 2021;70(6S):S1–6.

211. Heidenreich PA, Bozkurt B, Aguilar D, et al. 2022 AHA/ACC/HFSA guideline for the management of heart failure: a report of the American College of Cardiology/American Heart Association Joint Committee on clinical practice guidelines. *Circulation*. 2022;145(18):e895–1032.

212. He Z, Yang L, Nie Y, et al. Effects of SGLT-2 inhibitors on health-related quality of life and exercise capacity in heart failure patients with reduced ejection fraction: a systematic review and meta-analysis. *Int J Cardiol*. 2021;345:83–8.

213. Lebovitz HE. Thiazolidinediones: the forgotten diabetes medications. *Curr Diab Rep*. 2019;19(12):151.

214. Vadher K, Patel H, Mody R, et al. Efficacy of tirzepatide 5, 10 and 15 mg versus semaglutide 2 mg in patients with type 2 diabetes: an adjusted indirect treatment comparison. *Diabetes Obes Metab*. 2022;24(9):1861–8.

215. Karagiannis T, Avgerinos I, Liakos A, et al. Management of type 2 diabetes with the dual GIP/GLP-1 receptor agonist tirzepatide: a systematic review and meta-analysis. *Diabetologia*. 2022;65(8):1251–61.

216. Frias JP, Davies MJ, Rosenstock J, et al; SURPASS-2 Investigators. Tirzepatide versus semaglutide once weekly in patients with type 2 diabetes. *N Engl J Med*. 2021;385(6):503–15.

217. Gastaldelli A, Cusi K, Fernández Landó L, Bray R, Brouwers B, Rodríguez Á. Effect of tirzepatide versus insulin degludec on liver fat content and abdominal adipose tissue in people with type 2 diabetes (SURPASS-3 MRI): a sub-study of the randomised, open-label, parallel-group, phase 3 SURPASS-3 trial. *Lancet Diabetes Endocrinol*. 2022;10(6):393–406.

218. Ruan Z, Zou H, Lei Q, Ung COL, Shi H, Hu H. Pharmacoeconomic evaluation of dipeptidyl peptidase-4 inhibitors for the treatment of type 2 diabetes mellitus: a systematic literature review. *Expert Rev Pharmacoecon Outcomes Res*. 2022;22(4):555–74.

219. Campbell RK. Rationale for dipeptidyl peptidase 4 inhibitors: a new class of oral agents for the treatment of type 2 diabetes mellitus. *Ann Pharmacother*. 2007;41(1):51–60.

220. Chen Y, Men K, Li XF, Li J, Liu M, Fan ZQ. Efficacy and safety of dipeptidyl peptidase-4 inhibitors in the treatment of type 2 diabetes patients with moderate to severe renal impairment: a meta-analysis. *Eur Rev Med Pharmacol Sci*. 2018;22(11):3502–14.

221. Deacon CF. Dipeptidyl peptidase 4 inhibitors in the treatment of type 2 diabetes mellitus. *Nat Rev Endocrinol*. 2020;16(11):642–53.

222. Singh-Franco D, Perez A, Harrington C. The effect of pramlintide acetate on glycemic control and weight in patients with type 2 diabetes mellitus and in obese patients without diabetes: a systematic review and meta-analysis. *Diabetes Obes Metab*. 2011;13(2):169–80.

223. Krentz AJ, Bailey CJ. Oral antidiabetic agents: current role in type 2 diabetes mellitus. *Drugs*. 2005;65(3):385–411.

224. Defronzo RA. Bromocriptine: a sympatholytic, d2-dopamine agonist for the treatment of type 2 diabetes. *Diabetes Care*. 2011;34(4):789–94.

225. Arslanian S, El Ghormli L, Bacha F, et al; TODAY Study Group. Adiponectin, insulin sensitivity, β-cell function, and racial/ethnic disparity in treatment failure rates in TODAY. *Diabetes Care*. 2017;40(1):85–93.

226. Kelsey MM, Hilkin A, Pyle L, et al. Two-year treatment with metformin during puberty does not preserve β-cell function in youth with obesity. *J Clin Endocrinol Metab*. 2021;106(7):e2622–32.

227. Bjornstad P, Drews KL, Caprio S, et al; TODAY Study Group. Long-term complications in youth-onset type 2 diabetes. *N Engl J Med*. 2021;385(5):416–26.

228. Teede HJ, Misso ML, Costello MF, et al; International PCOS Network. Recommendations from the international evidence-based guideline for the assessment and management of polycystic ovary syndrome. *Fertil Steril*. 2018;110(3):364–79.

229. Legro RS, Arslanian SA, Ehrmann DA, et al; Endocrine Society. Diagnosis and treatment of polycystic ovary syndrome: an Endocrine Society clinical practice guideline. *J Clin Endocrinol Metab*. 2013;98(12):4565–92.

230. Martin KA, Anderson RR, Chang RJ, et al. Evaluation and treatment of hirsutism in premenopausal women: an Endocrine Society clinical practice guideline. *J Clin Endocrinol Metab*. 2018;103(4):1233–57.

231. Goodman NF, Cobin RH, Futterweit W, Glueck JS, Legro RS, Carmina E; American Association of Clinical Endocrinologists (AACE); American College of Endocrinology (ACE); Androgen Excess and PCOS Society. American Association of Clinical Endocrinologists, American College of Endocrinology, and Androgen Excess and PCOS Society Disease State clinical review: guide to the best practices in the evaluation and treatment of polycystic ovary syndrome—part 2. *Endocr Pract*. 2015;21(12):1415–26.

232. Goodman NF, Cobin RH, Futterweit W, Glueck JS, Legro RS, Carmina E; American Association of Clinical Endocrinologists (AACE); American College of Endocrinology (ACE); Androgen Excess and PCOS Society (AES). American Association of Clinical Endocrinologists, American College of Endocrinology, and Androgen Excess and PCOS Society Disease State clinical review: guide to the best practices in the evaluation and treatment of polycystic ovary syndrome—part 1. *Endocr Pract*. 2015;21(11):1291–300.

233. Rosenfield RL, Ehrmann DA. The Pathogenesis of Polycystic Ovary Syndrome (PCOS): the hypothesis of PCOS as functional ovarian hyperandrogenism revisited. *Endocr Rev*. 2016;37(5):467–520.

234. Dapas M, Lin FTJ, Nadkarni GN, et al. Distinct subtypes of polycystic ovary syndrome with novel genetic associations: an unsupervised, phenotypic clustering analysis. *PLoS Med*. 2020;17(6):e1003132.

235. Walters KA, Gilchrist RB, Ledger WL, Teede HJ, Handelsman DJ, Campbell RE. New Perspectives on the pathogenesis of PCOS: neuroendocrine origins. *Trends Endocrinol Metab.* 2018;29(12):841–52.

236. Coutinho EA, Kauffman AS. The role of the brain in the pathogenesis and physiology of Polycystic Ovary Syndrome (PCOS). *Med Sci (Basel).* 2019;7(8):84.

237. Altintas KZ, Dilbaz B, Cirik DA, et al. The incidence of metabolic syndrome in adolescents with different phenotypes of PCOS. *Ginekol Pol.* 2017;88(6):289–95.

238. Andrisse S, Garcia-Reyes Y, Pyle L, Kelsey MM, Nadeau KJ, Cree-Green M. Racial and ethnic differences in metabolic disease in adolescents with obesity and polycystic ovary syndrome. *J Endocr Soc.* 2021;5(4):bvab008.

239. Baranova A, Tran TP, Birerdinc A, Younossi ZM. Systematic review: association of polycystic ovary syndrome with metabolic syndrome and non-alcoholic fatty liver disease. *Aliment Pharmacol Ther.* 2011;33(7):801–14.

240. Akgul S, Bonny AE. Metabolic syndrome in adolescents with polycystic ovary syndrome: prevalence on the basis of different diagnostic criteria. *J Pediatr Adolesc Gynecol.* 2019;32(4):383–7.

241. Cassar S, Misso ML, Hopkins WG, Shaw CS, Teede HJ, Stepto NK. Insulin resistance in polycystic ovary syndrome: a systematic review and meta-analysis of euglycaemic-hyperinsulinaemic clamp studies. *Hum Reprod.* 2016;31(11):2619–31.

242. Arslanian SA, Lewy VD, Danadian K. Glucose intolerance in obese adolescents with polycystic ovary syndrome: roles of insulin resistance and beta-cell dysfunction and risk of cardiovascular disease. *J Clin Endocrinol Metab.* 2001;86(1):66–71.

243. Cree-Green M, Rahat H, Newcomer BR, et al. Insulin resistance, hyperinsulinemia, and mitochondria dysfunction in nonobese girls with polycystic ovarian syndrome. *J Endocr Soc.* 2017;1(7):931–44.

244. Cerda C, Pérez-Ayuso RM, Riquelme A, et al. Nonalcoholic fatty liver disease in women with polycystic ovary syndrome. *J Hepatol.* 2007;47(3):412–7.

245. Dunaif A. Insulin resistance and the polycystic ovary syndrome: mechanism and implications for pathogenesis. *Endocr Rev.* 1997;18(6):774–800.

246. Hudnut-Beumler J, Kaar JL, Taylor A, et al. Development of type 2 diabetes in adolescent girls with polycystic ovary syndrome and obesity. *Pediatr Diabetes.* 2021;22(5):699–706.

247. Teede HJ, Tay CT, Joham AE. Polycystic ovary syndrome: an intrinsic risk factor for diabetes compounded by obesity. *Fertil Steril.* 2021;115(6):1449–50.

248. Joham AE, Kakoly NS, Teede HJ, Earnest A. Incidence and predictors of hypertension in a cohort of Australian women with and without polycystic ovary syndrome. *J Clin Endocrinol Metab.* 2021;106(6):1585–93.

249. Cree-Green M, Bergman BC, Coe GV, et al. Hepatic steatosis is common in adolescents with obesity and PCOS and relates to de novo lipogenesis but insulin resistance. *Obesity (Silver Spring).* 2016;24(11):2399–406.

250. Stepto NK, Patten RK, Tassone EC, et al. Exercise recommendations for women with polycystic ovary syndrome: is the evidence enough? *Sports Med.* 2019;49(8):1143–57.

251. Moore JM, Waldrop SW, Cree-Green M. Weight management in adolescents with polycystic ovary syndrome. *Curr Obes Rep.* 2021;10(3):311–21.

252. Pirotta S, Lim SS, Grassi A, et al. Relationships between self-management strategies and physical activity and diet quality in women with polycystic ovary syndrome. *Patient Educ Couns.* 2022;105(1):190–7.

253. Santos IKD, Nunes FASS, Queiros VS, et al. Effect of high-intensity interval training on metabolic parameters in women with polycystic ovary syndrome: a systematic review and meta-analysis of randomized controlled trials. *PLoS One.* 2021;16(1):e0245023.

254. Teede H, Tassone EC, Piltonen T, et al. Effect of the combined oral contraceptive pill and/or metformin in the management of polycystic ovary syndrome: a systematic review with meta-analyses. *Clin Endocrinol (Oxf).* 2019;91(4):479–89.

255. Al Khalifah RA, Florez ID, Dennis B, Thabane L, Bassilious E. Metformin or oral contraceptives for adolescents with polycystic ovarian syndrome: a meta-analysis. *Pediatrics.* 2016;137(5):e20154089.

256. Buyers E, Sass AE, Severn CD, Pyle L, Cree-Green M. Twelve-month continuation of the etonogestrel implant in adolescents with polycystic ovary syndrome. *J Pediatr Adolesc Gynecol.* 2021;34(1):33–9.

257. Ibanez L, Diaz M, Sebastiani G, et al. Treatment of androgen excess in adolescent girls: ethinylestradiol-cyproteroneacetate versus low-dose pioglitazone-flutamide-metformin. *J Clin Endocrinol Metab.* 2011;96(11):3361–6.

258. Ezzat RS, Abdallah W, Elsayed M, Saleh HS, Abdalla W. Impact of bariatric surgery on androgen profile and ovarian volume in obese polycystic ovary syndrome patients with infertility. *Saudi J Biol Sci.* 2021;28(9):5048–52.

259. Fernandez RC, Moore VM, Van Ryswyk EM, et al. Sleep disturbances in women with polycystic ovary syndrome: prevalence, pathophysiology, impact and management strategies. *Nat Sci Sleep.* 2018;10:45–64.

260. Franik G, Krysta K, Madej P, et al. Sleep disturbances in women with polycystic ovary syndrome. *Gynecol Endocrinol.* 2016;32(12):1014–17.

261. Chatterjee B, Suri J, Suri JC, Mittal P, Adhikari T. Impact of sleep-disordered breathing on metabolic dysfunctions in patients with polycystic ovary syndrome. *Sleep Med.* 2014;15(12):1547–53.

262. Kumarendran B, Sumilo D, O'Reilly MW, et al. Increased risk of obstructive sleep apnoea in women with polycystic ovary syndrome: a population-based cohort study. *Eur J Endocrinol.* 2019;180(4):265–72.

263. Benson J, Severn C, Hudnut-Beumler J, et al. Depression in girls with obesity and polycystic ovary syndrome and/or type 2 diabetes. *Can J Diabetes.* 2020;44(6):507–13.

264. Coban OG, Tulacı ÖD, Adanır AS, Önder A. Psychiatric disorders, self-esteem, and quality of life in adolescents with polycystic ovary syndrome. *J Pediatr Adolesc Gynecol.* 2019;32(6):600–4.

265. Greenwood EA, Yaffe K, Wellons MF, Cedars MI, Huddleston HG. Depression over the lifespan in a population-based cohort of women with polycystic ovary syndrome: longitudinal analysis. *J Clin Endocrinol Metab.* 2019;104(7):2809–19.

266. Banting LK, Gibson-Helm M, Polman R, Teede HJ, Stepto NK. Physical activity and mental health in women with polycystic ovary syndrome. *BMC Womens Health.* 2014;14(1):51.

267. Kahaly GJ, Kampmann C, Mohr-Kahaly S. Cardiovascular hemodynamics and exercise tolerance in thyroid disease. *Thyroid.* 2002;12(6):473–81.

268. Shojaeifard M, Davoudi Z, Erfanifar A, et al. Comparison of myocardial deformation indices during rest and after activity in untreated hyperthyroid patients with normal population. *Am J Cardiovasc Dis.* 2020;10(3):230–40.

269. Cutovic M, Konstantinovic L, Stankovic Z, Vesovic-Potic V. Structured exercise program improves functional capacity and delays relapse in euthyroid patients with Graves' disease. *Disabil Rehabil.* 2012;34(18):1511–8.

270. Brusseau V, Tauveron I, Bagheri R, et al. Heart rate variability in hypothyroid patients: a systematic review and meta-analysis. *PLoS One.* 2022;17(6):e0269277.

271. Stuenkel CA, Davis SR, Gompel A, et al. Treatment of symptoms of the menopause: an Endocrine Society clinical practice guideline. *J Clin Endocrinol Metab.* 2015;100(11):3975–4011.

272. Bhasin S, Brito JP, Cunningham GR, et al. Testosterone therapy in men with hypogonadism: an Endocrine Society clinical practice guideline. *J Clin Endocrinol Metab.* 2018; 103(5):1715–44.

273. Bornstein SR, Allolio B, Arlt W, et al. Diagnosis and treatment of primary adrenal insufficiency: an Endocrine Society clinical practice guideline. *J Clin Endocrinol Metab.* 2016; 101(2):364–89.

274. Speiser PW, Arlt W, Auchus RJ, et al. Congenital adrenal hyperplasia due to steroid 21-hydroxylase deficiency: an Endocrine Society clinical practice guideline. *J Clin Endocrinol Metab.* 2018;103(11):4043–88.

275. Weise M, Mehlinger SL, Drinkard B, et al. Patients with classic congenital adrenal hyperplasia have decreased epinephrine reserve and defective glucose elevation in response to high-intensity exercise. *J Clin Endocrinol Metab.* 2004;89(2):591–7.

276. Riepe FG, Krone N, Krüger SN, et al. Absence of exercise-induced leptin suppression associated with insufficient epinephrine reserve in patients with classic congenital adrenal hyperplasia due to 21-hydroxylase deficiency. *Exp Clin Endocrinol Diabetes.* 2006;114(3):105–10.

277. Simunkova K, Jovanovic N, Rostrup E, et al. Effect of a pre-exercise hydrocortisone dose on short-term physical performance in female patients with primary adrenal failure. *Eur J Endocrinol.* 2016;174(1):97–105.

278. Weise M, Drinkard B, Mehlinger SL, et al. Stress dose of hydrocortisone is not beneficial in patients with classic congenital adrenal hyperplasia undergoing short-term, high-intensity exercise. *J Clin Endocrinol Metab.* 2004;89(8):3679–84.

279. Green-Golan L, Yates C, Drinkard B, et al. Patients with classic congenital adrenal hyperplasia have decreased epinephrine reserve and defective glycemic control during prolonged moderate-intensity exercise. *J Clin Endocrinol Metab.* 2007;92(8):3019–24.

280. Kim MS, Ryabets-Lienhard A, Dao-Tran A, et al. Increased abdominal adiposity in adolescents and young adults with classical congenital adrenal hyperplasia due to 21-hydroxylase deficiency. *J Clin Endocrinol Metab.* 2015;100(8):E1153–9.

281. Tamhane S, Rodriguez-Gutierrez R, Iqbal AM, et al. Cardiovascular and metabolic outcomes in congenital adrenal hyperplasia: a systematic review and meta-analysis. *J Clin Endocrinol Metab.* 2018;103(11):4097–103.

Musculoskeletal Concerns

INTRODUCTION

Individuals participating in exercise often have preexisting musculoskeletal issues, such as arthritis, muscle or joint pain, or back pain, as well as previous injuries or surgeries. As musculoskeletal pain and dysfunction are among the leading causes of disability, it is essential to consider these when working with any client. Exercise prescription must incorporate modifications for preexisting conditions and be designed in such a way as to address client needs and at the same time decrease the possibility of developing setbacks secondary to the exercise program.

This chapter identifies some of the most prevalent musculoskeletal concerns, including arthritis, osteoporosis, joint injuries and replacements, and neck and back pain. For each, it discusses the role of exercise prescription, including the benefits, contraindications, precautions, modifications, and components of the program.

COMMONALITIES

Two topics are relevant for all musculoskeletal concerns. Thus, it seems logical to discuss these prior to addressing specific concerns. The first of these is posture. Whereas each chapter section may still refer to specific postural concerns, a general overview of posture related to exercise assessment and prescription is important. The second common topic is medications and supplements. Although some medications are specific to a disease, such as those for osteoporosis, others — such as nonsteroidal anti-inflammatory drugs (NSAIDs) — are used for multiple musculoskeletal conditions, even though the mechanism of action may differ.

Posture

Poor posture has been identified as a contributor to many musculoskeletal problems and is even related to balance (1, 2). Good posture is classically defined as "the optimal alignment of the individual's body that allows the neuromuscular system to perform actions requiring the least amount of energy to achieve the desired effect" (3); thus, poor posture is loss of optimal alignment of body segments. Proper posture is usually identified using a top-down analysis, starting with vertical alignment of the head and the spine. When viewed from the side, a client's head should be centered over the trunk, and the normal curves of the spine should be what is called "mid-range," meaning the curve is not absent, but is not so concave or convex as to affect the spinal nerve foramen. The accepted bony landmarks for standing posture (viewed from the side) include the external auditory meatus, acromioclavicular joint, greater trochanter, fibular head, and anterior aspect of the lateral malleolus (4).

Good postural alignment supports normal joint range of motion (ROM), which is movement that occurs at specific joints. It also helps place the limbs in appropriate positions for functional activity and protects the musculoskeletal system from excessive force (5).

Although little actual muscle exertion is required to maintain good upright posture, endurance in the postural muscles is necessary to maintain postural control. These postural control muscles consist of the deep cervical flexors (longus capitis and longus colli), the transversus abdominis (TrA), and the multifidus muscles. When these muscles fatigue or are put into positions that reduce the normal length–tension ratio, the mechanics of their performance changes and the load is shifted to the inert tissues supporting the spine at the end ranges (2, 6). These stresses to the tissues lead to the stimulation of pain receptors (2, 6), as depicted in Figure 11.1. Relieving the mechanical stress (*i.e.*, correcting the posture) to these pain-sensitive structures should theoretically relieve the pain (1, 7).

In the adult population, one of the most common postural faults for the upper trunk is rounded shoulders and

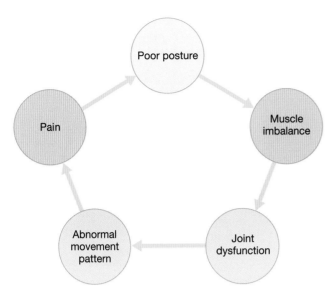

FIGURE 11.1 Theoretical cycle depicting effects of poor posture on pain. (Reprinted from Hoogenboom BJ, Voight ML, Prentice WE. *Musculoskeletal Interventions: Techniques for Therapeutic Exercise*. 3rd ed. Whitby (ON): McGraw-Hill; 2014.)

forward head during sitting (8). As the head alignment comes forward from the trunk, the work of the head and neck extensor muscles against gravity is increased (4, 8). This poor sitting posture places the muscles of the upper back in an overstretched position and the suboccipital muscles (short neck extensors) in a shortened position, as illustrated in Figure 11.2. The posterior scapular muscles are overstretched and weak, the pectoralis muscles are shortened and weakened force producing ability, whereas the neck extensors are constantly contracting to hold the

weight of the head up. In a systematic review, Côté et al. (8) noted that working with this prolonged posture is related to chronic upper back and neck pain, as well as frequent headaches. Similarly, a greater thoracic angle and a smaller cervical angle (forward head position) has been shown to be greater in those with neck pain (9).

Although education regarding the importance of proper posture and the balance of the head over the spine is important, rarely will it be enough to correct poor posture habits (10). An exercise program should be accompanied by a home exercise prescription and some simple ergonomic changes at work and at home in order to provide the best chances for longitudinal changes in posture.

To improve poor sitting posture, the following ergonomic changes and exercises may be helpful. Placing a small rolled-up towel at the belt line will provide some tactile feedback to encourage proper posture when sitting. Other cues might include instructions to change a computer monitor position, or to take regular breaks during work and change positions or move, in order to decrease the amount of time a client maintains the head in a forward position. Exercises that can be performed at home daily are essential to retrain the muscles and correct the faulty posture. Although some daily activities might use these muscle actions, the activities will probably not be of the frequency or intensity needed to provide a training stimulus. The pectoralis muscle can be stretched with a door stretch (Figure 11.3), and the deep neck extensor endurance can be improved with a chin tuck exercise (Figure 11.4). The scapular rotators can be strengthened

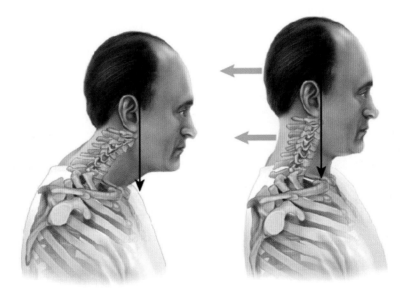

FIGURE 11.2 Forward head posture with rounded shoulders. (Adapted with permission from Muscolino JE. Seven keys to healthy neck posture. *Massage Therap J.* 2010:93–7. Artwork by Giovanni Rimasti. Available from: www.learnmuscles.com.)

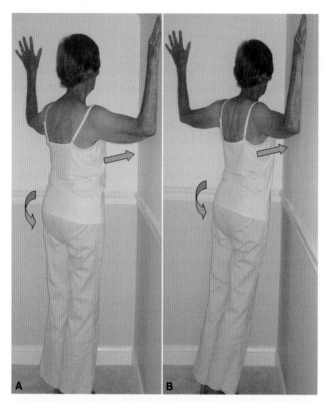

FIGURE 11.3 A. Starting position for a wall stretch. Hands at shoulder height, with upper arms and elbows at 90 degrees. **B.** Hips and trunk pressed forward, while upper arms move back, placing a stretch on the anterior chest. (Adapted with permission from Muscolino JE. Seven keys to healthy neck posture. *Massage Therap J.* 2010:93–7. Artwork by Giovanni Rimasti. Available from: www.learnmuscles.com.)

by performing scapular retraction pinches, adding resistance with an elastic band in order to further strengthen the posterior postural muscles and improve their endurance (Figures 11.5 and 11.6). The resistance should be

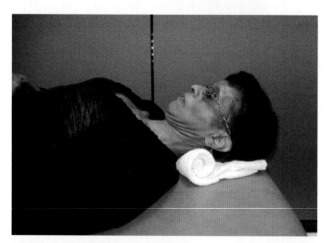

FIGURE 11.4 Chin tuck exercise for strengthening deep cervical flexors. (From Thompson W, editor. *ACSMs Clinical Exercise Physiology.* 1st ed. Philadelphia (PA): Wolters Kluwer; 2019.)

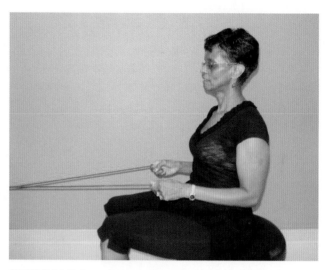

FIGURE 11.5 Scapular retraction exercises with tubing, shoulders in neutral position. (From Thompson W, editor. *ACSMs Clinical Exercise Physiology.* 1st ed. Philadelphia (PA): Wolters Kluwer; 2019.)

kept low enough so that the client can maintain proper posture throughout execution of the exercise. Because the scapular muscles are postural muscles, which need to generate a low level of muscle tension intermittently over a prolonged period of time, they need to be trained to resist fatigue as well as to increase strength and endurance.

Often, clients do not perform enough repetitions to truly improve the endurance of these muscles. Whereas starting at 10 repetitions may provide a training stimulus

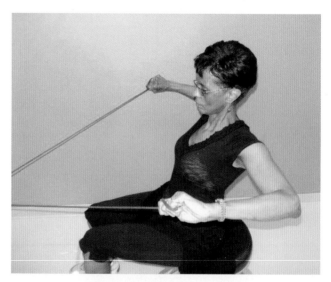

FIGURE 11.6 Scapular retraction exercises with tubing, shoulders in 90 degrees of abduction. (From Thompson W, editor. *ACSMs Clinical Exercise Physiology.* 1st ed. Philadelphia (PA): Wolters Kluwer; 2019.)

for someone who has been sedentary, some rehabilitation experts suggest that clients should progress to working with the elastic bands and increasing the number of repetitions to between 25 and 50 in one set. Progression is critical.

Medications and Supplements

Medications for arthritis, soft tissue issues, post joint replacement, and neck and back pain are generally used to decrease pain and inflammation. Table 11.1 shows the primary classifications of medications used for pain relief and inflammation control.

Table 11.1	Medications for Pain Relief and Inflammation Control
Category	**Examples (Trade Names)**
NSAIDs	Aspirin
	Ibuprofen (Advil, Motrin IB)
	Ketoprofen (Orudis)
	Naproxen (Naprosyn)
	Celecoxib (Celebrex)
DMARDs	Gold, injectable or oral
	Antimalarials (Plaquenil)
	Penicillamine (Cuprimine, Depen)
	Sulfasalazine (Azulfidine)
	Methotrexate (Rheumatrex)
	Azathioprine (Imuran)
	Cyclosporine (Sandimmun, Neoral)
	Leflunomide (Arava)
Glucocorticoids (steroids)	Prednisone (Deltasone, Orasone)
	Methylprednisolone (Medrol)
Biologic therapy	Etanercept (Enbrel)

DMARDs, disease-modifying antirheumatic drugs; NSAIDs, nonsteroidal anti-inflammatory drugs.

Source: Adapted from *ACSM's Resource Manual for Guidelines for Exercise Testing and Prescription.* 7th ed. Philadelphia (PA): Wolters Kluwer Health; 2014. 723 p.

The anti-inflammatories are among the first line of pharmacological intervention for many musculoskeletal issues. For osteoarthritis (OA), the American College of Rheumatology has recommended topical NSAIDs (for knee OA), oral NSAIDs, with conditional recommendations for topical NSAIDs, topical capsaicin (knee OA), duloxetine, and tramadol (see Chapter 7) (11–13). The potential side effects of these medications include gastrointestinal (GI) bleeding or liver damage. Naproxen sodium can increase blood pressure and cause lower extremity swelling. There is controversy regarding the use of NSAIDs for soft tissue inflammation or pain relief. NSAIDs have been shown to be effective for pain relief with chronic back pain (14); however, current recommendations for NSAID use with acute injuries are mixed, as there is evidence showing delayed healing for fractures or tendon-to-bone injuries. Findings regarding the effects of NSAID use on tendon healing are mixed, and factors such as patient age and general health may affect the response (15). Wilder and Barrett (16) examined the interaction between medication use and dropout from exercise in those with OA. They found that those individuals with greater medication use were four times more likely to drop out of exercise programs. Thus, different strategies may be needed for the clinical exercise physiologist (CEP) when working with someone who is on multiple medications.

In addition to anti-inflammatory medications, pharmacologic treatment of rheumatoid arthritis (RA) and other types of systemic arthritis includes several drugs that work on the immune system. These include disease-modifying antirheumatic drugs (DMARDs), glucocorticoids (steroids), and biologic drugs (17–21). Although these medications are effective for pain relief and decreasing joint deterioration, potential side effects include liver and kidney damage, and increased risk for infections. See Chapter 7 for a more thorough presentation of these medications. As osteoporosis is more prevalent in individuals with RA, there are management recommendations specific to individuals with both diseases (22).

Antiresorptive agents are prescribed for patients with osteoporosis. The initial treatment focuses on the use of bisphosphonate to reduce the risk of fracture (23, 24). Bisphosphonates improve bone mineral density (BMD) and as noted by Zhao et al. (25), there are some side effects to estrogen and phytoestrogen; thus, bisphosphonates are being used more frequently, as they have fewer side effects. A meta-analysis showed that the use of bisphosphonates in conjunction with exercise improves BMD. Dietary supplements recommended for patients with osteopenia or osteoporosis include calcium and vitamin D, which are more effective when taken together (23, 26).

Dietary supplements have been promoted for the treatment of arthritis. However, a recent systematic review (27) only identified ω-3 fatty acid supplementation as beneficial for clients with RA. A review of dietary supplements for RA showed that the Mediterranean diet, some specific spices, and antioxidants demonstrated reduced disease activity scores in individuals with RA (28).

ARTHRITIS

More than 100 forms of arthritis affect joints, surrounding muscles, and even body systems. OA is the most prevalent, accounting for almost 85% of arthritis diagnoses (29). Other common forms include RA and fibromyalgia. In addition, ankylosing spondylitis (AS), a spondyloarthropathy (SA), is a less common form of arthritis that requires specific exercise modifications (30). All forms of arthritis have an inflammatory component; however, OA is primarily joint specific, whereas the others, many of which are immune system dysfunctions, affect several systems.

The hallmark symptoms of arthritis are stiffness, joint or muscle pain, and fatigue. Arthritis is the leading cause of impaired functioning in adults and affects more than 58.5 million Americans. Importantly, arthritis is also the most common cause of activity limitation, with approximately 44% of those with arthritis reporting activity limitations. This accounts for over 10% of the total U.S. population (29). This number is projected to increase throughout the next few decades, as the "baby boomer generation" ages. Unfortunately, many clients with arthritis pain stop exercising, believing the activity worsens the symptoms and disease. However, appropriate exercise decreases the pain, does not speed up the joint degeneration, and most importantly, helps the client maintain normal function.

Risk Factors and Etiology

Risk factors vary by type of arthritis, but some common factors contribute to an increased risk for most types. These include sex and age, which cannot be altered. Females are more likely than males to have arthritis, with some exceptions, such as AS, which is more prevalent in males (30). The prevalence of arthritis increases with advancing age, becoming much greater in individuals over the age of 65 years. Excess body weight is also a risk factor for the development and progression of arthritis, and weight loss results in decreased pain associated with OA.

An individual's activity and medical history may also be related to the risk of OA development.

Damage to the joint surface as a result of trauma, abnormal biomechanics (movement), or repetitive joint stress can lead to OA. Figure 11.7 depicts the potential effects of biomechanical changes on OA and disability. It should be noted that there is an inflammatory component to OA, and increased inflammatory markers predict progression of the disease (31, 32). Some research suggests that biochemical changes in the cartilage may be the stimulus initiation of the inflammatory process (31, 32). Both function and severity of the arthritis are correlated with the level of inflammatory marker in the blood (33, 34). With the systemic forms of arthritis, an abnormal immune system response is the typical cause of the joint destruction (34).

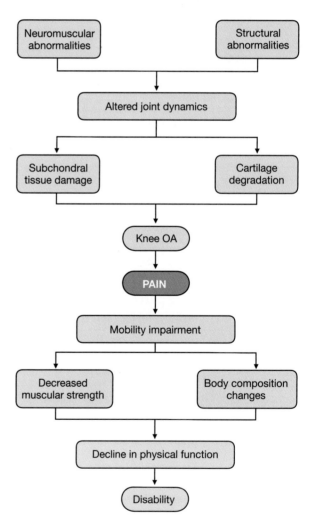

FIGURE 11.7 Theoretical biomechanical pathways for knee osteoarthritis (OA) and subsequent disability. (From *ACSM's Resource Manual for Guidelines for Exercise Testing and Prescription.* 7th ed. Philadelphia (PA): Wolters Kluwer Health; 2014.)

Regardless of the initial cause, as the damage progresses and the joint space narrows, the bone underlying the cartilage experiences abnormal stresses and deforms. Figures 11.8 and 11.9 depict the changes within the knee joint as a result of OA or RA.

Clinical Diagnosis

Osteoarthritis can be diagnosed through self-diagnosis or clinically, especially during the early stages (35). Initial diagnosis is often based on the individuals' age and symptoms.

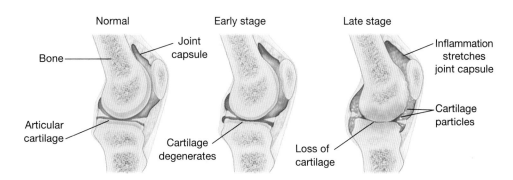

FIGURE 11.8 Progressive joint changes seen in knee arthritis (vault). (From Nath J. *Stedman's Medical Terminology*. 2nd ed. Philadelphia (PA): Wolters Kluwer; 2016.)

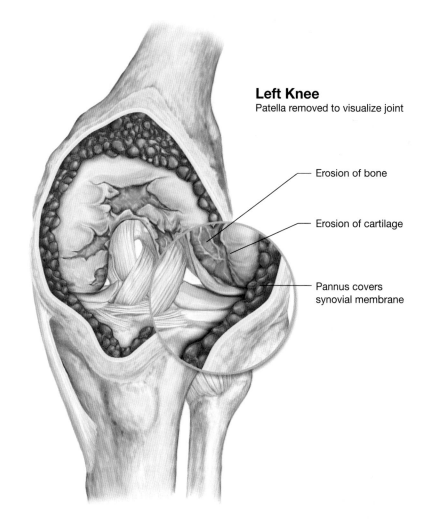

FIGURE 11.9 Joint and bone changes with knee rheumatoid arthritis (vault). (From Anatomical Chart Company. *Understanding Arthritis Anatomical Chart*. 1st ed. Philadelphia (PA): Wolters Kluwer; 2004.)

Damen et al. (36) found that a large percentage of those with symptoms who did not meet all of the diagnostic criteria developed diagnostic OA within a few years. Physicians may also use x-rays and laboratory tests, especially to diagnose systemic involvement (35, 37). Unfortunately, the relationship between pain and functional impairment and the amount of joint damage present in an x-ray is not consistent (38). Clients with arthritis who are involved in regular activity report less pain and better function when compared to those who are more sedentary.

As stiffness is the hallmark of arthritis, it is one of the most common symptoms used in the diagnosis, especially stiffness first thing in the morning. It was thought that morning stiffness that lasts less than 30 minutes is associated with OA (usually presenting initially in an individual joint) (35), whereas morning stiffness that lasted for an hour or more was thought to be part of the diagnosis of systemic arthritis. However, although this may be helpful for some clients, the newer criteria for diagnosis of RA focus on earlier detection, using a formula that includes definite clinical synovitis in one or more joints, the number of joints involved, serology results, duration of symptoms (months), and presence of systemic acute-phase reactants "(*i.e.,* markers of inflammation)" (34, 37). If a client presents with joint swelling and a complaint of stiffness, but no previous diagnosis, the client should be referred to a physician for a definitive diagnosis prior to implementation of an exercise program.

Fibromyalgia is unique as the symptoms are chronic muscular pain (>3 months), but not specific joint pain. In 2010, the diagnostic criteria were published for fibromyalgia (39) and later reviewed with recommendations on proposed revisions (40). The new criteria include a Symptom Severity (SS) scale, which includes ratings of somatic symptoms, waking unrefreshed, cognition, fatigue, sleep problems, and mood combined with the Widespread Pain Index (WPI). Fibromyalgia is then determined by either the combination of a WPI greater than or equal to 7 AND SS greater than or equal to 5 or a WPI 3–6 AND SS greater than or equal to 9 (40). These criteria recognize the complexity of fibromyalgia.

Management of Arthritis

When working with clients with arthritis, it is important to consider the type, the client's surgical and injury history, and current medications. A reliable functional questionnaire should be used to help determine baseline concerns and screen for comorbidities. Statistics regarding individuals with arthritis (41) show that 24% also have heart disease, 19% have chronic respiratory disease, 16% have diabetes, and 6.9% have had a stroke. More than half of those with arthritis have hypertension.

Exercise is one of the primary recommendations for all older clients, especially those with chronic conditions such as arthritis (11–13, 42). In addition to exercise, the recommendations for management of arthritis include weight control, pharmacologic interventions, and education in self-management (11). Maintenance of proper body weight can help reduce joint pain. In fact, losing as little as 10% of body weight has been shown to decrease pain (43). Referring your client to a registered dietitian (RD) who can provide nutritional advice and help with a weight loss plan may be essential for those who are overweight or obese.

Benefits of Exercise for Patients With Arthritis

Many people with arthritis limit or stop activity completely because of joint pain. Unfortunately, inactivity leads to muscle atrophy, loss of joint ROM, and increased pain. Systematic reviews regarding exercise and knee OA found that exercise results in decreased pain and improved function and quality of life (44–46). Similarly, both function and pain are improved by exercise in those with hip OA (15, 45, 47, 48). These reviews note limited adverse events reported in the studies that were reviewed.

Even one session of mild activity can prompt an immediate decrease in OA pain, with greater pain reductions seen with regular exercise (46). In fact, some studies have shown a reduction in pain medication use when regular activity is added to a client's routine. Given the potential side effects of some medications, a reduction in use is important.

Muscle atrophy and stiffness can lead to a reduced ability to perform some activities of daily living (ADL). Because exercise improves strength and mobility, function is usually improved. Low-intensity activities will slow the loss of function, whereas higher intensity activity has been shown to have greater strength and functional benefits (49–52). Clinicians previously advised against anything but low-intensity activity, suggesting that higher intensity activity would speed the progression of joint deterioration. However, numerous studies have shown that higher intensity activity does not worsen symptoms or cause joint destruction. In fact, higher intensity exercise has a strong positive effect, as long as the program has been progressed slowly and the joints are protected as needed (53).

Many of the systemic forms of arthritis are associated with an increase in cardiovascular risk. Thus, activity for these clients should help reduce their arthritis symptoms and should also have the additional benefit of reducing systemic disease risks.

Contraindications, Precautions, and Modifications to Exercise

There are very few contraindications to exercise for people with arthritis. The most significant are previous injury and acute inflammation. Even in such cases, modification of the activity is often preferable to complete cessation of activity. A primary contraindication for any client is the presence of a fever, which may be reported by the client during the initial assessment. Typically, a temperature over 100°F is considered a fever; however, body temperature decreases with aging, which means that a "normal" or slightly elevated temperature may actually represent fever in an older client (54). In a client with a systemic form of arthritis, the immune system may already be compromised, thus exercising when ill could endanger the client.

Although there are few contraindications to exercise, modifications to an exercise program are often required to improve client safety and effectiveness. Modifications are based on the clients' impairments and needs; some common issues include flare-ups, joint instability, excessive fatigue, and poor balance.

A flare-up is a time when the joints or muscles are more symptomatic than normal and may even be swollen. With RA and other systemic forms of arthritis, blood chemistries will often show an increased inflammatory response. An increase in inflammation is not a contraindication to exercise, but modification may be necessary. The client may need to reduce the intensity of activities or eliminate a particular exercise that aggravates the symptoms. The client should make sure to get more rest throughout the day during a flare-up, especially with a compromised immune system.

As arthritis progresses, the joint space narrows, causing the stabilizing tissues around the joint to slacken. Joint alignment also becomes an issue. These factors combine to produce the sensation of a loss of stability around the joint (55). Some patients report the sensation of giving way of the joint with certain activities. Unfortunately, the research into this problem is varied; thus, the recommendations are usually to modify the activity (56). The incidence of falls in older adults with arthritis is twice that of their age-matched counterparts who do not have arthritis (56, 57). Hayashibara et al. (56) assessed the incidence of falls

in women with RA, as previous research had found a relationship between falls and musculoskeletal dysfunction. The authors looked specifically at women with RA because, although strength has been shown to be reduced in all types of arthritis, the reduction is greater in those with RA. They found a 50% incidence of falls (40 of 80 patients) during the study. Characteristics that were related to an increased risk of falls included specific medications, severity of disease (swollen joint count), and single limb stance (time).

Some clients will need a brace to improve joint alignment or provide stability during activities. Clients who report feeling that the joint is unstable or gives way should be referred back to their physician or to a physical therapist for an evaluation.

Another treatment used to address alignment problems is an orthotic placed in the shoe (58). The research regarding orthotics for those with arthritis is mixed: most studies find a reduction in pain, but the effect on gait and biomechanical changes is varied (58). While on the topic of alignment, proper shoes are a must for a client with lower extremity arthritis, especially for weight-bearing activities. The clients' shoes should provide proper support and have good cushioning. Extremely worn shoes may aggravate pain and discomfort during activity.

Proper progression should help improve exercise effectiveness for those with excessive fatigue. The CEP should advise clients to intersperse regular rest periods into the day and into their exercise program. When having an exacerbation of symptoms, the client should reduce the intensity and sometimes the duration of the session. Importantly, the client should be reminded that increasing rest does not equate to stopping all activity. However, clients should also be told that a small amount of discomfort in the muscles or joints during or immediately after exercise is common following the performance of an unfamiliar exercise (59).

Poor balance should be addressed as part of a thorough exercise program. However, until the balance has improved, it should be determined whether the client can safely perform unsupported activities. For example, if the balance deficit is significant, recumbent cycling or activities in the water might be used to build fitness. Some facilities have harness systems to use while walking on the treadmill, which are effective in protecting against falls. Some activities, such as yoga, offer modified programs, during which the client uses a chair or other device for balance support.

The components of a proper exercise program for those with arthritis include aerobic and resistance training, flexibility, and balance activities, which are often referred to as neuromotor training. The training components should follow the guidelines of the American College of Sports Medicine (ACSM) and the guidelines for older adults and those with significant chronic conditions (42, 59, 60). Tables 11.2 and 11.3 highlight the frequency, duration or time, type, and intensity (FITT) guidelines from ACSM (59).

In addition, Vliet Vlieland and van den Ende (60) note that self-management interventions should be taught and supervised for at least 6 weeks for the best long-term adherence. A home-based 2-year strength-training program in early RA led to good long-term compliance in a 5-year follow-up (61, 62). Similarly, Lange et al. (51) found that a "guided intervention" at a gym had more benefits than a home program. Importantly, a review regarding exercise for OA included feedback from clients, making the recommendation to "provide better information and advice about the safety and value of exercise; provide exercise tailored to individual's preferences, abilities and needs; challenge inappropriate health beliefs and provide better support" (52; page 2).

Aerobic Activity

Aerobic fitness of individuals with arthritis has been shown to be 10%–25% lower than the same-aged individuals without arthritis. Although most of this loss appears to be due to reduced activity levels, in those with systemic arthritis, some may be due to a loss of muscle tissue and cardiovascular system compromise associated with the disease itself. A higher risk of heart disease has been identified in individuals with RA and AS. Individuals with RA have an increased mortality and a greater risk of coronary artery disease (CAD) when compared to age-matched individuals without RA (63). Recent evidence suggests that the risk of heart disease may be lower for those taking certain medications, but still higher than those in their age bracket (64). It has been recommended that cardiovascular risk scores should reflect a higher risk for individuals with inflammatory disease (65).

The duration of aerobic activity should be short if the client has been sedentary or has severe lower extremity pain (*e.g.*, two or three 10-min sessions a day). It should progress based on the clients' response. In addition to following the normal recommendations for progression and developing success (self-efficacy), starting with short bouts allows clients to develop their lower extremity strength. Biomechanical research suggests that improved lower extremity strength will in turn help absorb joint stress and reduce joint pain. Individuals with arthritis demonstrate normal responses to aerobic activity, unless

Table 11.2	FITT Recommendations for Individuals With Arthritis		
Frequency	**Aerobic** *3–5 d·wk^{-1}*	**Resistance** *2–3 d·wk^{-1}*	**Flexibility** *Daily*
Intensity	Moderate (40%–59% $\dot{V}O_2R$ or HRR) to vigorous (≥60% $\dot{V}O_2R$ or HRR)	60%–80% 1RM. Initial intensity should be lower (*i.e.*, 50%–60% 1RM) for those unaccustomed to resistance training	Move through ROM feeling tightness/stretch without pain. Progress ROM of each exercise only when there is little or no joint pain.
Time	Accumulate 150 min·wk^{-1} of moderate intensity, or 75 min·wk^{-1} of vigorous intensity, or an equivalent combination of the two, in bouts of ≥10 min.	Use healthy adult values and adjust accordingly (*i.e.*, 8–12 repetitions for 1–3 sets); include all major muscle groups.	Up to 10 repetitions for dynamic movements; hold static stretches for 10–30 s and repeat two to four times.
Type	Activities with low joint stress, such as walking, cycling, swimming, or aquatic exercise	Machine, free weights, resistance bands, tubing. Body weight exercises are also appropriate for most individuals with arthritis.	A combination of active, static, and proprioceptive neuromuscular facilitation stretching (see Box 5.5) of all major joints with a focus on affected joints and muscles crossing these joints.

1RM, one repetition maximum; HRR, heart rate reserve; ROM, range of motion; $\dot{V}O_2R$, oxygen uptake reserve.

Source: Reproduced from: Liguori G. *ACSM's Guidelines for Exercise Testing and Prescription*. 11th ed. Philadelphia (PA): Wolters Kluwer/Lippincott Williams & Wilkins; 2022. p. 310.

Table 11.3	FITT Recommendations for Individuals With Fibromyalgia		
	Aerobic	Resistance	Flexibility
Frequency	Begin with 1–2 d·wk^{-1} and gradually progress to 2–3 d·wk^{-1}	2–3 d·wk^{-1} with a minimum of 48 h between sessions	2–3 d·wk^{-1}
Intensity	Begin with light (30%–39% $\dot{V}O_2R$ or HRR). Gradually progress to moderate intensity (40%–59% $\dot{V}O_2R$ or HRR).	40%–80% 1RM. Gradually increase to 60%–80% concentric 1RM for strength. For muscle endurance, use ≤50% 1RM.	Stretch within limits of pain to the point of tightness or slight discomfort.
Time	Begin with 10 min·d^{-1} and progress to a total of 30–60 min·d^{-1} as soon as tolerated.	Strength: Gradually progress, as tolerated, from 4–5 to 8–12 repetitions, increasing from 1 to 2–4 sets per muscle group with at least 2–3 min between sets; endurance: 15–20 repetitions, increasing from 1 to 2 sets with a shorter rest interval.	Hold each stretch for 10–30 s.
Type	Low impact (*e.g.*, aquatic exercise, walking, dance, and other aerobic movement to music, swimming, cycling)	Body weight, elastic bands, dumbbells, cuff/ankle weights, weight machines. For resistance in water, use devices to manipulate turbulence (velocity, surface area)..	Static stretches (passive and/or active), for all major muscle tendon groups. Dynamic stretches may also be used.

1RM, one repetition maximum; HRR, heart rate reserve; $\dot{V}O_2R$, oxygen uptake reserve.

Source: Reproduced from: Liguori G. *ACSM's Guidelines for Exercise Testing and Prescription.* 11th ed. Philadelphia (PA): Wolters Kluwer/Lippincott Williams & Wilkins; 2022. P.329.

there is a comorbidity influencing the cardiovascular response, or medications that alter response.

The proper intensity of aerobic exercise has been the topic of several studies, as it was feared that higher intensity exercise would cause symptoms to be exacerbated or the joint deterioration to progress more rapidly. However, a systematic review examining the effects of exercise with either hip or knee OA found that those participating in higher intensity exercise rated their pain lower and their function better than those who participated in the lower intensity programs (66). They identified high intensity as additional time, sessions, and/or greater resistance as noted in the original studies. Many of the individual studies use 80% of 1RM as the base for higher intensity resistance. The authors noted that none of the reviewed studies reported any serious adverse events and those that reported adverse events reported them for both high and low intensity and these were usually related to increased knee pain. Furthermore, some studies started with lower intensity for resistance (60% of 1RM, then progressed to 80% 1RM over several weeks).

In keeping with ACSM recommendations (59), a comprehensive session should start with a warm-up. In addition to the normal progressive physiological changes, a warm-up will decrease the sensation of stiffness and improve the available motion at the involved joints. As with any warm-up, the activity should start with low-intensity movements and increase the intensity and ROM.

Any exercise mode that is used for those without arthritis can be used with clients with arthritis. The most common forms used in research include walking, cycling, and "dynamic" exercises (rhythmic activities using large muscle groups). One question that is often raised is the safety of jogging/running and its effect on progression of arthritis. Longitudinal studies have shown that running will not increase joint deterioration (67). One study noted that runners reported less arthritis pain as compared to an age-matched cohort. If weight-bearing activities are used for aerobic training, clients with arthritis in their feet may need more supportive shoes, with larger toe boxes. Although modifications for cycling may not be needed, padded gloves for those with arthritis affecting the hands may be helpful. Others may need to use cycles with padded forearm rests.

Although aquatic exercise has not demonstrated the same magnitude of change in cardiovascular fitness, it is a good option, especially if the client has severe lower extremity pain, pain that worsens with weight bearing, joint instability, or balance issues (68). Unloading the joints in the water helps the client to tolerate activity and to work on balance and ROM. Although there is not much supporting evidence, many clinicians discourage patients with shoulder arthritis from swimming laps, as the shoulder joint is less stable than other joints. If the client wishes to swim, stability exercises for the shoulder are typically recommended prior to starting a lap-swimming program.

For clients who prefer group activities, tai chi has numerous positive attributes. It is slow moving, provides a social network, and can improve several health/fitness components without aggravating arthritis symptoms. Tai chi has been shown to improve lower extremity strength, flexibility, and cardiovascular fitness among low-fit individuals (69). In addition, a recent review of tai chi and chronic pain found the same benefits for people with arthritis, as well as decreased pain and an improved sense of well-being (70).

Resistance Training

As noted earlier, resistance training has been shown to be very effective in reducing the pain and dysfunction associated with arthritis (44, 71–74). Resistance training may help address two specific issues common to patients with arthritis. One issue is the common sensation of the muscle "giving way" in people with knee arthritis. Although the problem appears to be due more to pain than to loss of strength, it is believed that a strengthening program may reduce such instances. The best effects appear to be from programs that combine strength with balance and movement activities (75, 76). Sul et al. (77) found improved strength and quality of life for individuals, with RA after a 12-week training program of only one time per week. Another issue that occurs with RA is cachexia — loss of muscle mass and associated strength, with an increase in fat mass. Resistance training has been shown to help reverse some of this loss (74). However, this review noted that high-intensity training is not advised when joint damage is advanced. Fitzgerald et al. (78) have reported that quadriceps activation failure interacts with strength and function for those with OA, thus both should be addressed.

Resistance training should follow ACSM guidelines for healthy adults or guidelines for those with chronic disease (42, 59). Some studies have found that a few individuals with arthritis were not able to tolerate high intensities initially; thus, lower intensities were used in the early sessions, and the program progressed appropriately, based on reassessment and the client's pain. Such recommendations are consistent with the recommended starting intensities for previously sedentary clients. For example, Jan et al. (53) reported using 60% of 1RM (repetitions maximum)/eight repetitions/three sets for the initial intensity. They retested every 2 weeks and increased the resistance by 5% of the new RM.

The modes used in resistance training studies with individuals with arthritis include machines, free weights, rubber tubing, and body weight, among many options. Most of the home exercise program studies used rubber tubing and body weight, while the supervised studies consisted of free weights and machines. Resistance band sets are useful for home exercise programs as they allow the client to progress the intensity of the program. Body weight activities have been used in a number of studies and in a variety of ways. Thus, strengthening for the quadriceps can be accomplished using a knee press machine, partial squats with free weights or tubing, or even partial squats without resistance. A simple home exercise for improving quadriceps strength is a wall squat (sometimes called a wall sit) as illustrated in Figure 11.10. Although this exercise is not optimal for those with patellofemoral pain, it is useful for those with arthritis who have decreased strength in their quadriceps.

Some modifications to a resistance activity may be necessary, depending on the site of arthritis and the severity. The most common modifications are limitations of the motion. Extreme ranges of motion are most likely to cause pain, and loss of full range in joint motion is one of the typical findings. For example, in the earlier example of quadriceps strengthening, squats were recommended. Many clients with moderate arthritis will prefer partial squats. In fact, some will not have the range to perform a full squat and may even be lacking the ability to completely straighten the knee. Padded gloves for grip will help when using free weights or using machines for the upper extremities. Finally, some clients may require splints. Usually, braces or splints would have been prescribed by the physician or by a therapist earlier in treatment.

Flexibility and ROM

Flexibility and ROM have been shown to be reduced in individuals with arthritis. This loss of motion is exacerbated by the typical response to pain and stiffness — the individual stops moving the joint. This leads to a cycle of increased pain and decreased ROM. Fortunately, regular ROM activities and stretching have been shown to increase joint ROM and reduce pain and the sensation of stiffness.

ROM focuses on moving the joint through the available range. Unlike stretching, ROM does not emphasize an end position, nor does it require that an end position be held for a period of time. Frequent movement through a joint range

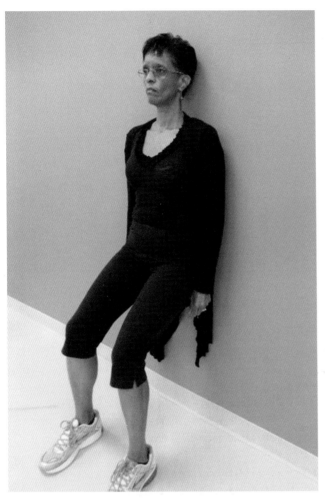

FIGURE 11.10 Partial wall squat. (From Thompson W, Ed. *ACSMs Clinical Exercise Physiology*. 1st ed. Philadelphia (PA): Wolters Kluwer; 2019.)

decreases stiffness and is best done several times daily, as stiffness never completely disappears (4, 6). In fact, stiffness can increase after even an hour of sedentary activity. For example, if the client sits for prolonged periods, the knees and/or hips may stiffen. The client will notice this when moving to a standing position. To decrease this sensation, the client should be counseled to stand and move around on a regular basis. Movement of the major joints, as well as any joint that is stiff, through their full ROM should be encouraged. ROM activities are contraindicated, however, if there is excessive pain with motion.

Stretching is performed to increase the extensibility of tight muscles. It can follow ACSM guidelines (3 d per wk). Static, dynamic, and proprioceptive stretching techniques have been shown to be effective, although some may be more comfortable than others for those with arthritis. Stretching should not cause pain, and clients should not be encouraged to stretch to an extreme range (past normal), especially if joint instability is present. Patients with AS require special

consideration. This disease causes a gradual loss of trunk flexion; thus, activities should focus on maintaining available trunk flexion. In an unpublished study, researchers showed better improvements in older individuals, with and without arthritis, when a prolonged stretch (several minutes) was used. The researchers had the subjects find a comfortable, supported position and emphasized that the stretch should not elicit pain. A gentle warm-up has been shown to improve the response to stretching.

ROM can also be addressed in activities that use large movements, such as tai chi. Both yoga and tai chi improve flexibility and balance (69, 76). Many aquatic classes also use large movements, and clients with arthritis have shown good improvements in ROM in these classes (68).

Neuromotor Training

One of the findings with any injury to a joint, including with arthritis, is a loss of proprioception. This decreased neural feedback regarding joint position is believed to be part of the reason for the previously mentioned 50% increase in falls in women with OA and RA (56, 57). Predictors of this risk included swollen joint count, use of specific medications (primarily antihypertensives and diuretics), single limb stance time, and increased sway area. Another issue that affects balance and function in clients with arthritis is quadriceps activation failure (78). Thus, recommendations for neuromotor training specific to arthritis are similar to those for older adults and those with chronic disease (11, 59). ACSM guidelines for neuromotor training identify a frequency of 2–3 days per week (59). Clinicians often recommend daily balance activities as this improves neural adaptation.

Neuromotor training includes agility exercises, balance activities, and other types of activities that stimulate feedback from the muscles and joints to the brain. These activities have been shown to improve balance and decrease pain (49, 78–80). Balance activities can be progressed from two-legged stance to tandem stances, single-leg stance, and activities on foam, which challenge balance further. Some of these balance activities are illustrated in Figures 11.11–11.14. Tai chi and yoga, in addition to boosting flexibility as mentioned earlier, have been shown to improve balance, as well as reduce disability and pain (69, 76). Many researchers observe that participants prefer the slow, controlled movements of these exercise forms, as well as the social interaction within the classes. When starting a program with a new client who has arthritis or osteoporosis, a quick assessment of balance is recommended to determine the safety of unsupported activities.

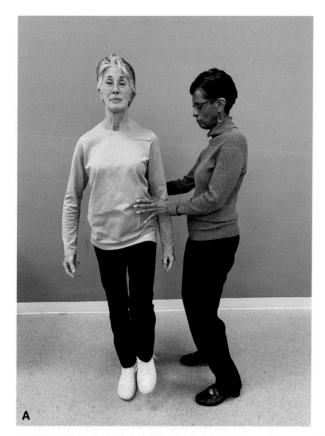
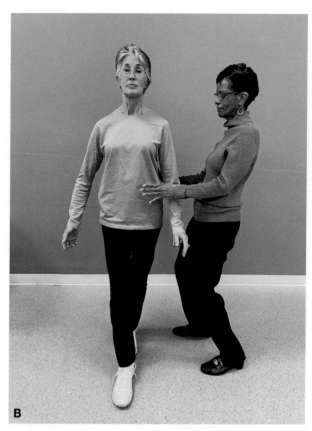

FIGURE 11.11 A. Single-leg stance — keep trunk and hips upright and level. **B.** Tandem stance — one heel immediately in front of the other toe. This narrows the stance and challenges balance.

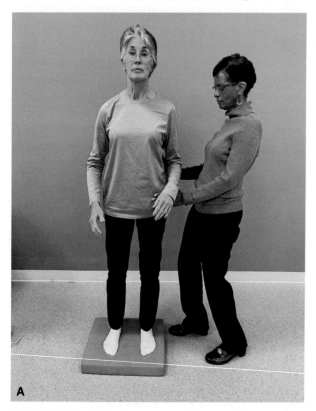
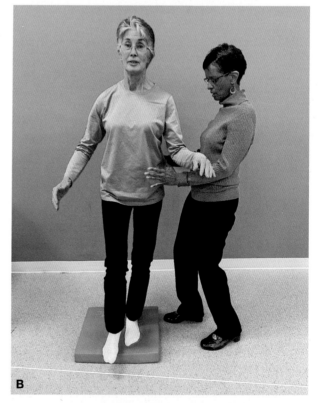

FIGURE 11.12 A. Two-leg stance — balance on foam or unstable surface. **B.** Single-leg stance on foam to further challenge balance.

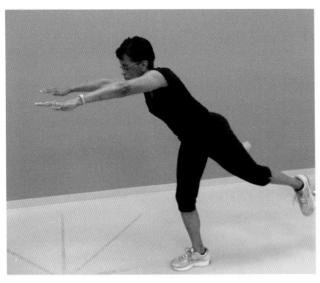

FIGURE 11.13 Single-leg balance with trunk and leg movement (modified airplane). (From Thompson W, Ed. *ACSM's Clinical Exercise Physiology.* 1st ed. Philadelphia (PA): Wolters Kluwer; 2019.)

OSTEOPENIA AND OSTEOPOROSIS

Osteopenia and osteoporosis are dysfunctions of bone modeling. Osteopenia is identified as low BMD, and osteoporosis is low BMD accompanied by "bone fragility and susceptibility to fracture" (81). Although initial changes may be in the trabecular component of the bone, later changes may involve the cortical layer. The most recent statistics show that 9% of those over the age of 50 years have osteoporosis in the lumbar spine or the neck of the femur (82). Furthermore, approximately 50% of adults aged 50 years or older have low BMD at one of the two sites. When BMD drops below a critical mass, the risk of fractures increases significantly, as illustrated in Figure 11.15. Perry and Downey (26) note that the long-term effects of sustaining a fracture often involve chronic pain and impaired mobility and posture. There is also an increased mortality associated with osteoporotic fractures (83, 84).

Risk Factors and Etiology

Risk factors for osteopenia and osteoporosis include increasing age (greater after age 50 years) and sex (women have twice the risk of men for low BMD and four times the risk for osteoporosis). Genetics — including both body size and race/ethnicity — also influences risk.

Non-Hispanic white, Mexican American, and other (other racial or ethnic groups not included in the three identified) women are at the highest risk of osteoporosis, whereas non-Hispanic Black women have a lower risk (84).

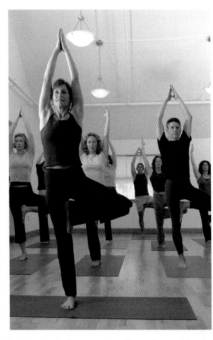

FIGURE 11.14 Yoga balance. (From McArdle WD, Katch FI, Katch VL. *Exercise Physiology.* 8th ed. Philadelphia (PA): Wolters Kluwer; 2014.)

In addition, a history of certain diseases, including OA, RA, and hypertension, increases the risk of low BMD and related fractures. Yang et al. (85) found that hypertension was a risk factor for fracture; women who had hypertension had lower BMD and a 50% greater risk of fractures when compared to age-matched cohorts. The long-term use of some medications, such as glucocorticoids, can also increase the risks of osteopenia and osteoporosis (81).

Another set of risk factors are considered modifiable, as they are primarily lifestyle related. These include

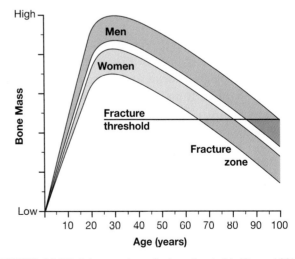

FIGURE 11.15 Osteoporosis — fracture threshold. (From *ACSM's Resource Manual for Guidelines for Exercise Testing and Prescription.* 7th ed. Philadelphia (PA): Wolters Kluwer Health; 2014.)

smoking, alcohol and caffeine use, calcium and vitamin D intake, and physical activity.

As noted earlier, osteoporosis is defined in part by susceptibility to fractures. Factors besides low BMD that increase the risk of fractures in this population include falls, balance problems, and reduced mobility. Falls are the most significant cause of fractures, and impaired balance and reduced mobility in those with osteopenia and osteoporosis contribute to the potential for a fall. Balance can in turn be impaired by medications, an association that highlights the importance of assessing patients for interactions between disease, medications, and other lifestyle factors.

Clinical Diagnosis

Diagnosis of osteopenia and osteoporosis is primarily made through the use of dual x-ray absorptiometry (DXA). Fracture without trauma is also used to clinically diagnose both, although DXA is used to confirm a diagnosis. Changes in BMD can be classified according to the etiology of bone loss (trabecular or cortical) and by the percentage of BMD as compared to "normal." The types and categories are identified in Box 11.1 (86, 87).

Reflecting the multifactorial nature of fracture risk, several risk assessment tools have been developed for use when screening older clients. The Fracture Risk Assessment Tool (FRAX) was developed based on data from a World Health Organization (WHO) subgroup and includes 12 risk factors to determine the risk of osteoporotic fracture (81). If a client has several risk factors, a thorough health history is recommended.

Management of Osteopenia and Osteoporosis

The National Osteoporosis Foundation has developed a guide for the prevention and treatment of osteoporosis (66). Pharmacologic guidelines for the treatment of osteoporosis focus on early intervention with bisphosphonates to reduce fracture risk (23, 24). In concert with pharmacologic treatment, recommendations include risk education, nutritional counseling regarding calcium and vitamin D needs, exercise prescription, fall risk assessment, counseling regarding alcohol reduction, and smoking cessation. Exercise recommendations specify weight-bearing and strengthening activities. Activities should focus on agility, strength, posture, and balance, with the ultimate goal of improving BMD and reducing fall risk. Thus, exercise prescription aligns with ACSM recommendations, illustrated in Table 11.4.

Benefits of Exercise for Patients With Osteopenia or Osteoporosis

The cardiovascular and musculoskeletal benefits of exercise for those with osteopenia and osteoporosis parallel findings for individuals without these diseases. In addition, many studies have focused on the effect of exercise on BMD, fracture reduction, and mobility and quality of life. A meta-analysis examining BMD preservation and exercise reported that resistance training significantly improved BMD, and the combination of resistance training with weight-bearing exercises had a more extensive impact on BMD (88). Another meta-analysis examined the effects of exercise on fracture reduction (89) and reported that the overall risk of fractures was reduced with the exercise groups. The findings regarding quality of life and mobility are inconsistent, with a recommendation for more studies (90).

Giangregorio et al. (90) published exercise recommendations either for those with osteoporosis or for those who had suffered a fracture based on a systematic review of literature and expert consensus. The strongest evidence for exercise showed a reduction in falls; however, the authors noted that these findings may vary by the type of exercise. The findings regarding the effect of exercise on fractures were mixed. Although the research tends to show a reduced risk of fractures, with exercise, the authors reported a U-shaped curve according to which the greatest risk of fractures was among those in the lowest and highest activity groups. These groups were not doing multicomponent programs, however. Thus, the authors' first recommendation is for clients with osteoporosis or osteoporotic fracture

Box 11.1	Types and Categories of Bone Loss
Type	**Categories**
Type I = loss of trabecular bone after menopause	Normal ± 1 SD below mean
Type II = loss of trabecular or cortical bone due to abnormal reabsorption	Osteopenia 1–2.5 SD below mean
	Osteoporosis ≥2.5 SD below mean
	Severe = 1 or more fractures

Table 11.4	FITT Recommendations for Individuals With Osteoporosis		
	Aerobic	**Resistance**	**Flexibility**
Frequency	4–5 d·wk^{-1}	Start with 1–2 nonconsecutive d·wk^{-1}; may progress to 2–3 d·wk^{-1}	5–7 d·wk^{-1}
Intensity	Moderate intensity (40%–59% V̇O$_2$R or HRR). Use of the CR-10 scale with ratings of 3–4 might be a more appropriate method of establishing intensity.	Adjust resistance so that last two repetitions are challenging to perform. High-intensity and high-velocity training can be beneficial for those who can tolerate it.	Stretch to the point of feeling tightness or mild discomfort.
Time	Begin with 20 min; gradually progress to a minimum of 30 min (with a maximum of 45–60 min). Increase time initially to a minimum of 10 min before increasing intensity. Progress to 30–60 min as tolerated.	Begin with 1 set of 8–12 repetitions; increase to 2 sets after ~2 wk; no more than 8–10 exercises per session	Hold static stretch for 10–30 s; 2–4 repetitions of each exercise
Type	Walking, cycling, or other individually appropriate aerobic activity (weight bearing preferred). Impact loading exercises such as jumping or bench stepping can be used in those with low or moderate risk for fracture.	Standard equipment can be used with adequate instruction and safety considerations. Compound movement exercises are best.	Static stretching of all major joints

HRR, heart rate reserve; V̇O$_2$R, oxygen uptake reserve.

Source: Liguori G. *ACSM's Guidelines for Exercise Testing and Prescription.* 11th ed. Philadelphia (PA): Wolters Kluwer/Lippincott Williams & Wilkins; 2022. p. 350.

to participate in multicomponent exercise programs with aerobic, resistance, and balance training. Their second recommendation emphasized that these clients should not participate in aerobic exercise alone because those who only walked had more fractures than those who also performed resistance training. Similarly, Kemmler et al. (89) reviewed 10 controlled studies on exercise and fracture reduction in clients with osteoporosis. Considerable variations in exercise intensity were noted; however, those who participated in exercise interventions had half the overall rate of fractures when compared to controls.

Contraindications, Precautions, and Modifications to Exercise

Contraindications to exercise are usually related to the presence of a fracture, previous injury, or acute severity of osteoporosis. Even in such cases, modification of the activity is often preferable to complete cessation of activity. As with arthritis and many other diseases, a primary precaution for activity is the presence of a fever. Clinical guidelines regarding exercise when febrile are broad, and they are usually based on the comorbidities and other signs of infection (91). In the

hospital, the health care staff will be able to ascertain whether the fever is under control to participate in an activity.

Modifications to an exercise program are often required to improve client safety and effectiveness and will be based on client issues such as decreased strength, poor balance, and impaired resting posture (extreme kyphosis). Giangregorio et al. (90) noted a potential for fractures with twisting motions when transitioning positions, thus implying that one precaution prior to exercise is thorough education before starting an activity. Importantly, the authors noted that the risk of adverse events during activity was outweighed by the benefits of activity and exercise. If the client also has RA, then precautions may follow those identified for that disease. Prior to the initiation of a program for an individual with diagnosed osteoporosis, the client should consult with their physician to determine precautions and contraindications for exercise.

Aerobic Activity

Few studies have examined cardiovascular responses to aerobic exercise, without concurrent resistance training, for those with osteoporosis or osteopenia. One early study showed good improvements in muscular endurance in a group that did treadmill walking and step training (92). More recent research focuses on multimodal programs. Prescription of aerobic training should follow recommendations for older adults (42) or ACSM guidelines (59). Any mode may be utilized, depending on the client's preference, although research shows that weight-bearing activities are most beneficial (89). As noted earlier, aerobic exercise alone is not recommended, as there appears to be a greater risk of fracture in those who do only aerobic exercise such as walking (90). Perry and Downey (26) identified some of the high-impact activities that have been used successfully, including such examples as running, jumping, skipping rope, and stair-climbing. Caution should be used with the initial-level jumping activities, such as low box jumps or obstacle hopping, especially with those who have already had a fracture. Initiation at too high of an impact level may lead to the development of fractures.

Kemmler and von Stengel (93) examined the BMD response to two different exercise frequencies over a 12-year period. Although nonsignificant, they found that those exercising greater than or equal to two to four times a week had better BMD. The lumbar spine density for the exercise group improved 0.009 ± 0.04 g·cm^{-2} versus a loss of 0.035 ± 0.029 g·cm^{-2} for those who exercised less than 2 days per week.

Resistance Training

Several guidelines have emphasized that resistance training is a crucial component. It has been shown to increase both femoral neck and lumbar spine BMD, with the magnitude of improvement greater when combined with a high-impact weight-bearing program (88). Hinton (94) found that both resistance and impact training (jump-type training) improved BMD at the lumbar spine. A consensus statement from the International and National Osteoporosis Foundation recommends a minimum of two times per week for resistance training. The recommendations also identify the one exercise for each major muscle group with 8–12 repetitions, which may be considered as high intensity (90). However, the authors caution that the use of machines "should be avoided in individuals at high risk of vertebral fracture," with the caveat that this may be allowable if clients can perform the exercise with good form and under supervision (90; page 829). Furthermore, slow, controlled movements are recommended, and twisting motions should be avoided. Similarly, Perry and Downey (26) identify resistance guidelines of two

to three times per week, 70%–90% of 1RM, two to three sets, though they did not identify a recommendation for the number of repetitions. Watson et al. (95) had subjects start with body weight and low-load activities, then progressed toward more than 80% 1RM after 1 month. They also included a small "drop" jump exercise to increase the impact. Montgomery et al. (96) found that jump activities had the greatest potential impact on spinal density. Thus, the recommended guidelines follow ACSM (59) resistance training guidelines, with the addition of some form of high-impact activity.

Another component of the resistance training recommendations includes the emphasis on strengthening postural muscles (90). The authors specifically noted the need to work such muscles as the spinal extensor muscles and discuss research showing that hyperkyphotic posture (Figure 11.16) is associated with decreased balance and an increased risk of falls. There is some evidence that specific resistance exercise can decrease hyperkyphosis and improve posture (97).

Flexibility and ROM

Recent studies only report flexibility training as part of a multicomponent program. Thus, flexibility training can follow ACSM guidelines or guidelines for those with chronic disease (42, 59). With clients who have had a fracture, most clinicians recommend caution in stretching the associated

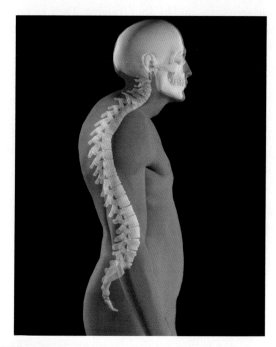

FIGURE 11.16 Hyperkyphosis. (From LifeART. *3D Super Anatomy 7.* 1st ed. Philadelphia (PA): Wolters Kluwer; 2000.)

joints and the use of static stretching versus dynamic or assisted. If one of the recommendations regarding resistance training is extrapolated to stretching, twisting stretches should be done with caution or avoided completely.

Flexibility may be part of a postural improvement program when used in association with resistance training. As hyperkyphosis is common in clients with osteoporosis, the postural program should include strengthening of the upper back and scapular stabilizers, with stretching of the anterior chest muscles. A forward head posture (FHP) is often associated with hyperkyphosis. Exercise training to address this was discussed earlier and will be addressed again in the Back and Neck Pain and Dysfunction section of this chapter.

Neuromotor Training

As noted, the risk of falls and ensuing fractures is a significant concern for those with osteopenia and osteoporosis. Thus, emphasis is given to balance training in all guidelines (90). The authors recommended daily balance training with 15–20 minutes per day (2 hours accumulated weekly). They emphasize that exercises should challenge balance in order to be beneficial. Numerous activities can be used, including those identified in the section on Arthritis. It is important to progress the difficulty and to use lifestyle-integrated exercises, such as stepping up and down a stair or curb, while emphasizing control of the movement. Another activity that can be done is to shift weight completely from one leg to the other, then back, while doing chores such as dishwashing.

Tai chi, a modality that incorporates weight-bearing activity with focused, controlled balance, is a recommended method of training balance (26, 90). Tai chi has been shown to improve stride width, which suggests improved gait and dynamic balance. In addition, for individuals with osteopenia, tai chi improves performance on the vestibular component of the Sensory Organization Test, which is considered evidence of improved balance (98).

Summary

Exercise is important for those with arthritis and/or osteoporosis. When an individual has a known diagnosis, the CEP should first determine if the physician has indicated any activity restrictions. If the CEP suspects an undiagnosed musculoskeletal issue with significant symptoms, the individual should be encouraged to consult their physician prior to initiating a program. A program for an individual with arthritis or osteoporosis should follow ACSM guidelines (59), with modifications based on the individual joint restrictions and symptoms. The CEP should be mindful of symptoms that the individual is having a "flare-up" or progression of symptoms and modify the program accordingly.

JOINT REPLACEMENTS

When arthritis has progressed to the point of severe pain or the individual can no longer function normally, joint replacement is often the next step. After the replacement, many of these clients may participate in exercise; however, specific modifications may be needed. This section will address the types of joint replacement, as well as some of the issues that should be considered when working with a client who has had a joint replacement.

Total joint arthroplasty (TJA), or more commonly total joint replacement (TJR), is a common surgical intervention for late-stage musculoskeletal conditions. The joints most frequently replaced are the knee, hip, shoulder, and elbow (99). Recent advances in joint replacement materials and design have also made the ankle a viable joint for replacement (100). In 2014, an estimated 3.7 million Americans were living with a knee TJR and another 2.5 million were living with a hip TJR (99). In general, joint replacement surgeries are successful, and patients lead active lives following rehabilitation.

Overview of TJR

Although the anatomy differs according to the joint involved, all TJR surgeries have a few commonalities. A TJR is a major orthopedic surgery requiring sawing bones, releasing tight soft tissue, removing the inflamed joint capsule, and sometimes removing ligaments around the joints. The articular surfaces of the bones are replaced with an implant made from metal alloys or ceramic and high-density plastic components with unique designs. Components are secured to the bone either with cement or a long stem in the middle of the bone or with a combination of both. This type of fixation allows immediate joint movement, weight bearing (if a weight-bearing joint), and ambulation.

The primary goal for any patient undergoing a TJR is to diminish or entirely resolve joint pain. Secondary goals are to improve function and maintain independent living. TJR is a treatment of last resort, meaning it is only offered to patients after a long course of failed conservative management. Delayed TJR in weight-bearing joints is typical because of the relatively short life of prosthetic materials. In 2021, the American Joint Replacement Registry (AJRR) reported knee replacements lasting more than 15 years (101). Better prosthetic design, surgical techniques, improved polyethylene wear characteristics, and rehabilitation strategies have pushed the life of a TJR beyond these estimates. Nevertheless, most physicians recommend that patients who develop joint damage in their 40s or 50s manage their symptoms pharmacologically and with activity modification until they are in their 60s. Over the past 8 years (2012–2020), the mean age of people undergoing total knee replacement was 69 years.

Revision surgeries are much more complicated because they involve removing the old implant(s) before replacing it with a new one. Not only is the surgery more difficult, but an older patient tends to have more comorbidities (hypertension, cardiac problems, etc.), which complicate the surgery itself as well as the rehabilitation after surgery.

This delayed treatment mentality creates several problems. First, people who have suffered debilitating pain and decreased function for a very long time are likely to have become deconditioned, with limited ROM and muscle atrophy around the affected joint. Second, people with chronic pain limit their movement secondary to fear of exacerbating the pain. Therefore, they do not reap the benefits of exercise. Third, because of their relative inactivity and a decrease in normal metabolism that may occur with aging, this population tends to become overweight. For these reasons, a physician may suggest a period of "prehabilitation" prior to surgery. The goals of a "prehab" program should be to normalize joint ROM and increase the muscular strength surrounding the joint. In the case of lower extremity joint replacement, it is also a good idea to strengthen both upper arms (biceps, triceps, and latissimus). After surgery, the upper arms will be instrumental in getting in and out of bed and for using any assisted device (walker, crutches). It is not unusual for a person with this type of chronic pain and dysfunction to consult a fitness trainer to get in shape prior to surgery or to lose weight to become a candidate for surgery.

Two different surgical techniques are commonly used for a TJR. An open procedure requires a large incision that crosses the joint being replaced. It also requires detachment of muscles surrounding the joint. These are later reattached. The advantage of an open procedure is that it allows the surgeon an unrestricted view and access to the joint. A disadvantage is the amount of soft tissue damage, which must also be repaired after placement of the implant. This type of surgical approach has led to restrictive

postoperative rehabilitation precautions, which may last from 3 to 6 months after surgery.

In order to speed up the postoperative rehabilitation, many physicians are now using a minimally invasive surgical procedure. An important benefit of this type of surgery is minimal soft tissue damage around the joint. This allows an accelerated postoperative rehabilitation plan. Another benefit is a reduced risk for postoperative complications. A drawback of this procedure is that the view of the joint during surgery is severely restricted, requiring an increase in the skill and training of the surgeon. Increased physician training and the addition of robotic tools and three-dimensional magnetic resonance imaging (MRI) during surgery have advanced the surgical techniques, which in turn has advanced the outcomes.

Good outcomes have been reported with fast-track postoperative care, with most TJR patients discharged from the acute hospital within 1.5 days (101). Most people attend either physical therapy in an outpatient setting or have a therapist come to their home for rehabilitation. Either way, it is common for someone to join a gym or seek a personal trainer's advice within 3–4 months after a TJR.

Complications of TJR

Postoperative complications of TJR are rare but can be serious. Deep vein thrombosis (DVT) usually occurs as an immediate complication of a total knee arthroplasty (TKA); however, it can occur any time after surgery and is more likely to occur after a lower extremity surgery. A common place for a DVT to occur is in the calf of the surgical leg. If a person has symptoms such as pain, a sensation of tightness (usually in the calf), whole leg swelling, or skin that is warm to touch, the Wells DVT Criteria should be used. The Wells DVT Criteria (102) is an evidence-based clinical decision rule, which estimates the pretest clinical probability of a DVT (Table 11.5). A Well's Criteria score of 1–2 indicates a moderate risk and a score of 3 or greater indicates a high risk of having a DVT. A deadly complication can occur if the DVT dislodges and becomes a pulmonary embolus. Because of the potentially fatal consequences of a DVT if left untreated, someone demonstrating symptoms of a DVT should be counseled to seek medical attention immediately.

Other complications that can occur after TJR are dislocation of the joint, which is more common in the hip and shoulder, and/or loosening of the implant. Loosening may occur even 5–10 years after the original surgery. Common signs of these rarer complications include severe joint pain, usually with functional activities such as

Table 11.5	Wells DVT Criteria Scoring	Points
Criteria		
Active cancer		1
Bedridden recently >3 d or major surgery within 4 wk		1
Calf swelling >3 cm compared to the other leg (measured 10 cm below tibial tuberosity)		1
Collateral (nonvaricose) superficial veins present		1
Entire leg swollen		1
Localized tenderness along deep venous system		1
Pitting edema, greater in symptomatic leg		1
Paralysis, paresis, or recent plaster immobilization of the lower extremity		1
Previously documented DVT		1
Alternative diagnosis to DVT as likely or more likely		−2
A score ≥2 indicates that probability of DVT is likely. A score <2 indicates that probability of DVT is unlikely.		

DVT, deep vein thrombosis.

walking and standing from a seated position, and pain referred down the extremity. In the case of a shoulder replacement, joint instability is a hallmark sign of prosthesis loosening. If a person with a history of TJR exhibits any of these symptoms, it would be wise to refer to a physician prior to beginning any exercise program.

Total Knee Arthroplasty

As previously mentioned, the knee is by far the most common joint replaced, with over 700,000 performed annually (103). The knee is a multi-joint complex (medial and lateral tibiofemoral joints and patellofemoral joint). A knee TJR replaces the articulating surfaces of the tibia and the femur as well as the posterior patella with artificial components. The most common surgical complication of a TKA, knee stiffness, occurs in 15%–20% of patients (104). A loss of knee extension (>15 degrees) is the most detrimental on mobility, whereas a decrease in knee flexion (<75 degrees) will interfere with ADL. It is very important to attempt to restore as much knee extension as possible. Walking with a bent knee increases the forces across the knee in both limbs (105) and can be a source of anterior knee pain. In addition, the literature supports that following a unilateral knee total knee replacement (TKR), there is an increase in the knee joint forces in the opposite knee during gait (106). Sixty-two

percent of individuals who received a unilateral TKA already had evidence of OA in the opposite knee at the time of surgery (107) and 37% of people who have a knee TKR have a TKA in the opposite knee within 10 years (108). This information warrants being mindful of the opposite knee during exercise programs.

Recent medical advances now allow surgeons to replace only the affected parts of the joint. Unicompartmental knee replacement only replaces the diseased part of the joint. Medial knee joint osteoarthritis is more prevalent than all three (medial, lateral, and patellar) and therefore is the most common site for a unicompartmental replacement. These unicompartmental joint replacements are more often performed on younger (64 years) and more active patients. A meta-analysis of medial (n = 32,083) and lateral (2,636) unicompartmental knee replacements reported a 92.8% and 86.6%, respectively, lasting greater than 10 years (109).

Activities to be avoided after any sort of knee replacement include high-impact activities such as jumping, running, or any activity with repetitive high axial loading. Likewise, kneeling on the surgical knee has been linked with an increase in wear of the contact area of the implant and may lead to wear on the plastic components (110).

There is a very strong relationship between quadriceps strength and functional performance after a TKA (111). Quadriceps weakness commonly persists even a year after surgery (112). A strengthening program focusing on the large muscle groups (gluteals, hip abductors, hamstrings, and quadriceps) of the lower legs performed two to three times per week is recommended. Weight-bearing exercises concentrating on eccentric control should be part of the exercise program. Single-leg stance and other balance exercises should be performed on all surfaces as strength and pain allow. Higher level activities such as athletic activities should only be attempted after the quadriceps strength is equal to that of the nonsurgical leg and then should be performed with caution (112).

Total Hip Arthroplasty

According to the AJRR (101), which has access to over 2,244,587 reported joint replacements in its database, total hip arthroplasty (THA) is less common in 34.6% of procedures versus TKA (52%). The most common reasons for a THA are OA, RA, or traumatic femoral neck fracture, all of which occur more often in the elderly. The average age for those undergoing elective hip replacement is 66 years versus those having a hip replacement as a treatment after a hip fracture (72.3 years). The hip is also susceptible to congenital deformities, which can lead to early-onset OA and early (second decade) THA to maintain quality of life. Because these patients require THA performed much earlier in life, harder, longer-lasting materials have been developed, such as ceramic-on-ceramic versus the traditional metal-on-plastic designs (113).

Regardless of prosthetic makeup, a THA typically replaces the femoral head and the acetabulum of the pelvis. Hemiarthroplasties, in which only one component, either the femoral head or the acetabulum, is replaced, make up only about 9% of hip replacements (101). Hip resurfacing is an option for those with only femoral head involvement and is often performed on young active adults with degenerative hip disease (Figure 11.17). The advantage of hip resurfacing is that the femoral head is not removed but is trimmed and capped with a smooth replacement. This is a new but growing trend in the U.S., accounting for only 0.2% of joint replacements (AJRR). One of the major indications for this surgery is strong, healthy bone. For that reason, hip resurfacing is much more common in males (101).

The hip is made for mobility and is inherently a stable joint. It relies on extremely strong ligaments and an extensive joint capsule, which provide passive stability in all directions. Any surgery to replace the hip requires postsurgical motion precautions, which may last longer than 6 months. It is important to know which surgical approach was taken to complete the THA procedure. The approach describes the location of the surgical incision and gives some indication of the structures that have been disturbed.

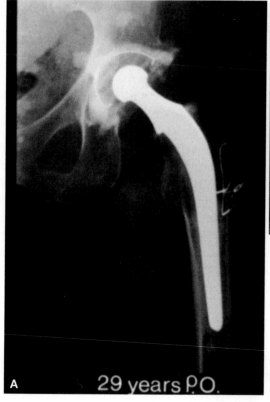

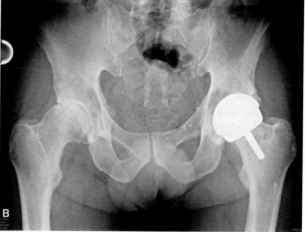

FIGURE 11.17 Types of hip replacement. **A.** Traditional hip implant in which both the femoral head and neck and the acetabulum of the pelvis are replaced. **B.** Hip resurfacing in which the head is reshaped and capped with an implant, whereas the neck of the femur is left intact with a hip-resurfacing procedure. (**A:** From Morrey BF, Berry DJ, An K-N, Kitaoka HB, Pagnano MW. *Joint Replacement Arthroplasty*. Philadelphia (PA): Wolters Kluwer; 2011. **B:** From Callaghan JJ, Rosenberg AG, Rubash HE, Clohisy J, Beaule P, DellaValle C. *The Adult Hip (Two Volume Set)*. 3rd ed. Philadelphia (PA): Wolters Kluwer; 2015.)

Of the three common approaches, the posterior lateral approach is the most popular (114). This procedure sacrifices the joint capsule, but the very important hip abductors are not cut. Motion precautions following this procedure include no hip flexion past 90 degrees, no crossing of midline with the surgical extremity, and no internal rotation (IR) past neutral. Physicians vary with the length of time for the precautions, but it is universally recommended to avoid performing all of the restricted movements at the same time for the life of the implant.

An anterolateral approach requires a small part of the hip abductors to be cut. This results in significant weakness of the hip abductors, which may affect walking ability. Protected movements are the same as above but also should avoid flexion with external rotation (ER) for at least 6 weeks postsurgical. Also, hip abductor strengthening may be delayed depending on the surgeon. This results in severe weakness of the hip abductor. Residual hip abductor weakness will result in the patient leaning side to side during ambulation.

Medical advances and increased surgeon training have led to the direct anterior approach. This surgical procedure does not cut or detach any muscles around the hip. This results in faster rehabilitation, mobility, and most importantly, no postsurgical movement precautions. The reasons this procedure is not performed more often are that it requires a great deal of surgical training to avoid common complications such as intraoperative fractures and inadequate femoral stem positioning resulting in early revision procedures (115).

Consider the appropriate mobility precautions when designing an exercise program for a patient who has had a THA. It is easy to adapt open-chain exercises to avoid restricted motions. Depending on the surgical approach, some stretches, such as the hurdle stretch (hip IR) or butterfly (hip ER) stretch, may need to be avoided. Closed-chain exercises are an important component of any strengthening program but require planning to avoid prohibited motions. When using weight machines where the seat can be adjusted, it is important to make sure the hips are never below the knees in a sitting or reclined position. Maintain an upright trunk position during squats and limit squats to 90 degrees of knee flexion to avoid excessive flexion of the hip. When performing single-leg balance activities with the surgical leg, remember that turning the torso away from the surgical leg is hip ER, while turning the torso toward the surgical leg is hip IR. Extremes of these motions should be avoided. It is best to seek guidance from the surgeon as to when ROM restrictions can be lifted.

Total Shoulder Arthroplasty

A total shoulder arthroplasty (TSA) is indicated in cases of severe glenohumeral OA, which causes severe pain and functional limitations in the upper extremity. This surgery involves the removal of the humeral head and replacement with a metal implant, and the replacement of the glenoid fossa with a high-density polyethylene component mimicking the normal anatomy of the shoulder. An intact rotator cuff musculature is paramount to the success of this surgery. Hemiarthroplasty can be used when the humeral head articular surface has deteriorated but the glenoid fossa is still intact.

A reversed TSA is a unique implant that is used in patients with a severely deficient rotator cuff. This design places the larger ball-shaped component on the glenoid surface and the flattened component on the humerus, as depicted in Figure 11.18. This design allows the deltoid muscle to be used to do the work of the rotator cuff muscles. A side-by-side comparison of those who received a standard TSA with those who received a reversed TSA found no differences in function or adverse events (116). However, those with a standard TSA did have a significantly greater external ROM compared to a standard TSA.

Although physician protocols vary, most people will have motion restrictions for 6–8 weeks after TSA, depending on the integrity of the rotator cuff. Usually, by

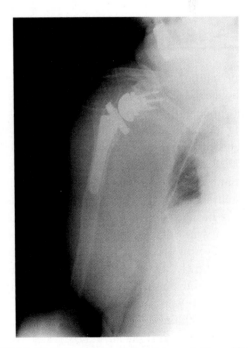

FIGURE 11.18 A reverse shoulder replacement. (From Morrey BF, An KN, Sperling JW. *Joint Replacement Arthroplasty*. 4th ed. Philadelphia (PA): Wolters Kluwer; 2010.)

3–4 months, they are working more independently and may be ready to resume presurgical activities such as exercise classes; however, full recovery may take 2 years or longer (117). Emphasis should be placed on restoring full-active pain-free ROM. Precaution should be taken to progress exercises slowly and to avoid any exercise that causes pain in the anterior or superior part of the shoulder. One position that should be avoided is horizontal abduction in combination with ER, especially with weights until specifically allowed by the surgeon. An easy reminder for the client is to instruct them to keep their elbow in front of the body with all exercises.

Summary

In general, clients recovering from a TJR will have some postoperative restrictions for 6 months or longer. Restoring ROM within allowed parameters is paramount to regaining full function of the extremity. However, care should be taken in all suggested exercises to make sure the client is not performing a prohibited action. Likewise, it is important to set up all weight machines to stay within ROM parameters. High-impact activities should be avoided with these clients as the joint replacement materials are not built for high-impact activities. It is very important to modify the exercise regimen with any reports of joint pain. With proper instruction, clients with a joint replacement can return to a pain-free active lifestyle.

SOFT TISSUE INJURIES

Soft tissue injuries are extremely common, especially in those who exercise. Most of these injuries are caused by some sort of repetitive motion or overusing a muscle by exercising too much or performing some exercise incorrectly. Tendonitis is an acute inflammation of the tendon. Many soft tissue injuries that don't involve the tendon at all are commonly but incorrectly referred to as tendonitis. A strain is an injury to the musculotendinous unit. A sprain is an injury to either the ligament or the joint capsule. Tenosynovitis is an inflammation of the synovial tissue covering the tendon. Tendinosis is a chronic condition in which the tendon has degenerated, usually because of repetitive use, but with very little inflammation. Bursitis is inflammation of the bursae. Synovitis is inflammation of the synovial membrane lining the inside of the joint capsule. Generally, all of these issues can be resolved with rest and correction of abnormal posture and/or movement pattern.

Posture

As noted in the beginning of the chapter, poor posture is a common trait associated with many musculoskeletal concerns and can be associated with many soft tissue injuries. The forward head with rounded shoulders position that was discussed has been related to shoulder dysfunction and pain (see Figure 11.2). These symptoms are due not only to strain on the muscles of the upper back and shoulders but also to the altered position of the cervical spine and scapula. When the cervical spine is not in optimal alignment, the nerves exiting the spinal column may be impinged, causing referred pain to the shoulder. Many jobs are sedentary, requiring sitting for long periods of time and often using a computer mouse. The rounded shoulders sitting posture causes the scapula to abduct (slide forward) and downwardly rotate. This long-term posture can result in weak and overstretched scapular stabilizers such as the middle trapezius and rhomboid muscles, and a tight pectoralis major. Even short periods of time with rounded shoulders and an abducted scapula can significantly decrease the amount of shoulder ROM (118). Thus, posture should be addressed when working with a client with upper back, neck, and/or shoulder issues.

Upper Limb Injuries

Shoulder

The shoulder complex refers to several joints (acromioclavicular, sternoclavicular, and glenohumeral) and the articulation between the scapula and thorax which moves like a joint (Figure 11.19). Most people blame shoulder

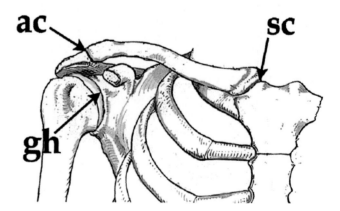

FIGURE 11.19 Front view of the shoulder complex consisting of the glenohumeral (gh), acromioclavicular (ac), and the sternoclavicular (sc) joints. (From Chila A, American Osteopathic Association. *Foundations of Osteopathic Medicine.* 3rd ed. Philadelphia (PA): Wolters Kluwer; 2010.)

pain on the glenohumeral joint, but it is important to incorporate flexibility and strength training of all the muscles which cross all the joints of the shoulder complex.

The shoulder anatomy is set up in such a way that it requires a concert of both passive (ligament) and dynamic (muscles) structures working in harmony to produce both the ROM and the stability required to perform ADLs. For example, the rotator cuff is made up of four different muscles (supraspinatus, infraspinatus, teres minor, and subscapularis), all originating on the scapula and inserting on the humerus, and they function as guidewires for the humeral head during overhead motion. The much larger deltoid muscles (anterior, middle, and posterior heads) are responsible for abducting the humerus while the rotator cuff produces a downward glide (depression) of the humeral head to keep the humerus centered in the glenoid, as depicted in Figure 11.20. This important force couple allows a large arc of arm motion with very little muscle movement. It is easy to see that even the slightest abnormality (muscular weakness, tightness, abnormal positioning) may cause shoulder dysfunction and pain. It is no wonder that shoulder pain is an extremely common complaint in the general population.

One of the most common causes of soft tissue injury in the shoulder is impingement syndrome. Primary impingement occurs when something protrudes into the subacromial space and compresses or rubs the rotator cuff tendons and/or the subacromial bursae both of which lie between the acromion and the humeral head (Figure 11.21). A common cause of primary impingement is a hook-shaped distal end of the acromion, referred to as a type III acromion (Figure 11.22). This structural abnormality cannot be changed by exercise; however, it can be made worse with chronic poor posture (rounded shoulders) or exercising with poor posture. Secondary impingement occurs when the muscles of the shoulder do not work in synchrony to allow the glenohumeral joint to glide normally. This usually occurs due to joint capsule tightness, muscle imbalance, or poor posture. Symptoms of impingement syndrome include lateral shoulder pain, which may radiate into the arm; limited overhead reach; and a painful arc of motion. A painful arc is characterized by shoulder pain that occurs or worsens in the middle portion of the overhead reach with or without pain at rest (Figure 11.23).

Another tendon that can be impinged when the scapula is in a poor position is the long head of the biceps.

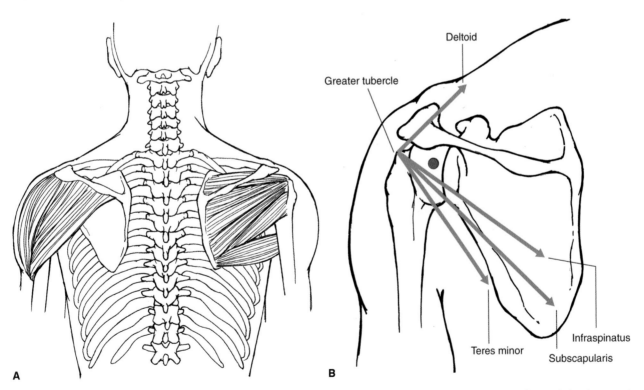

FIGURE 11.20 Force couples of the shoulder. **A.** The lines depict the pull of the deltoid in an upward direction and the downward direction of the rotator cuff (infraspinatus, subscapularis, and teres minor). **B.** The deltoid (left shoulder) and the posterior rotator cuff (right shoulder) form an important force couple in the shoulder. (**A:** From Hendrickson T. *Massage for Orthopedic Conditions.* 1st ed. Philadelphia (PA): Wolters Kluwer; 2002. **B:** From Oatis CA. *Kinesiology: The Mechanics and Pathomechanics of Human Movement.* 3rd ed. Philadelphia (PA): Wolters Kluwer; 2016.)

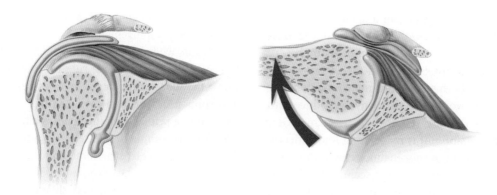

FIGURE 11.21 During overhead motions, impingement of the subacromial structures can occur if the humerus does not stay centered in the glenoid. (From Anatomical Chart Company. *Shoulder and Elbow*. 1st ed. Philadelphia (PA): Wolters Kluwer.)

It attaches to the supraglenoid tubercle of the humerus, which also glides under the coracoacromial arch with shoulder flexion. Irritation of this tendon would cause pain to be located more on the anterior shoulder.

If a person is unable to raise their arm overhead without pain, the problem could be a tight joint capsule. If they have less than a 10-degree deficit, it is possible to correct this with slow, sustained stretching. However, greater deficits are best treated with more aggressive manual therapy and should be referred to a physical therapist.

Muscle imbalances are common in those who regularly lift weights. The deltoid muscles get bigger and stronger, and the smaller rotator cuff muscles often are neglected in strength-training regiments. As noted, the function of the rotator cuff muscles is to guide the humeral head in a downward direction to allow the proper movement of the humerus in the glenoid cavity. If the deltoid overpowers the rotator cuff, the humeral head glides in an upward direction and invades the subacromial space. Muscle imbalances respond well to a proper exercise regimen.

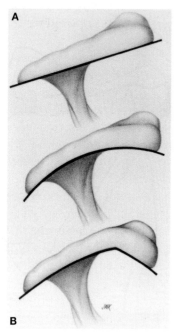

FIGURE 11.22 Acromial shapes. **A.** A normal shaped acromion (type I). **B.** A hook-shaped acromion (type III) often associated with the primary impingement syndrome. (From Iannotti JP, Williams GR. *Disorders of the Shoulder*. 2nd ed. Philadelphia (PA): Wolters Kluwer; 2006.)

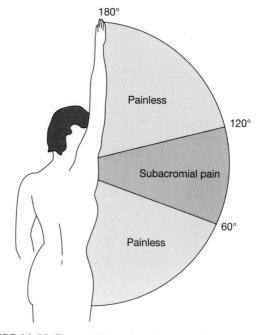

FIGURE 11.23 The painful arc is a characteristic symptom of rotator cuff impingement. Pain occurs primarily between 60 and 120 degrees of overhead shoulder motion. (From Bachur RG, Shaw KN. *Fleisher & Ludwig's Textbook of Pediatric Emergency Medicine*. 7th ed. Philadelphia (PA): Wolters Kluwer; 2015.)

Eliminating rounded shoulders and practicing good posture is one easy way to ensure the maximum amount of subacromial space is available. Another way to increase this space and reduce irritation is to externally rotate the arm when performing overhead movements. This rotates the greater tubercle of the humerus away from the acromion, thereby opening the subacromial space. An easy reminder for clients is to always start with the thumb pointed toward the ceiling when performing overhead motions.

It is important to correct the scapular posture, prior to embarking on a strengthening program. Muscles that have been chronically shortened need to be stretched, and muscles that have been overstretched need to be placed in a shortened position and strengthened in the range where they typically work.

Strengthening the Rotator Cuff

Often specific strengthening of the rotator cuff musculature will alleviate both muscle imbalance and poor posture and thereby relieve secondary impingement. For reasons already discussed, postural dysfunctions should be corrected prior to performing shoulder strengthening exercises (see the previous section on Posture).

When working with someone with possible impingement syndrome of the shoulder, use the following commonsense precautions: Do not have the client exercise through the painful arc ROM, and make sure the client performs overhead motions in the "thumb-up" position. The client also should avoid performing deltoid exercises above 90 degrees of shoulder abduction until they are able to perform full overhead reach without pain. In general, the client should avoid performing any exercises with the shoulder in 90 degrees of abduction. All of these activities may cause impingement of the tissues in the subacromial space.

The shoulder position for rotator cuff strengthening requires some consideration. The safest way to strengthen the rotator cuff is to abduct the arm approximately 30 degrees away from the torso. Place a towel or small roll between the torso and the upper arm to maintain this space (Figure 11.24). This position puts the coracohumeral ligament on slack, maximizes the subacromial space, and allows maximal vascularity to the rotator cuff, thereby decreasing the risk of injury (119). However, maximal infraspinatus activation Electromyography (EMG) has recently been described with the shoulder in zero degrees of abduction (120). If the client has shoulder pain, start rotator cuff strengthening in the safest position (15 degrees abduction). Once the upper arm is in this position, then proceed with external and IR strengthening exercises.

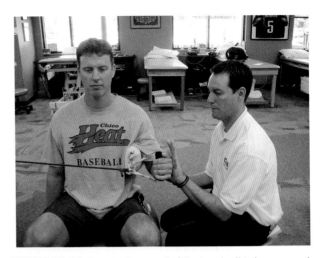

FIGURE 11.24 Proper placement of the towel roll to increase subacromial space with external rotation strengthening. (From Dines JS, Altchek DW, Andrews J, ElAttrache NS, Wilk KE, Yocum LA. *Sports Medicine of Baseball.* Philadelphia (PA): Wolters Kluwer; 2012.)

Because the rotator cuff muscles have small muscle bellies, the amount of weight or resistance used for these muscles should be significantly smaller than the weight used for the deltoids.

Rotator Cuff Surgical Repairs

Partial thickness tears of the rotator cuff and chronic primary rotator cuff impingement syndrome of the shoulder are often surgically managed by an arthroscopic subacromial decompression and repair. An arthroscopic procedure requires only small incisions by which surgical instruments and a camera are inserted into the joint space. The surgeon performs the entire procedure while looking at a monitor; therefore, a large incision is not required. Although the incision is small, the inflamed synovitis surrounding the joint and the coracoacromial ligament is still removed. The coracoacromial ligament both originates and inserts on the scapula, so sacrificing this ligament enlarges the subacromial space without resulting in any instability of the shoulder. In addition, the anterior, inferior one-third of the distal end of the acromion is often removed, further opening the space for the tendons of the rotator cuff to move through.

Large or full-thickness rotator cuff tears are often repaired using a more invasive open technique, which cuts more muscles and has a longer rehabilitation time. Some surgeons use an arthroscopic technique for even full-thickness tears. Research supports good outcomes using this less invasive technique as long as the surgeon is adequately trained in minimally invasive shoulder surgery (121). The important thing is to not judge the extent of the surgery by the scars. It is possible that the client had an extensive surgical repair with a small incision or arthroscopic incisions.

Post Rotator Cuff Surgery

Resistive exercises after a rotator cuff repair are progressed slowly to ensure the integrity of the repair. Most physicians do not allow progressive resistive exercises to begin until 12–16 weeks postoperatively. Nevertheless, it is important to continue with stretching exercises focusing on returning pain-free shoulder ROM. Clinical guidelines suggest starting resistive exercises with very low weights (2 lb) and high repetitions (122). ROM should be limited to the shoulder level in the scapular plane. The scapular plane (Figure 11.25) is the neutral plane of the scapula and is located 30 degrees anterior to the frontal plane. Performing exercises in the scapular plane maximizes the subacromial space. Scapular strengthening, bicep curls, triceps curls, scapular rows, and lat pull-downs can be performed as long as they are pain free. Any overhead strengthening should be taken slowly, with only one new exercise added per week. If shoulder pain develops, counsel the client to seek medical advice and not "push" through the pain.

Shoulder Instability

Shoulder instability is a common problem among young athletes and is associated with joint laxity. Glenohumeral

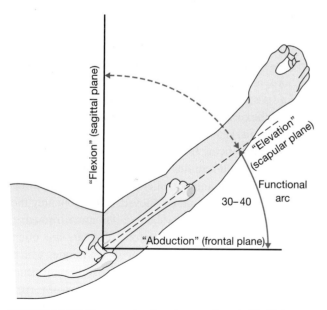

FIGURE 11.25 The scapular plane is approximately 30–40 degrees anterior to the frontal plane and is in line with the glenoid of the scapula when using good posture. (From Brody LT, Hall CM. *Therapeutic Exercise*. 3rd ed. Philadelphia (PA): Wolters Kluwer; 2010.)

laxity is present when the humeral head can translate on the glenoid of the scapula more than 50% of the size of the humeral head in any direction. Normally, anterior translation is greater than posterior translation. Instability occurs when unwanted humeral translation causes shoulder pain. A subluxation occurs when an abnormal amount of humeral translation occurs but is spontaneously returned to a normal resting position; it may or may not be painful. However, over time, these repetitive translations damage articular surfaces and ligament/capsule structure, leading to pain. Joint instabilities can be experienced in one direction (most common is anterior) or multidirectional (most common is anterior and inferior). Common complaints include anterior shoulder pain with arm heaviness, or a sensation of the shoulder "popping" out. Strengthening exercises are recommended to control the instability, but about 50% of patients end up having a capsular tightening surgery for long-term management of the injury (123).

A dislocation occurs when the humerus translates to the point that it no longer maintains contact with the glenoid fossa and usually does not spontaneously relocate. This requires immediate medical attention to "relocate" the humerus and to ensure integrity of the arm's neurovascular supply. Anterior dislocation is the most common and usually happens secondary to a traumatic injury. The most common position of dislocation is abduction to 90 degrees with full ER and horizontal abduction. Patients with this type of dislocation almost always have a better outcome with a surgical procedure to correct any problems versus exercise and immobilization alone. Sixty to eighty percent of people who do not have a surgical fixation report another shoulder dislocation, as opposed to 12% of those with a surgical repair (124).

Exercise precautions for clients dealing with shoulder instability should focus on strengthening the muscles while protecting the joint. This includes avoiding the highly provocative position of shoulder abduction to 90 degrees combined with ER and horizontal extension. Many times, limiting the ROM of an exercise is all that is required. For example, for the chest press and bench press, keeping the elbow from going behind the body limits horizontal extension.

Elbow

The elbow joint is a transitional link from the shoulder to the hand. Therefore, forces generated from the shoulder (*e.g.*, throwing) or from the hand (*e.g.*, falling on an outstretched hand) impact the elbow. In addition, the elbow allows precise movements of the hand by allowing pronation (palm down) and supination (palm up) of the hand to occur. The musculature and ligaments surrounding the elbow are smaller than those at other joints. These factors make the elbow susceptible to overuse injuries.

Overuse injuries are the most common maladies of the elbow. Lateral epicondylitis (tennis elbow) is an inflammation of the common extensor tendons of the forearm. However, lateral epicondylosis is the more appropriate term for describing a more chronic problem in which the tendon is deteriorated but little inflammation is present (125). A poorly executed backhand stroke (as in tennis) can cause this problem in those who play racket sports. Ideally, the arm and racket swing as a unit; however, sometimes the wrist "breaks" when the ball makes contact, causing a forceful eccentric contraction of the wrist extensors. Eccentric contractions are known to cause micro-tears in the muscle (126). Although those who play racket sports are more prone to this injury, it can occur at any time the wrist extensors are overworked. Some common activities that overwork the wrist extensors include typing or using a computer mouse and repetitive gripping such as when pulling weeds from the garden, painting, or using a screwdriver or other tool for an extended period. Symptoms include painful palpation of the lateral epicondyle and the associated extensor tendons located along the top of the forearm. Symptoms are made worse by gripping and other actions that stretch the wrist extensors.

Medial epicondylitis/epicondylosis (golfer's elbow) involves the common flexor tendons of the wrist. It is associated with repetitive wrist flexion, such as swinging a golf club, throwing a ball, and grasping small objects as in assembly-line work. The symptoms include pain along the medial portion of the forearm down the flexor tendons. The pain is made worse by wrist extension (active or passive) with the elbow straight or by forceful contraction of the wrist flexors.

Treatment of Elbow Overuse Injuries

Treatment recommendations for both conditions vary with the degree of severity. Stretching the involved musculature within pain limits, and cross-friction massage over the involved tendons should help restore the blood supply to the tendon, which will facilitate healing. The use of a counterforce brace (Figure 11.26) has good anecdotal evidence, but a recent review of the clinical effectiveness of conservative management did not offer support (127, 128). Severe symptoms may be relieved by wrist splints, which limit the movement of the wrist for extended periods of time. However, the hands and wrist are used for so many daily tasks that it is difficult to completely rest the tendons involved. Therefore, clients commonly ignore

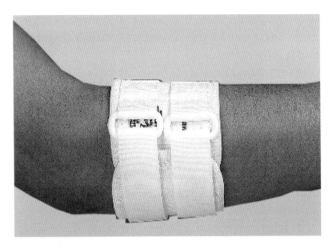

FIGURE 11.26 An example of a counterforce brace. The pad can be worn over the inflamed tendons of either the lateral side (tennis elbow) or the medial side (golfer's elbow), depending on the area of inflammation. (Courtesy of Medical Sports, Inc. Available from: https://www.countrforce.com/literalelbow.html.)

the symptoms and experience even more severe pain and limitation of ADL. Because the affected tendon is likely damaged, referral to a physical therapist for evaluation and recommendation of the best exercise and intensity is warranted.

Lower Limb Injuries

Soft tissue injuries of the hip are usually either muscle strains or bursitis. Hamstring strains are common in the active person and have a high recurrence rate, especially with injury to the biceps femoris (129). Symptoms have a rapid onset and often are severe enough that continuing the activity is not possible. The most common mechanism of injury is overstriding during sprinting when the muscle must eccentrically contract during a lengthened position to control knee extension. However, the hamstring can also be injured during a high kick or sagittal split. This stretch type of injury has been associated with a longer time to return to activity (129). Strengthening exercises after proper healing should include eccentric exercises when the hamstring is in a lengthening position (129).

Femoroacetabular impingement (FAI) is the name given to dysfunctions that involve the acetabular labrum. There could be extra boney formation on either the femur or the acetabulum or there could be a tear in the labrum. Common complaints are clicking or catching when performing a certain activity along with hip pain. Anterior or groin pain is closely associated with anterior or superior labral dysfunctions while posterior pain is associated with posterior labrum tears. If consistent popping or clicking occurs along with hip pain, referral for further diagnostic testing is warranted.

A common cause of posterior hip or buttock pain is the piriformis muscle. The piriformis is responsible for hip ER and assists with abduction when the hip is in neutral. If someone demonstrates a valgus collapse (hip IR and adduction) during athletic activities such as landing from a jump or running, then the piriformis may be overworked, resulting in pain and tightness. Stretching of the piriformis is recommended as well as correcting the faulty movement.

Trochanteric bursitis is a common cause of lateral hip pain. It is an inflammation of one of the peritrochanteric bursae by either direct trauma (fall on that side) or friction from a tight iliotibial band (ITB) (130). When the hip moves from extension to flexion, the ITB glides over the greater trochanter from posterior to anterior, and vice versa when the hip goes from flexion to extension. A tight ITB increases compression over the bursae with repetitive hip flexion and extension, thereby irritating the bursae. This irritation is exacerbated when concurrent hip adductor tightness moves the hip into adduction during running or walking. Pain, which can be quite debilitating, is typically localized in the area of the greater trochanter but can also extend distally into the lateral thigh. Ice, rest, and gentle stretching should begin immediately. Stretching of both the hip abductors and adductors is important, as is correcting any biomechanical abnormalities such as the foot crossing the midline during running. Once inflamed, direct pressure, such as from lying on the painful side, should be avoided. Modifications of exercise programs may be required. Persistent symptoms should be referred for medical testing to rule out limb-length inequalities, the need for orthotic intervention, or a gluteus medius tear (130).

Knee

The primary role of the knee in exercise is to act as a shock absorber. In that capacity, the knee is vulnerable to injuries involving the musculotendinous units. The knee is actually a two-joint complex (three if both the medial and lateral sides of the tib-fib joint are included). The patella is a free-floating sesamoid bone, which is encased by the patellar ligament (called patellar tendon by some) and joint capsule. There are several bursae around the knee, and these can also become inflamed.

Anterior Knee Pain

Anterior knee pain is by far the most common knee complaint. The myriad of causes all have very similar symptoms, identified in Box 11.2. Anterior knee pain that is aching in nature, knee popping, and pain with prolonged sitting and with stairs are characteristic of patellofemoral pain syndrome (PFPS). These symptoms develop over a period of time and affect ADL. It is a common diagnosis in both young active females (18–35 years old) accounting for 12%–13% of knee complaints and 7.3% in females aged 50-59 years (131, 132).

Women's broader pelvis, smaller muscle mass, and increased femoral anteversion account for the higher incidence of PFPS in females. Both broader pelvis and increased femoral anteversion directly increase the overall lateral pull from the quadriceps on the patella, which is a major contributor to anterior knee pain.

Patellar Causes of Anterior Knee Pain

Chondromalacia patellae specifically refer to the softening of the articular cartilage on the undersurface of the patella. Symptoms include patellar grinding and anterior knee pain, especially when going down stairs or

---

Box 11.2   Causes and Symptoms of Anterior Knee Pain

Causes
Patellofemoral compression syndrome
Patellar instability
Biomechanical dysfunction
Direct patellar trauma
Soft tissue lesions
Overuse syndromes

Osteochondritis dissecans
Chondromalacia patellae

Common Symptoms
Anterior knee pain
Tenderness under the surface of the patella
Tight musculature
Pain after prolonged sitting, stair-climbing, or squatting

Source: Data from Wilk KE, Davies GJ, Mangine RE, Malone TR. Patellofemoral disorders: a classification system and clinical guidelines for nonoperative rehabilitation. *J Orthop Sports Phys Ther*. 1998;28(5):307–22.

after prolonged sitting. Articular cartilage does not have a nerve supply; therefore, abnormal forces are placed on the underlying subchondral bone of the patella. It is likely that the cause of a young person's anterior knee pain is not chondromalacia patellae, but some other factor.

Abnormal patellar tracking is a common biomechanical cause of anterior knee pain. During knee flexion and extension, the patella must glide in the femoral groove. The articular cartilage is thicker on the facets on the patella's posterior surface, which should come in contact with the femur. A balance of soft tissue — including the lateral pull of the quadriceps and the medial pull of the vastus medialis oblique (Figure 11.27) — ensures that the patella stays centered and follows the intrachondral groove of the femur. This is the "train on the track" theory. If the lateral structures, such as the ITB and lateral joint retinaculum, pull too hard on the lateral side of the patella, or the vastus medialis obliquus (VMO) is weak and cannot generate enough force medially, then the patella will glide laterally instead of sitting in the intrachondral groove. This abnormal patellar tracking results in an abnormal amount of force on a relatively small portion of the lateral patella.

Femoral and Hip Causes of Anterior Knee Pain

Misalignment of the femur is also thought to cause PFPS. Powers (133) reported that clients with PFPS demonstrated IR of the femur during a squat, while the patella stayed in the correct position. This resulted in abnormal patellar tracking, but the cause was that the "track" itself was misaligned.

In addition, hip external rotator (134) and abductor weakness (135), which cause a more adducted position of the knee during a squat, have been demonstrated in clients with PFPS. A simple step-down test can be used to identify proximal hip weakness. During this test, the knee should stay in line with the supporting foot. Any amount of knee adduction (valgus collapse) is indicative of hip abductor muscle weakness as illustrated in Figure 11.28.

Abnormal Foot Biomechanics Causing Anterior Knee Pain

There is also a "bottom-up" theory of biomechanical abnormalities that may contribute to PFPS. When the

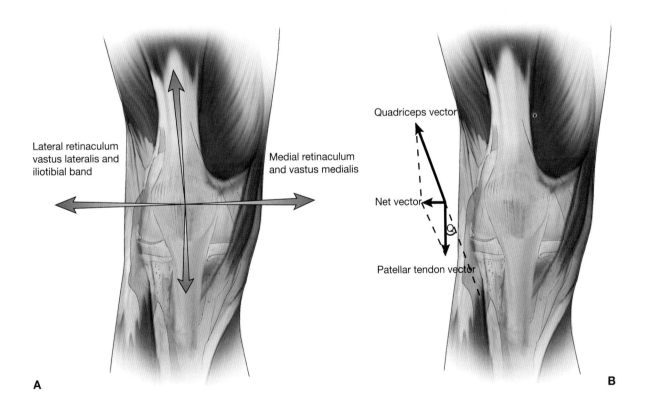

FIGURE 11.27 Patellar forces. **A.** There is a careful balance of the soft tissues surrounding the knee, with forces on the patella in both medial and lateral directions. **B.** However, because of the amount of lateral force, there is a net lateral force on the patella with knee extension. (From Weinstein SL, Flynn JM. *Lovell and Winter's Pediatric Orthopaedics.* 7th ed. Philadelphia (PA): Wolters Kluwer; 2013.)

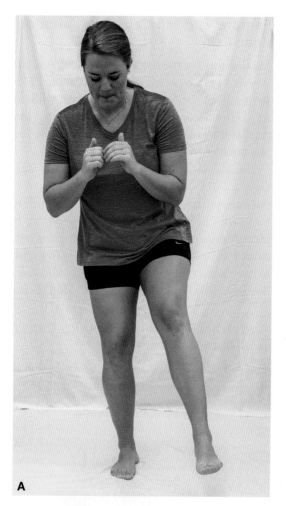
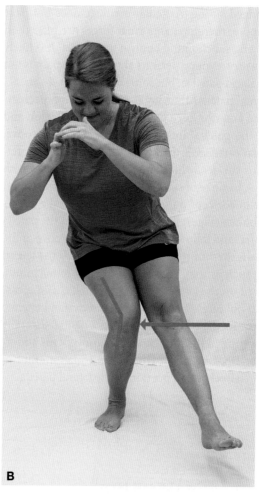

FIGURE 11.28 A step-down test demonstrating knee adduction, which is indicative of proximal hip musculature weakness. Ideally, the knee would remain aligned with the hip and foot. **A.** Normal alignment at knee prior to bending. **B.** Knee adduction occurring with increased flexion. (From Donnelly JM, Fernandez-de-Las-Penas C, Finnegan M, Freeman JL. *Travell, Simons & Simons' Myofascial Pain and Dysfunction.* Philadelphia (PA): Wolters Kluwer; 2018.)

medial arch of the foot collapses, the foot falls inward, or overpronates, causing the tibia to excessively internally rotate. This in turn causes the femur to internally rotate and leads to a valgus collapse (Figure 11.29). People with PFPS demonstrated 22% higher medial foot-loading during a drop-landing task and 32% higher medial foot-loading during a single-leg squat compared to those without PFPS (136). The end result of this adducted knee posture is an increase in the quadriceps' lateral pull.

Treatment of Anterior Knee Pain

If a client complains of anterior knee pain, address the inflammation and pain initially by icing and decreasing the intensity of exercises. Determining and addressing the biomechanical causes via exercise is usually very successful. An exercise program should include quadriceps and ITB stretching combined with VMO, hip ER, and hip

abductor strengthening (137). No exercises isolate the VMO; however, closed-chain exercises, such as a squat with isometric hip adduction and a forward lunge, cause more muscle activity in the VMO when compared to the other quadriceps muscles (138). Some evidence suggests that proximal hip strengthening may prevent PFPS in high school runners (134). These studies all suggest that both VMO and proximal hip strengthening are essential for PF rehabilitation.

Precautions include avoiding exercising through the ROM where there is significant compression force on the patella. For example, deep squats, leg extensions, stair-climbing (descending), and direct kneeling should be avoided. If the client seems to walk more on the inside of the foot (excessive pronation), a foot orthotic may be indicated to reduce the extreme pronation (139). For severe and chronic cases, where there has been adaptive

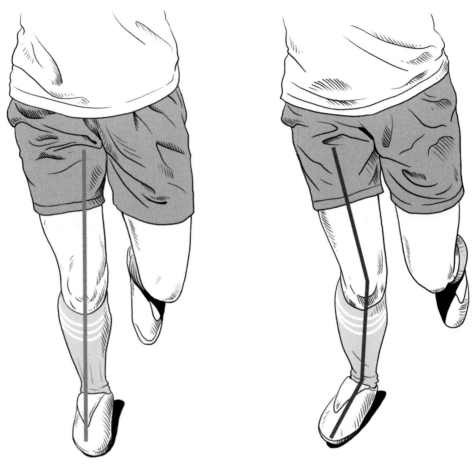

FIGURE 11.29 Excessive (over) pronation during a single-leg squat can lead to knee adduction. This is another possible cause of valgus collapse of the knee, which can lead to abnormal forces at the patellofemoral joint. (From Liebenson C. *Functional Training Handbook.* 1st ed. Philadelphia (PA): Wolters Kluwer; 2014.)

shortening of soft tissues, the client may need to be referred to a physical therapist for manual patellar mobilizations.

Inflammatory Knee Disorders

Localized pain around the knee is common and tends to have a more defined mechanism of injury than anterior knee pain. These soft tissue injuries develop quickly and, with the right care, will dissipate quickly.

Prepatellar bursitis is an inflammation of the bursa located between the skin and the patella. It is inflamed by direct trauma brought on by repetitive kneeling on a fully bent knee. This condition will resolve quickly just by avoiding putting weight directly over the bursae.

Jumper's knee is an inflammation of the patellar tendon typically caused by repetitive loading of the knee extensor mechanism such as in jumping, running, or climbing. It is characterized by anterior knee pain, especially after activity. Tenderness to palpation will be localized to the proximal portion of the patella tendon. Pain

usually alleviates with rest but returns with any activity that stresses the extensor mechanism. The fundamental problem in jumper's knee is that the quadriceps is not strong enough to complete the task; therefore, strengthening the quadriceps or decreasing the intensity of the task should alleviate the symptoms. In the acute phase, direct icing and rest will help the pain. Quadriceps stretching will help prevent the development of a chronic problem. Eccentric exercises have also proved to be beneficial in returning strength; however, no clear dose-response relationship has been established (140).

Sinding-Larsen and Johansson syndrome is an inflammation of the bone at the inferior pole of the patella. It is also caused by jumping and running activities but tends to be more common in the skeletally immature. Likewise, Osgood–Schlatter disease is an inflammation of the tibial tubercle and only occurs in the skeletally immature, typically during a growth spurt. It is caused by excessive traction from the patellar tendon on the tibial tubercle when the bones grow faster than the muscles. For that reason, it is often referred to as growing pains. It is characterized by enlargement of the tibial tuberosity, anterior knee pain with tenderness on the tibial tuberosity, and severe muscle tightness of the quadriceps and hamstrings. Treatment consists of quadriceps and hamstring flexibility, moderate-intensity quad strength, and ice. Some have used a strap around the knee at the mid-patellar level for pain relief during activity; however, there is little evidence to support its efficacy.

Ligament Injuries of the Knee

The most common ligament injury around the knee is rupture of the anterior cruciate ligament (ACL). According to the most recent assessments by the National Collegiate Athletic Association, ACL injuries continue to be significantly higher in women, especially in those who play basketball, volleyball, or lacrosse, whereas the highest rate of injury in men is in those who play football or soccer (141). Anatomical, hormonal, and muscular strength differences in women are thought to explain their higher risk of ACL injury (141).

ACL Surgery

The management of ACL tears is almost always surgical. The surgery replaces the torn ACL with a graft, which assumes the duties of the original ACL. The bone–patellar tendon–bone (BTB) graft, which uses the patient's own patellar tendon with bone attached at each end, is most often used in those who wish to return to sports. The BTB graft has the advantage of bone healing to bone in the drill holes, which can translate into an earlier return to full activity. However, there is the cost of pain and weakness from the patellar tendon graft site. A four-strand hamstring tendon graft harvested from the patient appears to provide equal joint stability with lower postoperative complications (142).

Regardless of type, the graft immediately loses tensile strength. There is a period of regeneration during which the body reestablishes the blood supply of the newly inserted graft and it slowly gains strength. Animal models suggest the entire process takes 8–12 months to gain 80% of the original ACL tensile strength (143).

Post-ACL Surgery Rehabilitation

Rehabilitation after surgery varies by surgeon but usually involves regular exercises to restore mobility, progressive weight bearing, and stretching and strengthening of all the major muscle groups of the lower leg. Three months

after surgery, the tensile strength of the graft is only 60%. Nevertheless, ROM is nearly normal, strength is returning, and walking looks and feels good. As a result, patients want to start doing more, such as running and jumping. Instead, patients should take extreme caution to restrict all activities not recommended by their physician. Patients who are athletes will probably be on an accelerated rehabilitation protocol, with return to sports by 6–8 months. If the patient is not an athlete, it is much safer to complete 10–12 months of rehabilitation and activity restriction in order to avoid rupture of the new graft.

Special precautions should be taken to avoid shearing forces in the knee for at least the first 6 months after ACL repair. Shear force on the ACL occurs with everyday activities such as descending stairs that cannot be entirely avoided, so instruction in proper form is important. Using a poor form with a squat exercise also can cause a high degree of shear force on the ACL. When the knees go anterior to the toes, the body weight force is directed in such a way that the femur is encouraged to "slide" off the tibia (Figure 11.30). To minimize this shear stress, keep the knees in line with the foot during squatting. In addition, squatting should be limited to 60 degrees of knee flexion to avoid excessive shear force (144). When performing open-chain exercises, leg weights or the resistance pad should be placed closer to the knee. Contraction of the quadriceps in open chain through the knee ROM from 45 to 15 degrees causes the greatest amount of shear force and should be avoided (144).

The most common complication after an ACL repair is anterior knee pain. It is especially likely in those with a BTB graft. The patellar tendon at the graft site is only two-thirds the size of the patellar tendon in the nonsurgical leg. Almost always the reason for the anterior knee pain is overloading the quadriceps. For that reason, wherever the graft was taken (patellar tendon or hamstring), progress that muscle group more slowly with resistive exercises. If pain does occur, the patient should rest, directly ice the tendon, and decrease the amount of force on the muscle group. Ignoring and pushing through the pain does not usually lead to good outcomes.

Meniscal Lesions

The menisci attached to the superior surface of the tibia play an important role in the stability and shock absorption capabilities of the knee. They are C-shaped wedges with a wider periphery compared to the thinner inside. This wedge shape helps keep the femoral condyles centered on the tibia with knee movement. This anatomy has a high tolerance for direct axial compression but does not tolerate torsion stresses well.

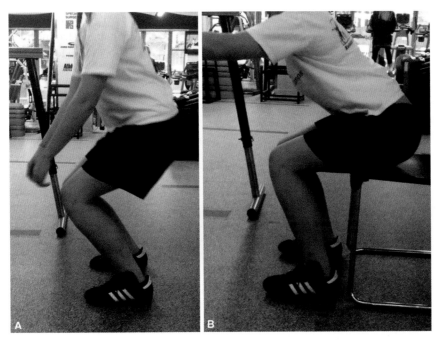

FIGURE 11.30 Squat technique and forces on knee. **A.** Increased shear force on the anterior cruciate ligament (ACL) during a squat in which the knee moves anterior to the toes. **B.** A safer squat technique to decrease anterior shear force on the ACL. Notice the tibia is in a much more vertical position compared to **A.** (From Cordasco F, Green D. *Pediatrics and Adolescent Knee Surgery.* 1st ed. Philadelphia (PA): Wolters Kluwer; 2015.)

The medial meniscus is injured more often than the lateral meniscus for two reasons. First, the medial meniscus is more firmly attached to the tibia. When the femur internally rotates, the medial meniscus is stressed in a radial fashion. The lateral meniscus is able to give more because of its looser attachment to the tibia. Second, the medial collateral ligament (MCL) attaches to the medial meniscus, and both are often injured when a valgus stress (typically a blow from the outside of the knee) causes a medial collapse of the knee.

The most common mechanism of meniscal injury involves rotation, axial compression, and knee flexion, such as occurs in a side-cutting maneuver. Symptoms include joint line pain, joint popping/clicking with movement, and an increase in pain with weight bearing and rotation. It is impossible to know if a meniscus is torn without an MRI scan. Therefore, a person with these symptoms should be referred to a medical professional immediately.

Only the outside portions of the menisci have a blood supply; therefore, only injuries in this portion can heal without surgery. If surgery is warranted, the surgical goal is to save as much of the meniscus as possible. It has long been known that removing as little as 20% of a meniscus increases the joint compression forces on the tibia by 350% (145). After surgery, there will be a period of restricted ROM and weight bearing. In general, open-chain exercises are appropriate to build strength; however, deep squats and rotary motions should not be attempted until they are cleared by the physician (146).

Leg, Foot, and Ankle

The functions of the lower leg and ankle are twofold. First, they serve to dampen the ground reaction forces received from weight-bearing activities, as well as to accommodate uneven terrain. Second, they serve to propel the body forward during ambulation. This requires strength and endurance of the lower leg musculature and ankle flexibility. Because of the repetitive and cyclic nature of walking and running, any deficit in the lower leg/ankle can quickly cause injuries.

Medial Tibial Stress Syndrome

Medial tibial stress syndrome (shin splints) is a very common complaint in runners with an incidence rate of 13.6%–20% in long-distance runners (147). It is characterized by diffuse pain over the medial two-thirds of the tibial border. This pain originates as inflammation of the posterior tibialis tendon at its broad attachment into the medial tibia. There can also be inflammation of the anterior tibialis tendon attachment, which would cause pain over the anterior aspect of the shin.

The most common mechanism of injury is overpronation. During gait, the posterior tibialis eccentrically decelerates pronation of the foot (148). Immediately after the maximum amount of pronation is reached, the posterior tibialis concentrically contracts to rapidly supinate the foot and make the foot into a rigid lever for push-off. With overpronation, the posterior tibialis is overstretched and is at a mechanical disadvantage to supinate the foot. This means the muscle has to generate more force. Over time, this may prompt inflammation of the tendon.

The best treatment for medial tibial stress syndrome is to control the overpronation with shoes or, in some cases, foot orthotics. Referral to a medical professional is indicated to determine which treatment is best for each client. Ice for pain control, stretching of the inflamed tissue, and rest from aggravating activities are other recommended treatments. Once the acute pain has resolved, progressive strengthening of the muscles can begin.

Achilles Tendon Conditions

The Achilles tendon is the common tendon formed with the union of the gastrocnemius and the soleus. It attaches to the posterior calcaneus. The gastrocnemius/soleus muscles are the most powerful muscles of the ankle and are used for any activity that requires propulsion of the body through space. Therefore, tremendous forces are passed through the tendon at great frequency. Achilles tendonitis/tendinopathy is an inflammation and/or damage to the Achilles tendon that causes pain and stiffness in the posterior lower leg. It is present in 10% of runners and is most common in those who play racket sports such as tennis (147).

Achilles injury can be a biomechanical problem. As previously discussed, the foot undergoes rapid pronation immediately after foot strike and then immediately supinates for push-off. During pronation, the tibia internally rotates; however, if rotation continues beyond midstance, then the femur will begin to externally rotate with knee extension. Because the gastrocnemius is a two-joint muscle, this opposite movement of the femur causes the Achilles tendon to "bow string" (149), wringing out the tendon. Other factors that have been associated with Achilles injury are running downhill and failure to stretch prior to sports.

Symptoms include localized pain over the Achilles tendon, usually in the middle of the tendon (midsubstance) or at the insertion onto the calcaneus. A lack of dorsiflexion ROM (<20 degrees) with the knee straight indicates tightness in the gastrocnemius, whereas a limitation in dorsiflexion with the knee bent indicates soleus tightness. The plantar flexors will be weak and painful with muscle contraction. Ice to the painful areas and rest will help alleviate the symptoms; however, until the biomechanical problem is fixed, Achilles pain will most likely return. A referral may be necessary to correct abnormal pronation. Stretching the plantar flexors with both knee bent and knee straight is important. Anyone who demonstrates symptoms of Achilles tendinopathy should avoid higher level exercises such as repetitive jumping, bounding, and plyometrics.

Ankle Sprains

Ankle sprains are common among athletes. Lateral ankle sprains, which injure the ligaments on the lateral side of the foot, are more common than medial ankle sprains. They are caused by extreme motions of plantarflexion and inversion (150). Medial ankle sprains are caused by extreme eversion, which injures the medial deltoid ligaments. The most common mechanism of injury is an instance of "rolling" the ankle when landing from a jump, walking/running over uneven ground, or stepping into a hole. Symptoms are pain and swelling on the side of the injury with painful weight bearing.

Recovery time varies according to the severity of the sprain. A grade I (minimal injury to only some of the ligaments) might be better in 1 week, whereas a grade III (complete rupture of the ligaments) might take 3 months for full recovery.

A high ankle sprain is an injury to the syndesmosis ligament, which is between the tibia and the fibula, and is responsible for the stability of the ankle mortise. This injury usually occurs when the foot is forced into extreme dorsiflexion and ER. The anterior body of the talus is wider than the posterior portion of the talus; therefore, in extreme dorsiflexion, the wider portion of the talus is forced between the tibia and the fibula, spreading the mortise. Pain and swelling are anterior and superior to the ankle joint. Because the syndesmosis ligament is responsible for the stability of the ankle mortise, weight bearing and gait with a high ankle sprain are typically very painful. Injuries to this ligament tend to take much longer to heal than a lateral ankle sprain and often lead to surgical fixation.

Lateral ankle sprains can contribute to chronic ankle instability, which in turn increases the risk for recurrent ankle sprains. Evidence indicates that the ankle continues to experience strength and mobility deficits 4 weeks after grade I or II lateral ankle sprain (151). Decreased neuromuscular control and balance deficits further contribute to functional instability of the ankle (150). Neuromuscular control describes the efficiency of the neuromuscular system when called upon to act. One theory of how poor neuromuscular control contributes to ankle instability suggests that the damaged joint capsule and ligaments are not able to produce strong enough reflex responses in the evertor muscles (150). In short, the evertors are not able to contract quickly enough when needed, leaving the ankle unprotected.

Many people do not regard an ankle sprain as a serious injury and simply wait for it to heal on its own. However, lack of proper restoration of ROM and ankle strength has been associated with chronic instability (152). Therefore, exercises incorporating strengthening and ROM should be part of the extended recovery. In addition, single-leg balancing on progressively unstable surfaces will improve not only balance but also neuromuscular control and endurance of the ankle musculature (150).

Plantar Fasciitis

Plantar fasciitis is the most common foot injury resulting in a doctor's visit, affecting approximately 2 million Americans annually (153). It is defined as inflammation of the plantar aponeurosis (fascia), which runs from the calcaneus to the metatarsals on the bottom surface of the foot. As the body weight is distributed on the talus, forces are split between the anterior and posterior columns of the foot. The plantar fascia both maintains the arch of the foot and helps the foot become a rigid lever during push-off, as illustrated in Figure 11.31.

Abnormal foot pronation, inadequate big toe extension and/or a tight gastrocnemius/soleus complex predisposes the foot to excessive tension in the plantar fascia. This tension can lead to an inflammatory response at the attachment on the body of the calcaneus. Other risk factors associated with the development of plantar fasciitis include rapid weight gain (pregnancy), pes planus (flat-foot) foot type, wearing shoes with little arch support, a sudden increase in weight-bearing activity (increase in training), or prolonged standing on hard surfaces (153).

Symptoms appear slowly but can be very painful and limit walking, running, and jumping. A hallmark symptom is point-tender medial-plantar heel pain, which may radiate to the entire plantar surface of the foot. Pain is typically worst in the morning or when weight bearing after sitting. Morning pain is thought to occur because, during sleep, the foot is in plantarflexion, which places the gastrocnemius/soleus complex and the fascia in a shortened position. Pain is felt when initial weight bearing places excessive stress on the shortened fascia, especially during

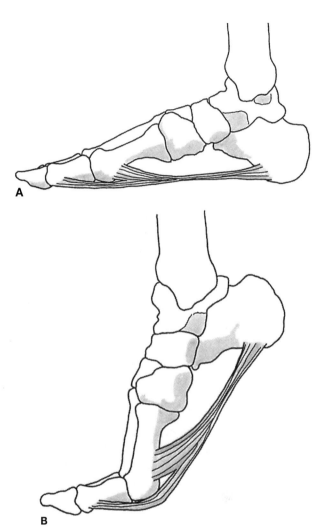

FIGURE 11.31 Plantar fascia. **A.** The plantar fascia maintains the integrity of the anterior and posterior columns of the foot. **B.** The plantar fascia tightens with toe off, raising the arch and adding stability to the foot to propel the body forward during walking or running. (From Hertling D. *Management of Common Musculoskeletal Disorders.* 4th ed. Philadelphia (PA): Wolters Kluwer; 2005.)

the push-off phase of gait. A night splint to hold the foot in a neutral position has been found to be effective in reducing pain over an 8-week period (154). Patients unable to put weight on the heel should be referred for a radiograph to rule out a bone spur.

Exercise precautions for this injury include avoiding exercises requiring the person to be on the balls of the feet. Running, jumping, and bounding should be limited until the pain subsides. Concentrated gastrocnemius and soleus stretching should be performed. Specific stretching of the plantar fascia can also be performed by passively extending the great toe. Rolling the plantar surface of the foot on a frozen water bottle can relieve pain at home. Patients also benefit from an orthotic evaluation (155), especially if they have an abnormal foot type (flatfoot or high arch).

Summary

Many soft tissue injuries occur with repetitive motions. Sometimes these repetitive motions occur because there is a restricted motion at that joint or a nearby joint. The human body will always take the path of least restriction. Restoring ROM of a joint after injury is important; however, it is good practice to ensure that joints above and below the injured area have an adequate ROM as well. Injured tissues go through a remodeling process and take time to heal. During this time, pain should not be ignored and should be a sign to the CEP that exercise modifications in intensity or activity are needed.

BACK AND NECK PAIN AND DYSFUNCTION

Musculoskeletal impairments are a major source of pain affecting the spine. This pain can occur in different areas of the back and neck and in different degrees of intensity. Some individuals experience an occasional dull pain, whereas others suffer constant agonizing pain that makes even the simplest movements difficult. Either way, back and neck pain can prevent people from performing normal ADL fulfilling work responsibilities and engaging in recreational pursuits. From a biomechanical standpoint, the spine is one of the most complex regions of the body. Intersecting nerve fibers, bones, joints, ligaments, and muscles all play integrated roles in spinal movement, making it difficult to pinpoint the exact offending structure when trying to determine the cause of a patient's back or neck pain.

Incidence and Prevalence

Most people will experience back and neck pain at some point in their lifetime. Experts describe the frequency of low back pain (LBP) as an "epidemic," an assessment that is supported consistently in the literature (156). Global estimates for the 1-year prevalence for a first episode of LBP range between 1.44% and 20% (157, 158). LBP is the leading cause of activity limitation and work absence throughout much of the world (157–159) and is the fifth most common reason for all visits to the medical doctor (159, 160). Moreover, an estimated 24%–80% of individuals who have experienced activity-limiting LBP suffer

recurrence (157). Although a troubling trend, recent evidence found approximately 50% increase in reported LBP during the last 20 years (160).

The prevalence of lower back and neck pain varies based on factors such as sex, age, education, and occupation. Women tend to have a higher prevalence of back and/or neck pain than men, although the difference reported varies in magnitude (161, 162). An increase in age and lower educational status are associated with an increased prevalence of LBP as well as a longer episode duration and worse outcome (156, 161, 163). Occupational differences in LBP prevalence have also been reported. Workers who perform physically demanding tasks such as repetitive lifting and carrying have an LBP prevalence of 39%, whereas workers in sedentary jobs have a prevalence of 18.3% (156, 164).

Risk Factors

Risk factors for LBP fall between two broad categories: intrinsic and extrinsic factors. Intrinsic risk factors include, but are not limited to, genetics, female sex, increased age, overweight or obesity, and possibly strength and flexibility (156). Smoking also increases the risk (165). Although an increase in age is associated with an increased prevalence of LBP (and neck pain), this risk factor tends to peak between 60 and 65 years (157). Although trunk muscle strength and/or mobility of the lumbar spine has been associated with increased back pain risk, the evidence is inconclusive (156, 166).

Key activity–related extrinsic risk factors for LBP (as well as neck pain) include a sedentary lifestyle and occupations that require either heavy physical demands such as repetitive lifting and/or twisting or awkward postures such as standing or sitting for long periods of time (167). Recent evidence suggests that psychosocial factors such as distress/depression or fear about resuming activity and work may impede recovery from an LBP episode and increase the risk for chronic back pain (156, 168). For a complete list of risk factors, see Box 11.3.

Pathoanatomical Features

A variety of causes of back and neck pain have been described. These include, but are not limited to, osteoarthritis, discogenic disorders, tumors, infection, myofascial pain syndrome, and traumatic injury. Whiplash, for example, is a common injury involving the impairment of muscles, ligaments, nerve roots, zygapophyseal joints, and vertebrae of the cervical pain. The identification of a

Box 11.3	Risk Factors for Low Back and Neck Pain

Intrinsic Risk Factors	**Extrinsic Risk Factors**
History of previous injury	Excessive load on spine — repetitive lifting, repetitive
Inadequate physical conditioning/Core (muscular	forward bending often combined with twisting
control) control	Speed and type of movement
Body composition	Number of repetitions
Bony alignment°	Surface
Limited strength or flexibility	Adverse environment conditions
Joint or ligamentous laxity	Fatigue
Psychosocial factors: fear, beliefs, depression	Sedentary lifestyle

Source: Delitto A, George S, Van Dillen L, et.al. Low back pain: clinical practice guidelines linked to the International Classification of Functioning, Disability, & Health from the Orthopaedic Section of the American Physical Therapy Association. *J Ortho Sports Phys Ther.* 2012;42(4):1–57; European Agency for Safety and Health at Work. Research on work-related low back disorders. 2000. Available from: https://osha.europa.eu/en/tools-and-publications/publications/reports/204; Valat JP, Goupille P, Vedere V. Low back pain: risk factors for chronicity. *Rev Rhum Engl Ed.* 1997;64(3):189–94. Available from: http://www.ncbi.nlm.nih.gov/pubmed/9090769.

pathoanatomical cause of back or neck pain is challenging, and in most causes a pathoanatomical cause cannot be determined (156, 161, 169). For example, some studies show that in up to 85%–90% of individuals with LBP, no clear cause is ever determined (156–160, 169).

Medical imaging can sometimes reveal the pathoanatomical basis for symptoms and guide treatment; however, the relationship between a medical imaging finding and a diagnosis is not always clear. For example, imaging confirmation of a herniated disc is shown in 20%–76% of persons with no sciatica or complaint of back pain (156, 170). Further, it has been shown that over 99% of patients presenting with acute or chronic back pain do not have serious conditions that require imaging (171). The lack of a clear relationship between most imaging findings and symptoms has created a dilemma for the health care provider.

Low Back Pain

Idiopathic and nonspecific LBP have emerged as catch-all terms in the diagnosis of LBP. The difficulty in determining a specific diagnosis stems from the fact that multiple structures in one or more spinal segments may be involved (4, 156). These structures could include ligaments, intervertebral discs, zygapophyseal joints, vertebral bodies, paravertebral musculature, blood vessels, and spinal nerve roots (4). Because so many structures are typically involved, most LBP is thought to be mechanical in nature; that is, back pain is triggered when the spine is overloaded or when abnormal stress and strain are placed on the spine and its surrounding tissues (156, 172). This

type of pain results from cumulative aggravating factors related to poor posture, faulty lifting and bending motions, age, and physical workload. These factors can lead to degenerative changes over time and may be associated with muscle impairments, joint restrictions, and deterioration within the articular surfaces, together resulting in a gradual loss of ROM and a decline in neuromuscular trunk control (4, 172).

Clients who sit at a desk or worktable for the majority of their work shift need to have seating that is properly aligned to their specific structural needs. Otherwise, faulty sitting will place abnormal stresses on the neck and back (173, 174). This can also be the case when clients are required to stand for long periods in a forward flexed position, or are required to lift heavy loads, especially if combined with twisting. These positions and movements cause significant loading on the spine and can be major contributors to LBP. Muscle impairments between agonists and antagonists can exist, some muscles become adaptively shortened and become tight while the opposing muscles may become lengthened and weak creating an imbalance in the system. This type of impairment contributes to LBP, and neck pain symptoms as well (4, 175). Thus, it is necessary to understand the underlying effects of faulty posture on flexibility, strength, and the pain the client may be experiencing. For example, proper alignment of the lumbar spine and pelvis helps minimize stress on the lumbar discs and facet joints (5). When postural adaptations occur in the low back, they can increase lordosis or pelvic tilt (Figure 11.32). Posture differs between clients and can change over time based on body type, activity level, work task performed, physical fitness levels, and aging (5).

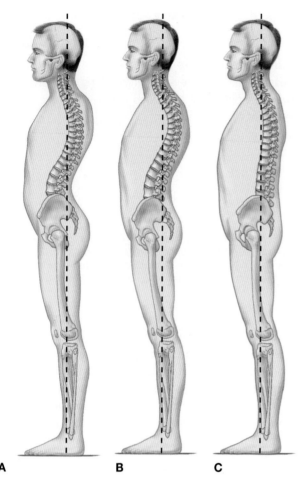

FIGURE 11.32 Postural anomalies. **A.** Exaggerated lordosis. **B.** Swayback. **C.** Flat back. (From Anderson MK. *Foundations of Athletic Training.* 6th ed. Philadelphia (PA): Wolters Kluwer; 2016.)

A growing body of evidence finds that weaknesses in the core muscles may be a major risk factor for chronic back symptoms. The core is defined as the lumbo-pelvic-hip complex (176) and is divided into two subsets, the local (or primary) system and the global (or secondary) system (177). Active engagement of both systems during functional activities is paramount to pain-free movement.

Local Core Muscle System and LBP

The local system includes the TrA, lumbar multifidus (LM), and the pelvic floor and diaphragm muscles (4). This local system is responsible for fine motor control.

Transverse Abdominis

As shown in Figures 11.33 and 11.34, the TrA attaches in a lattice-type arrangement that merges with the middle layer of the thoracolumbar fascia, making it the only abdominal muscle with an attachment onto the spine (5, 6). Although fitness guidelines have traditionally

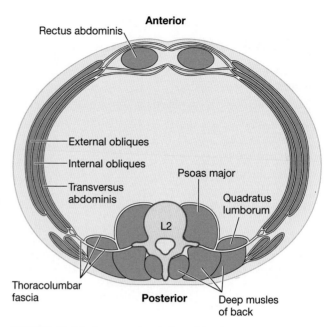

FIGURE 11.33 Cross-sectional view of lumbar spine. Notice the orientation of the transversus abdominis muscle. This is the only abdominal muscle with an attachment on the lumbar spine.

recommended strengthening the rectus abdominis muscle, commonly referred to as the "6-pack," recent evidence suggests that health care practitioners should additionally perform exercises that focus on the contraction of the TrA. Activating this muscle creates a rigid cylinder that enhances the stiffness and stabilization of the lumbar spinal segments via tensioning of the thoracolumbar fascia (4, 178, 179). Activation of this muscle serves as a feed-forward mechanism for limb movement (180). Researchers believe that, when an arm or leg is raised, the local core system of muscles is actively engaged prior to limb movement, thus serving to stabilize the spine and reducing painful shear stress on the vertebrae (180).

Lumbar Multifidus

Another group of muscles that serves a vital role in achieving spinal stability is the LM (Figure 11.35). This group of muscles originates on the mammillary process of the lumbar vertebrae and inserts on the spinous process of the higher vertebrae and may span two to four vertebrae (181). Numerous studies over the past several decades have looked at the relationship of this muscle group to LBP and its importance in lumbar spine stabilization. Biomechanical studies have shown that the LM supports lumbar segmental stabilization by providing segmental stiffness and controlling motion between individual vertebrae (182). Some researchers have concluded that the LM is responsible for two-thirds of the stiffness of the

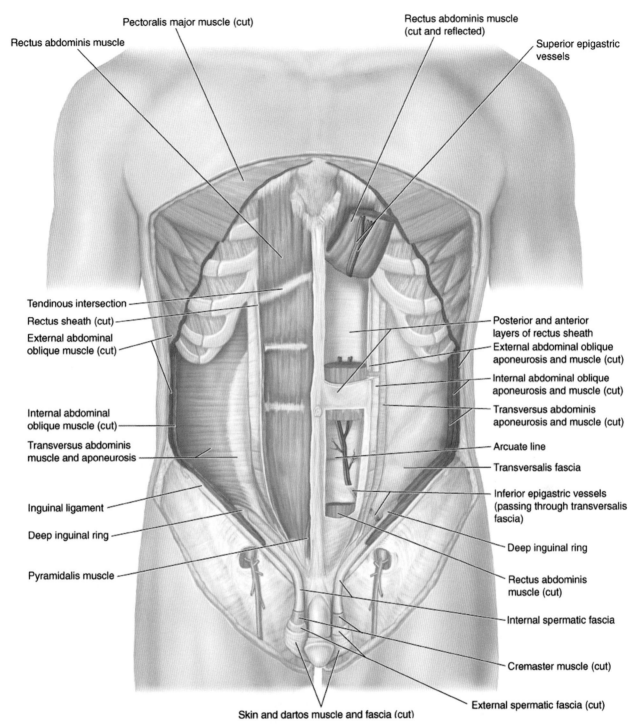

Pectoralis major muscle (cut)

Rectus abdominis muscle

Rectus abdominis muscle
(cut and reflected)

Superior epigastric
vessels

Tendinous intersection

Rectus sheath (cut)

External abdominal
oblique muscle (cut)

Internal abdominal
oblique muscle (cut)

Transversus abdominis
muscle and aponeurosis

Inguinal ligament

Deep inguinal ring

Pyramidalis muscle

Posterior and anterior
layers of rectus sheath

External abdominal oblique
aponeurosis and muscle (cut)

Internal abdominal oblique
aponeurosis and muscle (cut)

Transversus abdominis
aponeurosis and muscle (cut)

Arcuate line

Transversalis fascia

Inferior epigastric vessels
(passing through transversalis
fascia)

Deep inguinal ring

Rectus abdominis
muscle (cut)

Internal spermatic fascia

Cremaster muscle (cut)

External spermatic fascia (cut)

Skin and dartos muscle and fascia (cut)

FIGURE 11.34 Muscles comprising the global core: the external oblique, internal oblique, and rectus abdominis. (From Stephenson SR. *Diagnostic Medical Sonography: Obstetrics and Gynecology*. 3rd ed. Philadelphia (PA): Wolters Kluwer; 2015.)

lumbar spine and is active in nearly all antigravity activities, creating spinal stability by compressing the vertebrae together (183). This local core muscle group is needed for low-load strategies, such as when neuromuscular control is needed for the maintenance of upright postures during sitting, standing, and walking (177).

Evidence Supporting the Role of the TrA and LM

The local core muscle system is asked to function for long periods of time with relatively low-load muscle activation when endurance is needed. Recent evidence finds that in subjects with chronic LBP, activity of the TrA is

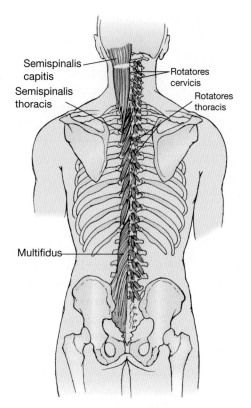

Semispinalis capitis

Rotatores cervicis

Semispinalis thoracis

Rotatores thoracis

Multifidus

FIGURE 11.35 The multifidus muscle provides segmental stabilization between vertebral bodies. (From Oatis CA. *Kinesiology: The Mechanics and Pathomechanics of Human Movement*. 3rd ed. Philadelphia (PA): Wolters Kluwer; 2016.)

delayed with movements of the arms even when the pain symptoms are in remission. This finding supports the importance of the TrA to spinal stabilization (178, 180). In addition, ultrasound imaging has shown that, following an acute episode of LBP, there is atrophy of the LM either at one specific level or at multiple levels (184, 185). Additionally, full muscle recovery function of the LM does not spontaneously occur on remission of painful symptoms either (185). Researchers have hypothesized that the absence of the local core muscle system — either through delayed activation patterns or through muscle atrophy — may be a key contributor to the high incidence of recurrence of back pain (186).

Pelvic Floor Muscles

The muscles that make up the pelvic floor work in a coordinated fashion to increase intraabdominal pressure, provide rectal support during defecation, inhibit bladder activity, support the pelvic organs, and assist in lumbopelvic stability (187). These muscles include the levator ani, a group composed of the pubococcygeus, puborectalis, and iliococcygeus that joins the coccygeus muscle to complete the pelvic floor (Figure 11.36). The pelvic floor muscles act in concert with the TrA and LM. These muscles are active during repetitive arm movement tasks regardless of the direction of movement. Maximal contraction of

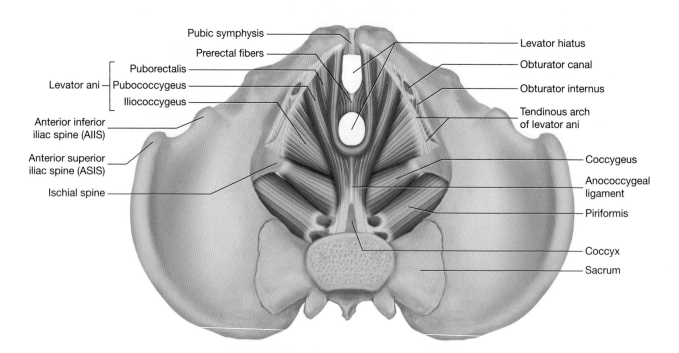

Pubic symphysis

Prerectal fibers

Puborectalis

Levator ani — Pubococcygeus

Iliococcygeus

Anterior inferior iliac spine (AIIS)

Anterior superior iliac spine (ASIS)

Ischial spine

Levator hiatus

Obturator canal

Obturator internus

Tendinous arch of levator ani

Coccygeus

Anococcygeal ligament

Piriformis

Coccyx

Sacrum

FIGURE 11.36 Superficial muscles of the pelvic floor, superior view. (From Muscolino JE. *Manual Therapy for the Low Back and Pelvis: A Clinical Orthopedic Approach*. 1st ed. Philadelphia (PA): Wolters Kluwer; 2014.)

the pelvic floor is associated with activity of all abdominal muscles while a submaximal contraction of the pelvic floor is associated with a more isolated contraction of the TrA muscle (188). These muscles need to be targeted and activated to enhance the local core muscle control.

Global Core Muscles and LBP

As shown in Figure 11.37, the global core muscle system consists of the rectus abdominis, internal and external oblique, and the erector spinae (177). These muscles act on the trunk and spine but are not directly attached to the spine. They can develop considerable force when high-load strategies are needed and muscle strength is required, such as when having to lift an object or push a heavy load (177). Again, for balanced trunk posture and strength, both the global and local core muscle systems need to be active and engaged (189).

Conditions That Impact the Thoracic Spine

Although clients can have pain in the thoracic spine, conditions in this area of the spine are not as predominate as in the cervical and lumbar regions. The thoracic spine is thought to be quite stable because of the rib attachments both to the spinous processes and sternum. This shell protects the thoracic spine but does not however exclude this area from injury and pain. A major concern in the thoracic spine, especially in older adults, is the impact of osteoporosis, which can lead to spinal compression fractures. Compression fractures can cause severe physical limitations, including back pain, functional disability, and progressive kyphosis of the thoracic spine that ultimately results in decreased appetite, poor nutrition, impaired

pulmonary function, and spinal cord compression with motor and sensory deficits (190). Whether the client has undergone surgery, the most common procedures are balloon kyphoplasty and vertebroplasty or not, exercise is a mainstay of management in clients with osteoporosis and vertebral fracture. Rehabilitation measures are of particular importance to restore the quality of life in these clients. Specific aspects of a program should include individualized exercises to address flexibility, muscle strength, especially spinal extensor strengthening, core stability, cardiovascular fitness, and gait steadiness (190, 191).

Neck Pain

As with LBP, finding a pathoanatomical cause of a client's neck pain is not possible in most cases (169, 192). Once serious medical conditions have been ruled out (see Box 11.4), clients are most often classified as having a nerve root compression or a mechanical neck disorder (169). Like the local core muscle system in stabilizing the lumbar spine, the deep cervical flexor muscles (longus capitis and longus colli) are thought to play a significant role in stabilizing the neck (Figure 11.38). At the same time, faulty muscle activation patterns and poor endurance in these muscles can lead to chronic neck pain.

The Role of Posture in Neck Pain

As noted in the beginning of the chapter, posture is a problem common to most musculoskeletal issues. An abnormal position of the head as related to the spine can place abnormal strains throughout the spine and neck muscles (193), leading to chronic neck pain (4, 194, 195).

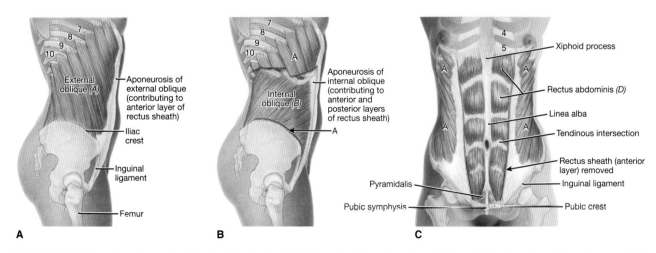

FIGURE 11.37 Muscles of the anterolateral abdominal wall. **A.** External oblique, **B.** Internal oblique, **C.** Rectus abdominis and pyramidalis. (From Agur AR, Dalley AF. *Grant's Atlas of Anatomy.* 14th ed. Philadelphia (PA): Wolters Kluwer; 2016.)

Box 11.4   Red Flags for a Serious Undetected Condition Presenting as Low Back Pain

Red Flags for Spine Cancer

Previous history of cancer

Night pain or pain at rest

Age > 50 yr or <17 yr old

Unexplained weight loss > 4.5 kg in 6 mo

Failure of conservative management in the past month

Red Flags for Spinal Fracture

Mild trauma, age > 50 yr

Age > 70 yr

Major trauma — fall from height >5′, moving vehicle accident, direct blow to spine

Known history of osteoporosis

Prolonged use of corticosteroids

Red Flags for Infection Within the Disc (Diskitis) or Vertebrae (Osteomyelitis)

The patient is immunosuppressed.

A prolonged fever with a temperature over 100.4°F

History of intravenous drug abuse

History of a recent urinary tract infection, cellulitis, or pneumonia

Red Flags for Cauda Equina Syndrome

Urine retention

Saddle anesthesia

Fecal incontinence

Sensory and motor deficits in the feet (L4, L5, Sl distribution)

A clinical finding in many clients, particularly those age 60 years or older, is a postural abnormality referred to as FHP (196). This postural dysfunction is associated with muscle shortening and tightness of the suboccipital musculature primarily consisting of the rectus capitis posterior major and

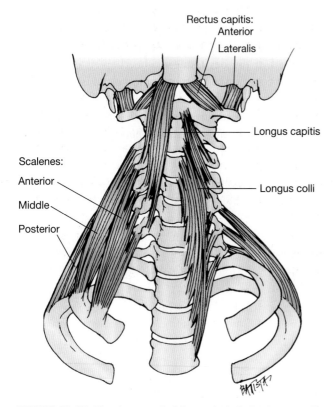

FIGURE 11.38 The deep cervical flexors include the longus colli, longus capitis, rectus capitis anterior, and lateralis. (From Oatis CA. *Kinesiology: The Mechanics and Pathomechanics of Human Movement.* 3rd ed. Philadelphia (PA): Wolters Kluwer; 2016.)

minor and the obliquus capitis superior and inferior. The cervical erector spinae muscles may also be shortened. These include the semispinalis and splenius capitis and cervicis, iliocostalis cervicis, longissimus cervicis, and spinalis cervicis. FHP is also associated with weakness of the deep cervical flexors — longus colli and capitis as well as the rectus capitis anterior and lateralis. Activation of the deep cervical flexors using a chin tuck (as illustrated in Figure 11.39) helps to reposition the head and decrease pain.

Other postural adaptations associated with FHP may include protracted scapulae with tight anterior muscles, specifically the pectoralis major and minor. The posterior muscles, the rhomboids and the middle trapezius, become stretched and weakened, a condition that often contributes to the development of a cervicothoracic kyphosis between C4 and T4 (197). This combination of tight muscles with weakened antagonists is sometimes referred to as "upper cross syndrome" (Figure 11.40). For example, the use of an ill-fitting chair that does not allow adequate upper extremity support can cause considerable stress affecting the upper trapezius, scalenes, pectoralis major and minor muscles, and other muscles of the upper quarter (4).

Other Causes of Neck Pain and Stiffness

A common cause of neck pain is muscle or soft tissue strain/sprain. This can result from multiple factors from sleeping with the neck in an awkward position, sleeping with several pillows under the cervical spine, or lifting a heavy object. Muscles can be strained during a traumatic injury such as a fall or a motor vehicle accident that forces the spine to extremes of ROM (4). Lastly, holding the neck

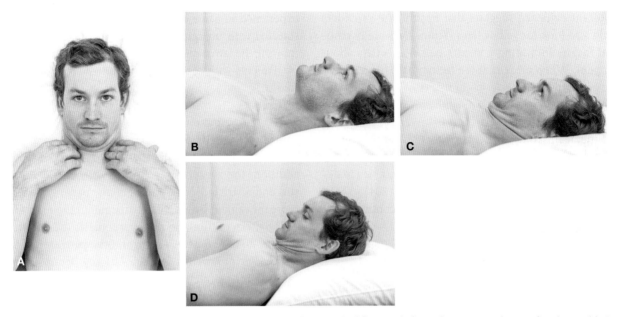

FIGURE 11.39 Chin tuck exercise to increase endurance of the deep cervical flexors. A–C are the same, patient performing a chin tuck: A. Forward position; B. A sideview of starting position; C. Performing the chin tuck with head supported; D. Patient further challenged by maintaining the chin tuck position while raising the crown of the head off pillow. (From Donnelly JM, Fernandez-de-Las-Penas C, Finnegan M, Freeman JL. *Travell, Simons & Simons' Myofascial Pain and Dysfunction.* Philadelphia (PA): Wolters Kluwer; 2018.)

in an abnormal position for a long period, such as when cradling a phone between the neck and the shoulder, can contribute to neck pain symptoms. Each of these situations can create abnormal stress on the muscles along the

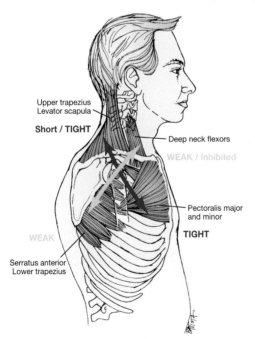

FIGURE 11.40 Forward head posture (FHP) may be associated with the "upper cross syndrome," which is characterized by short and tight suboccipitals, cervical extensors, upper trapezii, levator scapulae, and pectoral muscles and by weak and inhibited deep cervical flexors, middle and lower trapezii, and serratus anterior. (From Hendrickson T. *Massage and Manual Therapy for Orthopedic Conditions.* 2nd ed. Philadelphia (PA): Wolters Kluwer; 2009.)

back of the neck and extend into the scapular region, producing pain in the neck, the upper back, and even into the thoracic spine.

Stiffness in the neck can occur as a reaction to a more complex underlying condition such as a herniated disc or degenerative disc disease in the cervical spine (4, 169). Although not common, a potentially serious cause of stiffness in the cervical spine is meningitis. Clients who report a stiff neck that is associated with a high fever, headache, nausea, vomiting, or sleepiness should be advised to seek immediate medical attention (4, 198). Spondylosis is a chronic degenerative condition affecting the contents of the spinal canal, including the spinal nerve roots, spinal cord, and the vertebral bodies and intervertebral discs (4). Spondylosis and cervical disc herniation are most commonly linked to cervical radiculopathy and myelopathy (199, 200); however, the bony and ligamentous tissues affected by these conditions are themselves pain generators and are capable of giving rise to some of the referred symptoms observed in patients with neck pain (201, 202).

Warning Signs and Contraindications to Exercise

Red flags are warning signs that may indicate a potentially serious medical condition (203). The warning signs listed in Box 11.4 may present as a musculoskeletal complaint. When these signs are present, the client should be referred to their physician for further evaluation (156, 170, 172, 203).

Recent evidence suggests that health care providers should also look for yellow flags. Yellow flags are psychosocial factors indicating a client's personal beliefs about back pain. When present, these factors have been shown to be indicative of long-term chronicity of symptoms and disability (172). Yellow flags include, for example, an attitude that back pain is harmful or potentially severely disabling, fear, avoidance behavior that results in reduced activity levels; an expectation that passive rather than active interventions will be beneficial; and a tendency to depression, low morale, and social withdrawal (204).

A few primary signs or symptoms are contraindications to exercise for which the patient should be screened by a medical doctor. These include the following:

- Complaints of major neck trauma resulting from a recent history of a fall from a 5′ height or a motor vehicle accident.
- Reports of dizziness, drop attacks (a sudden fall without loss of consciousness), or blackouts.
- Signs of spinal cord compression, complaints of gait disturbance, or clumsy or weak hands.
- Stiff neck with high fever, nausea, or vomiting, especially if associated with headache.

Clients with any of these signs or symptoms need to be referred for medical follow-up, preferably to their personal physician.

Clinical Course of Back and Neck Pain

Classically, the course of back and neck pain is described as consisting of acute, subacute, and chronic phases. Understanding this continuum is especially important when working with patients with LBP, as intervention may need to be related to the phase of chronicity.

Acute LBP is defined as pain that has been present less than 1 month; subacute LBP has been present between 2 and 3 months; and chronic LBP has been present more than 3 months since the onset of the episode (160, 172). Because LBP is often recurrent in nature, time-based definitions should not be used exclusively (169) but in conjunction with other findings from the history.

Characteristically, an acute episode involves an inflammatory process with signs and symptoms of pain, swelling, and limited ROM with or without protective muscle guarding. Research suggests that the majority (~80%) of patients with acute LBP will fully recover within 6–8 weeks, requiring very little extensive treatment (205, 206). However, many clients present with an acute episode of a chronic condition. That is, people with a chronic condition such as lumbar disc herniation or degenerative disc disease often experience an acute episode of back pain that may be associated with unaccustomed activities such as gardening, mowing the lawn, and spring cleaning.

Patients with chronic LBP experience persistent pain that may or may not be associated with an inflammatory process. In response, they often reduce their activity level, becoming more sedentary. This relative immobility contributes greatly to muscle atrophy and poor neuromuscular control of the local and global core muscles. In addition, the zygapophyseal joints of the spine become stiff and restricted, contributing to the patient's belief that more movement would be detrimental to their condition. This pattern of thinking then perpetuates the notion that there is no cure for their pain, and the patient may experience a vicious cycle of low self-efficacy, depression, pain catastrophizing (an overestimation of the negative impact of the pain), and disability (170). Although such patients may represent fewer than 5% of all patients with LBP, they account for a substantial portion of LBP care (207, 208). The burden and psychosocial impact of chronic LBP is depicted in Figure 11.41.

Knowing where patients fall along the acute-to-chronic continuum is vitally important in helping them return to activity as usual. See Chapter 15 which addresses psychological and behavioral models related to exercise. Although exercise is necessary and appropriate for patients with back or neck pain, those in the acute phase of an injury should be discouraged from vigorous

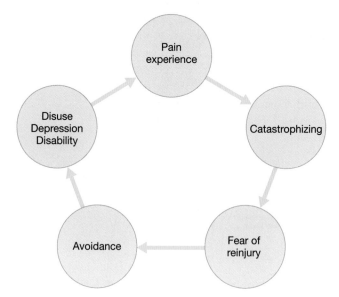

FIGURE 11.41 Psychosocial influences that can lead to chronic pain. (Data from Fritz J, George S, Delitto A. The role of fear-avoidance beliefs in acute low back pain: relationships with current and future disability and work status. *Pain*. 2001(94):7–15; Beattie PF. *The Lumbar Spine: Physical Therapy Patient Management Using Current Evidence. Current Concepts of Orthopaedic Physical Therapy*, 3rd ed.; 2011.)

exercise to avoid the negative impact it can have on the inflammatory process and tissue healing (6). For patients in the chronic phase of an injury, exercise is highly recommended. In fact, based on the highest classification of evidence, exercise to manage both chronic neck and back pain is strongly supported (156, 169). This includes exercises that address motor control impairments, muscle weakness, and decreased endurance.

Exercise Testing and Prescription for Back and Neck Pain

Most clients with back or neck pain should be able to participate in exercise testing. The evaluation should consider the impact that possible pain and fatigue may have on the test results and thus should proceed armed with this information.

Exercise recommendations for a client with neck or back pain follow ACSM guidelines (59). The spine program includes exercises for the cervical, thoracic, and lumbar spine, including the local and global core muscle stabilizers. It also includes flexibility training. The overall continued progression of a spine program includes movements that incorporate both the shoulder and the hip/pelvic girdle complex. A variety of machines and exercises can be used to train these areas, including seated rows and lateral pull-downs, which are great exercises that incorporate the shoulder girdle. The upper body ergometer poses a great challenge for building stability through the upper back. Resistance exercises that challenge the hip and the pelvic girdle include lunges, squats, and lateral walking (with resistance bands), and a leg press. The use of a recumbent bike, stepper, or treadmill for aerobic training is appropriate, although proper posture should be monitored. General advice to give regarding exercise includes several concepts presented in Box 11.5.

Targeted Cervical Spine Exercise

When working with clients who have predominate neck conditions, maintaining postural control is a primary consideration. Encourage a neutral position through the cervical spine with an exercise called a chin tuck (as shown in Figures 11.4 and 11.39). This exercise is key to recruiting and improving endurance of the longus colli and capitis, the deep cervical flexors. A neutral spine position should be encouraged with all upper extremity and trunk exercise positions including seated row, latissimus dorsi pull-down, trunk extension, abdominal flexion, and biceps curl, to name a few. A quick way to assess the presence of FHP is a simple finger test. First, have the client sit or stand in their natural and comfortable upright posture. Place one finger at the bottom of the ear lobe and one on the acromion process at the shoulder. The two fingers should be in a straight line. If they are not, the chin tuck exercise should be encouraged.

The client should initially perform the chin tuck exercise in a seated position. This position reduces the potential of using the sternocleidomastoid (SCM) muscle, which can easily overpower the targeted muscles, longus capitis, and longus colli. The endurance function of the muscle should be emphasized within the exercise prescription. Higher repetitions should be performed while maintaining the contraction for a longer duration (*e.g.,* hold position for 10 seconds and repeat 10 times) (4). The exercise should be very deliberate in the beginning, avoiding undesired movement patterns such as cervical side bending, rotation, or shoulder elevation. Resist the temptation to progress too rapidly if the endurance function has not been developed; for example, if the client is unable to maintain a chin tuck position when transitioning between exercise machines. As neuromuscular control improves, the client should be transitioned to more demanding positions such as performing the chin tuck while in quadruped, as illustrated in Figure 11.42.

Targeted Thoracic Spine Exercise

As the head moves anteriorly, the rest of the spine will follow, resulting in increased thoracic kyphosis or a flexed thoracic spine. The combination of FHP and thoracic kyphosis is often accompanied by weakness of the interscapular

Box 11.5	General Advice for Exercise and Back Pain

- Staying physically active is likely to be beneficial for those recovering from chronic back or neck pain (5).
- Many forms of exercise are good for back pain relief. These include aerobic exercise, strength training, flexibility training, and CORE strengthening (149).
- Participation in group exercises such as tai chi, yoga, and Pilates is effective in improving the overall health of the spine.

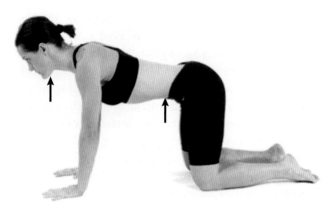

FIGURE 11.42 Activate deep cervical flexors in quadruped. Add more of a challenge by drawing in the transversus abdominis muscle. (From Williams A. *Massage Mastery: From Student to Professional.* 1st ed. Philadelphia (PA): Wolters Kluwer; 2012.)

muscles (the middle trapezius and rhomboid muscles). Exercises such as the seated row (Figures 11.5 and 11.6), lateral pull-down, and trunk extension help to strengthen this area. As mentioned earlier, when one muscle becomes weak, the opposing muscle adaptively shortens. In this case, the pectoralis major and minor may be tight; thus, exercises that facilitate the lengthening or stretching of these muscles should be included as part of the program.

Activation of the Core Stabilizers

All core stabilization exercises should start with the "drawing-in" maneuver (Figure 11.43). This exercise is said to provide specific activation of the TrA muscle. A good way to begin is to have the client in a hook-lying position (supine with knees 70–90 degrees and feet resting on the floor). They should place their fingers about an inch medial to the iliac crest. The verbal cues that have been shown to be helpful are to "draw your navel or belly button back toward the spine without moving your spine or tilting your pelvis." As demonstrated in Figure 11.44, the client should avoid tilting the pelvis posteriorly. Another cue that might be helpful is to "tighten the muscles in the pelvic floor, such as when needing to stop the flow of urine." When performing this exercise, the client should not hold their breath. The exercise can be performed in several positions, including quadruped, prone, and standing. The drawing-in maneuver should not be abandoned as the client progresses with the exercise plan.

Another baseline position used when teaching the client to activate the TrA is the quadruped position. Encourage the client to keep the trunk straight while drawing the abdomen up toward the spine. Endurance of the muscle is increased by having the client hold the contraction for 10 seconds and progressing in time up to 30–60 seconds for a count of 10 repetitions. This activation pattern should be encouraged and incorporated into all other forms of exercise and functional training, regardless of the level or intensity (*e.g.*, activating TrA while weightlifting, walking, running, or participating in aerobics classes). It is vital to maintaining a healthy and stable spine.

Selected activation of the LM muscles can be challenging. These muscles can best be targeted in the prone or side-lying positions. Clients commonly have difficulty contracting the LM, and tactile input can cue them as to which muscle they are being asked to contract.

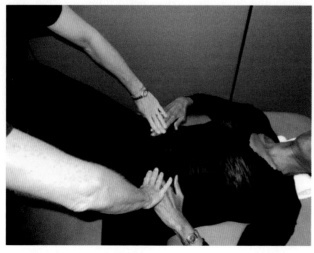

FIGURE 11.43 The "drawing-in" maneuver; fingers should be placed slightly medial and inferior to the anterior superior iliac crest. The client should pull the navel toward the spine without movement of the pelvis.

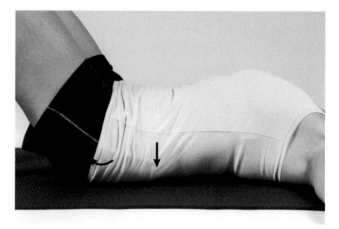

FIGURE 11.44 The posterior pelvic tilt provides a strong contraction of the rectus abdominis muscle causing actual posterior rotation of the pelvis, see arrow. (From Muscolino JE. *Manual Therapy for the Low Back and Pelvis: A Clinical Orthopedic Approach.* 1st ed. Philadelphia (PA): Wolters Kluwer; 2014.)

The muscle can best be palpated at the L5 level just medial to the spinous process. With the client in the prone position, a verbal cue that may help is to have the client think of initiating a *very tiny* tilt of the sacrum; for example, "Move your tailbone away from your body as if to arch your back, but do not actually let your back move." The LM can also be activated in prone by having the client lift the contralateral upper extremity (if raising the right arm, you should feel for the contraction on the left side of the spine) 5 cm (2 inches) with the shoulder abducted to 120 degrees and with the elbow flexed to 90 degrees (209).

With TrA and LM activation, the biggest obstacle is resisting the temptation to move on to more challenging positions before the foundation has been adequately laid, trained, and developed. Progressive exercise positions that train both TrA and LM can be found in Figures 11.45 through 11.50.

Progressing the Core Stabilization Program

The next step involves progression to a more comprehensive core stabilization approach as illustrated in Figures 11.51

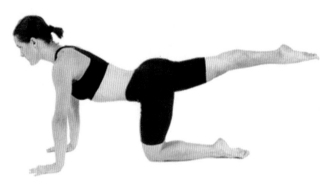

FIGURE 11.45 Increased demand on the core by continued activation of deep cervical flexors and the transversus abdominis while lifting one leg off the floor, extending it straight out from the hip. (From Williams A. *Massage Mastery: From Student to Professional.* 1st ed. Philadelphia (PA): Wolters Kluwer; 2012.)

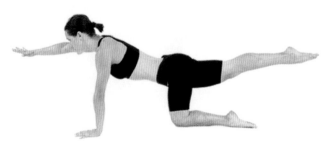

FIGURE 11.46 Increase the demand by having the client alternate lifting one leg and the opposite arm while maintaining a neutral spine position. (From Williams A. *Massage Mastery: From Student to Professional.* 1st ed. Philadelphia (PA): Wolters Kluwer; 2012.)

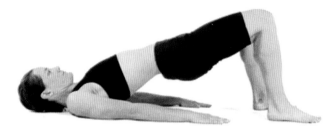

FIGURE 11.47 The "bridge" exercise is preceded by first engaging the local core muscles, before extending the hips. (From Williams A. *Massage Mastery: From Student to Professional.* 1st ed. Philadelphia (PA): Wolters Kluwer; 2012.)

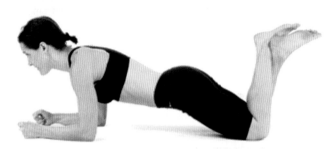

FIGURE 11.48 Modified front plank. (From Williams A. *Massage Mastery: From Student to Professional.* 1st ed. Philadelphia (PA): Wolters Kluwer; 2012.)

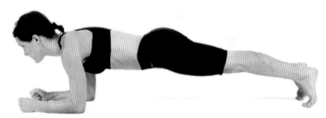

FIGURE 11.49 Front plank. (From Williams A. *Massage Mastery: From Student to Professional.* 1st ed. Philadelphia (PA): Wolters Kluwer; 2012.)

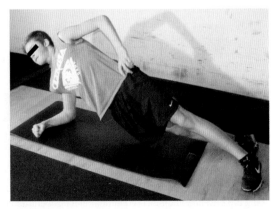

FIGURE 11.50 Side plank. (From Liebenson C. *Functional Training Handbook.* Philadelphia (PA): Wolters Kluwer; 2014.)

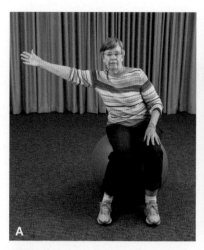
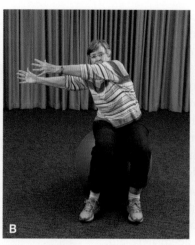
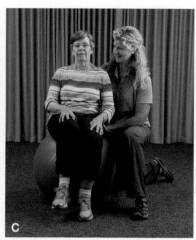

FIGURE 11.51 The unstable surface of the therapeutic ball adds an additional challenge. Encourage core activation through the cervical and lumbar spine with controlled single-leg lifts. Alternate right and left leg. **A.** Trunk control is challenged with weight shift and unilateral reaching with one arm. **B.** Increased trunk stability is required when challenged using both arms. **C.** The trunk is further challenged by removing one support surface. (From Brody L, Hall C. *Therapeutic Exercise*. Philadelphia (PA): Wolters Kluwer; 2017.)

and 11.52, which should be both progressive and functional. The core stabilization program should begin in the most challenging environment the client can control (5). The program can be manipulated by changing the plane of motion, the number of repetitions performed, and the loading parameter by using handheld weights, physioballs, medicine balls, tubing, body position, and duration of exercise. When building and progressing the program, always start with slow movements, which allow for controlled muscle recruitment patterns, before transitioning to movements in which the velocity in recruiting muscles is increased. Likewise, exercises should start with simple movement patterns and progress to more complex movements, from lower force output demand to exercise positions that require higher forces.

Training using therapeutic balls is a good way to progress the demands of the core stabilizers. Clients who have demonstrated improved neuromuscular control on the floor in supine or when sitting may be ready to transition into training their core on a therapeutic ball. A general rule of thumb is that the farther away the ball is from the core or center of the body (Figures 11.52, 11.53, and 11.54), the greater the demand placed on the core musculature. For example, when doing a push-up on the ball, placing the ball underneath the thigh makes doing the push-up much easier because the ball is closer to the trunk. To increase the difficulty, have the client roll the ball out to the feet; with the ball further away from the center of the body, the maintenance of balance is harder, increasing the requirements of the core muscles.

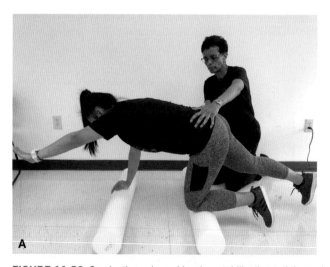
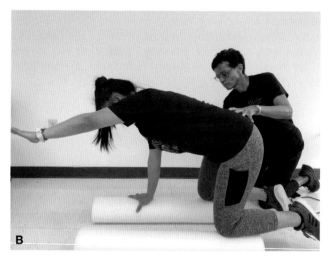

FIGURE 11.52 Cervicothoracic and lumbar stabilization training using foam rollers. **A.** Foam rollers perpendicular to body, quadruped with one hand and knee on each roller. Increased challenge to stabilizers by lifting arm. **B.** Foam rollers parallel to body. Quadruped with knees on one roller and hands on another roller. Lift alternate leg and arm to increase challenge to stability.

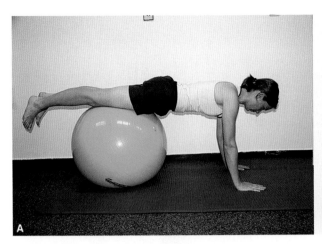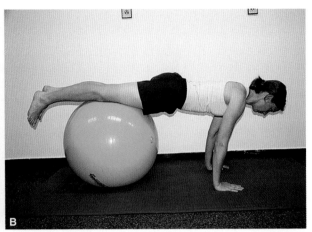

FIGURE 11.53 These positions encourage core control but primarily focus on the spinal extensors. **A.** Starting position with ball under thighs, hands directly under shoulders. **B.** Roll body slightly forward so that shoulders are forward of hands. This increases stability challenge at shoulders and upper trunk. (From Liebenson C. *Functional Training Handbook*. 1st ed. Philadelphia (PA): Wolters Kluwer; 2014.)

Flexibility Training

Another component of exercise that we have not discussed relates to exercise focused on improving joint ROM. Normal spinal mobility includes movements in flexion, extension, side bending, and rotation. When movement occurs across joint surfaces, many other structures such as muscles, ligaments, blood vessels, and nerves in the surrounding area are also affected. As mentioned earlier, muscle imbalances resulting from faulty posture, aging, or degenerative process may result in a loss or a decrease in spinal flexibility or ROM. Many other factors can lead to decreased ROM, including neurological or joint impairments, certain muscular diseases, surgery, traumatic injury, or simply inactivity (6). Clients with a history of chronic back or neck pain may also have impairments affecting their ROM. Although they may need a stabilization approach, these clients also need exercises that help to improve flexibility.

A simple exercise for overall back and joint flexibility is illustrated in Figure 11.55. A more difficult total flexion exercise is depicted in Figure 11.56; however, not all

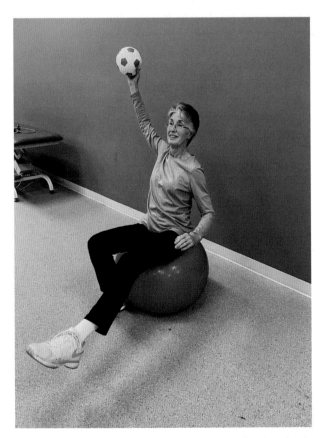

FIGURE 11.54 Sitting on therapeutic ball and performing simultaneous arm and leg exercises while catching an object is an example of an advanced spine stabilization exercise.

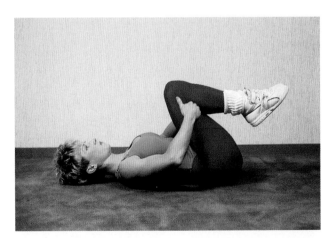

FIGURE 11.55 Increasing flexion mobility in the spine can be achieved as depicted by bringing single and double knees to chest. (From Brody L, Hall C. *Therapeutic Exercise: Moving Toward Function*. 3rd ed. Philadelphia (PA): Wolters Kluwer; 2010.)

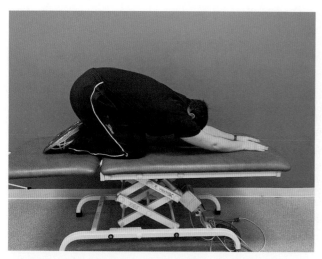

FIGURE 11.56 This flexion-based exercise (often called the "child's pose") combines flexion in the thoracic and lumbar spine and hips and knees. The degree of movement the client is able to achieve may depend on impairments in other joints, that is, hips and knees.

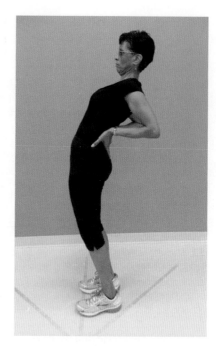

FIGURE 11.58 Standing back extension. (From Thompson W, Ed. *ACSMs Clinical Exercise Physiology.* 1st ed. Philadelphia (PA): Wolters Kluwer; 2019.)

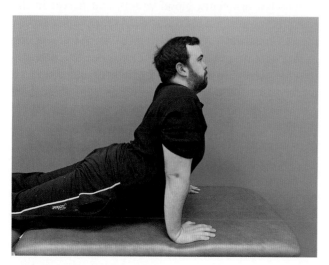

FIGURE 11.57 Prone extension.

clients will be able to perform this complete motion. Exercises that promote improved extension ROM include prone propping on elbows and the standing back bend, as depicted in Figures 11.57 and 11.58.

Flexion ROM can be improved with an exercise in the quadruped position, with the hands directly aligned under the shoulders, and the hips aligned with the knees. The client bows the spine upward "like a scary cat," then reverses the movement by allowing the spine to arch downward, commonly referred to as the camel, as illustrated in Figure 11.59.

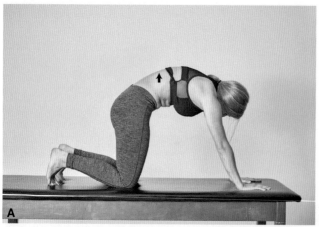

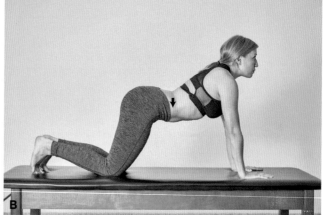

FIGURE 11.59 Lumbar flexion **(A)** and extension **(B)** mobility exercise in quadruped position. (From DiGiovanna E, Amen C, Burns D. *An Osteopathic Approach to Diagnosis and Treatment.* Philadelphia (PA): Wolters Kluwer; 2020.)

If, as a direct result of any of these movements, the client reports increased pain or numbness, especially in the lower extremity or extremities, the client should be referred to a health care provider such as a physical therapist or a medical doctor for further evaluation (6).

SUMMARY

Exercise is a very important component of a rehab program for those with musculoskeletal problems affecting the back and neck. Given recent projections that back pain has risen by as much as 50% during the last 20 years (161), there is a need for health care providers to promote a healthier lifestyle that includes exercise as a means of prevention of and controlling the severity of chronic symptoms. A balanced exercise program should include aerobic activities, resistance training, stretching, and neuromotor training (*i.e.*, balance and agility). As noted in each section, specific precautions, contraindications, or modifications must be considered when assessing, designing, or supervising an exercise program for a client with a musculoskeletal condition. As with all clients, a program should be individualized to meet the client's goals and limitations.

CHAPTER REVIEW QUESTIONS

1. What are the potential implications of a client's use of NSAIDs on exercise and healing?
2. What is the relevance of pathologic changes with arthritis to exercise prescription?
3. What risks should be screened for when working with a client with osteoporosis or RA? How are they similar or dissimilar?
4. What is the relevance of lower extremity dysfunction for balance?
5. Identify the two types of shoulder impingement and describe the causes of each.
6. What exercise modifications should be made for someone who reports she had a total hip replacement (posterior lateral approach) 3 months ago?
7. Describe two prevailing theories of malalignment that might explain the mechanism behind PFPS.
8. What is the clinical relevance of the local and global core as it relates to the prevention of LBP?
9. How does FHP impact the spine?
10. Why is LBP so prevalent in society today?

Case Study 11.1

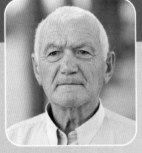

Edward is a 65-year-old man who came to the fitness center asking for an exercise program. He has been "somewhat active," having played golf two times per week and doing home activities, such as lawn mowing. He reports knee stiffness in the morning or after prolonged sitting, which improves as he gets moving. He currently takes ibuprofen several times a day to help control the pain. He reported that he is having problems walking the hills on the course, with his right knee sometimes "giving out," especially on the downhill. A fitness evaluation shows he has reduced extension and flexion in the right knee, a 1RM in the leg press that is 25% below his age group norms, and poor flexibility. His 6-minute walk time is 10% below his age group average.

Case Study 11.1 Questions

1. What is his probable diagnosis and what exercise needs are most important based on his diagnosis and his current status?
2. How will you modify the exercise prescription to accommodate the lack of range in the knees?

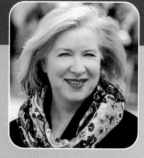

Case Study 11.2

Melissa, a 50-year-old woman, comes to you and wants to "get her back stronger." She is slightly overweight (body mass index [BMI] 26 placing her in the overweight category), stands 165.1 cm (65 inches), and weighs 74.8 kg (156 lb). She reports having experienced bouts of LBP when working in her yard and garden. This occurs about twice a year. She is employed as the administrative assistant for a seven-person law firm. She spends the majority of her shift answering the telephone and writing briefs; thus, she sits without interruption for long periods of time. She experiences intermittent bouts of back and neck pain, especially at the end of her work shift. Lately, she is taking over-the-counter medications to help with the discomfort. A friend mentioned that she should consider starting an exercise program. She says she has never been one to exercise, even during her school-age years, was never interested in physical fitness, and recalls being chubby when she was younger. She has recently become a grandmother. This has prompted her interest in working out. "I want to be able to lift my grandchildren without hurting myself."

Case Study 11.2 Questions

1. How would you advise this client on the safest approach when starting an exercise program?
2. What instructions can you provide this client that she could implement at work and that would help reduce her pain?
3. Name and describe four exercises that would be most appropriate for her as she embarks on this program.

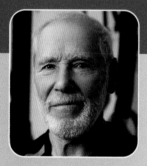

Case Study 11.3

Dan, a 50-year-old man, has been lifting weights one to two times per week for the past 6 weeks. He has had some left shoulder pain and is concerned about the exercises he is performing with his shoulders. He does not remember a specific instance when he hurt his shoulder, but now he is having pain even at work and having trouble sleeping on his left side. He even mentions having trouble doing simple tasks like reaching behind his back or reaching overhead to put on a shirt because of pain in the left shoulder. He is right-hand dominant and does not seem to have this trouble in his right shoulder. While he is sitting, you notice that he sits with rounded shoulders and FHP. He has primarily completed his weightlifting routine using the machines located at the gym. His upper body routine consists of chest press, military press, deltoid lateral raises to about 110 degrees of shoulder abduction, bicep curls, and triceps curls.

Case Study 11.3 Questions

1. What recommendations do you have to modify his existing exercise routine and why?
2. What are some recommendations for additional exercises?

REFERENCES

1. McGill SM. Linking latest knowledge of injury mechanisms and spine function to the prevention of low back disorders. *J Electromyogr Kinesiol*. 2004;14(1):43–7.

2. O'Sullivan P. Diagnosis and classification of chronic low back pain disorders: maladaptive movement and motor control impairments as underlying mechanism. *Man Ther*. 2005;10(4):242–55.

3. Ayub E. Posture and the upper quarter. In: Donatelli R, editor. *Physical Therapy of the Shoulder*. 2nd ed. New York (NY): Churchill Livingstone; 1991. p. 81–90.

4. Dutton M. *Dutton's Orthopaedic Examination, Evaluation, and Intervention*. 4th ed. New York (NY): McGraw-Hill Medical; 2018. p. 326–33, 1276, 1303–11, 1442–5, 1481–6, 1501–11.

5. Hoogenboom BJ, Voight ML, Prentice WE. *Musculoskeletal Interventions: Techniques for Therapeutic Exercise*. 3rd ed. New York (NY): McGraw-Hill Education/Medical; 2014. p. 137–8, 421–3.

6. Kisner C, Colby LA, Borstad J. *Therapeutic Exercise Foundations and Techniques*. 7th ed. Philadelphia (PA): F.A. Davis Co.; 2018. p. 321–34, 422–7, 453–64, 493–6, 513–28.

7. Scannell JP, McGill SM. Lumbar posture — should it, and can it, be modified? A study of passive tissue stiffness and lumbar position during activities of daily living. *Phys Ther*. 2003;83(10):907–17.

8. Côté P, van der Velde G, Cassidy JD, et al; Bone and Joint Decade 2000–2010 Task Force on Neck Pain and Its Associated Disorders. The burden and determinants of neck pain in workers: results of the Bone and Joint Decade 2000–2010 Task Force on Neck Pain and Its Associated Disorders. *Spine*. 2008;33(4 Suppl):S60–74.

9. Lau KT, Cheung KY, Chan KB, Chan MH, Lo KY, Chiu TT. Relationships between sagittal postures of thoracic and cervical spine, presence of neck pain, neck pain severity and disability. *Man Ther*. 2010;15(5):457–62.

10. Pillastrini P, de Lima ESRF, Banchelli F, et al. Effectiveness of global postural re-education in patients with chronic nonspecific neck pain: randomized controlled trial. *Phys Ther*. 2016;96(9):1408–16.

11. Hochberg MC, Altman RD, April KT, et al; American College of Rheumatology. American College of Rheumatology 2012 recommendations for the use of nonpharmacologic and pharmacologic therapies in osteoarthritis of the hand, hip, and knee. *Arthritis Care Res*. 2012;64(4):465–74.

12. Bannuru RR, Osani MC, Vaysbrot EE, et al. OARSI guidelines for the non-surgical management of knee, hip, and polyarticular osteoarthritis. *Osteoarthritis Cartilage*. 2019;27:1578–89.

13. Kolasinski SL, Neogi T, Hochberg MC, et al. 2019 American College of Rheumatology/Arthritis Foundation guideline for the management of osteoarthritis of the hand, hip, and knee. *Arthritis Rheumatol*. 2020;72(2):220–33.

14. White AP, Arnold PM, Norvell DC, Ecker E, Felhings MG. Pharmacologic management of chronic low back pain: synthesis of the evidence. *Spine*. 2011;36(21 Suppl):S131–43.

15. Su B, O'Connor JP. NSAID therapy effects on healing of bone, tendon, and the enthesis. *J Appl Physiol*. 2013;115(6):892–9.

16. Wilder FV, Barrett JP Jr. The association between medication usage and dropout status among participants of an exercise study for people with osteoarthritis. *Phys Ther*. 2005;85(2):142–9.

17. Singh JA, Saag KG, Bridges SL Jr, et al. 2015 American College of Rheumatology guideline for the treatment of rheumatoid arthritis. *Arthritis Rheumatol*. 2016;68(1):1–26. doi:10.1002/art.39480.

18. Allen A, Carville S, McKenna F; Guideline Development Group. Diagnosis and management of rheumatoid arthritis in adults: summary of updated NICE guidance. *BMJ*. 2018;362:k3015.

19. Janke K, Biester K, Krause D, et al. Comparative effectiveness of biological medicines in rheumatoid arthritis: systematic review and network meta-analysis including aggregate results from reanalysed individual patient data. *BMJ*. 2020;370:m2288. doi:10.1136/bmj.m2288.

20. Mian A, Ibrahim F, Scott DL. A systematic review of guidelines for managing rheumatoid arthritis. *BMC Rheumatol*. 2019;3:42. doi:10.1186/s41927-019-0090-7.

21. Köhler BM, Günther J, Kaudewitz D, Lorenz H-M. Current therapeutic options in the treatment of rheumatoid arthritis. *J Clin Med*. 2019;8(7):938.

22. Raterman HG, Lems WF. Pharmacological management of osteoporosis in rheumatoid arthritis patients: a review of the literature and practical guide. *Drugs Aging*. 2019;36:1061–72.

23. Eastell R, Rosen CJ, Black DM, Cheung AM, Murad MH, Shoback D. Pharmacological management of osteoporosis in postmenopausal women: an Endocrine Society* clinical practice guideline. *J Clin Endocrinol Metab*. 2019;104:1595–622.

24. Shoback D, Rosen CJ, Black DM, Cheung AM, Murad MH, Eastell R. Pharmacological management of osteoporosis in postmenopausal women: an Endocrine Society guideline update. *J Clin Endocrinol Metab*. 2020;105(3):587–94. doi:10.1210/clinem/dgaa048.

25. Zhao R, Xu Z, Zhao M. Antiresorptive agents increase the effects of exercise on preventing postmenopausal bone loss in women: a meta-analysis. *PLoS One*. 2015;10(1):e0116729.

26. Perry SB, Downey PA. Fracture risk and prevention: a multidimensional approach. *Phys Ther*. 2012;92(1):164–78.

27. Senftleber NK, Nielsen SM, Andersen JR, et al. Marine oil supplements for arthritis pain: a systematic review and meta-analysis of randomized trials. *Nutrients*. 2017;9(1):42. doi:10.3390/nu9010042.

28. Nelson J, Sjöblom H, Gjertsson I, Ulven SM, Lindqvist HM, Bärebring L. Do interventions with diet or dietary supplements reduce the disease activity score in rheumatoid arthritis? A systematic review of randomized controlled trials. *Nutrients*. 2020;12(10):2991. doi:10.3390/nu12102991.

29. Barbour KE, Helmick CG, Boring M, Brady TJ. Vital signs: prevalence of doctor-diagnosed arthritis and arthritis-attributable activity limitation — United States, 2013–2015. *MMWR Morb Mortal Wkly Rep*. 2017;66(9):246–53.

30. American College of Rheumatology. *Spondyloarthritis*. Atlanta (GA): American College of Rheumatology; 2013. Available from: https://www.rheumatology.org/I-Am-A/Patient-Caregiver/Diseases-Conditions/Spondyloarthritis.

31. Boehme K, Roulaffs B. Onset and progression of human osteoarthritis — can growth factors, inflammatory cytokines, or

differential miRNA expression concomitantly induce proliferation, ECM degradation, and inflammation in articular cartilage? *Int J Mol Sci.* 2018;19:2282. doi:10.3390/ijms19082282.

32. Chow YY, Chin K-Y. The role of inflammation in the pathogenesis of osteoarthritis. *Mediators Inflamm.* 2020;2020:8293921. doi:10.1155/2020/8293921.

33. Nees TA, Rosshirt N, Zhang JA, et al. Synovial cytokines significantly correlate with osteoarthritis-related knee pain and disability: inflammatory mediators of potential clinical relevance. *J Clin Med.* 2019;8(9):1343. doi:10.3390/jcm8091343.

34. van der Woude D, van der Helm-van Mil AHM. Update on the epidemiology, risk factors, and disease outcomes of rheumatoid arthritis. *Best Pract Res Clin Rheumatol.* 2018;32:174–87.

35. Altman R, Asch E, Bloch D, et al. Development of criteria for the classification and reporting of osteoarthritis. Classification of osteoarthritis of the knee. Diagnostic and Therapeutic Criteria Committee of the American Rheumatism Association. *Arthritis Rheum.* 1986;29(8):1039–49.

36. Damen J, van Rijn RM, Emans PJ, et al. Prevalence and development of hip and knee osteoarthritis according to American College of Rheumatology criteria in the CHECK cohort. *Arthritis Res Ther.* 2019;21(1):4. doi:10.1186/s13075-018-1785-7.

37. Aletaha D, Neogi T, Silman AJ, et al. 2010 Rheumatoid arthritis classification criteria: an American College of Rheumatology/European League Against Rheumatism collaborative initiative. *Ann Rheum Dis.* 2010;69(9):2569–81. doi:10.1002/art.27584.

38. Barker K, Lamb SE, Toye F, Jackson S, Barrington S. Association between radiographic joint space narrowing, function, pain and muscle power in severe osteoarthritis of the knee. *Clin Rehabil.* 2004;18(7):793–800.

39. Wolfe F, Clauw DJ, Fitzcharles MA, et al. The American College of Rheumatology preliminary diagnostic criteria for fibromyalgia and measurement of symptom severity. *Arthritis Care Res.* 2010;62(5):600–10.

40. Galvez-Sánchez CM, Reyes del Paso GA. Diagnostic criteria for fibromyalgia: critical review and future perspectives. *J Clin Med.* 2020;9(4):1219. doi:10.3390/jcm9041219.

41. Centers for Disease Control and Prevention. *Arthritis Data and Statistics.* Atlanta (GA): Centers for Disease Control & Prevention; 2016. Available from: https://www.cdc.gov/arthritis/data_statistics/index.htm.

42. Nelson ME, Rejeski WJ, Blair SN, et al. Physical activity and public health in older adults: recommendation from the American College of Sports Medicine and the American Heart Association. *Med Sci Sports Exerc.* 2007;39(8):1435–45.

43. Messier SP, Loeser RF, Miller GD, et al. Exercise and dietary weight loss in overweight and obese older adults with knee osteoarthritis: the arthritis, diet, and activity promotion trial. *Arthritis Rheum.* 2004;50(5):1501–10.

44. Fransen M, McConnell S, Harmer AR, Van der Esch M, Simic M, Bennell KL. Exercise for osteoarthritis of the knee: a Cochrane systematic review. *Br J Sports Med.* 2015;49(24):1554–7.

45. Goh SL, Persson MSM, Stocks J, et al. Efficacy and potential determinants of exercise therapy in knee and hip osteoarthritis: a systematic review and meta-analysis. *Ann Phys Rehabil Med.* 2019;62:356–65.

46. Brosseau L, Pelland L, Wells G, et al. Efficacy of aerobic exercises for osteoarthritis (part II): a meta-analysis. *Phys Ther Rev.* 2004;9(3):125–45.

47. Fransen M, McConnell S, Hernandez-Molina G, Reichenbach S. Exercise for osteoarthritis of the hip [Update of *Cochrane Database Syst Rev.* 2009;(3):CD007912]. *Cochrane Database Syst Rev.* 2014;(4):CD007912.

48. Skou ST, Pederson BK, Abbott JH, Patterson B, Barton C. Physical activity and exercise therapy benefit more than just symptoms and impairments in people with hip and knee osteoarthritis. *J Orthop Sports Phys Ther.* 2018;48(6):439–47.

49. Fitzgerald GK, Piva SR, Gil AB, Wisniewski SR, Oddis CV, Irrgang JJ. Agility and perturbation training techniques in exercise therapy for reducing pain and improving function in people with knee osteoarthritis: a randomized clinical trial. *Phys Ther.* 2011;91(4):452–69.

50. Hakkinen A, Pakarinen A, Hannonen P, et al. Effects of prolonged combined strength and endurance training on physical fitness, body composition and serum hormones in women with rheumatoid arthritis and in healthy controls. *Clin Exp Rheumatol.* 2005;23(4):505–12.

51. Lange E, Kucharski D, Svedlund S, et al. Effects of aerobic and resistance exercise in older adults with rheumatoid arthritis: a randomized controlled trial. *Arthritis Care Res.* 2019;71(1):61–70.

52. Hurley M, Dickson K, Hallett R, et al. Exercise interventions and patient beliefs for people with hip, knee or hip and knee osteoarthritis: a mixed methods review. *Cochrane Database Syst Rev.* 2018;4(4):CD010842.

53. Jan MH, Lin JJ, Liau JJ, Lin Y-F, Lin D-H. Investigation of clinical effects of high- and low-resistance training for patients with knee osteoarthritis: a randomized controlled trial. *Phys Ther.* 2008;88(4):427–36.

54. Amella EJ. Presentation of illness in older adults. *Am J Nurs.* 2004;104(10):40–51; quiz 52.

55. Schmitt LC, Fitzgerald GK, Reisman AS, Rudolph KS. Instability, laxity, and physical function in patients with medial knee osteoarthritis. *Phys Ther.* 2008;88(12):1506–16.

56. Hayashibara M, Hagino H, Katagiri H, Okano T, Okada J, Teshima R. Incidence and risk factors of falling in ambulatory patients with rheumatoid arthritis: a prospective 1-year study. *Osteoporos Int.* 2010;21(11):1825–33.

57. Barbour KE, Stevens JA, Helmick CG, et al; Centers for Disease Control and Prevention. Falls and fall injuries among adults with arthritis — United States, 2012. *MMWR Morb Mortal Wkly Rep.* 2014;63(17):379–83.

58. Riskowski J, Dufour AB, Hannan MT. Arthritis, foot pain and shoe wear: current musculoskeletal research on feet. *Curr Opin Rheumatol.* 2011;23(2):148–55.

59. Liguori G. *ACSM's Guidelines for Exercise Testing and Prescription.* 11th ed. Philadelphia (PA): Wolters Kluwer/Lippincott Williams & Wilkins; 2022. p. 166–79, 208–9, 211–5, 260–3, 315–7. FITT tables — p. 310, 329, 350.

60. Vliet Vlieland TP, van den Ende CH. Nonpharmacological treatment of rheumatoid arthritis. *Curr Opin Rheumatol.* 2011;23(3):259–64.

61. de Jong Z, Munneke M, Kroon HM, et al. Long-term follow-up of a high-intensity exercise program in patients with rheumatoid arthritis. *Clin Rheumatol.* 2009;28(6):663–71.

62. Hakkinen A, Sokka T, Hannonen P. A home-based two-year strength training period in early rheumatoid arthritis led to good long-term compliance: a five-year followup. *Arthritis Rheum.* 2004;51(1):56–62.

63. Naranjo A, Sokka T, Descalzo MA, et al; Theodore Pincus; QUEST-RA Group. Cardiovascular disease in patients with rheumatoid arthritis: results from the QUEST-RA study. *Arthritis Res Ther.* 2008;10(2):R30.

64. Peters MJ, Symmons DP, McCarey D, et al. EULAR evidence-based recommendations for cardiovascular risk management in patients with rheumatoid arthritis and other forms of inflammatory arthritis. *Ann Rheum Dis.* 2010;69(2):325–31.

65. Chung CP, Oeser A, Avalos I, et al. Utility of the Framingham risk score to predict the presence of coronary atherosclerosis in patients with rheumatoid arthritis. *Arthritis Res Ther.* 2006;8(6):R186.

66. Regnaux JP, Lefevre-Colau MM, Trinquart L, et al. High-intensity versus low-intensity physical activity or exercise in people with hip or knee osteoarthritis. *Cochrane Database Syst Rev.* 2015;2015(10):CD010203.

67. Bruce B, Fries JF, Lubeck DP. Aerobic exercise and its impact on musculoskeletal pain in older adults: a 14 year prospective, longitudinal study. *Arthritis Res Ther.* 2005;7(6):R1263–70.

68. Cochrane T, Davey RC, Matthes Edwards SM. Randomised controlled trial of the cost-effectiveness of water-based therapy for lower limb osteoarthritis. *Health Technol Assess.* 2005;9(31):iii–iv, ix–xi, 1–114.

69. Hall A, Maher C, Latimer J, Ferreira M. The effectiveness of Tai Chi for chronic musculoskeletal pain conditions: a systematic review and meta-analysis. *Arthritis Rheum.* 2009;61(6):717–24.

70. Peng PW. Tai Chi and chronic pain. *Reg Anesth Pain Med.* 2012;37(4):372–82.

71. Ettinger WH Jr, Burns R, Messier SP, et al. A randomized trial comparing aerobic exercise and resistance exercise with a health education program in older adults with knee osteoarthritis. The Fitness Arthritis and Seniors Trial (FAST). *JAMA.* 1997;277(1):25–31.

72. Farr JN, Going SB, McKnight PE, Kasle S, Cussler EC, Cornett M. Progressive resistance training improves overall physical activity levels in patients with early osteoarthritis of the knee: a randomized controlled trial. *Phys Ther.* 2010;90(3):356–66.

73. Hurkmans E, van der Giesen FJ, Vliet Vlieland TP, Schoones J, Van den Ende EC. Dynamic exercise programs (aerobic capacity and/or muscle strength training) in patients with rheumatoid arthritis. *Cochrane Database Syst Rev.* 2009;2009(4):CD006853.

74. Metsios GS, Stavropoulos-Kalinoglou A, Veldhuijzen van Zanten JJ, et al. Rheumatoid arthritis, cardiovascular disease and physical exercise: a systematic review. *Rheumatology (Oxford).* 2008;47(3):239–48.

75. Fitzgerald GK, Childs JD, Ridge TM, Irrgang JJ. Agility and perturbation training for a physically active individual with knee osteoarthritis. *Phys Ther.* 2002;82(4):372–82.

76. Bosch PR, Traustadottir T, Howard P, Matt KS. Functional and physiological effects of yoga in women with rheumatoid arthritis: a pilot study. *Altern Ther Health Med.* 2009;15(4):24–31.

77. Sul B, Lee KB, Joo YB, et al. Twelve weeks of strengthening exercise for patients with rheumatoid arthritis: a prospective intervention study. *J Clin Med.* 2020;9(9):2792. doi:10.3390/jcm9092792.

78. Fitzgerald GK, Piva SR, Irrgang JJ, Bouzubar F, Starz TW. Quadriceps activation failure as a moderator of the relationship between quadriceps strength and physical function in individuals with knee osteoarthritis. *Arthritis Rheum.* 2004;51(1):40–8.

79. Diracoglu D, Aydin R, Baskent A, Celik A. Effects of kinesthesia and balance exercises in knee osteoarthritis. *J Clin Rheumatol.* 2005;11(6):303–10.

80. Lin DH, Lin CH, Lin YF, Jan MH. Efficacy of 2 non-weight-bearing interventions, proprioception training versus strength training, for patients with knee osteoarthritis: a randomized clinical trial. *J Orthop Sports Phys Ther.* 2009;39(6):450–7.

81. Kanis JA, Johnell O, Oden A, Johansson H, McCloskey E. FRAX and the assessment of fracture probability in men and women from the UK. *Osteoporos Int.* 2008;19(4):385–97.

82. Sarafrazi N, Wambogo EA, Shepherd JA. *Osteoporosis or Low Bone Mass in Older Adults: United States, 2017–2018.* NCHS Data Brief, No. 405. Hyattsville (MD): National Center for Health Statistics; 2021. doi:10.15620/cdc:103477.

83. Cosman F, de Beur SJ, LeBoff MS, et al. Clinician's guide to prevention and treatment of osteoporosis [Published correction appears in *Osteoporos Int.* 2015;26(7):2045–7]. *Osteoporos Int.* 2014;25(10):2359–81.

84. Leslie WD, Morin SN. Osteoporosis epidemiology 2013: implications for diagnosis, risk assessment, and treatment. *Curr Opin Rheumatol.* 2014;26(4):440–6.

85. Yang S, Nguyen ND, Center JR, Eisman JA, Nguyen TV. Association between hypertension and fragility fracture: a longitudinal study. *Osteoporos Int.* 2014;25(1):97–103.

86. WHO Study Group. *Assessment of Fracture Risk and Its Application to Screening for Postmenopausal Osteoporosis.* WHO Technical Report Series 843. Geneva (Switzerland): World Health Organization; 1994. Available from: http://apps.who.int/iris/bitstream/handle/10665/39142/WHO_TRS_843_eng.pdf.

87. Kanis JA. Assessment of fracture risk and its application to screening for postmenopausal osteoporosis: synopsis of a WHO report. WHO Study Group. *Osteoporos Int.* 1994;4(6):368–81. doi:10.1007/BF01622200.

88. Zhao R, Zhao M, Xu Z. The effects of differing resistance training modes on the preservation of bone mineral density in postmenopausal women: a meta-analysis. *Osteoporos Int.* 2015;26(5):1605–18.

89. Kemmler W, Haberle L, von Stengel S. Effects of exercise on fracture reduction in older adults: a systematic review and meta-analysis. *Osteoporos Int.* 2013;24(7):1937–50.

90. Giangregorio LM, Papaioannou A, Macintyre NJ, et al. Too fit to fracture: exercise recommendations for individuals with osteoporosis or osteoporotic vertebral fracture. *Osteoporos Int.* 2014;25(3):821–35.

91. Nieman DC. Is infection risk linked to exercise workload? *Med Sci Sports Exerc.* 2000;32(Suppl 7):S406–11.

92. Chien MY, Wu YT, Hsu AT, Yang RS, Lai JS. Efficacy of a 24-week aerobic exercise program for osteopenic postmenopausal women. *Calcif Tissue Int.* 2000;67(6):443–8.

93. Kemmler W, von Stengel S. Dose-response effect of exercise frequency on bone mineral density in post-menopausal, osteopenic women. *Scand J Med Sci Sports.* 2014;24(3):526–34.

94. Hinton PS, Nigh P, Thyfault J. Effectiveness of resistance training or jumping-exercise to increase bone mineral density in men with low bone mass: a 12-month randomized, clinical trial. *Bone.* 2015;79:203–12.

95. Watson SL, Weeks BK, Weis LJ, Harding AT, Horan SA, Beck BR. High-intensity resistance and impact training improves bone mineral density and physical function in postmenopausal women with osteopenia and osteoporosis: the LIFTMOR randomized controlled trial. *J Bone Miner Res.* 2018;33(2):211–20.

96. Montgomery G, Abt, G, Dobson C, Smith T, Evans W, Ditroilo M. The mechanical loading and muscle activation of four common exercises used in osteoporosis prevention for early postmenopausal women. *J Electromyogr Kinesiol.* 2019;44:124–31. doi:10.1016/j.jelekin.2018.12.004.

97. Sinaki M, Brey RH, Hughes CA, Larson DR, Kaufman KR. Balance disorder and increased risk of falls in osteoporosis and kyphosis: significance of kyphotic posture and muscle strength. *Osteoporos Int.* 2005;16(8):1004–10.

98. Chyu MC, James CR, Sawyer SF, et al. Effects of tai chi exercise on posturography, gait, physical function and quality of life in postmenopausal women with osteopaenia: a randomized clinical study. *Clin Rehabil.* 2010;24(12):1080–90.

99. Maradit-Kremers H, Crowson CS, Larson D, Jiranek WA, Berry DJ. Prevalence of total hip (THA) and total knee (TKA) arthroplasty in the United States. In: *AAOS 2014 Annual Meeting*; New Orleans (LA): American Academy of Orthopaedic Surgeons; 2014.

100. Daniels TR, Mayich DJ, Penner MJ. Intermediate to long-term outcomes of total ankle replacement with the Scandinavian Total Ankle Replacement (STAR). *J Bone Joint Surg Am.* 2015;97(11):895–903.

101. American Joint Replacement Registry. *2021 Annual Report.* Rosemont (IL): American Academy of Orthopaedic Surgeons; 2021.

102. Hegsted D, Gritsiouk Y, Schlesinger P, Gardiner S, Gubler KD. Utility of the risk assessment profile for risk stratification of venous thrombotic events for trauma patients. *Am J Surg.* 2013;205(5):517–20; discussion 520.

103. Williams SN, Wolford ML, Bercovitz A. Hospitalization for total knee replacement among inpatients aged 45 and over: United States, 2000–2010. *NCHS Data Brief.* 2015;(210):1–8.

104. Su EP, Su SL, Della Valle AG. Stiffness after TKR: how to avoid repeat surgery. *Orthopedics.* 2010;33(9):658.

105. Harato K, Nagura T, Matsumoto H, Otani T, Toyama Y, Suda Y. Knee flexion contracture will lead to mechanical overload in both limbs: a simulation study using gait analysis. *Knee.* 2008;15(6):467–72.

106. Alnahdi AH, Zeni JA, Snyder-Mackler L. Gait after unilateral total knee arthroplasty: frontal plane analysis. *J Orthop Res.* 2011;29(5):647–52.

107. Chitnavis J, Sinsheimer JS, Suchard MA, Clipsham K, Carr AJ. End-stage coxarthrosis and gonarthrosis. Aetiology, clinical patterns and radiological features of idiopathic osteoarthritis. *Rheumatology.* 2000;39(6):612–9.

108. McMahon M, Block JA. The risk of contralateral total knee arthroplasty after knee replacement for osteoarthritis. *J Rheumatol.* 2003;30(8):1822–4.

109. Han S-B, Lee S-S, Kim K-H, Im J-T, Park P-S, Shin Y-S. Survival of medial versus lateral unicompartmental knee arthroplasty: a meta-analysis. *PLoS One.* 2020;15(1):e0228150. doi:10.1371/journal.pone.022815.

110. Lee TQ. Biomechanics of hyperflexion and kneeling before and after total knee arthroplasty. *Clin Orthop Surg.* 2014;6(2):117–26.

111. Mizner RL, Petterson SC, Snyder-Mackler L. Quadriceps strength and the time course of functional recovery after total knee arthroplasty. *J Orthop Sports Phys Ther.* 2005;35(7):424–36.

112. Meier W, Mizner RL, Marcus RL, Dibble LE, Peters C, Lastayo PC. Total knee arthroplasty: muscle impairments, functional limitations, and recommended rehabilitation approaches. *J Orthop Sports Phys Ther.* 2008;38(5):246–56.

113. D'Antonio JA, Capello WN, Naughton M. Ceramic bearings for total hip arthroplasty have high survivorship at 10 years. *Clin Orthop Relat Res.* 2012;470(2):373–81.

114. Smith TO, Blake V, Hing CB. Minimally invasive versus conventional exposure for total hip arthroplasty: a systematic review and meta-analysis of clinical and radiological outcomes. *Int Orthop.* 2011;35(2):173–84.

115. Kyriakopoulos G, Poultsides L, Christofilopoulos P. Total hip arthroplasty through an anterior approach: the pros and cons. *EFORT Open Rev.* 2018;3:574–83. doi:10.1302/2058-5241.3.180023.

116. Kiet TK, Feeley BT, Naimark M, et al. Outcomes after shoulder replacement: comparison between reverse and anatomic total shoulder arthroplasty. *J Shoulder Elbow Surg.* 2015;24(2):179–85.

117. Seitz W, Michaud E. Rehabilitation after shoulder replacement: be all you can be! *Semin Arthro.* 2012;23:106–13.

118. Kanlayanaphotporn R. Changes in sitting posture affect shoulder range of motion. *J Bodyw Mov Ther.* 2014;18(2):239–43.

119. Cyriax J. The shoulder. *Br J Hosp Med.* 1975;19:185–92.

120. Ryan G, Johnston H, Moreside J. Infraspinatus isolation during external rotation exercise at varying degrees of abduction. *J Sport Rehabil.* 2018;27(4):334–9.

121. Shin SJ. A comparison of 2 repair techniques for partial-thickness articular-sided rotator cuff tears. *Arthroscopy.* 2012;28(1):25–33.

122. Nikolaidou O, Migkou S, Karampalis C. Rehabilitation after rotator cuff repair. *Open Orthop J.* 2017;11:154–62. doi:10.217/1874325001711010154.

123. Longo UG, Rizzello G, Loppini M, et al. Multidirectional instability of the shoulder: a systematic review. *Arthroscopy.* 2015;31(12):2431–43.

124. Eljabu W, Klinger HM, von Knoch M. The natural course of shoulder instability and treatment trends: a systematic review. *J Orthop Traumatol.* 2017;18(1):1–8.

125. Pitzer ME, Seidenberg PH, Bader DA. Elbow tendinopathy [Published correction appears in *Med Clin North Am.* 2015;99(1):xix]. *Med Clin North Am.* 2014;98(4):833–49, xiii.

126. Faulkner JA, Brooks SV, Opiteck JA. Injury to skeletal muscle fibers during contractions: conditions of occurrence and prevention. *Phys Ther.* 1993;73(12):911–21.

127. Long L, Briscoe S, Cooper C, Hyde C, Crathorne L. What is the clinical effectiveness and cost-effectiveness of conservative interventions for tendinopathy? An overview of systematic reviews of clinical effectiveness and systematic review of economic evaluations. *Health Technol Assess.* 2015;19(8):1–134.

128. Oken O, Kahraman Y, Ayhan F, Canpolat S, Yorgancioglu ZR, Oken OF. The short-term efficacy of laser, brace, and ultrasound treatment in lateral epicondylitis: a prospective, randomized, controlled trial [Published correction appears in *J Hand Ther.* 2008;21(3):303]. *J Hand Ther.* 2008;21(1):63–7; quiz 68.

129. Brukner P. Hamstring injuries: prevention and treatment-an update. *Br J Sports Med.* 2015;49(19):1241–44. doi:10.1136/bjsports-2014-094427.

130. Redmond JM, Chen AW, Domb BG. Greater trochanteric pain syndrome. *J Am Acad Orthop Surg.* 2016;24(4):231–40.

131. Glaviano NR, Kew M, Hart JM, et al. Demographic and epidemiological trends in patellofemoral pain. *Int J Sports Phys Ther.* 2015;10(3):281–90.

132. Roush JR, Bay RC. Prevalence of anterior knee pain in 18–35 year-old females. *Int J Sports Phys Ther.* 2012;7(4): 396–401.

133. Powers CM. The influence of altered lower-extremity kinematics on patellofemoral joint dysfunction: a theoretical perspective. *J Orthop Sports Phys Ther.* 2003;33(11):639–46.

134. Finnoff JT, Hall MM, Kyle K, Krause DA, Lai J, Smith J. Hip strength and knee pain in high school runners: a prospective study. *PM R.* 2011;3(9):792–801.

135. Esculier JF, Roy JS, Bouyer LJ. Lower limb control and strength in runners with and without patellofemoral pain syndrome. *Gait Posture.* 2015;41(3):813–9.

136. Rathleff MS, Richter C, Brushoj C, et al. Increased medial foot loading during drop jump in subjects with patellofemoral pain. *Knee Surg Sports Traumatol Arthrosc.* 2014;22(10):2301–7.

137. Fukuda TY, Rossetto FM, Magalhaes E, Bryk FF, Lucareli PR, de Almeida Aparecida Carvalho N. Short-term effects of hip abductors and lateral rotators strengthening in females with patellofemoral pain syndrome: a randomized controlled clinical trial. *J Orthop Sports Phys Ther.* 2010;40(11):736–42.

138. Irish SE, Millward AJ, Wride J, Haas BM, Shum G. The effect of closed-kinetic chain exercises and open-kinetic chain exercise on the muscle activity of vastus medialis oblique and vastus lateralis. *J Strength Cond Res.* 2010;24(5):1256–62.

139. Gross MT, Foxworth JL. The role of foot orthoses as an intervention for patellofemoral pain. *J Orthop Sports Phys Ther.* 2003;33(11):661–70.

140. Murtaugh B, Ihm JM. Eccentric training for the treatment of tendinopathies. *Curr Sports Med Rep.* 2013;12(3):175–82.

141. Agel J, Rockwood T, Klossner D. Collegiate ACL injury rates across 15 sports: National Collegiate Athletic Association injury surveillance system data update (2004–2005 through 2012–2013). *Clin J Sport Med.* 2016;26(6):518–23.

142. Xie X, Liu X, Chen Z, Yu Y, Peng S, Li Q. A meta-analysis of bone-patellar tendon-bone autograft versus four-strand hamstring tendon autograft for anterior cruciate ligament reconstruction. *Knee.* 2015;22(2):100–10.

143. Panni AS, Milano G, Lucania L, Fabbriciani C. Graft healing after anterior cruciate ligament reconstruction in rabbits. *Clin Orthop Relat Res.* 1997;(343):203–12.

144. Wilk KE, Reinold MM, Hooks TR. Recent advances in the rehabilitation of isolated and combined anterior cruciate ligament injuries. *Orthop Clin North Am.* 2003;34(1):107–37.

145. Voloshin AS, Wosk J. Shock absorption of meniscectomized and painful knees: a comparative in vivo study. *J Biomed Eng.* 1983;5(2):157–61.

146. Lin DL, Ruh SS, Jones HL, Karim A, Noble PC, McCulloch PC. Does high knee flexion cause separation of meniscal repairs? *Am J Sports Med.* 2013;41(9):2143–50.

147. Lopes AD, Hespanhol Junior LC, Yeung SS, Costa LOP. What are the main running-related musculoskeletal injuries? A systematic review. *Sports Med.* 2012;42(10):891–905.

148. Simoneau G. Kinesiology of walking. In: Neumann DA, editor. *Kinesiology of the Musculoskeletal System: Foundations for Rehabilitation.* 2nd ed. St. Louis (MO): Mosby/Elsevier; 2010. p. 627–70.

149. McCrory JL, Martin DF, Lowery RB, et al. Etiologic factors associated with Achilles tendinitis in runners. *Med Sci Sports Exerc.* 1999;31(10):1374–81.

150. Holmes A, Delahunt E. Treatment of common deficits associated with chronic ankle instability. *Sports Med.* 2009;39(3):207–24.

151. Punt IM, Ziltener JL, Laidet M, Armand S, Allet L. Gait and physical impairments in patients with acute ankle sprains who did not receive physical therapy. *PM R.* 2015;7(1):34–41.

152. Kobayashi T, Gamada K. Lateral ankle sprain and chronic ankle instability: a critical review. *Foot Ankle Spec.* 2014;7(4):298–326.

153. Martin RL, Davenport TE, Reischl SF, et al. Heel pain-plantar fasciitis: revision 2014. *J Orthop Sports Phys Ther.* 2014;44(11):A1–33.

154. Lee WC, Wong WY, Kung E, Leung AK. Effectiveness of adjustable dorsiflexion night splint in combination with accommodative foot orthosis on plantar fasciitis. *J Rehabil Res Dev.* 2012;49(10):1557–64.

155. Walther M, Kratschmer B, Verschl J, et al. Effect of different orthotic concepts as first line treatment of plantar fasciitis. *Foot Ankle Surg.* 2013;19(2):103–7.

156. Delitto A, George SZ, Van Dillen LR, et al. Low back pain. *J Orthop Sports Phys Ther.* 2012;42(4):A1–57.

157. Hoy D, Brooks P, Blyth F, Buchbinder R. The epidemiology of low back pain. *Best Pract Res Clin Rheumatol.* 2010;24(6):769–81.

158. Francis F, Gebrye T, Odyemi I. Real-world incidence and prevalence of low back pain using routinely collected date. *Rheumatol Int.* 2019;39:619–26.

159. Della-Giustina D. Acute low back pain: recognizing the "Red Flags" in the workup. *Consultant.* 2013;53(6):436–40.

160. Chou R, Qaseem A, Snow V, et al; Clinical Efficacy Assessment Subcommittee of the American College of Physicians; American College of Physicians; American Pain Society Low Back Pain Guidelines Panel. Diagnosis and treatment of low back pain: a joint clinical practice guideline from the American College of Physicians and the American Pain Society [Published correction appears in *Ann Intern Med.* 2008;148(3):247–8]. *Ann Intern Med.* 2007;147(7):478–91.

161. Mattiuzzi C, Lippi G, Boni C. Current epidemiology of low back pain. *J Hosp Manag Health Policy.* 2020;4:15. doi:10.21037/jhmhp.20-17.

162. Bener A, Alwash R, Gaber T, Lovasz G. Obesity and low back pain. *Coll Antropol.* 2003;27(1):95–104.

163. Dionne CE, Von Korff M, Koepsell TD, Deyo RA, Barlow WE, Checkoway H. Formal education and back pain: a review. *J Epidemiol Community Health.* 2001;55(7):455–68.

164. Matsui H, Maeda A, Tsuji H, Naruse Y. Risk indicators of low back pain among workers in Japan. Association of familial and physical factors with low back pain. *Spine.* 1997;22(11):1242–7.

165. Shiri R, Karppinen J, Leino-Arjas P, et al. Cardiovascular and lifestyle risk factors in lumbar radicular pain or clinically defined sciatica: a systematic review. *Eur Spine J.* 2007;16(12):2043–54.

166. Hamberg-van Reenen HH, Ariens GA, Blatter BM, van Mechelen W, Bongers PM. A systematic review of the relation between physical capacity and future low back and neck/shoulder pain. *Pain.* 2007;130(1–2):93–107.

167. Samanta J, Kendall J, Samanta A. 10-minute consultation: chronic low back pain. *BMJ.* 2003;326(7388):535.

168. Waddell G, Newton M, Henderson I, Somerville D, Main CJ. A fear-avoidance beliefs questionnaire (FABQ) and the role of fear-avoidance beliefs in chronic low back pain and disability. *Pain.* 1993;52(2):157–68.

169. Childs JD, Cleland JA, Elliott JM, Teyhen DS, Wainner RS. Neck pain: clinical practice guidelines linked to the International Classification of Functioning, Disability, and Health from the Orthopedic Section of the American Physical Therapy Association [Published correction appears in *J Orthop Sports Phys Ther.* 2009;39(4):297]. *J Orthop Sports Phys Ther.* 2008;38(9):A1–34.

170. Beattie PF. Current understanding of lumbar intervertebral disc degeneration: a review with emphasis upon etiology,

pathophysiology, and lumbar magnetic resonance imaging findings. *J Orthop Sports Phys Ther.* 2008;38(6):329–40.

171. Henschke N, Maher CG, Refshauge KM, et al. Prevalence of and screening for serious spinal pathology in patients presenting to primary care settings with acute low back pain. *Arthritis Rheum.* 2009;60(10):3072–80.

172. Stetts DM, Carpenter JG. *Physical Therapy Management of Patients with Spinal Pain: An Evidence-Based Approach.* Thorofare (NJ): Slack Incorporated; 2014. p. 113–5, 455–64, 466.

173. European Institute for Occupational Safety and Health. *Research on Work-Related Low Back Disorders.* Brussels (Belgium): European Agency for Safety and Health at Work; 2000. Available from: https://osha.europa.eu/en/publications/report-work-related-low-backdisorders.

174. Lis AM, Black KM, Korn H, Nordin M. Association between sitting and occupational LBP. *Eur Spine J.* 2007;16(2):283–98.

175. Macfarlane GJ, Thomas E, Papageorgiou AC, Croft PR, Jayson MI, Silman AJ. Employment and physical work activities as predictors of future low back pain. *Spine.* 1997;22(10):1143–9.

176. Porterfield JA, DeRosa C. *Mechanical Low Back Pain: Perspectives in Functional Anatomy.* Philadelphia (PA): Saunders; 1991.

177. Bergmark A. Stability of the lumbar spine. A study in mechanical engineering. *Acta Orthop Scand Suppl.* 1989;230:1–54.

178. Hodges PW, Richardson CA. Inefficient muscular stabilization of the lumbar spine associated with low back pain. A motor control evaluation of transversus abdominis. *Spine.* 1996;21(22):2640–50.

179. Richardson C. *Therapeutic Exercise for Spinal Segmental Stabilization in Low Back Pain: Scientific Basis and Clinical Approach.* New York (NY): Churchill Livingstone; 1999.

180. Hodges PW, Richardson CA. Feedforward contraction of transversus abdominis is not influenced by the direction of arm movement. *Exp Brain Res.* 1997;114(2):362–70.

181. Hislop HJ, Avers D, Brown M. *Daniels and Worthingham's Muscle Testing: Techniques of Manual Examination and Performance Testing.* 9th ed. St. Louis (MO): Elsevier; 2014.

182. Panjabi M, Abumi K, Duranceau J, Oxland T. Spinal stability and intersegmental muscle forces. A biomechanical model. *Spine.* 1989;14(2):194–200.

183. Farfan HF. *Mechanical Disorders of the Low Back.* Philadelphia (PA): Lea & Febiger; 1973.

184. Cleland J, Schulte C, Durall C. The role of therapeutic exercise in treating instability-related lumbar spine pain: a systematic review. *J Back Musculoskelet Rehabil.* 2002;16(2):105–15.

185. Hides JA, Richardson CA, Jull GA. Multifidus muscle recovery is not automatic after resolution of acute, first-episode low back pain. *Spine.* 1996;21(23):2763–9.

186. Hides JA, Stokes MJ, Saide M, Jull GA, Cooper DH. Evidence of lumbar multifidus muscle wasting ipsilateral to symptoms in patients with acute/subacute low back pain. *Spine.* 1994;19(2):165–72.

187. Markwell SJ. Physical therapy management of pelvi/perineal and perianal pain syndromes. *World J Urol.* 2001;19(3):194–9.

188. Sapsford RR, Hodges PW, Richardson CA, Markwell SJ, Jull AG. Co-activation of the abdominal and pelvic floor muscles during voluntary exercises. *Neurourol Urodyn.* 2001;20(1):31–42.

189. Richardson C, Hodges PW, Hides J. *Therapeutic Exercise for Lumbopelvic Stabilization: A Motor Control Approach for the Treatment and Prevention of Low Back Pain.* 2nd ed. New York (NY): Churchill Livingstone; 2004.

190. Hoyt D, Urits I, Orhurhu V, et al. Current concepts in the management of vertebral compression fractures. *Curr Pain Headache Rep.* 2020;24(5):16. doi:10.1007/s11916-020-00849-9.

191. Sinaki M. Exercise for patients with osteoporosis: management of vertebral compression fractures and trunk strengthening for fall prevention. *Phys Med Rehab.* 2012;4:882–8. doi:10.1016/j.pmrj.2012.10.008.

192. Borghouts JA, Koes BW, Bouter LM. The clinical course and prognostic factors of non-specific neck pain: a systematic review. *Pain.* 1998;77(1):1–13.

193. Cailliet R. *Neck and Arm Pain.* 3rd ed. Philadelphia (PA): F.A. Davis Co.; 1990.

194. Janda V, Frank C, Liebenson C. Evaluation of muscular imbalance. In: Liebenson C, editor. *Rehabilitation of the Spine: A Practitioner's Manual.* 2nd ed. Philadelphia (PA): Lippincott Williams & Wilkins; 2007. p. 203–25.

195. Willford CH, Kisner C, Glenn TM, Sachs L. The interaction of wearing multifocal lenses with head posture and pain. *J Orthop Sports Phys Ther.* 1996;23(3):194–9.

196. Kuo YL, Tully EA, Galea MP. Video analysis of sagittal spinal posture in healthy young and older adults. *J Manipulative Physiol Ther.* 2009;32(3):210–5.

197. Refshauge K. The relationship between cervicothoracic posture and the presence of pain. *J Man Manip Ther.* 1995;3(1):21–4.

198. Attia J, Hatala R, Cook DJ, Wong JG. The rational clinical examination. Does this adult patient have acute meningitis? *JAMA.* 1999;282(2):175–81.

199. Bernhardt M, Hynes RA, Blume HW, White AA. Cervical spondylotic myelopathy. *J Bone Joint Surg Am.* 1993;75(1):119–28.

200. Radhakrishnan K, Litchy WJ, O'Fallon WM, Kurland LT. Epidemiology of cervical radiculopathy. A population-based study from Rochester, Minnesota, 1976 through 1990. *Brain.* 1994;117(Pt 2):325–35.

201. Bogduk N. The anatomy and pathophysiology of neck pain. *Phys Med Rehabil Clin N Am.* 2011;22(3):367–82, vii.

202. Bogduk N, Marsland A. The cervical zygapophysial joints as a source of neck pain. *Spine.* 1988;13(6):610–7.

203. Leerar PJ, Boissonnault W, Domholdt E, Roddey T. Documentation of red flags by physical therapists for patients with low back pain. *J Man Manip Ther.* 2007;15(1):42–9.

204. Costa Lda C, Maher CG, McAuley JH, et al. Prognosis for patients with chronic low back pain: inception cohort study. *BMJ.* 2009;339:b3829.

205. Gatchel RJ, Bernstein D, Stowell AW, Pransky G. Psychosocial differences between high-risk acute vs. chronic low back pain patients. *Pain Pract.* 2008;8(2):91–7.

206. Main CJ, Foster N, Buchbinder R. How important are back pain beliefs and expectations for satisfactory recovery from back pain? *Best Pract Res Clin Rheumatol.* 2010;24(2):205–17.

207. Deyo RA, Mirza SK, Martin BI. Back pain prevalence and visit rates: estimates from U.S. national surveys, 2002. *Spine.* 2006;31(23):2724–7.

208. Woolf AD, Erwin J, March L. The need to address the burden of musculoskeletal conditions. *Best Pract Res Clin Rheumatol.* 2012;26:183–224.

209. Kiesel KB, Uhl TL, Underwood FB, Rodd DW, Nitz AJ. Measurement of lumbar multifidus muscle contraction with rehabilitative ultrasound imaging. *Man Ther.* 2007;12(2):161–6.

CHAPTER

12 Physical, Sensory, and Intellectual Impairments

INTRODUCTION

"Exercise is Medicine" applies to all persons across the lifespan, including individuals with physical, sensory, and/or intellectual impairments (Box 12.1). Therefore, it is important for the clinical exercise physiologist (CEP) to understand the unique challenges to exercise these individuals face. This chapter provides an overview of common impairments as they impact acute and chronic responses to exercise. The conditions discussed here include amputation, cerebral palsy (CP), multiple sclerosis (MS), Parkinson disease (PD), spinal cord injury (SCI), autism spectrum disorder (ASD), vision and hearing loss, and intellectual disabilities (ID). For organizational purposes, each condition includes the following sections:

- Description of the impairment (including prevalence, incidence, and economic impact),
- Pathology, and
- Clinical application (including effects on the exercise response, benefits of exercise, and considerations for both exercise testing and programming).

This chapter addresses how health conditions impact body functions and associated activities that a person can participate in, but the chapter does not explore social and environmental factors that result in activity limitations and restrictions; therefore, this text prioritizes the term *impairment* instead of *disability*.

COMMON CONSIDERATIONS FOR WORKING WITH CLIENTS WITH IMPAIRMENTS

Despite the variety of conditions presented, several common themes are consistent throughout this chapter. First, although the U.S. Department of Health and Human Services recommends the same activity intensity and volume for special populations as for the general population to the extent possible (1), individuals with physical, sensory, and/ or intellectual impairments are much less active than the general population. Less than 15% of adults with disabilities meet both aerobic and muscular fitness guidelines for good health (2). Persons with impairments face multiple barriers to physical activity, ranging from personal barriers, such as low levels of self-concept and self-efficacy, to environmental barriers, such as restricted program access, facility accessibility, transportation, and social support. As a consequence, individuals with physical, sensory, and/or intellectual impairments are at a greater risk for secondary conditions such as coronary heart disease (CHD), obesity, and hypertension than the general population (2).

Another common theme is that health-related physical fitness and motor function vary greatly across individuals with the same diagnosis. For example, one individual with CP may be able to run independently whereas another may be dependent on an electric wheelchair for mobility. To select and administer effective and meaningful assessments and programs, the CEP must understand not only the pathology of individual impairments but also the range of functional abilities among people with a given diagnosis. No single exercise program is appropriate for all persons with the same diagnosis. The CEP must select

---

Box 12.1	Disability Versus Impairment According to the World Health Organization

- Disability — Term used to address impairments, activity limitations, and restrictions
- Impairment — Term used to describe body functions and structures, activities, and participation, including atypical functioning of body systems such as nervous, circulatory, and musculoskeletal.

Source: World Health Organization. *International Classification of Functioning, Disability and Health (ICF)*. World Health Organization; 2001. Available from: http://www.who.int/classifications/icf/en/.

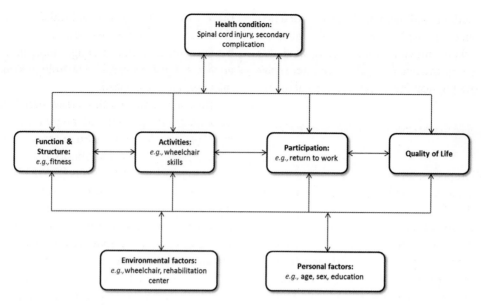

FIGURE 12.1 Exercise can lead to an improvement in fitness (*e.g.*, increase in peak power output and peak oxygen uptake), which influences almost all domains of the International Classification of Functioning (ICF).

assessments and prescriptions that fit the profiles of individual clients.

Finally, exercise can have meaningful physical and psychosocial benefits for persons with varied types of impairments. Physical activity and therapeutic exercise can prevent or delay the development of secondary conditions and functional regression associated with impairment. Exercise and physical activity can also improve the motor ability of persons with impairments and contribute to several important personal and social outcomes, identified in each section throughout this chapter.

In summary, individuals with physical, sensory, and/ or intellectual impairment benefit from activity but face greater challenges to participating in home, community, and leisure activities associated with good health. The International Classification of Functioning, Disability and Health (ICF) is a framework used to describe an individual's health status as it is influenced by impairment as well as involvement in home and community environments (3, 4). Impairment, as defined by the ICF and this chapter, refers to acute or chronic changes to *Body Functions* (*e.g.*, cardiorespiratory functioning) and *Body Structures* (*e.g.*, nerves, spinal cord). Involvement, on the other hand, reflects both *Activity* (*e.g.*, execute aerobic exercises) and *Participation* in the home, work, or community environment (*e.g.*, choice to play on a local sports team). Also, important to consider are the environmental factors (*i.e.*, physical, social, attitudinal) that affect activity and participation, and whether these factors are facilitators or barriers. A practical example of the ICF model, which can be

used as a framework for all health conditions, is shown in Figure 12.1. As depicted, the ICF views disability and functioning as outcomes resulting from the interaction between health conditions (diseases, disorders, and injuries) and contextual factors (*i.e.*, external environmental factors; internal personal factors) (3).

Although this chapter focuses on the ability of individuals with specific impairments to maximize their health and quality of life by engaging in physical activity in home and community settings, each section discusses the impaired body functions and structures that limit an individual's ability to do so. These limitations promote physical inactivity, which accelerates functional decline and thereby increases morbidity and mortality risk. The CEP is thus a critical agent of change for promoting healthy lifestyles in persons with physical, sensory, and/or intellectual impairments.

PHYSICAL IMPAIRMENTS

AMPUTATION

Amputation of a limb(s) can result from a traumatic event (injury, accident) or surgical removal following infection, diabetes mellitus (DM), peripheral vascular disease, cancer, or other diseases (5). In addition, congenital amputation may result from anomalies (dysmelias) in the embryo or fetus before birth. The physical, psychological, and vocational consequences of amputation commonly lead to social participation restrictions, and therefore limited interaction with the environment (3; see Figure 12.1). To reduce activity limitation and possible comorbidities associated with amputation and to improve quality of life, a comprehensive program to improve physical fitness is fundamental (6, 7).

Prevalence, Incidence, and Economic Impact

In 2005, 1.9 million people with a limb amputation were living in the U.S., and this number is estimated to more than double to 3.6 million by the year 2050 (8, 9). DM is the number one cause of limb loss in the U.S., with more than 65,000 amputations due to DM performed annually. In the U.S., $8.3 billion per year is spent on limb amputations, not including prosthetic costs (8). Global amputation statistics are more difficult to obtain.

Pathology and Presentation

An upper limb (UL) amputation can be shoulder disarticulation, transradial (forearm amputation through the ulna and radius), transhumeral (arm amputation through the humerus), elbow disarticulation, hand amputation, or metacarpal amputation.

A lower extremity amputation can be at the hip level and lower — hip disarticulation, transfemoral amputation, knee disarticulation, transtibial amputation, amputation through the ankle joint saving the heel pad, foot, partial foot, and toe.

By definition, limb amputation implies impairments in proprioception and the muscle structure of the affected limb. Lower limb (LL) amputations are primarily due to vascular complications of diabetes and peripheral vascular disease, whereas UL amputations are mostly due to injury from machinery or frostbite (10, 11). UL amputees for trauma-related reasons are, in general, younger than those with vascular disorders and diabetes (*e.g.*, persons with LL amputations).

One of the most common health concerns following amputation is a phenomenon known as "phantom limb pain," a sensation of pain where the limb used to be (12). Phantom limb pain can be differentiated from that deriving from the stump itself, which is typically caused by hair follicle infections, excessive pressure by the prosthetic device, blisters, or scar tissue breakdown (13). A strong correlation of long-standing phantom limb pain with depression has been shown in people with an amputation (14). Acroangiodermatitis, a cutaneous condition related to chronic venous insufficiency, may also be present together with several local dermatological conditions such as bulbous diseases, eczema, cysts, epidermal hyperplasia, bacterial or fungal infection, discoloration, and scarring. Periodical dermatological assessment and management are advised.

Risk for comorbidities varies based on the type of amputation. People with UL amputation have no greater risk for hypertension, cardiovascular disease (CVD), Type 2 DM (T2DM), and obesity than individuals of the same age without amputations (7, 10). However, the main concern for individuals with LL amputation is their high prevalence of ischemic heart disease and DM and their increased mortality rate for CVD, even in individuals who acquired their amputation from a war event (10, 15, 16). The prevalence of DM (22.6%) and ischemic heart disease (32.1%) has been reported to be significantly higher in people with LL traumatic amputation aged between 41 and 72 years (mean 57.2) than in age-matched able-bodied controls, in whom it was 9.4% and 18.2%, respectively (17).

Complications resulting from amputation must be differentiated by "preprosthetic" and "postprosthetic" types (7). Among the preprosthetic complications, flexure contractures in lower (*i.e.*, hip or knee) and upper (*i.e.*, shoulder and elbow) limbs are typical in transfemoral, transtibial, transhumeral, and transradial amputations, respectively. To prevent these contractures, flexibility exercises to increase range of motion (ROM) must be carried out as soon as the postoperative pain has become tolerable, naturally or with pain therapy, and specific sleeping postures (prone) are recommended.

Early postprosthetic complications such as residual limb pain, skin adherence to bone, sensitive skin, and poor prosthetic fit make walking difficult for people with recent limb loss. Depending on the level of the LL amputation, walking energy cost is greater in individuals with an amputation (18) and may increase from 10% to 20% in people with foot amputation to 60%–100% in those with bilateral transtibial amputation, and up to 90%–100% in people with transfemoral amputation (19). Despite technological progress in prosthetic feet to imitate almost completely the biomechanics of the ankle joint during walking, no currently available prosthesis is capable of significantly decreasing gait asymmetries and walking energy cost (20).

Clinical Application

An appropriate rehabilitative and exercise program utilizing multiple medical, surgical, rehabilitative, and exercise specialists can enable people with limb loss to reach a better quality of life (7, 10, 11).

Medical Interventions

Pharmacology is part of the clinical rehabilitation strategy. Because most LL amputations are a direct result of peripheral vascular disease and diabetes, many people with an amputation take drugs specific to these diseases. The CEP should review all medications the client is taking and the effects that these medications have on the exercise response. For example, drugs used to treat phantom limb pain include those prescribed to counteract epilepsy or depression (*i.e.*, a combination of antidepressants and narcotics, including methadone). These drugs may affect alertness, compromising motor skill, performance, and safety.

As soon as pain tolerance allows prosthetic use for UL amputation is encouraged to enable prehension (grabbing or seizing of an object) from the involved limb to restore body image and to rapidly gain functional use of the upper extremity. Normal functioning dexterity and coordination of the prosthetic arm and hand require daily training. Functional ability is proportional to the length of the residual UL.

The two main kinds of lower extremity prosthetic devices are the transfemoral prosthesis and the transtibial prosthesis. People with transfemoral amputation typically face significant difficulty regaining normal movement, especially walking. The speed and comfort of their walking is low, whereas the energy cost is high (21). This high energy cost is due to the complexity in movement associated with an artificial knee. In new and improved designed prostheses, hydraulics, carbon fiber, mechanical linkages, motors, computer microprocessors, and innovative combinations of these technologies are employed to give more control to the user.

Individuals with transtibial amputation are usually able to regain normal movements more readily than those with an upper-level amputation. This greater ease is due in large part to their intact knee joint that reduces the effort and energy expenditure required for ambulation.

In the early phases of LL postprosthetic rehabilitation, exercise on a treadmill, possibly equipped with a partial body-weight unloading apparatus to reduce walking energy expenditure, can be very useful to recover the walking pattern and gradually improve efficiency (22, 23).

Therapeutic Interventions

Rehabilitation carried out by physical and occupational therapists should include therapeutic exercise to reduce pain and swelling, increase muscular strength, and improve flexibility, agility, coordination, and balance.

To treat the chronic low back pain prevalent in people with LL amputation (24), therapeutic strength and flexibility exercises that target the lower back, abdomen, hip-pelvic girdle, and upper thigh musculature are recommended. Stretching and strengthening exercises are essential to provide both static and dynamic stability. The lower back and hip muscles can be manipulated with single and double knee-to-chest stretches, lower trunk rotation stretches, and hip flexor, quadriceps, and hamstring stretches. Trunk and hip stability and strength can be enhanced with abdominal curl-ups, pelvic tilts, straight-leg raises, and core stability training exercises. Proprioception and balance training may progress from a stable base to a dynamic surface such as a dynadisc or theraball (*i.e.*, Swiss ball). Use of devices, such as elastic tubing, medicine balls, or manual resistance movements under supervision is encouraged (18, 25, 26).

CEPs should also consider the biomechanics of an altered center of gravity. This point moves from a place approximately anterior to the sacral vertebra in the able-bodied population toward the side of the body opposite the amputated limb. Because this change impacts activities of daily living (ADL), affecting posture, balance, and walking, physical exercise to improve muscular strength, balance, and proprioception is recommended. Weight-shifting exercises such as side-to-side, forward-backward, and diagonal movements, as well as advanced activities such as timed single-leg stance, side-stepping, and forward and backward walking should be prescribed. These exercises should be recommended also to athletes with an amputation, especially those involved in weight-bearing sports. Because different types of LL prostheses may have a huge impact on athletic performance, the CEP should prescribe specific training with the prosthesis.

Beneficial Effects of Exercise on Clients With Amputation

Physical activity, exercise, sport participation, and reduced sedentary time have been demonstrated to be "determining factors for health-related quality of life among veterans with lower-limb amputation" (27). Clinical management includes a preparticipation screening (28) that addresses CVD (29) and risk of secondary cardiomyopathies, especially among individuals with an amputation from bone cancer who received antineoplastic therapy (30). Physical benefits in this population include improvements in strength, aerobic fitness, and balance (31).

Improvement in aerobic fitness was found to be also beneficial for improving walking efficiency (32). Psychological benefits include improved quality of life, coping, mood, self-esteem, cognitive function, community reintegration, independent living, and employment (33).

Improvements in cardiovascular fitness specifically have been demonstrated in people with LL amputation with different characteristics and etiology of amputation using different modalities of training, such as one-legged stationary cycling ergometer (34), arm cycling (35), or combined arm and leg cycling (32). Bernardi et al. (36) showed that athletes with LL amputation, SCI, or other locomotor impairments have no increased risk for atherosclerosis when their aerobic fitness is high (averaging $\dot{V}_{2max}$ of 36 mL·kg^{-1}·min^{-1}). However, a review aimed at determining activity and sport participation in persons with limb amputation showed that a sedentary lifestyle, due to activity and participation barriers rather than motivation, is unfortunately typical, especially in those with LL amputation (37).

Considerations for Health-Related Fitness Testing

All health and skill-related components of physical fitness should be tested in people with an amputation. Manual muscle testing is necessary to quantify the strength of the residual limb and the proximal joint (38). As with any client, testing should be carried out with appropriate communication, visual observation, palpation, and instruments (*e.g.*, goniometers, tape measures, and inclinometers). Active ROM tests the distensibility of the joint capsule and the muscle viscosity ("flexibility"), as well as the client's willingness and ability to move the limb. Passive ROM, to evaluate ligaments, bursa capsules, and cartilage, also should be assessed.

Muscle strength and endurance testing protocols for individuals with LL amputation depend on the level of amputation and involvement of limb loss. Most techniques used to evaluate upper body muscular strength and endurance can be performed in people with LL amputation in a sitting or lying posture (7). However, the "lowering shoulder" test (Figure 12.2), a population-specific assessment for UL muscles, may also be beneficial (36). Testing the lower part of the body in individuals with LL amputation, however, is also an essential part of the rehabilitative program.

A cycle ergometer, as opposed to a treadmill, is the best modality to use for aerobic fitness testing when functional evaluation includes an electrocardiogram (ECG) for cardiac disorder assessment and to minimize artifacts on the ECG. This exercise testing modality is most appropriate

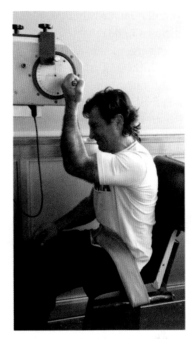

FIGURE 12.2 Individual with above-knee amputation on both legs performing the "lowering shoulders" test. (Photo credit Marco Bernardi.)

when assessment of ventilatory thresholds is required for an accurate and comprehensive aerobic fitness evaluation to assess appropriate workloads for exercise prescription. To assess the highest values of oxygen, uptake rowing ergometers (Figure 12.3), which utilize both upper and

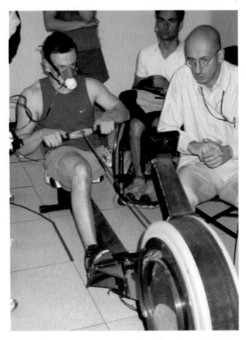

FIGURE 12.3 $\dot{V}O_{2peak}$ test conducted on a rowing ergometer. (Photo credit Marco Bernardi.)

lower body musculature, are another option for testing, and have been shown to be reliable and effective (39).

An arm cycling ergometer (ACErg) is preferred when testing the aerobic fitness of athletes with LL amputation competing in sports performed in a sitting posture (*e.g.*, wheelchair basketball, ice sledge hockey). The progression of power increases during the warm-up, and effort phases should be adjusted to result in a cardiopulmonary exercise test (CPET) approximately 13 minutes long (*i.e.*, the warm-up lasting about 2–3 minutes, and a total of 10 minutes for the following effort phases).

The use of sophisticated new prostheses results in a running energy cost similar to that of individuals without amputations (40). For clients with such prostheses, the CEP can evaluate aerobic fitness with traditional maximal exercise tests carried out on a treadmill.

Although resources exist to describe population-specific anaerobic power and capacity assessments (41), no differences in anaerobic metabolism are found between individuals with and without limb loss therefore no variations in the tests are needed. However, in elderly individuals with an amputation, and in individuals with limb loss who also have very low fitness or peripheral vascular disease, modifications of the tests such as the sit-to-stand test should be carried out to assess LL maximal explosive power (42). Evaluation utilizing the upper extremities can be carried out with ACErg 10-second Wingate tests to assess explosive power and with high-intensity ACErg (130% of the power reached in the ACErg CPET) tests to exhaustion to assess glycolytic capacity (36).

When an appropriate and comprehensive evaluation is planned, the client's energy expenditure should be measured in both the rehabilitative and the sport environments. Walking energy expenditure and energy cost can be measured with portable metabolic systems (43) to evaluate improvements in walking efficiency. During simulation of sport (30) and in training, not only energy expenditure but also the specific sources of energy should be investigated, integrating portable metabolic (and) and blood lactate measurements (Figure 12.4) to be able to optimize training.

In conclusion, functional evaluation tests similar to those for people without disabilities should be used for people with UL and LL amputations.

Considerations for Exercise Programming

Because postprosthetic complications can limit weight-bearing activities such as walking, all components of physical fitness can deteriorate (7). Exercises with no or partial weight-bearing activities (*i.e.*, upper or lower body

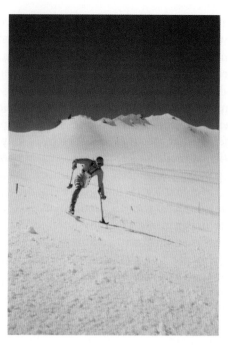

FIGURE 12.4 Aerobic fitness of a single above-knee amputee alpine skier being tested using a portable metabolic system. (Photo credit Marco Bernardi.)

ergometers, such as rowing ergometers, air-resistance ergometers, ACErg, and swimming) should be implemented in a comprehensive exercise program as soon as possible and integrated with weight-bearing activities when the complication is solved.

When the patient is stabilized, a complete medical review should be considered the first step in an exercise program regardless of the fitness status and the preamputation activity level. Adapted exercise programs should target all possible active muscles. A balanced training is important to prevent asymmetry and muscular imbalance. Cross-training, alternating different ergometers (ACErg, rowing, kayaking), and swimming and other water-based exercises are vital to improving aerobic and anaerobic fitness. Water-based training is particularly useful as it eliminates issues with the prosthesis and problems associated with wear on the stump (*e.g.*, skin integrity; 27). Population-specific resources are available to guide exercise training in individuals with LL amputations for both health and sport purposes (6, 44).

In agreement with *ACSM's Guidelines for Exercise Testing and Prescription* (44), people with an amputation should improve all components of health and the skill-related components of physical fitness. In the first phase of the exercise program, together with rehabilitation therapy, flexibility exercise should be included. Also, calisthenics routines are a fundamental part of a comprehensive exercise program. Calisthenics should be practiced with flexibility exercises in the warm-up phase, and again during the cool-down phase of both a resistance training activity and a sport training activity.

Because prostheses may limit the normal ROM, stretching exercises are essential. Examples of stretching exercises are overhead stretches for arm, shoulder, and upper body muscles, overhead bent-arm stretches for the muscles of the side of the trunk, shoulder/arm stretches for the shoulders, which are of capital importance for people with UL amputation, and standing calf stretches for the gastrocnemius and soleus muscles. To improve balance and develop flexibility in the hamstring muscles, standing toe touches are strongly recommended.

In preparation for prosthetic use, strength training for the residual limb is important. A gradual program progressing from manual resistive isometric exercises ("hold techniques") to isotonic training carried out throughout the full ROM contributes to improved prosthetic use for both individuals with UL and LL amputation (38).

When the person with an amputation has reached a reasonable physical fitness level, the preliminary exercises can be expanded with stair-climbing and rope jumping. Stretching exercises, both static and dynamic, are important for preventing injuries and should be included in both exercise training sessions and sport activities in the warm-up and cool-down phases. The use of ergometers during training is recommended and should be based on the previous aerobic and anaerobic fitness evaluations aimed at assessing the specific intensities useful to determine appropriate adaptations to exercise. *ACSM's Guidelines for Exercise Testing and Prescription* (44) should be followed for improving the health-related physical fitness components. Total volumes of training should be carefully evaluated, as it has been shown that athletes with LL amputations, together with those with SCI, are at higher risk of muscle injuries than athletes with other motor impairments (45).

High-intensity interval training (HIIT) improves both aerobic and anaerobic fitness and is very popular among Paralympic athletes competing in different endurance and power sports. However, even though HIIT is highly recommended in different sports (36, 46), no systematic prospective training studies using HIIT have been carried out on individuals with LL amputation.

Synopsis

In the next 25 years, the number of individuals with limb deficiencies will increase by almost 50% in the U.S. primarily because of increasing rates of DM. Similar increases are anticipated worldwide. Individuals with limb deficiencies need exercise training pre- and postrehabilitation. As for anyone, exercise for those with amputations will improve physical fitness, reduce morbidity, increase longevity, and improve quality of life. With minor adaptations to exercise testing and prescription, all health and skill-related components of physical fitness can improve.

CEREBRAL PALSY

CP is "a disorder of movement and posture due to a defect or lesion of the immature brain" (47). Since this classic definition, CP has been operationally defined to include activity limitations (Box 12.2); however, the essence of the description still emphasizes atypical motor control that results from damage to regions of the developing central nervous system (CNS), such as the cerebral cortex. Rather than one specific condition, CP refers to a collection of morbidities that cause atypical brain structure or function, ultimately interfering with voluntary movement (48). The effects of CP range in severity, allowing some persons to function completely independently while others are completely dependent on support care.

Box 12.2   Formal Definition of Cerebral Palsy

"Cerebral palsy describes a group of permanent disorders of the development of movement and posture, causing activity limitations that are attributed to non-progressive disturbances that occurred in the developing fetal or infant brain (cerebrum, cerebellum, or brainstem). The motor disorders of cerebral palsy are often accompanied by disturbances of sensation, perception, cognition, communication, and behavior, by epilepsy, and by secondary musculoskeletal problems."

Source: Rosenbaum P, Paneth N, Leviton A, et al. A report: the definition and classification of cerebral palsy. *Dev Med Child Neurol Suppl.* 2007;109:8–14.

Multiple approaches are used to determine CP "type." The most common classification models are based on the type of motor involvement, the location or topographical distribution of the involvement, or overall motor function (functional ability) of the individual (Table 12.1). Typically, clinicians use a combination of approaches to describe a person with CP (*e.g.*, an individual with spastic diplegia). Assessing and evaluating persons with CP is challenging because movement and posture vary within, as well as across, classification strata. Functionally, the majority of persons with CP walk independently, but approximately 30% of children with CP have limited or no walking ability during childhood (49, 50). Unfortunately, this percentage increases as children age into adulthood, especially in response to reduced physical activity over the lifespan.

Prevalence, Incidence, and Economic Impact

CP is considered the most common physical disability in childhood, and muscle spasticity, or increased muscle tone, is its most common motor manifestation. The incidence ranges between 1.5 and 3.5 per 1,000 live births across industrialized countries, but this figure is starting to increase due to medical advances for premature births

Table 12.1	Clinical Classification Strata for Cerebral Palsy	
Classification Strata	**Classification Categories**	**Category Descriptions**
Type of motor involvement[a]	Spasticity	Increased muscle tone that stiffens with movement speed
	Dystonia[b]	Involuntary contractions resulting in slow, repetitive movements, and/or atypical posture
	Ataxia	Atypical muscle coordination that typically affects balance
Topographical distribution	Diplegia	Primary involvement in the lower limbs but some (although less) involvement in the upper limbs
	Hemiplegia	Primary involvement on one side of the body
	Quadriplegia	Involvement similar among all four limbs and trunk
Motor function (gross motor function classification system)[c]	GMFCS I	Children are community walkers, but balance and coordination are affected.
	GMFCS II	Children walk but are limited, especially over long distances.
	GMFCS III	Children typically ambulate with walkers or wheelchairs.
	GMFCS IV	Children typically require powered mobility.
	GMFCS V	Children are transported by others.

[a]The term "mixed" type is often used to describe a person who exhibits multiple motor impairments (*e.g.*, both spasticity and dystonia); however, its use as a diagnosis is not recommended (266).

[b]Also referred to as dyskinesia, athetosis, or choreoathetosis.

[c]The Gross Motor Function Classification System (GMFCS) is the most common functional assessment for individuals with cerebral palsy (see https://cerebralpalsy.org.au/our-research/about-cerebral-palsy/what-is-cerebral-palsy/severity-of-cerebral-palsy/gross-motor-function-classification-system/ and https://canchild.ca/system/tenon/assets/attachments/000/000/058/original/GMFCS-ER_English.pdf).

and labor complications (51–53). The prevalence of CP has been stable over the past two decades and is more common in men than in women (54). The economic impact of CP can be burdensome to individuals and family members. Medical costs vary by severity and comorbidity but, in general, exceed the direct and indirect costs of any other congenital disability (52).

Pathology and Presentation

CP results from damage to the brain, before (most common), during, or shortly after birth. The resulting insult to the nervous system can lead to excessive muscle tone, contractures (permanent tightening and shortening of muscles), and ataxia (Table 12.1). It is important to recognize, however, that atypical brain development or brain structure may actually precede and potentially cause the peri- or postnatal events traditionally thought to cause CP (48).

CP is nonprogressive, meaning that the severity of the underlying impairment typically does not change. However, it is important to understand that an individual's movement and balance may vary over time due to therapeutic intervention and lifestyle, dramatically affecting an individual's participation in life activities (Figure 12.1). For example, the ability to walk independently and perform self-care skills can decline without sufficient physical activity or health-related behaviors. Therefore, practitioners play a vital role in improving an individual's ability to engage in ADLs and maximizing quality of life despite the limited ability to affect change in the underlying condition (55).

Hallmark signs of CP can include any combination of excessive muscle stiffness, muscle flaccidity, balance difficulty, writhing or repetitive gross motor movements, a crouch or scissor gait, drooling, delays in achievement of motor milestones (*e.g.*, crawling), and toe-walking. Diagnosis is essentially clinical and is made by a neurologist in early childhood (2–5 years) after reviewing symptoms, progress toward motor milestones, and possibly imaging such as magnetic resonance imaging (MRI) (53, 56). Because motor skill development is delayed in persons with CP, assessment of walking ability and predictive community ambulation in adulthood are not confirmed until late childhood. Risk factors for CP include premature birth, low birth weight, labor trauma, multiple births, infection (*e.g.*, meningitis), and maternal illness (*e.g.*, hypothyroidism), among others. Usually, however, multiple risk factors, rather than strictly one, contribute to CP (57).

Because CP is caused by damage to the developing brain, multiple comorbidities are often present. Epilepsy occurs in as many as 40% of persons with CP (51). ID and communication disorders (*e.g.*, ASD) are also common comorbidities. Pain and fatigue are common secondary conditions in persons with CP (58, 59), a fact that partly explains why exercise and physical activity levels are typically and chronically low in these clients. Pain can result from several factors, including muscle spasms, contractures, orthopedic issues, and loss of mobility with aging. The high energy cost for movement, sometimes referred to as physical strain (60), is a common cause of fatigue in persons with CP. Individuals with spasticity, the most common muscular manifestation of CP, expend a great deal of energy overcoming exaggerated muscle tone, increasing the intensity of effort required to complete ADL and to participate in physical activity and exercise.

Clinical Application

CP is managed with medical and therapeutic interventions to limit its effects on movement and balance (61).

Medical Interventions

Medical interventions include surgery, pharmacology, and orthoses. Tendon lengthening is a common surgical option to reduce the effect of contractures. For persons with severe spasticity, dorsal rhizotomy is a neurosurgical treatment that involves sectioning (cutting) highly active afferent nerves so that fewer signals for muscle contraction reach the spinal cord, thereby limiting excessive contractions (or hypertonicity). Additionally, misalignment of limbs, which is often due to contractures, may require sectioning of bone to reposition or realign long bones.

Botulinum toxin A (*i.e.*, Botox) is commonly administered for muscle-specific spasticity. Oral anti-spasm medications and muscle relaxants such as baclofen and diazepam (Valium), respectively, may also be used. Baclofen, in particular, may be delivered through an indwelling pump (62). Medications may also be used to decrease drooling, especially in persons with dystonia. Because of the high rate of epilepsy in this population, anti-seizure medications are also common.

Various orthoses for the foot and ankle are commonly prescribed to manage the effects of CP on movement and posture. In addition, walkers, canes, wheelchairs, and powered mobility devices may be used to promote improved functional ability and mobility.

Therapeutic Interventions

Therapeutic interventions may include physical therapy, occupational therapy, speech and language therapy, and therapeutic recreation. Therapy for the ULs typically focuses upon fine motor activities, whereas LL activities integrate gross motor exercises that incorporate physical fitness training (63). In general, therapeutic interventions produce modest improvements in function (64) and more meaningful improvements in postural outcomes (65). Most interventions continue to focus on body structures and functions, with relatively few addressing the outcomes associated with participation in community life such as sport and recreation (66, 67). Depending on the severity of impairment, these direct therapeutic services may be needed across the lifespan, thereby contributing to the high medical costs reported previously.

Effects of CP on the Exercise Response

Acute exercise responses are affected by a number of neuromuscular manifestations, such as atypical agonist–antagonist synchronization (68). As a result, the exercise effort is greater, as demonstrated by increased oxygen consumption, heart rate (HR), blood pressure (BP), and lactate production during acute submaximal exercise. This increased energy demand for submaximal work can be a major barrier to an individual's ability or motivation to exercise. Increased submaximal energy expenditure, in turn, results in reduced energy reserves to sustain exercise. Additionally, reduced force generation is common among persons with CP. Force reduction may be due to a number of mechanisms, including smaller muscle volume (69, 70), reduced neural drive (71, 72), altered motor-unit activation (69), distinctions in the extracellular matrix (73), and atrophy of type II muscle fibers (74). Consequently, anaerobic energy output during submaximal work is typically reduced. Strength training is therefore one of the most common interventions in persons with CP (75).

Health-related physical fitness values, especially for aerobic and muscular fitness, are lower in clients with CP (68, 76). Peak aerobic exercise can be limited by reduced venous return (77), reduced lactate clearance, and reduced muscle volume (70). It is important to note, however, that the peak potential for exercise is also blunted as a result of the client's inability to engage in coordinated and efficient gross motor movements (52). Deficits in muscle activation, coordination, and co-activation limit the client's ability to reach high exercise intensities, regardless of the cardiorespiratory system's ability to do so (78).

Benefits of Exercise for Clients With CP

Exercise results in several important benefits for persons with CP, including improved health-related physical fitness and reduced risk for secondary conditions such as CVD, obesity, and DM. The risk of mortality stemming from heart disease is two to three times greater in adults with CP than in the general population, and exercise has an important preventive effect. Exercise is also essential to maintaining function across the lifespan as a sedentary lifestyle can result in a loss of independent walking in adulthood.

Persons with CP typically have low levels of aerobic fitness but demonstrate short-term improvements similar to those of the general population (68, 79). Improvements in peak aerobic capacity of 10%–20% have been documented in both children and adults following 8–12 weeks of exercise intervention (80, 81). Greater gains in children, ranging from 25% to 40%, have been documented for interventions lasting more than 6 months (82, 83). However, the ability to retain aerobic benefits after an exercise intervention is quite low (63, 80). Additionally, there has been little evidence to suggest that aerobic training increases physical activity levels (80).

In adults with CP, motor function regresses earlier and faster than the rate demonstrated by adults without physical disabilities. Aerobic and resistance exercises, offered through a variety of rehabilitation settings, are essential to offset this rapid decline (64, 68). Depending on impairment level (see Table 12.1), walking ability may regress as early as adolescence, whereas both aerobic and resistance exercises can help maintain and/or reduce decline in this important function (68, 84, 85).

Exercise also has a great number of affective benefits. Persons with CP report reduced pain and fatigue (86), improved fitness (87, 88), increased activity level (89), enhanced social interaction (87, 90), and some improvement in self-concept (91) with regular exercise. Despite these important benefits, it is clear that exercise does not always improve the quality of life in this population, which may be due to ICF *Participation* barriers (83, 88, 92, 93).

Considerations for Health-Related Fitness Testing

Voluntary movement control is extremely heterogeneous in persons with CP. As a result, testing must be individualized to each client's movement and cognitive capabilities. Field tests of aerobic capacity, anaerobic capacity, and function are good options, despite the limited normative values for comparison. Field tests of aerobic capacity include 10-meter shuttle runs and pushes (for persons using wheelchairs) and may include real-time assessment of physiological responses via portable metabolic equipment

(Figure 12.5). These tests have been shown to be effective for evaluation purposes and compare favorably to laboratory-based tests of cycle and arm ergometry (83). They are often preferred, as treadmill walking may be difficult due to coordination and balance issues (94).

Field tests of muscular fitness typically consist of functional tasks (*e.g.*, timed stairs test, sit-to-stand, lateral step-ups) rather than muscle strength tasks. Laboratory tests of muscular fitness typically consist of 6–10 repetition maximum (RM) for multi-joint exercises (*e.g.*, leg press) or the use of isokinetic dynamometry to assess the strength of the hip flexors/extensors/abductors, knee flexors/extensors, and ankle plantar flexors (95).

Considerations for Exercise Programming

Effective interventions to improve physical activity are warranted in persons with CP but are lacking (63, 66, 76, 81). Regular physical activity across the lifespan is essential to maintain ICF activities such as walking and to reduce the risk of secondary conditions. To complement ACSM prescription guidelines (44), exercise interventions should start early before motor patterns have been established (*i.e.*, before the age of 7 years) (49, 55, 96). Also, because aerobic capacity is related to time spent in vigorous-intensity activity, the prescription should not be limited to moderate-intensity activities relative to an individual's capacity (76).

Individuals with CP typically have low levels of muscular fitness, with LL strength approximately 50%–90% of age-matched controls (55, 97, 98). Progressive

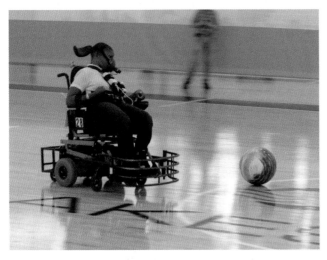

FIGURE 12.5 Assessment of energy expenditure during power soccer in a player with cerebral palsy. (Photo courtesy of Dr. Laurie Malone.)

resistance training results in short-term improvements (84, 99) through possible mechanisms such as improved muscle thickness, cross-sectional area, pennation angle, fascicle length, and motor-unit activation (100–104). As a result, isometric, isokinetic, and isotonic muscle strength can all increase following exercise training. However, because the effect of movement impairment is permanent in persons with CP, improved muscular fitness does not necessarily yield improvements in ICF activities or participation (105). Similar to aerobic exercise programs, resistance training programs reported in the literature have been relatively short (6–8 weeks) and temporary gains have typically been lost within 4 months of follow-up. Therefore, long training program durations are warranted to elicit sustained improvements in muscular strength (85, 92).

The effectiveness of resistance training programs has been demonstrated across a variety of settings (*e.g.*, home, community, and schools). Many effective modifications, such as weighted vests and backpacks, have been used to progress intensity for clients with balance and coordination difficulty (106). Weighted vests or backpacks can be worn on the trunk rather than on the extremities, allowing increased resistance while maintaining the center of gravity over a base of support among individuals with impaired balance. Strength improvement is important in this population as strength is related to the performance of ADL (107), but there may be a point of diminishing returns (85, 95, 99, 108, 109). Walking, for example, is not linearly related to strength, but requires rapid force generation more than maximal strength (110, 111). Muscle signaling and synchronization of agonist–antagonist muscles are more important for this skill, as is the case in most ADLs. As a result, anaerobic exercise may be more specific to the short duration, high-intensity daily functioning of persons with CP and may be a good complement to discontinuous resistance training (66, 79, 83, 100). Single-joint exercise (rather than multi-joint) and mechanically assisted walking (without body-weight support) may also be programming options that effectively address motor pattern limitations (112).

Synopsis

CP results from damage to the developing brain and affects voluntary movement, coordination, and balance. Aerobic and muscular fitness is typically lower in persons with CP than in the general population but can be improved through regular training. CP is nonprogressive but permanent, indicating that impairments such as muscle spasticity remain for the lifespan. For clients with CP, there is a tremendous need to increase health-related physical fitness and physical activity levels to slow the potentially rapid regression of functional skills and to reduce the risk of secondary conditions.

MULTIPLE SCLEROSIS

MS is a chronic inflammatory disease, causing sclerotic lesions in multiple areas of the CNS, including the brain, spinal cord, and optic nerve. In MS, an inflammatory immune-mediated process damages the myelin sheaths (Figure 12.6) that insulate neuronal axons, the underlying axons, and the myelin-producing oligodendrocytes (113–115). These changes interrupt or slow the transmission of neural impulses within the CNS, impairing bodily functions that the CNS controls and eventually resulting in a wide array of associated conditions, disability, and shorter than normal lifespan (113–115).

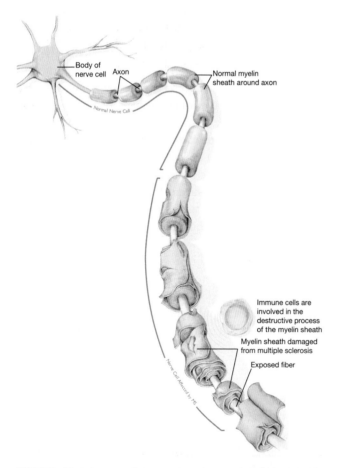

FIGURE 12.6 Nerve cell in multiple sclerosis. (From Anatomical Chart Company. *Understanding Multiple Sclerosis Anatomical Chart.* 1st ed. Philadelphia (PA): Wolters Kluwer; 2006.)

Prevalence, Incidence, and Economic Impact

There have been difficulties in evaluating the prevalence and incidence of MS. Data indicate that MS incidence and prevalence have been increasing (116–118). Consequently, newer prevalence estimates are significantly higher than previous ones, raising the number of people who live with MS in the U.S. to almost 1 million and those worldwide to nearly 3 million (118, 119). MS tends to be more common in parts of the world that are further away from the equator (113, 115).

Inpatient and outpatient health services, emergency room visits, and costly drugs make the economic impact of MS on the person and the health care system significant (120). Costs are generally higher among those with more advanced disease, those who experience disease exacerbations, and those who take disease-modifying drugs (121–123). One study found that annual health care costs per person for individuals with MS taking different disease-modifying drugs ranged between US$38,509 and US$81,627 (123). Aside from direct health costs, there are significant indirect costs such as from lost work time, especially during relapses (122). Total costs related to MS in the U.S. for 2019 were estimated at US$85 billion (https://www.nationalmssociety.org/).

Pathology and Presentation

The exact causes of MS are not known; however, research points to interactions among genetic, environmental, and immunologic factors (113–115). It appears that some people have a genetic predisposition, as some alleles associated with MS have been identified (124). In addition, first-degree relatives of people with MS have a 2%–5% risk for developing MS themselves. Caucasians, especially of Northern European descent, have higher risk for developing MS than members of other races/ethnicities (125). Genetics, however, does not explain most cases with MS, and even the identical twin of a person with MS has only a 25% chance of developing the disease (113).

A variety of environmental factors have been explored. As noted earlier, the risk seems to be higher among people living in regions that are further away from the equator (113, 115, 125, 126). Low sunlight exposure in these regions may promote deficiencies in vitamin D, which supports immune function. Existing data support the role of vitamin D deficiency in the pathogenesis of MS (127, 128). Viral infections, especially with the Epstein–Barr virus, may also contribute to pathogenesis (113, 115, 127, 129, 130). In addition, sex plays a role, with women having a two to three times higher probability of developing MS than men (117, 131). Finally, smoking seems to increase the risk for developing MS (127, 129).

MS is an immune-mediated condition in which immune cells infiltrating the CNS and CNS-resident cells damage the myelin sheaths, the myelin-producing oligodendrocytes, and nerve axons (113–115, 132). A virus (such as the Epstein–Barr virus mentioned earlier) or other environmental factors may trigger this autoimmune response in genetically predisposed people. Cells of the immune system, including autoreactive lymphocytes and monocytes, penetrate the blood–brain barrier. Within the CNS, autoreactive lymphocytes become activated and promote the formation of inflammatory cytokines, while monocytes differentiate into macrophages. Cells from within the CNS, such as microglia and astrocytes, contribute to the production of inflammatory mediators (114). Collectively, factors extrinsic and intrinsic to the CNS cause inflammation, eventually leading to demyelination and neurodegeneration (113–115, 132).

MS can impact many bodily functions controlled by the CNS; thus, persons with MS may experience a wide array and extent of symptoms. Common symptoms include dysesthesia, fatigue, numbness or tingling, weakness, dizziness and vertigo, sexual problems, walking and balance difficulties, spasticity, vision problems, bowel and bladder problems, pain, itching, emotional changes, cognitive impairment, and depression. Less common symptoms are speech problems, tremor, breathing problems, swallowing problems, loss of taste, seizures, and hearing loss (https://www.nationalmssociety.org/).

Although most of these symptoms are inherent in MS, several of them may have a component that can be considered secondary to other factors and, thus, be preventable. For example, fatigue — a major problem in MS — results from the direct impact of MS on the CNS but can also result from other factors such as deconditioning, sleep problems, medications, or depression. Similarly, depression may have a primary component, but may also be partly secondary to quality-of-life changes that a person with MS experiences as the condition progresses. Other secondary conditions in persons with MS include urinary tract infections, sleep problems, pressure sores, and inactivity (113–115).

People with MS typically experience a worsening of symptoms and disability over time. This worsening can be continuous or come in episodes known as disease exacerbations, relapses, or attacks. During relapses, there is active inflammation and demyelination resulting in exacerbations of previously experienced symptoms or presentation of new symptoms. However, neurons are capable of remyelination, which can promote partial or full recovery (remission) (113–115). The pattern of symptoms, together with imaging findings, allows neurologists to classify individual cases according to one of the following clinical courses (133):

- *Clinically isolated syndrome* (*CIS*) is the first clinical presentation of neurologic symptoms indicative of inflammation and demyelination in the CNS. Some people with CIS may not develop MS, especially if there is no MRI evidence of lesions in the brain.
- *Relapsing–remitting MS* (*RRMS*) is characterized by clearly defined relapses followed by partial or full remissions. During periods of remission, there is no evidence of worsening symptoms. RRMS is the initial diagnosis for about 85% of MS cases.
- *Primary progressive MS* (*PPMS*) is characterized by progressive worsening of neurologic function and disability from the onset of symptoms, without relapses or remissions early in the course. About 15% of individuals with MS are initially diagnosed as following this clinical course.
- *Secondary progressive MS* (*SPMS*) follows the RRMS course, and most people with RRMS transition into this course. SPMS is characterized by a progressive worsening of neurologic function; however, the individual may have periods without progression.

Although MS is more common in women, men are more likely to be diagnosed as having PPMS and to experience severe disease, lower recovery from relapses, and faster progression, and lower recovery from relapses than women (134). Most people with MS are diagnosed as having the condition between 20 and 50 years of age (114, 115). Pediatric MS is also possible, but less common than MS in adults (113, 135). Diagnosing MS requires the following (136):

1. Evidence of lesions in at least two separate areas of the CNS (dissemination in space),
2. Evidence that lesions have occurred at least 1 month apart (dissemination in time), and
3. Exclusion of other demyelinating conditions.

Evidence for MS diagnosis is gathered through a medical history, MRI of the CNS, cerebrospinal fluid analysis for detection of markers suggestive of abnormal immune responses or demyelination, testing of visual evoked potentials for measuring transmission speed of impulses along the optic nerve, and tests for excluding other conditions causing demyelination. Neurologists typically classify the disability level of an individual with MS using the Kurtzke Functional Systems Score and the Expanded Disability Status Scale (EDSS; Figure 12.7), which provide a numerical rating of functioning (137).

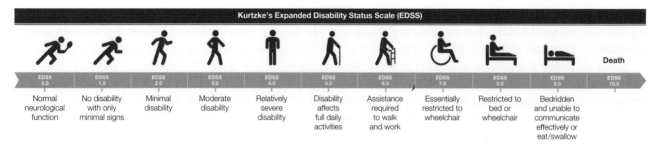

FIGURE 12.7 Functional decline as represented by scores on the Expanded Disability Status Scale. (With permission of My-MS.org. © 2008–2017. Available from: https://my-ms.org/legal_disability.htm.)

Clinical Application

Presently, there is no cure for MS. The management is multifactorial and includes medication, rehabilitation, and psychosocial support. An excellent source of information is the National Multiple Sclerosis Society (https://www.nationalmssociety.org/).

Medications can slow the disease course, reduce the frequency and severity of relapses, and manage relapses. Commonly prescribed medications for slowing the disease course and managing relapses include immunomodulators, such as β interferons and glatiramer acetate, and corticosteroids for reducing inflammation. Many patients with MS also take medications for symptoms such as fatigue, spasticity, pain, bowel and bladder problems, and depression. However, several MS medications have adverse effects. For example, the disease-modifying β interferons may cause fatigue and flu-like symptoms; medications for spasticity may also cause fatigue; and some corticosteroids may cause fluid and electrolyte disturbances and cardiac arrhythmias.

Rehabilitation may include physical and occupational therapy, exercise training, use of assistive devices, speech therapy, and vocational rehabilitation. Psychological and mental health services are also important for managing depression, stress, and cognitive changes associated with MS.

Benefits of Exercise for Clients With MS

Physical activity and exercise are important components of rehabilitation as well as of overall health promotion in persons with MS. Exercise training favorably impacts cardiorespiratory and muscular fitness, fatigue, depression, mobility, and health-related quality of life (138–140). Unfortunately, persons with MS — especially those with greater mobility problems — have low physical activity levels and high levels of sedentary behaviors (141–144). Therefore, there is a need to promote physical activity and exercise among persons with MS.

Effects of MS on the Exercise Response

The physiologic responses to exercise differ widely among people with MS. In general, persons with MS have low cardiovascular and muscular fitness levels (138, 145, 146). The peak rate of oxygen uptake ($\dot{V}O_{2peak}$) is lower in persons with than without MS, and it is inversely related to disability status (147). Peak work rate, HR_{peak}, and peak minute ventilation are also lower in people with MS (145). Furthermore, the submaximal rate of oxygen uptake during walking is higher (148, 149); possible causes include spasticity (150), altered gait patterns (151), and mitochondrial dysfunction (152).

Some people with MS show blunted HR and BP responses to exercise. These responses are thought to be due to autonomic nervous system dysfunction (153).

MS alters temperature regulation (154); thus, without counteractive measures, the client's temperature during exercise may increase to a greater extent than expected. This presents a special consideration because overheating may increase MS symptoms; however, this possible effect of exercise is not long lasting (138). Importantly, there is no evidence to suggest that exercise training triggers MS relapses (138).

Considerations for Health-Related Fitness Testing

The standard procedures for testing health-related physical fitness also apply to persons with MS (44). Graded exercise testing for aerobic fitness has diagnostic and therapeutic value. From a diagnostic standpoint, a graded exercise test in a client with MS aids in determining the presence of deconditioning, the appearance of symptoms during exercise, the extent to which the HR and BP responses to exercise have been affected by the disease, as well as the presence of CVD. From a therapeutic standpoint, graded exercise testing may help the CEP to develop an appropriate exercise rehabilitation program.

Graded exercise testing should include an assessment of the HR, BP, ECG, and oxygen uptake responses. Leg cycling is the most used mode for clients with MS because it reduces balance and coordination concerns during testing; however, treadmill walking may also be used in those with minor mobility problems, whereas arm exercise may be more appropriate with those with significant mobility limitations. Submaximal cycling tests appear accurate in predicting aerobic capacity in persons with MS with minimal disability levels (145). Muscular fitness, flexibility, balance, and functional tasks should also be evaluated using standard techniques.

A variety of assessment tools for physical functioning can be helpful. These include the EDSS score, which reflects the functional level of an individual with MS (Figure 12.7). In addition, disability and ambulation levels can be easily assessed with the 12-item Multiple Sclerosis Walking Scale (MSWS-12; Figure 12.8) or the Patient Determined Disease Steps (PDDS) scale (155, 156). Notably, the MSWS-12 score is associated with oxygen uptake during walking in persons with MS (157, 158).

Experts also recommend a holistic approach to evaluating core outcome measures for research on exercise in individuals with MS (159). Recommended assessments include the MS Impact Scale (MSIS-29); the MS Quality of Life-54 (MSQoL54); the Modified Fatigue Impact Scale (MFIS) or Fatigue Severity Scale (FSS); the 6-Minute Walk Test (6MWT); the Timed Up and Go (TUG); and body mass index (BMI) or waist–hip ratio (WHR). Although these are recommendations for outcome measures in

multidisciplinary research, they could also be considered by the CEP prior to developing exercise programs (44).

Considerations for Exercise Programming

Developing an exercise program for an individual with MS should start with an assessment of current physical activity levels, perhaps by using accelerometry and an analysis of the factors that determine physical activity in that individual. Physical activity in persons with MS is associated with disability level, ambulation difficulties, fatigue, self-efficacy, self-regulation, employment, level of education, and environmental factors including availability, accessibility, and cost of exercise programs, exclusion, level of support, and familial constraints (160, 161). Therefore, the CEP should be aware of each client's functional, psychosocial, and sociodemographic profile.

Based on research findings on the benefits of exercise training in adults with MS, experts recommend that individuals with MS should be encouraged to perform at least 150 minutes per week of exercise or other lifestyle physical activities (162). These experts further recommend that the frequency, intensity, duration, mode, and progression of the exercise program be individualized to fit the goals and the functional and mobility profiles of each person with MS based on EDSS scores.

Individuals with mild to moderate impairments (EDSS scores 0–6.5) may perform moderate-intensity aerobic exercise two to three times per week for 10–30 minutes and progressively increase to higher levels of frequency,

In the past 2 weeks, how much has your MS...	Not at all	A little	Moderately	Quite a bit	Extremely
1. Limited your ability to walk?	1	2	3	4	5
2. Limited your ability to run?	1	2	3	4	5
3. Limited your ability to climb up and down stairs?	1	2	3	4	5
4. Made standing when doing things more difficult?	1	2	3	4	5
5. Limited your balance when standing or walking?	1	2	3	4	5
6. Limited how far you are able to walk?	1	2	3	4	5
7. Increased the effort needed for you to walk?	1	2	3	4	5
8. Made it necessary for you to use support when walking indoors (e.g., holding onto furniture, using a stick)?	1	2	3	4	5
9. Made it necessary for you to use support when walking outdoors (using a stick, a frame, etc.)?	1	2	3	4	5
10. Slowed down your walking?	1	2	3	4	5
11. Affected how smoothly you walk?	1	2	3	4	5
12. Made you concentrate on your walking?	1	2	3	4	5

FIGURE 12.8 The 12-Item Multiple Sclerosis Walking Scale (MSWS-12). The MSWS-12 score is calculated by adding the numbers circled, giving a total out of 60, and then transforming this to a scale with a range from 0 to 100. Higher scores indicate a greater impact of MS on walking. (From Hobart JC, Riazi A, Lamping DL, Fitzpatrick R, Thompson AJ. Measuring the impact of MS on walking ability: the 12-Item MS Walking Scale (MSWS-12). *Neurology*. 2003;60(1):31–6.)

intensity, and duration (162). The recommendations are lower for those with higher EDSS scores. Intensity could be monitored based on HR and rating of perceived exertion (RPE) responses observed during graded exercise testing. The CEP should avoid selecting exercise intensities using formulas for predicting the rate of oxygen uptake that have been developed in healthy people; these formulas under-predict the intensity of exercise in persons with MS (163) and researchers are beginning to develop MS-specific formulas (157, 158). Interval aerobic exercise training may be particularly useful for persons with MS, especially those with lower functional profiles and especially in the initial stage of exercise progression. Preliminary evidence also suggests that HIIT is safe and effective for improving fitness in people with MS, but more research is needed (164). Aerobic activities may include walking, cycling, upper body ergometry, and aquatic exercise. Improving muscular fitness is important for counteracting the progression of disability and for improving balance, and it is generally recommended that individuals with MS perform strength training two to three times per week (162).

Flexibility training with stretching or yoga performed daily may aid in managing spasticity and contractures and inducing relaxation (138, 162). Neuromotor exercise for improving balance three to six times per week is also recommended (162). Individuals with MS should also be encouraged to perform functional activities and everyday skills while avoiding sedentary behaviors.

In summary, the CEP should consider the following factors in fitness testing and training for persons with MS:

1. Consider the clinical course of MS and the client's functional profile.
2. Avoid exercise testing during relapses.
3. Reduce the volume of exercise training during relapses.
4. Avoid excessive increases in core temperature by regulating the temperature of exercise rooms and by using additional strategies such as rehydration, fans, cooling vests, and evaporative garments.
5. Use simple instructions in the event of cognitive impairment.
6. Promote safety and fall prevention during exercise.
7. Conduct exercise sessions earlier in the day because MS symptoms tend to worsen as the day progresses.
8. Consider group exercise sessions to promote social interactions.

Synopsis

MS is an inflammatory disease damaging the CNS. It can lead to mobility problems, disability, lower quality of life, and early mortality. MS can be managed with medication, rehabilitation, and psychosocial support. Exercise is an important component of rehabilitation in individuals with MS. Carefully designed exercise programs increase fitness, reduce symptoms, and improve quality of life in persons with MS.

PARKINSON DISEASE

PD is a progressive neurodegenerative disorder associated with aging.

Prevalence, Incidence, and Economic Impact

PD is the second most common neurodegenerative disorder (after Alzheimer disease) in the U.S.. The prevalence of PD among persons 45 years or older is estimated to be 572 per 100,000 or approximately 1 million people (165). It is estimated that more than 10 million people are currently living with PD worldwide. Approximately 60,000 Americans are diagnosed with PD annually, and several thousand more are assumed to have the disease but go undiagnosed (165). The incidence of PD is greater in men as compared to women, and the typical age at onset of PD is between 65 and 70 years, with less than 5% of people with PD diagnosed prior to 40 years of age (166). As the number of people over the age of 65 years is growing faster than other age groups, the number of people with PD will likely increase.

PD treatments, which may include prescription medications, surgery, hospitalizations, and long-term care, are costly. Individuals with PD have significantly higher out-of-pocket medical expenses than those without PD, and the total economic impact of PD in the U.S. is estimated to be as high as $23 billion (167).

Pathology and Presentation

The primary area of the brain that is impacted in PD is the substantia nigra pars compacta in the midbrain. The neurons in this area of the brain utilize the neurotransmitter dopamine and have been well-documented to be affected in people with PD. Figure 12.9 illustrates the normal and diseased dopaminergic pathway.

The precise function of dopamine in the midbrain is complex and not fully understood, but the loss of neurons in this region results in multiple clinical symptoms. The four hallmark signs of PD include bradykinesia, resting

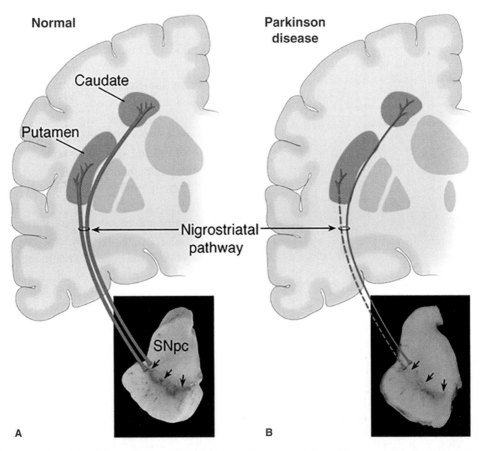

FIGURE 12.9 Neuropathology of Parkinson disease (PD). **A.** Schematic representation of the normal nigrostriatal pathway (in dark gray). It is composed of dopaminergic neurons whose cell bodies are located in the substantia nigra pars compacta (SNpc; see arrows). These neurons project (thick solid gray lines) to the basal ganglia and synapse in the striatum (*i.e.*, putamen and caudate nucleus). The photograph demonstrates the normal pigmentation of the SNpc produced by neuromelanin within the dopaminergic neurons. **B.** Schematic representation of the diseased nigrostriatal pathway (in dark gray). In PD, the nigrostriatal pathway degenerates. There is a marked loss of dopaminergic neurons that project to the putamen (dashed line) and a much more modest loss of those that project to the caudate (thin gray solid line). The photograph demonstrates depigmentation (*i.e.*, loss of dark pigment neuromelanin; arrows) of the SNpc due to the marked loss of dopaminergic neurons. (From Dauer W, Przedborski S. Parkinson's disease: mechanisms and models. *Neuron.* 2003;39(6):889–909 with permission from Elsevier.)

tremor, rigidity, and postural instability (Figure 12.10). Bradykinesia is slowness of movement and can impact multiple ADLs. Resting tremor, or "pill-rolling tremor," is most often found to occur in the arms and hands but does occur in other body structures and tends to disappear with intentional movement. Rigidity is a passive resistance to movement that can be observed in multiple areas of the body. Postural instability is the loss of postural reflexes and one of the primary reasons people with PD are at a high risk for falling.

Other motor signs commonly associated with PD include shuffling gait, freezing, lack of facial expression, and a flexed posture. Motor signs often start out unilaterally and may progress bilaterally over time. Nonmotor symptoms, which also may increase over time, include cognitive impairment, fatigue, depression, loss of smell, autonomic dysfunction, sleep disorders, and many others (168). Symptoms related to autonomic dysfunction include orthostatic hypotension, increased sweating, and constipation (168). PD dementia is known to occur in about 30% of patients; however, the cumulative prevalence is as high as 75% for those who survive greater than 10 years with PD (169). Signs and symptoms of PD are highly variable; however, each person will present in a unique manner.

Currently, no biomarkers or imaging studies are available to definitively diagnose PD (170). The diagnosis is typically based on clinical criteria, assessing both the motor and/or nonmotor signs and symptoms associated with PD that are present in the individual. A diagnostic biomarker would be advantageous because it is suggested

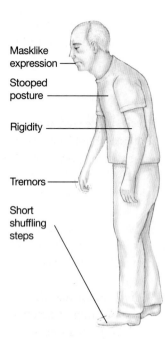

FIGURE 12.10 Characteristics of Parkinson disease. (From Anatomical Chart Company. *Understanding Parkinson's Disease Anatomical Chart.* 1st ed. Philadelphia (PA): Wolters Kluwer; 2009.)

that 60% of the neurons in the substantia nigra may be lost prior to the manifestation of clinically observed symptoms (171). Also, because several other conditions have signs and symptoms similar to those of PD, the diagnostic error rate is as high as 25% in medical practitioners with limited exposure to people with PD (170). However, recent advances have been made in the validation of criteria for clinical diagnosis and progress is being made in the development of diagnostic biomarkers (172). The initiation of prescription medications is typically delayed until symptoms are interfering with the individual's daily life, and many patients report having signs and symptoms well before seeking medical consultation. Once diagnosed with PD, the disease typically progresses in severity and number of symptoms, albeit at different rates for each individual.

The greatest independent risk factor for developing PD is age, with a higher incidence in males (166). Other than age and gender, several genetic mutations have been identified as contributing to the development of PD, although only 5%–15% of cases are considered inherited (168). There is also evidence that exposure to environmental factors like pesticides or other pollutants at younger ages may contribute to the development of PD (173). It should be noted that epidemiological studies investigating environmental risk factors for the development of PD or even factors that may protect one from developing PD are often inconsistent and additional work in the area is ongoing (174).

Clinical Application

To combat the loss of dopamine-producing neurons in the midbrain, the primary medical management for PD is typically some type of dopamine replacement therapy. Levodopa was first introduced over 50 years ago and has been the primary medical treatment for people with PD for decades (175). Chronic usage of levodopa is known to have significant side effects, including dyskinesias and other motor fluctuations. In an effort to reduce side effects, different formulations and delivery methods have been and are currently under investigation (176).

In addition to pharmacological management, focused ultrasound, stem cell therapy, and surgical interventions have been utilized for the treatment of PD. The most common, currently used surgical intervention for the treatment of PD is deep brain stimulation (177). In this procedure, the surgeon implants permanent stimulating electrodes in a specific region of the brain to deliver continuous, high-frequency electrical stimulation (ES) (Figure 12.11). Not all patients are appropriate for this intervention, but it is often used when medications can no longer control motor symptoms.

Effects of PD on the Exercise Response

The signs and symptoms experienced by individuals with PD are highly variable in both number and severity,

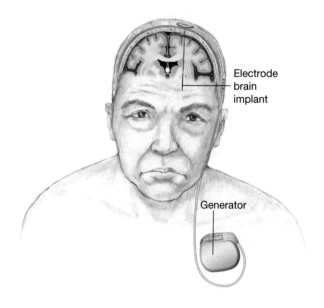

FIGURE 12.11 Deep brain stimulator in persons with Parkinson disease. (From Anatomical Chart Company. *Understanding Parkinson's Disease Anatomical Chart.* 1st ed. Philadelphia (PA): Wolters Kluwer; 2009.)

making it difficult to generalize about the impact of PD on the exercise response. However, people with PD are typically older and therefore are likely to experience the expected age-related changes to their body systems. One primary consequence to consider is sarcopenia, the age-related loss in skeletal muscle mass and function (178). It has been well-documented that people lose skeletal muscle at a rate of about 1%–2% per year after the age of 50 years (179). One of the single best counter-measures to both sarcopenia and the motor deficits associated with neurodegeneration in PD is high-intensity resistance training. Recent studies suggest that individuals with PD respond favorably to high-intensity exercise, showing gains in strength, function, and cardiorespiratory fitness (180).

Benefits of Exercise for Clients With PD

The benefits of exercise in people with PD have received considerable attention in recent years. Exercise interventions have been shown to impact multiple physiological systems, improve quality of life, and demonstrate the improved motor function on the Unified Parkinson's Disease Rating Scale (UPDRS; Figure 12.12), the gold standard scale used in clinical care and research for assessing PD (181).

Multiple studies have investigated the impact of resistance training, aerobic exercise, and other nontraditional exercise programs on people with PD. Resistance training has been clearly shown to improve muscle strength in PD, with endurance training producing increases in $\dot{V}_{2max}$ (178). Overall, these improvements lead to improved functional capacity. Although the underlying mechanisms are not fully understood and warrant further investigation, increasing evidence generally suggests that physical

Part 1: Nonmotor Aspects of Experiences of Daily Living

Part 2: Motor Aspects of Experiences of Daily Living

Part 3: Motor Examination

Part 4: Motor Complications

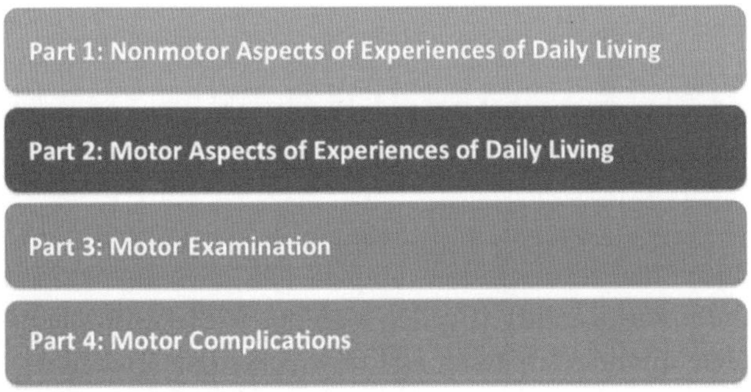

FIGURE 12.12 The four parts of the Movement Disorder Society–Sponsored Unified Parkinson's Disease Rating Scale (MDS–UPDRS), the most widely used clinical rating scale used for both clinical care and research for people with Parkinson disease. (From Goetz CG, Tilley BC, Shaftman SR, et al. Movement Disorder Society-Sponsored Revision of the Unified Parkinson's Disease Rating Scale (MDS-UPDRS): scale presentation and clinimetric testing results. *Mov Disord.* 2008;23(15): 2129–70. Available from: https://www.movementdisorders.org/MDS-Files1/PDFs/Rating-Scales/MDS-UPDRS_Vol23_Issue15_2008.pdf)

function, quality of life, and many other symptoms can be improved with exercise in persons with PD (180).

Considerations for Health-Related Fitness Testing

When conducting health-related fitness testing, special procedures/instructions should be considered for people with PD. As mentioned previously, people with PD have significant motor deficits that may include postural instability and a high risk of falls. If treadmill testing is indicated, the CEP will need to ensure that the participant is physically able to safely participate. An adaptation such as the use of a treadmill harness may be necessary, or another mode of testing such as cycle ergometry may be used.

Another consideration for the CEP to consider is the timing of medications. Testing of clients with PD should be conducted when the participant is "on" medications. Each person with PD will have a personalized regimen of specific medications that are more effective at certain times after taking the medication ("on"). The CEP should make note of the time of day and ask if the client is optimally medicated.

Considerations for Exercise Programming

Resistance training has been used in an effort to combat the losses in muscle mass and strength known to occur with aging and exaggerated with PD. In addition to strength gains, it may improve some of the motor and functional deficits associated with PD (182). One of the early studies that incorporated a progressive resistance training program for people with PD demonstrated that training two times per week for 8 weeks with initial training loads starting at 60% of 1RM was sufficient to increase strength to a level similar to the average level in individuals without PD (183). Since that time, several other studies of the impact of resistance training have found that individuals with PD can improve strength and function (182). In some cases, resistance training has been shown to improve UPDRS (motor section) scores and quality of life (184, 185). In a 2-year randomized controlled trial investigating the impact of supervised resistance training on people with PD, investigators used a two times per week training program with initial training loads of lower body exercises starting at 50%–60% of 1RM (185). Loads were progressively increased throughout the training program, and participants showed significant improvements in UPDRS (motor section) scores, strength, and quality of life without significant adverse events. Kelly et al. have reported similar improvements, and both studies reported very high adherence rates, suggesting people with PD can participate in, and adhere to, intensive exercise programs (184, 185).

Aerobic endurance training has also been utilized in people with PD. Although the age-related losses in muscle strength and function have been well-documented and publicized, there are also significant cardiorespiratory adaptations that occur with age. For example, it has been suggested that maximal oxygen consumption declines about 5%–10% per decade after age 45 years and maybe as high as 20% after age 70 years in sedentary older adults (186, 187). As the current public health guidelines suggest, adults should accumulate at least 150–300 minutes of moderate-intensity or 75–150 minutes of vigorous-intensity aerobic physical activity each week (1). A study by Shulman et al. (188) compared the effects of three different exercise programs on people with PD. For comparison were two aerobic endurance programs, a lower intensity (40%–50% HR reserve) treadmill training program and a higher intensity (70%–80% HR reserve) treadmill training program, and a stretching and resistance training program. The investigators found that each treadmill training program (three times per wk for 3 mo) increased peak oxygen uptake by about 8%, with improvements in gait speed and 6MWT distance also seen. Other studies have also reported improvements in aerobic capacity when using moderate-to-vigorous training intensities (189–191).

It is clear that people with PD can achieve significant improvements through conventional resistance and aerobic exercise training programs engaged in consistently and at intensities known to evoke physiological change. In addition, several studies have investigated multimodal exercise programs that utilize dance, boxing, and forced exercise to challenge the musculoskeletal, cardiorespiratory, and balance systems (189, 192–195). Multimodal exercises have significant potential to positively impact deficits associated with PD, alleviate symptoms, and improve quality of life. One study investigated a novel, high-intensity exercise prescription that utilized progressive resistance training (three sets of 8–12 repetitions at ~70% of 1RM) but also incorporated endurance, balance, and functional mobility exercises in lieu of rest periods between resistance training sets (184). This was done to maintain an HR > 50% of HR reserve during the entire 45-minute exercise training session. This study was supervised by a fitness professional and demonstrated improved strength, power, balance, and multiple measures of quality of life, thereby supporting the notion that a multimodal exercise program may be appropriate for people with PD.

Synopsis

PD is a neurodegenerative disease associated with aging. Individuals who are diagnosed with PD will likely experience all the typical age-related declines in physical function in addition to disease-specific conditions; therefore, they will likely benefit from participating in regular exercise. Multiple studies of different exercise programs have shown benefits to body systems and physical functional status in individuals with PD. However, there is no consensus on what mode or dosage of exercise is most effective. The CEP should prescribe clients with PD an exercise program that they are willing to adhere to that utilizes sufficient exercise intensities to evoke physiological adaptations. When done consistently, the literature suggests improvements will be obtained for most individuals.

SPINAL CORD INJURY

The spinal cord lies within the vertebral canal and consists of nerve fibers that transmit impulses to and from the brain. The spinal cord and the brain constitute the CNS. The spinal cord is very sensitive to injury and, in contrast to other body structures, does not have the ability to repair itself if it is damaged. An SCI occurs when there is damage to the spinal cord due to trauma (*e.g.*, a traffic accident, diving in shallow water), loss of normal blood supply, or situations such as a tumor, bleeding, or infection causing compression (196).

People with an SCI are often classified into two distinct categories based on the level of injury. Injuries below thoracic level 1 (T1) result in paraplegia. With paraplegia, all or part of the trunk, legs, and pelvic organs are affected. An SCI at or above T1 is classified as tetraplegia. This means that not only the trunk, legs, and pelvic organs are affected but the arms and hands as well (196; Figure 12.13).

The completeness of the lesion is also important. An injury that results in the complete loss of function below the point of injury is called a complete SCI. An incomplete injury refers to an SCI in which some sensation or movement is still evident below the point of injury. There are varying degrees of incomplete injury (196). For example, individuals with a high-level SCI (*e.g.*, at the cervical level) might still be able to walk after suffering a motor-incomplete SCI. Damage to the central part of the spinal cord (*i.e.*, central cord syndrome) results in an incomplete SCI that is characterized by impairment in the arms and hands while the legs might be impaired to a lesser extent.

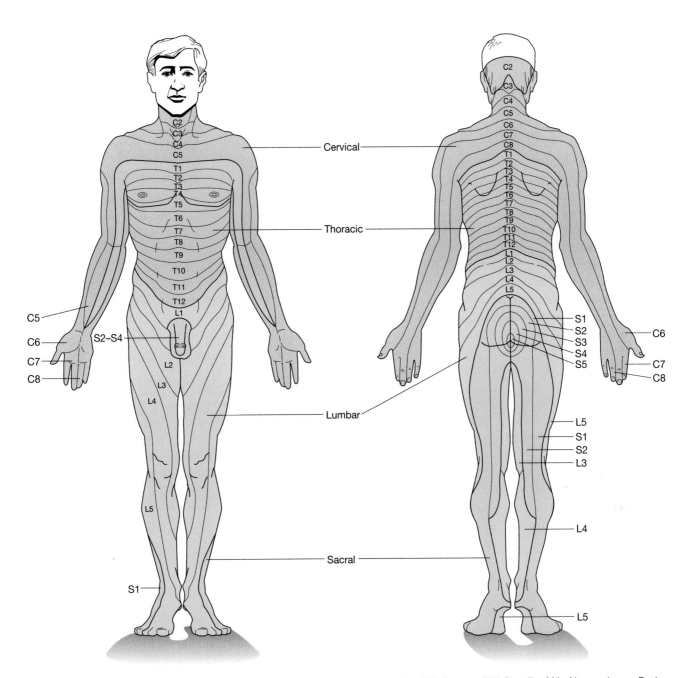

FIGURE 12.13 Lesion levels associated with tetraplegia and paraplegia. (From Bear MF, Connors BW, Paradiso MA. *Neuroscience: Exploring the Brain*. 4th ed. Philadelphia (PA): Wolters Kluwer; 2015.)

Prevalence, Incidence, and Economic Impact

Worldwide, between 250,000 and 500,000 people sustain an SCI annually. The prevalence or estimated proportion of the population living with an acute traumatic SCI varies around the world, reportedly highest in the U.S. (906 per million; 197). Incidence (*i.e.*, number of new cases per year) also varies around the world; New Zealand has the highest incidence (49 per million) whereas the incidence

in the U.S. is 40 per million, Spain having the lowest reported incidence at 8.0 per million (197).

According to the WHO, existing data do not allow for global cost estimates of SCI; however, they do offer a general picture (198). People with a higher lesion level generally have higher costs. For example, the estimated lifetime costs for a person who is 25 years old at injury range from $2.3 million for someone with complete paraplegia to $4.7 million for a person with a high complete tetraplegia (199). Much of the cost is borne by people with SCI and their families. Because exercise can improve the health of people with SCI (*e.g.*, by diminishing the risk factors for CVD and other comorbidities; 200, 201), it can also have an economic impact in this group.

Pathology and Presentation

Damage to the spinal cord impairs motor, sensory, and autonomic functions below the level of the lesion. The SCI is classified in terms of the level and completeness of the lesion by the International Standards for Neurological Classification of Spinal Cord Injury on the American Spinal Injury Association (ASIA) Impairment Scale, which leads to a standardized score (202). This scoring tool is available at https://asia-spinalinjury.org/international-standards-neurological-classification-sci-isncsci-worksheet/ (203). The higher the lesion level, the more the functional ability and autonomic control are impaired (Figure 12.14).

An SCI may result in one or more of the following symptoms: loss of movement and sensation below the lesion level, loss of bladder and bowel control, exaggerated reflex activities or spasms, and either pain or an intense stinging sensation caused by damage to the nerve fibers in the spinal cord. People with a high-level SCI may also have difficulty breathing, coughing, or clearing secretions from the lungs (204).

An SCI is first diagnosed by a medical history and physical examination. The individual's physician will obtain a medical history asking questions about the details of the injury. The physical examination will include testing to see if sensation to touch is intact in the arms and legs, as well as testing to determine muscle strength and the presence or absence of reflexes in the arms and legs. The next step is an x-ray or computed tomography (CT) scan to identify a fracture or dislocation of the vertebrae or MRI to assess damage to the spinal cord itself (204).

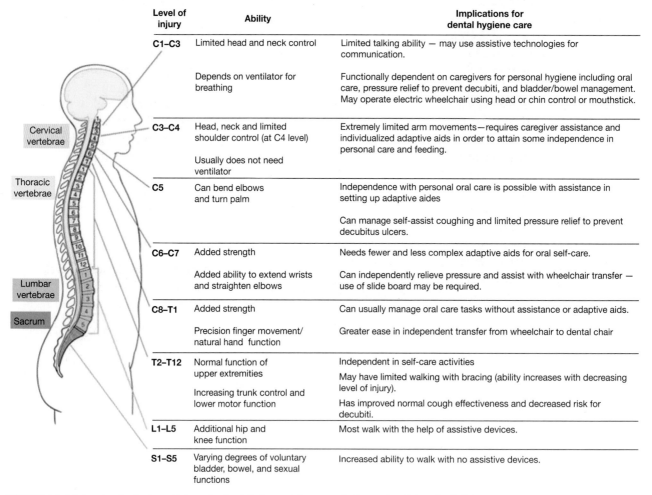

Level of injury	Ability	Implications for dental hygiene care
C1–C3	Limited head and neck control	Limited talking ability — may use assistive technologies for communication.
	Depends on ventilator for breathing	Functionally dependent on caregivers for personal hygiene including oral care, pressure relief to prevent decubiti, and bladder/bowel management. May operate electric wheelchair using head or chin control or mouthstick.
C3–C4	Head, neck and limited shoulder control (at C4 level)	Extremely limited arm movements—requires caregiver assistance and individualized adaptive aids in order to attain some independence in personal care and feeding.
	Usually does not need ventilator	
C5	Can bend elbows and turn palm	Independence with personal oral care is possible with assistance in setting up adaptive aides
		Can manage self-assist coughing and limited pressure relief to prevent decubitus ulcers.
C6–C7	Added strength	Needs fewer and less complex adaptive aids for oral self-care.
	Added ability to extend wrists and straighten elbows	Can independently relieve pressure and assist with wheelchair transfer — use of slide board may be required.
C8–T1	Added strength	Can usually manage oral care tasks without assistance or adaptive aids.
	Precision finger movement/ natural hand function	Greater ease in independent transfer from wheelchair to dental chair
T2–T12	Normal function of upper extremities	Independent in self-care activities
		May have limited walking with bracing (ability increases with decreasing level of injury).
	Increasing trunk control and lower motor function	Has improved normal cough effectiveness and decreased risk for decubiti.
L1–L5	Additional hip and knee function	Most walk with the help of assistive devices.
S1–S5	Varying degrees of voluntary bladder, bowel, and sexual functions	Increased ability to walk with no assistive devices.

FIGURE 12.14 Levels of spinal cord injury. On the left, the vertebrae are designated as C (cervical), T (thoracic), L (lumbar), and S (sacral). The effects of spinal cord injury on functional ability depend on the level of injury. (From Wilkins EM. *Clinical Practice of the Dental Hygienist.* 12th ed. Philadelphia (PA): Wolters Kluwer; 2016.)

Unintentional injury is often the cause of an SCI, but certain factors may increase the risk of such injury. Men are more at risk for an SCI than women, as 80% of the people with SCI are men (197, 205). Furthermore, people are most likely to suffer a traumatic SCI between the ages of 16 and 30 years. Engaging in risky behavior, like diving into shallow water, mountain biking, or riding a motorbike, are leading causes for SCI in people under 65 years. In people older than 65 years of age, falls are the cause of the majority of SCIs (197). Lastly, persons having a bone or joint disorder, such as arthritis or osteoporosis, are more susceptible to SCI after a relatively minor incident (196).

After an SCI, a person will typically experience numerous secondary complications. A longitudinal study, from 1 to 5 years, post discharge among wheelchair-dependent people with SCI showed that neuropathic pain (84%–92%), musculoskeletal pain (62%–87%), urinary tract infection (57%–59%), and pressure ulcers (29%–41%) were the most frequently reported secondary health conditions. The occurrence of several secondary health conditions was higher among women and individuals with a complete lesion, tetraplegia, and a high BMI (206).

Pressure ulcers are among the most serious complications in wheelchair users with SCI. They require immediate treatment because they often become infected and can lead to sepsis and become fatal. Pressure ulcers also often lead to bed rest and, therefore, interfere with ADL and exercise programs. Unfortunately, because of the loss of blood flow to the region and the patient's inability to shift positions, pressure ulcers are often very difficult to treat. This results in great discomfort and significant medical costs (207). Although there is a lack of controlled studies on the effects of ES on the incidence of pressure ulcers, moderate evidence suggests that ES-induced muscle activation has a favorable effect on several risk factors for developing pressure ulcers in people with an SCI (e.g., ischial tuberosity pressure, muscle volume, blood circulation, and tissue oxygenation; 207).

Clinical Application

Effects of SCI on the Exercise Response

In people with SCI, the exercise response can vary greatly depending on the level and completeness of the lesion. These different exercise responses between, for example, people with a high complete SCI and those with a low-level incomplete SCI are explained later.

The cardiovascular and autonomic consequences of an SCI affect several exercise responses, including HR, BP, and temperature regulation (208). The heart is under control of the parasympathetic and sympathetic nervous systems. The parasympathetic control of the heart is via the vagus nerve, which exits at the level of the brainstem and remains intact after SCI. However, the sympathetic innervation of the heart comes from thoracic vertebrae 1–5 and may be affected depending on the lesion level and completeness. This means that in people with complete tetraplegia, the HR can only increase by withdrawal of the parasympathetic tone (i.e., to a maximal HR of about 100–120 beats per min; 208). Furthermore, the relationship of HR to the rate of oxygen consumption is often not linear in people with tetraplegia (209). Consequently, HR cannot be used to quantify exercise intensity in this group. Using an RPE or power output for monitoring training intensity is, therefore, advised.

The BP response to exercise is also impaired in people with SCI due to loss of cardiovascular control and loss of reflexive vasoconstriction below the lesion level. For people with tetraplegia, the loss of abdominal muscle tone and the loss of supraspinal control to the splanchnic bed, which contains the largest blood volume, lead to blood pooling, which has a negative effect on the redistribution of blood during exercise (208).

Lastly, SCI results in impaired thermoregulation. There is a reduced afferent input to the thermoregulatory center and a disruption of both vasomotor control and sweating capacity below the SCI level (210). People with complete tetraplegia generally show little or no sweating response. Depending on the level and completeness of the lesion, people with an SCI might be more susceptible to heat strain due to environment (temperature and humidity) and exercise (intensity and duration) conditions (208).

Benefits of Exercise for Clients With SCI

Because of muscle paralysis below the lesion level, the active muscle mass of an individual with SCI is diminished. In consequence, the resting metabolic rate can be up to 25% lower than in the general population (211). A physically active lifestyle combined with a properly balanced diet is, therefore, very important to prevent overweight and obesity in this population. Various forms of exercise can also lead to an improvement in physical fitness (e.g., increase in peak power output, peak oxygen uptake, muscle strength; 212), which has a beneficial effect on almost all domains of the ICF model (Figure 12.1). Fitness, in turn, is positively related not only to multiple aspects of physical health, such as a favorable lipid profile (213) or respiratory function (214), but also to wheelchair-related ADL (215), return to work (216), and overall quality of life (217, 218).

Considerations for Health-Related Fitness Testing

The selection of specific tests and protocols to use is dependent on the aim of the assessment. Because 80% of people with SCI are dependent on a wheelchair (219), a graded arm ergometer exercise test (Figure 12.15) is the most commonly used assessment for cardiovascular endurance in this group. When evaluating exercise capacity for ADL or wheelchair sports, the graded exercise test can be performed using a wheelchair ergometer or on a treadmill using the client's own wheelchair.

Another modality to consider is arm crank exercise. In general, arm crank exercise, such as handcycling, is more physiologically efficient than handrim wheelchair propulsion (220) and leads to less load on the upper extremity (221). Handcycling is, therefore, a good exercise mode for people with SCI, especially for those with tetraplegia (222). When testing persons with SCI to set up a good handcycling training program (223), a graded handcycle exercise test, because of its task specificity, is more suitable than a wheelchair-graded exercise test. Regardless of the test used, it is important to remember that peak HR will be lower for arm exercise in general (224) and especially lower in people with tetraplegia or high paraplegia because of the disruption of the sympathetic nervous system (Figure 12.16).

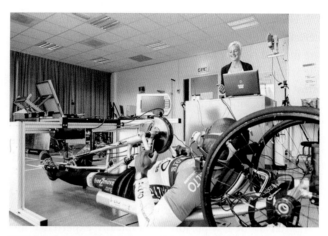

FIGURE 12.16 A graded exercise test performed in the participants' own handcycle. (Photo credit Marieke van der Heijden.)

Autonomic dysreflexia is a condition in which the autonomic nervous system overreacts to external or bodily stimuli. It is often observed in people with SCI above thoracic level six (T6). Because it reduces perceived exertion, autonomic dysreflexia can enhance endurance time-trial performance in athletes with SCI and may result in a 9.7% improvement of wheelchair race time in people with tetraplegia (225). Intentional induction of autonomic dysreflexia, called boosting, is classified as a doping method by the International Paralympic Committee (226). Despite its performance benefits, autonomic dysreflexia can trigger a high HR and BP and subsequently cerebral hemorrhage, blindness, aphasia, seizure, cardiac dysrhythmia, and even death (225). Therefore, it is important to prevent autonomic dysreflexia by, for example, regular and timely intermittent catheterization, a regular bowel program, and routine weight shifts and skin checks to prevent pressure ulcers. It is also important to monitor the SCI client for autonomic dysreflexia throughout the exercise test.

Lastly, individuals with SCI often have reduced sweating capacity. This might lead to an increased risk of heat strain during fitness testing and training (210). Cooling strategies, such as ice vest prior to exercise and water sprays during rest periods, may be highly beneficial, especially for people with tetraplegia (227).

Considerations for Exercise Programming

Few systematic reviews describe the effects of exercise training among people with an SCI (209, 212, 228). Among these, the most recent review by Van der Scheer et al. (212) found insufficient evidence to draw meaningful conclusions regarding the effects of exercise on people with an acute SCI. In contrast, 189 studies reported

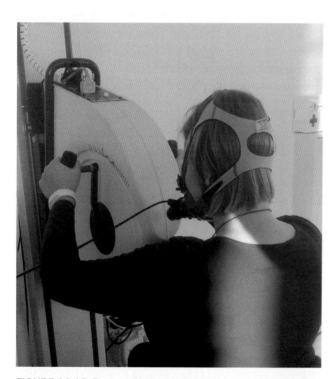

FIGURE 12.15 Person with spinal cord injury undergoing a graded exercise test on an arm ergometer. (Photo credit Sonja de Groot.)

on changes in fitness (cardiorespiratory fitness, power output, or muscle strength) and cardiometabolic health (body composition or cardiovascular risk factors) in people with a chronic SCI. Van der Scheer et al. (212) concluded that there was moderate to high confidence in the evidence showing exercise can improve cardiorespiratory fitness, power output, muscle strength, body composition, and cardiovascular risk factors in individuals with chronic SCI. This inference regarding the effect on fitness was supported by the conclusions of previous systematic reviews (209, 228).

Hicks et al. (228) also showed that exercise training can increase muscle strength. Their systematic review indicated that a variety of resistance training paradigms are effective, with consistent evidence for the effectiveness of training performed two to three times per week, at 50%–80% 1RM.

Based on the systematic review of Hicks et al. (228), the first exercise guidelines for people with an SCI were developed in 2011 (229). An update of these guidelines was performed in 2018 (230) based on the review of Van der Scheer et al. (212). The new guidelines consist of two parts: one for fitness and one for cardiometabolic health benefits. The guidelines can be downloaded (in different languages): https://www.ncsem-em.org.uk/sciguidelineseurope/. The effect of following the guidelines for fitness benefits was investigated in a 16-week randomized controlled trial, which showed a significant increase in peak oxygen uptake and muscle strength in the group that trained according to these guidelines (231).

Forms of exercise that can be performed by persons with SCI depend on the level and completeness of the injury. For people with tetraplegia, wheelchair rugby (Figure 12.17) was specifically developed in 1977 (232).

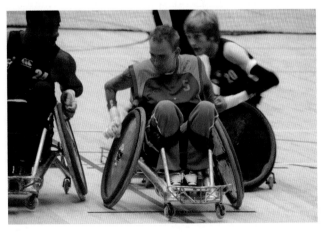

FIGURE 12.17 Wheelchair rugby athletes competing in a tournament. (Photo credit Sonja de Groot.)

Furthermore, handcycling is a great sport for those with tetraplegia as well, even during inpatient rehabilitation (222), because it is a physiologically more efficient form of exercise compared to handrim wheelchair sports (220).

People with lower level injury have good arm/hand function and therefore can participate in several wheelchair sports, such as athletics, basketball, and tennis, but also in non-wheelchair sports like alpine skiing, kayaking, and swimming (233). Furthermore, leisure-time wheelchair sports like wheelchair tennis and basketball have been found to generate a high enough energy expenditure to prevent CVD in people with SCI (234).

However, it is important to keep in mind that individuals who rely on a wheelchair for daily mobility do not have the large muscle mass of the legs available for exercise. Following the exercise training guidelines for the general population can, therefore, easily lead to overuse injuries of the musculoskeletal system. The shoulders in particular are at risk during wheelchair propulsion, which is shown by the high prevalence of shoulder pain among persons with SCI (235). Handcycling and other cyclical forms of exercise, or movements in the reverse direction of wheelchair pushing (e.g., rowing), are typically better alternatives than handrim wheelchair propulsion activities to minimize the risk of shoulder overuse injury. For clients with SCI who have a low level of fitness, the CEP should choose the best exercise mode and adapt the training intensity and frequency to prevent overuse injuries (201) and keep the client motivated (236).

For an improvement in cardiovascular fitness, it is an advantage to activate a larger muscle mass (237). For people with a complete lesion, functional electrical stimulation (FES) (i.e., applying small electrical pulses to paralyzed muscles) is a good method by which to activate the large, paralyzed muscle mass of the legs for activities such as cycling, walking, or rowing (238). Electrically stimulated leg exercise can also be combined with voluntary arm exercise (so-called hybrid exercise [e.g., rowing and handcycling]) to exercise an even larger muscle mass (200, 239). It is important to keep in mind that this exercise modality may not be an option due to lack of availability and/or appropriateness for each person. Furthermore, when starting this kind of exercise, professional guidance is warranted to prevent possible adverse events like skin problems or a femur fracture due to severe osteoporosis below the lesion.

Ambulatory people with an SCI, who use gait aids, are less active than manual wheelchair users with SCI (240). Intuitively, people who can walk might be expected to be more active, given their higher level of physical functioning. However, these findings suggest the importance of physical activity and exercise among people with SCI who are marginal household or community ambulators. Limited studies have been performed regarding exercise in ambulatory people with SCI. However, results showed that aerobic exercise training on a recumbent cross-trainer is safe, feasible, and effective for improving aerobic capacity and walking-related outcomes in ambulatory adults with chronic motor-incomplete SCI (241).

Synopsis

Although an SCI can be a devastating injury, exercise is a key factor in helping clients with an SCI become and stay fit. Fitness in turn improves associated and secondary conditions, as well as ADL, participation in life roles, and overall quality of life. Rehabilitation professionals play an important role in assisting people with an SCI to engage in an active lifestyle as soon as possible and over their lifespan. The CEP has the unique opportunity to promote exercise to extend the client's recovery from rehabilitation to community-based exercise (*e.g.*, rehabilitation-based fitness facilities or specialized fitness centers and programs for people with SCI; 242). A well-designed exercise program, based on outcomes of a peak exercise test and keeping autonomic dysfunction and overuse injuries in mind, is essential to preventing deconditioning in this group.

SENSORY IMPAIRMENTS

AUTISM SPECTRUM DISORDER

ASD is a developmental disorder that is recognized through impaired communication or atypical social/reciprocal interaction with associated repetitive behaviors that are typically fixated or inflexible (243). ASD reflects a continuum of disorders that previous editions of the *APA Diagnostic Manual* separated into different diagnoses, including autistic disorder, Asperger syndrome (colloquially called high-functioning autism), or pervasive developmental disorder. ASD is now the summary diagnosis that identifies individuals with impaired behavior and/or communication and may impact multiple domains of human development including social, emotional, cognition/learning, and sensory processing (244). Severity is reflected by the level of support required and, although the exact causes of ASD are not fully elucidated, genetic factors and environmental agents possibly contribute to the etiology (245).

Prevalence, Incidence, and Economic Impact

ASD affects approximately 1 in 44 children (or 23 per 1,000) born in the U.S. with prevalence estimates of 1.5%–2% of the population across industrialized countries (245–247). The incidence of ASD has increased over the past decade as the Autism and Developmental Disabilities Monitoring Network estimated that 1 in 150 children were affected in 2000 and as many as 1 in 54 were identified as recently as 2016. Males are four times more likely to be diagnosed with ASD than females but incidence rates no longer appear to be heavily influenced by race or socioeconomic status (246). In short, disparities by cultural factors are dissipating but still exist for sex. Because incidence is increasing and the care needs of persons with ASD may require multiple community resources across the lifespan, the direct and indirect costs are approaching $500 billion annually in the U.S., which approximates to $1.5–2.5 million per individual with ASD, depending on the level of intellectual impairment (248, 249).

Pathology and Presentation

ASD is typically identified by an inability to achieve language and communication milestones in childhood or regression from previously achieved levels. Common characteristics include restricted interests, repetitive behaviors, need for sameness, and sensory deficits. Screening can occur in early childhood with clinical diagnoses typically made after 36 months of age. Two hallmark criteria for diagnosis include impaired social communication and repetitive patterns of behavior that interfere with daily living (245, 248). Although ASD is nonprogressive, severity of symptoms can improve depending on the age of the first diagnosis and early intervention opportunities.

ASD is a brain-based disorder and, as a result, comorbidities are often present. Manifestations that impact mental health can include anxiety, depression, atypical behavior (including attention-deficit hyperactivity disorder [ADHD], impulse control disorder, and oppositional defiant disorder), and poor intra- and interpersonal engagement. Medical complications such as epilepsy (seizures), sleep disorders, and gastrointestinal complications are also common (250–252). An intellectual impairment is present in approximately 35% of cases (246); however, communication difficulty and repetitive movements are not directly related to intelligence quotient (IQ). Additionally, up to 40% of individuals are nonverbal, with approximately 25% demonstrating self-injurious behavior (251).

Clinical Application

Effects of ASD on the Exercise Response

ASD does not directly affect the acute responses or chronic adaptations to exercise, but it does impact the ICF *Participation* domain, especially physical activity behavior. Individuals with ASD are more likely to be over- or underweight than other children (with or without disabilities), and narrow food interests and repetitive eating habits can make proper nutrition intake difficult (253, 254). Consequently, obesity is a common health morbidity that limits physical activity behavior and drives chronic disease risk in this population. Obesity is directly related to ASD severity (254), and impaired motor skill development is a major correlate (253). Additionally, communication difficulty and dependence on rigid and inflexible routines disproportionately increase preference for screen time in adolescents with ASD, creating additional *Participation* barriers and further exacerbating the consequences of insufficient physical activity (243, 254–256).

Atypical social skills among persons with ASD also detract from participation in team and group exercise activities. As the competitiveness and abstract thinking requirements (strategy) increase developmentally in youth sports, the opportunities for persons with ASD to remain included in these settings become much less likely (254). Whereas many young people may achieve their moderate-to-vigorous physical activity (MVPA) through organized team sports, it is unlikely that these opportunities remain viable for many adolescents with ASD. It is clear that age is inversely related to physical activity in this population. As a result, interest in physical activity and group exercise is typically low which, in turn, increases chronic disease risk and exacerbates the effects of obesity experienced in childhood (243).

Benefits of Exercise for Clients With ASD

Fortunately, for individuals with ASD who are active, there are several meaningful outcomes relative to health and symptom severity. Health-related physical fitness can be consistent to persons without disabilities; therefore, training adaptations in persons with ASD are consistent with the general population. Additionally, exercise yields important improvements in motor skills among children and adolescents with ASD. Enhanced gross motor function, fine motor control, balance, and coordination have been demonstrated across a variety of school-based and recreation-based programs (256–262). Motor skill interventions are effective across the lifespan but typically have the greatest impact during childhood assuming they are

intentional and structured to meet specific goals (256, 263). Delays in meeting motor milestones are common in children with ASD, and structured exercise interventions that address motor and activity-specific functions are clearly warranted due to their effectiveness (259).

Exercise interventions for children with ASD positively impact a number of ICF *Personal Factors* related to communication and self-regulatory behavior (256, 258, 262, 264). Researchers have found positive benefits to a broad array of social factors such as eye contact, social interaction, and appropriate communication, all of which increase the ability to participate in community activities (Figure 12.1). Improvements following intervention seem to be most effective during childhood and positive adaptations tend to remain postintervention (263, 265). Although not fully elucidated, improved social function due to exercise interventions may be the result of additional practice in interpersonal settings as well as a byproduct of improved motor ability which, in turn, yields more participation opportunities in activity, sport, and play settings. Improvements in social function may also derive from neurological adaptations to exercise, specifically enhanced production and metabolism of the neurotransmitters serotonin and oxytocin (260, 265). The effect of exercise training on negative or detrimental behaviors, however, is less clear. Reductions in antisocial behavior, including repetitive stereotypical movements (*e.g.*, body rocking, repetitive finger or hand gestures) and self-injurious behaviors, have been noted in multiple experimental studies (254, 258, 265, 266) and confirmed through meta-analysis of nonrandomized interventions (267). However, a recent meta-analysis of strictly randomized controlled trials found that physical activity had no effect on stereotyped behavior among children or adolescents (263).

Considerations for Health-Related Fitness Testing

Deficits in walking/ambulation, motor programming, limb coordination, and posture are common in persons with ASD (268). These deficits may be due to increased motor rigidity, which negatively affects balance and gait (269). Therefore, testing modes that maximize balance or provide a wide base of support are useful assessment options (*e.g.*, recumbent bike). Treadmills are appropriate aerobic testing modes; however, CEPs should be mindful that reliance on handrails will cause an overestimation of maximum capacity which nullifies the use of submaximal prediction equations. Fine and gross motor skills are inversely related to IQ (270) so open-skill assessments such as aerobic walk, balance, and machine-based muscular strength tests are most appropriate for individuals with high levels of cognitive functioning assuming sufficient motivation is present.

The ability of persons with ASD to mirror skills and perform on-demand synchronous movements is directly related to symptom severity but not IQ (268, 270). Therefore, multiple demonstrations and more hands-on guidance than traditionally used in clinical exercise testing are appropriate. Individuals with ASD want to know what to expect from testing (271) so instructions about, and acclimation to, testing protocols may take multiple trials before an individual feels comfortable with the environment and expectation.

Considerations for Exercise Programming

There are multiple considerations that must be addressed to create an effective exercise program for individuals with ASD.

Environment

A major priority required for a successful program is the creation of a physical and social environment that persons with ASD will embrace. From an organizational standpoint (physical environment), multiple researchers have successfully used a "structured" teaching environment as an effective blueprint for exercise delivery. Structured teaching, or the TEACCH® method, includes a developmentally appropriate routine that leads individuals from one task to the next (272). Structured teaching includes the use of exercise schedules, work tasks, and use of visual cards to create step-by-step instructions and tasks for participants (264). Individuals with ASD want the activity environment to be predictable and want to know what is expected before participating (271). The use of structured teaching strategies, such as the use of a schedule, and clarifying expectations through physical boundaries and visual supports can clearly impact the emotional security experienced by participants, thereby making continuation in a program more likely. A Picture Exchange Communication System (PECS) is a common educational tool that uses visual cues to outline structured teaching directions and tasks, and an activity schedule board is a common PECS support that will benefit CEPs when organizing a therapy, exercise, or program session (Figures 12.18).

Socially, individuals with ASD may have very specific ideas about peer partners and teammates, so it is important to proactively organize peer interaction that may be different from random partner groups associated with typical exercise sessions (271). Cognitive development in youth with ASD does not necessarily match the tempo

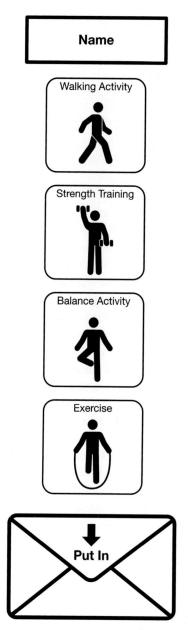

FIGURE 12.18 Activity schedule board. Clinical exercise physiologist (CEP) should arrange pictures in order of task.

or increased capacity observed in able-bodied peers. As a result, strategic partnering with exercise partners or parents may be necessary to ensure compliance. Parents are often needed to support integration into a new exercise program. Overcoming barriers to MVPA is a serious task as youth with ASD have reported that physical activity is their least favorite recreational option (273). As adolescents with ASD transition out of recreational play, the motor requirements, abstract rules (strategy), and social relationships of youth sport and activity all become challenges; as a result, parents have to take on more responsibility for participating in, or creating, physical activity opportunities because of the safe environment perceived by the individual with ASD (255).

Motor Confidence

One of the primary intrinsic factors that must be developed to encourage regular exercise training is motor confidence. Youth with ASD must believe in their ability to be successful in exercise to pursue or continue an exercise opportunity. Additionally, the activity must be both enjoyable and meaningful. Connecting physical activity settings with the expected benefits of participation, such as better health or strong muscles, is important to maintaining participation (271).

Characteristics of Intervention

The most promising physical activity interventions are typically over 10 weeks in duration (274, 275) with very high meeting frequency or intervention intensity (*i.e.*, >3 d per wk and potentially multiple hours per day; 257, 263, 274). Short interventions are less likely to yield benefits, especially in terms of emotional behavior (267, 276). Interventions are typically most effective in children (compared to adolescents) and require rigorous adherence to scheduling and planning in this population (255). Additionally, open exercise environments are not typically recommended. Adjusting to unexpected, external stimuli and conceptually difficult strategies are difficult for persons with ASD. As a result, individual closed-skill exercise programs such as yoga, tai chi, and swimming have become viable intervention strategies.

Synopsis

Physical activity levels are very low in this population due to involvement in both social and motor domains. ASD affects individuals across the lifespan, but motor and exercise interventions should be implemented during childhood to maximize effectiveness. Persons with ASD need a very organized testing and programming environment and may require exercise partners or parents to be involved. Because the incidence of ASD continues to climb at a fast rate, exercise interventions are urgently needed to offset the effects of obesity and other chronic diseases that impact this population.

VISION AND HEARING LOSS

Visual impairment (VI) and hearing loss are two of the most common sensory impairments worldwide. Both disorders occur on a spectrum; that is, from low vision to blindness and from hard of hearing to deafness. Deaf-blindness is a combination of vision and hearing impairment at varying levels (277).

Vision is measured using a visual acuity ratio, which is a comparison of the distance from which a person can identify an object with clarity (*e.g.*, 20 feet [6.1 meter]) relative to the distance a person without VI can identify the same object (*e.g.*, 400 feet [122 meter]). Individuals with a best-corrected visual acuity less than 20/40 in the better-seeing eye are considered to have a low vision (278). The World Health Organization (279) defines blindness as a visual acuity below 20/400 (3/60 in metric notation), whereas the U.S. definition is slightly lower at 20/200 best-corrected visual acuity in the better-seeing eye (280). Persons with VI may vary from being completely deprived of visual information, to perceiving light, color, and form, with limitations in the perception of space, details, movement, and three-dimensional shapes.

Hearing loss can be described in terms of severity, with loudness or volume of a sound measured in decibels (dB). Mild hearing loss is defined as 20–40 dB, moderate 41–60, and severe 61–80 (281). A hearing impairment is defined as a loss of more than 40 dB, with profound hearing loss or deafness as a loss of more than 81 dB (281). From a functional perspective, deafness is defined as a hearing disorder that limits the performance of oral communication to the extent that the primary sensory input for communication may be other than the auditory channel. Individuals who are hard of hearing, with hearing loss from mild to severe, may benefit from the use of assistive devices such as hearing aids, cochlear implants, and captioning (282).

Prevalence, Incidence, and Economic Impact

Recent reports from the WHO indicate that at least 2.2 billion people live with VI worldwide (279), whereas 430 million people experience disabling hearing loss (282). In the U.S., approximately 12 million people over age 40 years have a visual impairment, with 1 million classified as being blind (283). In addition, approximately 3% of children under the age of 18 years are classified as being blind or visually impaired (283). Figure 12.19 shows the projected increase in blindness through the year 2050.

Estimates for the number of people in the U.S. who are deaf or hard of hearing, however, are difficult to determine because there is no legal definition of deafness as there is for blindness. The available statistics come from people who reported themselves as deaf or hard of hearing.

Blindness

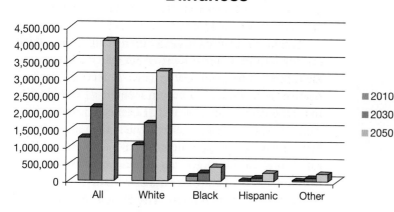

FIGURE 12.19 U.S. Projections for Blindness by year (2010–2030–2050). (Courtesy of the National Eye Institute, National Institutes of Health (NEI/NIH). Available from: https://nei.nih.gov/eyedata/blind)

Approximately 15% of American adults (37.5 million) aged 18 years and older report some trouble hearing (284, 285), with age being the strongest predictor of hearing loss (285). Estimates by the National Institute on Deafness and Other Communication Disorders suggest that about 2% of adults aged 45–54 years have disabling hearing loss, 8.5% for adults aged 55–64 years, and 25% for those aged 65–74 years. Nearly 50% of those who are 75 years and older have disabling hearing loss. Women are half as likely to experience hearing loss compared to men (285). The increase in bilateral speech frequency hearing loss is shown in Figure 12.20.

Reports indicate a considerable incremental economic cost associated with VI and hearing loss; however, the costs are much lower than those of impairments such as CP or ID. Health care costs associated with hearing loss are lower than the costs for persons with VI (286).

Pathology and Presentation

Disability resulting from a sensory impairment is directly associated with the age of onset, severity, and region of the sensory system affected by the disease. Different combinations of these factors make sensory conditions very heterogeneous among those affected. Both the visual and hearing systems have an external signal-capturing mechanism that decodes the signals so that they may be analyzed. To understand the impairment's impact, it is important to understand the compromised area and the resulting disability.

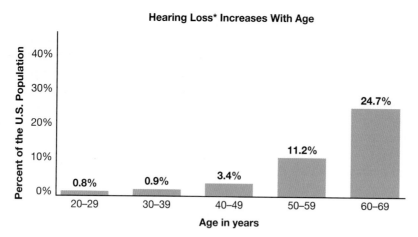

*Speech-frequency hearing loss in both ears (bilateral). The figure shows the percent of the U.S. population aged 20–69 with speech-frequency hearing loss in both ears. Hearing loss is defined as when the average threshold across four speech frequencies (0.5–1–2–4 kHz) is greater than 25 decibels hearing level. A loss of 25 decibels in the speech-frequency range is equal to very soft speech in a quiet room.

Source: National Health and Nutrition Examination Survey, 2011-2012. Analysis reported in *JAMA Otolaryngology - Head & Neck Surgery*, December 2016. Available from: https://www.nidcd.nih.gov/

Press release: https://www.nidcd.nih.gov/news/2016/hearing-loss-prevalence-declining-us-adults-aged-20-69

FIGURE 12.20 Bilateral speech frequency hearing loss in the U.S. increases with age.

The leading causes of VI worldwide are uncorrected refraction errors, glaucoma, age-related macular degeneration, cataracts, diabetic retinopathy, trachoma, and corneal opacity (279). Causes of VI vary by country and are associated with factors such as eye care literacy and availability and cost of eye care services. Distance vision impairment is 4× more prevalent in low- and middle-income regions (279). Although near vision impairment that has not been addressed (*e.g.*, corrective lenses) is estimated to be 10% in high-income regions, estimates are as high as 80% or greater in regions of Africa.

VI may be the result of problems in the ocular globe, optic nerve, and/or cortical brain. The ocular globe's structures form a tunnel through which light passes to the retina (Figure 12.21). Damage here blocks the path of light coming in (*e.g.*, cataract or corneal opacities) or will affect the focus of an image on the retina (*e.g.*, uncorrected refraction errors). Degeneration of the retina has several different causes (*e.g.*, diabetic retinopathy and retinal detachment) and limits the reception of visual information either partially (tunnel or island vision) or completely. Diseases of the optic nerve and cortical brain limit neural conduction or interpretation of the information coming in through the eye.

The causes of disabling hearing loss (>35 dB) and deafness may include genetic factors, maternal infections (*e.g.*, rubella), and childhood illnesses (*e.g.*, measles, mumps, and chronic ear infections). Other causes over the lifespan include low birth weight, meningitis, chronic diseases, smoking, excessive noise, head trauma, and nutritional deficiencies (282). The most frequent cause of hearing loss across the lifespan is exposure to loud noise (Figure 12.22), with unsafe listening practices putting

many young adults at risk of permanent, avoidable hearing loss. Estimates indicate that 1 in every 10 people will have disabling hearing loss by 2050 (282).

Lesions or other damage in different structures of the ear will lead to different types of hearing loss. The inner ear (cochlea) is particularly sensitive to loud noise. Conductive hearing loss occurs when sound cannot effectively pass through the outer or middle ear; treatment may include medicine or surgery. Sensorineural hearing loss, the most common type, happens when structures of the inner ear or auditory nerve are damaged or have deteriorated. Mixed hearing loss includes the combination of conductive and sensorineural losses. The degree of hearing loss can range from mild to profound (283).

Clinical Application

Medical management of visual and hearing impairments is critical. For those with VI, two factors that may impact physical activity must be considered. First, medications to control certain diseases of the eye (*e.g.*, β-adrenergic antagonist medicine for glaucoma) have a direct impact on physical performance that must be considered during exercise testing and prescription. Medications prescribed directly for hearing loss typically do not impact physical performance. However, medications for secondary conditions associated with hearing loss such as ADHD (287) or hypertension (288) may enhance or reduce physical performance depending on the specific drug taken.

Engagement in certain types of physical activity by individuals with specific vision or hearing disorders may be contraindicated. For example, contact sports should not be recommended to clients at risk for retinal detachment (289). In some severe cases, jump training can induce retinal detachment. For clients with diabetic retinopathy, strength training should not include heavy weightlifting, which dramatically increases BP and may cause retinal bleeding (290).

Various assistive technologies can be used to enhance the residual function of vision or hearing. Persons with blindness typically rely on auditory or tactile information, and systems to convert text to speech in computers and mobile devices are helpful. Persons with low vision can use binoculars, telescopes, or glasses to improve their perception of the environment; however, binoculars and telescopes may restrict physical activity. In contrast, walking canes, talking wristwatches, pacer systems, mobile devices with GPS, and environments with high contrast colors may facilitate physical activity. In addition to being

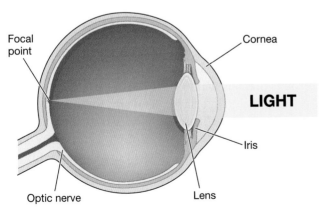

FIGURE 12.21 The ocular globe's structures form a tunnel through which light passes to the retina. (© The National Keratoconus Foundation. How the eye works. Available from: https://www.nkcf.org/how-the-eye-works/.)

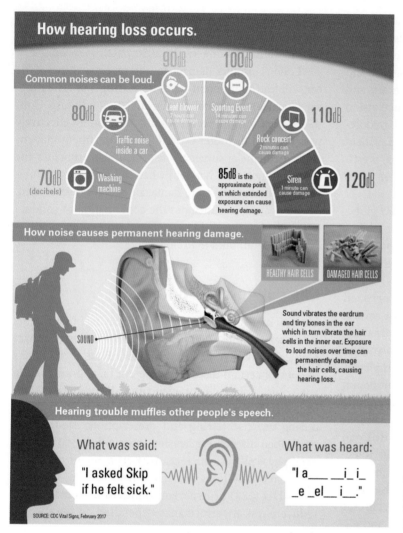

FIGURE 12.22 Many common noises can result in permanent hearing loss. (Centers for Disease Control and Prevention. Vital signs. 2017. Available from: https://www.cdc.gov/vitalsigns/hearingloss/)

assistive, glasses can help to protect the eye from impacts. Furthermore, persons with blindness due to loss of an eye or both eyes can use prosthetics for improving aesthetics and for protection of the ocular orbit.

To improve residual hearing, persons with hearing loss can use a hearing aid, the purpose of which is to capture and amplify sound using a system that is worn behind the ear, on the ear, and/or in the ear canal. The use of hearing aids may improve listening ability, as well as health-related quality of life in persons with mild to moderate hearing loss (291). Individuals with sensorineural impairment often require a cochlear implant (Figure 12.23), which receives sound and converts it to electrical impulses that are sent via an electrical array to the auditory nerve fibers within the cochlea (292). The device is surgically implanted on the outside of the skull behind the ear adjacent to the auditory nerve fibers.

Communication with persons who are deaf or have hearing loss may include different forms, such as speech, finger-spelling, manual signs, sign language, gestures, speechreading, cued speech, and augmentation of residual hearing.

Effects of Vision and Hearing Impairments on the Exercise Response

The performance of physical exercise in persons with VI is not directly associated with the impairment itself, but much more with the disability and associated limitations. For example, persons with VI may report issues with balance and have a fear of falling (293). VI often leads to compensations within the walking cycle (*e.g.*, shorter strides) to maintain balance. Similarly, various strategies are used to improve/maintain balance (*e.g.*, wider stance, arms out) during the execution of physical activity and sport skills. A very common strategy to compensate for VI during running is the use of a guide-runner (Figure 12.24). The guide runs together with the person with VI connected by a tether (hand/hand, arm/hand, or arm/arm) and provides an orientation to the environment, pace, motivation, and safety during the activity.

Greater impairment is typically associated with lower aerobic fitness in persons with VI. This relationship may be explained by the need for greater assistance and

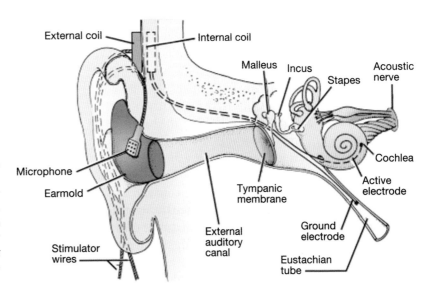

FIGURE 12.23 A cochlear implant has an internal coil with a stranded electrode lead that's surgically inserted into the scala tympani of the cochlea (as shown). The external coil (the transmitter) aligns with the internal coil (the receiver) by a magnet. When the microphone receives sound, the stimulator wires receive the signal after it's been filtered. This filtering allows the sound to transmit comfortably for the patient. Sound is then passed by the external transmitter to the inner coil receiver by magnetic conduction and is finally carried by the electrode to the cochlea. (From Smeltzer SC, Bare BG, Cheever KH, Hinkle JL. *Brunner & Suddarth's Textbook of Medical Surgical Nursing.* 11th ed. Philadelphia (PA): Wolters Kluwer; 2006.)

support during exercise, which in turn limits access and adherence to training, thereby reducing overall physical activity engagement. Also, the visual acuity of persons with low vision may decrease during high-intensity exercise due to physiologic adjustments of blood flow and the relationship between sympathetic and parasympathetic control (294). Persons with no light perception (full blindness) experience a disruption in their circadian rhythms. This condition may impact muscle strength, and simple reaction time, peak performance, and body temperature regulation throughout the day (295).

For those with hearing loss, issues with balance and mobility may occur (296), which may in turn impact the level of physical activity (297) and aerobic performance. The individual may perform more poorly during dynamic exercise as compared with exercise in a stationary position (*e.g.,* test on a treadmill compared with a bicycle ergometer) (298).

Benefits of Exercise for Clients With Vision and Hearing Impairments

Exercise has important benefits for persons with sensory impairments. Particularly important are the improvements in balance that exercise can promote. Individuals with VI often experience vestibular problems, which affect postural stability. Exercise training can mediate this condition and improve balance and mobility (299). Visual, proprioceptive, and exteroceptive cues can compensate for vestibular deficiency during postural control. Physical training can improve balance as well as neural integration of feedback from pressor receptors in the feet, proprioceptors, and visual cues (300). Moreover, in clients with severe VI, balance training can have a positive effect on vestibular function and proprioception (301).

Persons with and without VI show similar gains in maximal strength following a strength-training program, but muscle power performance is lower in those with VI (302). However, persons with VI may achieve physical performance similar to that of persons without disabilities provided that they are properly trained (303).

Considerations for Health-Related Fitness Testing

Clients With Vision Impairment

For effective testing of persons with VI, the CEP begins by orienting the client to the testing space. For example, in a jump test using a plyometric box for the development of a power-training program, the client should touch the box to identify the height, dimensions, and distance of any possible obstacles before the start of the test. For clients with low vision, objects and environments with highly contrasting colors (*e.g.,* black against white, red against white) improve testing conditions.

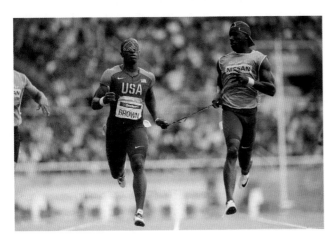

FIGURE 12.24 David Brown (left) runs the men's 100 meters T11 round 1 on day 3 of the Rio 2016 Paralympic Games on September 10, 2016, in Rio de Janeiro, Brazil.

Offering sounds and/or tactile instructions may help the client learn the movements required for the test. The CEP may also offer feedback during testing through verbal (e.g., directional cues such as "take two steps to the right") and/or auditory signals (e.g., orientation by a buzzer or clapping hands). As for tactile instruction, the CEP may provide the hand manipulated by the tester or demonstration of the movement with the hands; during tests on a treadmill, for example, a client with blindness can hold the handrails; alternately, an elastic band can be placed around the treadmill, offering tactile cues and defining the walking/running area. For field tests, a sighted guide and tether, caller, or guidewire system can be used. For assessing muscular strength and endurance in persons with VI, exercise professionals can use a variety of modalities including resistance machines, dumbbells, as well as activities such as push-ups and squats.

Clients With Hearing Loss

Before testing begins, it is important to ensure that the individual understands the protocol and performance goals. The CEP should explain the test protocol using a variety of communication methods including gestures, visual cues, pictures, and videos. Another valuable resource for improving communication is the support of an interpreter.

While conducting a test, the CEP should stay in the field of vision, keep continuous eye contact, and offer instructions in a normal voice and tone. In addition, the testing site should be equipped with visual information like flags, strobe lights, or a vibration system to ensure proper starting and finishing of a test or to indicate a possible need for adjustments to the participant. Precautions should be taken to ensure a safe testing environment for persons with sensorineural hearing impairment. Visual and proprioception stimulation strategies to compensate for limitations in balance control can be used during balance or treadmill testing. During strength testing, persons with balance issues should execute closed kinetic chain exercises.

Clients With Deaf-Blindness

The CEP must use alternative forms of communication when working with clients with deaf-blindness. To be most effective, instructions and explanations should incorporate presymbolic communication (i.e., communication without symbols such as words or signs) including body movements, touch, and objects. However, symbolic communication forms can also be used, including signed communication and fingerspelling (both visual and tactile), print, braille, computer-activated voice-output devices, and speech. When preparing for testing persons who are deaf-blind, allow extra time to ensure testing procedures are fully understood and any necessary modifications are made.

Considerations for Exercise Programming

Standard exercise recommendations, such as *ACSM Guidelines* (44) or the U.S. Physical Activity Guidelines for Americans (1) can be used for individuals with sensory impairments. However, balance training should be emphasized in the exercise program. To better enable individuals with sensory impairments to engage in their home and community environments, neuromuscular training, which combines balance, agility, and proprioceptive training, is recommended 2–3 days per week. Gradual progression to difficult postures, which reduce the base of support and sensory input, should be included in the exercise program. General adaptations or modifications to health-related exercise programming can be found in Table 12.2.

Synopsis

Sensory impairment limits the interaction between a person and their environment. Systematic physical activity can minimize the effect of sensory deprivation on physical performance. However, the quality of instruction is fundamental for improving the physical profiles and the motivation of clients with sensory impairments.

Table 12.2	Exercise Adaptations for Persons With Sensory Impairments		
	Adaptation		
Training Type	Person With Visual Impairment	Person With Hearing Loss	Deaf-Blindness
Aerobic	Run with a guide or bike/treadmill	No adaptations required	Guide or stationary bicycle
Strength	Quantity or velocity of movement support by an instructor or closed kinetic chain exercises		
Balance	Support by an instructor	Visual resources or support by an instructor	Support by an instructor

INTELLECTUAL IMPAIRMENTS

INTELLECTUAL DISABILITY

The American Association on Intellectual and Developmental Disabilities (AAIDD) defines intellectual disability (ID), also referred to as intellectual impairment, as a condition characterized by significant limitations in both intellectual functioning and adaptive behavior. *Intellectual functioning* (or intelligence) is a general mental ability with many components such as reasoning, planning, problem-solving, abstract thinking, and experiential learning, among others. *Adaptive behavior* is a set of skills that people learn through experience and that allow them to function in their daily lives. These include (304):

- Conceptual skills, such as language and literacy
- Social skills, such as interpersonal skills and social responsibility
- Practical skills, such as personal care and work responsibilities

Similarly, the *Diagnostic and Statistical Manual of Mental Disorders* (*DSM-5*) of the American Psychiatric Association (244) defines ID as impairment of general mental abilities that impact *adaptive functioning* in the conceptual, social, and practical domains. ID is a developmental disability, which means that it must have an onset during childhood or adolescence. ID should be differentiated from cognitive impairments that may result later in adulthood from a variety of causes (*e.g.*, MS, Alzheimer disease).

Prevalence, Incidence, and Economic Impact

Estimates of the prevalence of ID vary widely between countries and even between different states of the U.S., apparently due to differences in defining and identifying cases (305, 306). According to the *DSM-5*, about 1% of the population has ID (244). Research findings support a worldwide prevalence around 1%, but with variation between countries and studies (54, 306).

A common cause of ID that has been studied by exercise scientists to a relatively large extent is Down syndrome (DS). Although estimates of the prevalence of DS in the U.S. vary between 6.7 and 8.3 per 10,000 people, the available data indicate that more than 206,000 individuals with DS live in the U.S. and about 417,000 in Europe (307–309). These numbers would have been higher in the absence of a significant increase in elective prenatal terminations (308).

People with ID experience health disparities (310, 311). They live shorter lives than the general population, and life expectancy decreases as the level of ID increases (312–316). The leading cause of death among adults with ID is heart disease, and those with mild/moderate levels of ID have a higher risk of dying from DM than adults without ID (315). Those with DS die at younger ages than individuals with ID or the general population, and common causes are heart disease, dementia and Alzheimer disease, cancer, influenza, pneumonia, and respiratory failure (315, 316). Risk factors for mortality among persons with ID and other developmental disabilities include lower functional and motor skills, non-ambulation, behavioral issues, IQ level, communication problems, difficulties with self-help, parental death, and the presence of DS (317). Furthermore, people with ID are at high risk for multiple mental and physical health comorbidities (244, 312).

Not surprisingly, managing ID and its associated conditions incurs significant economic costs. Studies from around the world confirm that the economic impact of dealing with ID can stress the financial resources of society, as well as those of the person with ID and their family (318–321). Economic costs are driven by health care needs and are higher for people with greater levels of ID and more associated conditions (319, 320, 322, 323). Notably, obesity increases health care costs for individuals with ID (322). Arguably, physical activity and exercise may reflect cost-effective approaches to improving the client's health and reducing the total economic impact of ID.

Etiology and Presentation

The cause of ID can be (244, 304):

- Prenatal, including genetic and chromosomal syndromes, brain malformations, maternal disease, maternal alcohol abuse, and other environmental influences;
- Perinatal, such as prematurity and problems with labor; and
- Postnatal, including traumatic brain injury, infections, demyelinating disorders, seizure disorders, malnutrition, and social deprivation among others.

However, the cause of ID is not known in about 30%–50% of cases (312). Causes and risk factors for ID can be not only biomedical but also social, behavioral, and educational; and complex interactions among these factors may contribute to the etiology (324).

The most common prenatal causes of ID are DS, fragile-X syndrome, and fetal alcohol syndrome, which together account for nearly one-third of cases of the more severe forms of ID. DS (324), the most common of these three syndromes, is a set of symptoms that result from a chromosomal abnormality in which there is an extra whole or partial chromosome 21 in the individual's karyotype (325). The chromosomal abnormality accounting for 95% of DS cases is trisomy 21, followed by translocation (4%–5% of cases) and mosaicism (1%–2% of cases; 85). In trisomy 21, all body cells have an extra chromosome 21, whereas in mosaicism only some body cells have the extra chromosome 21. In translocation, an extra chromosome 21 is attached to another chromosome. The most important risk factor for giving birth to a child with DS is older maternal age. Physical features of DS include short stature, slanted eyes, small mouth, loose ligaments, and hypotonic muscles.

ID is diagnosed with assessments of intellectual functioning and adaptive behavior while considering the cultural and linguistic background of the person (244, 304). An IQ score of two or more standard deviations below the population mean (*i.e.*, a score of about 65–75) is indicative of ID. Adaptive behavior is also assessed with standardized methods. Additional diagnostic tools include medical history, physical examination, and psychological evaluation. DS is diagnosed at birth with a physical examination and can be confirmed by chromosomal analysis, but it can also be diagnosed prenatally with specific screening tests (325).

The severity of ID, which may change during a person's lifetime, is classified by different approaches. The World Health Organization's International Classification of Diseases — 11th revision classifies ID as mild, moderate, severe, and profound based on standardized assessments of intellectual functioning and adapted behavior against normative scores; in this classification system, severity is assigned by the level at which most assessments fall (4). The *DSM-5* proposes a model based on a general evaluation of the conceptual, social, and practical domains of adaptive functioning. Finally, AAIDD uses a different approach for assessing the severity of ID based on the intensity of support a person needs to fulfill all aspects of their functioning (304). The diagnostic and classification systems for ID have evolved over the years and are likely to continue to evolve.

ID is often co-occurring with a wide spectrum of other conditions that tend to be more frequent and of greater intensity among persons with more severe forms of ID (324). Associated conditions include CP, ADHD, seizure disorders, psychiatric/behavior disorders, sensory and neuromotor disorders, communication disorders, and ASD

among others, all of which make the diagnosis of ID more difficult (244, 324). Persons with DS often have several of the abovementioned conditions as well as congenital heart defects, hematologic disorders, endocrine abnormalities, gastrointestinal malformations, orthopedic complications, dental problems, delayed motor development, and early onset of Alzheimer disease (325). The number and intensity of these associated conditions differ widely among people with ID; thus, considerations for exercise testing and programming must be evaluated on a case-by-case basis. Two of the most common secondary conditions among persons with ID, especially those who have DS, are obesity and physical deconditioning (326–331). Other secondary conditions include hypertension (not common in those with DS), high blood cholesterol, DM, depression, loneliness, and limited friendships (332–335). Classifying a condition as associated or secondary in persons with ID can be difficult. Nevertheless, it is important to be aware of the complexity that coexisting conditions introduce to health management and exercise training.

Clinical Application

Presently, there is no cure for ID. Persons with ID are evaluated and treated for associated and secondary conditions. Typically, management of these conditions does not differ to a significant extent between people with and without ID. Persons with ID, however, need some level of support to facilitate their physical and psychosocial functioning, and some may live in assisted living settings.

About 40%–50% of persons with DS have congenital heart defects and undergo heart surgery early in life (336, 337). The introduction of heart surgery has dramatically increased the life expectancy of persons with DS (307).

Persons with ID often take medications for physical and mental health problems. Polypharmacy is common and may be partially due to multiple comorbidities (338).

Early intervention for addressing comorbidities, as well as the educational, recreational, and social needs of children with ID, can improve their physical and intellectual functioning (324). Furthermore, physical activity and exercise can contribute to the management of the physical and psychosocial health concerns of persons with ID (324, 339–341).

People with ID, however, have lower physical activity levels than the general population, high levels of sedentary behavior, and most do not meet the recommendations for health-promoting physical activity (342–344). Those with DS have even lower physical activity levels than people with ID without DS (342, 345). Commonly reported barriers to physical activity in persons with ID across the lifespan include (346–349) the following:

- Medical and physiologic issues;
- Negative attitudes toward exercise;
- Lack of accessible, inclusive, and appropriately designed programs;
- Low support from others;
- Costs;
- Transportation barriers;
- Competing family responsibilities;
- Parental education; and
- Lack of friends.

In turn, factors that facilitate physical activity among persons with ID are enjoyment, support, socialization, friendship, and familiarity with the program (348–350). Evaluating the barriers and facilitators of physical activity in an individual with ID is critical for effectively promoting their physical activity levels and developing a suitable exercise program. One outstanding program is the Special Olympics, which provides a variety of sports programs worldwide for children and adults with ID (Figure 12.25).

Effects of ID on the Exercise Response

The physiologic responses to acute exercise of persons with ID have not been thoroughly explored (351). Some differences are observed in the presence of conditions that alter metabolism or movement patterns. For example, persons with DS have a gait pattern that causes an increase in the rate of oxygen uptake at a given walking speed (352, 353).

Individuals with ID have lower performance in functional tasks than persons without ID. Those with DS specifically have even lower levels of performance (326, 327, 354). Notably, individuals with ID have low aerobic and muscular fitness. One possible physiologic explanation for the extremely low aerobic fitness of persons with ID, especially those with DS, is chronotropic incompetence (low peak heart rate [HR_{peak}]), which is thought to be due to problems in autonomic nervous system responses (331, 355, 356). For this reason, researchers have developed formulas for predicting HR_{peak} from age for persons with ID, with and without DS (356, 357); these formulas, however, have relatively large error in predicting the HR_{peak} of individual persons with ID, and thus limited utility for exercise prescription. Researchers have also suggested that additional causes for the low aerobic fitness of individuals with ID may include ventilatory limitations and peripheral muscle hypoperfusion (351).

Benefits of Exercise for Client With ID

Well-designed exercise programs improve aerobic and muscular fitness, body composition, functional performance, balance, and psychosocial outcomes in persons with ID (339–341, 354, 358–361). Appropriate goals of exercise programs for persons with ID include:

1. improving physical fitness
2. improving balance and preventing falls
3. lowering the risk for mortality
4. preventing or alleviating secondary health conditions, especially overweight and obesity

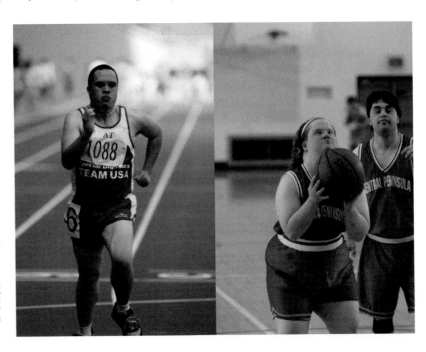

FIGURE 12.25 Special Olympics Alaska track and field athlete competing at World Summer Games in Shanghai, China (left). Special Olympics Alaska athlete playing basketball during State Summer Games (right). (Photo credit Fitzgerald Photography [compliments of Nicolle Egan, Special Olympics Alaska.])

Exercise programs for persons with ID should be designed in ways that promote independence and lifelong maintenance. To achieve these goals, exercise professionals should systematically educate persons with ID on how to participate in safe and effective exercise training. In designing exercise programs, exercise professionals should consider the individual preferences of persons with ID as well as their needs for social interaction and enjoyment. Importantly, exercise programs should be physically, socially, and economically accessible to persons with ID.

Considerations for Health-Related Fitness Testing

Health-related fitness testing in people with ID follows the same general principles as for the general population. Prior to assessments, clearance by a physician may be required because some conditions may limit the types of activities and movements that can be performed; for example, many people with DS have atlantoaxial instability (337), and therefore hyperextension or hyperflexion of the neck is not recommended. Another consideration in persons with DS requiring physician clearance is congenital heart disease. The validity of fitness assessments for participants with ID largely depends on thorough familiarization with the testing procedures, usually in a separate session; multiple sessions may be necessary for some persons (362). For successful testing, exercise professionals should offer demonstrations of techniques, simple instructions, and motivation, and should conduct testing on equipment that allows adjustments for body size and proportions. In addition, having more than one testing professional increases safety and supervision and thereby effectiveness of the testing.

Laboratory assessments of aerobic and muscular fitness are feasible, valid, and reliable in persons with ID (44). Treadmill walking is typically the first choice for aerobic fitness assessment. Cycle ergometry requires significantly more familiarization than treadmill exercise and has not been validated in individuals with ID. Combined arm and leg ergometry, however, is more feasible and could be used for individuals with ID who cannot perform treadmill exercise. As with the general population, protocols of aerobic fitness testing should be individualized. Field assessments of peak oxygen consumption ($\dot{V}O_{2peak}$) with the 20-meter shuttle run, 600-yard run per walk, or the 1-mile walking test using population-specific formulas are also valid in persons with ID without DS, but not in those with DS (44, 363). However, the 16-meter shuttle run has been found to provide a valid prediction of $\dot{V}O_{2peak}$ and can be used in those with DS (364).

Muscular strength can effectively be measured with isokinetic and isometric devices, as well as 1RM testing. Safety, however, may be a consideration during 1RM testing and, for this reason, experts recommend using weight machines for this population rather than free weights (44, 363). Alternatively, strength assessments of the 6RM or 12RM could be used (44).

The high prevalence of obesity among individuals with ID indicates a need to assess body composition and weight status. Apart from routinely assessing weight, BMI, and waist circumference, the CEP should prefer laboratory assessments of body composition such as dual x-ray absorptiometry (DXA) and air-displacement plethysmography, which have been successfully conducted in individuals with ID (365). Although field-based assessments are feasible and reliable, their validity in people with ID is still questionable, especially in those with DS (366, 367).

Assessments of flexibility with direct (e.g., goniometers) or indirect (e.g., sit-and-reach) methods are feasible. Assessments of functional performance and balance using standard techniques are also recommended because persons with ID have a high risk of falling (368). To this end, the short physical performance battery has successfully been utilized in individuals with ID (369, 370).

Considerations for Exercise Programming

The basic principles of exercise programming apply to persons with ID. Individuals with ID should be encouraged to meet the general recommendations for aerobic as well as muscle- and bone-strengthening activities and avoid sedentary behaviors. People with ID should participate in programs to improve aerobic and muscular fitness because both are typically low in these individuals. Flexibility training is also appropriate but should be conducted with caution in those with DS because these persons may have joint hypermobility (44). Improving body composition with multifactorial programs that facilitate weight loss is important, given the high rates of obesity in this population. Importantly, neuromotor exercise training should be conducted for improving balance and preventing falls. Combinations of aerobic, resistance, and balance training improve physical fitness, balance, and functional measures in people with ID (361). Exergames may also increase physical fitness and motor skills in individuals with ID (371–373).

During the initial phase of training, the focus should not be on intensity but on learning exercise techniques and safety. Proper supervision, simple instructions, and demonstrations can facilitate safety.

The CEP can design an individualized program based on the results of fitness assessments. However, the CEP should also consider group exercise training for promoting social interactions and enjoyment, while ensuring that intensity is high enough to elicit positive exercise adaptations. Importantly, exercising under the guidance of a peer mentor without a disability may provide the motivation and supervision required to ensure that participants with ID perform exercise at the prescribed intensities. This approach applied to resistance exercise training has been effective in increasing strength and physical activity levels in young people with DS when mentored by undergraduate physiotherapy students in Australia (374).

Synopsis

ID is a common developmental disability characterized by limitations in intellectual functioning and adaptive behavior and caused by a variety of biological and social factors. Persons with ID experience health disparities, often have multiple comorbidities, and have a shorter life expectancy than that of the general population. Physical activity and exercise can alleviate comorbidities and improve the physical and psychosocial health of clients with ID.

SUMMARY

It is clear that physical activity and exercise are beneficial for persons with a variety of physical, sensory, and/or intellectual impairments, improving their physical and psychosocial health and reducing their secondary disease risk. Exercise training is therefore an important component of multifactorial therapeutic management of these clients. The acute and chronic responses to exercise differ widely among persons with different conditions and even among persons with the same impairment. The CEP should carefully consider these differences when conducting fitness assessments and when developing effective exercise programs to best meet the needs of individual clients.

This chapter documented population-specific ICF *Body Function* improvements such as improved aerobic fitness, muscular fitness, and body composition that result from regular exercise and physical activity. Unfortunately, a variety of barriers continue to impede healthy physical activity levels among persons with varied health conditions. Effective exercise prescriptions are essential to reduce the risk of secondary diseases such as CVD and DM in these populations. Less clear, however, are the most effective strategies to improve ICF *Activity* and *Participation* domains. Exercise can improve impaired clients' physical function and participation in the community; however, effective physical activity interventions have yet to be sufficiently developed and integrated into the continuum of care as people transition from the medical model to community health and wellness programs.

CHAPTER REVIEW QUESTIONS

1. How are physical activity recommendations for individuals with physical, sensory, and intellectual impairments similar or different from recommendations for the general population?
2. Consider the World Health Organization's International Classification of Functioning. What are the differences among structures, activities, and participation?
3. How should an exercise program differ for a child with cerebral palsy compared to a typically developing child?
4. What does the statement "exercise programs should be physically, economically, and socially accessible to persons with ID" mean? How can this be achieved?
5. Sensory impairment (loss of vision or hearing) may affect balance. What is the impact of such impairment on the performance of other physical skills?
6. What specific characteristics of the SCI must the CEP consider when prescribing exercise for clients with SCI? What three physiological factors might differ in the SCI client's response to exercise as compared to the response of a nonimpaired client?
7. How can physical activity and exercise aid in reducing the economic impact of MS?
8. Identify an exercise intervention shown to counter both sarcopenia and the motor deficits associated with neurodegeneration in PD, and three ways in which it improves fitness.
9. What components of a clinical rehabilitation program should be listed in a visual session schedule for persons with ASD?
10. What is meant by functional variations across and within impairments?

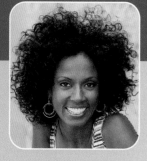

Case Study 12.1

Gemma is a 39-year-old female with CP. She describes herself as having spastic diplegia and she walks with a cane outside the house. She takes anti-spasm and pain medications but lately feels that her walking ability and general fitness level are becoming worse. She reports individual and environmental barriers that keep her from exercising more than she would like. "I need to have set times or set places where I can join people for exercise. If I don't have an appointment or a commitment, I usually just stay in my apartment. But I think I can do anything that anybody else can if I have the right equipment. A lot of places don't have the equipment that I need to exercise. Sometimes I need accessible equipment to do things at 'regular' gyms, but I can do it [exercise] if I have the right equipment." She also has limited experience with resistance exercise and prefers a cycle or arm ergometer over a treadmill.

Based on baseline assessments, Gemma's BMI is 22.6 kg·m^{-2}; she has a resting HR of 78 beats per minute and a resting BP of 121/78 mm Hg. She completed a cycle ergometry test and her end-test score was 1.60 L·min^{-1} or 26.67 mL·kg^{-1}·min^{-1}. She walks about 4,800 steps per day during weekdays and 2,700 steps per day during weekends. She also completed a series of 8–12 RM assessments on the seated leg press, overhead press, chest press, and machine row; her scores were 55, 9, 23, and 13.5 kg (121, 20, 51, and 30 pounds), respectively.

One of Gemma's primary goals will be to increase her physical activity level. Given that accessibility and personal motivation are barriers to Gemma's physical activity, it is essential that the CEP identify group exercise opportunities or personal training/partner activities that are available and accessible. Simply documenting an effective exercise program is unlikely to change Gemma's actual activity level, given the individual and environmental barriers she faces. A second goal is to improve aerobic capacity. To achieve this goal, be sure to include vigorous physical activity as part of her program, careful not to prescribe too low an intensity for her. A final exercise goal is to improve muscular fitness. Specifically, improving muscular strength should contribute to improved anaerobic capacity, which in turn is an important contributor to functional ability in persons with CP.

Case Study 12.1 Questions

1. What would an effective aerobic prescription include relative to exercise intensity and mode? What is the work-to-rest ratio that should be used?
2. Gemma wants to add resistance training to her exercise routine, but she is not able to access machine weights on a regular basis. What are some ways to increase the intensity of functional exercises that Gemma may complete at home?
3. What are some leisure activities available to persons with CP?

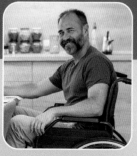

Case Study 12.2

Lucas is a 40-year-old man who sustained an SCI 10 years ago in a ski accident. The motor level of his injury is at C6, and his ASIA Impairment Scale is B, meaning that sensory, but not motor, function is preserved below the neurologic level. Lucas cannot walk, and he also has impairments in the arms and hands. Despite the impairment of his upper limbs, he is able to use a manual wheelchair.

In the last 5 years, Lucas has been increasingly busy with work and family and therefore has not made exercise a priority. However, he wants to become fit again because he knows that his daily activities would be easier to perform if he were fit. Because of his impaired arms and hands, he thinks about handcycling as an exercise mode. When asking for advice at a rehabilitation center, he is invited to train to participate in the HandbikeBattle (see: https://www.youtube.com/user/HandbikeBattle). The HandbikeBattle is a race on a mountain (12.5 miles and almost 0.6-mile elevation or 20 km and 1 km elevation) among handcycle teams of several rehabilitation centers. The HandbikeBattle is organized to encourage wheelchair users to keep training after rehabilitation to boost their fitness as well as their self-confidence when they reach the finish after their tough climb in the handcycle. Although Lucas might need a power-assisted handcycle, he agrees to participate in this challenge and have a training goal.

Before the start of the training, Lucas undergoes a medical screening and performs a graded peak exercise test on an arm crank ergometer in the rehabilitation center. Lucas' BMI is 20.2 $kg \cdot m^{-2}$, his resting HR is 60 beats per minute (bpm), and his resting BP is 110/65 mm Hg. After completion of the graded peak exercise test, he knows that his peak oxygen uptake is 1.14 $L \cdot min^{-1}$, his peak power output is 55 W, and his peak HR is 117 bpm.

Because Lucas wants to participate in the HandbikeBattle, he would like a training program that helps him become optimally fit without getting overuse injuries. He has his own handcycle and a bicycle computer with HR monitoring. In addition, he purchases a roller system that also gives an indication about power output, to train indoors when the weather is bad.

Case Study 12.2 Questions

1. What should be the minimal training prescription to start with for Lucas, who has been quite inactive in the last years, to become fit without getting overuse injuries?

2. How can Lucas monitor his handcycling training intensity best?

3. How can the CEP play a role in assisting Lucas to engage in exercise and enjoy an active lifestyle?

Case Study 12.3

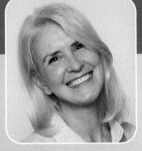

Penelope is a 48-year-old post office clerk who has MS. She was initially diagnosed with relapsing–remitting MS 8 years ago, but for the last 2 years, she has had secondary progressive MS. She presently experiences significant spasticity, pain, fatigue, depression, and drop foot (right foot), and she has some balance problems. Her symptoms usually get worse in the afternoon. She is taking medications for slowing the disease course and for managing spasticity, pain, fatigue, and depression. She is also using an ankle–foot orthotic and a cane, which have helped her with ambulation, but she cannot walk quickly. Her score on the EDSS is 6, and her score on the PDDS scale is 4, indicating significant walking impairment and the need for a cane for ambulation. The progressive nature of the disease has had a significant impact on her lifestyle, and, over the last 2 years, her quality of life has deteriorated. Penelope used to be active and enjoyed hiking and jogging, but she has had to gradually withdraw from these activities.

She describes herself as very deconditioned, and she is currently inactive.

Penelope decided to enroll in an exercise rehabilitation program, where a set of fitness evaluations were conducted. Penelope's weight is 80 kg (176 pounds); her height is 170 cm (67 inches); and her BMI is 27.7 $kg \cdot m^{-2}$, putting her in the overweight category. Using a leg cycle ergometer test, it was determined that her $\dot{V}O_{2\ Peak}$ is 1.50 $L \cdot min^{-1}$ or 18.75 $mL \cdot kg^{-1} \cdot min^{-1}$; her peak power is 95 W; and her peak HR is 152 beats per minute (bpm). On the day of the test, Penelope's resting $\dot{V}O_2$ was 4.0 $mL \cdot kg^{-1} \cdot min^{-1}$ and her resting HR was 72 bpm. Penelope has low muscular strength based on the 12RM, which was determined for several resistance exercises. Her flexibility level is also low.

Penelope's goals for her exercise program are to gradually increase her physical activity level; improve fitness; lose weight; reduce her fatigue, spasticity, and depression; and improve her overall quality of life. Based on this information and Penelope's preferences, the CEP determined that her initial exercise training program for the first 2 weeks will consist of aerobic exercise 2 days

(continued)

Case Study 12.3 *(continued)*

per week, strengthening exercises 2 days per week (on days there is no aerobic training), and stretching exercises daily.

Penelope will be performing interval aerobic exercise on the leg cycle (two bouts of exercise at 35 W [~50% of reserve], each lasting 5 minutes and separated by 3–5 minutes of rest). After another 3–5 minutes of rest, she will be exercising on the arm cycle at 25 W for another 5 minutes. The target RPE for aerobic exercise will be 12–13. Penelope's strength-training program for the first 2 weeks

will consist of five resistance exercises for major muscle groups (one set with 12 repetitions at the 12RM), and it will also include the performance of functional activities (*e.g.*, stepping up and down a block; sit-to-stand). Finally, Penelope will be performing static stretching exercises for 15 minutes daily. Adequate time for warm-up and cool-down will be included. The frequency, intensity, and duration of the exercise program will gradually increase following *ACSM Guidelines*. Penelope will be training early in the morning.

Case Study 12.3 Questions

1. What would be the primary concern regarding the progression of Penelope's training program?

2. Why will Penelope be exercising in the morning?
3. How can exercise help Penelope manage her fatigue?

REFERENCES

1. 2018 Physical Activity Guidelines Advisory Committee. 2018 *Physical Activity Guidelines Advisory Committee Scientific Report*. Washington, DC: U.S. Department of Health and Human Services; 2018..

2. Centers for Disease Control and Prevention. Increasing physical activity among adults with disabilities. 2016. Available from: https://www.cdc.gov/ncbddd/disabilityandhealth/pa.html.

3. World Health Organization. Towards a common language for functioning, disability and health: ICF — The International Classification of Functioning, Disability, and Health. 2002. Available from: https://cdn.who.int/media/docs/default-source/classification/icf/icfbeginnersguide.pdf.

4. World Health Organization. ICD-11: International Classification of Diseases 11th revision: the global standard for diagnostic health information. 2018. Available from: https://icd.who.int/en.

5. Amputee Coalition. Limb loss resource center. 2016. Available from: https://www.amputee-coalition.org/limb-loss-resource-center/.

6. Burgess E, Rappoport A. *Physical Fitness: A Guide for Individuals with Lower Limb Loss*. Baltimore (MD): Department of Veterans Affairs, Veterans Health Administration, Rehabilitation Research and Development Service; 1991.

7. Pitetti KH, Manske R. Amputation. In: Myers J, Nieman DC; American College of Sports Medicine, editors. *ACSM's Resources for Clinical Exercise Physiology: Musculoskeletal, Neuromuscular, Neoplastic, Immunologic, and Hematologic Conditions*. 2nd ed. Philadelphia (PA): Wolters Kluwer Health/Lippincott Williams & Wilkins Health; 2010. p. 197–204.

8. Amputee Coalition. Roadmap for limb loss prevention and amputee care improvement: a report of the Limb Loss Task Force. 2011. Available from: https://www.amputee-coalition.org/wp-content/uploads/2015/03/Roadmap-for-Limb-Loss-Prevention-and-Amputee-Care-Improvement-2011.pdf.

9. Ziegler-Graham K, MacKenzie EJ, Ephraim PL, Travison TG, Brookmeyer R. Estimating the prevalence of limb loss in the United States: 2005 to 2050. *Arch Phys Med Rehabil*. 2008;89(3):422–9. doi:10.1016/j.apmr.2007.11.005.

10. Kurichi J, Bates B, Stineman M. Amputation. In: *International Encyclopedia of Rehabilitation*. Buffalo (NY): Center for International Rehabilitation Research Information and Exchange; 2010.

11. World Health Organization. EXPERT Committee on medical rehabilitation; first report. *World Health Organ Tech Rep Ser*. 1958;108(158):1–51.

12. Gallagher, Allen D, Malcolm M. Phantom limb pain and residual limb pain following lower limb amputation: a

descriptive analysis. *Disabil Rehabil.* 2001;23(12):522–30. doi:10.1080/09638280010029859.

13. Ephraim PL, Wegener ST, MacKenzie EJ, Dillingham TR, Pezzin LE. Phantom pain, residual limb pain, and back pain in amputees: results of a national survey. *Arch Phys Med Rehabil.* 2005;86(10):1910–9. doi:10.1016/j.apmr.2005.03.031.

14. Lindesay JEB. Multiple pain complaints in amputees. *J R Soc Med.* 1985;78(6):452–5. doi:10.1177/014107688507800606.

15. World Health Organization. International Classification of Functioning, Disability and Health (ICF). 2001. Available from: http://www.who.int/classifications/icf/en/.

16. Bakalim G. Causes of death in a series of 4738 Finnish war amputees. *Artif Limbs.* 1969;13(1):27–36.

17. Yekutiel M, Brooks ME, Ohry A, Yarom J, Carel R. The prevalence of hypertension, ischaemic heart disease and diabetes in traumatic spinal cord injured patients and amputees. *Paraplegia.* 1989;27(1):58–62. doi:10.1038/sc.1989.9.

18. Gailey RS, Wenger MA, Raya M, et al. Energy expenditure of trans-tibial amputees during ambulation at self-selected pace. *Prosthet Orthot Int.* 1994;18(2):84–91. doi:10.3109/03093649409164389.

19. Ward KH, Meyers MC. Exercise performance of lower-extremity amputees. *Sports Med.* 1995;20(4):207–14. doi:10.2165/00007256-199520040-00001.

20. Versluys R, Beyl P, Van Damme M, Desomer A, Van Ham R, Lefeber D. Prosthetic feet: state-of-the-art review and the importance of mimicking human ankle–foot biomechanics. *Disabil Rehabil Assist Technol.* 2009;4(2):65–75. doi:10.1080/17483100802715092.

21. Vllasolli TO, Zafirova B, Orovcanec N, Poposka A, Murtezani A, Krasniqi B. Energy expenditure and walking speed in lower limb amputees: a cross sectional study. *Ortop Traumatol Rehabil.* 2014;16(4):419–26. doi:10.5604/15093492.1119619.

22. Felici F, Bernardi M, Rodio A, Marchettoni P, Castellano V, Macaluso A. Rehabilitation of walking for paraplegic patients by means of a treadmill. *Spinal Cord.* 1997;35(6):383–5. doi:10.1038/sj.sc.3100403.

23. Gazzani F, Bernardi M, Macaluso A, et al. Ambulation training of neurological patients on the treadmill with a new Walking Assistance and Rehabilitation Device (WARD). *Spinal Cord.* 1999;37(5):336–44. doi:10.1038/sj.sc.3100821.

24. Kušljugić A, Kapidžić-Duraković S, Kudumović Z, Čičkušić A. Chronic low back pain in individuals with lower-limb amputation. *Bosn J of Basic Med Sci.* 2006;6(2):67–70. doi:10.17305/bjbms.2006.3177.

25. Gailey R. *Balance, Agility, Coordination and Endurance for Lower Extremity Amputees.* Midlothian (VA): Advanced Rehabilitation Therapy, Inc; 1996. Available from: http://www.advancedrehabtherapy.com/.

26. Gailey R. *Stretching and Strengthening for Lower Extremity Amputees.* Midlothian (VA): Advanced Rehabilitation Therapy, Inc; 1994. Available from: http://www.advancedrehabtherapy.com/.

27. Christensen J, Ipsen T, Doherty P, Langberg H. Physical and social factors determining quality of life for veterans with lower-limb amputation(s): a systematic review. *Disabil Rehabil.* 2016;38(24):2345–53. doi:10.3109/09638288.2015.1129446.

28. Egidi F, Faiola F, Guerra E, Marini C, Sardella F, Bernardi M. Sport for disabled individuals: from rehabilitation to Paralympic Games. *Med Sport.* 2009;62(4):597–601.

29. Pelliccia A, Quattrini FM, Squeo MR, et al. Cardiovascular diseases in Paralympic athletes. *Br J Sports Med.* 2016;50(17):1075–80. doi:10.1136/bjsports-2015-095867.

30. Palmieri V, Spataro A, Bernardi M. Cardiovascular eligibility in specific conditions: the paralympic athlete. *Med Sport (Roma).* 2010;63(1):95–101.

31. Pepper M, Willick S. Maximizing physical activity in athletes with amputations. *Curr Sports Med Rep.* 2009;8(6):339–44. doi:10.1249/JSR.0b013e3181c1db12.

32. Pitetti KH, Snell PG, Stray-Gundersen J, Gottschalk FA. Aerobic training exercises for individuals who had amputation of the lower limb. *J Bone Joint Surg Am.* 1987;69(6):914–21.

33. Bragaru M, Dekker R, Geertzen JHB, Dijkstra PU. Amputees and sports: a systematic review. *Sports Med.* 2011;41(9):721–40. doi:10.2165/11590420-000000000-00000.

34. James U. Effect of physical training in healthy male unilateral above-knee amputees. *Scand J Rehabil Med.* 1973;5(2):88–101.

35. Davidoff GN, Lampman RM, Westbury L, Deron J, Finestone HM, Islam S. Exercise testing and training of persons with dysvascular amputation: safety and efficacy of arm ergometry. *Arch Phys Med Rehabil.* 1992;73(4):334–8. doi:10.1016/0003-9993(92)90006-I.

36. Bernardi M, Carucci S, Faiola F, et al. Physical fitness evaluation of paralympic winter sports sitting athletes. *Clin J Sport Med.* 2012;22(1):26–30. doi:10.1097/JSM.0b013e31824237b5.

37. Deans S, Burns D, McGarry A, Murray K, Mutrie N. Motivations and barriers to prosthesis users participation in physical activity, exercise and sport: a review of the literature. *Prosthet Orthot Int.* 2012;36(3):260–9. doi:10.1177/0309364612437905.

38. Clarkson HM. *Musculoskeletal Assessment: Joint Motion and Muscle Testing.* 3rd ed. Philadelphia (PA): Wolters Kluwer/Lippincott Williams & Wilkins Health; 2013.

39. Van Alsté JA, La Have MW, Huisman K, de Vries J, Boom HBK. Exercise electrocardiography using rowing ergometry suitable for leg amputees. *Int Rehabil Med.* 1985;7(1):1–5. doi:10.3109/03790798509165968.

40. Brown MB, Millard-Stafford ML, Allison AR. Running-specific prostheses permit energy cost similar to nonamputees. *Med Sci Sports Exerc.* 2009;41(5):1080–7. doi:10.1249/MSS.0b013e3181923cee.

41. Hutzler Y, Meckel Y, Berzen J. Aerobic and anaerobic power. In: Vanlandewijck YC, Thompson WR, editors. *The Paralympic Athlete: Handbook of Sports Medicine and Science.* Chichester, UK: Wiley-Blackwell; 2011. p. 137–55.

42. Bernardi M, Rosponi A, Castellano V, et al. Determinants of sit-to-stand capability in the motor impaired elderly. *J Electromyogr Kinesiol.* 2004;14(3):401–10. doi:10.1016/j.jelekin.2003.09.001.

43. Bernardi M, Macaluso A, Sproviero E, et al. Cost of walking and locomotor impairment. *J Electromyogr Kinesiol.* 1999;9(2):149–57. doi:10.1016/S1050-6411(98)00046-7.

44. American College of Sports Medicine; Liguori G, Feito Y, Fountaine C, Roy B, editors. *ACSM's Guidelines for Exercise Testing and Prescription.* 11th ed. Philadelphia, USA: Wolters Kluwer; 2021.

45. Bernardi M, Castellano V, Ferrara MS, Sbriccoli P, Sera F, Marchetti M. Muscle pain in athletes with locomotor disability:

Med Sci Sports Exerc. 2003;35(2):199–206. doi:10.1249/01.MSS.0000048635.83126.D4.

46. Bernardi M, Guerra E, Di Giacinto B, Di Cesare A, Castellano V, Bhambhani Y. Field evaluation of paralympic athletes in selected sports: implications for training. *Med Sci Sports Exerc.* 2010;42(6):1200–8. doi:10.1249/MSS.0b013e3181c67d82.

47. Bax M. Terminology and classification of cerebral palsy. *Dev Med Child Neurol.* 1964;6:295–7.

48. Rosenbaum P. What causes cerebral palsy? *BMJ.* 2014;349:g4514. doi:10.1136/bmj.g4514.

49. Eek MN, Tranberg R, Zügner R, Alkema K, Beckung E. Muscle strength training to improve gait function in children with cerebral palsy. *Dev Med Child Neurol.* 2008;50(10):759–64. doi:10.1111/j.1469-8749.2008.03045.x.

50. Paneth N, Hong T, Korzeniewski S. The descriptive epidemiology of cerebral palsy. *Clin Perinatol.* 2006;33(2):251–67. doi:10.1016/j.clp.2006.03.011.

51. Christensen D, Van Naarden Braun K, Doernberg NS, et al. Prevalence of cerebral palsy, co-occurring autism spectrum disorders, and motor functioning — Autism and Developmental Disabilities Monitoring Network, USA, 2008. *Dev Med Child Neurol.* 2014;56(1):59–65. doi:10.1111/dmcn.12268.

52. Priego Quesada J, Lucas-Cuevas A, Llana-Belloch S, Perez-Soriano P. Effects of exercise in people with cerebral palsy. A review. *JPES.* 2014;14(1):36–41.

53. Dy R, Frando M, Voto H, Baron K. Pediatric rehabilitation. In: Maitin IB, Cruz E, editors. *Current Diagnosis & Treatment: Physical Medicine & Rehabilitation.* New York, USA: McGraw Hill; 2014. [cited 2021 Oct 20]. Available from: https://accessmedicine.mhmedical.com/content.aspx?bookid=1180&sectionid=70379270.

54. Van Naarden Braun K, Christensen D, Doernberg N, et al. Trends in the prevalence of autism spectrum disorder, cerebral palsy, hearing loss, intellectual disability, and vision impairment, Metropolitan Atlanta, 1991–2010. *PLoS One.* 2015;10(4):e0124120. doi:10.1371/journal.pone.0124120.

55. Jung JW, Her JG, Ko J. Effect of strength training of ankle plantarflexors on selective voluntary motor control gait parameters, and gross motor function of children with cerebral palsy. *J Phys Ther Sci.* 2013;25(10):1259–63. doi:10.1589/jpts.25.1259.

56. Messer R, Schreiner T, Walleigh D, Yang M, Martin J, Demarest S. Neurologic & muscular disorders. In: Hay WW, Levin MJ, Abzug MJ, Bunik M, editors. *Current Diagnosis & Treatment: Pediatrics.* 25th ed. New York, USA: McGraw Hill; 2020. [cited 2021 Oct 29]. Available from: https://accessmedicine.mhmedical.com/content.aspx?bookid=2815&sectionid=244263666.

57. Nelson KB. Causative factors in cerebral palsy. *Clin Obstet Gynecol.* 2008;51(4):749–62. doi:10.1097/GRF.0b013e318187087c.

58. Malone LA, Vogtle LK. Pain and fatigue consistency in adults with cerebral palsy. *Disabil Rehabil.* 2010;32(5):385–91. doi:10.3109/09638280903171550.

59. Peterson MD, Lukasik L, Muth T, et al. Recumbent cross-training is a feasible and safe mode of physical activity for significantly motor-impaired adults with cerebral palsy. *Arch Phys Med Rehabil.* 2013;94(2):401–7. doi:10.1016/j.apmr.2012.09.027.

60. Dallmeijer AJ, Brehm MA. Physical strain of comfortable walking in children with mild cerebral palsy. *Disabil Rehabil.* 2011;33(15-16):1351–7. doi:10.3109/09638288.2010.531374.

61. Maltais D. Cerebral palsy. In: Moore GE, Durstine JL, Painter PL, editors. *ACSM's Exercise Management for Persons with Chronic Diseases and Disabilities.* 4th ed. Champaign (IL): Human Kinetics; 2016. p. 259–66.

62. Laskin J. Cerebral palsy. In: Larry DJ, editor. *ACSM's Exercise Management for Persons with Chronic Diseases and Disabilities.* 3rd ed. Champaign (IL): Human Kinetics; 2009 p. 343–9.

63. Rogers A, Furler BL, Brinks S, Darrah J. A systematic review of the effectiveness of aerobic exercise interventions for children with cerebral palsy: an AACPDM evidence report. *Dev Med Child Neurol.* 2008;50(11):808–14. doi:10.1111/j.1469-8749.2008.03134.x.

64. Damiano DL. Activity, activity, activity: rethinking our physical therapy approach to cerebral palsy. *Phys Ther.* 2006;86(11):1534–40. doi:10.2522/ptj.20050397.

65. Dewar R, Love S, Johnston LM. Exercise interventions improve postural control in children with cerebral palsy: a systematic review. *Dev Med Child Neurol.* 2015;57(6):504–20. doi:10.1111/dmcn.12660.

66. Noorduyn SG, Gorter JW, Verschuren O, Timmons B. Exercise intervention programs for children and adolescents with cerebral palsy: a descriptive review of the current research. *Crit Rev Phys Rehabil Med.* 2011;23(1):31–47.

67. Rosenbaum P, Gorter JW. The "F-words" in childhood disability: I swear this is how we should think! *Child Care Health Dev.* 2012;38(4):457–63. doi:10.1111/j.1365-2214.2011.01338.x.

68. Hombergen SP, Huisstede BM, Streur MF, et al. Impact of cerebral palsy on health — related physical fitness in adults: systematic review. *Arch Phys Med Rehabil.* 2012;93(5):871–81. doi:10.1016/j.apmr.2011.11.032.

69. Mcnee AE, Gough M, Morrissey MC, Shortland AP. Increases in muscle volume after plantarflexor strength training in children with spastic cerebral palsy. *Dev Med Child Neurol.* 2009;51(6):429–35. doi:10.1111/j.1469-8749.2008.03230.x.

70. Shortland A. Muscle deficits in cerebral palsy and early loss of mobility: can we learn something from our elders? *Dev Med Child Neurol.* 2009;51:59–63. doi:10.1111/j.1469-8749.2009.03434.x.

71. Rose J, McGill KC. Neuromuscular activation and motor-unit firing characteristics in cerebral palsy. *Dev Med Child Neurol.* 2005;47(5):329–36. doi:10.1017/S0012162205000629.

72. Stackhouse SK, Binder-Macleod SA, Lee SCK. Voluntary muscle activation, contractile properties, and fatigability in children with and without cerebral palsy. *Muscle Nerve.* 2005;31(5):594–601. doi:10.1002/mus.20302.

73. Peterson MD, Gordon PM, Hurvitz EA, Burant CF. Secondary muscle pathology and metabolic dysregulation in adults with cerebral palsy. *Am J Physiol Endocrinol Metab.* 2012;303(9):E1085–93. doi:10.1152/ajpendo.00338.2012.

74. Unnithan VB, Clifford C, Bar-Or O. Evaluation by exercise testing of the child with cerebral palsy: *Sports Med.* 1998;26(4):239–51. doi:10.2165/00007256-199826040-00003.

75. Martin L, Baker R, Harvey A. A systematic review of common physiotherapy interventions in school-aged children with cerebral palsy. *Phys Occup Ther Pediatr.* 2010;30(4):294–312. doi:10.3109/01942638.2010.500581.

76. Ryan JM, Forde C, Hussey JM, Gormley J. Comparison of patterns of physical activity and sedentary behavior between children with cerebral palsy and children with typical

development. *Phys Ther.* 2015;95(12):1609–16. doi:10.2522/ptj.20140337.

77. Lundberg Å. Maximal aerobic capacity of young people with spastic cerebral palsy. *Dev Med Child Neurol.* 1978;20(2):205–10. doi:10.1111/j.1469-8749.1978.tb15205.x.

78. Leunkeu AN, Gayda M, Nigam A, Lecoutre N, Ahmaidi S. Cardiopulmonary exercise data during quadriceps isometric contraction sustained to fatigue in children with cerebral palsy. *Isokinet Exercise Sci.* 2009;17(1):27–33. doi:10.3233/IES-2009-0328.

79. Maltais DB, Wiart L, Fowler E, Verschuren O, Damiano DL. Health-related physical fitness for children with cerebral palsy. *J Child Neurol.* 2014;29(8):1091–100. doi:10.1177/0883073814533152.

80. Butler JM, Scianni A, Ada L. Effect of cardiorespiratory training on aerobic fitness and carryover to activity in children with cerebral palsy: a systematic review. *Int J Rehabil Res.* 2010;33(2):97–103. doi:10.1097/MRR.0b013e328331c555.

81. Verschuren O, Peterson MD, Balemans ACJ, Hurvitz EA. Exercise and physical activity recommendations for people with cerebral palsy. *Dev Med Child Neurol.* 2016;58(8):798–808. doi:10.1111/dmcn.13053.

82. Van Den Berg-Emons RJ, Van Baak MA, Speth L, Saris WH. Physical training of school children with spastic cerebral palsy: effects on daily activity, fat mass and fitness. *Int J Rehabil Res.* 1998;21(2):179–94. doi:10.1097/00004356-199806000-00006.

83. Verschuren O, Ketelaar M, Gorter JW, Helders PJM, Uiterwaal CSPM, Takken T. Exercise training program in children and adolescents with cerebral palsy: a randomized controlled trial. *Arch Pediatr Adolesc Med.* 2007;161(11):1075–81. doi:10.1001/archpedi.161.11.1075.

84. Fowler EG, Kolobe TH, Damiano DL, et al; Section on Pediatrics Research Summit Participants; Section on Pediatrics Research Committee Task Force. Promotion of physical fitness and prevention of secondary conditions for children with cerebral palsy: section on pediatrics research summit proceedings. *Phys Ther.* 2007;87(11):1495–510. doi:10.2522/ptj.20060116.

85. Ross SM, MacDonald M, Bigouette JP. Effects of strength training on mobility in adults with cerebral palsy: a systematic review. *Disabil Health J.* 2016;9(3):375–84. doi:10.1016/j.dhjo.2016.04.005.

86. Vogtle LK, Malone LA, Azuero A. Outcomes of an exercise program for pain and fatigue management in adults with cerebral palsy. *Disabil Rehabil.* 2014;36(10):818–25. doi:10.3109/09638288.2013.821181.

87. Barfield JP, Malone LA. Perceived exercise benefits and barriers among power wheelchair soccer players. *J Rehabil Res Dev.* 2013;50(2):231–8. doi:10.1682/JRRD.2011.12.0234.

88. Malone LA, Barfield JP, Brasher JD. Perceived benefits and barriers to exercise among persons with physical disabilities or chronic health conditions within action or maintenance stages of exercise. *Disabil Health J.* 2012;5(4):254–60. doi:10.1016/j.dhjo.2012.05.004.

89. Slaman J, Roebroeck M, van der Slot W, et al; LEARN 2 MOVE Research Group. Can a lifestyle intervention improve physical fitness in adolescents and young adults with spastic cerebral palsy? A randomized controlled trial. *Arch Phys Med Rehabil.* 2014;95(9):1646–55. doi:10.1016/j.apmr.2014.05.011.

90. Slaman J, van den Berg-Emons H, van Meeteren J, et al. A lifestyle intervention improves fatigue, mental health and social support among adolescents and young adults with cerebral palsy: focus on mediating effects. *Clin Rehabil.* 2015;29(7):717–27. doi:10.1177/0269215514555136.

91. Unger M, Faure M, Frieg A. Strength training in adolescent learners with cerebral palsy: a randomized controlled trial. *Clin Rehabil.* 2006;20(6):469–77. doi:10.1191/0269215506cr961oa.

92. Jeng SC, Yeh KK, Liu WY, et al. A physical fitness follow-up in children with cerebral palsy receiving 12-week individualized exercise training. *Res Dev Disabil.* 2013;34(11):4017–24. doi:10.1016/j.ridd.2013.08.032.

93. Mulroy SJ, Winstein CJ, Kulig K, et al; Physical Therapy Clinical Research Network. Secondary mediation and regression analyses of the PTClinResNet Database: determining causal relationships among the International Classification of Functioning, Disability and Health levels for four physical therapy intervention trials. *Phys Ther.* 2011;91(12):1766–79. doi:10.2522/ptj.20110024.

94. Nsenga A, Shephard R, Ahmadi S. Aerobic training in children with cerebral palsy. *Int J Sports Med.* 2012;34(6):533–7. doi:10.1055/s-0032-1321803.

95. Scholtes VA, Becher JG, Comuth A, Dekkers H, Van Dijk L, Dallmeijer AJ. Effectiveness of functional progressive resistance exercise strength training on muscle strength and mobility in children with cerebral palsy: a randomized controlled trial. *Dev Med Child Neurol.* 2010;52(6):e107–13. doi:10.1111/j.1469-8749.2009.03604.x.

96. Park EY, Kim WH. Meta-analysis of the effect of strengthening interventions in individuals with cerebral palsy. *Res Dev Disabil.* 2014;35(2):239–49. doi:10.1016/j.ridd.2013.10.021.

97. Auld ML, Johnston LM. "Strong and steady": a community-based strength and balance exercise group for children with cerebral palsy. *Disabil Rehabil.* 2014;36(24):2065–71. doi:10.3109/09638288.2014.891054.

98. Thompson N, Stebbins J, Seniorou M, Newham D. Muscle strength and walking ability in diplegic cerebral palsy: implications for assessment and management. *Gait Posture.* 2011;33(3):321–5. doi:10.1016/j.gaitpost.2010.10.091.

99. Taylor NF, Dodd KJ, Baker RJ, Willoughby K, Thomason P, Graham HK. Progressive resistance training and mobility-related function in young people with cerebral palsy: a randomized controlled trial. *Dev Med Child Neurol.* 2013;55(9):806–12. doi:10.1111/dmcn.12190.

100. Gillett JG, Lichtwark GA, Boyd RN, Barber LA. FAST CP: protocol of a randomised controlled trial of the efficacy of a 12-week combined functional anaerobic and strength training programme on muscle properties and mechanical gait deficiencies in adolescents and young adults with spastic-type cerebral palsy. *BMJ Open.* 2015;5(6):e008059. doi:10.1136/bmjopen-2015-008059.

101. Lee JA, You JH, Kim DA, et al. Effects of functional movement strength training on strength, muscle size, kinematics, and motor function in cerebral palsy: a 3-month follow-up. *NeuroRehabilitation.* 2013;32(2):287–95. doi:10.3233/NRE-130846.

102. Lee M, Ko Y, Shin MMS, Lee W. The effects of progressive functional training on lower limb muscle architecture and

motor function in children with spastic cerebral palsy. *J Phys Ther Sci*. 2015;27(5):1581–4. doi:10.1589/jpts.27.1581.

103. Lee DR, Kim YH, Kim DA, et al. Innovative strength training-induced neuroplasticity and increased muscle size and strength in children with spastic cerebral palsy: an experimenter-blind case study — three-month follow-up. *NeuroRehabilitation*. 2014;35(1):131–136. doi:10.3233/NRE-131036.

104. Olsen JE, Ross SA, Foreman MH, Engsberg JR. Changes in muscle activation following ankle strength training in children with spastic cerebral palsy: an electromyography feasibility case report. *Phys Occup Ther Pediatr*. 2013;33(2):230–42. doi:10.3109/01942638.2012.723116.

105. Ryan JM, Cassidy EE, Noorduyn SG, O'Connell NE. Exercise interventions for cerebral palsy. *Cochrane Database Syst Rev*. 2017;6(6):CD011660. doi:10.1002/14651858.CD011660.pub2.

106. Liao H-F, Liu Y-C, Liu W-Y, Lin Y-T. Effectiveness of loaded sit-to-stand resistance exercise for children with mild spastic diplegia: a randomized clinical trial. *Arch Phys Med Rehabil*. 2007;88(1):25–31. doi:10.1016/j.apmr.2006.10.006.

107. Ross SA, Engsberg JR. Relationships between spasticity, strength, gait, and the GMFM-66 in persons with spastic diplegia cerebral palsy. *Arch Phys Med Rehabil*. 2007;88(9): 1114–20. doi:10.1016/j.apmr.2007.06.011.

108. Damiano DL, Arnold AS, Steele KM, Delp SL. Can strength training predictably improve gait kinematics? A pilot study on the effects of hip and knee extensor strengthening on lower-extremity alignment in cerebral palsy. *Phys Ther*. 2010;90(2):269–79. doi:10.2522/ptj.20090062.

109. Salem Y, Godwin EM. Effects of task-oriented training on mobility function in children with cerebral palsy. *NeuroRehabilitation*. 2009;24(4):307–13. doi:10.3233/NRE-2009-0483.

110. dos Santos AN, da Costa CSN, Golineleo MTB, Rocha NACF. Functional strength training in child with cerebral palsy GMFCS IV: case report. *Dev Neurorehabil*. 2013;16(5):308–14. doi:10.3109/17518423.2012.731085.

111. Moreau NG, Falvo MJ, Damiano DL. Rapid force generation is impaired in cerebral palsy and is related to decreased muscle size and functional mobility. *Gait Posture*. 2012;35(1): 154–8. doi:10.1016/j.gaitpost.2011.08.027.

112. Chiu HC, Ada L, Bania TA. Mechanically assisted walking training for walking, participation, and quality of life in children with cerebral palsy. *Cochrane Database Syst Rev*. 2020;11(11):CD013114. doi:10.1002/14651858.CD013114.pub2.

113. Compston A, Coles A. Multiple sclerosis. *Lancet*. 2008;372(9648):1502–17. doi:10.1016/S0140-6736(08)61620-7.

114. Dendrou CA, Fugger L, Friese MA. Immunopathology of multiple sclerosis. *Nat Rev Immunol*. 2015;15(9):545–58. doi:10.1038/nri3871.

115. Thompson AJ, Baranzini SE, Geurts J, Hemmer B, Ciccarelli O. Multiple sclerosis. *Lancet*. 2018;391(10130):1622–36. doi:10.1016/S0140-6736(18)30481-1.

116. Alonso A, Hernan MA. Temporal trends in the incidence of multiple sclerosis: a systematic review. *Neurology*. 2008;71(2): 129–35. doi:10.1212/01.wnl.0000316802.35974.34.

117. Koch-Henriksen N, Sørensen PS. The changing demographic pattern of multiple sclerosis epidemiology. *Lancet Neurol*. 2010;9(5):520–32. doi:10.1016/S1474-4422(10)70064-8.

118. Walton C, King R, Rechtman L, et al. Rising prevalence of multiple sclerosis worldwide: insights from the Atlas of MS, third edition. *Mult Scler*. 2020;26(14):1816–21. doi:10.1177/1352458520970841.

119. Wallin MT, Culpepper WJ, Campbell JD, et al; US Multiple Sclerosis Prevalence Workgroup. The prevalence of MS in the United States: a population-based estimate using health claims data. *Neurology*. 2019;92(10):e1029–40. doi:10.1212/WNL.0000000000007035.

120. Asche CV, Singer ME, Jhaveri M, Chung H, Miller A. All-cause health care utilization and costs associated with newly diagnosed multiple sclerosis in the United States. *J Manag Care Pharm*. 2010;16(9):703–12. doi:10.18553/jmcp.2010.16.9.703.

121. Karampampa K, Gustavsson A, Miltenburger C, Eckert B. Treatment experience, burden and unmet needs (TRIBUNE) in MS study: results from five European countries. *Mult Scler*. 2012;18(Suppl 2):7–15. doi:10.1177/1352458512441566.

122. Parisé H, Laliberté F, Lefebvre P, et al. Direct and indirect cost burden associated with multiple sclerosis relapses: excess costs of persons with MS and their spouse caregivers. *J Neurol Sci*. 2013;330(1–2):71–7. doi:10.1016/j.jns.2013.04.007.

123. Carroll CA, Fairman KA, Lage MJ. Updated cost-of-care estimates for commercially insured patients with multiple sclerosis: retrospective observational analysis of medical and pharmacy claims data. *BMC Health Serv Res*. 2014;14(1):286. doi:10.1186/1472-6963-14-286.

124. Zuvich RL, McCauley JL, Oksenberg JR, et al; International Multiple Sclerosis Genetics. Genetic variation in the IL7RA/IL7 pathway increases multiple sclerosis susceptibility. *Hum Genet*. 2010;127(5):525–35. doi:10.1007/s00439-010-0789-4.

125. Kingwell E, Marriott JJ, Jetté N, et al. Incidence and prevalence of multiple sclerosis in Europe: a systematic review. *BMC Neurol*. 2013;13(1):128. doi:10.1186/1471-2377-13-128.

126. Noonan CW, Williamson DM, Henry JP, et al. The prevalence of multiple sclerosis in 3 US communities. *Prev Chronic Dis*. 2010;7(1):A12.

127. Ascherio A, Munger KL. Environmental risk factors for multiple sclerosis. Part I: the role of infection. *Ann Neurol*. 2007;61(4):288–99. doi:10.1002/ana.21117.

128. Pierrot-Deseilligny C, Souberbielle JC. Contribution of vitamin D insufficiency to the pathogenesis of multiple sclerosis. *Ther Adv Neurol Disord*. 2013;6(2):81–116. doi:10.1177/1756285612473513.

129. Belbasis L, Bellou V, Evangelou E, Ioannidis JPA, Tzoulaki I. Environmental risk factors and multiple sclerosis: an umbrella review of systematic reviews and meta-analyses. *Lancet Neurol*. 2015;14(3):263–73. doi:10.1016/S1474-4422(14)70267-4.

130. Bjornevik K, Cortese M, Healy BC, et al. Longitudinal analysis reveals high prevalence of Epstein–Barr virus associated with multiple sclerosis. *Science*. 2022;375(6578)296–301.

131. Dilokthornsakul P, Valuck RJ, Nair KV, Corboy JR, Allen RR, Campbell JD. Multiple sclerosis prevalence in the United States commercially insured population. *Neurology*. 2016;86(11):1014–21. doi:10.1212/WNL.0000000000002469.

132. Wu GF, Alvarez E. The immunopathophysiology of multiple sclerosis. *Neurol Clin*. 2011;29(2):257–78. doi:10.1016/j.ncl.2010.12.009.

133. Lublin FD, Reingold SC, Cohen JA, et al. Defining the clinical course of multiple sclerosis: the 2013 revisions. *Neurology*. 2014;83(3):278–86. doi:10.1212/WNL.0000000000000560.

134. Coyle P. What can we learn from sex differences in MS? *J Pers Med.* 2021;11(10):1006.
135. Chabas D, Strober J, Waubant E. Pediatric multiple sclerosis. *Curr Neurol Neurosci Rep.* 2008;8(5):434–41. doi:10.1007/s11910-008-0067-1.
136. Polman CH, Reingold SC, Banwell B, et al. Diagnostic criteria for multiple sclerosis: 2010 revisions to the McDonald criteria. *Ann Neurol.* 2011;69(2):292–302. doi:10.1002/ana.22366.
137. Kurtzke JF. Rating neurologic impairment in multiple sclerosis: an expanded disability status scale (EDSS). *Neurology.* 1983;33(11):1444–52. doi:10.1212/WNL.33.11.1444.
138. White LJ, Dressendorfer RH. Exercise and multiple sclerosis: *Sports Med.* 2004;34(15):1077–100. doi:10.2165/00007256-200434150-00005.
139. Latimer-Cheung AE, Pilutti LA, Hicks AL, et al. Effects of exercise training on fitness, mobility, fatigue, and health-related quality of life among adults with multiple sclerosis: a systematic review to inform guideline development. *Arch Phys Med Rehabil.* 2013;94(9):1800–28.e3. doi:10.1016/j.apmr.2013.04.020.
140. Motl RW, Sandroff BM. Benefits of exercise training in multiple sclerosis. *Curr Neurol Neurosci Rep.* 2015;15(9):62. doi:10.1007/s11910-015-0585-6.
141. Rietberg MB, van Wegen EEH, Kollen BJ, Kwakkel G. Do patients with multiple sclerosis show different daily physical activity patterns from healthy individuals? *Neurorehabil Neural Repair.* 2014;28(6):516–23. doi:10.1177/1545968313520412.
142. Ezeugwu V, Klaren RE, Hubbard EA, Manns PT, Motl RW. Mobility disability and the pattern of accelerometer-derived sedentary and physical activity behaviors in people with multiple sclerosis. *Prev Med Rep.* 2015;2:241–6. doi:10.1016/j.pmedr.2015.03.007.
143. Veldhuijzen van Zanten JJ, Pilutti LA, Duda JL, Motl RW. Sedentary behaviour in people with multiple sclerosis: is it time to stand up against MS? *Mult Scler.* 2016;22(10):1250–6. doi:10.1177/1352458516644340.
144. Motl RW, Sandroff BM, Kwakkel G, et al. Exercise in patients with multiple sclerosis. *Lancet Neurol.* 2017;16(10):848–56. doi:10.1016/S1474-4422(17)30281-8.
145. Motl RW, Fernhall B. Accurate prediction of cardiorespiratory fitness using cycle ergometry in minimally disabled persons with relapsing-remitting multiple sclerosis. *Arch Phys Med Rehabil.* 2012;93(3):490–5. doi:10.1016/j.apmr.2011.08.025.
146. Guerra E, di Cagno A, Mancini P, et al. Physical fitness assessment in multiple sclerosis patients: a controlled study. *Res Dev Disabil.* 2014;35(10):2527–33. doi:10.1016/j.ridd.2014.06.013.
147. Klaren RE, Sandroff BM, Fernhall B, Motl RW. Comprehensive profile of cardiopulmonary exercise testing in ambulatory persons with multiple sclerosis. *Sports Med.* 2016;46(9):1365–79. doi:10.1007/s40279-016-0472-6.
148. Olgiati R, Jacquet J, Di Prampero PE. Energy cost of walking and exertional dyspnea in multiple sclerosis. *Am Rev Respir Dis.* 1986;134(5):1005–10. doi:10.1164/arrd.1986.134.5.1005.
149. Motl RW, Snook EM, Agiovlasitis S, Suh Y. Calibration of accelerometer output for ambulatory adults with multiple sclerosis. *Arch Phys Med Rehabil.* 2009;90(10):1778–84. doi:10.1016/j.apmr.2009.03.020.
150. Olgiati R, Burgunder JM, Mumenthaler M. Increased energy cost of walking in multiple sclerosis: effect of spasticity, ataxia, and weakness. *Arch Phys Med Rehabil.* 1988;69(10):846–9.
151. Sosnoff JJ, Sandroff BM, Motl RW. Quantifying gait abnormalities in persons with multiple sclerosis with minimal disability. *Gait Posture.* 2012;36(1):154–6. doi:10.1016/j.gaitpost.2011.11.027.
152. Kent-Braun JA, Ng AV, Castro M, et al. Strength, skeletal muscle composition, and enzyme activity in multiple sclerosis. *J Appl Physiol (1985).* 1997;83(6):1998–2004. doi:10.1152/jappl.1997.83.6.1998.
153. Huang M, Jay O, Davis SL. Autonomic dysfunction in multiple sclerosis: implications for exercise. *Auton Neurosci.* 2015;188:82–5. doi:10.1016/j.autneu.2014.10.017.
154. Davis SL, Wilson TE, White AT, Frohman EM. Thermoregulation in multiple sclerosis. *J Appl Physiol (1985).* 2010;109(5):1531–7. doi:10.1152/japplphysiol.00460.2010.
155. Hohol MJ, Orav EJ, Weiner HL. Disease Steps in multiple sclerosis: a simple approach to evaluate disease progression. *Neurology.* 1995;45(2):251–5. doi:10.1212/WNL.45.2.251.
156. Hobart JC, Riazi A, Lamping DL, Fitzpatrick R, Thompson AJ. Measuring the impact of MS on walking ability: the 12-Item MS Walking Scale (MSWS-12). *Neurology.* 2003;60(1):31–6. doi:10.1212/WNL.60.1.31.
157. Agiovlasitis S, Motl RW. Cross-validation of oxygen uptake prediction during walking in ambulatory persons with multiple sclerosis. *NeuroRehabilitation.* 2016;38(2):191–7. doi:10.3233/NRE-161310.
158. Agiovlasitis S, Sandroff BM, Motl RW. Prediction of oxygen uptake during walking in ambulatory persons with multiple sclerosis. *J Rehabil Res Dev.* 2016;53(2):199–206. doi:10.1682/JRRD.2014.12.0307.
159. Paul L, Coote S, Crosbie J, et al. Core outcome measures for exercise studies in people with multiple sclerosis: recommendations from a multidisciplinary consensus meeting. *Mult Scler.* 2014;20(12):1641–50. doi:10.1177/1352458514526944.
160. Learmonth YC, Motl RW. Physical activity and exercise training in multiple sclerosis: a review and content analysis of qualitative research identifying perceived determinants and consequences. *Disabil Rehabil.* 2016;38(13):1227–42. doi:10.3109/09638288.2015.1077397.
161. Streber R, Peters S, Pfeifer K. Systematic review of correlates and determinants of physical activity in persons with multiple sclerosis. *Arch Phys Med Rehabil.* 2016;97(4):633–45.e29. doi:10.1016/j.apmr.2015.11.020.
162. Kalb R, Brown TR, Coote S, et al. Exercise and lifestyle physical activity recommendations for people with multiple sclerosis throughout the disease course. *Mult Scler.* 2020;26(12):1459–69. doi:10.1177/1352458520915629.
163. Agiovlasitis S, Motl R, Fernhall B. Prediction of oxygen uptake during level treadmill walking in people with multiple sclerosis. *J Rehabil Med.* 2010;42(7):650–5. doi:10.2340/16501977-0570.
164. Campbell E, Coulter EH, Paul L. High intensity interval training for people with multiple sclerosis: a systematic review. *Mult Scler Relat Disord.* 2018;24:55–63. doi:10.1016/j.msard.2018.06.005.
165. Marras C, Beck JC, Bower JH, et al; Parkinson's Foundation P4 Group. Prevalence of Parkinson's disease across North America. *NPJ Parkinsons Dis.* 2018;4(1):21. doi:10.1038/s41531-018-0058-0.
166. Tysnes OB, Storstein A. Epidemiology of Parkinson's disease. *J Neural Transm (Vienna).* 2017;124(8):901–5. doi:10.1007/s00702-017-1686-y.

167. Boland DF, Stacy M. The economic and quality of life burden associated with Parkinson's disease: a focus on symptoms. *Am J Manag Care*. 2012;18(Suppl 7):S168–75.

168. Balestrino R, Schapira AHV. Parkinson disease. *Eur J Neurol*. 2020;27(1):27–42. doi:10.1111/ene.14108.

169. Aarsland D, Kurz MW. The epidemiology of dementia associated with Parkinson's disease. *Brain Pathol*. 2010;20(3):633–9. doi:10.1111/j.1750-3639.2009.00369.x.

170. Miller DB, O'Callaghan JP. Biomarkers of Parkinson's disease: present and future. *Metabolism*. 2015;64(3 Suppl 1):S40–6. doi:10.1016/j.metabol.2014.10.030.

171. Jankovic J, Sherer T. The future of research in Parkinson disease. *JAMA Neurol*. 2014;71(11):1351–2. doi:10.1001/jamaneurol.2014.1717.

172. Tolosa E, Garrido A, Scholz SW, Poewe W. Challenges in the diagnosis of Parkinson's disease. *Lancet Neurol*. 2021;20(5):385–97. doi:10.1016/S1474-4422(21)00030-2.

173. Tranchant C. Introduction and classical environmental risk factors for Parkinson. *Rev Neurol (Paris)*. 2019;175(10):650–1. doi:10.1016/j.neurol.2019.04.006.

174. Polito L, Greco A, Seripa D. Genetic profile, environmental exposure, and their interaction in Parkinson's disease. *Parkinsons Dis*. 2016;2016:6465793. doi:10.1155/2016/6465793.

175. Ovallath S, Sulthana B. Levodopa: history and therapeutic applications. *Ann Indian Acad Neurol*. 2017;20(3):185–9. doi:10.4103/aian.AIAN_241_17.

176. Cabreira V, Soares-da-Silva P, Massano J. Contemporary options for the management of motor complications in Parkinson's disease: updated clinical review. *Drugs*. 2019;79(6):593–608. doi:10.1007/s40265-019-01098-w.

177. Tsuboi T, Lemos Melo Lobo Jofili Lopes J, Moore K, et al. Long-term clinical outcomes of bilateral GPi deep brain stimulation in advanced Parkinson's disease: 5 years and beyond. *J Neurosurg*. 2021;135(2):601–10. doi:10.3171/2020.6.JNS20617.

178. Cruz-Jentoft AJ, Baeyens JP, Bauer JM, et al; European Working Group on Sarcopenia in Older People. Sarcopenia: European consensus on definition and diagnosis: report of the European Working Group on Sarcopenia in Older People. *Age Ageing*. 2010;39(4):412–23. doi:10.1093/ageing/afq034.

179. Marcell TJ. Sarcopenia: causes, consequences, and preventions. *J Gerontol A Biol Sci Med Sci*. 2003;58(10):M911–6. doi:10.1093/gerona/58.10.M911.

180. Gamborg M, Hvid LG, Dalgas U, Langeskov-Christensen M. Parkinson's disease and intensive exercise therapy — an updated systematic review and meta-analysis. *Acta Neurol Scand*. 2022;145(5):504–28. doi:10.1111/ane.13579.

181. Goetz CG, Fahn S, Martinez-Martin P, et al. Movement Disorder Society-sponsored revision of the Unified Parkinson's Disease Rating Scale (MDS-UPDRS): process, format, and clinimetric testing plan. *Mov Disord*. 2007;22(1):41–7. doi:10.1002/mds.21198.

182. Chung CLH, Thilarajah S, Tan D. Effectiveness of resistance training on muscle strength and physical function in people with Parkinson's disease: a systematic review and meta-analysis. *Clin Rehabil*. 2016;30(1):11–23. doi:10.1177/0269215515570381.

183. Scandalis TA, Bosak A, Berliner JC, Helman LL, Wells MR. Resistance training and gait function in patients with Parkinson's disease. *Am J Phys Med Rehabil*. 2001;80(1):38–43. doi:10.1097/00002060-200101000-00011.

184. Kelly NA, Ford MP, Standaert DG, et al. Novel, high-intensity exercise prescription improves muscle mass, mitochondrial function, and physical capacity in individuals with Parkinson's disease. *J Appl Physiol (1985)*. 2014;116(5):582–92. doi:10.1152/japplphysiol.01277.2013.

185. Corcos DM, Robichaud JA, David FJ, et al. A two-year randomized controlled trial of progressive resistance exercise for Parkinson's disease. *Mov Disord*. 2013;28(9):1230–40. doi:10.1002/mds.25380.

186. Fleg JL, Morrell CH, Bos AG, et al. Accelerated longitudinal decline of aerobic capacity in healthy older adults. *Circulation*. 2005;112(5):674–82. doi:10.1161/CIRCULATIONAHA.105.545459.

187. Jackson AS, Sui X, Hébert JR, Church TS, Blair SN. Role of lifestyle and aging on the longitudinal change in cardiorespiratory fitness. *Arch Intern Med*. 2009;169(19):1781–7. doi:10.1001/archinternmed.2009.312.

188. Shulman LM, Katzel LI, Ivey FM, et al. Randomized clinical trial of 3 types of physical exercise for patients with Parkinson disease. *JAMA Neurol*. 2013;70(2):183–90. doi:10.1001/jamaneurol.2013.646.

189. Ridgel AL, Vitek JL, Alberts JL. Forced, not voluntary, exercise improves motor function in Parkinson's disease patients. *Neurorehabil Neural Repair*. 2009;23(6):600–8. doi:10.1177/1545968308328726.

190. Schenkman M, Hall DA, Barón AE, Schwartz RS, Mettler P, Kohrt WM. Exercise for people in early- or mid-stage Parkinson disease: a 16-month randomized controlled trial. *Phys Ther*. 2012;92(11):1395–410. doi:10.2522/ptj.20110472.

191. Dağ F, Çimen ÖB, Doğu O. The effects of arm crank training on aerobic capacity, physical performance, quality of life, and health-related disability in patients with Parkinson's disease. *Ir J Med Sci*. 2022;191(3):1341–8. doi:10.1007/s11845-021-02772-3.

192. Beall EB, Lowe MJ, Alberts JL, et al. The effect of forced-exercise therapy for Parkinson's disease on motor cortex functional connectivity. *Brain Connect*. 2013;3(2):190–8. doi:10.1089/brain.2012.0104.

193. Combs SA, Diehl MD, Staples WH, et al. Boxing training for patients with Parkinson disease: a case series. *Phys Ther*. 2011;91(1):132–42. doi:10.2522/ptj.20100142.

194. Hackney ME, Earhart GM. Effects of dance on gait and balance in Parkinson's disease: a comparison of partnered and nonpartnered dance movement. *Neurorehabil Neural Repair*. 2010;24(4):384–92. doi:10.1177/1545968309353329.

195. Pereira APS, Marinho V, Gupta D, Magalhães F, Ayres C, Teixeira S. Music therapy and dance as gait rehabilitation in patients with Parkinson disease: a review of evidence. *J Geriatr Psychiatry Neurol*. 2019;32(1):49–56. doi:10.1177/0891988718819858.

196. Field-Fote E. Spinal cord injury: an overview. In: Field-Fote E, editor. *Spinal Cord Injury Rehabilitation*. Philadelphia (PA): F.A. Davis; 2009.

197. Singh A, Tetreault L, Kalsi-Ryan S, Nouri A, Fehlings MG. Global prevalence and incidence of traumatic spinal cord injury. *Clin Epidemiol*. 2014;6:309–31. doi:10.2147/CLEP.S68889.

198. World Health Organization. Spinal cord injury. 2013. Available from: http://www.who.int/en/news-room/fact-sheets/detail/spinal-cord-injury.

199. Cao Y, Chen Y, DeVivo M. Lifetime direct costs after spinal cord injury. *Top Spinal Cord Inj Rehabil.* 2011;16(4):10–6. doi:10.1310/sci1604-10.

200. Bakkum A, Paulson T, Bishop N, et al. Effects of hybrid cycle and handcycle exercise on cardiovascular disease risk factors in people with spinal cord injury: a randomized controlled trial. *J Rehabil Med.* 2015;47(6):523–30. doi:10.2340/16501977-1946.

201. Cowan R, Malone L, Nash M. Exercise is Medicine™: exercise prescription after SCI to manage cardiovascular disease risk factors. *Top Spinal Cord Inj Rehabil.* 2009;14(3):69–83. doi:10.1310/sci1403-69.

202. Kirshblum SC, Burns SP, Biering-Sorensen F, et al. International standards for neurological classification of spinal cord injury (revised 2011). *J Spinal Cord Med.* 2011;34(6):535–46. doi:10.1179/204577211X13207446293695.

203. American Spinal Injury Association. International Standards for Neurological Classification of Spinal Cord Injury (ISNCSCI) worksheet. 2019. Available from: https://asia-spinalinjury.org/international-standards-neurological-classification-sci-isncsci-worksheet/.

204. Eck J. Spinal cord injury: treatments and rehabilitation. 2015. [cited 2022 Mar 28]. Available from: https://www.medicinenet.com/spinal_cord_injury_treatments_and_rehabilitation/article.htm.

205. National Spinal Cord Injury Statistical Center. *Spinal Cord Injury: Facts and Figures at a Glance.* Birmingham (AL): University of Alabama at Birmingham; 2016. Available from: https://www.nscisc.uab.edu/public_pages/FactsFiguresArchives/SCI%20Facts%20and%20Figures%20at%20a%20Glance%202016.pdf.

206. Adriaansen J, Post M, Groot S, et al. Secondary health conditions in persons with spinal cord injury: a longitudinal study from one to five years post-discharge. *J Rehabil Med.* 2013;45(10):1016–22. doi:10.2340/16501977-1207.

207. Smit CAJ, de Groot S, Stolwijk-Swuste JM, Janssen TWJ. Effects of electrical stimulation on risk factors for developing pressure ulcers in people with a spinal cord injury: a focused review of literature. *Am J Phys Med Rehabil.* 2016;95(7):535–52. doi:10.1097/PHM.0000000000000501.

208. Krassioukov A, West C. The role of autonomic function on sport performance in athletes with spinal cord injury. *PM R.* 2014;6(Suppl 8):S58–65. doi:10.1016/j.pmrj.2014.05.023.

209. Valent L, Dallmeijer A, Houdijk H, Talsma E, van der Woude L. The effects of upper body exercise on the physical capacity of people with a spinal cord injury: a systematic review. *Clin Rehabil.* 2007;21(4):315–30. doi:10.1177/0269215507073385.

210. Price MJ. Thermoregulation during exercise in individuals with spinal cord injuries. *Sports Med.* 2006;36(10):863–79. doi:10.2165/00007256-200636100-00005.

211. Price M. Energy expenditure and metabolism during exercise in persons with a spinal cord injury. *Sports Med.* 2010;40(8):681–96.

212. van der Scheer JW, Martin Ginis KA, Ditor DS, et al. Effects of exercise on fitness and health of adults with spinal cord injury: a systematic review. *Neurology.* 2017;89(7):736–45. doi:10.1212/WNL.0000000000004224.

213. de Groot S, Dallmeijer AJ, Post MWM, Angenot ELD, van der Woude LHV. The longitudinal relationship between lipid profile and physical capacity in persons with a recent spinal cord injury. *Spinal Cord.* 2008;46(5):344–51. doi:10.1038/sj.sc.3102147.

214. Postma K, Haisma JA, de Groot S, et al. Changes in pulmonary function during the early years after inpatient rehabilitation in persons with spinal cord injury: a prospective cohort study. *Arch Phys Med Rehabil.* 2013;94(8):1540–6. doi:10.1016/j.apmr.2013.02.006.

215. Kilkens OJ, Dallmeijer AJ, Nene AV, Post MW, van der Woude LH. The longitudinal relation between physical capacity and wheelchair skill performance during inpatient rehabilitation of people with spinal cord injury. *Arch Phys Med Rehabil.* 2005;86(8):1575–81. doi:10.1016/j.apmr.2005.03.020.

216. Velzen J, Leeuwen C, Groot S, Woude L, Faber W, Post M. Return to work five years after spinal cord injury inpatient rehabilitation: is it related to wheelchair capacity at discharge? *J Rehabil Med.* 2012;44(1):73–9. doi:10.2340/16501977-0899.

217. Hicks AL, Martin KA, Ditor DS, et al. Long-term exercise training in persons with spinal cord injury: effects on strength, arm ergometry performance and psychological well-being. *Spinal Cord.* 2003;41(1):34–43. doi:10.1038/sj.sc.3101389.

218. van Koppenhagen CF, Post M, de Groot S, et al. Longitudinal relationship between wheelchair exercise capacity and life satisfaction in patients with spinal cord injury: a cohort study in the Netherlands. *J Spinal Cord Med.* 2014;37(3):328–37. doi:10.1179/2045772313Y.0000000167.

219. Post MWM, van Asbeck FWA, van Dijk AJ, Schrijvers AJP. Services for spinal cord injured: availability and satisfaction. *Spinal Cord.* 1997;35(2):109–15. doi:10.1038/sj.sc.3100362.

220. Dallmeijer AJ, Zentgraaff IDB, Zijp NI, van der Woude LHV. Submaximal physical strain and peak performance in handcycling versus handrim wheelchair propulsion. *Spinal Cord.* 2004;42(2):91–8. doi:10.1038/sj.sc.3101566.

221. Arnet U, vanDrongelen S, Scheel-Sailer A, van der Woude LH, Veeger DH. Shoulder load during synchronous handcycling and handrim wheelchair propulsion in persons with paraplegia. *J Rehabil Med.* 2012;44(3):222–8. doi:10.2340/16501977-0929.

222. Valent LJM, Dallmeijer AJ, Houdijk H, et al. Effects of hand cycle training on physical capacity in individuals with tetraplegia: a clinical trial. *Phys Ther.* 2009;89(10):1051–60. doi:10.2522/ptj.20080340.

223. Hoekstra S, Valent L, Gobets D, van der Woude L, de Groot S. Effects of four-month handbike training under free-living conditions on physical fitness and health in wheelchair users. *Disabil Rehabil.* 2017;39(16):1581–8. doi:10.1080/09638288.2016.1200677.

224. Goosey-Tolfrey V. BASES physiological testing guidelines: the disabled athlete. In: Winter EM, Jones AM, Davison RCR, Bromley PD, Mercer TH, editors. *Sport and Exercise Physiology Testing Guidelines: Volume 1—The British Association of Sport and Exercise Sciences Guide.* London, UK: Routledge; 2007. p. 358–67.

225. Burnham R, Wheeler G, Bhambhani Y, Eriksson P, Steadward R. Intentional induction of autonomic dysreflexia among quadriplegic athletes for performance enhancement: efficacy, safety, and mechanism of action. *Clin J Sport Med.* 1994;4(1):1–10.

226. Bhambhani Y, Mactavish J, Warren S, et al. Boosting in athletes with high-level spinal cord injury: knowledge, incidence and attitudes of athletes in paralympic sport. *Disabil Rehabil.* 2010;32(26):2172–90. doi:10.3109/09638288.2010.505678.

227. Griggs KE, Price MJ, Goosey-Tolfrey VL. Cooling athletes with a spinal cord injury. *Sports Med.* 2015;45(1):9–21. doi:10.1007/s40279-014-0241-3.

228. Hicks AL, Martin Ginis KA, Pelletier CA, Ditor DS, Foulon B, Wolfe DL. The effects of exercise training on physical capacity, strength, body composition and functional performance among adults with spinal cord injury: a systematic review. *Spinal Cord.* 2011;49(11):1103–27. doi:10.1038/sc.2011.62.

229. Ginis KAM, Hicks AL, Latimer AE, et al. The development of evidence-informed physical activity guidelines for adults with spinal cord injury. *Spinal Cord.* 2011;49(11):1088–96. doi:10.1038/sc.2011.63.

230. Martin Ginis KA, van der Scheer JW, Latimer-Cheung AE, et al. Evidence-based scientific exercise guidelines for adults with spinal cord injury: an update and a new guideline. *Spinal Cord.* 2018;56(4):308–21. doi:10.1038/s41393-017-0017-3.

231. Pelletier CA, Totosy de Zepetnek JO, MacDonald MJ, Hicks AL. A 16-week randomized controlled trial evaluating the physical activity guidelines for adults with spinal cord injury. *Spinal Cord.* 2015;53(5):363–7. doi:10.1038/sc.2014.167.

232. International Wheelchair Rugby Federation. Introduction to wheelchair rugby. 2016. Available from: https://worldwheelchair.rugby/about-the-sport/.

233. International Paralympic Committee. Paralympic sports. 2016. Available from: https://www.paralympic.org/sports.

234. Abel T, Platen P, Rojas Vega S, Schneider S, Strüder HK. Energy expenditure in ball games for wheelchair users. *Spinal Cord.* 2008;46(12):785–90. doi:10.1038/sc.2008.54.

235. Eriks-Hoogland IE, Hoekstra T, de Groot S, Stucki G, Post MW, van der Woude LH. Trajectories of musculoskeletal shoulder pain after spinal cord injury: identification and predictors. *J Spinal Cord Med.* 2014;37(3):288–98. doi:10.1179/2045772313Y.0000000168.

236. Haskell WL. J.B. Wolffe Memorial Lecture. Health consequences of physical activity: understanding and challenges regarding dose-response. *Med Sci Sports Exerc.* 1994;26(6):649–60. doi:10.1249/00005768-199406000-00001.

237. Raymond J, Davis GM, Climstein M, Sutton JR. Cardiorespiratory responses to arm cranking and electrical stimulation leg cycling in people with paraplegia. *Med Sci Sports Exerc.* 1999;31(6):822–8. doi:10.1097/00005768-199906000-00010.

238. Davis GM, Hamzaid NA, Fornusek C. Cardiorespiratory, metabolic, and biomechanical responses during functional electrical stimulation leg exercise: health and fitness benefits. *Artif Organs.* 2008;32(8):625–9. doi:10.1111/j.1525-1594.2008.00622.x.

239. Wilbanks SR, Rogers R, Pool S, Bickel CS. Effects of functional electrical stimulation assisted rowing on aerobic fitness and shoulder pain in manual wheelchair users with spinal cord injury. *J Spinal Cord Med.* 2016;39(6):645–54. doi:10.1179/2045772315Y.0000000052.

240. Martin Ginis KA, Latimer AE, Arbour-Nicitopoulos KP, et al. Leisure time physical activity in a population-based sample of people with spinal cord injury part I: demographic and injury-related correlates. *Arch Phys Med Rehabil.* 2010;91(5):722–8. doi:10.1016/j.apmr.2009.12.027.

241. DiPiro ND, Embry AE, Fritz SL, Middleton A, Krause JS, Gregory CM. Effects of aerobic exercise training on fitness and walking-related outcomes in ambulatory individuals with chronic incomplete spinal cord injury. *Spinal Cord.* 2016;54(9):675–81. doi:10.1038/sc.2015.212.

242. Rimmer JH. Getting beyond the plateau: bridging the gap between rehabilitation and community-based exercise. *PM R.* 2012;4(11):857–61. doi:10.1016/j.pmrj.2012.08.008.

243. Jones RA, Downing K, Rinehart NJ, et al. Physical activity, sedentary behavior and their correlates in children with autism spectrum disorder: a systematic review. *PLoS One.* 2017;12(2):e0172482. doi:10.1371/journal.pone.0172482.

244. American Psychiatric Association, editor. *Diagnostic and Statistical Manual of Mental Disorders: DSM-5.* 5th ed. Washington (DC): American Psychiatric Association; 2013.

245. Lyall K, Croen L, Daniels J, et al. The changing epidemiology of autism spectrum disorders. *Annu Rev Public Health.* 2017;38(1):81–102. doi:10.1146/annurev-publhealth-031816-044318.

246. Maenner MJ, Shaw KA, Bakian AV, et al. Prevalence and characteristics of autism spectrum disorder among children aged 8 years — autism and developmental disabilities monitoring network, 11 sites, United States, 2018. *MMWR Surveill Summ.* 2021;70:1–16. Available from: https://www.cdc.gov/mmwr/volumes/70/ss/ss7011a1.htm#suggestedcitation.

247. Hyman SL, Levy SE, Myers SM; Council on Children with Disabilities, Section on Developmental and Behavioral Pediatrics. Identification, evaluation, and management of children with autism spectrum disorder. *Pediatrics.* 2020;145(1):e20193447. doi:10.1542/peds.2019-3447.

248. Buescher AVS, Cidav Z, Knapp M, Mandell DS. Costs of autism spectrum disorders in the United Kingdom and the United States. *JAMA Pediatr.* 2014;168(8):721–8. doi:10.1001/jamapediatrics.2014.210.

249. Leigh JP, Du J. Brief report: forecasting the economic burden of autism in 2015 and 2025 in the United States. *J Autism Dev Disord.* 2015;45(12):4135–9. doi:10.1007/s10803-015-2521-7.

250. Masi A, DeMayo MM, Glozier N, Guastella AJ. An overview of autism spectrum disorder, heterogeneity and treatment options. *Neurosci Bull.* 2017;33(2):183–93. doi:10.1007/s12264-017-0100-y.

251. Autism Speaks. Autism statistics and facts. [cited 2022 Jan 15]. Available from: https://www.autismspeaks.org/autism-statistics-asd.

252. Lai MC, Kassee C, Besney R, et al. Prevalence of co-occurring mental health diagnoses in the autism population: a systematic review and meta-analysis. *Lancet Psychiatry.* 2019;6(10):819–29. doi:10.1016/S2215-0366(19)30289-5.

253. Liu T, Kelly J, Davis L, Zamora K. Nutrition, BMI and motor competence in children with autism spectrum disorder. *Medicina.* 2019;55(5):135. doi:10.3390/medicina55050135.

254. McCoy SM, Jakicic JM, Gibbs BB. Comparison of obesity, physical activity, and sedentary behaviors between adolescents with autism spectrum disorders and without. *J Autism Dev Disord.* 2016;46(7):2317–26. doi:10.1007/s10803-016-2762-0.

255. Arnell S, Jerlinder K, Lundqvist LO. Parents' perceptions and concerns about physical activity participation among adolescents with autism spectrum disorder. *Autism.* 2020;24(8):2243–55. doi:10.1177/1362361320942092.

256. Healy S, Nacario A, Braithwaite RE, Hopper C. The effect of physical activity interventions on youth with autism spectrum disorder: a meta-analysis. *Autism Res.* 2018;11(6):818–33. doi:10.1002/aur.1955.

257. Ketcheson L, Hauck J, Ulrich D. The effects of an early motor skill intervention on motor skills, levels of physical activity, and socialization in young children with autism spectrum disorder: a pilot study. *Autism.* 2017;21(4):481–92. doi:10.1177/1362361316650611.

258. Pan CY. Effects of water exercise swimming program on aquatic skills and social behaviors in children with autism spectrum disorders. *Autism*. 2010;14(1):9–28. doi:10.1177/1362361309339496.

259. Pan CY. The efficacy of an aquatic program on physical fitness and aquatic skills in children with and without autism spectrum disorders. *Res Autism Spectr Disord*. 2011;5(1):657–65. doi:10.1016/j.rasd.2010.08.001.

260. Najafabadi MG, Sheikh M, Hemayattalab R, Memari AH, Aderyani MR, Hafizi S. The effect of SPARK on social and motor skills of children with autism. *Pediatr Neonatol*. 2018;59(5):481–7. doi:10.1016/j.pedneo.2017.12.005.

261. Rafie F, Ghasemi A, Zamani Jam A, Jalali S. Effect of exercise intervention on the perceptual-motor skills in adolescents with autism. *J Sports Med Phys Fitness*. 2017;57(1–2):53–9. doi:10.23736/S0022-4707.16.05919-3.

262. Sansi A, Nalbant S, Ozer D. Effects of an inclusive physical activity program on the motor skills, social skills and attitudes of students with and without autism spectrum disorder. *J Autism Dev Disord*. 2021;51(7):2254–70. doi:10.1007/s10803-020-04693-z.

263. Huang J, Du C, Liu J, Tan G. Meta-analysis on intervention effects of physical activities on children and adolescents with autism. *Int J Environ Res Public Health*. 2020;17(6):1950. doi:10.3390/ijerph17061950.

264. Zhao M, Chen S. The effects of structured physical activity program on social interaction and communication for children with autism. *Biomed Res Int*. 2018;2018:1825046. doi:10.1155/2018/1825046.

265. Movahedi A, Bahrami F, Marandi SM, Abedi A. Improvement in social dysfunction of children with autism spectrum disorder following long term Kata techniques training. *Res Autism Spectr Disord*. 2013;7(9):1054–61. doi:10.1016/j.rasd.2013.04.012.

266. Tse ACY. Brief report: impact of a physical exercise intervention on emotion regulation and behavioral functioning in children with autism spectrum disorder. *J Autism Dev Disord*. 2020;50(11):4191–8. doi:10.1007/s10803-020-04418-2.

267. Ferreira JP, Ghiarone T, Cabral Júnior CR, et al. Effects of physical exercise on the stereotyped behavior of children with autism spectrum disorders. *Medicina*. 2019;55(10):685. doi:10.3390/medicina55100685.

268. National Research Council. *Educating Children With Autism*. Washington (DC): National Academies Press; 2001. p. 10017. doi:10.17226/10017.

269. Bojanek EK, Wang Z, White SP, Mosconi MW. Postural control processes during standing and step initiation in autism spectrum disorder. *J Neurodev Disord*. 2020;12(1):1. doi:10.1186/s11689-019-9305-x.

270. Kaur M, Srinivasan SM, Bhat AN. Comparing motor performance, praxis, coordination, and interpersonal synchrony between children with and without Autism Spectrum Disorder (ASD). *Res Dev Disabil*. 2018;72:79–95. doi:10.1016/j.ridd.2017.10.025.

271. Arnell S, Jerlinder K, Lundqvist LO. Perceptions of physical activity participation among adolescents with autism spectrum disorders: a conceptual model of conditional participation. *J Autism Dev Disord*. 2018;48(5):1792–802. doi:10.1007/s10803-017-3436-2.

272. Mesibov GB. Program for child with autism. *J Autism Dev Disord*. 2004;34(3):363. doi:10.1023/B:JADD.0000029673.75348.6a.

273. Potvin MC, Snider L, Prelock P, Kehayia E, Wood-Dauphinee S. Children's assessment of participation and enjoyment/preference for activities of children: psychometric properties in a population with high-functioning autism. *Am J Occup Ther*. 2013;67(2):209–17. doi:10.5014/ajot.2013.006288.

274. Case L, Yun J. The effect of different intervention approaches on gross motor outcomes of children with autism spectrum disorder: a meta-analysis. *Adapt Phys Activ Q*. 2019;36(4):501–26. doi:10.1123/apaq.2018-0174.

275. Toscano CVA, Carvalho HM, Ferreira JP. Exercise effects for children with autism spectrum disorder: metabolic health, autistic traits, and quality of life. *Percept Mot Skills*. 2018;125(1):126–46. doi:10.1177/0031512517743823.

276. Rivera P, Renziehausen J, Garcia JM. Effects of an 8-week judo program on behaviors in children with autism spectrum disorder: a mixed-methods approach. *Child Psychiatry Hum Dev*. 2020;51(5):734–41. doi:10.1007/s10578-020-00994-7.

277. Aitken SA, Buultjens M, Clark C, Eyre JT, Pease L, editors. *Teaching Children Who Are Deafblind: Contact, Communication and Learning*. London: Routledge; 2013.

278. National Eye Institute. Low vision data and statistics. Low vision defined. National Institutes of Health. 2019. [cited 2019 Jul 17]. Available from: https://www.nei.nih.gov/learn-about-eye-health/outreach-campaigns-and-resources/eye-health-data-and-statistics/low-vision-data-and-statistics.

279. World Health Organization. Blindness and vision impairment. 2021. [cited 2021 Oct 14]. Available from: https://www.who.int/news-room/fact-sheets/detail/blindness-and-visual-impairment.

280. National Eye Institute. Blindness data and statistics. Blindness defined. National Institutes of Health. 2019. [cited 2019 Jul 17]. Available from: https://www.nei.nih.gov/learn-about-eye-health/outreach-campaigns-and-resources/eye-health-data-and-statistics/blindness-data-and-statistics.

281. InformedHealth.org. Hearing loss and deafness: normal hearing and impaired hearing. Institute for Quality and Efficiency in Health Care (IQWiG). 2017. Available from: https://www.ncbi.nlm.nih.gov/books/NBK390300/.

282. World Health Organization. Deafness and hearing loss. 2021. [cited 2021 Apr 1]. Available from: https://www.who.int/news-room/fact-sheets/detail/deafness-and-hearing-loss.

283. Centers for Disease Control and Prevention. Vision health initiative: fast facts of common eye disorders. 2020. [cited 2020 Jun 9]. Available from: https://www.cdc.gov/vision-health/basics/ced/fastfacts.htm.

284. Blackwell DL, Lucas JW, Clarke TC. Summary health statistics for U.S. adults: national health interview survey, 2012. *Vital Health Stat 10*. 2014;(260):1–161.

285. National Institute on Deafness and Other Communication Disorders. Quick statistics about hearing. National Institutes of Health. 2021. [cited 2021 Mar 25]. Available from: https://www.nidcd.nih.gov/health/statistics/quick-statistics-hearing#3.

286. Centers for Disease Control and Prevention. Economic costs associated with mental retardation, cerebral palsy, hearing loss, and vision impairment — United States, 2003. *MMWR Morb Mortal Wkly Rep*. 2004;53(3):57–9.

287. Soleimani R, Jalali MM, Faghih HA. Comparing the prevalence of attention deficit hyperactivity disorder in hearing-impaired children with normal-hearing peers. *Arch Pediatr*. 2020;27(8):432–5. doi:10.1016/j.arcped.2020.08.014.

288. de Moraes Marchiori LL, de Almeida Rego Filho E, Matsuo T. Hypertension as a factor associated with hearing loss. *Braz J Otorhinolaryngol.* 2006;72(4):533–40. doi:10.1016/S1808-8694(15)31001-6.

289. Micieli JA, Easterbrook M. Eye and orbital injuries in sports. *Clin Sports Med.* 2017;36(2):299–314. doi:10.1016/j.csm.2016.11.006.

290. Dickerman RD, McConathy WJ, Smith GH, East JW, Rudder L. Middle cerebral artery blood flow velocity in elite power athletes during maximal weight-lifting. *Neurol Res.* 2000;22(4):337–40. doi:10.1080/01616412.2000.11740679.

291. Ferguson MA, Kitterick PT, Chong LY, Edmondson-Jones M, Barker F, Hoare DJ. Hearing aids for mild to moderate hearing loss in adults. *Cochrane Database Syst Rev.* 2017;9(9):CD012023. doi:10.1002/14651858.CD012023.pub2.

292. Yawn R, Hunter JB, Sweeney AD, Bennett ML. Cochlear implantation: a biomechanical prosthesis for hearing loss. *F1000Prime Rep.* 2015;7:45. doi:10.12703/P7-45.

293. Zetterlund C, Lundqvist L, Richter HO. Visual, musculoskeletal and balance symptoms in individuals with visual impairment. *Clin Exp Optom.* 2019;102(1):63–9. doi:10.1111/cxo.12806.

294. Oliveira Filho CW de, Almeida JJG de, Vital R, Carvalho KMM de, Martins LEB. A variação da acuidade visual durante esforços físicos em atletas com baixa visão, participantes de seleção brasileira de atletismo [The visual acuity variability during physical efforts in low vision athletes from the athletics Brazilian team]. *Rev Bras Med Esporte.* 2007;13(4):254–8. doi:10.1590/S1517-86922007000400009.

295. Squarcini CFR, Pires MLN, Lopes C, et al. Free-running circadian rhythms of muscle strength, reaction time, and body temperature in totally blind people. *Eur J Appl Physiol.* 2013;113(1):157–65. doi:10.1007/s00421-012-2415-8.

296. Carpenter MG, Campos JL. The effects of hearing loss on balance: a critical review. *Ear Hear.* 2020;41(Suppl 1):107S–19S. doi:10.1097/AUD.0000000000000929.

297. Kuo PL, Di J, Ferrucci L, Lin FR. Analysis of hearing loss and physical activity among US adults aged 60–69 years. *JAMA Netw Open.* 2021;4(4):e215484. doi:10.1001/jamanetworkopen.2021.5484.

298. Ellis MK, Darby LA. The effect of balance on the determination of peak oxygen consumption for hearing and nonhearing female athletes. *Adapt Phys Activ Q.* 1993;10(3):216–25. doi:10.1123/apaq.10.3.216.

299. Sweeting J, Merom D, Astuti PAS, Antoun M, Edwards K, Ding D. Physical activity interventions for adults who are visually impaired: a systematic review and meta-analysis. *BMJ Open.* 2020;10(2):e034036. doi:10.1136/bmjopen-2019-034036.

300. Majlesi M, Farahpour N, Azadian E, Amini M. The effect of interventional proprioceptive training on static balance and gait in deaf children. *Res Dev Disabil.* 2014;35(12):3562–7. doi:10.1016/j.ridd.2014.09.001.

301. Wiesmeier IK, Dalin D, Wehrle A, et al. Balance training enhances vestibular function and reduces overactive proprioceptive feedback in elderly. *Front Aging Neurosci.* 2017;9:273. doi:10.3389/fnagi.2017.00273.

302. Loturco I, Nakamura FY, Winckler C, et al. Strength-power performance of visually impaired paralympic and olympic judo athletes from the Brazilian national team: a comparative study. *J Strength Cond Res.* 2017;31(3):743–9. doi:10.1519/JSC.0000000000001525.

303. Malwina KA, Krzysztof M, Piotr Z. Visual impairment does not limit training effects in development of aerobic and anaerobic capacity in tandem cyclists. *J Hum Kinet.* 2015;48(1):87–97. doi:10.1515/hukin-2015-0095.

304. Schalock RL, Luckasson R, Tassé MJ. *Intellectual Disability: Definition, Diagnosis, Classification, and Systems of Supports.* 12th ed. Silver Spring (MD): American Association on Intellectual and Developmental Disabilities; 2021.

305. Maulik PK, Mascarenhas MN, Mathers CD, Dua T, Saxena S. Prevalence of intellectual disability: a meta-analysis of population-based studies. *Res Dev Disabil.* 2011;32(2):419–36. doi:10.1016/j.ridd.2010.12.018.

306. McKenzie K, Milton M, Smith G, Ouellette-Kuntz H. Systematic review of the prevalence and incidence of intellectual disabilities: current trends and issues. *Curr Dev Disord Rep.* 2016;3(2):104–15. doi:10.1007/s40474-016-0085-7.

307. Presson AP, Partyka G, Jensen KM, et al. Current estimate of Down syndrome population prevalence in the United States. *J Pediatr.* 2013;163(4):1163–8. doi:10.1016/j.jpeds.2013.06.013.

308. de Graaf G, Buckley F, Skotko BG. Estimates of the live births, natural losses, and elective terminations with Down syndrome in the United States. *Am J Med Genet A.* 2015;167A(4):756–67. doi:10.1002/ajmg.a.37001.

309. de Graaf G, Buckley F, Skotko BG. Estimation of the number of people with Down syndrome in Europe. *Eur J Hum Genet.* 2021;29(3):402–10. doi:10.1038/s41431-020-00748-y.

310. US Department of Health and Human Services. Closing the gap: a national blueprint to improve the health of persons with mental retardation. Office of the Surgeon General. 2002. Available from: https://stacks.cdc.gov/view/cdc/21851.

311. Krahn GL, Fox MH. Health disparities of adults with intellectual disabilities: what do we know? What do we do? *J Appl Res Intellect Disabil.* 2014;27(5):431–46. doi:10.1111/jar.12067.

312. Maulik P, Harbour C. Epidemiology of intellectual disability. In: *International Encyclopedia of Rehabilitation.* Buffalo (NY): Center for International Rehabilitation Research Information and Exchange; 2010.

313. Heslop P, Blair PS, Fleming P, Hoghton M, Marriott A, Russ L. The confidential inquiry into premature deaths of people with intellectual disabilities in the UK: a population-based study. *Lancet.* 2014;383(9920):889–95. doi:10.1016/S0140-6736(13)62026-7.

314. Lauer E, McCallion P. Mortality of people with intellectual and developmental disabilities from select US State disability service systems and medical claims data. *J Appl Res Intellect Disabil.* 2015;28(5):394–405. doi:10.1111/jar.12191.

315. Landes SD, Stevens JD, Turk MA. Cause of death in adults with intellectual disability in the United States. *J Intellect Disabil Res.* 2021;65(1):47–59. doi:10.1111/jir.12790.

316. Landes SD, McDonald KE, Wilmoth JM, Carter Grosso E. Evidence of continued reduction in the age-at-death disparity between adults with and without intellectual and/or developmental disabilities. *J Appl Res Intellect Disabil.* 2021;34(3):916–20. doi:10.1111/jar.12840.

317. Esbensen AJ, Seltzer MM, Greenberg JS. Factors predicting mortality in midlife adults with and without Down syndrome

living with family. *J Intellect Disabil Res.* 2007;51(Pt 12): 1039–50. doi:10.1111/j.1365-2788.2007.01006.x.

318. Polder JJ, Meerding WJ, Bonneux L, van der Maas PJ. Healthcare costs of intellectual disability in the Netherlands: a cost-of-illness perspective. *J Intellect Disabil Res.* 2002;46(2):168–78. doi:10.1046/j.1365-2788.2002.00384.x.

319. Crowder SA, Melton DJ. Individual and system-related factors associated with the costs of intellectual and developmental disabilities. *Tenn Med.* 2012;105(8):49–51.

320. Doran CM, Einfeld SL, Madden RH, et al. How much does intellectual disability really cost? First estimates for Australia. *J Intellect Dev Disabil.* 2012;37(1):42–9. doi:10.3109/13668250.2011.648609.

321. Salvador-Carulla L, Symonds S. Health services use and costs in people with intellectual disability: building a context knowledge base for evidence-informed policy. *Curr Opin Psychiatry.* 2016;29(2):89–94. doi:10.1097/YCO.0000000000000237.

322. Fujiura GT, Li H, Magaña S. Health services use and costs for Americans with intellectual and developmental disabilities: a national analysis. *Intellect Dev Disabil.* 2018;56(2):101–18. doi:10.1352/1934-9556-56.2.101.

323. Lunsky Y, De Oliveira C, Wilton A, Wodchis W. High health care costs among adults with intellectual and developmental disabilities: a population-based study: high health care costs. *J Intellect Disabil Res.* 2019;63(2):124–37. doi:10.1111/jir.12554.

324. Shapiro B, Batshaw M. Developmental delay and intellectual disability. In: Batshaw ML, Roizen NJ, Lotrecchiano GR, editors. *Children With Disabilities.* 7th ed. Baltimore (MD): Paul H. Brookes Publishing; 2013, p. 291–306.

325. Roizen N. Down syndrome (Trisomy 21). In: Batshaw ML, Roizen NJ, Lotrecchiano GR, editors. *Children With Disabilities.* 7th ed. Baltimore (MD): Paul H. Brookes Publishing; 2013 p. 307–18.

326. Croce RV, Pitetti KH, Horvat M, Miller J. Peak Torque, average power, and hamstring/quadriceps ratios in nondisabled adults and adults with mental retardation. *Arch Phys Med Rehabil.* 1996;77(4):369–72. doi:10.1016/S0003-9993(96)90086-6.

327. Fernhall B, Pitetti KH, Rimmer JH, et al. Cardiorespiratory capacity of individuals with mental retardation including Down syndrome. *Med Sci Sports Exerc.* 1996;28(3):366–71. doi:10.1097/00005768-199603000-00012.

328. Baynard T, Pitetti KH, Guerra M, Unnithan VB, Fernhall B. Age-related changes in aerobic capacity in individuals with mental retardation: a 20-yr review. *Med Sci Sports Exerc.* 2008;40(11):1984–9. doi:10.1249/MSS.0b013e31817f19a1.

329. Stancliffe RJ, Lakin KC, Larson S, et al. Overweight and obesity among adults with intellectual disabilities who use intellectual disability/developmental disability services in 20 U.S. states. *Am J Intellect Dev Disabil.* 2011;116(6):401–18. doi:10.1352/1944-7558-116.6.401.

330. Hsieh K, Rimmer JH, Heller T. Obesity and associated factors in adults with intellectual disability: obesity and ID. *J Intellect Disabil Res.* 2014;58(9):851–63. doi:10.1111/jir.12100.

331. Hilgenkamp TIM, Baynard T. Do individuals with intellectual disability have a lower peak heart rate and maximal oxygen uptake? *J Appl Res Intellect Disabil.* 2018;31(5):785–91. doi:10.1111/jar.12430.

332. Duvdevany I, Arar E. Leisure activities, friendships, and quality of life of persons with intellectual disability: foster homes vs community residential settings. *Int J Rehabil Res.* 2004;27(4):289–96. doi:10.1097/00004356-200412000-00006.

333. Draheim CC. Cardiovascular disease prevalence and risk factors of persons with mental retardation. *Ment Retard Dev Disabil Res Rev.* 2006;12(1):3–12. doi:10.1002/mrdd.20095.

334. Rimmer JH, Yamaki K, Lowry BMD, Wang E, Vogel LC. Obesity and obesity-related secondary conditions in adolescents with intellectual/developmental disabilities: obesity and youth with IDD. *J Intellect Disabil Res.* 2010;54(9):787–94. doi:10.1111/j.1365-2788.2010.01305.x.

335. de Winter CF, Bastiaanse LP, Hilgenkamp TIM, Evenhuis HM, Echteld MA. Cardiovascular risk factors (diabetes, hypertension, hypercholesterolemia and metabolic syndrome) in older people with intellectual disability: results of the HA-ID study. *Res Dev Disabil.* 2012;33(6):1722–31. doi:10.1016/j.ridd.2012.04.010.

336. Freeman SB, Bean LH, Allen EG, et al. Ethnicity, sex, and the incidence of congenital heart defects: a report from the National Down Syndrome Project. *Genet Med.* 2008;10(3): 173–80. doi:10.1097/GIM.0b013e3181634867.

337. Bull MJ; Committee on Genetics. Health supervision for children with Down syndrome. *Pediatrics.* 2011;128(2):393–406. doi:10.1542/peds.2011-1605.

338. O'Dwyer M, Peklar J, McCallion P, McCarron M, Henman MC. Factors associated with polypharmacy and excessive polypharmacy in older people with intellectual disability differ from the general population: a cross-sectional observational nationwide study. *BMJ Open.* 2016;6(4):e010505. doi:10.1136/bmjopen-2015-010505.

339. Carmeli E, Kessel S, Coleman R, Ayalon M. Effects of a treadmill walking program on muscle strength and balance in elderly people with Down syndrome. *J Gerontol A Biol Sci Med Sci.* 2002;57(2):M106–10. doi:10.1093/gerona/57.2.M106.

340. Tsimaras V, Giagazoglou P, Fotiadou E, Christoulas K, Angelopoulou N. Jog-walk training in cardiorespiratory fitness of adults with Down syndrome. *Percept Mot Skills.* 2003;96(3 Pt 2):1239–51. doi:10.2466/pms.2003.96.3c.1239.

341. Heller T, Hsieh K, Rimmer JH. Attitudinal and psychosocial outcomes of a fitness and health education program on adults with Down syndrome. *Am J Ment Retard.* 2004;109(2):175–85. doi:10.1352/0895-8017(2004)109<175:AAPOOA>2.0.CO;2.

342. Phillips AC, Holland AJ. Assessment of objectively measured physical activity levels in individuals with intellectual disabilities with and without Down's syndrome. *PLoS One.* 2011;6(12):e28618. doi:10.1371/journal.pone.0028618.

343. Harris L, McGarty AM, Hilgenkamp T, Mitchell F, Melville CA. Patterns of objectively measured sedentary behaviour in adults with intellectual disabilities. *J Appl Res Intellect Disabil.* 2019;32(6):1428–36. doi:10.1111/jar.12633.

344. Ghosh S, Choi P, Brown SP, Motl RW, Agiovlasitis S. Levels and patterns of sedentary behavior in men and women with intellectual disability. *Disabil Health J.* 2021;14(3):101059. doi:10.1016/j.dhjo.2020.101059.

345. Oreskovic NM, Cottrell C, Torres A, et al. Physical activity patterns in adults with Down syndrome. *J Appl Res Intellect Disabil.* 2020;33(6):1457–64. doi:10.1111/jar.12773.

346. Heller T, Hsieh K, Rimmer J. Barriers and supports for exercise participation among adults with Down syndrome. *J Gerontol Soc Work.* 2003;38(1–2):161–78. doi:10.1300/J083v38n01_03.

347. Bodde AE, Seo DC. A review of social and environmental barriers to physical activity for adults with intellectual disabilities. *Disabil Health J*. 2009;2(2):57–66. doi:10.1016/j.dhjo.2008.11.004.

348. Mahy J, Shields N, Taylor NF, Dodd KJ. Identifying facilitators and barriers to physical activity for adults with Down syndrome: facilitators and barriers to activity. *J Intellect Disabil Res*. 2010;54(9):795–805. doi:10.1111/j.1365-2788.2010.01308.x.

349. Pitetti K, Baynard T, Agiovlasitis S. Children and adolescents with Down syndrome, physical fitness and physical activity. *J Sport Health Sci*. 2013;2(1):47–57. doi:10.1016/j.jshs.2012.10.004.

350. Love A, Agiovlasitis S. How do adults with Down syndrome perceive physical activity? *Adapt Phys Activ Q*. 2016;33(3):253–70. doi:10.1123/APAQ.2015-0042.

351. Boonman A, Schroeder EC, Hopman, M, Fernhall BO, Hilgenkamp TIM. Cardiopulmonary profile of individuals with intellectual disability. *Med Sci Sports Exerc*. 2019;51(9):1802–8.

352. Agiovlasitis S, McCubbin JA, Yun J, Widrick JJ, Pavol MJ. Gait characteristics of adults with Down syndrome explain their greater metabolic rate during walking. *Gait Posture*. 2015;41(1):180–4. doi:10.1016/j.gaitpost.2014.10.004.

353. Agiovlasitis S, McCubbin JA, Yun J, Pavol MJ, Widrick JJ. Economy and preferred speed of walking in adults with and without Down Syndrome. *Adapt Phys Activ Q*. 2009;26(2):118–30. doi:10.1123/apaq.26.2.118.

354. Carmeli E, Barchad S, Masharawi Y, Coleman R. Impact of a walking program in people with Down syndrome. *J Strength Cond Res*. 2004;18(1):180–4. doi:10.1519/1533-4287(2004)018<0180:IOAWPI>2.0.CO;2.

355. Fernhall B, Mendonca GV, Baynard T. Reduced work capacity in individuals with down syndrome: a consequence of autonomic dysfunction? *Exerc Sport Sci Rev*. 2013;41(3):138–47. doi:10.1097/JES.0b013e318292f408.

356. Fernhall B, Mccubbin JA, Pitetti KH, et al. Prediction of maximal heart rate in individuals with mental retardation: *Med Sci Sports Exerc*. 2001;33(10):1655–60. doi:10.1097/00005768-200110000-00007.

357. Mendonca GV, Santos I, Fernhall B, Baynard T. Predictive equations to estimate peak aerobic capacity and peak heart rate in persons with Down syndrome. *J Appl Physiol (1985)*. 2022;132(2):423–33.

358. Rimmer JH, Heller T, Wang E, Valerio I. Improvements in physical fitness in adults with Down syndrome. *Am J Ment Retard*. 2004;109(2):165–74. doi:10.1352/0895-8017(2004)109<165:IIPFIA>2.0.CO;2.

359. Tsimaras VK, Fotiadou EG. Effect of training on the muscle strength and dynamic balance ability of adults with Down syndrome. *J Strength Cond Res*. 2004;18(2):343–7. doi:10.1519/R-12832.1.

360. Cowley PM, Ploutz-Snyder LL, Baynard T, et al. The effect of progressive resistance training on leg strength, aerobic capacity and functional tasks of daily living in persons with Down syndrome. *Disabil Rehabil*. 2011;33(22–23):2229–36. doi:10.3109/09638288.2011.563820.

361. Oviedo GR. Guerra-Balic M, Baynard T, Javierre C. Effects of aerobic, resistance and balance training in adults with intellectual disabilities. *Res Dev Disabil*. 2014;35(11):2624–34. doi:10.1016/j.ridd.2014.06.025.

362. Rintala P, McCubbin JA, Dunn JM. Familiarization process in cardiorespiratory fitness testing for persons with mental retardation. *Sports Med Training Rehabil*. 1995;6(1):15–27. doi:10.1080/15438629509512032.

363. Baynard T., Fernhall B, Intellectual disability. In: Ehrman JK, Gordon PM, Visich PS, Keteyian SJ, editors. *Clinical Exercise Physiology*. 4th ed. Champaign (IL): Human Kinetics Inc; 2023. p. 583–96.

364. Boer PH, Moss SJ. Validity of the 16-metre PACER and six-minute walk test in adults with Down syndrome. *Disabil Rehabil*. 2016;38(26):2575–83. doi:10.3109/09638288.2015.1137982.

365. Bertapelli F, Agiovlasitis S, Motl RW, et al. Development and cross-validation of a prediction equation for estimating percentage body fat from body mass index in young people with intellectual disability. *Adapt Phys Activ Q*. 2020;37(4):481–97. doi:10.1123/apaq.2019-0150.

366. Casey AF. Measuring body composition in individuals with intellectual disability: a scoping review. *J Obes*. 2013;2013:628428. doi:10.1155/2013/628428.

367. Patusco R, Matarese L, Ziegler J. Body composition in adults with intellectual disabilities: implications for practice. *Health Promot Pract*. 2018;19(6):884–95. doi:10.1177/1524839917748595.

368. Hsieh K, Rimmer J, Heller T. Prevalence of falls and risk factors in adults with intellectual disability. *Am J Intellect Dev Disabil*. 2012;117(6):442–54. doi:10.1352/1944-7558-117.6.442.

369. Choi P, Wei T, Motl RW, Agiovlasitis S. Risk factors associated with history of falls in adults with intellectual disability. *Res Dev Disabil*. 2020;106:103748. doi:10.1016/j.ridd.2020.103748.

370. Olsen MI, Halvorsen MB, Søndenaa E, et al. Factors associated with non-completion of and scores on physical capability tests in health surveys: the North Health in Intellectual Disability Study. *J Appl Res Intellect Disabil*. 2022;35(1):231–42. doi:10.1111/jar.12942.

371. Silva V, Campos C, Sá A, et al. Wii-based exercise program to improve physical fitness, motor proficiency and functional mobility in adults with Down syndrome. *J Intellect Disabil Res*. 2017;61(8):755–65. doi:10.1111/jir.12384.

372. Perrot A, Maillot P, Le Foulon A, Rebillat AS. Effect of exergaming on physical fitness, functional mobility, and cognitive functioning in adults with Down syndrome. *Am J Intellect Dev Disabil*. 2021;126(1):34–44. doi:10.1352/1944-7558-126.1.34.

373. Suarez-Iglesias D, Martinez-de-Quel O, Marín Moldes JR, Ayan Perez C. Effects of videogaming on the physical, mental health, and cognitive function of people with intellectual disability: a systematic review of randomized controlled trials. *Games Health J*. 2021;10(5):295–313. doi:10.1089/g4h.2020.0138.

374. Shields N, Taylor NF, Wee E, Wollersheim D, O'Shea SD, Fernhall B. A community-based strength training programme increases muscle strength and physical activity in young people with Down syndrome: a randomised controlled trial. *Res Dev Disabil*. 2013;34(12):4385–94. doi:10.1016/j.ridd.2013.09.022.

CHAPTER

13

Cancer

INTRODUCTION

Given that 40% of Americans will experience a cancer diagnosis during their lifetime (1), there is a high likelihood that clinical exercise physiologists (CEPs) will work with patients who have cancer many times throughout their career. Compelling randomized controlled trial evidence supports the use of exercise training throughout the cancer trajectory, from diagnosis, through treatment, to rehabilitation, survivorship, and end of life.

After presenting the fundamental pathophysiology of cancer, this chapter provides an overview of seven of the most common cancer diagnoses. It then discusses evidence that exercise may help or harm the patient, including the information a CEP needs to evaluate and prescribe appropriate exercise for adults who have been diagnosed with cancer. At the end of the chapter is a series of case studies that may be of assistance when working with people who are being actively treated for cancer or who have already finished treatment. Another excellent resource on this topic is "ACSM's Guide to Exercise and Cancer Survivorship" (2). In addition, the American College of Sports Medicine (ACSM) has a specialty certification related to cancer survivorship, entitled the "Cancer Exercise Trainer."

Individuals differ in their willingness to be identified as a patient with cancer and/or survivor as they move through the cancer trajectory. The National Coalition for Cancer Survivorship defines survivorship as beginning at the point of diagnosis. That said, some who have had a cancer diagnosis and are undergoing treatment do not feel they are yet a "survivor," and some who have survived many years since their last cancer treatments prefer not to be referred to as a cancer survivor. Therefore, the CEP is advised to ask those who have experienced cancer how they think of themselves. Sensitivity to the preferences of adults who have had a cancer diagnosis will help underscore the CEP's commitment to this growing population.

OVERVIEW AND PATHOPHYSIOLOGY OF CANCER

There are over 100 types of cancer. The common thread throughout all of these cancer types is abnormal cell growth and/or irregulation of normal cell senescence. Fundamentally, cancer is a breakdown in the normal regulation of cell growth, aging, and death.

Normally, cell division is carefully controlled by a variety of mechanisms. Cancer develops when these mechanisms break down. Cells that become damaged or abnormal survive when they should not. These abnormal cells then divide continually, evading the normal controls on cell growth (3). The term *hyperplasia* identifies a state in which cells divide faster than normal and extra cells accumulate, but the cells still look normal under a microscope (Figure 13.1). The term *dysplasia* is used when cells divide and proliferate more rapidly than normal and look abnormal under a microscope; moreover, there are changes in the organization of the cells within the tissue. An accumulation of abnormal cells is commonly called a tumor. A benign tumor is not invasive. The term *cancer* is used only for malignant tumors; that is, tumors in which the abnormal cells are capable of invading nearby tissue (see Figure 13.1).

In a process called metastasis, cancer cells can travel from the tumor (called the primary tumor) through the blood or lymphatic vessels to form a cancerous growth in another part of the body. Figure 13.2 demonstrates how cancer can metastasize (3).

The development of cancer is commonly thought of as a multistep process that starts with genetic changes to a cell. For only 5%–10% of cancers, genetic variants inherited from parents play a major role. One example is the *BRCA1* gene that is known to significantly elevate the risk for breast and ovarian cancer (4). The majority of genetic

DNA Structure

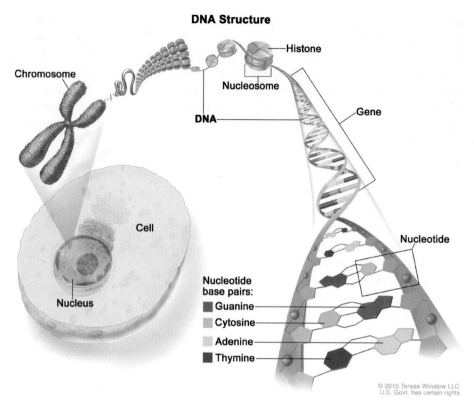

FIGURE 13.1 Development of cancer. Normal tissue undergoes a progression of abnormal changes from hyperplasia (increase in number of cells but cells still appear normal under a microscope), to dysplasia (cells look abnormal under a microscope but are not cancer), and finally to cancer. (© 2015 Terese Winslow LLC. Available from: http://www.teresewinslow.com/index.asp. U.S. Govt. has certain rights.)

Metastasis

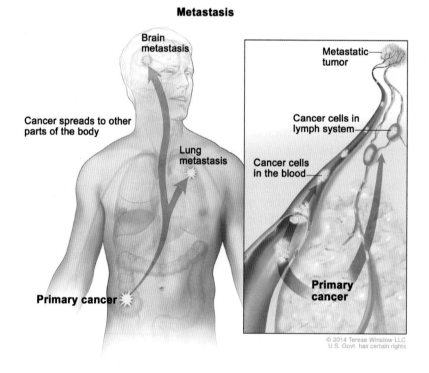

FIGURE 13.2 Metastasis. From the primary cancer, cells can break away and travel through the blood or lymph system to form new tumors (metastatic tumors) in another area of the body. (© 2014 Terese Winslow LLC. Available from: http://www.teresewinslow.com/index.asp. U.S. Govt. has certain rights.)

changes arise because of damage to DNA from aging or environmental factors, such as the chemicals in tobacco smoke or ultraviolet radiation from sun exposure. If this damage to the cell is not repaired or the cell does not undergo apoptosis (controlled cell death), this breakdown of normal regulation of cell growth can progress to cancer (4).

The exact amount of exposure to a specific environmental factor needed to cause cancer is unclear and likely varies person to person because of a variety of factors, but, in general, greater exposure results in greater risk. For example, with sun exposure, both increasing cumulative amount of total exposure and greater number of sunburns are linked to a higher risk of melanoma (a serious type of skin cancer) (5). Sun exposure also promotes the body's synthesis of vitamin D, which is crucial for bone health and many other body functions, so some exposure is necessary. The precise amount of time in the sun needed to produce enough vitamin D varies according to the individual's skin color, age, time of day, time of year, and geographical location, but usually just a few minutes is sufficient.

Classification of Cancer

Cancer can form in virtually any cell type in the body (3). The most common type of cell to develop cancer is the epithelial cell, which covers the inside and outside surfaces of the body. Cancers involving epithelial cells are called carcinomas. Carcinomas can be further broken down into the following types:

- Adenocarcinomas form in epithelial cells that produce fluids or mucus, such as glandular tissue (*i.e.*, breast, colon, or prostate cancer).
- Basal cell carcinomas form in epithelial cells in the base or basal level of the epidermis (*i.e.*, skin cancer).
- Squamous cell carcinomas form in epithelial cells that lie beneath the outer surface of the skin (*i.e.*, skin cancer).
- Transitional cell carcinomas form in epithelial cells that function to stretch an organ such as the bladder.

Cancers that form in connective tissues of the body, like bone or soft tissue (*i.e.*, muscle or fat), are called sarcomas. Blood cancers do not form solid tumors; instead, the abnormal cells circulate in the blood. Cancer can also arise from other cell types, such as the neural cells in the brain.

The types of cells and the organ in which the cancer begins to grow significantly influence the treatment and prognosis (prediction of the course of the disease). For example, a squamous cell carcinoma that starts on the skin

of the nose is far less aggressive and will be treated quite differently from a cancer with the same cell type that starts in the nasal mucosa or sinus cavity. As the abnormal cells grow and spread, they may begin to alter the function of the organ or tissue from which they originated or to which they spread. These factors influence the choices physicians will make regarding the therapies to treat the cancer.

Cancer staging is a process in which an oncologist (physician specializing in cancer) or other provider assesses the extent and severity of cancer in the patient's body. Staging for each cancer is unique, but typically requires consideration of the cell type and features, number of lymph nodes involved, evidence of metastasis, and other criteria. Box 13.1 provides an overview of the commonly used staging approaches for most cancers.

Cancer Treatment

Cancer treatment varies according to the type, stage, and other factors. The most common treatments are as follows:

- Surgery: Some cancers are removed by surgery (also called resection). Though typically performed with scalpels or lasers, other techniques involve the destruction of cells with extreme cold (cryosurgery) or heat (hyperthermia).
- Chemotherapy: This treatment involves the use of powerful medications to kill rapidly dividing cells in the body or slow their rate of growth. It can also be used to shrink tumors before surgery or in order to relieve pain and pressure.
- Radiotherapy: In this treatment, high doses of ionizing radiation are directed specifically at the tumor or, following surgery, to the area where cancer occurred. It damages and eventually destroys rapidly dividing cells in that region of the body.

Box 13.1 Cancer Staging

Stage 0, carcinoma in situ. This means that abnormal cells are present but are still contained within the initial basement membrane site where they started. This is not a cancer, but this may become a cancer.

Stage 1–3, Cancer is present. The higher the number, the larger the tumor. Stage 3 cancer indicates that it has spread to nearby tissues.

Stage 4, Cancer has spread to distant parts of the body.

- Targeted biologic, hormonal, or immune therapies: These treatments involve the use of monoclonal antibodies, hormones, vaccines, or bacteria to stimulate immune or other mechanisms to act against cancer cells. The term "targeted therapies" may be used to describe treatments that use drugs or other substances to identify and attack specific types of cancer cells with less harm to normal cells. Some targeted therapies block the action of certain enzymes, proteins, or other molecules involved in the growth and spread of cancer cells. Targeted therapy may have fewer side effects than other types of cancer treatment. Most targeted therapies are either small-molecule drugs or monoclonal antibodies. One example of a targeted therapy would be trastuzumab, a monoclonal antibody used to treat a specific subtype of breast cancer. Many patients receive more than one type of therapy. For example, a patient may undergo an initial surgery to remove a tumor, followed by radiation to the region to disable any cancer cells that may have been left behind, or by chemotherapy to destroy any cells that may have metastasized.

The goal of cancer treatment is complete remission, meaning that there is no evidence of disease; the signs and symptoms of the disease have disappeared. Even after several years of remission, cancer can return or the original treatments can produce adverse effects; thus, cancer survivors are often monitored for many years after active treatment ends.

BREAST CANCER

Epidemiology

Over 260,000 women are diagnosed with breast cancer in the U.S. every year (6). The median age at diagnosis is 62 (7). In addition, there are over 3.8 million breast cancer survivors alive in the U.S. Breast cancer survivors represent nearly one-fourth of the total number of cancer survivors in the U.S. at this time.

Common Presentation

The majority of breast cancers are first noticed by the woman herself (8). Her primary care provider (PCP) would then typically recommend mammography. The second most common method of detection is through screening mammography. In either case, the mammogram may be followed by an ultrasound or magnetic resonance imaging (MRI) to gather more data about the finding. Following

this, there will generally be a biopsy, sometimes guided by MRI or ultrasound. The tissue removed will be reviewed by a pathologist, who will determine whether there is a tumor. If there is a tumor, the pathologist will determine whether it is benign (*i.e.*, not cancerous) or malignant (*i.e.*, cancerous). In order to complete staging, the oncologist may have the woman undergo a full-body PET (positron emission tomography) scan, which will help reveal whether the cancer has spread to the lymph nodes or distant organs. However, the final diagnosis and staging is not definitive until after the surgery and pathological review are complete. During the surgery, the surgeon will evaluate the lymphatic structures adjacent to the tumor. If there is evidence of lymphatic involvement, lymph nodes from the axilla will be removed. After the surgery, the pathologist will review the microscopic presentation of the tumor cells. The combination of the surgeon's experience and the pathologists review will result in final staging.

When reviewing the surgical notes of a patient with breast cancer, it is important to distinguish between the numbers of lymph nodes that are found to have cancer (called "positive" nodes) versus the number of nodes removed from the body regardless of whether they are found to have cancer. The reason is that many women misunderstand that the number of "positive" nodes equates to the number of nodes removed, whereas the number of positive nodes is usually far fewer than the total number of nodes removed from the body. Lymph nodes are a vital component of the lymphatic circulatory system. Removal of lymph nodes is associated with the development of a chronic condition called lymphedema. Thus, it is important for the CEP to understand the total number of nodes removed when evaluating the potential risk to lymphatic function after cancer surgery.

Prognosis

The 5-year relative survival rate for breast cancer is 91% in the U.S. Women with localized breast cancer (no spread to lymph nodes, nearby structures, or other locations beyond the breast) have a 5-year survival rate of 99%. This represents 61% of all cases. Survival is lower for women with lymph node involvement or metastasis. Prognosis has improved over the past decade for all women, but Black women still lag behind White women. The 5-year survival rate has improved from 76% in the 1970s to 92% from 2009 to 2015 in White women. By comparison, among Black women, 5-year survival rate was 62% in the 1970s and increased to 83% by 2009–2015. The racial divide in survival has persisted over time (6).

Treatment

The choice of breast cancer treatments will be made based on the tumor characteristics, including stage, size, extent to which it has spread, and patient's preference. Surgical options may include lumpectomy, breast-conserving surgery, or mastectomy. Women who undergo mastectomy may also undergo reconstructive surgery. The types of reconstructive surgeries available today are evolving. Exercise professionals working with long-term survivors are likely to encounter women with a variety of reconstructive procedures, including free-flap reconstruction, which involves autologous transplantation from the latissimus dorsi or transverse abdominis muscles, or silicone implants that are often placed under the pectoral muscle. Treatments may also include chemotherapy, radiation therapy, hormonal therapy, or immunologic therapies. Targeted therapies are also available to women whose tumors overexpress specific genetic traits.

Health Implications for Survivors

The health implications for survivors of breast cancer have much more to do with the treatments than the cancer itself. The effects of surgery vary not just with the amount of tissue resected to remove the cancer in the breast, but the number of lymph nodes removed and the type of reconstructive surgery performed, if any.

There is a linear relationship between the number of lymph nodes removed and the risk for breast cancer–related lymphedema. Lymphedema is largely characterized by swelling in the affected body part. For breast cancer survivors, this may include the breast and torso as well as the arm on the affected side. Lymphedema occurs in 20%–30% of all breast cancer survivors but remains relatively mild for most women with early-stage disease. Black race, obesity, and a full axillary dissection of lymph nodes are all associated with increased risk for onset and worse clinical course of lymphedema. Examples of breast cancer–related lymphedema are depicted in Figure 13.3.

Surgical treatment of cancer may occur separately from reconstructive surgeries. Either the initial surgery or the reconstructive surgery can alter the way the latissimus dorsi, abdominal muscles, and/or pectoral muscles and shoulder girdle function. There may be imbalances and weakness after surgical recovery and multiple periods during which upper body exercise is not possible. This may result in an extended period of immobility, which is a major factor in the common outcome of shoulder immobility among breast cancer survivors.

In addition to surgery, there are implications of radiation, chemotherapy, and immunotherapies. Radiation may cause lymphedema or damage the soft tissues in the region irradiated. The damage from radiation continues for the balance of life and for breast cancer survivors that could include the heart and/or lungs.

Some of the chemotherapies (anthracyclines) and immunotherapies (trastuzumab) used for breast cancer can cause long-term damage to the heart, leading to cardiac myopathies and heart failure. The risk of cardiotoxicity is reliant on the type and dose of treatment received. It is reported that breast cancer survivors have lower maximal aerobic capacity than their age-matched peers (9). Some chemotherapy agents (taxanes) are associated with peripheral neuropathy, which may or may not resolve over time. This may adversely affect balance. Another very

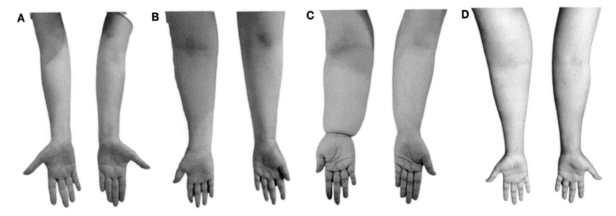

FIGURE 13.3 Lymphedema examples. **A and B.** Display mild stage of lymphedema, manifested by significant difference at the forearm area when compared to the other sites of the affected arms. **C and D.** Moderate to severe stage of lymphedema, characterized by swelling in major sites of the arms including metacarpal-phalangeal joint, wrist, forearm, and upper arm area. (Reprinted from Yusof KM, Avery-Kiejda KA, Ahmad Suhaimi S, et al. Assessment of potential risk factors and skin ultrasound presentation associated with breast cancer-related lymphedema in long-term breast cancer survivors. *Diagnostics.* 2021;11(8):1303. doi:10.3390/diagnostics11081303.)

common treatment-related side effect is arthritis-like arthralgias that are associated with the hormonal therapies that many breast cancer survivors are prescribed to take for up to 10 years' posttreatment. The cause of these aromatase inhibitor–associated arthralgias appears to be the reduction in female reproductive hormones, principally estrogen. Finally, many breast cancer survivors report weight gain as a result of their treatment. The specific causes of this weight gain are not yet clear, but are of concern given the link between obesity and cancer recurrence and mortality (10).

CEPs are urged to obtain as much information as possible about the treatments a breast cancer survivor has received and to research the short- and long-term adverse effects of those treatments prior to evaluation and exercise prescription. Contact with the cancer treatment team would be appropriate for this purpose. The oncology clinical team is focused on cure. As such, they may not communicate as extensively about short-term and long-term adverse treatment effects. CEPs may therefore find that they are the first to discuss with the survivor of these effects of treatment, which is important to do because they can influence exercise tolerance.

GYNECOLOGIC CANCERS

Epidemiology

It is estimated that 115,130 women were diagnosed with gynecologic cancers in the U.S. in 2021 (1). This includes ovarian, fallopian tube, endometrial corpus, endometrial cervix, vaginal, and vulvar cancers. The average age of diagnosis varies by tumor site: 50 years for cervical cancer, 60 for endometrial cancer, and 63 for ovarian cancer (11). In addition, there are over 1.34 million gynecologic cancer survivors in the U.S., representing approximately 8% of the total number of cancer survivors in the U.S. at this time. The most common gynecologic cancer diagnosis is endometrial corpus cancer, which accounts for nearly 66,000 of the annual gynecologic cancer diagnoses in the U.S. There are over 800,000 endometrial cancer survivors in the U.S., the second largest cancer survivor population among women.

Common Presentation

The common presentation for gynecologic cancers varies by tumor site. For endometrial corpus cancer, the cardinal presentation is abnormal uterine bleeding. For cervical, vaginal, and vulvar cancer, there may be no signs or symptoms at diagnosis, although some women do present with vaginal bleeding. Ovarian cancer signs and symptoms are diffuse and vague, and thus difficult to distinguish from intestinal symptoms (*e.g.*, bloating, abdominal swelling, pelvic pain, feeling full).

Prognosis

As with the presentation, the prognosis for women with gynecologic cancer varies broadly by the specific tumor site. The 5-year relative survival rate for endometrial cancer is 84%, and among the two-thirds of women diagnosed with early-stage disease, the 5-year relative survival rate is 95%. For cervical cancer, the 5-year relative survival rate is 66%. For ovarian cancer, the overall 5-year relative survival rate is 49% (1). Vaginal, vulvar, and other above-noted gynecologic cancers are too rare for the survival statistics to be as useful.

Treatments

The treatments used will vary by the specific tumor site, as well as the extent of disease. For example, for ovarian cancer, surgery and chemotherapy are common across all stages. However, radiation is only used in the treatment of small, localized recurrent tumors. By contrast, treatments for endometrial cancer commonly include a broad variety of approaches, including surgery, radiation, chemotherapy, hormonal therapy, and biological therapies to boost the immune system response to cancer. For cervical cancer, treatments commonly include surgery, radiation, and chemotherapy.

Health Implications for Survivors

Obesity is very strongly associated with the risk for endometrial cancer (12). As such, CEPs will likely have multiple obesity-related chronic conditions with which to contend when preparing to evaluate and prescribe exercise for endometrial cancer survivors, in addition to the issues specific to cancer treatment. Some of the surgeries for gynecologic cancers include removal of lymph nodes. Therefore, as with breast cancer, there is risk for lymphedema, in this case in the lower extremities and pelvis. This can be much more disfiguring and have a larger impact on function than lymphedema in the upper extremities. It is estimated that approximately 36% of gynecologic cancer survivors have lower extremity lymphedema (13, 14).

Radiation treatment of the pelvic area can contribute to the risk of lymphedema and may also result in long-term difficulties with urination and/or defecation, and bone or hip pain (possible avascular necrosis), as well as altered range of motion (ROM), nonbone pelvic pain, and sexual dysfunction. It would be wise for the CEP to ask about these and other posttreatment changes in symptoms or function prior to commencing with the evaluation and prescription (15).

Platinum-based chemotherapies (*e.g.*, carboplatin, cisplatin) are used in the treatment of many types of gynecologic cancers. The best described long-term side effects of these drugs include permanent peripheral neuropathy in the hands and feet and tinnitus or hearing loss (16). Patients treated with platinum-based chemotherapies will often exhibit poor balance and may require balance training or alterations to their exercise prescription to account for poor balance (*e.g.*, cycle ergometry rather than walking or treadmill exercise). Paclitaxel is also commonly used in treating gynecologic cancers. This drug is also associated with peripheral neuropathy in the hands and feet (17).

Finally, endometrial cancer chemotherapy regimens can include doxorubicin (18). This is the same drug associated with the increased risk for heart failure and cardiomyopathies in breast cancer survivors. Although there has been less research into the increased risk for adverse cardiovascular outcomes among endometrial than breast cancer patients, there is good reason for vigilance with regard to evaluation and monitoring of heart health among endometrial cancer survivors exposed to doxorubicin. CEPs are urged to gather medical records regarding the treatments that were used and investigate details on the effects of each treatment prior to evaluation and exercise prescription.

Hormonal therapies used for endometrial cancer include some of the same ones used for breast cancer. These have the same risk for arthralgias that may exacerbate or mimic arthritis.

PROSTATE CANCER

Epidemiology

Prostate cancer is the most common form of nonskin cancer diagnosed in men in the U.S. One in every eight men is expected to have a prostate cancer diagnosis in his lifetime. Prostate cancer is the second leading cause of cancer-related death for men, behind lung cancer. The American Cancer Society estimated that in 2023,

there will be 288,300 new cases of prostate cancer and 34,700 deaths from prostate cancer (1). Men are mostly older when diagnosed (mean age at diagnosis is 66), with 60% of men diagnosed after the age of 65. Prostate cancer rarely occurs in men younger than 40 years of age. Non-Hispanic Black men are at a disproportionately higher risk of prostate cancer, where the incidence rate is 73% higher in non-Hispanic Black men than in non-Hispanic White men (1).

Common Presentation

A blood-based prostate cancer screening test is available. It detects levels of prostate-specific antigen (PSA), which is secreted by the prostate gland. As prostate cancer develops, blood levels of PSA rise above 4 $ng \cdot mL^{-1}$. The risk of prostate cancer increases again if PSA exceeds a level of 10 $ng \cdot mL^{-1}$. Another method of detecting prostate cancer before symptoms occur is the digital rectal examination (DRE), in which the PCP palpates the prostate and checks for abnormalities. Both the PSA and DRE tests are likely to detect cancers in an early stage, before symptoms are present. Men whose prostate cancer is advanced or progressing may experience symptoms related to urination, erectile dysfunction, bone metastases (pain), or spinal cord compression. If prostate cancer is suspected based on PSA or DRE tests and/or symptoms, a biopsy of the prostate gland will be performed, and additional imaging may be done to detect spread of the cancer. Staging of prostate cancer is based on the results of these tests and is often also categorized as localized, regional, and distant disease based on whether and how far the cancer has spread outside of the prostate gland.

Prognosis

Even though prostate cancer is one of the leading causes of cancer-related deaths, most men will not die from the disease. The 5-year overall survival rate for prostate cancer approaches 99%. This rate decreases for men diagnosed with advanced prostate cancer. For instance, 5-year survival rates for men whose prostate cancer is localized or confined to a region near the prostate are close to 100%, but plummet to 31% if the cancer has spread to the bones or brain. Because men with localized or regional cancer can undergo a variety of treatments for their cancer and live for many years, if not decades, they may have to deal with the consequences of cancer and its treatment for a long time. As of 2022, there are an estimated 3.1 million prostate cancer survivors in the U.S.

Treatment

Depending on the stage of prostate cancer and other considerations (*e.g.*, age, cancer history, personal preference), a man may undergo one or more of the following standard treatments:

- Watchful waiting or active surveillance
- Surgery
- Radiation and radiopharmaceutical therapy
- Hormone therapy
- Chemotherapy
- Biologic therapy
- Bisphosphonate therapy

Watchful waiting and active surveillance are treatment approaches for early-stage, asymptomatic prostate cancers in older or otherwise healthy men. In both cases, men are followed for signs that the prostate cancer is growing, which for active surveillance includes regularly scheduled examinations and tests. Men should also self-monitor for the appearance of or changes in symptoms (*i.e.*, problems urinating, blood in urine or semen, erectile problems, or pain in the hips, back, or chest).

For men with tumors confined to the prostate, surgery to remove the prostate, seminal vesicles, and nearby tissue (including nearby lymph nodes), a *radical prostatectomy* is performed. Radiation therapy for prostate cancer can be applied externally or internally directly into the prostate, whereas radiopharmaceutical therapy delivers a radioactive substance (*i.e.*, radium-223) into the bloodstream to treat prostate cancer that has spread to the bones.

Hormone therapy for prostate cancer aims to reduce testosterone levels that can drive tumor growth and can be given for short or prescribed periods of time in conjunction with other treatments or for longer periods of time when cancer is progressing or advanced. Hormone therapy can include orchiectomy (*i.e.*, removal of testes); injections with luteinizing hormone–releasing hormone (LHRH) agonists or antagonists to stop the gonads from making testosterone; oral medications that inhibit the pathways involved in testosterone synthesis (CYP17 inhibition, adrenal inhibition); or the binding of testosterone to androgen receptors (antiandrogens).

For cancer that has metastasized, men may be treated with chemotherapy, biologic therapy with a cancer vaccine to boost immune function, and/or bisphosphonate therapy when cancer is in the bones.

Health Implications for Survivors

Radical prostatectomy can have side effects of impotence, urinary or bowel leakage or incontinence, and inguinal hernia. Radiation therapy can also have side effects of erectile problems and urinary or bowel leakage or incontinence, but may also cause fatigue and/or lower extremity lymphedema. Side effects of hormone therapy include vasomotor symptoms (hot flushes, night sweats), fatigue, impotence, breast tenderness, anemia, cognitive difficulties, vertigo, muscle and bone loss, fat gain, hyperlipidemia and hypercholesterolemia, and depression.

Most prostate cancers are detected at an early stage and are usually treated using surgery and/or radiation therapy and possibly short courses of hormone therapy. Although generally the side effects of these treatments wane over time, some men face residual side effects for years, chiefly a disruption in sexual function and urinary/bowel continence, and sometimes lingering fatigue. Men who have been treated with hormone therapy are more likely to develop osteoporosis, frailty (exhaustion, slowness, weakness, sarcopenia, and inactivity), diabetes, and cardiovascular disease (CVD), than men who don't receive this treatment possibly even if they discontinue therapy (19). Body image, masculinity, and self-esteem are also key factors impacting men with prostate cancer and are critical to understanding the prostate cancer experience.

All prostate cancer survivors have faced a life-threatening illness that may also threaten their masculinity; thus, attention to a man's emotional well-being across stages of disease and phases of treatment is important. Similarly, because most prostate cancer survivors are older when diagnosed, consideration of age-related conditions, comorbidities, and the interaction of these with treatment is an essential component of their care.

LUNG CANCER

Epidemiology

Lung cancer is the second most common type of cancer in men and women and the leading cause of cancer death in the U.S. A man's lifetime risk of developing lung cancer is 1 in 15 and a woman's is 1 in 17, regardless of smoking history, although the risk of lung cancer increases sharply among smokers. The American Cancer Society estimated that in 2022, there were 236,740 new cases of lung cancer and 130,180 deaths from lung cancer (1). Lung cancer is most commonly diagnosed at a later age (mean age at diagnosis is 70 years.), with two-thirds of men and women diagnosed after the age of 65. Lung cancer rarely strikes in persons younger than 45 years of age.

Of the three types of lung cancer, non–small cell lung cancer is the most common type, accounting for 84% of all cases. It is followed by small cell lung cancer and carcinoid tumors of the lung. Non–small cell lung cancer can be classified into the following three subtypes depending on the nature of the cancer and where it develops: adenocarcinoma, squamous cell carcinoma, and large cell (undifferentiated) carcinoma. Whereas non–small cell lung cancer can develop in nonsmokers, small cell lung cancer is strongly linked to smoking and is a fast-growing cancer. Carcinoid tumors of the lung are relatively rare (5% of all cases), slow growing, and unlikely to spread. Until recently, there have been no screening tests to detect lung cancer before symptoms arose, so lung cancer is typically already advanced when diagnosed. Low-dose computed tomography (LDCT) has been introduced as a screening tool for persons at risk of lung cancer and will be described in more detail below.

Common Presentation

Respiratory symptoms such as persistent coughing, wheezing, and shortness of breath, among others, may be signs of lung cancer or possibly other conditions like bronchial infection. Lung cancer can also be found on a routine chest x-ray that may or may not be performed on suspicion of cancer. Worth mentioning is the advent of a new screening tool for lung cancer that uses LDCT and may lead to earlier diagnoses and decreases in lung cancer death rates over time. Adoption of LDCT varies widely across the U.S. and is currently targeted at adults 55–74 years of age with a strong history of smoking.

A determination of the diagnosis, location, and extent of lung cancer is based on information obtained from biological samples, including a lung biopsy, and imaging tests. Staging of lung cancer, as with other solid tumors, is based on features of the tumor and whether and where the cancer has spread beyond the lungs.

Prognosis

Lung cancer is rarely diagnosed at a curable stage, but treatments can extend a person's life for many years. Survival from lung cancer (both non–small cell and small cell) depends on the stage that it is diagnosed. The 5-year overall survival rate for lung cancer regardless of stage is 22%; and 5-year survival rates for localized, regional, and distant-staged disease are 64%, 37%, and 8%, for non–small cell and 29%, 18%, and 3% for small cell lung cancers, respectively. As of 2022, there are an estimated 541,000 lung cancer survivors in the U.S. (1). Even though lung cancer has a serious prognosis and is treated aggressively, people with lung cancer can live for many years. They typically must not only face this difficult prognosis but also cope with the consequences of the disease and its treatment throughout their remaining lifetime.

Treatment

Treatment for lung cancer will vary depending on the stage of disease. For localized stage 1 disease, the typical treatments are surgery if the tumor is operable and radiation therapy. Techniques for surgical resection of lung tumors attempt to minimize excision of lung tissue, but lobectomy or pneumonectomy may be unavoidable, and, in any case, compromised pulmonary function is a common side effect that may or may not subside over time. Radiation therapy can be delivered conventionally or can be hypofractionated; that is, higher doses of radiation are delivered over a shorter period of time to improve outcomes and lower side effects such as scarring of lung tissues, pain, and fatigue.

For locally advanced or regionally spread lung cancers, tumors may or may not be resectable surgically; however, radiation is likely, and chemotherapy, either delivered presurgically (neoadjuvant) and/or postsurgically, is typically added to the treatment regimen. Platinum-based chemotherapy agents are used to treat lung cancer. In addition to the side effects such as fatigue common with most chemotherapy agents, platinum-based agents have numerous neurotoxic side effects, which may or may not persist long term, including peripheral neuropathy, vestibulotoxicity, ototoxicity, and potentially cognitive impairments.

Patients with distant disease (stage IV) are treated with platinum-based chemotherapy alone or in conjunction with other biologic therapies that target select pathways in the growth of the cancer.

Health Implications for Survivors

Most people will not be cured of lung cancer, but some can live for many years after treatment ends. Persons who had surgical resection of their tumors will likely experience some degree of compromised pulmonary function associated with either a reduced total lung capacity or damage to lung tissues and pulmonary structures. This can result in reduced exercise tolerance, exercise avoidance, low self-efficacy, and persistent fatigue. Exercise prescriptions for lung cancer survivors need to be tailored to accommodate spikes in breathlessness. Cardiotoxicity from chemotherapy and radiation treatment is likely. Treatment for lung cancers may accelerate aging. Because people are typically diagnosed with lung cancer survivors at an advanced age, consideration of age-related conditions, comorbidities, and the interaction of these with treatment is an essential component of care. Persons treated for metastatic disease may experience additional complications related to the impact on distant organs (*i.e.*, brain, bone). Even when lung cancer is detected early, the risk of recurrence is high; thus, lung cancer survivors live under the constant threat that their cancer will return and attention to their psychological state is prudent. There is still insufficient research into the long-term health of lung cancer survivors because survival rates are low, but with advances in early detection, opportunities to determine long-term and late effects of lung cancer will increase.

COLORECTAL CANCER

Epidemiology

Colorectal cancer is the third most common cancer diagnosed in both men and women in the U.S. and the third leading cause of cancer-related death in men and women. The lifetime risk of developing colorectal cancer is 1 in 24 for men and 1 in 25 for women (1). According to the American Cancer Society, there were an estimated 106,180 new cases of colon cancer and 44,850 new cases of rectal cancer in 2022 and 52,580 deaths from colorectal cancer. Although colorectal cancer is more common after age 50, 12% of cases will be diagnosed in individuals younger than age 50 years (1).

Common Presentation

Colorectal cancer commonly develops slowly, often over a period of up to 20 years (1). Many tumors start as polyps; noncancerous growths that develop on the inner lining of the colon or rectum (20). Although all polyps have the potential to become cancerous, especially if they enlarge, less than 10% progress to an invasive cancer. Therefore, screening, which aims to identify and remove these precancerous growths, plays an important part in the prevention of colorectal cancer. As there are often no symptoms of early-stage colorectal cancer, screening can also be effective in catching it earlier when treatment is less extensive and has the potential to be more successful.

Screening options include stool tests, which can detect cancer, and colonoscopy, which can both detect cancer and allow for the removal of precancerous growths. Regular screening for colorectal cancer using a high-sensitivity stool-based test or colonoscopy is recommended for all adults aged 45 years and older. All positive tests on noncolonoscopy tests should be followed up by a colonoscopy in a timely manner (21). The current screening guidelines in the U.S. lowered the recommended age of screening from 50 to 45 years because of increasing number of cases of younger people and aim to balance the availability of resources (i.e., access to colonoscopy) and

the greater potential willingness to be screened initially with less invasive stool tests (21). Although the number of Americans being screened continues to improve, currently only 66% of adults over 50 years of age in the U.S. are receiving the recommended screening (22).

Common signs and symptoms of colorectal cancer are blood in the stool or bleeding from the rectum, or bowel obstruction as the tumor grows large enough to block the intestine (i.e., cramping or discomfort in the lower abdomen, narrow stools), as well as constipation or diarrhea that lasts for more than a few days, or unintentional weight loss (23). Staging of colon cancer is similar to staging of other solid tumors and is based on features of the tumor and whether and where the cancer has spread.

Prognosis

Currently, the 5-year survival rate for colorectal cancer is 64%. For the 39% of colorectal cancers identified at the stage of localized disease, the 5-year survival rate is 90%. The 5-year survival for those diagnosed at a regional stage is 71%, and for those diagnosed at a distant stage, the 5-year survival drops to 14% (23).

Treatment

The primary treatment approach for colon cancer is surgery to remove the tumor. This requires an abdominal incision. For localized (stage 1) cancers, surgery may be the only treatment required. The tumor is removed along with a length of colon on either side and nearby lymph nodes. For regional stage cancers, if the tumor has grown through the wall of the colon, radiation therapy and/or chemotherapy may be added to a surgical resection. If the cancer has spread to nearby lymph nodes, chemotherapy is usually added after surgery to reduce the risk of the cancer returning.

The treatment for rectal cancer follows an approach similar to that for colon cancer. A key difference is that surgical resection of the tumor may be achieved through the anus, thus avoiding the need for an abdominal incision. Radiation and/or chemotherapy is sometimes neoadjuvant, meaning given before surgery.

Health Implications for Survivors

During chemotherapy or radiation treatment, individuals often suffer from diarrhea. This adverse effect may reduce patients' willingness to participate in physical activity, especially if there is no washroom easily accessible. Furthermore, fecal incontinence can be a side effect of surgery and radiation treatment, particularly for those treated for rectal cancer. Bladder irritation is also a common side effect of radiation treatment because of the location of the treatment. The CEP is encouraged to be aware of these issues.

In the case of an abdominal incision, it is advisable to follow recommendations provided by the surgeon regarding physical activity levels for the first 4–6 weeks after surgery to allow healing of the surgical site. This commonly involves avoiding activities that cause excessive intra-abdominal pressure or direct pressure on the incision. A unique potential health implication of colorectal cancer may be a temporary or permanent ostomy. If a section of colon or rectum is removed as part of surgical treatment, the surgeon can usually connect the healthy parts of the bowel again and waste can be eliminated normally. However, if reconnection is not possible, the surgeon will then complete an ostomy, in which the bowel is connected to an opening made in the skin of the abdomen (a stoma), thereby allowing waste to leave the body. The waste is commonly collected in a flat bag that is attached to the stoma and held in place by special adhesive tape. This may be temporary: once the area has healed from the initial surgery, another surgery may be performed to reconnect the bowel. In some cases, the ostomy may be permanent. If the ostomy is connected to the colon, it is called a colostomy, and if it is connected to the small intestine, it is called an ileostomy (1). ACSM recommends those with an ostomy to empty the ostomy bag before starting exercise, consider use of an ostomy protector/shield for contact sports or where there is a risk of a blow to the ostomy, and for those with an ileostomy to get medical advice on ways to maintain optimal hydration prior, during and after exercise because of increased risk of dehydration (24). ACSM also recommends starting with low resistance and progress slowly with weightlifting or resistance exercise, ideally under the guidance of a trained exercise professional. People with an ostomy may be at an increased risk of parastomal hernia. Avoid using the Valsalva maneuver is recommended as well as modification of any core exercises that cause excessive intra-abdominal pressure, namely the feeling of pressure in the abdomen or observed bulging of the abdomen (24) modify core exercises or other.

One of the most common chemotherapy agents used for colorectal cancer is oxaliplatin. A primary side effect is the development of peripheral neuropathy, which presents as numbness, tingling, and cramping of the hands or feet. Numbness of the feet may impair balance and cramping in the hands may impair hand grip. These symptoms tend to improve slowly following treatment, but they can sometimes persist.

HEAD AND NECK CANCER

Epidemiology

Head and neck cancer is a general term used for cancers that start in the oral cavity/tongue, lips, parts of the throat (oro-, naso-, or hypopharyngeal cancers), nasal cavity and paranasal sinuses, or salivary glands (25). According to the American Cancer Society, each year there are 54,000 new cancer cases of the oral cavity and pharynx in the U.S. and 11,230 people die from this type of cancer (1). The main risk factors for the development of head and neck cancers are tobacco (smoking and smokeless products) and alcohol, which have an additive effect when combined. These risk factors account for approximately 75% of cases. Human papillomavirus (HPV) is an emerging risk factor for head and neck cancers. Infection with HPV is currently linked to 70% of cancers of the oropharynx (25). Oral cancer prevention has now been added as an indication for the HPV vaccine; however, only 59% of adolescents (13–17 years) were up to date with HPV vaccination as of 2020 (1).

Common Presentation

The presentation of head and neck cancers varies depending on the function of the area where the cancer originates. For example, cancers of the larynx may present as hoarseness, whereas cancers of the pharynx may present as difficult swallowing (dysphagia). However, the symptoms commonly are nonspecific or general, such as ear pain or a sore throat, or painless enlarged lymph nodes in the neck area (26). This can make head and neck cancers difficult to detect or diagnose.

Currently, the only proposed screening for head and neck cancers is visual examination for oral cancer, such as by a dentist. However, there is limited evidence to support the benefits of this screening in the general population (27).

As with other solid tumors, staging of head and neck cancer is based on features of the tumor and whether and where the cancer has spread.

Prognosis

The 5-year survival rate is 66% for cancer of the oral cavity or pharynx (1). The 5-year survival rate for HPV-related cancers is higher, and, in recent studies, has approached 90%, even in more advanced cancer (*i.e.*, stage IV) and especially in people who have never smoked (28). A key feature is that cancers at these anatomical sites affect important functions such as speech, swallowing, taste, and smell. As a result, both the cancer and its treatment can considerably reduce quality of life (QOL) (26).

Treatment

Treatment for early-stage (stages I and II) head and neck cancers usually entails either surgery or radiation. The treatment decision is based on the location of the tumor, the extent of the tumor, and the functional/aesthetic outcome. For more advanced stage (*i.e.*, stage III, stage IV cancer), a multimodal approach to treatment is common, including surgery, radiation, and chemotherapy (25).

Health Implications for Survivors

The aesthetic impact of cancer surgery and radiation treatment may include significant disfigurement of the head and neck area. In addition, surgery can result in functional impairments, such as in the patient's ability to speak or swallow. Musculoskeletal issues are also common, especially when the surgery includes a neck dissection to examine surrounding lymph nodes for signs of cancer. Neck dissection and radiation can damage the muscles, nerves, and other structures of the neck and lead to spinal accessory-nerve palsy, spasms of cervical muscles, or neuropathies, shoulder dysfunction, and lymphedema. The current American Cancer Society Head and Neck Cancer Survivorship Care Guidelines recommend completion of a baseline assessment of shoulder ROM and muscular strength to monitor changes following treatment, and referral to a rehabilitation specialist, such as a physical therapist, to address pain, disability, and dysfunction in the neck or shoulder regions (25). Patients with head and neck cancer also typically experience significant weight loss in the year following treatment, particularly if treatment results in altered eating/swallowing capacity. A cancer exercise specialist may also be a member of the team and work in conjunction with a physical therapist to address issues of muscle strength and function.

HEMATOLOGICAL CANCER

Epidemiology

Cancers that begin in blood-forming tissue, such as the bone marrow, or in the cells of the immune system are called "blood" or hematological cancers. These are usually classified into three main categories: lymphoma arises in the tissues of the lymphatic system, myeloma (or multiple myeloma) is cancer of the plasma cells (antibody-producing B cells) in the bone marrow, and leukemias are cancers that affect blood-forming tissues and usually involve leukocytes (white blood cells). Within each of these three categories are different types of cancer with differing presentations, treatment, and prognosis. According to the American Cancer Society, each year there are 89,010 new cases of lymphoma. Of these, 90% were non-Hodgkin lymphoma, and the remainder were Hodgkin lymphoma. There were also 34,470 new cases of myeloma and 60,650 new cases of various types of leukemia (1).

Common Presentation

The presentation of hematological cancers stems from the impact of abnormal blood cells and their resulting functions. The common symptoms of lymphoma are swollen lymph nodes, shortness of breath, chest pain, abdominal fullness, loss of appetite, and intermittent fever. For myeloma and leukemia, common symptoms include fatigue, paleness, repeated infections, bleeding or bruising easily, bone or joint pain, and swelling in lymph nodes. These signs can appear suddenly in acute leukemia or more gradually in chronic leukemia. For myeloma, common symptoms also include bone pain, as myeloma cells make a substance that causes osteoclasts to speed up bone breakdown. This commonly presents as pain in the back, hip, and skull, as well as high levels of calcium in the blood (1).

Staging for each cancer is unique. It involves consideration of the number of abnormal cells, features of the abnormal cells, number of lymph nodes involved, and other criteria.

Prognosis

The prognosis depends on the type of hematological cancer. For non-Hodgkin lymphoma and Hodgkin lymphoma, the 5-year survival rate is 73% and 88%, respectively. For leukemia, the 5-year survival rate varies substantially by the subtype of leukemia and ranges from 27% for those diagnosed with acute myeloid leukemia (AML) to 87% for those diagnosed with chronic lymphocytic leukemia (CLL) (1).

Treatment

Because hematological cancers develop in blood-forming tissue, such as the bone marrow, or in the cells of the immune system, the primary treatment is chemotherapy, which is systemic. This typically involves combinations of chemotherapy agents, sometimes in combination with targeted drugs (1). If chemotherapy is not successful, the patient may undergo a stem cell transplant (29), in which high-dose chemotherapy is administered to ablate the patient's diseased bone marrow, followed by replacement with blood-forming (hematopoietic) stem cells that will produce normal hematological cells. Stem cell transplantations can be allogeneic (taken from one person and given to the recipient) or autologous (taken from the recipient's own bone marrow or blood). There is a higher chance of the cancer returning with an autologous transplant, because some cancer cells may escape the chemotherapy treatments and be returned to the host (29). However, the allogeneic transplant has a higher rate of complications, including graft-versus-host disease (GVHD), in which the recipient's immune system recognizes the donated stem cells as foreign and starts to destroy them. GVHD can be acute (within the first 100 days after transplant) or chronic. The signs and symptoms are commonly skin rash, abdominal pain or cramps, diarrhea, nausea, vomiting, and jaundice or other liver problems. These are commonly managed with immunosuppressant drugs (30).

Health Implications for Survivors

Individuals treated for hematological cancers typically experience the main side effects of chemotherapy treatment, such as fatigue, anemia, and nausea. The chemotherapy regimens may be longer than those associated with other cancer types, so patients may be more deconditioned than those with other types of cancer. The addition of aerobic and resistance exercise to the care plan for individuals with hematological cancers improves QOL, especially physical functioning, depression, and fatigue (31).

Of particular note for hematological cancers, stem cell transplantation is an extremely rigorous process (32). Patients often have extended hospital stays, commonly under isolation precautions because of their immunocompromised state, and suffer significant fatigue from the treatment itself. The result is significant reductions in physical activity and physical function (33). However, in systematic reviews and meta-analyses, exercise for those receiving a stem cell transplantation led to positive changes in cardiorespiratory fitness, muscle strength, and the functional mobility-state, along with higher QOL and less fatigue (34). During hospitalization, the safety of exercise is carefully monitored daily by checking hematological values and for signs of a potential infection, such as body temperature.

As noted earlier, a unique and common feature of myeloma is osteolytic bone destruction. This can result in long bone or vertebral fractures. Therefore, it is important for the CEP working with this population to understand the current extent of bone involvement and to monitor clients for any new symptoms, such as pain or changes in neurological function, which may suggest additional bone involvement or new fracture (35). The CEP must supervise exercises carefully and modify exercises to ensure safety (36, 37).

THE ROLE OF EXERCISE IN CANCER INCIDENCE AND RECURRENCE

Exercise is known to reduce the risk of a variety of chronic diseases, including cancer. Research also indicates a protective role of exercise in cancer recurrence and mortality.

Evidence That Exercise Reduces Cancer Incidence and Recurrence

Regular exercise is associated with a reduced risk of incidence for breast, colon, endometrial, kidney, bladder, esophageal, and stomach cancer (38). Moreover, epidemiologic evidence is rapidly growing for a potential protective effect of exercise after diagnosis to lower the risk of cancer-specific death of breast, colon, and prostate cancers (38). More research is needed, however, including corroboration from randomized controlled trials and elucidation of the underlying mechanisms and the exact dose of exercise needed to reduce cancer-specific and all-cause mortality. There is also emerging research that reducing sedentary time may also lower risk of endometrial, colon, and lung cancers (38). However, higher physical activity has been shown to be associated with a higher risk of melanoma, a serious form of skin cancer (38). This is thought to be because of higher sun exposure as many types of physical activity are done outside. So good sun safety with outdoor exercise is recommended.

Proposed Mechanisms for the Beneficial Effects of Exercise on Cancer Risk

Several hypotheses attempt to explain the effect of regular exercise on the risk of cancer progression. These include the following: alteration to metabolic pathways and growth factors (*i.e.*, insulin and insulin-like growth factor [IGF] axis pathways); reduction in sex-steroid synthesis; improved immune function; reduced systemic inflammation and oxidative damage; and interrupting angiogenesis in the tumor (39, 40). Interestingly, exercise may be more or less effective at altering tumorigenesis depending on the molecular characteristics of the tumor. This variability in effectiveness suggests a potential precision-medicine approach for exercise in the clinical management of cancer (41).

Exercise may exert a protective effect through changes in the amount and/or activity of adipose or skeletal muscle tissue. Excess adipose tissue can generate signals that the body is in a state of energy surplus, which supports cell proliferation and can contribute to an oncogenic state. Adipose tissue can also serve as an additional energy source if storage depots are located near cancer cells, fueling their growth and survival (42). Numerous studies report that reductions in metabolic hormones and adipocytokines from exercise training are mediated by reductions in body fat (43, 44), and alterations in these metabolic and inflammatory pathways interrupt or slow cancer progression.

Signaling cascades from skeletal muscle might also play a role in slowing cancer progression. Cytokines (myokines) and peptides are released by contracting skeletal muscle. Chronic exposure to these cytokines and peptides may play a protective role in chronic conditions fueled by low-grade inflammation or metabolic dysfunction, including cancer (45)

CLINICAL APPLICATIONS OF EXERCISE IN PATIENTS WITH CANCER AND SURVIVORS

Regular exercise plays an important role not only in reducing the risk of cancer recurrence, but also in supporting the cancer patient's recovery from treatment and increasing the health and fitness of cancer survivors.

Current Guidelines on Exercise After Cancer

In 2010, ACSM published the first exercise guidelines for cancer survivors, which were the results of a roundtable on exercise after cancer (46). The guidelines were first and foremost to "avoid inactivity" and then consistent with the 2008 U.S. Department of Health and Human Services Physical Activity Guidelines for health, namely, aim to achieve 150 minutes per week of moderate aerobic exercise or 75 minutes of vigorous aerobic exercise, along with two times per week or resistance exercise for major

muscle groups (47). The developers of ACSM roundtable guidelines looked for evidence that the advice to cancer survivors should be altered from the federal-wide guidelines and found none. In 2018, ACSM convened a second roundtable with an increased focus on international partners and multidisciplinary representation (i.e., in addition to exercise professionals and researchers, also included oncologists, physiatrist, physiotherapists, and nurses). The 2019 guidelines continued to support the recommendation to avoid inactivity. There was then sufficient evidence from meta-analyses, systematic reviews, and randomized controlled trials to provide specific exercise prescription recommendations to manage many of the common side effects of cancer treatments where benefit is seen with a lower amount of exercise than outlined in the 2010 guidelines (i.e., 90 min per wk moderate-intensity aerobic exercise alone or twice-weekly resistance training alone, or combined aerobic plus resistance training three times per wk for 30 min per session) (24). Once symptom management was achieved, cancer survivors are then advised to progress to the current 2018 U.S. Department of Health and Human Services Physical Activity Guidelines for health. These guidelines recommend 150–300 minutes of moderate aerobic exercise or 75–150 minutes of vigorous aerobic exercise, in addition to 2 days per week of resistance training for all major muscle groups. In addition, the second roundtable developed a framework to promote the use of "ask, advise, refer" as a way for health care providers working in the oncology setting to connect more people to exercise programming during and following cancer treatment (48). These guidelines are consistent with those published by the American Society of Clinical Oncology in 2022, which state that "oncology providers should recommend regular aerobic and resistance exercise during active treatment with curative intent" (49). The triage are provided in Table 13.1.

The Challenge of Triage

There is a range of levels of function and ability to exercise among those who have been diagnosed with cancer. Further, cancer is diagnosed at many ages, in people who vary broadly with regard to their athletic and health histories. The challenge is to get as many cancer survivors as possible active, while avoiding unnecessary risk to them. The 2019 ACSM guidelines on exercise and cancer (24) provide guidance around various adverse treatment effects specifically around recommendations, the appropriate setting, and level of supervision. These recommendations were based on the National Comprehensive Cancer Network

Table 13.1	Guidelines for Exercise After Cancer		
	Aerobic Activities	Muscle-Strengthening Activities	Flexibility Activities
Deemed safe during and after treatment	Yes	Yes	Yes
Special instructions	Note that aerobic exercise tolerance will vary during treatment.	Start low, progress slow, let symptoms guide. Be aware of risk or history of lymphedema, bone lesions, and peripheral neuropathy.	Effects of surgery and radiation may alter range of motion in the area of treatment. Proceed slowly in stretches.
Volume	Build to 150 min per wk.	Two to three times weekly, 1–3 sets of 8–15 repetitions. One exercise per major muscle group	Most days
Intensity	Moderate (*e.g.*, walking)	Moderate	N/A

The first two words of the guidelines are in keeping with the 2008 U.S. Department of Health and Human Services Federal Wide Physical Activity Guidelines (2008): Avoid Inactivity.

There has long been a misconception that patients with cancer should "rest, take it easy, and not push themselves." These first two words are vital to changing the language of oncology clinicians to recommend maintenance of normal activities during cancer treatment.

N/A, not applicable.

Source: ACSM (American College of Sports Medicine, 2013), American Cancer Society (Rock CL, Doyle C, Demark-Wahnefried W, et al. Nutrition and physical activity guidelines for cancer survivors. *CA Cancer J Clin.* 2012;62(4):242–74); National Comprehensive Cancer Network (Ligibel JA, Denlinger CS. New NCCN guidelines for survivorship care. *J Natl Compr Canc Netw.* 2013;11(5 Suppl):640–4.)

(NCCN) survivorship guidelines published in 2013 (50). Such effects include, for example, bone health issues among breast and prostate cancer survivors, lymphedema risk for breast and gynecologic cancer survivors, issues related to stomas among those with a history of gastrointestinal tumors, peripheral neuropathy for all survivors exposed to chemotherapy, and musculoskeletal morbidity for all cancer survivors. Finally, to decrease barriers to physical activity, there was specific language to avoid the need for any evaluation before walking, mild strengthening exercise, or flexibility exercises (46).

The triage guidelines are provided in Table 13.2.

Finally, there have been several attempts to create agreement on the list of issues that would suggest when exercise should be supervised (vs. unsupervised). One particular effort to separate patients with cancer and survivors into those needing medical supervision, general supervision, and no supervision is the EXCEEDS (Exercise in Cancer Evaluation and Decision Support) algorithm (51). This instrument, developed using a Delphi process, aims to provide a patient-facing tool that can clarify whether a given patient needs medicalized cancer rehabilitation delivered by an outpatient cancer rehabilitation professional, supervised exercise delivered by an exercise oncology professional, or general exercise recommendations similar to the general population. The instrument is provided in Table 13.3 and is being incorporated into the American College of Sports Medicine's Moving Through Cancer Directory to ease clinician's concerns by simplifying referral of patients to appropriate exercise.

There is a natural tension between the effort to connect as many cancer survivors as possible with exercise and the effort to minimize their exercise-related risks. Connecting all survivors with exercise would require community- and home-based programming that would minimize any prior evaluation, with given focus of resources. This would place some proportion of survivors in harm's way but would benefit a large number of survivors. At the other extreme, if requiring all survivors to attend a clinical evaluation with a physician or physical therapist prior to referral to exercise would ensure that those who needed rehabilitation or supervision would be appropriately referred, maximizing safety. Some in the field of exercise oncology see the need for evaluation as a barrier to starting exercise. One tool that could bridge these two options is a self-administered evaluation for survivors to accurately predict whether they need further evaluation and/or supervision. At this time, this self-administered evaluation for survivors does not exist. All exercise professionals are urged to keep survivors moving while keeping them safe.

Table 13.2	Adapted National Comprehensive Cancer Network Triage Approach Based on Risk of Exercise-Induced Adverse Events
Description of Patients	Evaluation, Prescription, and Programming Recommendation
No comorbidities	No further evaluation, follow general guidelines for exercise after cancer
Peripheral neuropathy, arthritis/musculoskeletal issues, poor bone health (*e.g.*, osteopenia or osteoporosis), lymphedema	Recommend preexercise medical evaluation[a] Modify general exercise recommendations based on assessments Consider referral to trained personnel[b]
Lung or abdominal surgery, ostomy, cardiopulmonary disease, ataxia, extreme fatigue, severe nutritional deficiencies, worsening/changing physical condition (*i.e.*, lymphedema exacerbation), bone metastases	Preexercise medical evaluation[a] and clearance by physician before exercise Referral to trained personnel[b]

[a]Medical evaluation — per NCCN guidelines for specific symptoms and side effects.

[b]Rehabilitation specialists (*i.e.*, physical therapists, occupational therapists, physiatrists) and certified exercise physiologists (*i.e.*, ACSM Certified Clinical Exercise Physiologist [ACSM-CEP], Canadian Society for Exercise Physiology Certified Exercise Physiologist [CSEP-CEP], Exercise & Sport Science Australia Accredited Exercise Physiologist [ESSA-AEP]).

Table 13.3	EXCEEDS Triage Algorithm	
Algorithm Domain	Criteria	References
Section 1: Medical Clearance Recommendation		
Physical activity level	Yes or no: currently meeting exercise guidelines (guidelines: ≥30 min of moderate-intensity exercise on ≥3 d per wk for ≥3 mo)[a]	• American College of Sports Medicine guidelines for exercise testing and prescription (52) • ActivOnco Model (53)
Chronic disease	Yes or no: presence of ≥1 chronic disease or related complications, including the following: • Heart failure • Kidney failure (or other renal disease) • Diabetes • Metastatic cancer to bones or brain or another major organ • Unstable angina • Dizziness resulting in loss of balance or consciousness • Major surgery with restrictions in past 3 mo • History of cardio-toxic treatment	• Physical Activity Readiness Questionnaire (PAR-Q) (54) • American College of Sports Medicine guidelines for exercise testing and prescription (52) • Cancer-specific exercise risk screening tool (55) • National Comprehension Cancer Network (NCCN): Survivorship Clinical Practice Guidelines V1.2020 (National Comprehensive Cancer Network, 2020) (56) • Macmillan Cancer Rehabilitation pathways (57)
	Yes or no: new, worsening, or difficulty managing any of the following conditions: lymphedema, ostomy, significant weight fluctuations, infection, ataxia, malnourishment, severe fatigue, bone/back/neck pain and unusual weakness	• ActivOnco Model (53) • Macmillan Cancer Rehabilitation pathways (57)

Table 13.3	EXCEEDS Triage Algorithm (*continued*)	
Algorithm Domain	**Criteria**	**References**
High-risk signs/ symptoms	Yes or no: presence of ≥1 complication or high-risk signs/symptoms associated with the following diseases: • Cardiovascular or respiratory disease • Previous stroke, neurological condition, or spinal cord injury • Musculoskeletal injury or degenerative conditions • Recent steroid injection and potential for steroid-induced myopathy • Uncontrolled diabetes mellitus	• Physical Activity Readiness Questionnaire (PAR-Q) (54) • National Comprehension Cancer Network (NCCN): Survivorship Clinical Practice Guidelines V1.2020 (56) • Macmillan Cancer Rehabilitation pathways (57) • Cancer-specific exercise risk screening tool (55) • ActivOnco Model (53)
Section 2: Triage Recommendations		
Cancer-specific factors	Yes or no, presence of ≥1 of the following factors: • Cancer type (head and neck, lung myeloma, sarcoma, or metastasis to bones, brain, or other organ) • Fracture risk or severe osteoporosis or osteopenia • History of blood clot, deep vein thrombosis, or pulmonary embolism • Lymphedema high risk or difficulty managing	• ActivOnco Model (53) • Macmillan Cancer Rehabilitation pathways (57) • National Comprehension Cancer Network (NCCN): Survivorship Clinical Practice Guidelines V1.2020 (56) • Focused review of safety considerations in cancer rehab (58) • The Interdisciplinary Rehabilitation Care Team and the Role of Physical Therapy in Survivor Exercise (59)
Level 2 functional factors	Yes or no, presence of ≥1 of the following factors: • Mobility aid required to complete daily activities • Able to mobilize 1 block of less • Limited upper extremity range of motion • ADL or IADL dependency • Moderate-to-severe general mobility pain (hip knee, back, etc.) • Ataxia or unusual weakness • Moderate cognitive declines that impair function • Peripheral neuropathy that is painful or limits function	• National Comprehension Cancer Network (NCCN): Survivorship Clinical Practice Guidelines V1.2020 (56) • NCCN Guidelines® Insights: Older Adult Oncology, Version 1.2021 (https://pubmed.ncbi.nlm.nih.gov/34551388/) • Exercise in Medicine in Oncology: ACSM 2019 Roundtable (48) • Macmillan Cancer Rehabilitation pathways (57) • ActivOnco Model (53) • Cancer-specific exercise risk screening tool (55) • Association of Clinical Oncology (ASCO) Management of Older Adults Guideline (61) • The Interdisciplinary Rehabilitation Care Team and the Role of Physical Therapy in Survivor Exercise (59) • International Society of Geriatric Oncology (SIOG) recommendation for management of cancer-related cognitive decline (62)

(*continued*)

Table 13.3	EXCEEDS Triage Algorithm *(continued)*	
Algorithm Domain	**Criteria**	**References**
Level 2 side effects	Yes or no, presence of ≥1 of the following factors: • Moderate-to-severe fatigue (4+) • Neurological symptoms (dizziness/lightheaded; disorientation) • Blurred vision • Dyspnea	• Macmillan Cancer Rehabilitation pathways (57) • ActivOnco Model (53) • The Interdisciplinary Rehabilitation Care Team and the Role of Physical Therapy in Survivor Exercise (59)
Level 1 functional factors	Yes or no, presence of ≥1 of the following factors: • Fall in previous 6 mo • Other mobility issues, including decreased balance, decreased gait speed, mild bodily pain when moving, difficulty with ADL/IADL	• Macmillan Cancer Rehabilitation pathways (57) • Association of Clinical Oncology (ASCO) Management of Older Adults Guideline (61) • Cancer and Aging Research Group Fall Risk Model (63) • Exercise in Medicine in Oncology: ACSM 2019 Roundtable (48) • The Interdisciplinary Rehabilitation Care Team and the Role of Physical Therapy in Survivor Exercise (59)
Level 1 side effects	Yes or no, presence of ≥1 of the following factors: • Active treatment or surgery in past 3 mo • Treatment side effects, including the following: • Daily mild fatigue • Mild neuropathy • Occasional cognitive difficulty • Orthostatic hypotension • Gastrointestinal (severe nausea; vomiting/diarrhea; dehydration; inadequate food/fluid intake) • Urinary or fecal incontinence • Managed lymphedema • Weakened immune system: thrombocytopenia (low platelets), anemia (low hemoglobin), or neutropenia (low white blood cell count)	• The Interdisciplinary Rehabilitation Care Team and the Role of Physical Therapy in Survivor Exercise (59) • Macmillan Cancer Rehabilitation pathways (57) • ActivOnco Model (53) • National Comprehension Cancer Network (NCCN): Survivorship Clinical Practice Guidelines V1.2020 (56)
Presence of a catheter	Yes or no, current or planned upcoming presence of catheter (including but not limited to: peripherally inserted central catheter [PICC], intraperitoneal catheter, or ostomy)	• National Comprehension Cancer Network (NCCN): Survivorship Clinical Practice Guidelines V1.2020 (56) • Macmillan Cancer Rehabilitation pathways (57)

Table 13.3	EXCEEDS Triage Algorithm (*continued*)	
Algorithm Domain	Criteria	References
Exercise self-efficacy	Yes or no, high confidence in ability to exercise at least three times per wk for at least 30 min per d over the next 3 mo without support from an exercise professional.	• Macmillan Cancer Rehabilitation pathways (57) • National Comprehension Cancer Network (NCCN): Survivorship Clinical Practice Guidelines V1.2020 (56) • The Interdisciplinary Rehabilitation Care Team and the Role of Physical Therapy in Survivor Exercise (59)

ADL, activities of daily living; IADL, instrumental activities of daily living.

aMeasure: Physical Activity Vital Sign (PAVS).

Source: Reprinted from Covington KR, Marshall T, Campbell G, et al. Development of the Exercise in Cancer Evaluation and Decision Support (EXCEEDS) algorithm. *Support Care Cancer.* 2021;29:6469–80.

Clinical Considerations for Working With Patients Currently in Treatment

Preexercise screening for participation in moderate to vigorous aerobic exercise or resistance exercise should follow ACSM guidelines (24). In this process, it is essential to obtain a health history, including preexisting comorbid chronic health conditions, preexisting musculoskeletal issues that may limit exercise participation, and any other exercise contraindications. Information on the current cancer treatment regimen should also be recorded, primarily the type of treatment (chemotherapy, radiotherapy) and treatment schedule (*i.e.*, 2- or 3-week cycle for chemotherapy and total number of anticipated cycles, or planned number of fractions of radiotherapy). An assessment of prior exercise history is also important to allow individualization of the exercise prescription (64).

The baseline physical assessment should include a comprehensive assessment of all components of health-related physical fitness. Standard exercise testing methods are generally safe and appropriate for patients with cancer, keeping in mind any modifications required based on the information obtained in the health history and the most common toxicities associated with cancer treatments (52). Of note, there is no evidence that the level of medical supervision required for symptom-limited or maximal exercise testing needs to be different for patients with cancer than for other populations, and there is evidence that 1-RM testing is safe among early-stage breast cancer survivors (52).

A key feature of exercise prescription during treatment is that an individual's exercise tolerance or ability to progress exercise volume may fluctuate with treatment cycles or with the accumulation of treatment side effects, such as increasing fatigue with serial radiation treatments. For clients who are not currently meeting ACSM guidelines of 150 minutes per week, it may be appropriate to start with 10- to 20-minute bouts, three times per week for 2–3 weeks, and assess how the individual is tolerating that dose, with the goal of gradually moving the individual toward meeting the target for cancer-related health outcomes (*i.e.*, 90 min per wk of moderate aerobic exercise) (24) or build up to at least 150 minutes per week of aerobic exercise if overall health is the goal (65). Of note, during active treatment, there are published approaches on how to progress exercise between chemotherapy cycles, including building in a 10% in reduction in exercise load (*i.e.*, reduced intensity) in the 3–5 days following chemotherapy and then progress exercise in weeks between chemotherapy cycles (66, 67).

Unique challenges of exercise during chemotherapy are changes in blood counts and dehydration and low-energy intake, the latter of which are common when chemotherapy triggers symptoms of nausea. If possible, it is helpful to review the client's recent blood counts either through approved access to the medical record or by asking the patient to provide the latest blood count values taken as part of routine medical care. Table 13.4 identifies blood values and symptoms for which exercise may be contraindicated. Review by a physician is warranted prior to continuing. Both resting and exercise heart rate may be less reliable during treatment (68), so it is advisable to teach clients to use rating of perceived exertion to monitor exercise intensity.

Resting and exercise blood pressure values may also vary more during treatment. Feeling lightheaded when changing position can be common because of dehydration, so clients are advised to change positions slowly, especially after exertion (*i.e.*, such as standing up from a leg press machine). Clients may also experience side effects that may reduce the ability to perform some or all modes of exercise, or they may require modifications. The CEP should also modify the exercise as necessary to ensure

Table 13.4	Factors to Monitor for Exercise Participation During Cancer Treatment	
	Precaution Requiring Physician Approval	Consideration
General	Pain	Investigate any new onset of pain; modify exercise to avoid exacerbations of existing pain.
Chemotherapy/ targeted therapy	Platelets <50,000	Avoid activities that increase risk of injury (falling), bruising, or bleeding. Check with physician on safety of exercise beyond activities of daily living.
	White blood cells <3,000	Avoid public facilities where risk of exposures to bacteria is high; adhere to infection control guidelines.
	Hemoglobin <10 g·dL^{-1}	Prescribe only low-intensity activities (*e.g.*, easy walking). Activities should be performed for shorter periods of time, more frequently. Allow for adequate rest/recovery.
	Febrile illness >100°F	No formal exercise training; avoid exercise until asymptomatic by >48 h.
		Vomiting or diarrhea
	Peripheral neuropathy: loss of sensation and poor balance	Avoid free weights and treadmill; use well-supported positions for exercise.
	Osteoporosis bone issues	Avoid high-impact exercise.
Radiotherapy	Cancer-related fatigue	Closely monitor response to exercise.
	Severe tissue reaction in region	Avoid exercises that compromise the skin and tissue in the region.

Source: Data from McNeely ML, Peddle CJ, Parliament M, Courneya KS. Cancer rehabilitation: recommendations for integrating exercise programming in the clinical practice setting. *Curr Cancer Ther Rev.* 2006;2(4):351–60.

safety, such as by moving aerobic exercise to a stationary bike or limiting the use of handheld free weights.

Specific Cancer and Treatment-Related Sequelae Affecting Exercise

Even if treated for the same type of cancer, cancer survivors vary in the nature and pattern of their responses to treatment. Even in the same patient, some side effects might subside within a short time after treatment is completed, others might gradually subside over many months, yet others might persist for years and potentially a lifetime. Given this variability in the nature and trajectory of cancer-related sequelae, individual consideration of conditions that might impact a person's safety and tolerance for exercise is strongly recommended. A thorough review of medical records (if accessible), a comprehensive client intake process, and performance assessment are advised.

Several of the most common sequelae that survivors experience is discussed in the following, along with their impact on exercise capacity. A summary of acute and long-term treatment-related sequelae is provided in Table 13.5.

Fatigue

Fatigue is the most common side effect during cancer treatment. Over 90% of patients experience fatigue during treatment, and in as much as 60% of survivors, fatigue will persist for many years past the cancer diagnosis (69). Cancer-related fatigue is described as being distinct from the tiredness that the average person feels at the end of a workday or after a long exercise session and as feeling "sick." The experience of cancer-related fatigue has been associated with elevated cytokines; however, whether it is centrally or peripherally mediated remains unclear, and the precise mechanisms may vary across individuals, treatments, and time. Universally, the impact of persistent fatigue could manifest as a reduced exercise tolerance and potentially reduced motivational drive. Thus, adjusting the exercise prescription to an individual's symptom level may improve compliance. To maintain effectiveness, yet accommodate

Table 13.5	Side Effects of Cancer Treatment That Influence Exercise Tolerance		
	Timing		
Therapy Type	Acute[a]	Long Term[b]	Late[c]
Surgery	• Swelling • Pain • Constipation	• Pain • Lymphedema[d] • Limited ROM	• Lymphedema • Difficulty communicating, swallowing, or eating • Sexual dysfunction • Hernia, bowel or bladder dysfunction • Difficulty breathing, pain, fatigue
Radiation therapy	• Fatigue • Nausea/vomiting • Hair loss • Skin changes	• Pain • Limited ROM • Fatigue • Lymphedema[d]	• Second cancers • Fibrosis in the area treated
Chemotherapy	• Fatigue • Nausea/vomiting • Hair loss • Peripheral neuropathy • Altered executive cognitive function	• Fatigue • Weakness • Neurotoxicities • Weight gain or weight loss[e]	• CVD • Frailty • Second cancers
Hormone therapy — antiestrogens	• Hot flashes • Cognitive impairment	• Arthralgias, myalgias • Weight gain	• Osteoporosis • Metabolic syndrome
Hormone therapy — antiandrogens	• Vasomotor flushing • Fatigue • Vertigo	• Fatigue • Weakness • Altered body composition ($\downarrow$muscle, $\uparrow$fat, $\downarrow$bone mass) • Depression	• Frailty • Osteoporosis • Metabolic syndrome

CVD, cardiovascular disease; ROM, range of motion.

[a]Onsets mainly during treatment and resolves when treatment is complete.

[b]Onsets during or shortly after treatment and does not resolve after completion of treatment.

[c]Onsets many months or years after completion of treatment.

[d]Most common in breast, gynecologic, and bladder cancer, but can occur in any type of cancer when and where lymph nodes are surgically resected.

[e]The direction of weight change during chemotherapy is dependent on the cancer type, but weight gain usually leads to a disproportionate increase in body fat, whereas weight loss usually leads to a disproportionate loss of muscle.

day-to-day fluctuations in fatigue levels, training programs should have both progression and flexibility for modifications built in. Regular symptom-limited exercise can be an effective countermeasure for treatment-related fatigue (70).

Pain

Pain can also result from surgery, radiation therapy, chemotherapy, and antiestrogen hormonal therapies. Pain related to surgery or radiation therapy is mostly localized to the treatment site and could limit a person's tolerance for exercises using the involved or proximal joints and musculature. Survivors may be able to exercise with pain that

is tolerable and not worsened by exercise; however, modification or omission of individual exercises that exacerbate pain may be necessary. For persons treated with chemotherapy, pain associated with peripheral neuropathy may also linger and impact mobility and function of both the lower and upper extremities (71). Arthralgias (joint pain) and myalgias (muscle pain) are common side effects of aromatase inhibitor therapy for breast cancer and may limit exercise tolerance. Although exercise may need to be modified to accommodate pain and improve compliance, it may also be an effective therapeutic strategy to reduce chronic musculoskeletal pain. In a randomized controlled trial of previously inactive breast cancer survivors, a yearlong program of combined moderate-intensity aerobic and resistance training was well tolerated and significantly decreased joint pain, pain severity, and pain interference (72). In head and neck cancer survivors, progressive resistance training reduced shoulder pain and upper extremity disability (73).

Cancer that has spread to the bones is often painful, and bone pain can be an initial sign of skeletal metastases. Exercise training may be safe and tolerated in persons with skeletal metastases when it is carefully prescribed, includes an element of supervised exercise instruction (74), or limits forces through involved skeletal sites (75, 76). A 2021 systematic review reported that there are now published exercise recommendations for people with bone metastases (35) which provide additional guidance for exercise professionals.

Limited ROM

ROM is often limited as a result of scarring that follows surgical resection of cancer and, in some cases, after radiation therapy. In particular, survivors of breast and head and neck cancers are often faced with considerable arm and shoulder morbidity that can limit upper extremity function. Indirectly, prolonged deconditioning could limit joint mobility. Limited ROM can affect a survivor's ability to fully participate in exercise, particularly resistance training, and thus improving ROM and correcting asymmetries may be an important initial goal of training. Flexibility exercise or low-intensity dynamic exercise, such as water aerobics or tai chi, may improve ROM even in persons who are many years past treatment completion (77–79).

Lymphedema

Lymphedema is a common sequel of surgery and, sometimes, radiation therapy. It results from removal and/or damage to lymph vessels and nodes. Disruption of the lymphatic system can weaken its ability to properly clear lymph fluid from surrounding tissues, causing fluid to build up in the affected areas. For example, upper limb lymphedema can occur in 10%–90% of breast cancer survivors who are treated with surgery and/or radiation therapy (80). The onset of lymphedema can vary and may even manifest several months or longer after treatment completion. Lymphedema is not a contraindication to exercise. Rather, resistance training may be helpful in restoring normal lymph function in affected limbs (81). However, exercise must be carefully approached to avoid exacerbation of symptoms. A program should begin at a low intensity, and progress slowly, and the CEP should monitor the patient

for exacerbation of symptoms (e.g., increased swelling or pressure in the affected limb). If prescribed, compression garments should be worn during exercise (82).

In the landmark Physical Activity and Lymphedema (PAL) trial, progressive low- to moderate-intensity resistance training did not increase the onset or worsening of lymphedema in breast cancer survivors who were at risk for or who already had lymphedema (83, 84). The PAL trial also noted improvements in muscular strength, functional status, body image, lymphedema symptoms, and QOL. As such, the study investigators translated the intervention into a clinical intervention taught by physical therapists, covered by insurance, and with exercises performed at home (85). This translated intervention remained effective, and an online course to train physical therapists (and clinical exercise professionals) to deliver this intervention is now available (86). Because research and guidelines for exercise in persons with lower extremity lymphedema is less abundant, similar safety precautions should be taken and symptoms should be aggressively tracked.

Muscle Weakness

Muscle weakness is common after cancer treatment because of overall deconditioning and other factors. Chemotherapy may cause a small loss of lean mass because of direct cytotoxic effects on skeletal muscle, whereas men with prostate cancer are particularly likely to develop weakness from loss of muscle caused by androgen deprivation therapy (ADT). Because most cancer survivors are older when diagnosed, treatment may compound age-related weakness and sarcopenia. Epidemiologic evidence from a case-control cohort from the study of osteoporotic fractures observed that grip strength declined faster in older women following a breast cancer diagnosis than in older noncancer controls (87). A sharp decline in quadriceps strength also occurred in the immediate postdiagnosis period, but gradually recovered; suggesting that older survivors may be particularly prone to weakness-related impairments and falls early in the postdiagnosis period. For patients with any degree of muscle weakness, the CEP should tailor the exercise programs to each person's relative capacity and progress the program gradually. Resistance training may be a particularly important modality; moreover, exercises that focus on functional movements should be considered so that neuromuscular adaptations directly translate to movement patterns used during activities of daily living.

Neurotoxicity

Cancer survivors may have been treated with a chemotherapy agent (e.g., platinum-based agents, vinca alkaloids, taxanes) that affects the central and peripheral nervous systems and results in neurotoxicity. Specific sequelae could include peripheral neuropathy, ototoxicity, vestibulotoxicity, and/or cognitive difficulties.

Chemotherapy-induced peripheral neuropathy (CIPN) results from damage to peripheral nerves and causes symptoms of numbness and/or tingling in the hands and/or feet that is often painful. CIPN may persist for many years in as much as 50% of people treated with chemotherapy and is associated with altered gait, reduced physical functioning, falls, and disability (88). In individuals with CIPN, exercise may need to focus on restoring normal gait and functional mobility while attending to safety precautions that minimize the risk of falls.

Some cancer survivors experience ototoxicity, vestibulotoxicity, and/or cognitive difficulties as a result of chemotherapy. These problems can affect survivors' ability to hear and follow exercise instructions, especially those involving complex movement sequences. Vestibulotoxicities are difficult to identify, but may manifest as vertigo, unsteadiness, or chronic dizziness. As such, safety precautions to reduce fall risk during exercise should be identified and implemented.

There is mixed evidence about whether exercise might alleviate neurotoxic symptoms and side effects, although this research is still in its infancy. Despite this, exercise training in persons with neurotoxicity is not contraindicated, especially if safety and tolerability are monitored.

LATE EFFECTS OF CANCER TREATMENT

Awareness is growing of the "late effects" of cancer treatment; that is, adverse effects that linger long after treatment ends. Now that cancer survivors are living considerably longer after initial diagnosis, follow-up surveillance studies of survivor health are providing opportunities to observe the incidence of conditions that are linked to cancer treatment but manifest later during the survivorship process. Furthermore, because cancer is typically diagnosed at a later age, late effects may act synergistically with age-related functional decline and other comorbidities to affect exercise tolerance. Awareness of these potential late effects and interactions can guide the CEP in monitoring patients for signs/symptoms of a new condition and incorporating appropriate safety precautions.

Cardiovascular Disease

As survival rates for cancer have improved, CVD has become a competing cause of morbidity and mortality for survivors of cancer with a favorable prognosis (89). Several pathological processes are known to increase the risk of CVD, including myocardial stress, endothelial dysfunction, atherosclerosis, and platelet activation. There is growing evidence that cancer treatments — including cytotoxic chemotherapy, targeted cancer therapies, and radiation — can contribute to these processes. Heart failure, for example, is increasingly recognized as a potential late effect of cancer treatment (90). In addition to its direct effects on cardiovascular health, cancer treatment may also elevate certain risk factors for CVD. For example, Weaver and colleagues reported that survivors of breast, prostate, and gynecologic cancers had significantly elevated rates of obesity, hypertension, diabetes, and physical inactivity compared with the general adult population (91).

CVD that is associated with cancer treatment can manifest many years or even decades after initial treatment is completed. Given the potential for underlying CVD, cancer survivors who are treated with chemotherapy and/or radiation therapy should be screened for cardiovascular risk factors and, if implicated, have a cardiopulmonary exercise test prior to beginning exercise (92). For individuals with known or suspected CVD, exercise training should follow appropriate guidelines. As with primary and secondary prevention of CVD, exercise may be a useful strategy to manage CVD risk in cancer survivors, although specific trials with clinical outcomes in the oncology setting have yet to be done (93).

Metabolic Disease

Rates of metabolic syndrome and Type 2 diabetes mellitus (T2DM) may also be elevated following cancer treatment and manifest several years after treatment ends. Obesity is both a risk factor for and consequence of cancer and may thus fuel progression of these conditions in survivorship. Some treatments may have more of a direct effect on metabolic health. ADT for prostate cancer, for example, is linked to dyslipidemia, hyperinsulinemia, and obesity (94), and rates of both CVD and T2DM increase after initiation of antiandrogen therapy (95). For cancer survivors at risk for or with T2DM, exercise training needs to follow the usual recommendations and precautions. Survivors with known or suspected obesity, dyslipidemia, and hypertension should follow exercise guidelines for persons at risk for CVD.

Frailty

Frailty is the culmination of declines in several physiologic systems and is usually associated with advanced age.

Fried et al. proposed five criteria to objectively measure frailty and demonstrated that older adults with at least three of the five frailty criteria (*i.e.*, unintentional weight loss, exhaustion, weakness, slow walking speed, low physical activity) were at increased risk of worsening mobility, hospitalization, and death (96, 97).

A growing body of evidence suggests that cancer treatment may hasten the development of frailty and thus place older cancer survivors at a particularly high risk of poor health outcomes. The physical problems reported by cancer survivors, such as cognitive difficulty, neuropathy, sarcopenia, muscle weakness, slowing, and fatigue, may be similar to those of older people without cancer, but cancer treatment can worsen these declines such that the trajectory toward frailty begins at an earlier age or is accelerated in an older survivor (98, 99). For example, childhood cancer survivors have an increased prevalence of frailty in adulthood at an age not typically associated with frailty (100). This increased prevalence of frailty is thought to be because of the effects of cancer treatment. Other studies have reported a higher prevalence and earlier onset of frailty among breast cancer survivors compared to women without cancer (101).

Objective assessment of frailty is within the scope of preexercise evaluation (96), but can also be obtained by self-report if objective assessment is not possible (102). By detecting frailty early, as a "prefrail" state (*e.g.*, presence of 1–2 frailty criteria using the Fried phenotype), the CEP can help the patient prevent this syndrome. It is also possible to move a patient along the frailty continuum to a lesser state, for example, from "frail" to "prefrail." Because inactivity is itself a component of frailty and affects other frailty components, exercise is a reasonable strategy to address this syndrome in any population. Cancer survivors, in particular, are prone to inactive lifestyles because of the impact of cancer and related treatments; thus, the CEP can play a key role in preventing or reversing frailty.

Bone Loss

Treatment for several cancers can accelerate bone loss, increasing the risk for osteoporosis and subsequent fractures. For example, breast and prostate cancer survivors on long-term hormonal therapies to reduce circulating estrogen or testosterone levels are at an elevated risk of fractures. Thus, the use of exercise to reduce fracture risk, along with appropriate precautions and modifications, should be a central consideration.

For individuals with known or suspected osteoporosis, contraindicated movements include those that place an excessively high load on fragile skeletal sites. These include the following: high-impact loads, hyperflexion or hyperextension of the trunk, flexion or extension of the trunk with added resistance, and dynamic twisting motion. Several research studies have aimed to determine whether exercise can slow bone loss in cancer survivors at risk for osteoporosis because of cancer treatment. In large part, the most effective interventions have followed ACSM exercise recommendations to preserve bone health in the general population (103). ACSM recommends that women engage in weight-bearing endurance exercise (*e.g.*, if walking, include intermittent jogging), appropriate impact activities (contraindicated for persons with known or suspected osteoporosis), and/or resistance exercise, or a combination thereof that produces moderate to high bone loading forces for 3–5 days per week for endurance exercise and 2–3 days per week for resistance and/or impact exercise. The sessions should last 30–60 minutes.

To reduce fracture risk in cancer survivors, preventing falls must also be a goal of therapy, because falls play an important role in fracture etiology (104). There is increasing evidence that men and women fall more frequently after cancer treatment than before and compared to persons who have never had cancer (105, 106); thus, for individuals for whom bone loading may be contraindicated because of age, orthopedic limitations, or balance disorders, a fall prevention program that focuses on lower body strength, balance, and mobility would be a reasonable strategy to lower fracture risk. Trials to determine whether the same types of exercise that reduce age-related falls (*e.g.*, strength training, tai chi training) are similarly effective at preventing falls associated with cancer treatment are underway (107).

Psychosocial Distress

Cancer and its diagnosis can cause significant distress to the patient and his/her loved ones, particularly caregivers. For some people, the emotional toll of cancer is severe enough to lead to posttraumatic stress disorder. Others don't quite reach the level of clinical syndromes but still have significant worries, fears, and other psychological sequelae. For example, a working mother who had a mastectomy for stage 3 breast cancer might experience distress around body image, fear of cancer recurrence, and worries about her ability to return to work or care for her children.

Additionally, the emotional stress and strain of cancer do not evaporate once treatment is over. In fact, the transition from oncological care back to the primary care setting can be a very difficult time psychologically for patients and families because there are few resources or systems to help people navigate back to their everyday lives. In a national survey of cancer survivors who were over 10 years beyond their diagnosis, 30%–40% stated their top health concerns were fear of illness, cancer recurrence, and/or their future, along with trouble sleeping (108).

Because a cancer diagnosis and lingering side effects, like cognitive difficulties, can socially isolate a cancer survivor from others, group exercise with other cancer survivors may be an effective way to reengage and energize a client. Likewise, because caregivers often suffer significant physical and emotional strain from caring for an ill-loved one, involving caregivers in a joint exercise or individual program can improve their health and caregiving abilities (109).

SUMMARY

There are over 100 different types of cancer, and cancer treatments vary broadly according to the site of the cancer, the stage, and many other factors. All forms of treatment — surgery, radiation, chemotherapy, and others — can have lingering effects on functional abilities, chronic disease risks, psychosocial health, and other aspects of the patient's QOL. This can be daunting to the CEP starting to work with cancer survivors. Nonetheless, interacting with and finding positive healthy lifestyle solutions for cancer survivors is a remarkably rewarding process. Further, because there is much still to be learned about the risks and benefits of exercise during and after cancer treatments, work with this population is on the cutting edge of clinical exercise practice.

ACSM and others have published exercise guidelines for those who have had a diagnosis of cancer. In general, the client should aim to avoid inactivity, follow physical activity guidelines for symptom management (*i.e.*, 90 min per wk of moderate aerobic exercise and/or 2 d per wk of resistance training) and progress to standard physical activity guidelines for general health, namely perform 150 minutes per week of aerobic activity, muscle-strengthening exercises two to three times weekly, and flexibility exercises on most days. That said, it is highly recommended that exercise prescriptions for cancer survivors take into account the precise diagnosis and treatment history of cancer survivors. As such, ACSM strongly advocates that cancer survivors should seek highly specialized certified exercise professionals to undergo individualized testing and prescription that will account for their individual needs. The questions of who needs evaluation and supervised exercise remain open at this time; however, evidence supports a brief evaluation prior to starting a new exercise program for all cancer survivors. The CEP should find ways to keep survivors moving while keeping them safe, regardless of the risk level within and for a specific client.

The evidence that exercise has benefits for cancer prevention, prevention of recurrence and mortality, and reduction of persistent adverse effects of treatment is compelling. The CEP, through exercise oncology programming, is urged to collaborate with and support clinical oncology specialists to help clients avoid inactivity, maintain normal daily activities, and improve outcomes during and after treatment across the cancer survivorship spectrum.

Exercise, which is known to help reduce depression and anxiety and elevate mood, is beneficial for someone with a history of cancer (110). However, it is important to recognize that psychological distress, in its many forms, may also impact a cancer survivor's self-efficacy, confidence, motivation, and willingness to begin an exercise program, in addition to his/her ability to stick with this lifestyle change over time. When working with cancer survivors, the CEP should be aware of the emotional burden caused by cancer, particularly when setting short- and long-term behavioral goals. Additional support and reinforcement may be necessary to improve adherence to a program. Even former athletes may have difficulty getting back to an exercise routine, because their expectations and self-image before cancer may be discordant from their current abilities.

CHAPTER REVIEW QUESTIONS

1. What are the three most common cancers your male and female clients are likely to have been diagnosed with?
2. With treatment for breast cancer, what are the main risk factors for developing lymphedema?
3. What are the main side effects of ADT used as part of treatment of prostate cancer?
4. What is an ostomy and what implications does this have for appropriate exercise prescription?

5. What is the most common side effect of cancer treatment and how can an exercise prescription be adapted to address this?
6. Individuals with cancer can experience various types of pain. Identify the main causes of pain and discuss how an exercise prescription should be adapted accordingly.

7. Why is CVD a competing cause of morbidity and mortality for survivors of cancer?
8. What is the current exercise recommendations for people with cancer from ACSM?
9. What does the process of triage refer to and why is it important in the setting of exercise and cancer?
10. What are contraindicated exercises in a patient with known or suspected osteoporosis?

Case Study 13.1

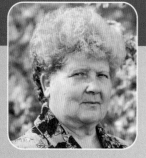

Joanne is 63 years old and had breast cancer 4 years ago. She underwent a mastectomy and reconstruction of the left breast. Ten lymph nodes were removed, and two were positive for cancer. Her reconstruction was performed using expanders that were inserted underneath the pectoral muscle to gradually make room for the silicone implant that matched the size of her right breast. She received doxorubicin, cytoxan, and taxol for her chemotherapy. Radiation of the left chest wall and axilla followed chemotherapy. She takes hormonal therapy (aromatase inhibitors) and will be taking these for 6 more years. Prior to cancer, she was obese (body mass index [BMI] 31 kg·m^{-2}), hypertensive, and had osteoarthritis in both knees.

The arthritis in her knees creates a challenge for her in her full-time occupation as a nurse's aide. She reports that the pain in her knees is worse because of the aromatase inhibitor her oncologist prescribed (*e.g.*, hormone therapy). When she comes to see you, she reports that she's "tired all the time" and is sure she gained 9.1 kg (20 lb) as a result of her breast cancer treatment (current BMI 35 kg·m^{-2}). She is having difficulty maintaining full-time employment as a nurse's aide, given her fatigue and knee pain. She's been referred to you for help regaining the strength and endurance needed to maintain her employment. She is the sole breadwinner for a household of three adults. You notice her left arm is bigger than the right one. When asked, she reports her left arm tires easily.

Your evaluation starts with taking the above history. You request that she sign documents allowing you access to her medical records so you can review her full cancer history. You have her complete a 6-minute walk test (she is at the 50th percentile for age/gender), grip strength test (she is at the 70th and 50th percentiles for age/gender on her right and left arms, respectively), and measure the circumference of her arms at four matched locations on both arms. The left arm sum of circumferences is 10% larger than the right arm. A balance test reveals she is unable to stand on one foot for more than a second or two.

Case Study 13.1 Questions

1. What further information do you need to gather to develop an exercise prescription for Joanne? Who might you want to call/consult for more information?
2. Given her goals, what elements of fitness will be the focus of your prescription?

3. How will you have Joanne start?
4. Will she need to see you for supervised exercise initially? Or will it be possible to prescribe at-home exercise for her?
5. What concerns do you have about unsupervised exercise?

Case Study 13.2

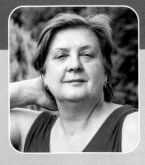

Dorothy is 54 years old and was diagnosed with endometrial cancer 1 year ago. She underwent a total hysterectomy, performed laparoscopically. Of the 30 lymph nodes removed, 15 were positive for cancer. She received doxorubicin, carboplatin, and paclitaxel for her chemotherapy. Radiation of the pelvis and lymph node bed followed chemotherapy. She takes progestins, luteinizing hormone–releasing hormones, and tamoxifen, and will take these for years. Prior to cancer, she was morbidly obese (BMI 45 kg·m^{-2}), diabetic, hypertensive, and had osteoarthritis in both knees.

When she comes to see you, she reports that she's just tired all the time and that she feels dizzy from the ringing in her ears. She cannot currently maintain a job, given her lack of energy, as well as lack of control over defecation. She's been referred to you because of hip pain. She wants help regaining the strength and endurance needed to resume her own self-care and to care for her family (husband and four kids). You notice her left leg is bigger than the right one.

Your evaluation starts with taking the above history. You request that she sign documents allowing you access to her medical records so you can review her full cancer history. You have her complete a 6-minute walk test (she is unable to complete it), a sit and stand test (she is unable to sit and stand from a chair 10 times without a rest), a grip strength test (she is at the 70th and 65th percentiles for age/gender on her dominant and nondominant arms, respectively), and measure the circumference of her legs at four matched locations on both legs. The left leg sum of circumferences is 40% larger than the right leg. A balance test reveals she is unable to stand with feet touching each other without holding on to a chair/wall.

Case Study 13.2 Questions

1. Are there other professionals who may need to evaluate Dorothy for possible other medical therapies before or while you are working with her? Who would they be? Who could you turn to in your professional network to help you discern next steps?
2. Given Dorothy's goal to care for herself and her family, what elements of fitness will be the focus of your prescription?
3. What additional information do you need to complete your evaluation and prescription?
4. How will you have Dorothy start? Will she need to see you for supervised exercise initially? Or will it be possible to prescribe at-home exercise for her?

Case Study 13.3

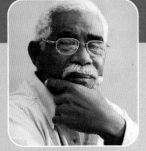

Wendell is 82 years old. He was treated for prostate cancer 10 years ago but is currently being treated for a biochemical recurrence of his disease. When he was first diagnosed with prostate cancer, he had a radical prostatectomy. He had five lymph nodes removed, but none were positive for cancer. The surgery resulted in a small amount of urinary stress incontinence and occasional bowel leakage, but no other bothersome symptoms. About 2 years ago, Wendell was put on ADT to treat a rising PSA level. He receives regular doses of a gonadotropin-releasing hormone agonist, leuprolide (*e.g.*, Lupron Depot), every 4 months. He has also had routine imaging tests, which show no evidence that his cancer has spread to any other organs. His oncologist ordered a follow-up bone density test last month that showed that he had lost bone density and now has osteopenia in his hip and spine. His blood lipids show an elevated low-density lipoprotein cholesterol and

(continued)

Case Study 13.3 (*continued*)

triglycerides and borderline high-fasting blood glucose. He has gained 9.1 kg (20 lb) in the past 2 years but still has a reasonable BMI (26 kg·m^{-2}). At age 65, Wendell had a mild heart attack, but completed cardiac rehabilitation and has been asymptomatic ever since.

When he comes to you, Wendell mentions that as soon as he started the leuprolide shots, he started to experience hot flushes and night sweats that make it difficult for him to sleep well, causing him to feel tired a lot. He has also noticed that he has difficulty climbing up and down the stairs of his two-story house and it takes him longer to complete household chores. This year it took him 3 days to get all of the holiday decorations out of the basement, a task he accomplished in 1 day before starting ADT. He fell a couple of times in the past few months when getting up to go to the bathroom at night, but only experienced bumps and bruises. He is feeling frustrated that he is not as strong and able as he used to be. His wife is worried

about his falls and that he might break his hip. As a former college athlete, Wendell knows he should exercise to get back in shape but is worried about controlling his bladder and his bowels during exercise and does not want to go to a gym. His fatigue makes it difficult for him to be motivated to exercise and he hasn't really done much in several years.

Your evaluation starts with taking the above history. You request that he sign documents allowing you to access his medical records so you can review his full cancer history. You have him complete a 6-minute walk test and he scores in the 50th percentile, a sit and stand test (he completes five chair stands in 15 seconds), and a grip strength test (he is at the 50th percentile for age/gender). A balance test reveals he is unable to stand on one foot for any length of time without losing his balance. His speed walking 4 m (4.4 yards) is 0.9 m·s^{-1} and you notice that he shuffles his feet and needs to take many short steps to complete the course.

Case Study 13.3 Questions

1. Are there other professionals who may need to evaluate Wendell before he starts an exercise program? Would you consult with other professionals about the challenges he is having in his home environment?
2. Given Wendell's health history and the concerns he and his wife have, what goals would you focus on for the initial phase of his exercise program and what program

would you design to meet them? How would you build and progress his program over time?
3. What additional information do you need to complete your evaluation and prescription?
4. How will you have Wendell start? Will he need to see you for supervised exercise initially? Or will it be possible to prescribe at-home exercise for him? How will you keep him motivated to exercise, especially when he is tired?

Case Study 13.4

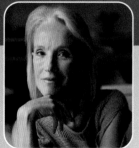

Cindy is 62 years old and was recently treated for non–small cell lung cancer. She was diagnosed just a couple of years before her retirement as a public school administrator. She started smoking at the age of 16 years and smoked 10–15 cigarettes a day, but she quit smoking about 10 years ago at the urging of her family. Her oncologic workup showed that she had a 3.8 cm (1.5-inches) tumor with hilar lymph node involvement, but no spread to distant organs.

She underwent a lobectomy and lymph node dissection, then underwent chemotherapy with cisplatin + vinblastine. During her initial evaluation, evidence of obstructive airway disease was discovered from spirometry, and she was put on an inhaler. Prior to cancer, Cindy was always thin and has unintentionally lost weight over the last year. Her current BMI is 18 kg·m^{-2}. She has no other chronic health conditions.

When she comes to see you, Cindy seems depressed and says she is really only doing this because her daughter thought exercise could help her regain some strength. After listening to Cindy more, you find that she feels tired and weak from the treatment and has a hard time keeping up at the same pace she did at work because she feels "foggy in the head" ever since chemotherapy. She stopped going to her social activities, like book club, and stopped cooking for herself and her husband because it is too taxing. She stopped going for her usual walks around the neighborhood, too, because the pain in her feet is too much and she has trouble not tripping on the bumps and cracks along the old sidewalks. She was told her neuropathy would go away after treatment, but it has not. Although she is not convinced that exercise can do anything for her at this point, she is willing to try working with you for her daughter's sake.

Your evaluation starts with taking the above history. You request that she sign documents allowing you access to her medical records so you can review her full cancer history. You have her complete a 6-minute walk test and she scores in the 25th percentile and is noticeably short of breath after the test. In her sit-to-stand test, she needs to use her hands to get out of the chair and also scores in the 25th percentile for her age. Her grip strength test is at the 50th percentile. A balance test reveals she is able to stand for 10 seconds in a side-by-side position but then can no longer maintain her balance with her eyes closed. She takes 3.2 seconds to walk a 4-m (4.4-yard) course.

Case Study 13.4 Questions

1. Are there other professionals that may need to evaluate Cindy before or while you are working with her? What additional screening, if any, would you want Cindy to undergo before starting an exercise program with you?
2. What additional information do you need to complete your evaluation and prescription? What would be the most important goals for the initial phase of her training program?
3. How will you have Cindy start? Will she need to see you for supervised exercise initially? Or will it be possible to prescribe at-home exercise for her? Are there other settings or environments that might be appropriate for Cindy?
4. Given that Cindy seems skeptical about exercise and is there for external reasons, how will you get her motivated and engaged about exercise? What resources could you enlist to help Cindy?

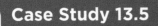

Case Study 13.5

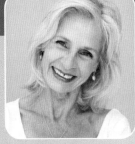

Donna is 58 years old and is undergoing treatment for stage II colon cancer. She underwent surgery 12 weeks ago and did *not* need a colostomy. She is currently receiving chemotherapy treatment every 2 weeks for eight cycles of a regimen called FOLFOX, which is folinic acid (leucovorin), fluorouracil, and oxaliplatin (Eloxatin). She just completed her third of six planned cycles.

Prior to cancer, she was normal weight (BMI 23 kg·m^{-2}) and engaged in some physical activity, namely occasional 30-minute walks with friends one to two times per week and some gardening. She has hypertension that is effectively managed with medications (β-blocker). She works as an administrative assistant at an elementary school and is currently off work on sick leave during her chemotherapy treatment. She is very fatigued from

treatment and is having issues with frequent diarrhea. She reports that since the second chemotherapy cycle she has had significant tingling and numbness in her feet and hands, which got worse after the third treatment she just had. These symptoms have interfered with her gardening as she is having difficulty holding the gardening tools. She also noticed that it is harder to walk on the uneven gravel path in her garden and she says she has tripped a few times but never fallen as a result. After surgery, she would go for walks around the block daily with her husband. She has not been going for many walks since she started chemotherapy because she is worried about being too far from a bathroom, and on one recent walk she did, her feet felt very sensitive and a bit painful with the friction of her socks and shoes on her feet. She has been referred to you by her oncology doctor to help her maintain her endurance and physical function during chemotherapy. However, she says she is not sure if exercise is safe or a good idea during

(*continued*)

Case Study 13.5 (*continued*)

chemotherapy and she doesn't think that any of her friends who have had cancer in the past have done exercise while on treatment.

Your evaluation starts with taking the above history. You request that she sign documents allowing you to access her medical records so you can review her full cancer history and

current treatment. You complete a 6-minute walk test (she is in the 40th percentile for age and gender), grip strength test (she is in the 30th percentile for age and gender and reports difficulty holding the dynamometer), and a sit-to-stand test (she is in the 30th percentile); a balance test reveals she is only able to stand on 1 foot for 2–3 seconds.

Case Study 13.5 Questions

1. What further information do you need to gather to develop an exercise prescription for Donna? Who might you want to call/consult for more information?
2. Given her concerns about safety, how would you approach patient education to address this concern?

3. Given her goals, what elements of fitness will be the focus of your prescription?
4. With Donna being on chemotherapy, what things would you want to keep track of each time Donna comes to see you?

Case Study 13.6

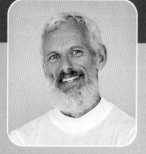

Aaron is 48 years old and was diagnosed with stage II oropharyngeal cancer last year. He received surgery, which included a neck dissection in which five lymph nodes were removed. None was positive for cancer. This was followed by radiation treatment, which he finished 2 months ago. He initially had some difficulty swallowing during radiation but currently has no difficulties. Prior to cancer he was very active and fit, and he had no other health issues. He played recreational hockey two times a week and ran 5–10 km (3–6 miles), three times per week, but he has not done either of these activities since his diagnosis. He used to do weight training at the gym when he was younger. He is an accountant, and the majority of his work time is spent sitting. One month ago, he started a graduated return to work, and

he is now back to working full-time. However, he reports that he has lost a lot of muscle mass and feels very weak. He was moving boxes in the garage last week and had a lot of difficulty lifting boxes off the higher shelves and putting them back up. Two weeks ago, he tried to go for a run for the first time. He ran for 20 minutes and was exhausted for the next 2 days. He shows you a picture of him prior to diagnosis and you can see the muscle mass loss he reports. He has been doing the shoulder ROM and strength training given to him by a physical therapist, and he says his shoulder function is getting better. He has come to see you for help to regain strength and endurance to get back to his recreational sports activities and general household activities.

Your evaluation starts with taking a history. You have him complete a 6-minute walk test (he is in the 90th percentile for age and gender), and grip strength test (he is at the 50th percentile for age and gender on both sides).

Case Study 13.6 Questions

1. What further information do you need to gather to develop an exercise prescription for Aaron? Who might you want to call/consult for more information?
2. Given his goals, what elements of fitness will be the focus of your prescription?

3. Given this client's exercise history and recent difficulty getting back to his usual activities, how will you counsel him about progressing his exercise levels?
4. How will you progress his exercise, keeping in mind his recent return to full-time work?

Case Study 13.7

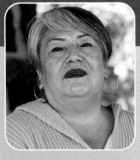

Jennifer is 65 years of age and was diagnosed and received treatment for chronic myeloid leukemia 4 years ago, which included treatment with chemotherapy (fludarabine and cyclophosphamide), steroids (dexamethasone), and targeted therapy (with a monoclonal antibody called rituximab). She states that her doctors say the initial treatment worked, and she goes to see them every 6 months for a checkup. She was employed as a landscaper at the time of her cancer diagnosis and decided to retire. She says she has gained some weight since her diagnosis and retirement and her BMI is now 29 kg·m⁻², but otherwise she has no health conditions. She used to rely on her job to keep her active and currently she does not do any recreational physical activity. Her grandchildren are now 8 and 10 years old and Jennifer wants to take them hiking but reports feeling too out of shape to do that. She was also recently diagnosed with low bone density, which the doctors said might be because of the steroids used to treat her cancer.

The evaluation starts with taking the above history. Request that Jennifer sign documents allowing you to access her medical records so you can review her full cancer history. You complete a 6-minute walk test (she is in the 60th percentile for age and gender), grip strength test (she is in the 50th percentile for age and gender), and sit-to-stand test (she is in the 50th percentile).

Case Study 13.7 Questions

1. What further information do you need to gather to develop an exercise prescription for Jennifer? Who might you want to call/consult for more information?
2. Given her goals, what elements of fitness will be the focus of your prescription?
3. How will you start Jennifer? Will you plan for supervised or unsupervised exercise initially? What concerns do you have about unsupervised exercise?
4. What signs and symptoms should you look for that might indicate Jennifer's cancer has returned?

REFERENCES

1. American Cancer Society. *Cancer Facts & Figures*. Atlanta (GA): American Cancer Society, Inc; 2022. Available from: https://www.cancer.org/research/cancer-facts-statistics/all-cancer-facts-figures/cancer-facts-figures-2022.html.
2. Irwin ML. *ACSM's Guide to Exercise and Cancer Survivorship*. Champaign (IL): Human Kinetics; 2012.
3. Murphy GP, Lawrence W, Lenhard RE. *American Cancer Society Textbook of Clinical Oncology*. 2nd ed. Atlanta (GA): American Cancer Society; 1995.
4. World Cancer Research Fund, American Institute for Cancer Research. *Food, Nutrition, Physical Activity and the Prevention of Cancer: A Global Perspective. Summary*. Washington (DC): World Cancer Research Fund, American Institute for Cancer Research; 2007.
5. Dennis LK, Vanbeek MJ, Beane Freeman LE, Smith BJ, Dawson DV, Coughlin JA. Sunburns and risk of cutaneous melanoma: does age matter? A comprehensive meta-analysis. *Ann Epidemiol*. 2008;18(8):614–27.
6. American Cancer Society. *Breast Cancer Facts & Figures 2019–2020*. Atlanta (GA): American Cancer Society, Inc; 2019. Available from: https://www.cancer.org/content/dam/cancer-org/research/cancer-facts-and-statistics/breast-cancer-facts-and-figures/breast-cancer-facts-and-figures-2019-2020.pdf.
7. Howlader N, Noone AM, Krapcho M, et al. *SEER Cancer Statistics Review, 1975–2010*. Bethesda (MD): National Cancer Institute; 2013. Available from: https://seer.cancer.gov/archive/csr/1975_2010/.
8. Roth MY, Elmore JG, Yi-Frazier JP, Reisch LM, Oster NV, Miglioretti DL. Self-detection remains a key method of breast cancer detection for U.S. women. *J Womens Health (Larchmt)*. 2011;20(8):1135–9.
9. Jones LW, Courneya KS, Mackey JR, et al. Cardiopulmonary function and age-related decline across the breast cancer survivorship continuum. *J Clin Oncol*. 2012;30(20):2530–7.
10. Playdon MC, Bracken MB, Sanft TB, Ligibel JA, Harrigan M, Irwin ML. Weight gain after breast cancer diagnosis and

all-cause mortality: systematic review and meta-analysis. *J Natl Cancer Inst.* 2015;107(12):djv275.

11. Altekruse S, Kosary C, Krapcho M, et al. *SEER Cancer Statistics Review, 1975–2007.* Bethesda (MD): National Cancer Institute; 2010. Available from: https://seer.cancer.gov/csr/1975_2007/.

12. Calle EE, Rodriguez C, Thun M. Obesity and cancer. *N Engl J Med.* 2003;349(5):502–4.

13. Brown JC, John GM, Segal S, Chu CS, Schmitz KH. Physical activity and lower limb lymphedema among uterine cancer survivors. *Med Sci Sports Exerc.* 2013;45(11):2091–7.

14. Dunberger G, Lindquist H, Waldenström AC, Nyberg T, Steineck G, Åvall-Lundqvist E. Lower limb lymphedema in gynecological cancer survivors — effect on daily life functioning. *Support Care Cancer.* 2013;21(11):3063–70.

15. Lind H, Waldenström A-C, Dunberger G, et al. Late symptoms in long-term gynaecological cancer survivors after radiation therapy: a population-based cohort study. *Br J Cancer.* 2011;105(6):737–45.

16. Matei D, Miller AM, Monahan P, et al. Chronic physical effects and health care utilization in long-term ovarian germ cell tumor survivors: a gynecologic oncology group study. *J Clin Oncol.* 2009;27(25):4142–9.

17. Scripture C, Figg W, Sparreboom A. Peripheral neuropathy induced by paclitaxel: recent insights and future perspectives. *Curr Neuropharmacol.* 2006;4(2):165–72.

18. Amant F, Moerman P, Neven P, Timmerman D, Van Limbergen E, Vergote I. Endometrial cancer. *Lancet.* 2005;366(9484):491–505.

19. Winters-Stone KM, Moe E, Graff JN, et al. Falls and frailty in prostate cancer survivors: current, past, and never users of androgen deprivation therapy. *J Am Geriatr Soc.* 2017;65(7):1414–9.

20. Stryker SJ, Wolff BG, Culp CE, Libbe SD, Ilstrup DM, MacCarty RL. Natural history of untreated colonic polyps. *Gastroenterology.* 1987;93(5):1009–13.

21. Wolf AMD, Fontham ETH, Church TR, et al. Colorectal cancer screening for average-risk adults: 2018 guideline update from the American Cancer Society. *CA Cancer J Clin.* 2018;68(4):250–81.

22. National Center for Health Statistics, Division of Health Interview Statistics. *National Health Interview Survey Public Use Data File 2018.* Hyattsville (MD): Centers for Disease Control and Prevention; 2019. Available from: https://www.cdc.gov/nchs/nhis/index.htm.

23. American Cancer Society. *Colorectal Cancer Facts & Figures 2020–2022.* Atlanta (GA): American Cancer Society; 2020. Available from: https://www.cancer.org/content/dam/cancer-org/research/cancer-facts-and-statistics/colorectal-cancer-facts-and-figures/colorectal-cancer-facts-and-figures-2020-2022.pdf.

24. Campbell KL, Winters-Stone KM, Wiskemann J, et al. Exercise guidelines for cancer survivors: consensus statement from international multidisciplinary roundtable. *Med Sci Sports Exerc.* 2019;51(11):2375–90.

25. Cohen EEW, LaMonte SJ, Erb NL, et al. American Cancer Society head and neck cancer survivorship care guideline. *CA Cancer J Clin.* 2016;66(3):203–39.

26. Mehanna H, Paleri V, West CML, Nutting C. Head and neck cancer — part 1: epidemiology, presentation, and prevention. *BMJ.* 2010;341:c4684.

27. Kujan O, Glenny AM, Oliver R, Thakker N, Sloan P. Screening programmes for the early detection and prevention of oral cancer. In: The Cochrane Collaboration, editor. *Cochrane Database of Systematic Reviews.* Chichester (UK): John Wiley & Sons, Ltd; 2006. [cited 2022 Jun 29]. Available from: https://doi.wiley.com/10.1002/14651858.CD004150.pub2.

28. Benson E, Li R, Eisele D, Fakhry C. The clinical impact of HPV tumor status upon head and neck squamous cell carcinomas. *Oral Oncol.* 2014;50(6):565–74.

29. Soiffer RJ, editor. *Hematopoietic Stem Cell Transplantation.* Totowa (NJ): Humana Press; 2008. [cited 2022 Jun 29]. Available from: http://link.springer.com/10.1007/978-1-59745-438-4.

30. Smith SR, Asher A. Rehabilitation in chronic graft-versus-host disease. *Phys Med Rehabil Clin N Am.* 2017;28(1):143–51.

31. Bergenthal N, Will A, Streckmann F, et al. Aerobic physical exercise for adult patients with haematological malignancies. *Cochrane Database Syst Rev.* 2014;2014(11). Available from: https://www.scopus.com/inward/record.uri?eid=2-s2.0-84922221660&doi=10.1002%2F14651858.CD009075.pub2&partnerID=40&md5=08f6246da99b313314a4ee-92acfcd94f.

32. Copelan EA. Hematopoietic stem-cell transplantation. *N Engl J Med.* 2006;354(17):1813–26.

33. Hacker ED, Ferrans C, Verlen E, et al. Fatigue and physical activity in patients undergoing hematopoietic stem cell transplant. *Oncol Nurs Forum.* 2006;33(3):614–24.

34. Morales-Rodriguez E, Pérez-Bilbao T, San Juan AF, Calvo JL. Effects of exercise programs on physical factors and safety in adult patients with cancer and haematopoietic stem cell transplantation: a systematic review. *Int J Environ Res Public Health.* 2022;19(3):1288.

35. Campbell KL, Cormie P, Weller S, et al. Exercise recommendation for people with bone metastases: expert consensus for health care providers and exercise professionals. *JCO Oncol Pract.* 2022;18(5):e697–709.

36. Groeneveldt L, Mein G, Garrod R, et al. A mixed exercise training programme is feasible and safe and may improve quality of life and muscle strength in multiple myeloma survivors. *BMC Cancer.* 2013;13(1):31.

37. Shallwani S, Dalzell MA, Sateren W, O'Brien S. Exercise compliance among patients with multiple myeloma undergoing chemotherapy: a retrospective study. *Support Care Cancer.* 2015;23(10):3081–8.

38. Patel AV, Friedenreich CM, Moore SC, et al. American College of Sports Medicine roundtable report on physical activity, sedentary behavior, and cancer prevention and control. *Med Sci Sports Exerc.* 2019;51(11):2391–402.

39. Betof AS, Dewhirst MW, Jones LW. Effects and potential mechanisms of exercise training on cancer progression: a translational perspective. *Brain Behav Immun.* 2013;30:S75–87.

40. McTiernan A. Mechanisms linking physical activity with cancer. *Nat Rev Cancer.* 2008;8(3):205–11.

41. Friedenreich CM, Neilson HK, Farris MS, Courneya KS. Physical activity and cancer outcomes: a precision medicine approach. *Clin Cancer Res.* 2016;22(19):4766–75.

42. Hopkins BD, Goncalves MD, Cantley LC. Obesity and cancer mechanisms: cancer metabolism. *J Clin Oncol.* 2016;34(35):4277–83.

43. Kang DW, Lee J, Suh SH, Ligibel J, Courneya KS, Jeon JY. Effects of exercise on insulin, IGF axis, adipocytokines, and

inflammatory markers in breast cancer survivors: a systematic review and meta-analysis. *Cancer Epidemiol Biomarkers Prev.* 2017;26(3):355–65.

44. Winters-Stone K, Dieckmann N, Maddalozzo G, Bennett J, Ryan C, Beer T. Resistance exercise reduces body fat and insulin during androgen-deprivation therapy for prostate cancer. *Oncol Nurs Forum.* 2015;42(4):348–56.

45. Pedersen BK, Febbraio MA. Muscles, exercise and obesity: skeletal muscle as a secretory organ. *Nat Rev Endocrinol.* 2012;8(8):457–65.

46. Schmitz KH, Courneya KS, Matthews C, et al; American College of Sports Medicine. American College of Sports Medicine roundtable on exercise guidelines for cancer survivors. *Med Sci Sports Exerc.* 2010;42(7):1409–26.

47. U.S. Department of Health and Human Services. *2008 Physical Activity Guidelines for Americans: Be Active, Healthy, and Happy!.* Washington (DC): U.S. Department of Health and Human Services; 2008. Available from: https://health.gov/paguidelines/pdf/paguide.pdf.

48. Schmitz KH, Campbell AM, Stuiver MM, et al. Exercise is medicine in oncology: engaging clinicians to help patients move through cancer. *CA Cancer J Clin.* 2019;69(6):468–84.

49. Ligibel JA, Bohlke K, May AM, et al. Exercise, diet, and weight management during cancer treatment: ASCO guideline. *J Clin Oncol.* 2022;40(22):2491–507.

50. Ligibel JA, Denlinger CS. New NCCN guidelines® for survivorship care. *J Natl Compr Canc Netw.* 2013;11(Suppl 5):640–4.

51. Covington KR, Marshall T, Campbell G, et al. Development of the Exercise in Cancer Evaluation and Decision Support (EXCEEDS) algorithm. *Support Care Cancer.* 2021;29(11):6469–80.

52. American College of Sports Medicine. *ACSM's Guidelines for Exercise Testing and Prescription.* 10th ed. Philadelphia (PA): Wolters Kluwer; 2018.

53. Dalzell N, Sateren W, Sintharaphone A, et al. Rehabilitation and exercise oncology program: translating research into a model of care. *Curr Oncol.* 2017;24:e191–8.

54. Warburton D, Jamnik V, Bredin S, Shephard RJ, Gledhill N. The 2019 physical activity readiness questionnaire for everyone (PAR-Q+) and electronic physical activity readiness medical examination (ePARmed-X+). *Health Fitness J Canada.* 2018;11(4). doi:10.14288/hfjc.v11i4.270.

55. Brown JC, Ko EM, Schmitz KH. Development of a risk screening tool for cancer survivors to participate in unsupervised moderate- to vigorous-intensity exercise: results from a survey study. *PM R.* 2015;7:113–22.

56. National Comprehensive Cancer Network. Survivorship. (Version 1.2023). 2020. [cited 2023 Mar 24]. https://www.nccn.org/professionals/physician_gls/pdf/survivorship.pdf.

57. Macmillan Cancer Support. Cancer rehabilitation pathways. 2020. [cited 2020 Dec 20]. Available from: https://www.macmillan.org.uk/healthcareprofessionals/news-andresources/guides/cancer-rehabilitationpathways-guidance.

58. Maltser S, Cristian A, Silver JK, Morris GS, Stout NL. A focused review of safety considerations in cancer rehabilitation. *PM R.* 2017;9:S415–28.

59. McNeely ML, Dolgoy N, Onazi M, Suderman K. The interdisciplinary rehabilitation care team and the role of physical therapy in survivor exercise. *Clin J Oncol Nurs.* 2016;20:S8–16.

60. National Comprehensive Cancer Network. Older adult oncology. (Version 1.2023). 2020. [cited 2023 Feb 14]. Available from: https://www.nccn.org/professionals/physician_gls/pdf/senior.pdf.

61. Mohile SG, Dale W, Somerfield MR, et al. Practical assessment and management of vulnerabilities in older patients receiving chemotherapy: ASCO Guideline for Geriatric Oncology. *J Clin Oncol.* 2018;36:2326–47.

62. Pergolotti M, Battisti NML, Padgett L, et al. Embracing the complexity: older adults with cancer-related cognitive decline — a Young International Society of Geriatric Oncology Position Paper. *J Geriatr Oncol.* 2019;11:237–43.

63. Wildes TM, Maggiore RJ, Tew WP, et al; Cancer and Aging Research Group. Factors associated with falls in older adults with cancer: a validated model from the Cancer and Aging Research Group. *Support Care Cancer.* 2018;26:3563–70.

64. Jones LW, Eves ND, Peppercorn J. Pre-exercise screening and prescription guidelines for cancer patients. *Lancet Oncol.* 2010;11(10):914–6.

65. Piercy KL, Troiano RP, Ballard RM, et al. The physical activity guidelines for Americans. *JAMA.* 2018;320(19):2020–8.

66. Bland KA, Kirkham AA, Bovard J, et al. Effect of exercise on taxane chemotherapy-induced peripheral neuropathy in women with breast cancer: a randomized controlled trial. *Clin Breast Cancer.* 2019;19(6):411–22.

67. Kirkham AA, Bland KA, Zucker DS, et al. "Chemotherapy-periodized" exercise to accommodate for cyclical variation in fatigue. *Med Sci Sports Exerc.* 2020;52(2):278–86.

68. Khouri MG, Douglas PS, Mackey JR, et al. Cancer therapy-induced cardiac toxicity in early breast cancer: addressing the unresolved issues. *Circulation.* 2012;126(23):2749–63.

69. Weis J. Cancer-related fatigue: prevalence, assessment and treatment strategies. *Expert Rev Pharmacoecon Outcomes Res.* 2011;11(4):441–6.

70. Mock V, Atkinson A, Barsevick A, et al; National Comprehensive Cancer Network. NCCN practice guidelines for cancer-related fatigue. *Oncology (Williston Park).* 2000;14(11A):151–61.

71. Stubblefield MD, McNeely ML, Alfano CM, Mayer DK. A prospective surveillance model for physical rehabilitation of women with breast cancer: chemotherapy-induced peripheral neuropathy. *Cancer.* 2012;118(Suppl 8):2250–60.

72. Irwin ML, Cartmel B, Gross CP, et al. Randomized exercise trial of aromatase inhibitor–induced arthralgia in breast cancer survivors. *J Clin Oncol.* 2015;33(10):1104–11.

73. McNeely ML, Parliament MB, Seikaly H, et al. Effect of exercise on upper extremity pain and dysfunction in head and neck cancer survivors: a randomized controlled trial. *Cancer.* 2008;113(1):214–22.

74. Weller S, Hart NH, Bolam KA, et al. Exercise for individuals with bone metastases: a systematic review. *Crit Rev Oncol Hematol.* 2021;166:103433.

75. Cormie P, Newton RU, Spry N, Joseph D, Taaffe DR, Galvão DA. Safety and efficacy of resistance exercise in prostate cancer patients with bone metastases. *Prostate Cancer Prostatic Dis.* 2013;16(4):328–35.

76. Hart NH, Galvão DA, Newton RU. Exercise medicine for advanced prostate cancer. *Curr Opin Support Palliat Care.* 2017;11(3):247–57.

77. Johansson K, Hayes S, Speck RM, Schmitz KH. Water-based exercise for patients with chronic arm lymphedema: a randomized controlled pilot trial. *Am J Phys Med Rehabil.* 2013;92(4):312–9.

78. Mustian KM, Palesh OG, Flecksteiner SA. Tai Chi Chuan for breast cancer survivors. *Med Sport Sci.* 2008;52:209–17.

79. Mustian KM, Sprod LK, Palesh OG, et al. Exercise for the management of side effects and quality of life among cancer survivors. *Curr Sports Med Rep.* 2009;8(6):325–30.

80. Hayes SC, Johansson K, Stout NL, et al. Upper-body morbidity after breast cancer: incidence and evidence for evaluation, prevention, and management within a prospective surveillance model of care. *Cancer.* 2012;118(Suppl 8):2237–49.

81. Schmitz KH. Balancing lymphedema risk: exercise versus deconditioning for breast cancer survivors. *Exerc Sport Sci Rev.* 2010;38(1):17–24.

82. National Lymphedema Network. *Exercise: Position Statement of the National Lymphedema Network.* San Francisco (CA): National Lymphedema Network; 2011. Available from: https://klosetraining.com/wpcontent/uploads/2015/05/NLNexercise.pdf

83. Schmitz KH, Ahmed RL, Troxel AB, et al. Weight lifting for women at risk for breast cancer-related lymphedema: a randomized trial. *JAMA.* 2010;304(24):2699–705.

84. Schmitz KH, Ahmed RL, Troxel A, et al. Weight lifting in women with breast-cancer-related lymphedema. *N Engl J Med.* 2009;361(7):664–73.

85. Beidas RS, Paciotti B, Barg F, et al. A hybrid effectiveness-implementation trial of an evidence-based exercise intervention for breast cancer survivors. *J Natl Cancer Inst Monogr.* 2014;2014(50):338–45.

86. Klose Training & Consulting LLC. *Klose Training Lymphedema Certification.* Lafayette (CO): Klose Training & Consulting LLC; 2016. Available from: https://klosetraining.com/course/online/strength-abc/.

87. Luo J, Carter SJ, Feliciano EMC, Hendryx M. Trajectories of objectively measured physical function among older breast cancer survivors in comparison with cancer-free controls. *Breast Cancer Res Treat.* 2022;193(2):467–76.

88. Winters-Stone KM, Horak F, Jacobs PG, et al. Falls, functioning, and disability among women with persistent symptoms of chemotherapy-induced peripheral neuropathy. *J Clin Oncol.* 2017;35(23):2604–12.

89. Patnaik JL, Byers T, DiGuiseppi C, Denberg TD, Dabelea D. The influence of comorbidities on overall survival among older women diagnosed with breast cancer. *J Natl Cancer Inst.* 2011;103(14):1101–11.

90. Haykowsky MJ, Beaudry R, Brothers RM, Nelson MD, Sarma S, La Gerche A. Pathophysiology of exercise intolerance in breast cancer survivors with preserved left ventricular ejection fraction. *Clin Sci (Lond).* 2016;130(24):2239–44.

91. Weaver KE, Foraker RE, Alfano CM, et al. Cardiovascular risk factors among long-term survivors of breast, prostate, colorectal, and gynecologic cancers: a gap in survivorship care? *J Cancer Surviv.* 2013;7(2):253–61.

92. Gilchrist SC, Barac A, Ades PA, et al. Cardio-oncology rehabilitation to manage cardiovascular outcomes in cancer patients and survivors: a scientific statement from the American Heart Association. *Circulation.* 2019;139(21):e997–1012. doi:10.1161/CIR.0000000000000679.

93. Chen JJ, Wu PT, Middlekauff HR, Nguyen KL. Aerobic exercise in anthracycline-induced cardiotoxicity: a systematic review of current evidence and future directions. *Am J Physiol Heart Circ Physiol.* 2017;312(2):H213–22.

94. Saylor PJ, Smith MR. Metabolic complications of androgen deprivation therapy for prostate cancer. *J Urol.* 2013;189(1S):S34–44. doi:10.1016/j.juro.2012.11.017.

95. Keating NL, O'Malley AJ, Freedland SJ, Smith MR. Diabetes and cardiovascular disease during androgen deprivation therapy: observational study of veterans with prostate cancer. *J Natl Cancer Inst.* 2010;102(1):39–46.

96. Fried LP, Tangen CM, Walston J, et al; Cardiovascular Health Study Collaborative Research Group. Frailty in older adults: evidence for a phenotype. *J Gerontol A Biol Sci Med Sci.* 2001;56(3):M146–56.

97. Gill TM, Gahbauer EA, Han L, Allore HG. Trajectories of disability in the last year of life. *N Engl J Med.* 2010;362(13):1173–80.

98. Clough-Gorr KM, Stuck AE, Thwin SS, Silliman RA. Older breast cancer survivors: geriatric assessment domains are associated with poor tolerance of treatment adverse effects and predict mortality over 7 years of follow-up. *J Clin Oncol.* 2010;28(3):380–6.

99. Maccormick RE. Possible acceleration of aging by adjuvant chemotherapy: a cause of early onset frailty? *Med Hypotheses.* 2006;67(2):212–5.

100. Ness KK, Armstrong GT, Kundu M, Wilson CL, Tchkonia T, Kirkland JL. Frailty in childhood cancer survivors: frailty in childhood cancer Survivors. *Cancer.* 2015;121(10):1540–7.

101. Bennett JA, Winters-Stone KM, Dobek J, Nail LM. Frailty in older breast cancer survivors: age, prevalence, and associated factors. *Oncol Nurs Forum.* 2013;40(3):E126–34.

102. Woo J, Yu R, Wong M, Yeung F, Wong M, Lum C. Frailty screening in the community using the FRAIL scale. *J Am Med Dir Assoc.* 2015;16(5):412–9.

103. Kohrt WM, Bloomfield SA, Little KD, Nelson ME, Yingling VR; American College of Sports Medicine. American College of Sports Medicine Position Stand: physical activity and bone health. *Med Sci Sports Exerc.* 2004;36(11):1985–96.

104. Frost HM. Should future risk-of-fracture analyses include another major risk factor? The case for falls. *J Clin Densitom.* 2001;4(4):381–3.

105. Huang M, Shilling T, Miller K, Smith K, Fredrickson K. History of falls, gait, balance, and fall risks in older cancer survivors living in the community. *Clin Interv Aging.* 2015;10:1497–503.

106. Spoelstra SL, Given BA, Schutte DL, Sikorskii A, You M, Given CW. Do older adults with cancer fall more often? a comparative analysis of falls in those with and without cancer. *Oncol Nurs Forum.* 2013;40(2):E69–78.

107. Winters-Stone KM, Li F, Horak F, et al. Comparison of tai chi vs. strength training for fall prevention among female cancer survivors: study protocol for the GET FIT trial. *BMC Cancer.* 2012;12(1):577.

108. Stein KD, Syrjala KL, Andrykowski MA. Physical and psychological long-term and late effects of cancer. *Cancer.* 2008;112(S11):2577–92.

109. Winters-Stone KM, Lyons KS, Dobek J, et al. Benefits of partnered strength training for prostate cancer survivors and spouses: results from a randomized controlled trial of the Exercising Together project. *J Cancer Surviv.* 2016;10(4):633–44.

110. Craft LL, VanIterson EH, Helenowski IB, Rademaker AW, Courneya KS. Exercise effects on depressive symptoms in cancer survivors: a systematic review and meta-analysis. *Cancer Epidemiol Biomarkers Prev.* 2012;21(1):3–19.

The Immune System and Exercise

INTRODUCTION

Exercise has a profound influence on the immune system (1, 2). The nature of the immune response to exercise is closely tied to the degree of physiological stress imposed by the exercise workload and regimen. As will be emphasized in this chapter, moderate exercise training has been consistently linked with improved immune function and lowered risk for acute respiratory infections. In contrast, exercise training pushed to the level of overreaching and overtraining can lead to immune dysfunction and elevated infection rates (1).

Exercise immunology is a relatively new area of scientific endeavor with the majority of papers published after 1990. Much has been learned about immune responses to varying exercise workloads, and this information will be summarized in this chapter. Emerging multiomics technologies are now being used by exercise immunologists, and an explosion in new findings is expected, which will more clearly define underlying mechanisms in exercise-induced immune changes (3).

This chapter provides a brief overview of the immune system and then discusses the acute and chronic effects of exercise on the immune system and infection risk.

OVERVIEW OF THE IMMUNE SYSTEM

The immune system is the primary physiologic system that mediates the response to harmful exogenous agents (*i.e.*, bacteria and other pathogenic microbes) and endogenous agents (*i.e.*, tumor cells). There is a growing awareness that the immune system is also functionally coupled to metabolism and that the exercise-induced metabolic responses influence immunity (3–5). Demanding exercise workloads cause large perturbations in metabolites, lipid mediators, and proteins that influence immune cell

activation, oxygen consumption, and function. This has opened up a new area of scientific endeavor called immunometabolism (3).

The thymus gland and bone marrow are the central "organs" of the immune system, as this is where most of the immune cells are generated. The spleen, tonsils, lymph nodes, lymph vessels, and skin and liver are considered secondary organs where immune cells interact with the body. In addition, the immune system is divided into both central and peripheral organs and tissues, cellular components, and soluble macromolecules (6). Functionally, it is divided into two systems: (a) the body's innate immune defenses, which are collectively referred to as natural or nonspecific immunity; and (b) the acquired host defenses, which are referred to as adaptive or specific immunity. These two systems interact and overlap in a coordinated fashion to neutralize or destroy pathogens, cells infected by viruses and tumor cells, and maintain health (6–9).

Cells and Organs of the Immune System

The immune system is primarily composed of leukocytes or white blood cells (WBCs), and the peripheral lymphoid tissue where leukocytes are garrisoned. Leukocytes are responsible for protecting the body from bacteria, viruses, or parasites and travel through the blood and tissues to identify and eliminate these harmful agents. Leukocytes are formed in the bone marrow and lymph tissue, where after formation they are transported throughout the body in blood and lymphatic tissue. Five main types of leukocytes exist, namely neutrophils, eosinophils, basophils, lymphocytes, and monocytes. Of these, neutrophils and lymphocytes are most abundant in the blood.

Of all leukocytes, neutrophils are considered the "first responders" to microbial infections, as they are mature cells and can attack and destroy bacteria in circulating blood via phagocytosis. Similarly, monocytes travel in the blood removing bacteria but live longer than neutrophils and are also able to travel into the tissue and become macrophages, which remove cell debris. Eosinophils are less abundant than neutrophils but play a significant role in the body's defense mechanism by attacking and eliminating parasites through special surface molecules that release substances that eliminate the parasites. These cells are rarely seen in the blood and are typically present in the mucous membrane of the respiratory, digestive, and urinary tracts. Basophils are the least abundant of the leukocytes but are responsible for releasing heparin, histamine, and bradykinin, which are part of the allergic and antigen response of the body.

Lymphocytes are the most common type of cell found in lymph and include natural killer cells (NK cells), T cells, and B cells. NK cells are part of the body's innate immune response, and T cells and B cells are involved in adaptive immune responses. NK cells attack and destroy tumor cells or cells that have been infected by viruses. Advances in immunology indicate that NK cells, neutrophils, and macrophages have functional attributes of both innate and adaptive immunity, calling into question the classical division of the immune system into two separate arms (10). There are two major subtypes of T cells: (1) the killer T cell, which also kills cells that are infected with pathogens or dysfunction, and (2) the helper T cell, which regulates both innate and adaptive immune responses to a particular pathogen. B cells recognize pathogens and produce specific antibodies that bind to pathogens and trigger a cascade of actions resulting in their elimination.

Innate Immune Responses

The innate immune system includes anatomic and physiologic barriers (skin, mucous membranes, body temperature, low pH, and special chemical mediators such as complement and interferon), specialized cells (NK cells, and phagocytes including neutrophils, monocytes, and macrophages, which can engulf, kill, and digest whole microorganisms), and inflammatory barriers. The innate immune system quickly defends the host from infection by pathogens in a nonspecific manner. This means that the cells of the innate system recognize, and respond to, pathogens in a generic way, but unlike the adaptive immune system, it does not confer long-lasting or protective immunity to the host. When the innate immune system fails to effectively combat an invading pathogen, the body mounts an acquired (specific) immune response.

Polymorphonuclear phagocytes (primarily neutrophils and eosinophils) arise from pluripotent stem cells in the bone marrow. These are characterized by the presence of cytoplasmic granules, which contain enzymes destructive to the pathogens such as acid hydrolases, neutral proteases, peroxidases, myeloperoxidase, cationic proteins, lysozyme, and lactoferrin (11). Mononuclear phagocytes (monocytes and macrophages) also develop from stem cells in the bone marrow but lose their granules during successive differentiation.

The enzymes found in the cytoplasmic granules of neutrophils are involved in oxygen-independent (*e.g.*, hydrolases and lysozyme) or oxygen-dependent (*e.g.*, myeloperoxidase) destruction of invaders during phagocytosis. Some of these enzymes trigger complement cascades, a form of innate immune defense that facilitates and mediates cytolysis of pathogenic and damaged body cells. Polypeptides, such as kinins (*e.g.*, bradykinin), circulate in the blood in an inactive form and can be activated by enzymes released from phagocytic granules. This activation indirectly enhances vascular permeability and chemotaxis of phagocytic and other immune cells to an area of infection.

Oxygen-dependent killing by phagocytic cells is an important pathway for the destruction of pathogens. During cellular respiration, the transfer of electrons from nicotinamide adenine dinucleotide phosphate ($NADP^+$) to oxygen results in the production of superoxide, peroxide, and hydroxyl radicals within the phagosome of neutrophils. Later in this chapter, we will discuss the possible regulatory roles of reactive oxygen species (ROS) in metabolism and exercise immunology.

Macrophages are large phagocytes found in all tissues and engulf and digest anything that does not have surface proteins specific to healthy body cells. Macrophages trap pathogens in phagosomes that fuse with lysosomes where enzymes and toxic peroxides digest the pathogen (11). Besides phagocytosis, macrophages help regulate inflammation. Macrophages that promote inflammation are called M1 macrophages in contrast to M2 macrophages that decrease inflammation and encourage tissue repair. Macrophages also initiate adaptive immune responses by presenting pathogen antigens to helper T cells. The antigen presentation by the macrophage is done by displaying it attached to a major histocompatibility complex (MHC) class II molecule to indicate to T cells that the macrophage is not a pathogen. T cells that recognize the antigen-MHC II complex cause B cells to produce specific antibodies that facilitate the process of elimination by phagocytes.

Acquired Immune Responses

The acquired immune system includes special cells called B and T lymphocytes that are capable of secreting a large variety of specialized chemicals (antibodies and cytokines) to regulate the immune response. T lymphocytes can also engage in direct cell-on-cell warfare. The immune system adapts its response during an infection to improve its recognition of the pathogen. This improved response is then retained after the pathogen has been eliminated, in the form of an immunological memory, and allows the adaptive immune system to mount faster and stronger attacks each time this pathogen is encountered.

The development of antibodies is triggered by the acquired immune system, which is characterized by three components:

1. Recognition of a specific antigenic determinant (or antigenic epitope), which is the portion of the antigen molecule that is recognized as foreign by the host's immune cells,
2. Proliferation of immune cells specific to the antigen, and
3. Immunologic memory, that is, the capacity of the immune system to recognize and defend against an antigen long after an initial encounter.

The cell type that mediates acquired immune responses is the lymphocyte. The most important lymphocytes involved are the thymus-derived (T) lymphocyte, the B lymphocyte, and the NK cell (Figure 14.1).

The immune cells are identified by cluster of differentiation (CD) antigens, which are markers on the surface of the cells. As such, different subsets of lymphocytes express different CD antigens at the cell surface. For example, T-helper cells (CD4) assist the T-cell receptor to communicate with other antigen-presenting cells (APCs) by amplifying the signal generated and recruiting CD8 killer cells. T lymphocytes with killer (cytotoxic) properties express the CD8 antigen, and B cells express the CD19 antigen. All lymphocytes — indeed, all leukocytes — express CD62L or L-selectin antigens, which are adhesion molecules that facilitate the lymphocyte's entry into secondary lymphoid organs (*e.g.*, lymph nodes, spleen). Lymphocytes are also further categorized within a given CD. For example, all leukocytes (WBCs) can be identified as CD45-positive cells (a marker for the common leukocyte antigen) and can be further divided into naive cells (CD45RA$^+$) and memory

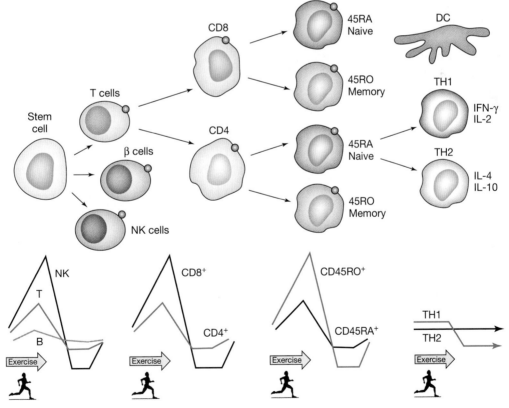

FIGURE 14.1 The major lymphocyte subpopulations involved in mediating specific immune responses. T lymphocytes are effector cells for cell-mediated reactions, and B lymphocytes are effector cells for antibody-mediated reactions. Natural killer (NK) cells are involved in cytolysis of target cells. (From Hoffman-Goetz L, Klarlund Pedersen B. Exercise and the immune system. In: Farrell PA, Joyner MJ, Caiozzo VJ, editors. *ACSM's Advanced Exercise Physiology.* 2nd ed. Philadelphia (PA): Wolters Kluwer; 2012. p. 507–28.)

cells (CD45RO+). Moreover, memory cells are subdivided into memory B cells, which are antibody-producing cells, and memory T cells, which are infection-fighting cells (8). Although naive cells (CD45RA+ lymphocytes) are the body's first response to an antigen, both B and T memory cells (CD45RO+ lymphocytes) enable the body to respond rapidly and potently to subsequent exposures to a specific antigen. Memory T and B cells are also formed in response to antigens introduced into the body through vaccines. Using flow cytometry — a laser- or impedance-based technology to count and sort cells — lymphocytes are frequently identified by the presence of multiple CD antigens, which provide information about their structure, development, and function. Table 14.1 provides a summary of CD antigens studied in relation to exercise training. The reader is encouraged to review immunology texts for a complete list of these CD antigens.

Lymphocytes circulate via lymphatic vessels, lodge in lymph nodes or specialized regions of lymphatic tissue, or enter the cardiovascular system through the major lymphatic ducts. The movement (extravasation) and recirculation of lymphocytes are both linked to the expression of numerous cell-adhesion molecules (CAMs). L-selectins (CD62L), which are found on all leukocytes, are involved in tethering and rolling of leukocytes in the bloodstream, whereas integrin molecules, LFA-1 (CD11a/CD18), are involved in the adhesion and arrest of these cells. It is after the activation of the endothelial cells and the adhesion and arrest of the lymphocytes that transendothelial migration occurs and the lymphocytes enter the lymphatic system. Therefore, CAMs not only enhance leukocyte adhesion to vascular and mucosal endothelium but also contribute to the interactions among lymphocytes, APCs, and target cells. Circulating levels of intercellular adhesion molecule-1 (ICAM-1) in healthy individuals are significantly elevated after exhaustive exercise, and it plays a role in skeletal muscle remodeling (12, 13).

The acquired immune response is described as either cell mediated, involving T cells, or antibody mediated (humoral), involving B cells and the production of antibodies.

Cell-Mediated Immunity

The first step in cell-mediated immunity is to initiate the proliferation of APCs, such as macrophages and dendritic cells. APCs are so named because they recognize, degrade, and present the antigen to T lymphocytes. Once an APC has recognized an antigen, its lysosomal vesicles engulf the antigen and break it down into peptides. These peptides are then recognized by MHC molecules.

In the human body, there are two main types of MHC glycoproteins, classes I and II. Class I MHC glycoproteins (MHC I) are found in all nucleated cells, along with platelets — but not red blood cells. MHC I are recognized by cytolytic T cells (CD8), also called MHC class I restricted T cells. Overall, the function of MHC I is to trigger an immediate response against nonself antigens. Class II MHC glycoproteins (MHC II) have a more restricted cell distribution but are constitutively expressed only on APCs. After APCs take up and degrade the antigen, they present the antigenic determinants attached to the MHC II on their surface. This processed antigen and MHC II complex are together known as a T-cell epitope and can be "seen" by CD4 T lymphocytes (also known as MHC class II restricted T cells). The T-cell epitope acts as an induction signal for CD4 lymphocytes, leading to mitosis, activation, and proliferation of memory and effector T cells. These effector CD4 T cells secrete growth factors, which recruit other immune cells to assist in the immune response. Naive CD4 lymphocytes, which respond to "new" pathogens not yet faced by the immune system, are divided into type 1 and type 2 helper cells (T_h1 and T_h2, respectively). T_h1 helper

Table 14.1	Common CD Markers Studied in Exercise Immunology
Type of Immune Cells	**CD Markers**
All leukocyte groups	CD45+
Granulocyte	CD45+, CD11b+, CD15+, CD24+, CD114+, CD182+
Monocyte	CD4+, CD45+, CD14+, CD114+, CD11a+, CD11b+, CD91+, CD16+
T lymphocyte	CD45+, CD3+
T-helper cell	CD45+, CD3+, CD4+
Cytotoxic T cells	CD45+, CD3+, CD8+
T regulatory cell	CD45+, CD3+, CD4+, CD25+, Foxp3+
B lymphocyte	CD45+, CD19+, CD20+, CD24+, CD38+, CD22+
Thrombocyte	CD45+, CD61+
Natural killer (NK) cell	CD16+, CD56+, CD3−, CD31+, CD30+, CD38+

Note: The human cluster of differentiation (CD) antigens are surface molecules detected on white blood cells (WBCs or leukocytes).

cells provide aid against intracellular bacteria, whereas T_h2 helper cells target extracellular parasites. In contrast to naive CD4 lymphocytes, naive CD8 lymphocytes respond to abnormal MHC I by producing an array of cytokines, which results in the killing of specific target cells.

Cytokines are low-molecular-weight proteins that are important in cell signaling and influence the direction, intensity, and duration of immune responses. Even though cytokine actions on target cells are limited by the expression of the specific cytokine receptors (e.g., IL-2 and its receptor IL-2R), cytokines have a range of actions and act on cells that secrete them (autocrine action), on nearby cells (paracrine action), or on distant cells (endocrine action). Although cytokines are produced by many cells in the body, helper T cells and macrophages are the most predominant. Most cytokines are classified as pro-inflammatory (e.g., IL-1B, IL-6, and tumor necrosis factor-α [TNF-α]), meaning they are involved in the regulation of inflammatory reactions or anti-inflammatory (e.g., IL-1, IL-4, IL-10, IL-13), which control the pro-inflammatory response. For a complete discussion on cytokines and their roles, the readers are referred to comprehensive immunology textbooks (13, 14).

Antibody-Mediated Immunity

Antibodies, also known as immunoglobulins (Ig), are y-shaped proteins produced by B lymphocytes. They have multiple functions. First, antibodies can bind antigens through precipitation or agglutination reactions and trigger its neutralization. Second, antibodies can promote phagocytosis of an antigen through a process known as opsonization, in which neutrophils and macrophages bind a portion of the antibody molecule at receptors found on their surface (FcR), and the entire antibody–antigen complex is then taken up by the phagocytic cell. Finally, certain antibodies (including IgG and IgM) activate the complement cascade, resulting in nonspecific lysis of pathogenic cells or infected body cells (14, 15).

Similar to the activation of T lymphocytes, B lymphocytes also require two signals to become activated. The first signal occurs in the B-cell receptor where the interaction between the antigen and surface Ig causes endocytosis and engulfs the antigen. The antigen fragments are then expressed on the cell membrane in conjunction with MHC II and the CD4 T_h2 lymphocytes interact with the T-cell epitope to provide the first signal for the synthesis of antibodies related to the antigen. A second signal is transmitted by the interaction of CD40 and CD40L, which, after activation and stimulation from growth and differentiation cytokines, allows B cells to differentiate into plasma cells

and secrete IgM, IgG, or IgA antibodies. Within 2 weeks of this initial exposure to an antigen, the primary antibody response peaks, and both effector and memory B cells are generated. Thereafter, subsequent exposure to the antigen results in faster production of antibodies and higher blood antibody concentrations (or titers).

In summary, the body's defenses entail physical and chemical barriers; specific innate responses involving neutrophils, macrophages, NK cells, and other nonspecific leukocytes; and an acquired immune response effected by T and B lymphocytes. Together, these cells provide the major pathways for recognizing and responding to infectious tumor antigens and other antigens.

IMMUNE SYSTEM RESPONSE TO ACUTE PHYSICAL ACTIVITY

The acute immune response to physical activity depends on the overall workload stress. For example, moderate-to-vigorous physical activity (MVPA) bouts lasting 20–60 minutes cause modest immune system perturbations in contrast to extensive changes measured in response to prolonged and intensive exercise bouts similar to marathon race events (1).

Immune System Response to MVPA

During MVPA, many beneficial, transient changes in immune system surveillance functions occur (1). For example, tissue macrophages are activated, and antipathogen functions increase. At the same time, an enhanced recirculation of important immune system components occurs. These include modestly higher blood levels of immunoglobulins, anti-inflammatory cytokines, neutrophils, NK cells, cytotoxic T cells, and immature B cells. Each of these plays critical role in immune defense activity (16–20). Acute MVPA bouts preferentially mobilize NK cells and CD8$^+$ T lymphocytes that exhibit high cytotoxicity and tissue-migrating potential. Stress hormones and pro-inflammatory cytokines, which can suppress immune cell function, do not reach high levels during MVPA bouts, especially when rest and low-intensity intervals are incorporated (similar to most sports).

As MVPA is repeated on a near-daily basis for weeks and months, these transient, exercise-induced increases in selective immune components enhance immunosurveillance against pathogens, lowering the risk for acute respiratory illnesses (ARIs). At the same time, resting-state systemic inflammation levels are decreased (1, 21). There is increasing evidence that regular exercise training has an overall anti-inflammatory influence mediated through multiple pathways. MVPA improves the control of inflammatory signaling pathways and helps reduce adipose tissue. The net effect is a chronic lowering of inflammatory biomarkers including acute phase proteins, cytokines such as IL-6, C-reactive protein (CRP), and inflammation-related lipids called oxylipins. The persistent increase in inflammation biomarkers is defined as chronic or systemic inflammation and is linked with multiple disorders and diseases including obesity, arthritis, atherosclerosis and cardiovascular disease (CVD), chronic kidney disease, liver disease, metabolic syndrome, insulin resistance and Type 2 diabetes mellitus, sarcopenia, arthritis, bone resorption and osteoporosis, chronic obstructive pulmonary disease (COPD), dementia, depression, and various types of cancers. Chronic inflammation can be countered through the combined effect of MVPA and keeping body fat at normal levels.

Metabolically, MVPA induces small, transient, acute elevations in IL-6 that improves glucose and lipid metabolism over time (22). Another benefit may include an enhanced antibody-specific response when vaccinations are followed by acute exercise bouts (1). Studies have been disappointing and inconsistent as to whether acute exercise just before vaccination increases the 2- to 4-week postvaccination antibody response. However, one study showed an impressive augmentation of the antibody response to both influenza and COVID-19 vaccinations when subjects engaged in 90-minute MVPA bouts after receiving the vaccination (23). When the exercise duration was cut down to 45 minutes, the improved antibody response did not occur. Although the investigators reasoned that the exercise intervention was feasible for people who exercised regularly at light intensities such as walking, it is doubtful that a meaningful proportion of the adult population is going to walk for 90 minutes after receiving a flu or COVID-19 shot. More research is needed to determine whether shorter and more intensive aerobic exercise bouts work just as well.

Taken together, MVPA can be regarded as an immune system adjuvant to stimulate the ongoing exchange of leukocytes between the circulation and tissues (16).

Immune System Response to Prolonged and Intensive Exercise

In contrast, physiologically stressful exercise training workloads, endurance running, cycling competitive events, and other endurance sports have been linked to immune dysfunction, inflammation, oxidative stress, and elevated risk for acute respiratory infections (1, 2, 24–26).

The "open window" model summarizes these findings as depicted in Figure 14.2.

Unusually demanding exercise workloads are accompanied by physiological, metabolic, and psychological stress, and the immune system reflects this stress. NK cell and neutrophil function, various measures of T and B cell function, salivary IgA output, skin delayed-type hypersensitivity (DTH) responses, macrophage MHC II expression, and other aspects of immune function are altered (1). These exercise-induced changes in immunity can last for several hours to weeks depending on the biomarker and magnitude of stress and occur in the skin, upper respiratory tract mucosal tissue, lung, blood, muscle, and peritoneal cavity.

Advances in technology have allowed hundreds of molecules to be measured at one time from blood or tissue samples collected before and after exercise (3, 5, 27–30). In a typical study with human athletes exercising intensely for more than 2 hours, significant increases in hundreds of metabolites (via metabolomics procedures), proteins (proteomics), and lipids (lipidomics) can be measured in response to the physiological stress. These studies based on a human systems biology approach have revealed that metabolism and immunity are intimately linked. This has led to a new area of research endeavor called immunometabolism (3). Exercise-induced perturbations in metabolites, lipid mediators, and proteins have direct influences on immune function (1, 3, 5). Immune activation is accompanied by oxygen and fuel substrate demands, and exercise-induced physiological stress competes for the

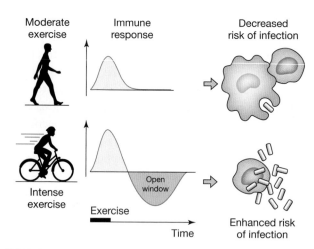

FIGURE 14.2 The open window model, which relates the intensity of exercise to increased or decreased risk of infection (and other clinical conditions). This increased or decreased risk presumably reflects intervening variables of immune system function. (From Hoffman-Goetz L, Klarlund Pedersen B. Exercise and the immune system. In: Farrell PA, Joyner MJ, Caiozzo VJ, editors. *ACSM's Advanced Exercise Physiology*. 2nd ed. Philadelphia (PA): Wolters Kluwer; 2012. p. 507–28.)

same resources. As a result, immune cell metabolic capacity is reduced during recovery from physiologically demanding bouts of intensive exercise, resulting in transient immune dysfunction (1, 3, 5).

PHYSICAL ACTIVITY AND ACUTE RESPIRATORY ILLNESS RISK

Animal and human studies support that regular MVPA reduces the risk for ARI. In contrast, unusually demanding exercise workloads and competitive events especially when combined with other stressors can increase ARI risk.

MVPA and Lowered ARI Risk

Randomized clinical trials (RCTs) and epidemiological studies support an inverse relationship between MVPA and ARI incidence. The RCTs (2–12 months in length) consistently demonstrate that participants assigned to MVPA experience reduced ARI incidence, duration, and symptomatology (31–41). The magnitude of reduction in ARI symptom days (40%–50% in some studies) with near-daily MVPA bolsters public health guidelines urging individuals to be physically active on a regular basis. The protective effect of MVPA on ARI contrasts with the increased ARI risk linked to prolonged and intensive exercise, as summarized in the J-curve model (Figure 14.3) (37).

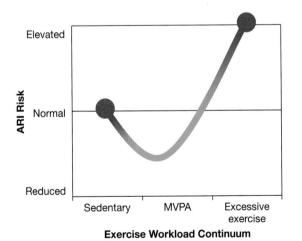

FIGURE 14.3 The "J-curve" depicts the relationship between acute respiratory illness (ARI) and the exercise workload continuum. Regular moderate-to-vigorous physical activity (MVPA) has been linked in many studies to a lowered ARI risk (green portion of the curve), whereas sedentary behavior and excessive exercise workloads have been linked to an elevated ARI risk. (Based on data from Nieman DC. Is infection risk linked to exercise workload? *Med Sci Sports Exerc.* 2000;32(Suppl 7):S406–11.)

In one epidemiological study, a group of 1,002 adults (aged 18–85 years, 60% female, 40% male) was studied for 12 weeks, with monitoring of ARI symptoms and severity using the validated Wisconsin Upper Respiratory Symptom Survey (40). The number of days with ARI was 43% lower in subjects engaging in an average of 5 or more days per week of aerobic exercise (20-minute bouts or longer) compared to those who were largely sedentary (≤1 day per week). This strong effect remained even after adjustment for age, education level, marital status, gender, body mass index (BMI), and perceived mental stress. These results are similar to other epidemiological studies supporting a linkage between MVPA and lowered risk for ARI (38, 39, 41).

Figure 14.4 summarizes the evidence supporting a beneficial effect of MVPA against viral and bacterial infections (40–44). Near-daily MVPA compared to inactivity has been linked to reduced incidence rates for influenza, the common cold, and severe cases of COVID-19, with diminished mortality rates for pneumonia and other viral and bacterial infections in the general population.

For example, in a large epidemiological study of 97,844 adults from England and Scotland, exercise training was linked to lowered risk for bacterial and viral infectious disease mortality by more than 50% over a 9-year period (43) (Figure 14.4). Data from the UK Biobank (UKBB) showed that physical inactivity was related to 32% increased risk for COVID-19 hospitalizations (44) (Figure 14.4). The lifestyle combination of physical inactivity, cigarette smoking, and obesity increased the risk of COVID-19 hospitalization 4.4-fold compared to optimal lifestyles and accounted for up to 51% of the population's attributable risk (44). Other data support that being both lean and fit is an effective lifestyle strategy to lower the odds of COVID-19 mortality (45). In another cohort study, individuals with low cardiorespiratory fitness had more than two times the risk of dying from COVID-19 compared to those with moderate or high fitness (46). These data complement findings from a retrospective observational study within the Henry Ford Medical Group that showed an independent and inverse association between maximal exercise capacity and the likelihood of COVID-19 hospitalization (47). Respiratory and circulatory failure are common causes of death among COVID-19 patients, and those with higher levels of cardiorespiratory fitness may possess the extra capacity needed for survival.

Other data support reductions in incidence and mortality rates for influenza and pneumonia (42, 48–51). The risk for severe influenza is higher in communities reporting a high prevalence of physical inactivity and obesity (52).

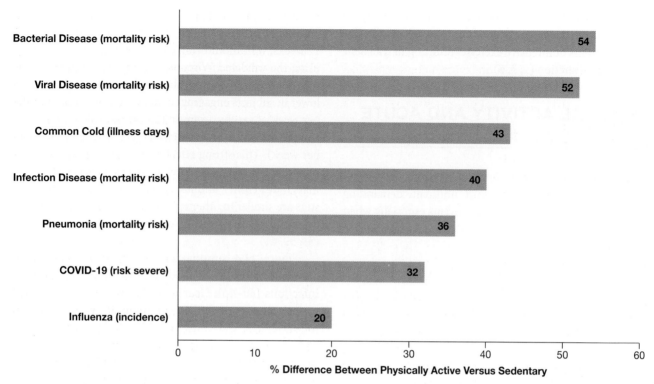

FIGURE 14.4 This chart illustrates the percent difference between incidence and mortality rates between physically active and sedentary individuals for a variety of respiratory infections. Epidemiological data consistently link MVPA with reduced risk for influenza, COVID-19, pneumonia, the common cold, and viral and bacterial diseases in general. (Adapted from Calabrese L, Nieman DC. Exercise, infection and rheumatic diseases: what do we know? *RMD Open.* 2021;7(2):e001644.)

Regular exercise training was associated with reduced influenza mortality in an epidemiological study of elderly individuals (53). Pneumonia is a serious lung infection caused by bacteria, viruses, or fungi and ranks with other lower respiratory infections as the fourth leading cause of death worldwide. One meta-analysis supported a robust and consistent 36% reduction in pneumonia-related mortality and an 18% reduction in incident pneumonia when comparing the most versus least physically active groups (48).

A community-based cohort study examined associations between multiple lifestyle factors with infectious disease mortality (median follow-up time of 11.3 years) (54). Lifestyle risk factors included physical activity, sedentary time, sleep quality, diet quality, alcohol drinking status, and smoking status. These six lifestyle behaviors were combined into an index and adjusted models contrasted the healthiest and least healthy groups. These contrasts showed 71%, 74%, and 58% lower mortality rates for infectious disease, pneumonia, and COVID-19, respectively, in the healthiest group. When each lifestyle behavior was examined separately, never smoking, keeping alcohol consumption within guidelines, and sufficient physical activity had the strongest effects in lowering risk for all types of infectious disease mortality.

These findings support the strategy of adopting positive lifestyle behaviors to lower the odds of severe infectious disease outcomes. Regular MVPA has emerged as one of the most important lifestyle habits to improve internal defenses against the wide variety of pathogens seeking entry into the body (1, 55–57). MVPA can be viewed as an immune system adjuvant and an important lifestyle strategy to complement vaccination protocols.

Prolonged and Intensive Exercise and ARI Risk

High-intensity, long-duration exercise causes extensive perturbations in the immune system and can elevate ARI risk especially when combined with other stressors such as mental stress, lack of sleep, travel, and malnutrition (1). As described earlier, this linkage between exercise workload stress, immune dysfunction, and elevated ARI risk has been captured in the "open window" and "J-curve" models (Figures 14.2 and 14.3).

Early epidemiological studies showed that ARI risk was elevated in individuals competing in marathon and ultramarathon race events (58, 59). In a large group of 2,311 endurance runners, the odds of ARI during the week following the Los Angeles Marathon (LAM) race were 5.9 times higher compared to a control group (58). Forty percent of the runners reported at least one ARI episode during the 2-month winter period before the LAM, and those running more than 96 km per week versus less than 32 km per week doubled their odds for ARI. A 1-year retrospective study of German athletes showed that ARI risk was highest in endurance athletes, especially in those who also reported significant stress and sleep deprivation (60). Several long-term studies of elite athletes linked ARI incidence with high-volume training and endurance competitive events (61–63).

The International Olympic Committee (IOC) and the International Association of Athletics Federation (IAAF) initiated acute illness surveillance systems to establish underlying risk factors for ARI (64–67). These studies showed that the significant ARI risk factors included female gender, high levels of depression or anxiety, engaging in unusually intensive training periods, heavy training during the winter and at high altitudes, increased training monotony, international travel across several time zones, lack of tapering before major events, participation in competitive events especially during the winter, lack of sleep, and low-energy diet intake (64–68). The IOC recommends that athletes and coaches focus on load management of both internal (*e.g.*, psychological responses) and external loads (*e.g.*, training and competition workloads) (64). Load management is a key strategy, according to the IOC, to reduce ARI incidence and associated downturns in exercise performance, interruptions in training, missed competitive events, and risk of serious medical complications.

Most elite athletes do everything possible to avoid ARI because episodes can interfere with training and competitive goals. One study, for example, showed that COVID-19 had a significant impact on sport participation for over a quarter of elite athletes who experienced symptoms for more than a month following infection (69), and 6% of athletes still have not fully recovered after 3 months. Excessive fatigue was a key symptom, as well as difficulty in breathing, chest pain, and cough. This symptom cluster predicted which athletes would experience long COVID and was preferred when compared to the "neck-check" rule that was proposed decades ago without proper evaluation. The old "neck-check" rule urged full exercise cessation if the athlete experienced symptoms below the neck, with permission to continue if symptoms were above the neck. This is no longer accepted as sound clinical advice for athletes. Why so many of the elite athletes in this study experienced COVID-19 symptoms for more than a month was not determined. There are multiple reports in the literature of athletes developing protracted chronic fatigue symptoms following an intensive

exercise training session during the time they were ill with an ARI episode (1, 70, 71).

Infection can have both acute and chronic effects on physical activity patterns and capacity. For example, many individuals experience reduced exercise capacity related to lung, heart, and muscle dysfunction for months after the initial COVID-19 infection (72). The morbidity aftermath of the COVID-19 pandemic turned out to be more serious than originally projected, with at least one-third of individuals testing positive for SARS-CoV-2 reporting not being fully recovered after an average of 8–12 months of recovery (72, 73). One in twenty reported severe limitations in their capacity to perform daily activities. Women experienced more severe postacute symptom persistence than men. Other risk factors for long COVID include older age and high disease severity during the initial infection. Long COVID or postacute sequelae of COVID-19 (PASC) may be due in part to aberrant immunity, viral infiltration into tissues, and systemic inflammation. Common PASC symptoms include fatigue, increased respiratory effort, postexertional malaise and/or poor endurance, "brain fog" or cognitive impairment, chest pain, headache, arthralgia and myalgia, diarrhea, insomnia, and mood changes. Many of these symptoms are similar to myalgic encephalomyelitis, chronic fatigue syndrome (ME/CFS), and postural orthostatic tachycardia syndrome. Physical activity with a gradual increase in the total workload is recommended for ME/CFS, but with care to target a decrease in fatigue, improvement in overall quality of life, and the avoidance of symptom aggravation. There is every reason to believe that these are prudent guidelines for individuals with PASC.

Load Management Strategies to Reduce ARI Risk

Athletes must train hard for the competition and are interested in strategies to counter ARI despite the physiologic stress experienced. The ultimate objective is to achieve performance goals with little interruption from ARI. Several training, hygienic, nutritional, and psychological strategies are recommended, and these require the coordinated involvement of the medical staff, coaches, and athletes (1, 37, 64, 74, 75). Here is a summary of the most important load management guidelines to lower ARI risk:

- Develop an individualized training and competition plan that provides for sufficient recovery, sleep, nutrition support, hydration, and psychological support.
- Use small increments when changing the training load (typically less than 10% weekly) and avoid monotony (*i.e.*, vary the load day-to-day and week-to-week).

- Monitor for early signs and symptoms of overreaching, overtraining, and ARI.
- Avoid intensive training when ill or experiencing the early signs and symptoms of illness.
- Minimize exposure to viruses and bacteria by avoiding close contact with infected individuals in crowded and enclosed spaces. Avoid exercise sessions in poorly ventilated clubs and gymnasium facilities.
- Practice good hygiene by limiting hand-to-face contact (*i.e.*, self-inoculation), washing hands regularly and effectively, and smothering sneezes and coughs.

- Maintain vaccinations needed for home and foreign travel, with a new focus on influenza and COVID-19.
- Prioritize regular, high-quality sleep.
- Consume a well-balanced diet with sufficient energy to maintain a healthy weight. Focus on plant foods to provide sufficient carbohydrates and polyphenols to reduce exercise-induced inflammation and support immunity.
- Follow stress management techniques to reduce the number and impact of life stressors.

SUMMARY

This chapter provided a basic introduction to the human immune system and the acute and chronic influence of exercise training.

The immune system is the primary physiologic system that mediates the response to harmful exogenous and endogenous agents. There is a growing awareness that the immune system is also functionally coupled to metabolism and that exercise-induced metabolic responses influence immunity.

The immune system is very responsive to exercise, with the extent and duration reflecting the degree of physiological stress imposed by the workload. Regular MVPA is an important habit to support immunity and to stimulate the ongoing exchange of distinct and highly active immune cell subtypes between the circulation and tissues. In particular, each exercise bout improves the antipathogen activity of tissue macrophages in parallel with an enhanced recirculation of immunoglobulins, anti-inflammatory cytokines, neutrophils, NK cells, cytotoxic T cells, and immature B cells. With near daily exercise, these acute changes operate through a summation effect to enhance immune defense activity and metabolic health.

RCTs and epidemiological studies consistently support the inverse relationship between moderate exercise training and incidence of upper respiratory tract infections. Several epidemiological studies also suggest that regular physical activity is associated with reduced mortality and incidence rates for influenza and pneumonia.

In contrast, high exercise training workloads; competition events; and the associated physiological, metabolic, and psychological stress are linked to transient immune perturbations, inflammation, oxidative stress, muscle damage, and increased ARI risk. Risk for ARI is increased when an athlete goes through repeated cycles of unusually heavy exertion and competitions and experiences other stressors to the immune system. These data led to the development of the J-curve model that links URTI (upper respiratory tract infection) risk with the exercise workload continuum.

ARI risk factors for athletes include being a female, training and competing in long endurance events, high levels of depression or anxiety, participation in unusually intensive training periods, international travel across several time zones, participation in competitive events especially during the winter, lack of sleep, and low-energy diet intake. Load management of both internal (*e.g.*, psychological responses) and external factors (*e.g.*, training and competition workloads) and lifestyle strategies (*e.g.*, hygiene, nutritional support, vaccination, regular sleep) can be used to reduce ARI risk.

CHAPTER REVIEW QUESTIONS

1. Describe the components of the innate immune system.
2. What are the three primary types of lymphocytes? What CD antigens can be used during flow cytometry to identify these lymphocytes in the blood?
3. Describe the "open window" concept within exercise immunology.
4. Describe the "J-curve" model within exercise immunology.
5. List at least five of the most important load management guidelines to lower ARI risk.
6. Describe the basic immune response to MVPA.
7. List five significant ARI risk factors for athletes.
8. What are the central and secondary organs of the immune system?
9. What are the five main types of leukocytes?
10. The development of antibodies is triggered by the acquired immune system and is characterized by what three components?

Case Study 14.1

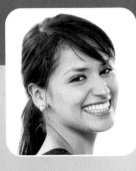

Erin is a 23-year-old woman who is an avid exerciser and has visited the clinical exercise physiologist (CEP) for advice on continuing her exercise program. Erin has a history of stable Type 1 diabetes mellitus for 10 years. Over the last 6 months, she has started to experience abdominal discomfort and diarrhea. She does not report any changes in her dietary intake but recalls attending a local microbrewery several months ago, and taking an ample sampling of their beer, which she thinks started her abdominal discomfort. She does not have any history of abnormal pelvic exams or Papanicolaou smear (also known as the Pap test). Hormone levels are within normal ranges, and she reports normal menstrual cycles. Recent immunological studies show higher than normal levels for some antibodies. She reports following a low-carbohydrate diet regularly.

Case Study 14.1 Questions

1. What should be Erin's first course of action based on the results of her blood work?

2. Is it possible her body is reacting to her sampling of the local brewery's beer?

Case Study 14.2

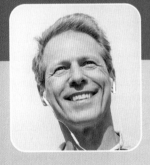

Jake is a 40-year-old marathon runner who clocks over 64.4 km (40 miles) per week. He has visited the CEP for advice on improving his exercise performance. Jake has been dealing with a chest cold, which has persisted for the last 2 months. He has taken multiple over-the-counter medications, but nothing seems to work. He feels his performance is starting to suffer.

Case Study 14.2 Questions

1. What may be considered the root cause of Jake's "chest cold"?

2. What recommendation would the CEP provide Jake in order to maintain his training and improve his performance?

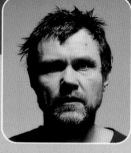

Case Study 14.3

Joe is a 50-year-old adventure athlete. He reports that currently he is having a hard time feeling good on any run. His times are slow and runs feel labored. Any intensity work causes Joe to get very fatigued and he often gets sick with acute respiratory illnesses. Joe ran in races since he was 13, and then starting training and competing in adventure races when he was 35 years old. He competed in many multiday adventure races in all environmental conditions. Recently, he was diagnosed with asthma and thinks this was a sign he was overtraining. Joe also experienced several life events in the last 7 years that have been difficult including a divorce, attendant issues with his children, shake-ups at work, and the passing of his dad from Parkinson disease.

Case Study 14.3 Questions

1. What recommendations would you give Joe regarding his health and training?

REFERENCES

1. Nieman DC, Wentz LM. The compelling link between physical activity and the body's defense system. *J Sport Health Sci.* 2019;8(3):201–17.
2. Simpson RJ, Campbell JP, Gleeson M, et al. Can exercise affect immune function to increase susceptibility to infection? *Exerc Immunol Rev.* 2020;26:8–22.
3. Nieman DC, Pence BD. Exercise immunology: future directions. *J Sport Health Sci.* 2020;9(5):432–45.
4. Pedersen BK, Febbraio MA. Muscle as an endocrine organ: focus on muscle-derived interleukin-6. *Physiol Rev.* 2008;88(4):1379–406.
5. Nieman DC, Lila MA, Gillitt ND. Immunometabolism: a multi-omics approach to interpreting the influence of exercise and diet on the immune system. *Annu Rev Food Sci Technol.* 2019;10:341–63.
6. Mak TW, Saunders ME, Jett BD. *Primer to the Immune Response.* 2nd ed. Burlington (MA): AP Cell Press; 2014.
7. Delves PJ, Martin SJ, Burton DR, Roitt IM. *Roitt's Essential Immunology.* 13th ed. Chichester (West Sussex): John Wiley & Sons, Ltd; 2017.
8. Hall JE. Resistance of the body to infection: I. Leukocytes, granulocytes, the monocyte-macrophage system, and inflammation. In: Hall JE, editor. *Guyton and Hall Textbook of Medical Physiology.* 13th ed. Philadelphia (PA): Elsevier; 2016. p. 455–64.
9. Kumar V, Abbas AK, Aster JC. *Robbins Basic Pathology E-Book.* 10th ed. Philadelphia (PA): Elsevier; 2017.
10. Vivier E, Raulet DH, Moretta A, et al. Innate or adaptive immunity? The example of natural killer cells. *Science.* 2011;331(6013):44–9.
11. Baldwin C. Constitutive host resistance. In: Kreier JP, editor. *Infection, Resistance and Immunity.* 2nd ed. New York (NY): Taylor & Francis; 2002.
12. Rehman J, Mills PJ, Carter SM, Chou J, Thomas J, Maisel AS. Dynamic exercise leads to an increase in circulating ICAM-1: further evidence for adrenergic modulation of cell adhesion. *Brain Behav Immun.* 1997;11(4):343–51.
13. Stromberg A, Rullman E, Jansson E, Gustafsson T. Exercise-induced upregulation of endothelial adhesion molecules in human skeletal muscle and number of circulating cells with remodeling properties. *J Appl Physiol.* 2017;122(5):1145–54.
14. Flajnik MF, Singh NJ, Holland SM. *Paul's Fundamental Immunology.* 8th ed. Philadelphia (PA): Lippincott Williams & Wilkins; 2022.
15. Punt J, Stranford S, Jones P, Owen J, Goldsby RA. *Kuby Immunology.* 8th ed. New York (NY): Macmillan; 2019.
16. Adams GR, Zaldivar FP, Nance DM, Kodesh E, Radom-Aizik S, Cooper DM. Exercise and leukocyte interchange among central circulation, lung, spleen, and muscle. *Brain Behav Immun.* 2011;25:658–66.
17. Bigley AB, Rezvani K, Chew C, et al. Acute exercise preferentially redeploys NK-cells with a highly-differentiated phenotype and augments cytotoxicity against lymphoma and multiple myeloma target cells. *Brain Behav Immun.* 2014;39:160–71.

18. Nieman DC, Henson DA, Austin MD, Brown VA. Immune response to a 30-minute walk. *Med Sci Sports Exerc.* 2005;37:57–62.

19. Turner JE, Spielmann G, Wadley AJ, Aldred S, Simpson RJ, Campbell JP. Exercise-induced B cell mobilization: preliminary evidence for an influx of immature cells into the bloodstream. *Physiol Behav.* 2016;164(Pt A):376–82.

20. Campbell JP, Riddell NE, Burns VE, et al. Acute exercise mobilizes CD8+ T lymphocytes exhibiting an effector-memory phenotype. *Brain Behav Immun.* 2009;23(6):767–75.

21. Pedersen BK. Anti-inflammatory effects of exercise: role in diabetes and cardiovascular disease. *Eur J Clin Invest.* 2017;47:600–11.

22. Karstoft K, Pedersen BK. Exercise and type 2 diabetes: focus on metabolism and inflammation. *Immunol Cell Biol.* 2016;94: 146–50.

23. Hallam J, Jones T, Alley J, Kohut ML. Exercise after influenza or COVID-19 vaccination increases serum antibody without an increase in side effects. *Brain Behav Immun.* 2022;102:1–10.

24. Nieman DC. Immune response to heavy exertion. *J Appl Physiol (1985).* 1997;82(5):1385–94.

25. Peake JM, Della Gatta P, Suzuki K, Nieman DC. Cytokine expression and secretion by skeletal muscle cells: regulatory mechanisms and exercise effects. *Exerc Immunol Rev.* 2015;21:8–25.

26. Siedlik JA, Benedict SH, Landes EJ, Weir JP, Vardiman JP, Gallagher PM. Acute bouts of exercise induce a suppressive effect on lymphocyte proliferation in human subjects: a meta-analysis. *Brain Behav Immun.* 2016;56:343–51.

27. Sakaguchi CA, Nieman DC, Signini EF, Abreu RM, Catai AM. Metabolomics-based studies assessing exercise-induced alterations of the human metabolome: a systematic review. *Metabolites.* 2019;9(8):164.

28. Nieman DC, Groen AJ, Pugachev A, et al. Proteomics-based detection of immune dysfunction in an elite adventure athlete trekking across Antarctica. *Proteomes.* 2020;8(1):4.

29. Signini ÉF, Nieman DC, Silva CD, Sakaguchi CA, Catai AM. Oxylipin response to acute and chronic exercise: a systematic review. *Metabolites.* 2020;10(6):264.

30. Nieman DC, Gillitt ND, Sha W. Identification of a select metabolite panel for measuring metabolic perturbation in response to heavy exertion. *Metabolomics.* 2018;14(11):147.

31. Nieman DC, Henson DA, Gusewitch G, et al. Physical activity and immune function in elderly women. *Med Sci Sports Exerc.* 1993;25(7):823–31.

32. Nieman DC, Nehlsen-Cannarella SL, Markoff PA, et al. The effects of moderate exercise training on natural killer cells and acute upper respiratory tract infections. *Int J Sports Med.* 1990;11:467–73.

33. Nieman DC, Nehlsen-Cannarella SL, Henson DA, et al. Immune response to exercise training and/or energy restriction in obese women. *Med Sci Sports Exerc.* 1998;30:679–86.

34. Chubak J, McTiernan A, Sorensen B, et al. Moderate-intensity exercise reduces the incidence of colds among postmenopausal women. *Am J Med.* 2006;119:937–42.

35. Barrett B, Hayney MS, Muller D, et al. Meditation or exercise for preventing acute respiratory infection: a randomized controlled trial. *Ann Fam Med.* 2012;10:337–46.

36. Barrett B, Hayney MS, Muller D, et al. Meditation or exercise for preventing acute respiratory infection (MEPARI-2): a randomized controlled trial. *PLoS One.* 2018;13:e0197778.

37. Nieman DC. Is infection risk linked to exercise workload? *Med Sci Sports Exerc.* 2000;32(Suppl 7):S406–11.

38. Matthews CE, Ockene IS, Freedson PS, Rosal MC, Merriam PA, Hebert JR. Moderate to vigorous physical activity and risk of upper-respiratory tract infection. *Med Sci Sports Exerc.* 2002;34:1242–8.

39. Fondell E, Lagerros YT, Sundberg CJ, et al. Physical activity, stress, and self-reported upper respiratory tract infection. *Med Sci Sports Exerc.* 2011;43(2):272–9.

40. Nieman DC, Henson DA, Austin MD, Sha W. Upper respiratory tract infection is reduced in physically fit and active adults. *Br J Sports Med.* 2011;45:987–92.

41. Zhou G, Liu H, He M, et al. Smoking, leisure-time exercise and frequency of self-reported common cold among the general population in northeastern China: a cross-sectional study. *BMC Public Health.* 2018;18:294.

42. Wu S, Ma C, Yang Z, et al. Hygiene behaviors associated with influenza-like illness among adults in Beijing, China: a large, population-based survey. *PLoS One.* 2016;11:e0148448.

43. Hamer M, O'Donovan G, Stamatakis E. Lifestyle risk factors, obesity and infectious disease mortality in the general population: linkage study of 97,844 adults from England and Scotland. *Prev Med.* 2019;123:65–70.

44. Hamer M, Kivimäki M, Gale CR, Batty GD. Lifestyle risk factors, inflammatory mechanisms, and COVID-19 hospitalization: a community-based cohort study of 387,109 adults in UK. *Brain Behav Immun.* 2020;87:184–7.

45. Hamrouni M, Roberts MJ, Thackray A, Stensel DJ, Bishop N. Associations of obesity, physical activity level, inflammation and cardiometabolic health with COVID-19 mortality: a prospective analysis of the UK Biobank cohort. *BMJ Open.* 2021;11(11):e055003.

46. Christensen RAG, Arneja J, St Cyr K, Sturrock SL, Brooks JD. The association of estimated cardiorespiratory fitness with COVID-19 incidence and mortality: a cohort study. *PLoS One.* 2021;16(5):e0250508.

47. Brawner CA, Ehrman JK, Bole S, et al. Inverse relationship of maximal exercise capacity to hospitalization secondary to Coronavirus Disease 2019. *Mayo Clin Proc.* 2021;96(1):32–9.

48. Song Y, Ren F, Sun D, et al. Benefits of exercise on influenza or pneumonia in older adults: a systematic review. *Int J Environ Res Public Health.* 2020;17(8):2655.

49. Williams PT. Reduced total and cause-specific mortality from walking and running in diabetes. *Med Sci Sports Exerc.* 2014;46:933–9.

50. Williams PT. Dose-response relationship between exercise and respiratory disease mortality. *Med Sci Sports Exerc.* 2014;46:711–7.

51. Wong CM, Lai HK, Ou CQ, et al. Is exercise protective against influenza-associated mortality? *PLoS One.* 2008;3(5):e2108.

52. Charland KM, Buckeridge DL, Hoen AG, et al. Relationship between community prevalence of obesity and associated behavioral factors and community rates of influenza-related hospitalizations in the United States. *Influenza Other Respir Viruses.* 2013;7:718–28.

53. Wong CM, Chan WM, Yang L, et al. Effect of lifestyle factors on risk of mortality associated with influenza in elderly people. *Hong Kong Med J.* 2014;20(Suppl 6):S16–9.

54. Ahmadi MN, Huang BH, Inan-Eroglu E, Hamer M, Stamatakis E. Lifestyle risk factors and infectious disease mortality,

including COVID-19, among middle aged and older adults: evidence from a community-based cohort study in the United Kingdom. *Brain Behav Immun.* 2021;96:18–27.

55. Calabrese L, Nieman DC. Exercise, infection and rheumatic diseases: what do we know? *RMD Open.* 2021;7(2):e001644.

56. Nieman DC. Exercise is medicine for immune function: implication for COVID-19. *Curr Sports Med Rep.* 2021;20(8):395–401.

57. Nieman DC. Coronavirus disease-2019: a tocsin to our aging, unfit, corpulent, and immunodeficient society. *J Sport Health Sci.* 2020;9(4):293–301.

58. Nieman DC, Johanssen LM, Lee JW, Arabatzis K. Infectious episodes in runners before and after the Los Angeles Marathon. *J Sports Med Phys Fitness.* 1990;30:316–28.

59. Peters EM, Bateman ED. Ultramarathon running and upper respiratory tract infections. An epidemiological survey. *S Afr Med J.* 1983;64:582–4.

60. Konig D, Grathwohl D, Weinstock C, Northoff H, Berg A. Upper respiratory tract infection in athletes: influence of lifestyle, type of sport, training effort, and immunostimulant intake. *Exerc Immunol Rev.* 2000;6:102–20.

61. Rama L, Teixeira AM, Matos A, et al. Changes in natural killer cell subpopulations over a winter training season in elite swimmers. *Eur J Appl Physiol.* 2013;113:859–68.

62. Hellard P, Avalos M, Guimaraes F, Toussaint JF, Pyne DB. Training-related risk of common illnesses in elite swimmers over a 4-yr period. *Med Sci Sports Exerc.* 2015;47:698–707.

63. Svendsen IS, Gleeson M, Haugen TA, Tønnessen E. Effect of an intense period of competition on race performance and self-reported illness in elite cross-country skiers. *Scand J Med Sci Sports.* 2015;25:846–53.

64. Schwellnus M, Soligard T, Alonso JM, et al. How much is too much? (Part 2) International Olympic Committee consensus statement on load in sport and risk of illness. *Br J Sports Med.* 2016;50:1043–52.

65. Timpka T, Jacobsson J, Bargoria V, et al. Preparticipation predictors for championship injury and illness: cohort study at the Beijing 2015 International Association of Athletics Federations World Championships. *Br J Sports Med.* 2017;51:271–6.

66. Alonso JM, Edouard P, Fischetto G, Adams B, Depiesse F, Mountjoy M. Determination of future prevention strategies in elite track and field: analysis of Daegu 2011 IAAF Championships injuries and illnesses surveillance. *Br J Sports Med.* 2012;46:505–14.

67. Derman W, Badenhorst M, Eken M, et al. Risk factors associated with acute respiratory illnesses in athletes: a systematic review by a subgroup of the IOC consensus on 'acute respiratory illness in the athlete'. *Br J Sports Med.* 2022;56(11):639–50.

68. Drew MK, Vlahovich N, Hughes D, et al. A multifactorial evaluation of illness risk factors in athletes preparing for the Summer Olympic Games. *J Sci Med Sport.* 2017;20:745–50.

69. Hull JH, Wootten M, Moghal M, et al. Clinical patterns, recovery time and prolonged impact of COVID-19 illness in international athletes: the UK experience. *Br J Sports Med.* 2022;56(1):4–11.

70. Parker S, Brukner P, Rosier M. Chronic fatigue syndrome and the athlete. *Sport Med Train Rehab.* 1996;6:269–78.

71. Roberts JA. Viral illnesses and sports performance. *Sports Med.* 1986;3:298–303.

72. Duggal P, Penson T, Manley HN, et al. Post-sequelae symptoms and comorbidities after COVID-19. *J Med Virol.* 2022;94(5):2060–6.

73. Zhang X, Wang F, Shen Y, et al. Symptoms and health outcomes among survivors of COVID-19 infection 1 year after discharge from hospitals in Wuhan, China. *JAMA Netw Open.* 2021;4(9):e2127403.

74. Walsh NP, Gleeson M, Pyne DB, et al. Position statement. Part two: maintaining immune health. *Exerc Immunol Rev.* 2011;17:64–103.

75. Bermon S, Castell LM, Calder PC, et al. Consensus statement immunonutrition and exercise. *Exerc Immunol Rev.* 2017;23:8–50.

Behavior and Mental Health

INTRODUCTION

Sedentary lifestyles contribute to leading causes of morbidity and mortality in the U.S. (1) and worldwide (2). Despite increased efforts to promote regular physical activity and exercise, only 53.3% of U.S. adults meet the Physical Activity Guidelines for aerobic activity, and only 23.2% meet the Guidelines for both aerobic and strengthening activities (3). For fitness professionals, assisting individuals in becoming and staying physically active is a challenge that requires understanding and applying theory-based principles of behavior change. It is also important for fitness professionals to have a basic understanding of mental health problems and their relationship to physical activity as well as the impact of chronic disease on both mental health and behavior.

PRACTICAL SKILLS FOR BEHAVIOR CHANGE

The clinical exercise physiologist (CEP) may find it helpful to use a "toolbox approach" to facilitate physical activity behavior change in their clients. By being familiar with a variety of "tools" derived from theory and research, the CEP can tailor recommendations and action plans to meet individual client needs, providing clients with the strategies and skills to manage their behavior long term.

Assessing the Client's Knowledge, Expectations, and Attitudes

Assessing the client's knowledge, expectations, and attitudes associated with physical activity can be helpful prior to initiating behavior change (4). Clients' knowledge about physical activity and past exercise experience often influences their expectations and perceptions, which in turn can provide early cues to guide education, problem-solving, and planning (5). Information can be gathered using interviews, questionnaires, or personal timeline methods, as part of a formal or informal assessment. This can help the CEP clarify participant expectations concerning physical activity (what can and cannot be accomplished and when results should be expected) and provide educational support to increase knowledge about physical activity and fitness.

Exploring Decisional Balance

Decisional balance is the evaluation of the potential positive and negative consequences of changing a behavior, such as physical activity (6). Advantages ("pros") can be emphasized for motivation, whereas identified disadvantages ("cons") can provide opportunities to learn more about the activity, tailor recommendations to address individual barriers, and develop coping strategies and problem-solving skills. Clients are typically encouraged to log advantages and disadvantages on a decisional balance worksheet so that they can analyze the costs and benefits of a potential change.

The CEP can assist the client in examining the actual and perceived advantages and disadvantages of increasing physical activity. This may help the client to:

1. establish the reasons and motives for behavior change.
2. set specific goals and avoid future pitfalls.
3. understand environmental supports and challenges for physical activity.
4. identify behaviors needed for adoption and maintenance of exercise.

Identifying Benefits of Physical Activity

There are numerous identified benefits to regular physical activity. Participating in regular physical activity can (1):

- reduce risk of chronic diseases including diabetes, hypertension, heart disease, and certain cancers.
- assist in weight management.

- promote healthy bones, muscles, and joints.
- improve cognitive functioning and mental health and reduce symptoms of depression, stress, and anxiety.
- improve body image, self-esteem, and self-concept.
- increase fitness, improve physical functioning, and enhance ability to perform activities of daily living (ADLs).
- provide opportunities to develop social contacts and relationships with others.

Although clients may have heard about or experienced multiple benefits of physical activity, certain benefits typically hold greater motivational influence or salience for each person. Therefore, it is worthwhile to consider the importance and personal relevance for each potential benefit for the individual client as a possible motivating factor for exercise (7). Fitness professionals can help clients to identify personal priorities so that benefits are meaningful.

Examining Barriers to Physical Activity

Most people recognize several benefits of regular exercise; however, clients may feel these benefits are outweighed by the disadvantages, barriers, and/or risks of physical activity. Whether real or imagined, barriers can have a significant impact on motivation and behavior. In addition, other factors such as the client's age, ethnicity, socioeconomic status, and current state of health may potentiate the significance of certain barriers. For example, health-related barriers and concerns about risks are particularly important among older individuals who may have fears of exercise-related injury (8). Individuals in groups at risk for physical inactivity may benefit from an emphasis on moderate-intensity activities that can be readily adapted for various fitness levels and abilities and incorporated into their daily routines.

Common barriers to adopting and maintaining physical activity include:

- lack of time
- fatigue
- physical limitations, low physical fitness, or medical conditions
- fear of becoming injured
- mental health concerns such as depression, anxiety, or stress
- accessibility, affordability, and convenience of safe facilities and equipment
- environmental and ecological factors such as geographical location or climate
- insufficient encouragement or lack of social support
- discomfort or anxiety exercising in front of others
- lack of enjoyment or boredom

Individuals in the early stages of exercise adoption typically report fewer benefits and more barriers than those in the latter stages (9). The CEP should work with clients to evaluate perceived benefits and barriers, highlighting the benefits of physical activity with an emphasis on those that have personal relevance for the client. In addition, problem-solving strategies can be very helpful in coping with specific barriers.

Encouraging Self-Management and Problem-Solving

Self-management strategies are important to successful behavior change. Forming a professional partnership that fosters the client's feelings of autonomy and control with respect to the physical activity program is important for long-term participation and maintenance of exercise behavior (10). Thus, participants should be encouraged to take a self-directed approach to all aspects of physical activity (*e.g.*, goal setting, planning, problem-solving) rather than relying on the CEP.

Because barriers arise at all stages of health-related behavior change, a critical behavioral skill is practical and systematic problem-solving to overcome these barriers (11). Box 15.1 demonstrates how to apply the four steps of the IDEA Method of practical problem-solving for overcoming barriers to physical activity. Barriers often change over time; therefore, self-management in problem-solving will be important to the maintenance of exercise over a lifetime.

Setting Goals, Shaping Behaviors, and Rewarding Effort

Once the benefits, barriers, and potential risks associated with exercise are recognized, short- and long-term goals can be established. Goal setting is a stepwise process that involves assessing an individual's current level of fitness or physical

Box 15.1	Steps for Practical Problem-Solving: The IDEA Method

1. **I**dentify and prioritize personal barriers for physical activity and select a specific barrier to address.
2. **D**evelop a list of possible solutions. Encourage creative brainstorming for multiple possibilities and alternative ways to address the barrier.
3. **E**valuate each solution and select one to try.
4. **A**ct on the plan and **a**ssess how well the plan worked. If it worked, continue using that solution. If it didn't work, select another solution to try. Whether or not the plan worked, it is a step in the right direction.

activity level, evaluating the individual's expected outcome, and considering best professional practices for exercise prescription. For sedentary clients, the major objective is to establish a successful physical activity habit that considers health and fitness goals while decreasing the likelihood for failure. The initial activity prescription should be well within the client's capabilities. Additionally, individual preferences, motivation, skills, and life circumstances should be considered.

SMART Goal Setting

Successful behavior change relies on the establishment of effective goals. Goals should provide the individual with a modest challenge, leading to increased self-efficacy when achieved. For some clients, the goal may simply be to take the stairs at work instead of using the elevator. For others, it may be to engage in 30 minutes of moderate-intensity structured exercise at a fitness center. Effective goals include the following "SMART" principles (11, 12):

- **S**pecific: The behavior should be clearly and precisely established, including mode, frequency, intensity, and duration of physical activity.

- **M**easurable: The behavior should be something that can be readily monitored such as by using logs or fitness trackers.
- **A**djustable: Physical activity should be able to be modified as needed. For example, frequency, duration, or intensity can be adjusted if injury, illness, or other life event occurs.
- **R**ealistic: The behavior should be somewhat challenging, but within the individual's capabilities, and readily achievable. For example, an incremental exercise prescription ensures that goals are appropriate for the client's health and fitness level.
- **T**ime frame specific: The behavior should specify a reasonable period (*e.g.*, 1 month, 6 months) to enable measurement of progress and appropriate acknowledgment or rewards.

Especially in the beginning, clients should set goals that are simple and easy to remember. Each goal should have an associated action plan with specific strategies for implementation. Keeping the goals, timeline, and strategies visible through a worksheet, calendar, journal, or poster can serve as a tangible reminder of the physical activity action plan (see Figure 15.1). There are a variety

Last Week's Average: _____7,700_____ steps per day

This Week's Goal: _____8,200_____ steps per day

Reminders:

- Wear tracker all day / keep charger by bed
- Walk 20 minutes after work on Tuesday and Thursday

Day	Steps	Notes
Monday		
Tuesday		
Wednesday		
Thursday		
Friday		
Saturday		
Sunday		

FIGURE 15.1 Sample goal sheet using steps.

of resources to assist people in developing a plan. Examples include mobile fitness apps and technology-assisted workouts that can be customized for fitness level and interests. Wearable technology such as GPS watches, accelerometers, and heart rate monitors can also be useful tools for goal setting and automated tracking and feedback.

As part of the goal-setting process, the CEP can help the client consider both short-term and long-term goals. This approach is important for building confidence and encourages sustainable motivation. In addition, it is important to model an expectation of intentionally revisiting and adjusting goals as part of long-term behavior change.

Shaping Behaviors

A key consideration in all physical activity program planning is the gradual shaping of the physical activity behavior toward the established goals agreed upon by the client and the CEP. When physical activity progresses too quickly, adherence may be negatively affected, particularly when client expectations and preferences are not considered. The risk of injury and dropout may increase when beginning exercisers are prescribed physical activities too high in intensity, duration, or frequency. A physical activity program should be gradually incremented, ensuring success at each stage. The CEP should assess clients' perceptions of their progress to gauge their readiness for adjustments in the exercise prescription and physical activity goals.

Together the CEP and client can consider psychosocial, behavioral, and fitness progression toward short- and long-term goals. The CEP should consider periodic fitness assessment as well as behavioral check-ins to encourage self-management skill development. This is a collaborative and iterative process that relies on ongoing tracking and measurement of observable behaviors and outcomes as well as client self-assessment of motivation and self-efficacy.

Rewards and Reinforcement

For many individuals, the initial steps involved in becoming more physically active may not be pleasant or intrinsically (internally) rewarding. Often, it is not until several months into a regular physical activity program that participants begin to report positive benefits from physical activity. In fact, the longer the period of inactivity and the more unfit the individual, the longer it may be before physical activity becomes intrinsically reinforcing. Therefore, external rewards may be needed for encouragement and motivation.

The CEP should encourage the client to select the rewards, as the incentives people find motivating vary from person to person. Some individuals may even find the use of external rewards uncomfortable or counterproductive. Smaller rewards (*e.g.*, watching a favorite show) for achieving short-term goals and larger rewards (*e.g.*, new running shoes or a massage) for achieving long-term goals may help the individual focus on the steps of the goal-setting process and provide incentives for sustained motivation (13). Many clients find that encouraging feedback from the CEP provides positive reinforcement that rewards physical activity. Ideally, as physical activity behaviors are established, participants' motivation will become more intrinsic, reducing the reliance on external factors.

Exercise professionals may also consider program-based incentives as a form of extrinsic motivation. Ideas include the use of point systems, competitions, and recognition. These should be based on readily achievable physical activity goals (*e.g.*, attendance or participation) during the early stages of physical activity adoption. As activity continues, accumulated points can be redeemed for material rewards such as exercise gear, a gift certificate, or a training session. Other strategies include requiring a monetary deposit that is returned upon achievement of goals, especially behavioral goals such as attendance and participation or a reduction in program fees with program adherence. Because some individuals spend significant time restarting physical activity, strategies for maintenance should be an integral component of programming.

Exercise professionals can also help individuals identify the intrinsically rewarding aspects of the physical activity itself such as enjoyment, increased energy, opportunities to socialize, or a chance to "get away." Intrinsic motivation may be learned when an individual experiences personal, self-identified rewards for behavior (*e.g.*, personal achievement, the satisfaction obtained in reaching one's physical activity goals) independent of extrinsic or external reinforcements (14). Self-determination theory indicates that intrinsic motivation may be positively related to continued participation in physical activity (15). Thus, the CEP can encourage self-directed and sustained physical activity by exploring the client's feelings about the proposed change, encouraging a personal rationale for the change, providing a choice of alternative behaviors to reduce conflicts, and recognizing the importance of individual preferences and experiences (16).

Self-Monitoring

Another important aspect of self-management for behavioral success is identifying physical activity patterns and receiving feedback, especially self-monitored feedback regarding progress. Such self-monitoring can have a positive effect on a wide variety of health-related behaviors. For example, short-term reduction in caloric intake usually results when caloric intake is monitored. Similarly, physical activity habits are frequently enhanced when attendance, physical activity behaviors, or the results of the exercise program are systematically monitored. Self-monitoring can be used to identify unhelpful patterns or sedentary activities, set goals, monitor progress, identify barriers, and improve physical activity choices (11). Methods include the use of activity journals, step counters, mobile apps, and automated body monitors. Reports of different physical activity variables (*e.g.*, steps, mileage, minutes, plotted heart rates, intensity levels, or attendance) can be used to monitor progress and provide feedback. Fitness assessments can be used to compare current measures with past levels of fitness and guide setting of future goals. Objective feedback can be a powerful motivating factor when used in conjunction with relevant short- and long-term goals.

Research continues to support the usefulness of regular self-monitoring of physical activity for long-term maintenance. However, few behavioral strategies evoke more resistance from participants than the prospect of ongoing self-monitoring. As with any goal-setting strategy, individuals should fully participate in designing the self-monitoring strategies that will be the easiest and most convenient for them to maintain.

Building Confidence

Self-efficacy, or the extent to which individuals feel capable of performing desired behaviors, appears to be a particularly potent predictor of physical activity participation in the early stages (17, 18). Self-efficacy can be enhanced by setting realistic personally tailored physical activity goals (see SMART goals), encouraging regular positive feedback, receiving social support, and tracking physical activity to measure progress and highlight success. Helping clients take charge of their physical activity behaviors leads to improved confidence in maintaining physical activity patterns over time.

To help build the client's self-efficacy, the CEP should explore with the client any previous experiences with physical activity, along with unreasonable or inaccurate beliefs about exercise. For example, many inactive individuals believe that exercise is inherently painful or aversive and may be unaware of the benefit of moderate activities that may be more appealing and comfortable than more vigorous activity regimens. Fitness professionals can provide specific instruction on how to perform specific activities at a safe, beneficial intensity to obtain health-related benefits while avoiding injury and minimizing unpleasant aspects of exercise (19). Table 15.1 presents different types of strategies for increasing physical activity self-efficacy.

Identifying and Recruiting Social Support

Identifying and recruiting social support is an important skill for behavior change, particularly a complex behavior like physical activity. Social support for physical activity can be obtained through fitness and health professionals, workout partners, family members, coworkers, and/or friends who encourage increased activity and assist in planning exercise. Many individuals also give and receive support through online communities and social networking groups formed around common interests.

There are two broad categories of social support: structural support and functional support. Structural support refers to social networks and includes such indices as marital status, number of friends, and participation in church or civic organizations. Functional support refers to the perception of support and includes instrumental support (*e.g.*, tangible acts like providing childcare or transportation) and emotional support (*e.g.*, complimenting a person on results).

Praise and encouragement are critical components of social support, especially for inexperienced or completely relapsed former exercisers. To be most effective, encouragement should be both immediate (during or very shortly after the physical activity episode, if possible) and specific. Informational support can be very helpful and is generally necessary, especially for beginners. This support can include providing the appropriate exercise prescription for the client's goals or something as simple as providing a list of parks with walking trails. Appraisal or validation support is another type of support that can be used to help individuals maintain an exercise program; it involves comparison with others or one's past to confirm one's thoughts, feelings, or experiences. A beginner in yoga class might reflect on her first session to confirm her progress or compare her progress with a friend who started the class at the same time. Friends and family members can also participate in physical activity to enhance support. However, others' physical activity pace must be appropriate and matched to that of the individual. When support from significant others is active and ongoing, individuals are more likely to continue physical activity (20).

Table 15.1	Strategies for Increasing Physical Activity Self-Efficacy
Information Sources for Self-Efficacy	**Strategies**
Past performances	• Assess past physical activity history and behavioral goals; use positive experiences and successes to build confidence; create activity timelines. • Set small goals and rehearse activity behaviors. • Use self-monitoring with fitness trackers or activity logs to track success.
Vicarious experiences	• Arrange workout/accountability partners tailored to the client. • Use videos and success stories of active peer role models. • Have peer role models lead group physical activity sessions.
Verbal persuasion	• Encourage and praise client for progress. • Enlist family and friends to support and reinforce the activity behavior. • Arrange additional support from other health professionals.
Physiological cues	• Help clients anticipate and positively interpret physical signs and discomforts related to physical activity (*e.g.*, fatigue, increased breathing, muscle soreness). • Use relaxation training to decrease stress and anxiety. • Use an incremental exercise prescription matched to client fitness.
Emotional state	• Help clients identify positive feelings associated with physical activity (accomplishment, pride, enjoyment). • Address and reframe negative feelings (frustration, shame, dislike).

Source: Adapted from Pekmezi D, Jennings E, Marcus BH. Evaluating and enhancing self-efficacy for physical activity. *ACSM's Health Fit J.* 2009;13(2):16–21; *ACSM's Behavioral Aspects of Physical Activity and Exercise.* 1st ed. Philadelphia (PA): Wolters Kluwer; 2013.

Appropriate and consistent physical activity role models can also provide social support for beginning or continuing exercise. Role models should be as similar as possible to the targeted individuals. For example, some programs use successful graduates as future participant assistants for maximal effectiveness (7). When possible, the CEP should set an appropriate example by exercising with participants and displaying other behaviors that are consistent with an active lifestyle such as taking the stairs, setting fitness goals, and making hydration and nutrition a priority.

The continued use of various social support mechanisms is valuable for continued physical activity maintenance (Box 15.2). For example, in group exercise formats, fitness professionals can contact absent participants to let them know that they are missed and that others care about them. Fellow exercisers can also assume this type of responsibility through a "buddy system." If physical activity is done outside of a formal setting, the exercise professional may continue support in the form of periodic telephone calls, texts, e-mails, or newsletters (21). Family members, coworkers, neighbors, and friends should

continue to encourage and support the physical activity program. It may be helpful to teach support persons how to provide continuing support through prompting, modeling, and reinforcing physical activity. Most importantly,

Box 15.2	Types of Social Support for Physical Activity

Encourage the participant to identify different people who can provide different types of support.
• Knowledge: Provide information and assist in practical advice about exercise and physical activity (*e.g.*, a CEP provides instruction on technique)
• Participatory: Participate in physical activity with the individual (*e.g.*, a friend serves as a workout partner)
• Motivational: Provide encouragement and accountability (*e.g.*, a family member provides positive feedback and acts as a "cheerleader")
• Practical: Assist in logistical arrangements to enable the participant to make and complete exercise plans (*e.g.*, spouse watches the kids)

individuals should be encouraged to be proactive in identifying and seeking out sources of support so that they can match their personal needs with available support resources in their environments (13). It is also important to remember that support needs can vary depending on the individual needs at a given time, and there is no one "best" type of support.

Employing Stimulus Control

Stimulus control, or structuring one's personal environment to remind or encourage behavior using visual or auditory reminders or prompts, can positively impact physical activity (22, 23). Experimental studies on the use of environmental changes to encourage stair use in public buildings consistently find that the placement of prompts increases the rate of stairway use. Research also indicates that making environments more pleasant using art and music further increases the use of stairs (24). Reminders such as setting calendar alarms, posting sticky notes, or leaving exercise shoes by the door can inspire some individuals to act. Prompts may also serve as automatic cues to promote sedentary behavior. Fitness professionals can work with clients to remove unhelpful cues and plan reminders that will be the most effective in promoting physical activity.

Because of the myriad dynamic influences on physical activity behavior, assisting clients in developing skills that can be adapted to facilitate physical activity over time is critical for successful behavior change and maintenance. A summary of behavioral skills and strategies to promote physical activity is given in Box 15.3.

MOTIVATIONAL CONSIDERATIONS FOR PHYSICAL ACTIVITY

Factors that influence initial adoption and early participation in physical activity may differ from those that affect subsequent long-term maintenance. One of the most important factors in maintaining physical activity is motivational readiness.

Stages of Change: Matching Skills to Motivational Readiness

The role of motivational readiness in changing and maintaining behavior has been widely applied to physical activity and exercise (25, 26). Stages-of-change models that acknowledge the role of readiness in supporting behavior change may help the CEP identify strategies that may be effective for individuals in different stages and at different levels of physical activity participation. One of the best known is the transtheoretical model (TTM) of behavior change (Figure 15.2), which proposes that individuals

---

Box 15.3	Behavioral Skills and Strategies to Promote Physical Activity

- **Decisional balance:** Identify personal benefits of physical activity and evaluate barriers for change. Relate benefits to personal meaning and core values to enhance motivational influence. Facilitate problem-solving skills for overcoming barriers.
- **Self-monitoring:** Record physical activity variables such as type of activity, intensity, minutes, and calories expended as well as sedentary behaviors, such as time spent sitting, watching television, or computer use. Use fitness trackers, particularly for individuals who have not begun structured exercise or find it difficult to keep written logs.
- **Goal setting:** Set SMART short-term and long-term goals for physical activity behaviors. Goals should target specific behaviors, be measurable to monitor progress, be adjustable, be realistic, and occur in a reasonable time frame. Include appropriate rewards for meeting goals.

- **Commitment:** Make a commitment to healthy behaviors; use behavioral contracts and incentives to enhance motivation.
- **Social support:** Identify and enlist social support to allow participants to share concerns, gain knowledge, receive encouragement, and practice new behaviors. Identify significant others who could hinder physical activity efforts, then develop strategies and assertiveness skills to deal with them.
- **Stimulus control:** Recognize and control physical, psychological, environmental, and social cues for physical activity behaviors.
- **Relapse prevention:** Identify high-risk situations and plan for potential lapses in physical activity. Practice cognitive restructuring to overcome unhelpful or negative thought patterns.

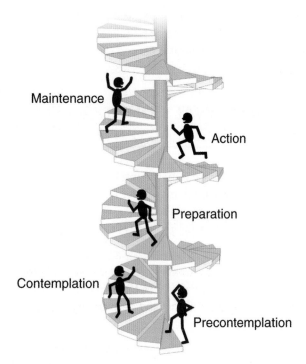

FIGURE 15.2 The stages-of-change model. (From *ACSM's Behavioral Aspects of Physical Activity and Exercise.* 1st ed. Philadelphia (PA): Wolters Kluwer; 2013.)

move through five stages of readiness for changing health behaviors (27, 28):

- Precontemplation (not thinking about changing physical activity)
- Contemplation (thinking about changing physical activity)
- Preparation (making small changes in physical activity but not to a degree that meets the desired target)
- Action (meeting physical activity goals but for fewer than 6 months)
- Maintenance (being physically active at the desired level for at least 6 months)

Movement through the stages may not progress in a stepwise, predictable fashion; instead, individuals often move back and forth through the stages.

By understanding and assessing the client's readiness for change, the CEP can tailor physical activity interventions and exercise programs to meet the client's current needs and level of motivation. See Table 15.2, for suggested strategies by stage of readiness for change.

Maximizing Enjoyment and Avoiding Boredom

For most individuals, enjoyment of the physical activity program is important to adherence. Methods for enhancing the client's enjoyment include customizing the mode, intensity, duration, format, and location. The CEP can also help clients develop individualized action plans that increase motivation and adherence. Exercise plans should consider activities, environments, goals, partners, settings, variety, and other aspects of physical activity that match client preferences and expectations.

Boredom is often a barrier to long-term maintenance. With a wide variety of physical activities and a diversity of programming options, boredom can often be minimized. For example, some individuals may prefer to do physical activity in multiple short bouts rather than in one long session. Pairing physical activity with another enjoyable activity (*e.g.*, listening to music, watching TV while on stationary equipment, or exercising with a friend) can serve as a distraction and increase enjoyment of exercise. Often, enjoyable competition such as fun runs, group fitness classes, or facility contests can help to stimulate maintenance and reinvigorate a stale program or routine. The CEP can work with clients to develop activity plans that maximize enjoyment and reduce boredom.

Preventing Relapse

A relapse is a stopping of the adopted behavior and return to the previous habit. One useful step in preventing relapse is to prepare in advance (both psychologically and behaviorally) for situations that commonly provoke lapses in exercise participation. A lapse is a break in activity that may lead to a full-blown relapse and a return to the previous sedentary lifestyle (7, 29). For example, a client may stop exercising completely after a break because of illness or injury, travel, holidays, a period of inclement weather, or increased work demands. The CEP can help clients anticipate such interruptions to physical activity. This is another means of enhancing clients' self-efficacy and resiliency while facilitating their adherence (7, 29). Individuals high in resiliency, cognitive coping skills, and behavioral strategies have fewer relapses. Resilient individuals can view setbacks as opportunities rather than failures.

The CEP can also assist clients in normalizing lapses and understanding that barriers and interruptions are part of the process of becoming more active and do not indicate failure. Occasional lapses are to be expected. Learning to overcome them will enable clients to experience greater behavioral control and know how to get back on track.

Strategies to prepare for lapses and to restart physical activity include planning ahead for high-risk situations, identifying alternate activities that can be done in place of

Table 15.2	Strategies for Moving to Next Stage of Motivational Readiness for Change	
Stage of Change	**Goal**	**Specific Strategies**
Precontemplation	To facilitate client thinking about becoming more active	• Encourage client to learn more about physical activity and options for physical activity (*e.g.*, read articles, watch videos, talk to others about physical activity). • Make a list of potential benefits of physical activity and identify those with personal meaning.
Contemplation	To facilitate client to consider and taking small steps toward being physically active	• Have the client observe a fitness class or training session; take a tour of the fitness facility to build familiarity and confidence. • Identify barriers to getting started and problem-solve strategies for overcoming them. • Set a small goal and develop an action plan for getting started.
Preparation	To support client in making progress toward meeting physical activity goals	• Help client experiment with different activities. • Explore different types of environmental and social support resources. • Have client self-monitor physical activity and track progress toward goals. • Consider appropriate reinforcement and rewards for meeting short-term, incremental goals of increased physical activity. • Use prompts as reminders to be more active (wear fitness tracker, keep walking shoes by the door). • Identify barriers to goals and problem-solve strategies for overcoming them.
Action	To support current physical activity and help client maintain physical activity over time	• Identify obstacles that might interfere with being active in the future and develop a plan for how to overcome them. • Help client train for a future event to encourage long-term goals (5K, hike a mountain trail).
Maintenance	To help client prepare for any future setbacks and increase enjoyment of physical activity	• Encourage planning of enjoyable physical activity (*e.g.*, new activities; listen to music or watch TV while on treadmill; walk with a friend). • Make a plan for getting back on track after a .break in physical activity. • Encourage client to mentor someone else who is interested in becoming more physically active.

Source: Adapted from Pekmezi D, Barbera B, Marcus BH. Using the transtheoretical model to promote physical activity. *ACSM's Health Fit J.* 2010;14(4):8–13.

the usual activity, planning to exercise as soon as possible after a break, enhancing accountability and support systems, and modifying goals to avoid discouragement (11).

Revisiting Benefits

Recognizing the relevant personal benefits of physical activity (physical, social, and psychological) is important for sustained motivation. The CEP should regularly ask clients about the benefits they are noticing from their current physical activity program. Clients who cannot identify any benefits of their physical activity or, alternatively, provide several negatives are at high risk of dropout. Such participants should be targeted for increased attention and support. Having participants regularly revisit their decisional balance worksheet can be useful for reinforcing their personal commitments to be active, as well as revising the physical activity plan to increase the benefits portion of the equation.

Generalization Training

Generalization training involves expanding a behavior (exercise) to a different setting to link the behavior with cues or stimuli in the second setting that may help to facilitate ongoing participation. For example, before discontinuing supervised or structured, facility-based sessions, the client's exercise program should be generalized to the future environment (*e.g.*, home, workplace, or community fitness center) (30). Generalization may be accomplished in several ways. Examples include beginning home exercise sessions at an early stage of the program, involving significant others in physical activity sessions, and adding additional exercises that are easily maintained in the new setting. Ideally, the responsibility for session monitoring, support, reinforcement, and feedback should be gradually transferred from the CEP to the client. This more closely approximates the conditions likely to be experienced in the maintenance setting.

Reassessment of Goals

Regular reassessment of physical activity goals provides an opportunity to verify that goals are relevant, realistic, and motivating. As noted earlier, goals that are too distant (*e.g.*, several months) or vague (*e.g.*, "I will exercise more") do not provide sufficient motivation or structure to maintain behavior through difficult periods. During the early stages of a physical activity program, goals should be adjusted as frequently as necessary to direct physical activity behavior.

As physical activity progresses, participants should understand the importance of continued goal reassessment and reinforcement to enhance long-term motivation. Additionally, along with exercise and fitness goals, it is important that clients reassess their personal vision, strengths, and values as they relate to their physical activity goals.

HELPING CLIENTS REACH AND MAINTAIN RECOMMENDED ACTIVITY LEVELS

As the CEP engages clients in behavioral skill building and exercise prescription, it is important to take steps to promote a productive professional relationship that facilitates behavior change. Applying basic counseling strategies can promote an atmosphere that increases the likelihood of long-term success by facilitating self-directed planning for physical activity.

Client-Centered Coaching

The client-centered approach to health counseling (31, 32) promotes a collaborative relationship between the client and the professional. The key elements of this partnership include genuineness, positive regard for the client, empathy, and understanding that the client is the primary driver of behavior change. In this approach, the client achieves their desired outcomes using skills and processes that are personally relevant and self-directed. The goals of the client-centered approach include encouraging clients to express concerns, helping them to be more active in the consultation, giving them more control of goal setting and decision-making (33). When used by health care providers, the approach has been associated with higher client satisfaction, increased medication compliance, a reduction in clients' concerns, and improvement in health-related variables such as blood pressure (34). Box 15.4 lists several of the key elements of the client-centered approach (33).

The Five A's Model (Assess, Advise, Agree, Assist, Arrange) has been used in client-centered counseling for physical activity to provide a framework for professionals (11, 35, 36). This model is useful to structure the physical activity counseling session, assess motivational readiness to be active, and tailor recommendations based on the individual's current physical activity level, goals, and stage of change.

In the Five A's Model, the CEP and the client work together as follows:

| Box 15.4 | Summary of Client-Centered Techniques |

- Create a collaborative relationship based on authenticity, empathy, and respect for client autonomy.
- Ask simple, open-ended questions (*i.e.*, questions that elicit details, not brief yes-or-no responses).
- Listen and encourage with verbal and nonverbal prompts.
- Clarify and summarize. Check your understanding of what the client said and verify that the client understood what you said.
- Use reflective listening. Include statements that bridge the gap between what the client is saying and the underlying meaning behind the statements.

■ Assess: The CEP assesses relevant aspects of the client's current health and physical activity level, including the type, frequency, intensity, and duration of current physical activity, as well as any contraindications to exercise. In addition, the CEP evaluates the client's stage of change, benefits and barriers, self-efficacy, and social support system.

■ Advise: The CEP advises the client based on the information gathered and the client's stage of change. The advice is client-centered, including individually tailored recommendations.

■ Agree: The CEP and the client agree on the type and level of intervention and establish exercise goals.

■ Assist: The CEP assists the client in crafting a specific action plan, developing skills and strategies to support the behavior change, and identifying resources to support the change.

■ Arrange: Lastly, the CEP arranges the next steps for the client. This could include scheduling subsequent sessions and follow-up visits, sending reminder messages, and/or making referrals to other health care providers or programs (37, 38).

Studies have indicated that even brief counseling can have an impact on changes in physical activity behaviors (39). To achieve the goals of the client-centered approach, practitioners should focus on creating a collaborative and cooperative partnership with their clients. Establishing professional rapport with trust and mutual respect is important for a successful working relationship. People want to feel heard and understood by others; communicating genuine interest and empathy helps to build rapport (33). Communicating empathy includes verbal and nonverbal acknowledgment of the other person's thoughts and feelings in a nonjudgmental, supportive manner.

Active listening is important to the CEP-client relationship. Active listening is a process wherein the practitioner tries to understand the underlying meaning of what the client is saying, then communicates the understanding back to the client through reflecting or repeating the information, summarizing client statements, and asking questions for clarification (33, 40). Reflecting back the underlying meaning can help to establish rapport and empathy in that it demonstrates understanding of the client's perspective. Summarizing statements can help review content and identify key themes and issues, not only to demonstrate an understanding of the client's perspective, but also to keep the session focused. Open-ended questions expand dialogue by allowing clients to continue the conversation and clarify their thoughts or meaning. Thoughtful and effective questions can elicit information that can be useful for intervention and for guiding the client toward behavior change (41). Attending to nonverbal communications, such as posture and facial expressions, can also be important to fill in the gaps between what the person might be saying and what they are feeling (40).

Considering Socioecological Factors

Exercise professionals should recognize that a client's physical activity behavior occurs within the larger context of behavioral determinants and influences. Considering the relationships among socioecological factors (intrapersonal, interpersonal, community, and organizational factors), physical activity is essential to support clients in successful behavior change (42).

It is important for fitness professionals to work with clients to explore how factors specific to the individual such as age, gender, race, culture, socioeconomic status, health, or family relationships might influence attitudes, behaviors, and motivations toward physical activity. The relative importance of each of these factors can vary widely from person to person. In addition, factors outside the individual such as policy, environmental features, or community infrastructure can also play an important role in inhibiting or promoting physical activity. For example, walkability, options for active transportation, availability of parks and public spaces, and safe environments for physical activity are environmental features that promote physical activity (Table 15.3) (43).

Using a client-centered approach, the CEP can elicit information about the personally relevant multiple determinants of the client's physical activity or inactivity across levels

Table 15.3	Sociological Factors That Contribute to Active Living
Element	Examples
Walkability and connectivity	Safe and easy active travel connections to local destinations; well-lit side-walks, even and well-maintained surfaces (for the elderly, to reduce fall risk)
Active travel alternatives	Efficient public transportation, well-marked biking and walking routes; safe routes to school for children
Quality and accessible public space	High-quality and safe parks, trails, open space for the community to use
Social interaction and inclusion	Mixed-use developments that encourage walking and cycling for local trips
Domestic environments can be made to be more active	Doing gardening, household chores, and using these as "energy expenditure opportunities" as well as tasks

Source: Adapted from *ACSM's Behavioral Aspects of Physical Activity and Exercise.* 1st ed. Philadelphia (PA): Wolters Kluwer; 2013.

of influence: individual, interpersonal, social environment, physical environment, and society. The CEP can guide the client in identifying strengths and weaknesses in each of the levels, which can provide greater insight into personal health behavior and create opportunities for change in physical activity. Together, the client and the exercise professional can conceptualize behavior patterns and develop action plans within a larger context in a way that makes sense for the client.

Group Coaching Techniques

Behavior change techniques can be readily integrated into a group setting. The CEP may even find that the group setting facilitates key behavioral strategies. A major advantage of groups for behavior change is the natural support system that it provides to clients. Other advantages of a group setting include the participants' ability to:

- provide feedback to each other based on experiences.
- develop self-efficacy from peer role models and emulate others' successful techniques.
- evaluate the practicality of desired goals, objectives, and plans.
- encourage commitment and accountability.
- develop solutions for barriers.
- provide additional resources.

To maximize the effectiveness of group programs and interventions, the facilitator needs to positively manage the group dynamics. Effective groups generally require purpose and structure, so members are successful both individually and collectively. The facilitator guides participants in identifying collective objectives and establishing group norms. This gives each participant ownership and fosters a unified purpose. An effective group facilitator also guides and controls the group process to ensure participation, mutual understanding, and shared responsibility for outcomes. Depending on the group and setting, the facilitator may need to take steps to manage difficult participants or sensitive topics to ensure that the group stays on task, individual needs are addressed, and each member's privacy and rights are protected.

HELPING CLIENTS WITH MENTAL HEALTH DISORDERS

Mental health and mental illness are considered part of a continuum of mental functioning. Mental disorders are characterized by disturbance in thoughts, emotions, or behaviors significant enough to affect the individual's functioning. They are common, occurring in nearly half of all people in the U.S. at least once in their lifetime (44). They can be transient or chronic and can range from mild to severe. Some may require referral to treatment by a mental health professional, or they may resolve over time (45).

Given the widespread prevalence of mental disorders, the CEP is likely to work with clients experiencing these conditions. An understanding of the most common mental disorders, especially anxiety and depression, and their effect on behavior, cognitive processes, emotional states, and physical health, is therefore important.

Impact of Mental Disorders on Exercise Participation

Mental health can affect physical health in several ways. There is consistent evidence of bidirectional influences of mental illness and chronic diseases (46), and some mental disorders are more prevalent in those with chronic disease (47). For example, people with depression are more likely to develop cardiovascular disease (CVD) and diabetes. Similarly, if individuals with heart disease or diabetes have depression, they are more likely to have worse outcomes compared with those with chronic disease without depressive symptoms (48, 49). Disruptions in mental health can affect glycemic control, immunity, and cardiovascular functioning (50). Behaviorally, mental health concerns can adversely affect medication adherence, treatment compliance, exercise and nutrition habits, sleep patterns, and substance use (51). Population studies consistently show that individuals with poor mental health are less likely to be physically active and have greater rates of early mortality (52, 53). Therefore, the CEP should be aware of clients' mental health concerns and the potential implications on their health-related behaviors. In addition to recognizing symptoms of mental disorders, the CEP should be ready to refer clients to appropriate treatment resources if needed. Often, the delay or failure to receive treatment results in worsening of symptoms and greater functional impairment (54). Mental health resources that provide evaluation and treatment services are identified in Box 15.5.

Exercise can help in the management of mental disorders. Overall, exercise is associated with reduced symptoms of depression and anxiety, improved self-esteem, better functioning and quality of life, improved sleep quality and less fatigue, reductions in pain and physical complaints, and improved cognitive function (1). Physical activity can have advantages over traditional mental health treatments in terms of convenience, accessibility, few negative side effects, and positive side effects of better fitness and improved health. With a variety of physical activity options to address individual needs and preferences and the ability to allow the client to control activity choices, exercise may be perceived as a positive treatment choice (55).

Helping Clients Manage Stress

Psychological stress is something everyone experiences to varying degrees. Acute stress is typically in response to an immediate, but short-term event or stressor, such as being stuck in traffic on the way to an important meeting or getting a reprimand at work. Chronic stress is longer term and is in response to situations that are persistent, such as financial strain or an unhealthy relationship. Symptoms of psychological stress often overlap those of depression and anxiety disorders (see Box 15.6).

Physical symptoms of acute stress reflect autonomic nervous system activation and include elevated heart rate and blood pressure. Prolonged stress may impair the immune system, resulting in susceptibility to illness. In addition, high levels of stress may be associated with higher pain ratings, feelings of anger and irritability, and increased risk of injury. Stress may also negatively influence health behaviors, including smoking, sleep, diet, medication compliance, and physical activity (56).

Interventions for stress include enhancing social support networks, self-help or support groups, and relaxation training including biofeedback, guided imagery, and progressive relaxation. Resilience training can enable individuals to identify solutions and reduce the risk of developing other serious mental or physical disorders (57, 58). Psychotherapy may be needed to help individuals develop appropriate coping strategies. The CEP can help clients identify professional resources in their community and facilitate outreach to qualified providers as appropriate.

The CEP should be able to recognize when stress is negatively affecting a client's daily functioning or is causing health problems. Many people find relief from stress by participating in physical activity, and the CEP can work with clients to determine the most appropriate types of activities and settings that will accomplish the purposes of both meeting fitness goals and reducing stress. For example, clients may prefer activities that are not overly

---

Box 15.5   Treatment Resources for Mental Health

Local mental health services include the following:

- Mental health practitioners, including psychiatrists, psychologists, social workers, or mental health counselors
- Family practice/internal medicine physicians
- Community mental health centers
- Hospital psychiatry departments and outpatient clinics
- Family service and social agencies
- Religious organizations and clergy

Box 15.6   Symptoms of Psychological Stress

Symptoms of psychological stress are often similar to symptoms of depression and anxiety and include the following:

- Feeling worried or keyed up
- Difficulty sleeping and fatigue
- Muscle tension and soreness
- Changes in appetite
- Headaches or gastrointestinal problems
- Irritability

competitive, noisy, or demanding or that incorporate relaxation techniques such as yoga or Tai Chi. Exercise can help to relieve acute stress and may provide a break from thinking about chronic stress. However, those experiencing chronic stress situations will likely have difficulty with adherence and need intervention beyond exercise to address their stress.

Helping Clients With Depression

Depression, or major depressive disorder, is a mood disorder characterized by discrete symptoms (Box 15.7) that are present most of the day, nearly every day, for at least 2 weeks. Of all mental disorders, the burden of depression is the most significant. According to the Global Burden of Disease Study conducted by the World Health Organization, major depression accounts for 8.3% of all years lived with disability in the U.S.. It ranks second behind ischemic heart disease in years lived with disability and is predicted to surpass ischemic heart disease by 2030 (59). An estimated one in five U.S. adults will experience a mood disorder sometime in their lifetime, with depression being the most common (60). In 2020, an estimated 21.0 million U.S. adults (8.4% of all U.S. adults) had at least one major depressive episode (61). Considering these vital statistics, it is likely that a CEP will work with a client who has depression at some point.

There are other common mood disorders that can affect exercise participation. Persistent depressive disorder is a more chronic depression characterized by less severe symptoms. It typically lasts at least 2 years and can occur with or without episodes of major depression (62).

Box 15.7	Signs and Symptoms of Major Depressive Disorder (MDD)

- Depressed mood; persistent feelings of sadness or irritability
- Loss of interest in previously enjoyed activities
- Feelings of guilt, worthlessness, or helplessness
- Fatigue or decreased energy
- Difficulty thinking or concentrating
- Sleep disturbances, including insomnia or oversleeping
- Changes in appetite; weight gain or loss
- Slowed movements/lethargy or restlessness/agitation
- Thoughts of death or suicide

Source: American Psychiatric Association. *Diagnostic and Statistical Manual of Mental Disorders.* 5th ed. Arlington (VA): American Psychiatric Association; 2013.

A related mood disorder is bipolar disorder, which is characterized by periods of both depression and mania. Symptoms of mania include extreme elation or irritability, increased energy and decreased need for sleep, grandiose ideas, inflated self-esteem, distractibility, increased goal-directed activity, physical agitation, and poor judgment or inappropriate behavior (62).

Risk Factors for Depression

Depression and other mood disorders can be triggered by stressful life events, such as the loss of a spouse or a job, or it can be triggered by physiological factors, such as having an acute or chronic disease, such as heart disease and diabetes. Genetic, biologic, social, and cognitive factors may all play a causal role in the development of depressive disorders (63). Being sedentary may also increase the risk for depression (64).

Treatment of Depression

Effective treatments for depression include antidepressant medications and psychotherapy, Common medications include selective serotonin reuptake inhibitors (SSRIs), serotonin and norepinephrine reuptake inhibitors (SNRIs), and older medications such as tricyclic antidepressants (TCAs) and monoamine oxidase inhibitors (MAOIs) (63, 65). These medications are not habit-forming and appear to work by influencing the balance of neurotransmitters in the brain. Finding the appropriate medication and dose is not always easy. Antidepressants take several weeks before a noticeable reduction in symptoms begins, and often the dosage must be adjusted for optimal therapeutic effect. The CEP should be aware of the type of medication and any side effects. Most antidepressant medications should not affect the response to exercise. However, some side effects, such as weight change, fatigue, or insomnia, may be relevant to exercise participation and affect exercise adherence or trigger a lapse.

Psychotherapy, including cognitive behavioral therapy (CBT) and interpersonal psychotherapy, has also been found to be effective in managing depression. Psychotherapy may be used alone or in combination with antidepressant medication to treat depression. In cases of severe depression or when depression persists despite treatment, electroconvulsive therapy (ECT) may be used and has been found to be effective (63).

Exercise can be helpful as an adjunctive treatment for individuals who have depressive disorders. In cases of mild depression, guidelines from the American Psychiatric Association suggest exercise may be a good alternative antidepressant treatment if symptoms are monitored (64).

Clinical research has demonstrated that exercise can be an important antidepressant therapy, with most research focusing on aerobic modes of exercise. However, resistance training and yoga may also be helpful in managing symptoms (66, 67). Current evidence supports a dose of exercise consistent with guidelines recommended for general fitness and health (1, 68). Participants should inform their mental health providers about their exercise participation.

Regardless of antidepressant treatment modality, it is important that patients are regularly assessed by a mental health professional throughout the course of treatment to evaluate symptoms. For individuals who do not respond to the initial course of treatment, it may be necessary to use a combination of treatments, change medication dose, or switch treatment modalities. This process often requires long-term follow-up and monitoring (65).

Clients at Risk for Suicide

The CEP may occasionally encounter a client who expresses such hopelessness or despair that the CEP suspects the client is at risk for suicide. In such cases, it is necessary to directly inquire if the client is thinking about suicide. Simply asking, "You seem pretty down. Have you had any recent thoughts of harming yourself?" may help determine the client's intent (69). People will usually respond honestly, giving the CEP the opportunity to gauge the seriousness of such thoughts. Immediate action is needed if the client communicates planned harmful or suicidal intentions. If the client is not under the care of a mental health provider, they can be referred to a local suicide or crisis center or be taken directly to a hospital emergency room. It is important to make sure that the client is accompanied to the treatment center and is not left alone until professional help is available. The National Hopeline Network (1-800-SUICIDE) is a 24-hour hotline that connects individuals to trained counselors at a local crisis center.

Suicide is an important public health issue, and all health professionals can assist in prevention efforts. Strategies for suicide prevention include addressing economic factors, improving access to and delivery of mental health care, creating protective environments, promoting connectedness, increasing coping and problem-solving skills, and identifying and supporting those at risk (70).

Helping Clients With Anxiety

Anxiety disorders are the most prevalent mental disorders. In the U.S., the estimated projected lifetime prevalence of anxiety disorders is 36% (44). Anxiety has high rates of comorbidity with other mental disorders and medical conditions. A feature of most anxiety disorders is unwarranted sympathetic nervous system (SNS) activation in response to anticipated risk or danger. Normal SNS activation is adaptive and even protective, as when a reflexive fight-or-flight reaction is triggered in a risky or dangerous situation. Elevated heart rate, peripheral vasodilation, altered breathing, and sweating are correlates of SNS activation (71). Activation of the SNS is normally counterbalanced with that of the parasympathetic nervous system (PNS), which exerts a calming effect. Either chronic or episodic SNS activation under circumstances that pose no immediate danger can be highly debilitating and lead to additional anxiety, typically in the form of worry (72), as well as have a negative impact on health (73).

Common Types of Anxiety Disorders

Some of the most common types of anxiety disorders include panic disorder, generalized anxiety disorder (GAD), obsessive-compulsive disorder (OCD), specific phobias, posttraumatic stress disorder (PTSD), and social anxiety disorder. The disorders are diagnosed according to specific diagnostic criteria (74).

Panic disorder is an anxiety disorder involving the experience of sudden, unexpected periods of intense fear. Common panic attack symptoms include accelerated heart rate, sweating, trembling, shortness of breath, sensation of choking, chest pain, nausea, dizziness, and tingling. Individuals with panic disorder feel out of control during panic attacks and worry about when the next attack will happen. Because these attacks can be very intense, individuals may mistake a panic attack for a heart attack. They may also avoid places where panic attacks have occurred (62, 74).

GAD is characterized by chronic, exaggerated worry that occurs more days than not for at least 6 months. The anxiety and worry involve several events and activities, and worry is out of proportion relative to the actual event. A person with generalized anxiety has at least three of the following six symptoms:

- Feeling restlessness or keyed up
- Having trouble concentrating
- Being irritable
- Unusual fatigue
- Muscle tension
- Sleep problems such as difficulty falling or staying asleep

OCD involves the experience of disturbing and irrational thoughts (obsessions) and the need to engage in repeated behaviors or rituals (compulsions) to prevent or relieve the anxiety. Individuals with OCD usually recognize that their thoughts and behaviors are senseless, but they are controlled by the troubling thoughts and the urgent need to engage in rituals. Rituals often involve counting, checking, or washing and may significantly interfere with daily functioning (74).

Specific phobias are intense fears triggered by the presence or anticipation of specific objects or situations (*e.g.*, excessive fear of heights). The fear prompts symptoms such as excessive sweating, heart pounding, shaking, shortness of breath, and/or nausea (74).

PTSD develops after experiencing or witnessing an intense, traumatic event, such as a violent attack, serious accident, natural disaster, armed conflict, or abuse. Symptoms include repeated disturbing thoughts of the trauma, nightmares, sleep disturbances, or feeling as if the event is recurring. A person with PTSD tries to avoid thoughts or feelings of the trauma and often has disinterest in activities that were once important, a restricted range of affect, and low expectations for a normal life. These individuals also tend to be hypervigilant and have sleep difficulties, irritability, and startle easily. PTSD causes significant impairment in daily functioning (74).

Social anxiety disorder is also known as social phobia. This disorder is characterized by intense anxiety and self-consciousness during normal social situations in which there is a possibility of scrutiny by others. Individuals with this disorder have a persistent, excessive fear of being watched and evaluated by others and worry of being embarrassed or humiliated. Social anxiety disorder can be specific to certain situations, such as speaking or eating in public, or be generalized to any social setting (74).

Diagnosis and Treatment of Anxiety Disorders

Diagnosis of anxiety disorders can only be made by trained professionals using standard diagnostic criteria. Referral to a mental health counselor, psychologist, psychiatrist, or physician is important to develop an appropriate treatment plan, which may include psychotherapy and/or medication. Common medications for anxiety include antidepressant medications, benzodiazepines, and β-blockers (75). Some medications, such as SSRIs, often take several weeks to achieve the full therapeutic effect. Benzodiazepines quickly reduce anxiety symptoms and are commonly used in the treatment of panic disorder, social phobia, and GAD. However, patients develop tolerance to benzodiazepines and may become dependent

on them; symptom rebound may occur when medication is discontinued. β-Blockers, typically used to treat heart conditions, may be used to minimize physical symptoms (rapid heart rate, shaking) when an anxiety-provoking event is anticipated (76).

Targeted psychotherapy is often indicated for anxiety disorders (77). CBT, in particular, has been found to be useful for the treatment of panic disorder and social phobia. Exposure therapy, a type of behavioral therapy, is often used to treat specific phobias, OCD, and PTSD. This technique involves exposing individuals to the feared object or situation in a safe environment so that individuals can practice controlling their anxiety and responding in more appropriate and productive ways (77). Relaxation training, including guided imagery, breathing exercises, and biofeedback, may also be used as a component of anxiety treatment (78). Treatment plans for an anxiety disorder should also include evaluation for, and treatment of, comorbid mental disorders because depression, substance abuse, or other anxiety disorders often co-occur (74). In addition to the mental health resources listed in Box 15.5, self-help groups can help individuals with anxiety share their concerns and solve problems related to daily functioning.

As with depression, population studies suggest that physical activity may reduce the risk of developing an anxiety disorder (1). In addition, research suggests that exercise may be useful in reducing symptoms of stress and anxiety among healthy individuals and those with chronic illness (1, 79, 80). Although individuals with panic disorder may avoid participating in exercise for fear of inducing a panic attack, the attacks are not more likely to occur during physical activity than during other daily activities (81). Despite limited research, evidence suggests that exercise may be helpful in reducing anxiety symptoms among patients with clinical anxiety disorders, including panic and other disorders (1).

When working with clients who may have anxiety, collaboration with the client's other health professionals can help ensure the safest and most effective treatment plan to manage anxiety symptoms. If individuals are taking anti-anxiety medication, the CEP should be aware of the type of medication and any potential side effects, as some types of medication may affect the physiological response to exercise so that heart rate or blood pressure may not increase as expected (82).

Working with the client, the CEP should consider factors related to the exercise prescription or setting that may influence a client's symptoms of anxiety. Exercise itself can cause physical responses that are sometimes associated with anxiety such as increased heart rate and breathlessness. In addition, there might be elements of the exercise setting that increase anxiety such as group settings, competitions, noise, or unpredictable events. The CEP who has identified the client's concerns can work to create a comfortable environment by minimizing potential exposure to anxiety-inducing situations.

Helping Clients With Eating Disorders

Disordered eating comprises a spectrum of behavioral, cognitive, and emotional symptoms involving disturbances in eating and body image. For example, frequently adopting, then discarding, fad diets may qualify as disordered eating. In contrast, eating disorders can cause significant distress, impairment in daily functioning and social relationships, physical health consequences, and even death. Therefore, recognition of the signs and symptoms and an understanding of appropriate treatment is critical. The general signs and symptoms of eating disorders are presented in Box 15.8.

Types of Eating Disorders

Eating disorders are diagnosed according to standard criteria and include anorexia nervosa, bulimia nervosa, and binge eating disorders (74). Signs of eating disorders are sometimes readily recognizable to outside observers. However, determining the severity of the disorder is often difficult because individuals with these disorders often hide their behaviors and resist intervention. There are also individuals who have disordered patterns of eating that do not meet the clinical diagnosis for eating disorders. Although these patterns are not as clearly identified as eating disorders, they are still concerning and need to

Box 15.8	**Signs and Symptoms of Eating Disorders**

- Extreme eating patterns, including restriction and overeating
- Body weight loss or gain
- Purging behaviors, including vomiting, laxative use, or excessive exercise
- Unusual eating behaviors, including preferences or phobias for certain foods and obsessive rituals
- Excessive weighing or avoidance of weighing
- Distorted body image, low self-esteem, or feelings of guilt and self-disgust

Source: American Psychiatric Association. *Diagnostic and Statistical Manual of Mental Disorders*. 5th ed. Arlington (VA): American Psychiatric Association; 2013.

be addressed. The CEP should be alert to signs of eating disorders and refer clients to treatment when appropriate.

Anorexia nervosa is an eating disorder in which a person has insufficient calorie intake to sustain a normal body weight for age and height. Individuals who have this disorder have intense fear of becoming "fat" and a distorted body image. Sometimes there are also disturbances in menstrual cycles in women. Health complications of this disorder include osteoporosis, muscle atrophy, electrolyte imbalances, cardiac arrhythmias, and sometimes early death. There is also a binge purge type of anorexia where individuals have episodes of binging and purging even though they have very restrictive caloric intake (74). This form of anorexia should not be confused with bulimia nervosa.

Bulimia nervosa involves episodes of binge eating and compensatory purging via self-induced vomiting, misuse of laxatives, or excessive exercise to prevent weight gain. Binge eating episodes are characterized by eating significantly more than what most individuals would eat in a discrete time period and a lack of control over the amount during the episode. Individuals with this disorder are often of normal body weight but may express intense body dissatisfaction and desire to lose weight. Health consequences of bulimia nervosa include gastrointestinal disturbances, electrolyte imbalances, esophageal ruptures, pancreatitis, and erosion of tooth enamel (74).

Binge eating disorder involves recurrent binge eating episodes during which the individual lacks control over how much they are eating and eat significantly more than what most people would eat in a similar time period. This behavior occurs at least once per week for 3 months and, unlike bulimia nervosa, does not involve compensatory behaviors to prevent weight gain. The episodes often involve rapid eating, feeling uncomfortably full, eating when not hungry, eating alone, and feelings of guilt or disgust (74). Those with binge eating disorder are often overweight. It is the most common eating disorder making up almost half of the cases of eating disorders.

Diagnosis and Treatment of Eating Disorders

Professional assessment of eating disorders involves multiple components:

1. Medical evaluation to assess body weight and health problems
2. Psychological evaluation to assess the severity of the eating disorder and presence of comorbid mental disorders
3. Nutritional consultation to evaluate current eating habits

Treatment of eating disorders is a multifaceted process that often involves a team of health care professionals, including mental health counselors, physicians, psychologists, and nutritionists. Eating disorders like anorexia nervosa are sometimes treated in an inpatient setting so that weight can be stabilized, and medical conditions can be treated. Psychotherapy is an important component of treatment to reduce inappropriate eating behaviors and explore psychological issues such as body image, self-esteem, and interpersonal relationships. Nutritionists and exercise professionals can play an important role in the intervention team to regulate energy balance through appropriate caloric intake and energy expenditure. Finally, SSRI medications may be helpful in the treatment of some eating disorders (83).

Disordered eating is often a contributing factor to the development of the female athlete triad. Low-energy availability because of high-energy expenditure and insufficient dietary energy intake (which may be because of restrictive eating behaviors as part of a clinical or subclinical eating disorder) can lead to disturbances in menstrual function (amenorrhea) and changes in bone density (osteoporosis) (84). When working with patients who have eating disorders, care should be taken to monitor energy balance and to modify exercise prescriptions to accommodate any medical problems. Furthermore, the CEP should use sensitivity when weighing or conducting body composition measurements and communicate appropriate messages to protect body image and self-esteem.

Helping Clients With Substance-Use Disorders

Substance-use disorders include any disorders associated with the use of alcohol, prescribed or over-the-counter medications, and toxins such as inhalants. The features of substance-use disorders include social impairment, risky use, impaired control, and pharmacological criteria (tolerance and withdrawal). Social impairment is indicated by use of the substance even when doing so interferes with the person's ability to fulfill role obligations. Risky use causes the individual to engage in behaviors resulting in legal, interpersonal, social, psychological, or health problems. Impaired control is indicated by an inability to stop using the substance; that is, trying to quit but being unable to do so. Pharmacological effects include tolerance to the substance, such as a need for a greater amount to achieve an effect, and withdrawal symptoms in the absence of the substance (62).

Professional assessment of substance-use disorders is critical to ensure the safety of the individual and

to implement appropriate treatment. Substance abuse commonly occurs with other mental disorders, such as depression, and treatment may involve a combination of individual therapy, group therapy, and/or medication (85). Local hospitals and substance-abuse centers can provide medical and psychological evaluation and treatment in inpatient or outpatient settings.

The CEP is most likely to recognize symptoms of substance use during acute intoxication or when the patient reports questionable behaviors, such as recurrent overindulgent behaviors or blackouts (86). Often, individuals with drug or alcohol problems may deny a problem and resist treatment; however, they may be open to a referral if the information is presented in a professional and caring manner. When working with athletes, fitness professionals should be alert to the possible use of performance-enhancing drugs, including androgens, growth hormones and growth factors, stimulants, β-agonists, β-blockers, diuretics, nutritional supplements, and other legal or illegal substances that may be used to improve physical performance (87). Athletes may also engage in substance abuse as a way of coping with mental illness or stress. The various mechanisms of action, potential side effects, and legal concerns make substance use in sports and exercise a particularly difficult issue to address.

Exercise has been used as a therapeutic treatment for substance use, often as an adjunctive therapy within an integrative treatment program for a variety of outcomes including smoking cessation, alcohol rehabilitation, and stimulant addiction (88). Evidence suggests that exercise may be helpful in promoting abstinence among illicit drug abusers and in reducing withdrawal symptoms and cravings among alcohol, nicotine, and illicit drug users (89). Physical activity has the potential to provide multiple relevant benefits including favorable neurobiological adaptations, distraction and coping, enhanced self-esteem, and sense of control, increased social support, and management of comorbid risk factors such as depression and anxiety (88, 90). Further research is needed to understand how exercise dose, mode (*i.e.*, aerobic, resistance, and mind-body), setting, and other prescription components influence benefits for the treatment of addiction and substance use (88, 89).

Behavioral Strategies for Working With Clients With Mental Health Concerns

When working with clients who are experiencing mental health concerns, it is critical that exercise professionals develop a professional relationship based on trust, open communication, and mutual respect. In addition, behavioral strategies to support physical activity behavior change can be even more important as common symptoms of psychological disorders—including low motivation, poor self-esteem, anxiety, fatigue, and somatic complaints—can interfere with physical activity plans. The skills and strategies discussed earlier in the chapter can be helpful in facilitating the implementation of exercise plans with the purpose of improving both physical and mental health. Additional recommendations are presented in Box 15.9.

BEHAVIOR CHANGE AND MENTAL HEALTH IN PATIENTS WITH CHRONIC DISEASE

The symptoms and functional limitations associated with chronic disease reduce quality of life and increase the risk for psychological distress and mental disorders. Here, we discuss the psychosocial and behavioral aspects of a few of the most common chronic diseases affecting the cardiovascular, endocrine, and respiratory systems.

Cardiovascular Disease

CVD has been the most prevalent chronic illness in the U.S. for several decades (91). CVD includes acute coronary syndrome (ACS), hypertension, peripheral artery disease, cerebrovascular disease (stroke), heart failure (HF), and many other disorders of the heart and blood vessels. Approximately 20.1 million Americans have coronary heart disease (CHD), which is the leading cause of death in the U.S. (92).

Stroke is a form of CVD that deserves special attention because of its characteristic psychological sequelae and the need for more effective poststroke interventions. Stroke is the fifth leading cause of death in the U.S. and the leading cause of long-term disability. Each year, 795,000 people experience a new or recurrent stroke (91).

HF is a form of CVD affecting more than 5.7 million patients in the U.S.. The prevalence of HF is expected to increase substantially as the population ages (93) such that, by 2030, it is expected to have increased by 25%. Like stroke, HF merits special consideration because of its prevalence and high level of associated disability and decline.

Mental health, psychosocial, and behavioral factors can influence the development, assessment, and treatment of CVD and are important considerations for professionals who work with clients with CVD.

Stress and Anxiety in CVD

Evidence indicates a relationship between chronic life stress, and both development and of CVD, myocardial infarction (MI), and sudden death. Stressful life events include the breakup of intimate personal relationships, death of a family member or friend, economic hardship, role conflict, work overload, racism and discrimination, poor physical health, accidental injury, and assault (94). Stressful life events may also reflect past events such as

---

Box 15.9	Recommendations for Working With Clients With Mental Health Concerns

- Be familiar with symptoms of common psychological disorders and medications used to treat them. Know where to refer clients for professional help if needed. Collaborate with other health professionals when appropriate.
- Build rapport using a nonjudgmental, client-centered approach. Involve clients in planning exercise programs to promote active collaboration and enhance feelings of autonomy and control.
- Assess physical fitness, health status, and motivational factors to individualize the physical activity plan.
- Consider psychological symptoms in exercise action plans to address barriers and maximize benefits.

- Encourage enjoyable, nonthreatening, convenient exercise.
- Identify and problem-solve barriers.
- Set reasonable goals and help clients integrate physical activity into their daily routine to build exercise self-efficacy.
- Adopt a nonjudgmental, problem-solving stance when difficulties with compliance arise. Emphasize immediate benefits rather than long-term outcomes; normalize and reframe lapses as part of the change process.

Source: Adapted from O'Neal HA, Dunn AL, Martinsen EW. Depression and exercise. *Int J Sport Psychol.* 2000;31:110–35.

childhood sexual and physical abuse. Past trauma may persist as long-term stressors or may make individuals more vulnerable to ongoing stress. Each person has a unique response to stressful life events that includes physiological, cognitive, emotional, and behavioral characteristics that may be harmful to susceptible individuals. Work stress, particularly, has been linked to the presence of CVD risk factors and the development of CVD. Work stress has been associated with higher levels of cholesterol, systolic blood pressure (SBP), and smoking behavior (95). Monotonous work, high-paced work, and job burnout have been correlated with an increased incidence of CHD (96). High-demand jobs with low decision latitude have been associated with a fourfold increased risk of cardiovascular-related death (97). Work stress associated with high demand and low reward has also resulted in an increase in cardiac events and the progression of carotid atherosclerosis (98). In the 20-year follow-up of the Framingham Heart Study, the incidence of angina was two times greater among those who exhibited higher levels of worry, dissatisfaction with work, feeling undue time pressure, and competitive drive (99).

Acute stress has been implicated in the triggering of cardiovascular events. Epidemiologic evidence has revealed that life-threatening situations such as earthquakes (100) and war (101) are associated with increased rates of MI and cardiac mortality. Intense, but non-life-threatening situations, such as important national soccer games, have also been associated with an increase in the rate of hospital admissions for MI (102).

Negative emotional states such as anger, anxiety, and frustration are associated with myocardial ischemia. In one study, risk of MI more than doubled after a bout of acute anger (103). Moreover, emotional stress may induce transient ischemia and disturb autonomic function leading to arrhythmias. Anxiety disorders can also impact a person's risk of CVD. As previously discussed, underlying all anxiety disorders is a state of heightened arousal or fear in relation to stressful events or feelings. The Harvard Mastery of Stress Study revealed that severe anxiety and conflict with hostility were significant predictors of CVD and risk of overall future illness (104). Together, research indicates a strong association between acute stress, chronic stress, and anxiety and the development of CVD.

Depression in Patients With CVD

The prevalence of depression among patients with CVD is three times higher than in the general population. Assessments among MI patients suggest that as many as 15%–20% of hospitalized patients meet the criteria for major depression (105). Similarly, depression is the most common psychological reaction in individuals suffering a stroke. The incidence of poststroke depression ranges from 25% to 79%, with most studies showing a rate of approximately 30% (106). Depression is also common in patients with HF. In a meta-analysis of 36 studies, depression was present in 21.5% of patients with HF.

Depression tends to be underdiagnosed and undertreated in patients with CVD. Fewer than 25% of CVD patients with major depression are recognized as being depressed by their cardiologists or general internists, and only about half of the patients diagnosed as depressed receive treatment. Depression is associated with a worse prognosis, and some studies suggest there is a doubling in risk of CVD events in the 1–2 years following an MI (107). Epidemiologic evidence demonstrates a significant prospective relationship between depression and the incidence of future cardiac events among both healthy (107) and CVD populations (108). Among stroke patients, depression can negatively impact recovery, resulting in greater health care utilization including inpatient hospitalization days and outpatient visits (109).

Assessment and treatment of depression is critical in this population. Assessing depression following cardiac events and stroke is complicated by the fact that patients may exhibit lethargy, memory impairment, and difficulties because of physical impairments, medications, or other disease or treatment-related factors. It is unclear whether depression among patients with CVD are the result of the psychosocial adjustment required by the disease, or a combination of biological and psychological mechanisms. In addition, multiple psychosocial factors may contribute to depression following a cardiac event or stroke, including medical complications and comorbidities, long-term care needs, impairment of ADLs, financial or family stress, and social support.

Depression has also been shown to be a predictor of poor adherence to a wide variety of medical treatments (103). A meta-analysis revealed that patients with chronic disease with depression were three times more likely to be nonadherent with medical treatment than patients without depression (110). Moreover, physical inactivity, tobacco use, and poor diet may also contribute to the development and progression of coronary artery disease (CAD) in patients with depression (106). Consequently, depression may indirectly promote the progression of chronic illness by negatively impacting health behaviors such as healthy eating, exercise, taking medications appropriately, abstaining from smoking, managing stress, limiting alcohol intake, and sleep habits.

Psychosocial and Behavioral Considerations for Patients With CVD

The role of exercise as a stand-alone intervention in the prevention and management of CVD is well documented. In addition to improved cardiovascular health and physiological benefits, exercise interventions can positively impact psychosocial predictors of CVD including depression, anxiety, and stress. Although the extent to which clinical outcomes may have been directly or indirectly affected by improved psychosocial status as a result of exercise is not clear, it is safe to conclude that exercise therapy added to a multi-intervention approach that includes behavioral cardiac risk modification, education, and counseling may improve CVD outcomes. The Lifestyle Heart Trial demonstrated that an intervention composed of exercise therapy, group support meetings, education and skills training in a low-fat diet, and daily stress management (*i.e.*, yoga-derived stretching, breathing, meditation, imagery, and relaxation techniques) could assist a highly motivated group of patients with CVD to make comprehensive changes in lifestyle. Arterial stenosis showed a regression from 40.0% to 37.8% in the intervention group compared with a progression from 42.7% to 46.1% in a usual care group at a 1-year follow-up (111). A 5-year follow-up showed continued progression in the control group and regression in the intensive lifestyle intervention group (112).

When working with patients with CVD, the CEP should keep in mind the potential impact of psychosocial and behavioral factors that could influence a client's physical health as well as adherence to the exercise intervention. The fitness professional can help educate clients on CVD risk factors and monitor for symptoms of excess stress, depression, or anxiety and refer clients to appropriate health care providers if there are concerns. The CEP should also consider behavioral strategies to address specific barriers and set appropriate goals for patients with CVD and adapt exercise programming to promote psychosocial as well as physical health benefits.

Because of the variability in disability and symptomatology in patients with CVD, tailoring the exercise intervention is of utmost importance. In addition to traditional exercise prescription and medical considerations, the fitness professional may need to assess and account for other factors such as cognitive limitations, communication needs, social support, barriers, goal setting, and

motivation. It may also be necessary to include family and caregivers in intervention planning to consider practical needs like scheduling appointments and transportation and assisting with adherence to home-based physical activity plans.

For patients with CVD, enhancing social support as part of the physical activity intervention may be particularly important. Social support has been widely recognized as an independent predictor of health and well-being in both general and clinical populations, especially among patients with CVD. Social isolation, indicating few close relationships or social ties, is associated with an increase in all-cause and CVD mortality and predicts 1-year mortality after MI as strongly as other more traditional risk factors (113). Low social support has also been prospectively associated with poor clinical prognosis among patients with HF and stable CVD (114).

Motivating patients with CVD to adopt and maintain comprehensive changes in lifestyle is a challenge that health care professionals face, and motivational interviewing is an innovative approach that has demonstrated efficacy in brief consultations. Compared with traditional cardiac rehabilitation, adding motivational interviewing coupled with brief skills-building sessions has been shown to significantly lower stress and enhance multiple health-related behaviors for patients with CVD (115).

Diabetes

Diabetes is a chronic disease caused by insulin deficiency, resistance to insulin action, or both. Type 2 diabetes (T2D) is the most common, accounting for 90%–95% of all cases. Diabetes prevalence in the U.S. is about 37.3 million. According to recent estimates, 14.7% of all U.S. adults and 29.2% of people aged 65 years or older have diabetes (116). It is the leading cause of new cases of blindness and kidney failure, and 60%–70% of individuals with diabetes mellitus (DM) have mild-to-severe forms of nervous system damage (117).

Psychosocial and Behavioral Considerations for Patients With Diabetes

Psychological reactions to diabetes include anger, denial, and stress. Depression is more common among people with diabetes compared to the general population (118). The challenge of managing a chronic illness places a high emotional and behavioral demand on patients. The need for ongoing blood sugar testing, medication management, and lifestyle modification can increase risk of depression, anxiety, or disordered eating. In addition, diabetes is associated with cognitive dysfunction including detrimental effects on attention, concentration, memory, processing speed, and executive function, and these deficits can then impact self-management of diabetes (119). Managing emotions and recognizing symptoms of mental disorders are therefore important for all individuals with diabetes.

The few studies involving psychosocial and behavioral interventions in patients with DM have involved CBT, coping skills, empowerment, and diabetes management training. These approaches have been found to decrease diabetes-related anxiety and avoidance behaviors; enhance quality of life, coping ability, and emotional well-being; and improve self-care and glycemic control (119).

The Diabetes Prevention Program (DPP) Research Group (120) demonstrated a strong benefit of physical activity and weight loss on preventing diabetes onset in high-risk adults. Compared with usual care, there was a 58% decrease at the onset of T2D over a period of approximately 3 years among individuals who were supported in their efforts to follow a healthy lifestyle. A recent American College of Sports Medicine (ACSM) consensus statement outlines key recommendations for physical activity in people with T2D. Relevant for physical activity behavior change include recommendations for greater energy expenditure and longer duration exercise as well as the benefit of activity throughout the day to break up time spent sitting (121). The CEP can assist clients by facilitating relevant behavior change skills including physical activity, nutrition, and healthy weight management; encouraging adherence to appropriate self-care including monitoring of glucose levels, medication adherence, and regular health care visits; and being aware of diabetes complications or other medical concerns that may require additional support or accommodations.

Chronic Obstructive Pulmonary Disease, Asthma, and Other Lung Diseases

Chronic obstructive pulmonary disease (COPD) is a common lung condition characterized by airflow obstruction resulting from chronic bronchitis and emphysema, two diseases that often coexist. COPD is the sixth leading cause of death in the U.S., currently affecting 12.5 million adults. Exposure to tobacco smoke is a main risk factor for developing COPD. Prevalence rates of a COPD diagnosis are 13% for current smokers and 9.4% for former smokers compared to 1.8% for those who never smoked (122).

Asthma is a chronic lung disease affecting approximately 25 million children and adults in the U.S. (123). It is characterized by recurrent exacerbations of airflow constriction, mucus secretion, and inflammation of the airways, resulting in reduced airflow that causes symptoms of wheezing, coughing, chest tightness, and difficulty breathing.

Psychosocial and Behavioral Considerations for Patients Lung Disease

Depression and anxiety are common mental health concerns for people with lung disease, including COPD and asthma. A cross-sectional study of 1,224 Veterans Administration patients with COPD found that 39% were diagnosed with depression (124). Similarly, in a study of hospitalized patients with COPD who were followed for 1 year, the prevalence of depression on admission to hospital was 44.4% (125). Further analysis revealed that depression was significantly associated with longer hospital stay, worse physical and social functioning, and higher mortality.

Numerous studies report that the prevalence of depression in those with asthma ranges from 14% to 41%. The variation in prevalence is likely because of three limitations affecting this research: symptoms of asthma linked to depression may be misinterpreted; many patients use corticosteroids, which has been hypothesized as a possible side effect between asthma and depression; and in some patients, depression may lead to nonadherence with asthma treatment, which then exacerbates asthma, increasing depression (126).

Anxiety is another common psychological concern among patients with lung disease. The prevalence of GAD in patients with COPD ranges from 10% to 33%, and the prevalence of panic attacks ranges from 8% to 67% (127). Dyspnea in conjunction with fear of suffocation and death is a source of significant anxiety in this population. Dyspnea increases during acute exacerbations of COPD with intractable dyspnea, being associated with anxiety. Moreover, feelings of anger and frustration are potent triggers of anxiety that may heighten dyspnea (127).

Among patients with asthma, research has demonstrated an association between emotional stress and various indices of impaired airway function, including increased breathlessness (dyspnea) and bronchoconstriction (126). As in patients with COPD, anxiety is common in patients with asthma, with panic disorder being particularly prevalent (128). The prevalence of anxiety is 16%–52%. Anxiety in patients with asthma appears to be associated with excessive use of bronchodilators, greater prescriptions for corticosteroid medication, more frequent hospital readmissions, and lengthier hospitalizations, independent of pulmonary impairment.

In addition to possible mental health concerns, the CEP should be alert to disease-related factors that might influence physical activity behavior or exercise adherence in clients with COPD, asthma, or other lung conditions. The fitness professional can explore specific barriers such as pulmonary symptoms, fears related to dyspnea or asthma attack, and medication management. Working together, the CEP and client can plan physical activity (*e.g.*, mode, intensity, setting) to minimize potential triggers of symptom exacerbation, ensure medication adherence, and tailor progression to increase self-efficacy and accommodate medical needs. For individuals with more advanced lung disease, worsening dyspnea, fatigue, or perceived poor health, may decrease functional capacity and exercise tolerance. Therefore, it is important for the CEP to monitor these factors over time and intervene appropriately.

Alzheimer Disease and Dementia

Dementia is defined as the loss of cognitive function to the extent that it interferes with a person's ability to carry out daily activities. Dementia can have various causes with a range of impact from mild to severe. Alzheimer disease is the most common type of dementia affecting approximately 6.5 million adults over age 65. It is the fifth leading cause of death among people 65 years or older (129). In addition to cognitive impairment, other symptoms include sleep disturbances, aggression, agitation, wandering, and anxiety. Although exact causes are not known, common cardiovascular disease risk factors have been associated with increased risk for Alzheimer disease. Hypertension, diabetes, dyslipidemia, obesity, depression, and smoking can increase the risk, so it is important to consider the possible comorbidities when working with those who have Alzheimer disease. Research also shows that regular exercise is associated with a lower risk of developing Alzheimer disease.

Psychosocial and Behavioral Considerations of Patients With Dementia

Individuals with Alzheimer disease or a related dementia (ADRD) can participate in regular physical activity. When planning a physical activity program for a client who has ADRD, it is important to communicate with the client's health care provider to understand medications, disease severity, and limitations to develop a safe and realistic program. Physical activity should be encouraged, as those with Alzheimer disease can see positive effects on health, mood, sleep, and physical function. Strength, balance, and cardiorespiratory fitness are likely to increase and improve the ability to perform ADLs. Simple activities such as walking can be used to increase physical activity and decrease sedentary time. Those living with ADRD can work toward meeting the recommended Physical Activity Guidelines for older adults. Keep programs simple and maintain consistency with exercises and time of day. The morning might be ideal, as symptoms tend to worsen throughout the day. Activities should incorporate multiple aspects of fitness, and as with older adults in general, exercise to improve balance and range of motion is important. Combination activities such as dance, Tai Chi, and yoga are good choices to target multiple fitness components. Setting SMART goals, using self-monitoring to track progress and symptoms, and providing positive reinforcement are behavioral strategies that help with the adoption and maintenance of regular physical activity. A strong support network is also recommended.

Cancer

In the U.S., new cancer diagnoses are expected to number over 1.9 million in 2022. Cancer is the second leading cause of death in the U.S., with over 600,00 cancer deaths reported in 2020 (130). There are over 100 different types of cancer. Among men, the three most common cancers are prostate, lung, and colorectal cancers, accounting for approximately 43% of all cancers diagnosed each year. Among women, breast, lung, and colorectal are the most common, accounting for approximately half of all new cancer diagnoses (131).

The cancer mortality rate has decreased significantly in recent years with a 32% decrease between 1991 and 2019. The lower death rate is attributed to several factors including a decrease in smoking, early screening and detection, and advances in treatment (132). It is estimated that there are almost 17 million cancer survivors in the U.S., and this number is expected to increase by 31.4% over the next decade (132).

It is estimated that approximately 40% of cancers could be prevented by modifying smoking behaviors and other unhealthy behaviors. An estimated 19% of cancers are attributed to smoking and tobacco use and another 18% are because of excess weight, diet, alcohol use, and/or physical inactivity (132). Exercise has gained increased attention as an integral part of cancer prevention, treatment, and survivorship. ACSM's *Moving Through Cancer* aims to "assure that all people living with and beyond cancer are assessed, advised, referred to and engaged in appropriate exercise and rehabilitation programming as a standard of care" (133). This collection of resources for exercise professionals, health care providers, and patients is available through the Exercise Is Medicine® website at www.exerciseismedicine.org.

Psychosocial and Behavioral Considerations of Patients With Cancer

The course of a cancer illness varies widely from person to person based on factors such as cancer type, stage of disease at diagnosis, availability of treatments, and other medical comorbidities. In addition, many patients experience a range of side effects during their therapy, and some side effects can be long term or develop later (late effects of treatment).

Common psychological reactions to cancer include denial, anger, fear, anxiety, and depression (134). Studies suggest that almost one-third of patients with cancer have a mental disorder. Depression and anxiety are common among patients with cancer (134) and cancer survivors (135). Certain cancer types and treatments may also increase the risk of depression and anxiety in patients with cancer (134). Additional factors that may increase risk of mental health problems among patients with cancer include pain, symptom burden, disability, fatigue, and history of mental illness (134). Among cancer survivors, financial problems, quality of life, and cognitive function have been associated with risk of depression and anxiety (136).

Physical activity can have many benefits for cancer patients and survivors including improved fatigue, mental health, sleep, appetite, and physical function (137). In addition to the usual benefits of physical activity, the CEP can explore the personal relevance of potential cancer-related benefits and how they might be important for physical activity motivation and behavior. In addition, the CEP should understand how the patient's cancer, treatments, and related symptoms could impact current and future physical activity. The fitness professional should also be aware of problems that can have multidimensional impact on physical activity through psychosocial, practical, and medical means. Examples include cancer-related concerns because of the disease or treatment include peripheral neuropathy, compromised immune function, lymphedema, cognitive impairment, and long-term damage to heart, lungs, or other organs (138). With appropriate medical guidance

and clearance, physical activity can be planned to maximize relevant benefits, address barriers, and accommodate health needs. Because the course of illness and treatment varies widely, it is important for the CEP to monitor these factors over time and work with the client and other medical professionals to adjust exercise goals and interventions as needed (138).

Reminders When Working With Clients With Health Conditions

The implications of behavioral adherence are even more significant when prescribing exercise for the prevention or management of disease. The complexities of physical activity in the context of medical needs presents special challenges for both the CEP and client. Therefore, establishing a CEP-client relationship based on trust, communication, and rapport is essential.

Practical steps for the CEP to consider when working with clients with medical needs include:

- Develop specialized knowledge, skills, and experience. This will foster a better understanding and appreciation of client needs to enable appropriate tailoring and safety.
- Complete a preparticipation screening and get appropriate medical clearance. A health care provider referral or exercise recommendation may increase initial buy-in or positive perception of exercise.
- Conduct a comprehensive assessment of the patient's medical, fitness, and behavioral status. Include assessment of benefits, barriers, social and environmental supports, and goals.
- Develop the exercise prescription in cooperation with the client and incorporate behavioral skills and strategies in the activity plan.
- Connect with the patient's health care provider and establish regular communication regarding status, progress, medical needs, and goals. Be alert for changes in medical status that may influence physical and/or mental health or may prompt other behavioral strategies.
- Develop a network of health care providers and community resources for appropriate referrals.
- Consider practical and social needs such as caregiver support, transportation, and assistive devices or modifications, especially when working with individuals who have advanced illness or disability.

Visit exerciseismedicine.org to download the Exercise Is Medicine® Exercise Professionals' Action Guide or to access the Rx for Health series of exercise prescription guidelines for specific health conditions.

EXERCISE FOR SPECIAL POPULATIONS

Although this chapter cannot address the specifics of working with all special populations, some general recommendations for working with individuals who fit into a category considered a special population should be considered. Research has provided evidence-based information about population-specific physical activity barriers and correlates for many populations. It is good to be familiar with those variables and to understand sociocultural and environmental influences on physical activity participation across populations, as these factors can influence exercise choice, exercise setting, self-efficacy, and goals. However, it is important to avoid a "one size fits all" approach. The CEP can use population-specific data and recommendations as a starting point to guide physical activity planning, but that should not replace getting to know the personal variables that support or impede physical activity. The behavioral strategies discussed in this chapter are tools that can be applied across all populations and subgroups. Understanding the individual and population-specific correlates and barriers will help to apply the behavioral strategies discussed in a way that will be most effective for each individual client.

Box 15.10 lists additional resources for the CEP seeking to learn how to include behavior change strategies in physical activity interventions.

Box 15.10 Behavior Change Resources for Fitness Professionals

- American College of Sports Medicine. *ACSM's Resource Manual for the Exercise Physiologist.* 3rd ed. Wolters Kluwer Health/Lippincott Williams & Wilkins; 2021.
- *ACSM's Guidelines for Exercise Testing and Prescription.* 11th ed. Wolters Kluwer; 2021. See Chapters 11 and 12.
- American College of Sports Medicine. *ACSM's Resource Manual for Exercise Testing and Prescription.* 7th ed. Philadelphia (PA): Wolters Kluwer Health/Lippincott Williams & Wilkins; 2014. See Chapters 16 and 17.
- American College of Sports Medicine. *ACSM's Complete Guide to Fitness & Health.* 2nd ed. Human Kinetics; 2016.
- Blair SN, Dunn AL, Marcus BH, Carpenter RA, Jaret P. *Active Living Every Day.* 3rd ed. Human Kinetics; 2021.
- Claudio NR; American College of Sports Medicine. *ACSM's Behavioral Aspects of Physical Activity and Exercise.* Wolters Kluwer Health/Lippincott Williams & Wilkins; 2014.

SUMMARY

Behavioral strategies are critical to facilitate adoption and long-term maintenance of physical activity, and CEPs play an important role in promoting behavioral skill building for clients. Expectations concerning physical activity–related benefits and outcomes should be addressed during the initial stage of a program. Exploring beliefs, attitudes, and barriers sets the stage for realistic goal setting and minimizes disappointment and frustration. To encourage sustained participation over time, self-management strategies should be encouraged. Skills to support behavior change include self-monitoring, goal setting, problem-solving, decisional balance, reward systems, stimulus control, relapse prevention, social support, and other self-management strategies.

CEPs should be able to recognize symptoms of mental disorders and refer patients to appropriate community resources for treatment. They should also be aware of how mental health can influence physical activity. Mental health problems can be effectively managed, and individuals can achieve significant improvements in psychological functioning, physical health, and quality of life. In most cases, exercise is a useful adjunctive therapy in the treatment of mental disorders and results in both physical and psychological benefits for clients.

Given the increased recognition of exercise as medicine in the treatment of chronic disease, exercise professionals should be knowledgeable about symptomatology, treatment, and exercise implications for clients with common medical conditions. In addition, the psychosocial aspects of chronic disease are important considerations, as these factors are likely to influence disease progression and adherence to treatment modalities, including exercise. CEPs should encourage self-directed planning as a means of tailoring physical activity programs to fit the needs and preferences of participants and promote personal control and autonomy. Using a client-centered approach can enhance the professional relationship and further support behavior change.

CHAPTER REVIEW QUESTIONS

1. What are elements of a SMART goal?
2. According to TTM of behavior change, what are the five stages of readiness for change, as applied to physical activity? Give some examples of behavioral skills to prioritize at different stages of motivational readiness.
3. What are the steps in the five A's Framework, and how can the CEP use them?
4. Why is the client-centered approach important when helping someone become more active? How can the CEP build rapport with clients?
5. What factors that facilitate the use of behavior change techniques in a group setting? What can the facilitator do to maximize the effectiveness of the group dynamics and interventions

6. Identify the three clinical eating disorders and the six common signs and symptoms they share.
7. How is chronic stress associated with the presence of CVD risk factors and development of CVD?
8. What are the three psychological or behavioral concerns to consider when working with patients with COPD or asthma?
9. What are the three psychological or behavioral concerns or recommendations to consider when working with patients with ADRD?
10. Discuss three practical steps to take when working with clients with medical conditions. How might the CEP incorporate specific behavioral skills and strategies?

Case Study 15.1

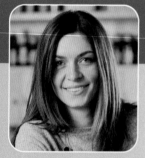

Kathryn is a 32-year-old woman who wants to be more active after giving birth to her first child 12 weeks ago. She recently started meeting a friend to walk on Saturday mornings. Because they both have young children in strollers, when the weather is bad or the baby has had a bad night, they often skip their walking session. Kathryn and her husband have a fitness facility membership, and she has gone a few times to work out by herself using the nursery for childcare. Kathryn used to do group exercise classes, but she is unsure how to start back after having a C-section. Kathryn reports having difficulty sleeping and worrying a lot about the baby. She also is frustrated by her pregnancy weight gain.

Case Study 15.1 Questions

1. What is Kathryn's stage of change for physical activity and how might her stage influence the exercise prescription?
2. How could you use the Five A's Model to help Kathryn be more active?
3. What behavioral skills stand out to you as being important for Kathryn?
4. What mental health concerns would you be aware of when working with Kathryn? What specific symptoms would you look for?

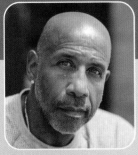

Case Study 15.2

John was recently diagnosed with Type 2 diabetes. His doctor told him that regular exercise would help to manage his diabetes and prevent weight gain. John has never been an exerciser, but he is very motivated to get started with exercise to improve his health.

He is not sure that he understands all of the exercise prescription he was given, and he is unsure about how to manage his blood glucose levels when he exercises. He has a flexible job, and his employer supports employee wellness. His family is also supportive of his desire to make lifestyle changes, but they are healthy and do not fully understand the impact of Type 2 diabetes.

Case Study 15.2 Questions

1. How could John use self-monitoring to address his concerns and barriers?
2. Write a reasonable initial short-term SMART for John.

3. What type of social support does John need and how can he best use the available support?
4. What psychological concerns related to diabetes will you have to consider when working with John?

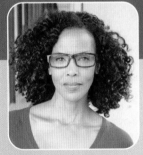

Case Study 15.3

Susan has been active on and off throughout her adult life. She turns 50 years old in 6 months and has the goal of completing a half marathon to celebrate her milestone birthday. She was excited about her goal at first, but she is now frustrated that the process is slow. This is

the first time she has made running her primary activity. She found a running program through a fitness app, which she started 3 weeks ago. She is only running 10 minutes at a time without having to walk. She thought she would be further along by now. She is starting to regret that she already registered for the event.

Case Study 15.3 Questions

1. What behavioral strategies could you use to help Susan increase her self-efficacy?
2. What are some ways you could help Susan develop and use a support network?
3. How might you and Susan develop a relapse prevention plan to adhere to her exercise program so she can meet her goal of completing a half marathon?

4. What types of rewards or reinforcement could be used to promote exercise adherence? How would you work with Susan to plan the timing of rewards?

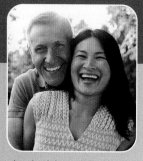

Case Study 15.4

The Smiths are a couple who want to start exercising to improve health. They both have a family history of at least one chronic disease that has physical inactivity as a risk factor. Additionally, each has had at least one extended family member die prematurely due a chronic disease. Although the Smiths are healthy now, they are both busy professionals with high stress jobs. They report work and stress are part of the reason they have not been successful at incorporating exercise into their lives. They do not know how to get started and are concerned about costs of a gym membership and/or personal training.

Case Study 15.4 Questions

1. Write a decisional balance evaluation for the Smiths. How could this evaluation be used to help them adopt an exercise program?
2. Apply the IDEA Method to help the Smiths address their challenges to getting started.

3. What psychological concerns need to be addressed with the Smiths considering their family history and work stress?

REFERENCES

1. U.S. Department of Health and Human Services. *Physical Activity Guidelines for Americans.* 2nd ed. Washington (DC): U.S. Department of Health and Human Services; 2018. Available from: https://health.gov/sites/default/files/2019-09/Physical_Activity_Guidelines_2nd_edition.pdf.
2. World Health Organization. *Physical Inactivity.* Geneva (Switzerland): World Health Organization; 2020. Available from: https://www.who.int/news-room/fact-sheets/detail/physical-activity.
3. Centers for Disease Control and Prevention, National Center for Health Statistics. *Exercise or Physical Activity.* Atlanta (GA): Centers for Disease Control; 2021. Available from: http://www.cdc.gov/nchs/fastats/exercise.htm.
4. Lewis BA, Marcus BH, Pate RR, Dunn AL. Psychosocial mediators of physical activity behavior among adults and children. *Am J Prev Med.* 2002;23(Suppl 2):26–35.
5. Neff KL, King AC. Exercise program adherence in older adults: the importance of achieving one's expected benefits. *Med Exerc Nutr Health.* 1995;4(6):355–62.
6. Pekmezi DW, Barbera BL, Markus B. Using the transtheoretical model to promote physical activity. *ACSM's Health Fit J.* 2010;14(4):8–13.
7. Marcus BH, Dubbert PM, Forsyth LH, et al. Physical activity behavior change: issues in adoption and maintenance. *Health Psychol.* 2000;19(1S):32–41.
8. King AC, Rejeski WJ, Buchner DM. Physical activity interventions targeting older adults. A critical review and recommendations. *Am J Prev Med.* 1998;15(4):316–33.
9. Myers RS, Roth DL. Perceived benefits of and barriers to exercise and stage of exercise adoption in young adults. *Health Psychol.* 1997;16(3):277–83.
10. King AC, Friedman R, Marcus B, et al. Harnessing motivational forces in the promotion of physical activity: the Community Health Advice by Telephone (CHAT) project. *Health Educ Res.* 2002;17(5):627–36.
11. Nigg CR. *ACSM's Behavioral Aspects of Physical Activity and Exercise.* Philadelphia (PA): Wolters Kluwer Health/Lippincott Williams & Wilkins; 2014.
12. Chambliss H. Motivating physical activity: skills and strategies for behavior change. In: Watson RR, editor. *Diet and Exercise in Cystic Fibrosis.* Amsterdam (Netherlands): Elsevier Inc.; 2014. p. 307–16.
13. Blair SN. *Active Living Every Day.* 3rd ed. Champaign (IL): Human Kinetics; 2021.
14. Deci EL, Ryan RM. *Intrinsic Motivation and Self-Determination in Human Behavior.* New York: Plenum; 1985.
15. Mullan E, Markland D, Ingledew DK. A graded conceptualisation of self-determination in the regulation of exercise behaviour: development of a measure using confirmatory factor analytic procedures. *Pers Individ Dif.* 1997;23(5):745–52.
16. Deci EL, Ryan RM. The support of autonomy and the control of behavior. *J Pers Soc Psychol.* 1987;53(6):1024–37.
17. Bandura A. *Self-Efficacy: The Exercise of Control.* New York: WH Freeman; 1997.
18. Oman RF, King AC. Predicting the adoption and maintenance of exercise participation using self-efficacy and

previous exercise participation rates. *Am J Health Promot.* 1998;12(3):154–61.

19. Jackson D. How personal trainers can use self-efficacy theory to enhance exercise behavior in beginning exercisers. *Strength Cond J.* 2010;32(3):67–71.

20. Trost SG, Owen N, Bauman AE, Sallis JF, Brown W. Correlates of adults' participation in physical activity: review and update. *Med Sci Sports Exerc.* 2002;34(12):1996–2001.

21. Castro CM, King AC. Telephone-assisted counseling for physical activity. *Exerc Sport Sci Rev.* 2002;30(2):64–8.

22. Andersen RE, Franckowiak SC, Snyder J, Bartlett SJ, Fontaine KR. Can inexpensive signs encourage the use of stairs? Results from a community intervention. *Ann Intern Med.* 1998;129(5):363–9.

23. Sallis JF, Bauman A, Pratt M. Environmental and policy interventions to promote physical activity. *Am J Prev Med.* 1998;15(4):379–97.

24. Boutelle KN, Jeffery RW, Murray DM, Schmitz MK. Using signs, artwork, and music to promote stair use in a public building. *Am J Public Health.* 2001;91(12):2004–6.

25. Marcus BH, Simkin LR. The transtheoretical model: applications to exercise behavior. *Med Sci Sports Exerc.* 1994;26(11):1400–4.

26. Young DR, King AC. Exercise adherence: determinants of physical activity and applications of health behavior change theories. *Med Exerc Nutr Health.* 1995;4(6):335–48.

27. Bandura A. The anatomy of stages of change. *Am J Health Promot.* 1997;12(1):8–10.

28. Prochaska JO, DiClemente CC. Transtheoretical therapy: toward a more integrative model of change. *Psychotherapy (Chic).* 1982;19(3):276–88.

29. King AC, Frederiksen LW. Low-cost strategies for increasing exercise behavior: relapse preparation training and social support. *Behav Modif.* 1984;8(1):3–21.

30. Rejeski W, Brawley L. Shaping active lifestyles in older adults: a group-facilitated behavior change intervention. *Ann Behav Med.* 1997;19(Suppl):S106.

31. Rogers CT. A theory of therapy, personality, and interpersonal relationships as developed in the client-centered framework. In: Koch S, editor. *Psychology: A Study of a Science.* New York: McGraw-Hill; 1959. p. 184–256.

32. Griffin JC. *Client-Centered Exercise Prescription.* 3rd ed. Champaign (IL): Human Kinetics; 2015.

33. Mason P. *Health Behavior Change: A Guide for Practitioners.* 3rd ed. New York: Elsevier; 2018.

34. Stewart M, Brown JB, Weston W, McWhinney IR, McWilliam CL, Freeman T. *Patient-Centered Medicine: Transforming the Clinical Method.* 3rd ed. CRC Press; 2014.

35. Meriwether RA, Lee JA, Lafleur AS, Wiseman P. Physical activity counseling. *Am Fam Physician.* 2008;77(8):1129–36.

36. Pinto BM, Lynn H, Marcus BH, DePue J, Goldstein MG. Physician-based activity counseling: intervention effects on mediators of motivational readiness for physical activity. *Ann Behav Med.* 2001;23(1):2–10.

37. Marcus B, Forsyth L. *Motivating People to Be Physically Active.* 2nd ed. Champaign (IL): Human Kinetics; 2009.

38. Marcus BH, Napolitano MA, King AC, et al. Telephone versus print delivery of an individualized motivationally tailored physical activity intervention: project STRIDE. *Health Psychol.* 2007;26(4):401–9.

39. Carroll JK, Fiscella K, Epstein RM, et al. Getting patients to exercise more: a systematic review of underserved populations. *J Fam Pract.* 2008;57(3):170–6.

40. Gavin J, McBrearty M. *Lifestyle Wellness Coaching.* 3rd ed. Champaign (IL): Human Kinetics; 2018.

41. Rollnick S, Miller WR, Butler C. *Motivational Interviewing in Health Care: Helping Patients Change Behavior.* New York: Guilford Press; 2008.

42. Sallis JF, Owen N. Ecological models of health behavior. In: Glanz K, Rimer BK, Viswanath K, editors. *Health Behavior: Theory, Research, and Practice.* 5th ed. San Francisco: Jossey-Bass/Wiley; 2015. p. 43–64.

43. Bauman AE, Macniven R, Gebel K. Influencing policy and environments to promote physical activity behavior change. In: Nigg CR, editor. *ACSM's Behavioral Aspects of Physical Activity and Exercise.* Philadelphia (PA): Wolters Kluwer Health/Lippincott Williams & Wilkins; 2014.

44. Kessler RC, Angermeyer M, Anthony JC, et al. Lifetime prevalence and age-of-onset distributions of mental disorders in the World Health Organization's World Mental Health Survey Initiative. *World Psychiatry.* 2007;6(3):168–76.

45. U.S. Public Health Service, Office of the Surgeon General. *Mental Health: A Report of the Surgeon General.* Rockville (MD): U.S. Department of Health and Human Services; 1999. Available from: https://profiles.nlm.nih.gov/ps/access/NNBBHS.pdf.

46. Katon W, Lin EH, Kroenke K. The association of depression and anxiety with medical symptom burden in patients with chronic medical illness. *Gen Hosp Psychiatry.* 2007;29(2):147–55.

47. Scott KM, Bruffaerts R, Tsang A, et al. Depression-anxiety relationships with chronic physical conditions: results from the World Mental Health Surveys. *J Affect Disord.* 2007;103(1-3):113–20.

48. Evans DL, Charney DS, Lewis L, et al. Mood disorders in the medically ill: scientific review and recommendations. *Biol Psychiatry.* 2005;58(3):175–89.

49. Pan A, Lucas M, Sun Q, et al. Bidirectional association between depression and type 2 diabetes mellitus in women. *Arch Int Med.* 2010;170(21):1884–91.

50. Katon WJ. Epidemiology and treatment of depression in patients with chronic medical illness. *Dialogues Clin Neurosci.* 2011;13(1):7–23.

51. Katon WJ. Clinical and health services relationships between major depression, depressive symptoms, and general medical illness. *Biol Psychiatry.* 2003;54(3):216–26.

52. Parks J, Svendsen D, Singer P, et al. *Morbidity and Mortality in People with Serious Mental Illness.* Alexandria (VA): National Association of State Mental Program Directors; 2006. Available from: https://www.nasmhpd.org/sites/default/files/Mortality%20and%20Morbidity%20Final%20Report%208.18.08_0.pdf.

53. Pan A, Lucas M, Sun Q, et al. Increased mortality risk in women with depression and diabetes mellitus. *Arch Gen Psychiatry.* 2011;68(1):42–50.

54. Wang PS, Angermeyer M, Borges G, et al. Delay and failure in treatment seeking after first onset of mental disorders in the World Health Organization's World Mental Health Survey Initiative. *World Psychiatry.* 2007;6(3):177–85.

55. Chambliss H, Greer TL. Depression. In: Bushman BA; American College of Sports Medicine, editors. *Complete Guide to Fitness and Health*. 2nd ed. Champaign (IL): Human Kinetics; 2017, p. 385–96.

56. Cohen S, Kessler RC, Underwood LG. *Measuring Stress: A Guide for Health and Social Scientists*. New York: Oxford University Press; 1995.

57. Cicchetti D. Resilience under conditions of extreme stress: a multilevel perspective. *World Psychiatry*. 2010;9(3):145–54.

58. Timmermans M, van Lier PA, Koot HM. The role of stressful events in the development of behavioural and emotional problems from early childhood to late adolescence. *Psychol Med*. 2010;40(10):1659–68.

59. Mathers C, Fat DM, Boerma JT. *Global Burden of Disease Update 2004*. Geneva (Switzerland): World Health Organization; 2008. Available from: http://www.who.int/healthinfo/global_burden_disease/GBD_report_2004update_full.pdf.

60. Kessler RC, Berglund P, Demler O, Jin R, Merikangas KR, Walters EE. Lifetime prevalence and age-of-onset distributions of DSM-IV disorders in the National Comorbidity Survey Replication. *Arch Gen Psychiatry*. 2005;62(6):593–602.

61. National Institute of Mental Health. *Major Depression*. Bethesda (MD): National Institute of Mental Health; 2022. Available from: https://www.nimh.nih.gov/health/statistics/major-depression.shtml.

62. American Psychiatric Association. *Diagnostic and Statistical Manual of Mental Disorders: DSM-5*. 5th ed. Arlington (VA): American Psychiatric Association; 2013.

63. National Institute of Mental Health. *Depression*. Bethesda (MD): National Institute of Mental Health; 2018. Available from: https://www.nimh.nih.gov/health/topics/depression/index.shtml.

64. Galper DI, Trivedi MH, Barlow CE, Dunn AL, Kampert JB. Inverse association between physical inactivity and mental health in men and women. *Med Sci Sports Exerc*. 2006;38(1):173–8.

65. Qaseem A, Barry MJ, Kansagara D; Clinical Guidelines Committee of the American College of Physicians. Nonpharmacologic versus pharmacologic treatment of adult patients with major depressive disorder: a clinical practice guideline from the American College of Physicians. *Ann Intern Med*. 2016;164(5):350–9.

66. Krogh J, Nordentoft M, Sterne JA, Lawlor DA. The effect of exercise in clinically depressed adults: systematic review and meta-analysis of randomized controlled trials. *J Clin Psychiatry*. 2011;72(4):529–38.

67. Mead GE, Morley W, Campbell P, Greig CA, McMurdo M, Lawlor DA. Exercise for depression. *Cochrane Database Syst Rev*. 2009;3:CD004366.

68. Dunn AL, Trivedi MH, Kampert JB, Clark CG, Chambliss HO. Exercise treatment for depression: efficacy and dose response. *Am J Prev Med*. 2005;28(1):1–8.

69. Meyer RE, Salzman C, Youngstrom EA, et al. Suicidality and risk of suicide — definition, drug safety concerns, and a necessary target for drug development: a consensus statement. *J Clin Psychiatry*. 2010;71(8):e1–21.

70. Stone DM, Holland KM, Bartholow B, Crosby AE, Davis S, Wilkins N. *Preventing Suicide: A Technical Package of Policies, Programs, and Practices*. Atlanta (GA): National Center for Injury Prevention and Control, Centers for Disease Control and Prevention; 2017. Available from: https://www.cdc.gov/violenceprevention/pdf/suicidetechnicalpackage.pdf.

71. Widmaier EP, Raff H, Strang KT. *Vander's Human Physiology: The Mechanisms of Body Function*. 15th ed. New York: McGraw-Hill; 2019.

72. Borkovec TD, Inz J. The nature of worry in generalized anxiety disorder: a predominance of thought activity. *Behav Res Ther*. 1990;28(2):153–8.

73. Grassi G. Sympathetic overdrive and cardiovascular risk in the metabolic syndrome. *Hypertens Res*. 2006;29(11):839–47.

74. National Institute of Mental Health. *Anxiety Disorders*. Bethesda (MD): National Institute of Mental Health; 2018. Available from: https://www.nimh.nih.gov/health/topics/anxiety-disorders/index.shtml.

75. Garakani A, Murrough JW, Freire RC, et al. Pharmacotherapy of anxiety disorders: current and emerging treatment options. *Front Psychiatry*. 2020;11:595584.

76. Hunot V, Churchill R, Silva de Lima M, Teixeira V. Psychological therapies for generalised anxiety disorder. *Cochrane Database Syst Rev*. 2007;(1):CD001848.

77. Norton PJ, Price EC. A meta-analytic review of adult cognitive-behavioral treatment outcome across the anxiety disorders. *J Nerv Ment Dis*. 2007;195(6):521–31.

78. Jorm AF, Christensen H, Griffiths KM, Parslow RA, Rodgers B, Blewitt KA. Effectiveness of complementary and self-help treatments for anxiety disorders. *Med J Aust*. 2004;181(Suppl 7):S29–46.

79. Herring MP, O'Connor PJ, Dishman RK. The effect of exercise training on anxiety symptoms among patients: a systematic review. *Arch Int Med*. 2010;170(4):321–31.

80. Cameron OG, Hudson CJ. Influence of exercise on anxiety level in patients with anxiety disorders. *Psychosomatics*. 1986;27(10):720–3.

81. Davidson JR. Pharmacologic treatment of acute and chronic stress following trauma: 2006. *J Clin Psychiatry*. 2006;67(Suppl 2):34–9.

82. Hainer V, Kabrnova K, Aldhoon B, Kunesova M, Wagenknecht M. Serotonin and norepinephrine reuptake inhibition and eating behavior. *Ann N Y Acad Sci*. 2006;1083:252–69.

83. Nattiv A, Loucks AB, Manore MM, Sanborn CF, Sundgot-Borgen J, Warren MP; American College of Sports Medicine. American College of Sports Medicine position stand. The female athlete triad. *Med Sci Sports Exerc*. 2007;39(10):1867–82.

84. Riggs PD, Mikulich-Gilbertson SK, Davies RD, Lohman M, Klein C, Stover SK. A randomized controlled trial of fluoxetine and cognitive behavioral therapy in adolescents with major depression, behavior problems, and substance use disorders. *Arch Pediatr Adolesc Med*. 2007;161(11):1026–34.

85. National Institute of Mental Health. *Substance Use and Co-occurring Mental Disorders*. Available from: https://www.nimh.nih.gov/health/topics/substance-use-and-mental-health.

86. Reardon CL, Creado S. Drug abuse in athletes. *Subst Abuse Rehabil*. 2014;5:95–105.

87. Watson CJ, Stone GL, Overbeek DL, Chiba T, Burns MM. Performance-enhancing drugs and the Olympics. *J Intern Med*. 2022;291(2):181–96.

88. Wang D, Wang Y, Wang Y, Li R, Zhou C. Impact of physical exercise on substance use disorders: a meta-analysis. *PLoS One*. 2014;9(10):e110728.

89. Smith MA, Lynch WJ. Exercise as a potential treatment for drug abuse: evidence from preclinical studies. *Front Psychiatry*. 2011;2:82.

90. U.S. Department of Health and Human Services. *Physical Activity Guidelines for Americans*. 2nd ed. Washington (DC): U.S. Department of Health and Human Services; 2018. Available from: https://health.gov/our-work/nutrition-physical-activity/physical-activity-guidelines.

91. Virani SS, Alonso A, Aparicio HJ, et al; American Heart Association Council on Epidemiology and Prevention Statistics Committee and Stroke Statistics Subcommittee. Heart disease and stroke statistics-2021 update: a report from the American Heart Association. *Circulation*. 2021;143(8):e254–743.

92. Centers for Disease Control and Prevention. Underlying Cause of Death, 1999–2018. *CDC WONDER Online Database*. Atlanta (GA): Centers for Disease Control and Prevention; 2018.

93. Centers for Disease Control and Prevention. *Heart Failure Fact Sheet*. Atlanta (GA): Centers for Disease Control and Prevention; 2016. Available from: https://www.cdc.gov/dhdsp/data_statistics/fact_sheets/fs_heart_failure.htm.

94. Krieger N, Rowley DL, Herman AA, Avery B, Phillips MT. Racism, sexism, and social class: implications for studies of health, disease, and well-being. *Am J Prev Med*. 1993;9(Suppl 6):82–122.

95. Pieper C, LaCroix AZ, Karasek RA. The relation of psychosocial dimensions of work with coronary heart disease risk factors: a meta-analysis of five United States data bases. *Am J Epidemiol*. 1989;129(3):483–94.

96. Appels A, Schouten E. Burnout as a risk factor for coronary heart disease. *Behav Med*. 1991;17(2):53–9.

97. Karasek R, Baker D, Marxer F, Ahlbom A, Theorell T. Job decision latitude, job demands, and cardiovascular disease: a prospective study of Swedish men. *Am J Public Health*. 1981;71(7):694–705.

98. Lynch J, Krause N, Kaplan GA, Salonen R, Salonen JT. Workplace demands, economic reward, and progression of carotid atherosclerosis. *Circulation*. 1997;96(1):302–7.

99. Eaker ED, Abbott RD, Kannel WB. Frequency of uncomplicated angina pectoris in type A compared with type B persons (the Framingham Study). *Am J Cardiol*. 1989;63(15):1042–5.

100. Leor J, Kloner RA. The Northridge earthquake as a trigger for acute myocardial infarction. *Am J Cardiol*. 1996;77(14):1230–2.

101. Bergovec M, Mihatov S, Prpic H, Rogan S, Batarelo V, Sjerobabski V. Acute myocardial infarction among civilians in Zagreb city area. *Lancet*. 1992;339(8788):303.

102. Carroll D, Ebrahim S, Tilling K, Macleod J, Smith GD. Admissions for myocardial infarction and World Cup football: database survey. *BMJ*. 2002;325(7378):1439–42.

103. Mittleman MA, Maclure M, Sherwood JB, et al. Triggering of acute myocardial infarction onset by episodes of anger. Determinants of Myocardial Infarction Onset Study Investigators. *Circulation*. 1995;92(7):1720–5.

104. Russek LG, King SH, Russek SJ, Russek HI. The Harvard Mastery of Stress Study 35-year follow-up: prognostic significance of patterns of psychophysiological arousal and adaptation. *Psychosom Med*. 1990;52(3):271–85.

105. Lichtman JH, Bigger JT Jr, Blumenthal JA, et al. Depression and coronary heart disease: recommendations for screening, referral, and treatment: a science advisory from the American Heart Association Prevention Committee of the Council on Cardiovascular Nursing, Council on Clinical Cardiology, Council on Epidemiology and Prevention, and Interdisciplinary Council on Quality of Care and Outcomes Research: endorsed by the American Psychiatric Association. *Circulation*. 2008;118(17):1768–75.

106. Kneebone II, Dunmore E. Psychological management of post-stroke depression. *Br J Clin Psychol*. 2000;39(Pt 1):53–65.

107. Barefoot JC, Schroll M. Symptoms of depression, acute myocardial infarction, and total mortality in a community sample. *Circulation*. 1996;93(11):1976–80.

108. Frasure-Smith N, Lesperance F, Juneau M, Talajic M, Bourassa MG. Gender, depression, and one-year prognosis after myocardial infarction. *Psychosom Med*. 1999;61(1):26–37.

109. Ghose SS, Williams LS, Swindle RW. Depression and other mental health diagnoses after stroke increase inpatient and outpatient medical utilization three years poststroke. *Med Care*. 2005;43(12):1259–64.

110. DiMatteo MR, Lepper HS, Croghan TW. Depression is a risk factor for noncompliance with medical treatment: meta-analysis of the effects of anxiety and depression on patient adherence. *Arch Int Med*. 2000;160(14):2101–7.

111. Ornish D, Brown SE, Scherwitz LW, et al. Can lifestyle changes reverse coronary heart disease? The Lifestyle Heart Trial. *Lancet*. 1990;336(8708):129–33.

112. Ornish D, Scherwitz LW, Billings JH, et al. Intensive lifestyle changes for reversal of coronary heart disease [Erratum appears in *JAMA*. 1999;281(15):1380]. *JAMA*. 1998;280(23):2001–7.

113. Mookadam F, Arthur HM. Social support and its relationship to morbidity and mortality after acute myocardial infarction: systematic overview. *Arch Int Med*. 2004;164(14):1514–8.

114. Murberg TA, Bru E. Social relationships and mortality in patients with congestive heart failure. *J Psychosom Res*. 2001;51(3):521–7.

115. Scales R, Lueker RD, Alterbom HE, et al. Motivational interviewing and skills-based counseling to change multiple lifestyle behaviors. *Ann Behav Med*. 1998;20:68.

116. American Diabetes Association. *Statistics about Diabetes*. Arlington (VA): American Diabetes Association; 2017. Available from: http://diabetes.org/diabetes-basics/statistics/.

117. CDC. *Living with Diabetes*; 2022. https://www.cdc.gov/diabetes/index.html

118. American Diabetes Association. *Mental Health: Living with Type 1*; n.d. Available from: diabetes.org/diabetes/type-1/mental-health.

119. Gonzalvo JD, Hamm J, Eaves S, et al. A practical approach to mental health for the diabetes educator. *AADE Practice*. 2019;7(2):29–44.

120. Knowler WC, Barrett-Connor E, Fowler SE, et al; Diabetes Prevention Program Research Group. Reduction in the incidence of type 2 diabetes with lifestyle intervention or metformin. *N Engl J Med*. 2002;346(6):393–403.

121. Kanaley JA, Colberg SR, Corcoran MH, et al. Exercise/physical activity in individuals with type 2 diabetes: a consensus statement from the American College of Sports Medicine. *Med Sci Sports Exerc*. 2022;54(2):353–68.

122. American Lung Association. *COPD Trends Brief*. Chicago (IL): American Lung Association; 2023. Available from: https://

www.lung.org/research/trends-inlung-disease/copd-trends-brief

123. Centers for Disease Control and Prevention. *Most Recently National Asthma Data*. Atlanta (GA): Centers for Disease Control and Prevention. Available from: https://www.cdc.gov/asthma/most_recent_national_asthma_data.htm.

124. Norwood R. Prevalence and impact of depression in chronic obstructive pulmonary disease patients. *Curr Opin Pulm Med*. 2006;12(2):113–7.

125. Ng TP, Niti M, Tan WC, Cao Z, Ong KC, Eng P. Depressive symptoms and chronic obstructive pulmonary disease: effect on mortality, hospital readmission, symptom burden, functional status, and quality of life. *Arch Int Med*. 2007;167(1):60–7.

126. Hill K, Geist R, Goldstein RS, Lacasse Y. Anxiety and depression in end-stage COPD. *Eur Respir J*. 2008;31(3):667–77.

127. Affleck G, Apter A, Tennen H, et al. Mood states associated with transitory changes in asthma symptoms and peak expiratory flow. *Psychosom Med*. 2000;62(1):61–8.

128. Lehrer P, Feldman J, Giardino N, Song HS, Schmaling K. Psychological aspects of asthma. *J Consult Clin Psychol*. 2002;70(3):691–711.

129. CDC. *Alzheimer's Disease and Healthy Aging*; 2020. Available from: https://www.cdc.gov/aging/aginginfo/alzheimers.htm.

130. American Cancer Society. *Cancer Facts & Figures 2022*. Atlanta (GA): American Cancer Society; 2022.

131. National Cancer Institute. *Cancer Statistics*. Rockville (MD): National Cancer Institute; 2020. Available from: https://www.cancer.gov/about-cancer/understanding/statistics.

132. American Cancer Society. *Cancer Treatment & Survivorship Facts & Figures 2019-2021*. Atlanta (GA): American Cancer Society; 2019.

133. American College of Sports Medicine. *Moving Through Cancer*; 2021. Available from: https://www.exerciseismedicine.org/eim-in-action/moving-through-cancer.

134. Singer S. Psychosocial impact of cancer. *Recent Results Cancer Res*. 2018;210:1–11.

135. Pitman A, Suleman S, Hyde N, Hodgkiss A. Depression and anxiety in patients with cancer. *BMJ*. 2018;361:k1415. doi:10.1136/bmj.k1415.

136. Götze H, Friedrich M, Taubenheim S, Dietz A, Lordick F, Mehnert A. Depression and anxiety in long-term survivors 5 and 10 years after cancer diagnosis. Support care. *Cancer*. 2020;28(1):211–20. doi:10.1007/s00520-019-04805-1.

137. Campbell KL, Winters-Stone KM, Wiskemann J, et al. Exercise guidelines for cancer survivors: consensus statement from International Multidisciplinary Roundtable. *Med Sci Sports Exerc*. 2019;51(11):2375–90.

138. American College of Sports Medicine. *Being Active When You Have Cancer*, 2021. Available from: https://www.exerciseismedicine.org/eim-in-action/health-care/resources/rx-for-health-series/.

d in those with a lower socioeconomic status, of age (2). Those in the lowest income bracket who lack access to reliable health care are to engage in harmful health behavior such as nadequate physical activity, and substandard 8).

e Factors

ctors can have pleiotropic downstream effects nultiple chronic conditions. Insufficient physical or dietary habits, smoking, chronic stress, poor air quality, and excessive alcohol intake are con- factors for cardiovascular disease (CVD), meta- e, and chronic respiratory disease. These factors oute to musculoskeletal degeneration, impaired stem function, chronic inflammation, neurode- cognitive decline, and accelerated aging (9–16). lifestyle behaviors can lead to the concurrent nt of multiple chronic diseases. For example, ial with a sedentary lifestyle may present with cardiovascular, musculoskeletal, and possibly tive multimorbidity. Skeletal muscle is the lin-sensitive tissue as well as a major site for posal and storage (17). Lack of adequate con- ivity and inadequate muscle mass contribute etabolic pathology as a result of loss of insu- ty, impaired glucose disposal, reduced skeletal od flow, and mitochondrial insufficiency and 1 (17–20). In addition, lack of mechanical stress cal activity can lead to loss of muscle and bone ig to sarcopenia, osteopenia, and osteoporosis. ve caloric intake and sub-optimal physical ac- to adipose tissue accumulation. A large body 1 significant adiposity increase stress on the lower body and can lead to arthritis of the hips s well as low back pain (21). Adequate physical nportant for maintenance of neurologic health ve function (12–14). Dietary factors, chronic ine dependence, and excessive alcohol intake similar cascades with deleterious downstream ing to multiple multimorbidity of the meta- ovascular, and musculoskeletal systems.

mental factors, genetics, and lifestyle fac- ute to the development of multimorbidity by changes in cellular function that occur sys- id thus affect multiple organ systems. These systemic changes include insulin resistance, v-grade inflammation, obesity (characterized ation and dysfunction of visceral and perivas- se tissue), oxidative stress, and mitochondrial

dysfunction, which together have been referred to as the "common soil" etiology of chronic disease (22). Impor- tantly, these changes tend to co-occur in the aging process. Older adults demonstrate more accumulation of fat in the liver and intramuscular compartment, as well as impaired glucose regulation and insulin sensitivity (23). Aging is also characterized by chronic inflammation, termed "inflam- maging" (24). As such, multimorbidity becomes increas- ingly common in older individuals. The following is a brief description of each of these shared mechanisms underlying the development of chronic disease.

Insulin Resistance

Skeletal muscle insulin resistance contributes to multi- morbid conditions (Figure 16.1). It is considered the ma- jor underlying pathology leading to the development of Type 2 diabetes mellitus (T2DM) (17). Insulin resistance is also thought to contribute to the development of obesity, dyslipidemia, and hypertension (19, 20, 25). Furthermore, insulin resistance in the brain, which occurs through mechanisms similar to those in the periphery, may be a major contributor to neurodegeneration and dementia (26). Loss of insulin signaling in the skeletal system may contribute to loss of bone mass and increased risk for

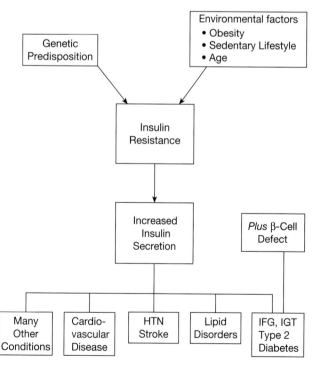

FIGURE 16.1 Schematic of insulin resistance and its relationship to comorbid conditions. (From Koda-Kimble MA, Young LY, Kradjan WA, et al. *Applied Therapeutics: The Clinical Use of Drugs*. 9th ed. Philadelphia (PA): Wolters Kluwer; 2008.)

CHAPTER

16 Persons With Multimorbidity

INTRODUCTION

There is an increased prevalence of individuals experiencing multiple simultaneous chronic conditions. The term "multimorbidity" refers to the coexistence of two or more chronic conditions, where one disease is not necessarily more central than others (1). Health care guidelines, exercise recommendations, and clinical trials tend to focus specifically on isolated medical conditions, when frequently, individuals experience multiple conditions simultaneously (2).

The term "multimorbidity" is preferred over "comorbidity," which was first used in 1970 to describe any additional disease or condition added to an index disease (3). Multimorbidity was defined in 1996 as "the co-occurrence of multiple chronic or acute diseases and medical conditions within one person" (4), and in 2010, additional clarification was provided to indicate that no condition was more central than others (5).

Ninety-two percent of older adults have at least two simultaneously occurring diseases and 77% have at least three. It is estimated that 50% of adults will be treated for multiple chronic conditions, like coronary heart disease, hypertension, metabolic diseases, cancer, or depression during the last 15 years of their life (6), making it more likely that the clinical exercise physiologist (CEP) will encounter patients with multimorbidity.

Multimorbidity is likely to complicate treatment, driving up health care costs, negatively impacting mobility, and reducing quality of life (6, 7). The CEP should be aware of the skills needed to implement a safe and effective exercise program for patients with a single condition and elevate their knowledge to be aware of additional considerations for patients with multimorbidity.

Medically complex patients can benefit from a safe and appropriate exercise evaluation, an individualized exercise program tailored to their goals, supervision during exercise, and support for ongoing exercise adherence. These patients require additional safety considerations. Thoughtful consideration should be used to evaluate the underlying environmental factors that contribute to th

This chapter will define nisms of pathophysiology f explore predictive tools for outline the process to creat view the communication to Situation, Background, As tion (SBAR) format, and u the process that the CEP s patients with complex med mat will be discussed in de

SHARED MECHA PATHOPHYSIOL

Detailed explanations of th dividual conditions have b book. The following is an in mechanisms of pathophys morbidity that commonly These mechanisms include

- Shared mechanisms of lin resistance, low-grade stress. These are related netics, lifestyle factors, a
- Secondary effects or comp sis or its treatment. These a

Contributing Facto Multimorbidity

There are many factors that mulating chronic condition increased prevalence of m ever, increased rates of ac

documente
regardless
and those
more likel
smoking,
nutrition (

Lifesty

Lifestyle fa
leading to
activity, po
sleep, poor
sidered ris
bolic disea
also contri
immune sy
generation,

Certai
developme
an individ
metabolic,
neurocogn
largest ins
glucose dis
tractile ac
to cardiom
lin sensitiv
muscle blo
dysfunctio
from physi
mass leadi

Excess
tivity lead
habitus an
joints of th
and knees
activity is i
and cognit
stress, nic
can lead to
effects lead
bolic, card

Enviro
tors contri
prompting
temically a
cellular an
chronic lo
by accumu
cular adip

osteopenia in those with diabetes (27). Moreover, insulin resistance leads to a compensatory increase in insulin production by the β cells of the pancreas, resulting in hyperinsulinemia. Hyperinsulinemia may be an important factor in the pathogenesis of cancer by promoting growth of abnormal precancerous cells (15). Insulin resistance in muscle and liver tissues leads to hyperglycemia, which has detrimental effects on the vascular endothelium, leading to diseases of the cardiovascular system, eyes, nervous system, and renal system (28).

A variety of factors are thought to lead to the development of insulin resistance. These include inflammatory signaling, particularly tumor necrosis factor-α (TNF-α) signaling; mitochondrial insufficiency and dysfunction; impaired glycogen synthesis, mainly from reduced glycogen synthase activity; endoplasmic reticulum stress; impaired lipid metabolism; and accumulation of intramuscular and intrahepatic lipids and lipid metabolites such as diacylglycerol, long-chain fatty acyl-coenzyme A, and ceramides (17, 23).

Chronic Low-Grade Inflammation

Chronic inflammation is characterized by a continual low-grade activation of the immune system evidenced by elevated levels of inflammatory markers such as C-reactive protein (CRP), TNF-α, monocyte chemotactic protein-1 (MCP-1), interleukin-8 (IL-8), and interleukin-6 (IL-6). It is an important factor in the pathophysiology of several chronic conditions, including insulin resistance, diabetes, obesity, atherosclerosis and CVD, neurodegenerative diseases, stroke, chronic obstructive pulmonary disease (COPD), cancer, sarcopenia, and autoimmune conditions (29, 30). For example, individuals with prediabetes and insulin resistance present with elevated levels of inflammatory markers such as high-sensitivity CRP (hsCRP) and increased erythrocyte sedimentation rate (31). Likewise, circulating levels of inflammatory factors, including intercellular adhesion molecules 1 (ICAM-1), P-selectin, TNF-α, and IL-6, are elevated in individuals with or at risk for hypertension, diabetes, and atherosclerosis (32–37). The pathophysiology of COPD involves lung tissue and systemic oxidative stress and inflammation, which is thought to partially explain the tendency for patients with COPD to develop CVD and experience greater risk for stroke (29).

Low-grade inflammation may additionally be explained by air pollution and particulate matter in the particulate matter (PM) 2.5 size range because of their ability to travel deeply into the respiratory tract, reaching the lungs and circulating through the blood (16). PM has been linked to pulmonary disease, myocardial infarction, arrhythmias, asthma, decreased pulmonary function, and a variety of respiratory symptoms including airway irritation, coughing, and dyspnea. Exposure to PM 2.5 increases heart rate (HR) and reduces HR variability and has a more profound reduction in those with obesity (38).

Obesity

Obesity, particularly accumulation of adipose tissues in the visceral region, abdominal cavity, and chest wall (*i.e.*, central obesity), may lead to multiple chronic cardiovascular, metabolic, respiratory, and musculoskeletal conditions. Abdominal obesity is a central feature of the metabolic syndrome, which is associated with multimorbidity (Figure 16.2). Central obesity leads to chronic inflammation by the secretion of proinflammatory cytokines (19). Visceral adipose tissue (VAT) secretes various hormones and cytokines, termed "adipokines," including leptin, MCP-1, TNF-α, IL-6, resistin, leptin, adiponectin, and angiotensinogen. These adipokines have systemic effects on inflammation, insulin sensitivity, and metabolism (39). Adipokines such as TNF-α, leptin, resistin, angiotensinogen, and adiponectin can also affect vascular function, endothelial homeostasis, and atherogenesis,

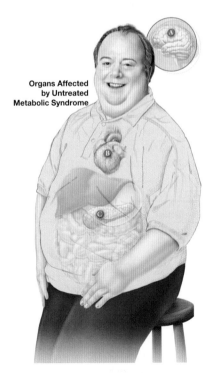

Organs Affected by Untreated Metabolic Syndrome

FIGURE 16.2 Organ systems harmed by metabolic syndrome and central obesity may include the (**A**) brain, (**B**) heart, and (**C**) pancreas. (From Anatomical Chart Company. *Metabolic Syndrome Anatomical Chart.* 1st ed. Philadelphia (PA): Wolters Kluwer; 2003.)

thus explaining one possible mechanism linking adiposity with CVD (40). VAT is more lipolytic than subcutaneous adipose tissue and releases nonesterified fatty acids (NE-FAs), which interfere with insulin signaling and promote the intracellular accumulation of lipid metabolites. This accumulation may in turn lead to skeletal muscle insulin resistance, fatty liver, and hepatic insulin resistance (19). Thus, central adiposity, through its effects on systemic inflammation and metabolic function, is considered an essential link between obesity and other chronic diseases, such as diabetes, heart disease, and neurodegenerative disorders.

Excessive adipose tissue mass can impair body functions. Accumulation of adipose tissue in the abdominal and chest cavity, for example, may impair respiratory mechanics and lung function, leading to respiratory conditions, particularly restrictive in nature, including exertional and resting dyspnea, obstructive sleep apnea, and obesity hypoventilation syndrome (41). Obesity may also exacerbate symptoms or increase mortality from existing respiratory conditions, such as asthma and COPD (41). The link between abdominal obesity, inflammation, and insulin resistance may explain much of the relationship between obesity and chronic disease (see Figure 16.3). In addition to the cardiometabolic consequences, obesity may also contribute to the development or accelerate the progression of existing musculoskeletal conditions including osteoarthritis of the knee and hip, gait disturbances, plantar fasciitis, and low back pain (21). The musculoskeletal effects of obesity should not be taken lightly, particularly by CEPs. Musculoskeletal impairments may reduce exercise enjoyment and adherence and can lead to deconditioning and worsened health.

Oxidative Stress

Reactive oxygen species (ROS) are unstable oxygen-containing molecules that easily react with other molecules in the cell. The formation of ROS is a normal and vital aspect of cellular function. Generation of ROS from the mitochondria is an important signal for adaptations to training, such as mitochondrial biogenesis, and cellular apoptosis (42, 43). However, the generation of ROS in excess of the cellular mechanisms available to neutralize them (*e.g.*, antioxidant vitamins and enzymes) leads to oxidative stress (Figure 16.4). The concentration of ROS and antioxidants determines beneficial or harmful effects. Increased oxidative stress can interfere with cellular function, leading to deoxyribonucleic acid (DNA) damage, endothelial dysfunction, and other detrimental effects. Oxidative stress is thereby implicated in the pathophysiology of many chronic conditions. One well-known example is the role of ROS in the vascular complications of diabetes. Hyperglycemia related to insulin resistance/insulin deficiency and diabetes leads to uptake of glucose by non-insulin-dependent tissues, such as endothelial cells, and subsequent increased production of ROS. This increase in ROS activates inflammatory pathways and is thought to be a major factor linking hyperglycemia to vascular disease (28, 44).

Mitochondrial Dysfunction

Reduced mitochondrial capacity for oxidative metabolism (because of reduced number of mitochondria or inadequate oxidative enzyme levels) contributes to chronic disease through impaired fatty acid metabolism and

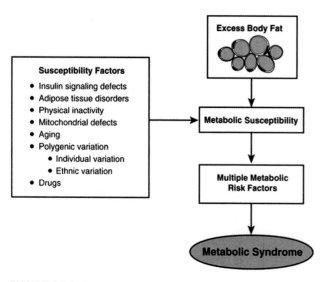

FIGURE 16.3 Factors that contribute to susceptibility to metabolic syndrome. (From Kaplan NM, Victor RG. *Kaplan's Clinical Hypertension*. 11th ed. Philadelphia (PA): Wolters Kluwer; 2014.)

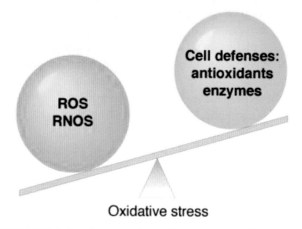

FIGURE 16.4 Development of oxidative stress caused by overproduction of reactive oxygen species (ROS) and reactive nitrogen oxide species (RNOS) can overwhelm antioxidant defenses in the cell and contribute to chronic disease. (From Lieberman MA, Marks A, Peet A. *Marks' Basic Medical Biochemistry*. 4th ed. Philadelphia (PA): Wolters Kluwer; 2012.)

subsequent accumulation of lipid metabolites, as well as increased generation of ROS and/or reduced antioxidant capacity (20). Mitochondrial dysfunction in skeletal muscle is considered an important factor in the development of insulin resistance and is also involved in the pathophysiology of endothelial dysfunction, cardiotoxicity from chemotherapy, and possibly cancer (17, 45). For example, the activity of oxidative enzymes, mitochondrial activity, and mitochondrial size were reduced in skeletal muscle from individuals with obesity and T2DM when compared with healthy controls. Impairments in mitochondrial structure and function were greater in T2DM than in nondiabetic individuals, and the activity of oxidative enzymes was correlated with insulin sensitivity (20).

MULTIMORBIDITY RESULTING FROM A PRIMARY DIAGNOSIS AND SECONDARY EFFECTS OR COMPLICATIONS

Multimorbidity can also result as a complication from a primary diagnosis or its treatment. The following section provides examples of secondary effects and complications, which are by no means exhaustive.

Metabolic Disease

Metabolic diseases are associated with increased risk for multimorbidity. Metabolic and cardiovascular pathologies are interrelated and may exacerbate each other through a feed-forward mechanism involving inflammation, hyperglycemia, oxidative stress, and endothelial dysfunction (Figure 16.5). The vascular complications associated with uncontrolled and long-term diabetes are well known. Diabetes increases the risk for large artery disease including coronary artery disease and peripheral artery disease (28). The microvascular complications from long-term/poorly regulated diabetes include retinopathy, nephropathy, and

neuropathy (28). Hyperglycemia leads to macro- and microvascular damage through increased production of ROS, reduced nitric oxide (NO) bioavailability, activation of inflammatory pathways, and endothelial dysfunction (46) (Figure 16.6). Likewise, adequate vascularization and perfusion of tissues is necessary for insulin and glucose delivery to insulin-sensitive tissues, primarily skeletal muscle. Reduced blood flow to skeletal muscle can contribute to or worsen insulin resistance and impair postprandial glucose disposal (47, 48).

Furthermore, metabolic diseases, including obesity and diabetes, are associated with an increased risk for neurologic disorders such as Alzheimer disease, vascular dementia, and Parkinson disease (26, 49–51). The relationship appears to be mediated by inflammation, insulin resistance, and mitochondrial dysfunction (50). Individuals diagnosed with neurodegenerative or musculoskeletal disorders, such as Parkinson disease, multiple sclerosis, and spinal cord injuries, may in turn reduce their physical activity levels. Physical inactivity leads to further deconditioning, negative effects on metabolism and vascular function, and the development of multimorbidity, including metabolic disease and CVDs (52). Lack of muscular activity also may lead to muscular weakness, reductions in cardiovascular endurance, reduced flexibility, reduced balance and stability, and loss of bone mass. Just as physical exercise has pleiotropic benefits, physical inactivity may lead to multiple downstream pathologies.

Multimorbidity Arising From Cancer Treatment

Cancer survivors may experience an increased risk for CVD or permanent cardiovascular damage as a result of the treatment modalities used. Chemotherapeutic agents can cause acute and chronic damage to the cardiovascular system. Short- and long-term effects include congestive heart failure (CHF), left ventricular (LV) systolic or diastolic dysfunction, myocardial ischemia and infarction, hypertension, thromboembolism,

Relationship between hyperglycemia markers and microvascular complication risk

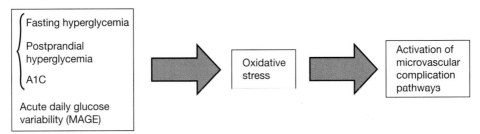

FIGURE 16.5 Oxidative stress resulting from poor glucose control can lead to microvascular complications associated with diabetes. (From Strayer DS, Rubin E. *Rubin's Pathology*. 7th ed. Philadelphia (PA): Wolters Kluwer; 2014.)

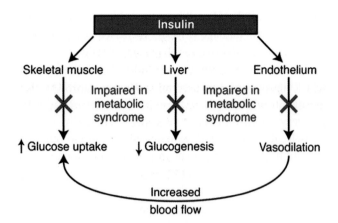

FIGURE 16.6 Insulin action in skeletal muscle, liver, and the vascular endothelium is impaired in metabolic syndrome leading to vascular dysfunction and impaired blood glucose regulation. (From Strayer DS, Rubin E. *Rubin's Pathology*. 7th ed. Philadelphia (PA): Wolters Kluwer; 2014.)

arrhythmias, and conduction disturbances, as well as damage to the vascular endothelium (53, 54).

Angiogenic inhibitors, medications that impair the activity of growth factors such as vascular endothelial growth factor to reduce blood supply to the tumor, may compromise normal vascular structural integrity and function. Angiogenic inhibitors may also limit the ability of cardiomyocytes to cope with stress, leading to apoptosis and impaired cardiac function (54). Certain forms of chemotherapy also appear to impair energy metabolism and increase oxidative stress, two cellular pathologies fundamental to cardiovascular dysfunction (55). Chemotherapy-induced damage to the cardiovascular system may be reversible or permanent. The nature and extent of damage depend on the combination and dose of chemotherapy agents used, the length of exposure, concomitant therapies (such as radiation), and the underlying health of the individual, such as age and multimorbidity (53–55).

Multimorbidity With Human Immunodeficiency Virus Infection

Individuals with chronic human immunodeficiency virus (HIV) infection are considered to be at increased risk for CVD (56–58). The HIV affects cardiovascular health through changes in body fat distribution and lipoatrophy, altered levels of adipokines (leptin and adiponectin), dyslipidemia (reduced high-density lipoprotein [HDL]-cholesterol and low-density lipoprotein [LDL]-cholesterol, increased triglyceride levels, decreased LDL particle size, and reduced LDL clearance), insulin resistance, and damage to the vascular endothelium (58). Altered activation of the immune system (CD4 T-cell depletion; CD8 T-cell and monocyte

activation) and subsequent chronic inflammation may explain many of the cardiovascular consequences of HIV, such as accelerated atherosclerosis (57, 58). The cardiovascular consequences of HIV and antiretroviral therapy (ART) appear to depend on the severity of immune system perturbation and the antiretroviral agents administered. Detrimental effects may also be seen in the musculoskeletal system in the form of muscle wasting sarcopenia, rheumatic conditions, and low bone mineral density, which are also thought to be partially mediated by inflammation (59, 60).

Chronic Illness and Mental Health

Physical and mental health are inextricably connected. A chronic physical illness such as COPD, cancer, diabetes, CVD, multiple sclerosis, HIV, or Parkinson disease can lead to anxiety and depression. Likewise, mental illness, including depression, anxiety disorders, bipolar disorder, untreated attention-deficit/hyperactivity disorder (ADHD), and schizophrenia, can lead to unhealthy behaviors including poor dietary habits, lack of physical activity, substance abuse disorders, sleep disturbances, or noncompliance with medications and treatments (61).

An example of this bidirectional relationship is between chronic stress and chronic disease. There are many stressors that one can experience after being diagnosed with a chronic disease. These stressors include a change in self-identity, relationship strain because of changes in roles, reduction in mobility or functional status, change in employment or financial status, for those with low health literacy it can feel like learning a new language, navigating a complex medical system and multiple health care appointments, fear of future health declines, and uncertainty surrounding medical bills. Unmanaged chronic stress, through modulation of autonomic nervous system activity and the hypothalamic–pituitary axis, can alter immune function, affect hemodynamics, lead to chronic low-grade inflammation, prompt endothelial dysfunction, and create a prothrombotic environment. Chronic stress may contribute to metabolic perturbations (insulin resistance, abdominal obesity, hyperglycemia), hypertension, and neurodegenerative, cognitive, and psychological disorders such as anxiety and depression (62). Chronic stress affects the cardiovascular system and may increase the risk for CVD and cardiac events (62).

It is essential to consider the interconnected relationship between physical and mental health. Exercise may be even more important for patients who have multiple conditions including physical and mental health because of the potential synergistic beneficial impact on emotional and physical well-being. Consider the effects of chronic disease and mental illness on lifestyle choices and be aware of other potential issues such as unmanaged, persistent high stress levels. Exercise prescriptions should consider environmental stimuli, anxiety triggers, and exercise enjoyment.

MEASUREMENT TOOLS FOR MORTALITY RISK

There are many tools available to support the CEP to manage a patient with multimorbidity. The two predictive tools presented below to evaluate mortality risk can help the CEP set reasonable expectations and meaningful goals during the patient discussion. The first tool can be used for patients with any diagnoses, and the second tool is intended to be used for patients with COPD.

The Charlson Comorbidity Index (CCI) is the most widely used matrix to determine 10-year mortality risk in patients who present with multiple comorbidities (63). Based on the responses to 17 questions, a final score is calculated and a percentage estimate of the 10-year survival is provided, as seen in Table 16.1. Scores range from 1 to 37, an example outcome is CCI = 6, with a 2.0% estimated 10-year survival.

The BODE Index was developed as a prognostic mortality risk tool. It is specifically created for patients with

Table 16.1	Charlson Comorbidity Index						
Variable							
	0	+1	+2	+3	+4	+6	Score
Age Years	<50 years	50–59	60–69	70–79	>80	–	
Myocardial infarction History of definite or probable MI (EKG changes and/or enzyme changes)	No	Yes					
CHF Exertional or paroxysmal nocturnal dyspnea and has responded to digitalis, diuretics, or afterload reducing agents	No	Yes					
Peripheral vascular disease Intermittent claudication or past bypass for chronic arterial insufficiency, history of gangrene or acute arterial insufficiency, or untreated thoracic or abdominal aneurysm (≥6 cm)	No	Yes					
CVA or TIA History of a cerebrovascular accident with minor or no residual and transient ischemic attacks	No	Yes					
Dementia Chronic cognitive deficit	No	Yes					
COPD	No	Yes					
Connective tissue disease	No	Yes					
Peptic ulcer disease Any history of treatment for ulcer disease or history of ulcer bleeding	No	Yes					

(continued)

Table 16.1	Charlson Comorbidity Index (*continued*)						
Variable							
	0	+1	+2	+3	+4	+6	Score
Liver disease Severe = cirrhosis and portal hypertension with variceal bleeding history; moderate = cirrhosis and portal hypertension but no variceal bleeding history; mild = chronic hepatitis (or cirrhosis without portal hypertension)	None	Mild	–	Moderate to severe	–	–	
Diabetes mellitus	None or diet controlled	Uncomplicated	End-organ damage	–			
Hemiplegia	No	–	Yes				
Moderate-to-severe CKD Severe = on dialysis, status/post kidney transplant, uremia; moderate = creatinine > 3 mg·dL^{-1} (0.27 mmol·L^{-1})	No	–	Yes				
Solid tumor	None	–	Localized	–	–	Metastatic	
Leukemia	None	–	Yes				
Lymphoma	None	–	Yes				
AIDS	None	–	–	–	–	Yes	
Total score = Charlson Comorbidity Index (CCI)							
Predicted 10-yr survival = 0.983^(e$^{CCI \times 0.9}$)							

CHF, congestive heart failure; COPD, chronic obstructive pulmonary disease; CVA, cerebrovascular accident; EKG, electrocardiogram; MI, myocardial infarction; TIA, transient ischemic attack.

COPD. It incorporates body mass index (BMI), lung obstruction, dyspnea, and a measure of exercise capacity through exercise walking tolerance (Table 16.2). The following values are those that can be assigned to determine the BODE Index. Scores range from 0 to 10. Variables include BMI, airway obstruction through FEV$_1$, dyspnea values as measured through the modified Medical Research Council (mMRC), and exercise tolerance as measured by a 6-minute walk test (6MWT).

Considerations for Multimorbidity and Exercise Prescription

The large majority of Americans are not performing adequate amounts of physical activity, and it is notably even lower for those with preexisting medical conditions. The U.S. National Health Interview Survey in 2016 indicated that 48% of adults are not meeting the physical activity guidelines for aerobic activity, and 78% of adults are not meeting the physical activity guidelines for both aerobic and strength training (64). Additional morbidity presence and frequency is associated with lower physical activity levels with respiratory and CVD comorbidities having the greatest impact on further reductions of exercise participation for those with osteoarthritis (65).

Patients with multimorbidity face significant barriers to physical activity and may have hesitancy to perform structured exercise. The barriers include, but are not limited to, a lack of knowledge or belief in the benefits of exercise, low self-efficacy, fatigue or low energy, concerns

Table 16.2	The BODE Index Table				
Variable	0	1	2	3	Score
Body mass index (kg·m⁻²)	≥21	<21			
FEV$_1$ (% predicted)	≥65	50–64	36–49	≤35	
mMRC dyspnea scale	0–1	2	3	4–5	
6-Minute walk test (m)	≥350	250–349	150–249	≤149	
BODE Index					

mMRC, modified Medical Research Council.

for safety, mobility and balance concerns, polypharmacy, schedule limitations because of multiple medical appointments, transportation or infrastructure challenges, and financial concerns because of the high costs of health care. For patients with multimorbidity who are not currently exercising, the initial focus of an exercise prescription is to encourage safe engagement in consistent exercise, working toward an optimal dose.

Because of the wide continuum of conditions that fall under the umbrella of multimorbidity, the initial exercise goal and prescription may vary greatly. Although both classified as multimorbid, a patient with mild osteoarthritis, prediabetes, and clinical anxiety will present very differently than a patient with Marfan syndrome and stage 4 melanoma with co-occurring heart failure as a result of chemotherapy. For some patients, the goal of engaging in exercise is to slow or reduce functional decline and to improve quality of life. For others, the goal may be to manage or improve function and to delay or eliminate onset of additional chronic conditions.

The benefits of exercise are well documented for those with preexisting and complex medical conditions. Significant improvements can be seen in reduction of disease-specific and all-cause mortality, decreased pain for many conditions, reduced risk of progression disease for many conditions, improved cognitive function, and an additive effect on weight loss when combined with moderate dietary restriction (66).

Exercise is not without risks, and extra caution should be taken for those with severe or complex medical conditions. The clinical management of one condition may compromise or complicate the management of another, for example, by affecting a patient's response or adherence to exercise. The following are some examples:

- Patients with chronic kidney disease (CKD) may be at increased risk for hypoglycemia during exercise because of decreased clearance of insulin in the kidneys. The risk may be greater if kidney function is acutely worsening or if they are taking hypoglycemic diabetic medications.

- Patients with diabetes who have been newly diagnosed with coronary artery disease may be advised to discontinue use of nonsteroidal anti-inflammatory drugs (NSAIDs) because of their potentially harmful cardiac effects (67). Because these patients cannot use NSAIDs to prevent or alleviate current or anticipated joint pain during exercise, exercise compliance may decline.

- As a final example, a patient with right-sided heart failure and gastroparesis secondary to diabetes may experience abdominal bloating. Determining the cause of the abdominal bloating is important for the CEP because exercise may alleviate bloating because of constipation but is contraindicated if the bloating is because of cor pulmonale, right ventricle enlargement as a result of pulmonary disease.

These are only some examples of how multimorbidity can complicate exercise prescription and supervision for the CEP. More examples are provided in the case studies later in this chapter. The CEP must be aware of the relationship between conditions, including complications that commonly arise from a primary diagnosis, as well as how the treatment or management of one condition may influence another.

CONDITIONS OCCURRING SIMULTANEOUSLY

Box 16.1 identifies the conditions that the CEP is likely to encounter. They are divided into three categories: frequently seen (>10% of the time), commonly seen (2%–9% of the time), and infrequently seen (<2% of the time).

BOX 16.1	Multimorbidities: The Clinical Exercise Physiologist Is Likely to Encounter

Frequently seen comorbidities:
- Type 2 diabetes
- Orthopedic issues
- Arthritis
- Low back pain
- Obesity
- Depression
- Hypertension
- Coronary artery disease (myocardial infarction, percutaneous coronary intervention, coronary artery bypass graft, angina)
- Sarcopenia
- Mental illness
- Gastroesophageal reflux disease (GERD)
- Tobacco use

Commonly seen multimorbidities:
- Valvular heart disease (aortic stenosis, mitral stenosis/regurgitation)
- Peripheral vascular disease
- Dementia
- Atrial fibrillation
- Chronic lung disease (chronic obstructive pulmonary disease, interstitial lung disease, asthma, cystic fibrosis)
- Chronic kidney disease
- Osteoporosis

- Hearing impairment
- Visual impairment
- Aneurysms
- Heart failure (heart failure with reduced ejection fraction, heart failure with preserved ejection fraction, right-sided failure)
- Type 1 diabetes
- Chronic liver disease
- Status/post (S/P) cerebrovascular accident (CVA), traumatic brain injury (TBI)
- Abdominal aortic aneurysm (AAA)
- Anemia
- Pulmonary embolus
- Autoimmune disorders (also immunocompromised patients)
- Pulmonary hypertension

Infrequently seen comorbidities:
- End-stage renal disease
- Multiple sclerosis
- Postpolio syndrome
- Bleeding dyscrasias
- Metastatic cancer
- Postural orthostatic tachycardia syndrome (POTS)
- Amyotrophic lateral sclerosis (ALS)
- Others too numerous to mention (research when they present)

CASE STUDY APPROACH

In this chapter, a number of case studies have been selected to demonstrate a recommended process by which the CEP can work with patients with multimorbidity. The steps involved in developing an appropriate exercise prescription for these complex patients will be reviewed.

The case studies are presented according to the SBAR format, which is commonly used for transitions in care from one provider to another within a health care system. It is designed to succinctly provide all necessary information for safe transitions. The basic information presented in each of the sections of the SBAR is identified below. The precise information varies by patient, facility, and provider, but is relatively consistent across care settings.

Situation — Describe why the patient is here. Items included: Presenting diagnosis, age, sex, chief complaint, and so on.

Background — Include pertinent medical history (PMH)

- History and physical/discharge summary from last hospitalization

- Clinical provider notes (This could include various providers, including, but not limited to medical doctor (MD), doctor of osteopathic medicine (DO), nurse practitioner (NP), physician assistant (PA), respiratory therapist (RT), physical therapist (PT), registered dietitian (RD), clinical exercise physiologist (CEP), and so on
- Labs — Important labs to note include basic metabolic panel (BMP), complete blood count (CBC), arterial blood gases (ABG), lipids, hemoglobin A1c (HbA1c), brain natriuretic peptide (BNP), cardiac enzymes (creatine kinase [CK], creatine kinase myocardial isozyme [CKMB], troponin)
- Pulmonary function tests (PFTs)
- Echocardiogram (ECHO)
- Catheterization (cath) reports
- Operative reports
- 12-Lead electrocardiogram (ECG)
- Imaging
- Stress test results

Assessment — Use the information from the medical record review, clinical interview, and exercise testing performed to conduct a clinical assessment. Include patient exercise preferences, exercise testing results, concerns, and fall risk evaluation.

Recommendation — Provide the exercise prescription including the mode of exercise, duration, intensity, frequency, and plan for progression for the major components of cardiovascular, strength, and flexibility training.

The SBAR approach allows the CEP to communicate effectively with other providers. The SBAR is useful for two potential roles: (1) receiving the handoff for a new patient or (2) providing the handoff to another clinician on patient graduation, transition to another team member, or discharge from your care. An example SBAR is included in the case study section of this chapter.

Steps for Developing the Exercise Prescription

The CEP follows six essential steps in developing a clinical exercise prescription for a patient with multimorbidity.

1. Obtain provider referral
2. Review medical records
3. Identify priority medical concerns
4. Complete the clinical interview
5. Perform appropriate exercise testing
6. Create the exercise prescription and supervise exercise

The First Step — Obtain Provider Referral

Requirements will vary by state depending on practice acts in your particular area. Some states allow advanced practice professionals (APPs), including PAs and NPs, to make referrals and determine eligibility and appropriateness prior to beginning an exercise program. In all states, physicians (MD, DO) can make referrals regardless of specialty. This referral is necessary prior to beginning an exercise program for clinically complex patients, both to promote the patient's safety and to reduce the CEP's legal liability.

The Second Step — Review Medical Records

Having obtained the appropriate referrals, the CEP will review all available medical records. At a minimum, the following should be available:

1. The discharge summary from last hospitalization or the most recent clinic visit note for patients that were not hospitalized.
2. A current medication list. The medication list should be reviewed during the clinical interview and verified for accuracy. Any significant discrepancies should be brought to the attention of the treating medical provider.
3. Additional records should be obtained to answer any questions not discussed in the above records. For example, if there is mention of "heart failure" in the clinic note, the most recent ECHO should be reviewed to determine the etiology of the failure. If there is

mention of "prediabetes," the most recent HBA1C% and fasting glucose should be reviewed. Blood glucose can change rapidly with exercise, and it is helpful to know in advance if the patient has elevated risk for post-exercise hypoglycemia. Another example is if a patient's last CBC showed the patient's hemoglobin and hematocrit as anemic or low, then follow-up lab work may be necessary prior to initiating activity.

The Third Step — Identify Priority Medical Concerns

Exercise safety is of critical importance. Prioritizing concerns can help the CEP focus on the factors that are crucial and create an exercise prescription that considers the most problematic factors, first. Priority concerns include pulmonary and hemodynamic instability, significant metabolic disturbances, mental health conditions that create an unsafe environment, acute infectious or inflammatory conditions, severe orthopedic issues or connective tissue disorders, and suspected or known dissecting aneurysm.

Pulmonary or hemodynamic instability is the primary concern prior to beginning an exercise program. If the patient is unable to maintain adequate oxygenation and peripheral perfusion at rest, activity will be poorly tolerated and unsafe. The main clinical issues that should be reviewed in such cases are heart failure, aortic stenosis, pulmonary hypertension, exercise-induced bronchoconstriction, angina, uncontrolled cardiac dysrhythmias, undertreated hypertension, and symptomatic hypotension.

Metabolic imbalances are also priority concerns. Examples that would fall into this category are high or low blood glucose levels, electrolyte abnormalities, anemia, and severe endocrine disorders such as unmanaged hyperthyroidism (68).

Primary mental health concerns focus on whether the patient can follow safety instructions and adequately communicate symptoms brought on or aggravated by physical activity. Patients with neurologic or mental disorders, including dementia, severe depression, bipolar disorder, anxiety disorders, untreated psychosis, or severe personality disorders, should be identified and evaluated and prioritized during the clinical interview. It can be challenging to maintain a safe environment if a patient with neurologic or mental illness has aggressive outbursts, incoherent language, acute episodes of severe anxiety, or displays violence with physical aggression. These issues should be prioritized, and a safety strategy should be in place prior to initiating exercise.

Patients with infectious or inflammatory conditions, including sepsis, myocarditis, pericarditis, or an acute infectious process, including COVID-19, would be precluded from participation in physical activity until their condition is resolved (68).

Other priority issues of note include but are not limited to severe orthopedic impairment that could be aggravated by activity or could limit activity, connective tissue disorders that are exacerbated by activity, and suspected or known dissecting aneurysm.

The Fourth Step — Complete the Clinical Interview

The clinical interview involves a discussion between the patient and the CEP. The CEP will perform an assessment of the disease burden using the information gleaned from the medical record review. Together they will discuss the patient's previous exercise experience and collaborate to create patient goals by asking and answering questions. This process provides an opportunity for the CEP to learn about the patient's personality, preferences, and concerns. It also creates an opportunity to provide education and to establish trust.

During the interview, a current functional status comparison is helpful to identify current baseline functional status in relationship to the functional status in the 1 year preceding the major event that led to referral to the CEP. Major complaints are the main issue for which the patient was referred. Often, this is not the limiting factor or major consideration in prescribing and supervising exercise but needs to be addressed during the intake appointment.

Assessing the patient's exercise history provides insight into their ability to accurately report signs and symptoms as well as to document perceived exertion. Patients with little or no experience with physical activity may have difficulty rating their effort or exertion level. Patients with a history of strenuous activity may struggle to accept that they can no longer perform as they did previously, because of deconditioning or an event that resulted in a functional limitation. An example is the resistance trained or endurance athlete who has a major myocardial infarction (MI) resulting in heart failure secondary to ischemic cardiomyopathy. These patients may try to perform beyond safe limits if they do not understand why they can no longer exercise as they did previously. Peripheral adaptations to previous exercise training degrade at a slower rate than cardiac function, and a mismatch may result between peripheral demands and central supply. When this happens during cardiovascular exercise, the patient becomes symptomatic, fatigued, or unable to tolerate activity consistent with the historical baseline. In resistance training, the consequences can be much more significant. Because of the development of high pressures during such exercise, the afterload that the heart needs to overcome becomes elevated, and as a result, the athlete may experience a cardiac dysrhythmia. The role of the CEP is to clearly communicate the safe limits of exercise and to educate the patient on the factors that are likely and unlikely to change with consistent exercise training.

In addition to major issues and exercise history, the CEP should discuss the goals of the exercise program with the patient, as discussed in detail in the next section. As part of the goal-setting process, the CEP addresses whether the patient is able to perform the physical tasks required for three major categories: (1) functional for activities of daily living (ADLs), (2) work or occupational demands, and (3) recreational pursuits. These considerations will inform the metabolic equivalent (MET) level required for the patient to return to prior level of function. The Compendium of Physical Activities (69) can be used as a guide to compare the MET level of the desired activity compared to the current functional level of the patient. This activity intensity comparison can support meaningful goal setting and help to set realistic expectations for physical performance. The compendium provides information regarding the type, intensity, and duration of activities in a systematic manner. It is noteworthy that the Compendium of Physical Activities records absolute MET levels and does not take into account individual differences that impact mechanical efficiency (e.g., those who use mobility aids or prosthetics), body weight that is significantly under or overweight, or for those with significantly high or low body fat percentages.

The three primary goal categories, functional, occupational, and recreational, should be evaluated using a collaborative approach during the clinical interview. Appropriate and meaningful goals should be set in each area.

Functional

The functional goal is for the patient to perform all of the necessary ADLs. Interview questions should address routine daily activities, including basic self-care, such as bathing, preparing meals, and housework, as patients with multimorbidity may find these activities difficult to perform. Specific questions should be posed in an attempt to discover nuances. For example, patients who have to carry laundry up and down two flights of stairs at their home will have a higher functional goal than one who does not need to climb stairs to complete the task. Another example is a patient who has to perform and care for a disabled spouse within the home and provide a moderate assist for transfers and bathing. These specific demands may be best addressed by focused flexibility work and strength training and will need to be identified during the clinical interview.

Occupational

The occupational requirements of the patient can vary widely. The U.S. Department of Labor publishes a list of occupations and the associated metabolic demand for each job class (70). Additional questions should be directed to strength and flexibility demands of various occupations. The principle of "specificity of training" should be followed as closely as possible.

Recreational

Recreational goals can vary widely. A patient may provide a clear goal such as "play a game of tennis with my family." The CEP can evaluate the necessary components to perform tennis safely. The expected duration of activity can be identified, balance and agility requirements can be reviewed, the needed MET level (as found in the Compendium of Physical Activities) can be compared to current exercise intensity, exercise environment and footwear can be discussed, and a reasonable exercise prescription can be created. Other patients may provide an ambiguous goal, such as "playing with the grandchildren." Upon further investigation, the CEP may learn that this means traveling by airplane, with all of the physical demands of navigating airports, handling luggage, close-quarters transfers, and repeatedly walking long distances. Upon arrival at the travel destination, the goal may include safely lowering to the floor to play with the children and then returning to a standing position multiple times. If the patient needs assistive devices to facilitate the performance of these activities or for energy conservation, then this need must be identified and included in the exercise prescription. Although some recreational goals require relatively low functional capacity requirements, other goals require a large functional capacity to perform safely. A patient with a goal of big game hunting in Alaska will require much higher physical demands than a game of basketball. Physical demands for this goal may require traveling, packing gear, hiking, carrying a weapon, and possibly additional weight in the cold over rough terrain for several days. Basic exercise physiology principles, including specificity of training, overload, and progression, will apply for goals with large and small energy requirements. The starting point and progression will vary greatly for each patient.

The Fifth Step — Exercise Testing

After the clinical interview, exercise testing should be performed. Testing is individualized to the functional capacity of the patient and may include cardiopulmonary exercise testing (CPET), graded exercise testing (GXT), 6MWT, or a submaximal ramped protocol on various modalities. Exercise modalities may include the treadmill, upright or recumbent bike, and seated stepper, rower, or elliptical depending on patient needs and functional limitations.

Fall risk should also be assessed using fall history and functional tests, such as the Timed Up and Go (TUG) test, 30-second chair sit-to-stand test, and 4-Stage Balance Test, as presented in Table 16.3. The Stopping Elderly Accidents, Death and Injuries (STEADI) Algorithm for Fall Risk Assessment & Interventions (71) may be used to classify fall risk.

Patients with multimorbidity may require creative solutions to safely perform exercise testing. A challenging example is a patient with a complex medical history, including sternal precautions for a recent coronary artery

Table 16.3	Fall Risk Assessment Methods	
Test	**Advantages**	**Considerations**
Fall history *Number of falls within the last 12 mo*	• Has face validity • Fall history is predictive of future falls	• Relies on patient recall • Not accurate if patient has cognitive impairment • Does not take into account recent significant changes in status
30-Second sit-to-stand	• Simple for patients to understand • Fast — *30 s* • Easy to administer	• Orthopedic limitations may limit ability to perform but test remains valid
Timed Up and Go (TUG)	• Validated • Fast • Used in a variety of settings for longitudinal tracking	• Patient must be able to transfer out of chair, walk, and transfer back to chair with a stand-by assist
4-Stage Balance Test	• Fast — *10 s per stage*	• Slightly more complicated to administer because of the four-stage process

bypass grafting (CABG) procedure who is currently using a wheelchair for a below knee amputation. Traditional exercise testing may not be possible. In these scenarios, the CEP should remain calm and curious as they seek creative solutions. Ask questions and consult other medical professionals who have experience in adaptive scenarios such as a PT, physiatrist, or other medical specialty. Use peer-reviewed resources to located established protocols that could be feasible. There will be times when no

established protocols are available. In these scenarios, use a conservative approach to administer a symptom-limited exercise bout to find an appropriate intensity and duration of exercise.

The results of these tests presented in Table 16.4 should include the duration of exercise completed, maximum METs performed during the exercise, maximum HR, maximum BP, lowest SpO_2%, rating of perceived exertion (RPE), supplemental oxygen used (if any), and

Table 16.4	Cardiovascular Exercise Testing Methods	
Test	**Advantages**	**Considerations**
Stress test *(Maximal test)*	• Significant information provided for diagnostic purposes • Performed under physician supervision	• Test can be difficult to administer and cost-prohibitive • May not provide incremental data for prescription services • Increased risk of a cardiac event or death
Cardiopulmonary exercise testing (CPET) *(Maximal test)*	• Prognostic information provided • Comprehensive cardiac and pulmonary information is provided during each stage of exercise • In complex patients with dyspnea of unknown etiology, the test can determine root cause • Often performed under physician supervision	• Not available in all locations • Can be complicated to administer • Can be cost-prohibitive • Patients may not tolerate the mask during exercise • Increased risk of a cardiac event or death
Submaximal ramped protocol *(Submaximal test)*	• Most widely used approach • Standardized protocols for specific populations are available • Ability to compare results to established norms and predictive values • Flexible and can be used with many exercise modalities if modifications are needed • Information can be used to create an initial exercise prescription or starting point	• Questionable validity depending on the protocol used — any modifications from established protocol is extremely important if the test is to be repeated later
6-Minute walk test (6MWT) *(Submaximal test)*	• Set time of 6 min • Safe to administer because of the self-limiting nature *The walking pace is self-selected and able to stop when fatigued or with development of symptoms* • Easy for patients to understand • Provides prognostic information if followed over time	• Difficult or impossible for those that struggle with upright ambulation • Will not give adequate information if patient has a functional capacity >3 METs

METs, metabolic equivalents.

reason for stopping the tests. These values are necessary to create a safe and meaningful exercise prescription. Additional information regarding exercise test evaluation and interpretation are discussed elsewhere in this text.

The Sixth Step — Exercise Prescription and Supervision

After reviewing the medical record, identifying priority concerns, completing the clinical interview, and exercise tests, the necessary information is available to create the initial exercise prescription. Every exercise prescription should include the components of cardiovascular exercise, strength training, and flexibility training, with a plan for progression.

The CEP should design the exercise program so as to mitigate potential side effects and also consider alternative activities in the event that the initial exercise prescription is poorly tolerated. When working with patients with multimorbidity, it is best to start off slowly and progress gradually.

Each exercise prescription should be individualized to meet the patient's goals, accommodate the clinical restrictions, and provide an adequate stimulus to create a training effect. If the CEP has a large case load, it can be tempting to use a standardized template and provide a generic exercise prescription with a warm-up, cardiovascular exercise, strength training, and flexibility completed during the cool-down for every patient. Although a template can save time, it is important to evaluate the areas that are providing the most significant functional limitations and adjust the components of the prescription accordingly.

Additional exercise prescription considerations include available exercise equipment, exercise setting (individual or a group setting), available monitoring equipment (ECG or HR monitor, oximeter, blood pressure [BP] cuff and stethoscope, glucometer, etc.), and availability of support staff.

Exercise supervision should provide direct observation of the patient during exercise to ensure safety. To support patients with limited exercise experience, it is recommended to use multiple methods to describe the exercise prescription. Recommended methods include using verbal cues, visual demonstrations, providing the exercise prescription in a written format with instructions to support learning retention, and providing prompt feedback once exercise has been initiated. The CEP should help the patient set up cardiovascular exercise equipment to accommodate their unique size and shape. This may include but is not limited to adjusting seat position, using technology to set the exercise duration, adjusting the walking speed, adjusting the treadmill incline, setting the

MET level or watts, or instructing the patient to hold the revolutions per minute (RPM) at a specific cadence. The CEP should evaluate exercise form and make adjustments as needed. During exercise, the CEP should prompt ongoing patient feedback through RPE and rating of perceived dyspnea (RPD) for those with pulmonary conditions. Additional measures of HR, BP, SpO_2%, and telemetry, when available, can provide insight into how well the exercise prescription is tolerated. At minimum these measures should be evaluated pre-, peak-, and post-exercise. A high priority of exercise supervision is to create a safe and enjoyable exercise environment. Identify any signs or symptoms that indicate the patient is not tolerating the exercise well. Effort should be taken to make the exercise environment enjoyable for the patient, as exercise adherence is notably poor in this population.

Medically complex patients tend to have poor exercise histories and may be intimidated by exercise. They may be less tolerant of the sensations of muscle exertion, delayed onset muscle soreness, or fatigue. Although proper progression is important to facilitate improvements in functional capacity, at some point the patient can move to a "maintenance dose" of exercise.

When patients meet the American College of Sports Medicine (ACSM) and the Centers for Disease Control and Prevention (CDC) physical activity guidelines, they can transition into the maintenance dose of exercise if they prefer to do so. Moderate-intensity aerobic exercise should be completed for 30-minute a day on 5 days per week, or vigorous intensity aerobic activity for a minimum of 20 minutes on 4 days per week and performing activities that maintain or increase muscular strength and endurance for a minimum of 2 days per week. Just as we encourage and support patients to take their pharmacological medication as prescribed, it is important for the proper dosing of exercise to be communicated and encouraged.

Goals of the Exercise Prescription

For patients with significant multimorbidity, the goals of exercise should be individualized to be meaningful and reasonably attainable, just as with patients who have less disease burden. The ultimate goal of exercise training is to return the patient to pre-event (for many, their pre-diagnosis) functional status. The secondary goal is to return to the level of function 1-year previously, and the tertiary goal is to return to a level of function that meets all of the patient's goals. In addition, goals of the exercise prescription fall into the three categories: functional, occupational, and recreational.

SUMMARY

Patients with multimorbidity are increasingly prevalent in a clinical setting and thus CEPs must be prepared to handle the nuances and complexities of exercise testing and prescription for these patients. Multimorbidity may result from shared underlying pathology or as secondary consequences of a primary diagnosis. Regardless of the etiology, prescribing exercise to a patient with multimorbidity can be challenging, and the CEP must take a systematic approach to assessment and exercise prescription. The CEP must be aware of complicating factors, such as medication interactions, reduced exercise tolerance, and interactions between disease processes that may affect exercise adherence or functional capacity. Although patients should approach exercise with caution, they should not avoid it, because ultimately, a well-designed exercise program will provide a multitude of benefits for most patients with multimorbidity.

CHAPTER REVIEW QUESTIONS

1. Name two indices that can be used to assess health status and mortality risk. Which index should only be used for patients with COPD?
2. Describe the shared mechanisms of chronic disease. Provide a specific example of one mechanism underlying many chronic conditions.
3. Provide two examples of how a primary diagnosis can lead to additional conditions.
4. What are frequently seen coexisting conditions? Why do these conditions tend to occur together?
5. What factors should be considered when creating an exercise prescription for patients who have chronic conditions for mental and physical health?
6. Describe the SBAR method for approaching an exercise prescription for patients with multimorbidity.

Use the case studies provided to give an example of each step.

7. Identify the six steps in designing a clinical exercise prescription for an individual with multimorbidity.
8. Name and provide examples of three types of goals in prescribing exercise for a patient with multimorbidity.
9. A fall risk assessment should be completed before performing cardiovascular exercise testing. What are the four methods that the CEP can use to evaluate fall risk?
10. It is very likely that a CEP will encounter new combinations of chronic conditions while working with patients with multimorbidity. What are the two strategies that a CEP can use when encountering rare conditions or a new combination of conditions?

CASE STUDIES

Note: The following case studies are used as examples of patient information that would be communicated in a clinical context. The first case study provides a lengthened format, for education purposes to describe the patient scenario in greater detail. Subsequent case studies are presented in a more succinct format that would be reflective of a clinical note.

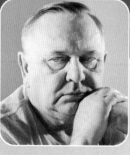

Case Study 16.1

Situation: Maurice is a 56-year-old male who was referred after percutaneous coronary intervention. The patient was referred to cardiology by his primary care provider (PCP) after several weeks of intermittent symptoms of breathlessness and indigestion unrelieved by antacids. The patient was taken electively to the cardiac catheterization laboratory where a drug-eluting stent was placed in the circumflex artery. Thrombolysis in myocardial infarction (TIMI) (72) score in the circumflex was grade 3 post-stenting. After the procedure, the patient had recurrent shortness of breath and indigestion similar to the presenting complaint, but further intervention was deferred because of poor renal function. The patient was referred to a cardiothoracic surgeon, who determined him to be a poor surgical candidate because of his high-risk status and referred him for evaluation and rehabilitation, medical management, and presurgical optimization.

Background: The patient has a long history of poorly controlled T2DM, with the most recent HbA1c = 8.5%, and a BMI of 45 $kg \cdot m^{-2}$. Maurice experienced an MI 3 years ago, but no records of coronary anatomy from that time are available. He also experienced a cerebrovascular accident (CVA) 3 years ago with no residual impairment. Other PMH: patient has stage III CKD, hypertension, S/P right great toe amputation (4 weeks ago), gastroparesis, chronic low back pain, and diabetic neuropathy. The most recent ejection fraction (EF) obtained by ECHO was 30%. The patient's medications include metoprolol succinate, clopidogrel, aspirin, atorvastatin, lisinopril, insulin glargine, insulin aspart (sliding scale), furosemide, gabapentin, trazodone, hydrocodone-acetaminophen 5-325, and nitroglycerin as needed (PRN). He is also a former smoker with a 35 pack-year history (quit 4 years ago). He underwent a Roux-en-Y gastric bypass surgery 2 years ago.

Assessment: The healing status of the great toe amputation was evaluated with no signs of infection or improper healing. *Footwear is challenging during the healing phase.* A backless shoe is currently being worn until a shoe fitting can take place upon discharge from the wound care clinic. The new change in gait and peripheral neuropathy will increase fall risk. The patient reported one fall in the past year and completed the first stage of the 4-Stage Balance Test, placing the patient at a high fall risk.

A recumbent cycle ramp protocol was used to evaluate functional capacity, resulting in 3.0 METs for 6 minutes of exercise completed. The test was stopped because of an RPE of 5 out of 10 reached and a simultaneous HR increase outside of calculated range. Patient exhibited normal HR and BP responses to exercise. The patient reported no exercise in the last 10 years and may need additional support for motivation and self-reported exertion level.

The blood glucose trends since his gastric bypass procedure were reviewed. Low blood glucose is difficult to treat with gastroparesis, and priority would be given to pre-exercise optimization of blood glucose to avoid symptomatic hypoglycemia. Hypoglycemia may be further exacerbated by this patient's history of gastric bypass surgery.

The patient is unable to walk comfortably and would like to return to grocery shopping and playing with his dog. There is a public track close to his home and his starting goal is to walk to the track, circle once (400 m) and walk back home. This course is estimated to be a 1-mile walk in

total. He is primarily limited by pain because of the healing status of his toe, with additional strength and endurance limitations. He is not currently using an assistive device.

Maurice reports that his functional capacity has greatly declined in the last year. Functional status 1-year prior to an event is predictive of the highest level of function that can be achieved in a rehabilitative setting and can guide reasonable expectations.

He has received focused education on sodium restriction, fluid restriction, signs and symptoms of decompensation, and the importance of medical adherence and of monitoring body weight daily, through the heart failure clinic. Assessment of daily body weight may be particularly difficult in this patient because small fluctuations in weight may be reflective of inconsistent bowel movements because of gastroparesis.

Other PMH: The patient is on multiple diuretics, and electrolyte abnormalities are common and potentially fatal. Trend of glomerular filtration rate (GFR) or HbA1c, dry weight, per cardiology, and recent labs, such as CBC and BMP should be obtained. Labs that would be specifically pertinent to exercise would be electrolytes, hemoglobin, and hematocrit. A CBC is important because patients with CKD often develop anemia. An ECHO would be helpful to review cardiac function (diastolic function and pulmonary arterial pressures). The patient's report of dyspnea could be because of pulmonary hypertension. It would be helpful to have a PFT for this patient. His smoking history predisposes him to chronic lung disease. If the patient has comorbid COPD, this will need to be addressed. Oxygen saturation (SpO_2%) will need to be closely monitored. Even if the patient has normal test results, it is possible that he could have obesity hypoventilation syndrome. With the patient's history and BMI and reported sleep disturbances, it is recommended that a STOP-BANG evaluation be performed to screen for sleep apnea (73, 74).

The primary goal of exercise training is to return the patient to pre-event functional status. The secondary goal is to return to the level of function 1 year previously, and the tertiary goal is to return to a level of function that meets all of the patient's goals.

Recommendation: The patient should continue to follow up with the wound care clinic until he is discharged from their care. Because of orthopedic concerns and back pain, non-weight bearing cardiovascular exercise is initially recommended with the goal of progressing to an interval walking program. Maurice expressed that his large lower abdomen weight is causing discomfort during exercise and would like to progress to standing exercise once his surgical site on his foot has healed.

(continued)

Case Study 16.1 (*continued*)

The upright upper body ergometer (UBE) can be considered as an alternative to the recumbent cycle if the discomfort is intolerable. He expressed concern about hydration during exercise for this bowel regime for gastroparesis. He will follow up with his PCP to discuss the use of stool softeners, adequate fiber intake, and possible laxative use.

The initial exercise prescription includes supervised exercise two to three times a week, and strength training for all major muscle groups two times a week, gradually progressing exercise duration and intensity. Flexibility training will be prioritized to help gain additional flexibility

to put on socks without the use of an assist device. An appropriate warm-up and cool-down will be implemented prior to starting and finishing exercise. The initial cardiovascular exercise prescription includes five, 2-minute bouts of recumbent cycling as tolerated with an MET range of 1.8–2.4. Exercise goal is to elicit an RPE of 4–6/10 and RPD of less than 6. Joint stabilization and mobility will be the focus 2 days a week, with consistent encouragement and support. Flexibility training will be included 5 days a week (2 days supervised and 3 days at home) with the goal of a 20- to 30-second hold for five lower body exercises.

Case Study 16.1 Questions

1. List at least four orthopedic concerns that should be factored into the initial exercise prescription for the patient. Describe how exercise prescription could be modified to accommodate these concerns.

2. List at least two reasons the patient may be at an increased risk for falls. Describe three tests that can be performed to assess fall risk.

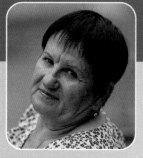

Case Study 16.2

Situation: Leslie is a 58-year-old woman who was admitted for COPD exacerbation and is being referred to pulmonary rehabilitation for sarcoidosis for medical management and to increase muscle strength and cardiovascular endurance. Recent PFT: forced expiratory volume in 1 second (FEV_1) 65%, the proportion of vital capacity expired in the first second of forced expiration (FEV_1/FVC; also known as the Tiffeneau-Pinelli index) is 110%; diffusing capacity or transfer factor of the lung for carbon monoxide (DLCO) is 18%.

Background: PMH: COPD, obstructive sleep apnea (on bilevel positive airway pressure therapy), T2DM (insulin dependent), hypertension, peripheral neuropathy, CKD stage 3 (creatinine 1.5), BMI = 42 $kg \cdot m^{-2}$, sarcoidosis, pulmonary hypertension, asthma, gout, hyperlipidemia, and heart failure with preserved EF (HFpEF; EF 65% upon last ECHO).

Assessment: Leslie is currently working as a data analyst, and she sits for the majority of her day. She would like to be able to breathe easier and spend more time with her adult children without feeling exhausted. She is able to perform her ADLs, but verbalized that it takes her much longer to do the same tasks than it did last year. She performed a 6MWT test, resulting in 690 feet (210 m) and 2.0 METs. Patient used a four-wheeled walker and was on 3L O_2 with desaturation to 88% during test. Patient completed TUG in 22.9 seconds, placing patient at high risk for falls at time of initial intake. BMI, airflow obstruction, dyspnea, and exercise capacity (together known as the BODE Index score, which gives an indication of how patients with COPD are likely to do in the future) is 4. Patient's mMRC scale for dyspnea is 3.

Recommendation: Patient will be placed on an interval walking program alternating work and rest bouts of 3 minutes. Progression will be attempted at weekly intervals, with the goal of being able to complete 15 minutes of continuous walking. Once that has been accomplished, the patient will be oriented to the treadmill and placed on moderate-intensity interval training with 2-minute work and 2-minute rest intervals with constant speed and variable elevation to elicit an RPE of 5–6/10 and RPD of less than 6. Oxygen flow rates will be titrated to maintain SpO_2 more than 90%. Patient will also be placed on an UBE initially for 6 minutes continuously and progressed to 10 minutes by increasing 1 minute per week. The initial strength training prescription will focus on challenging all major muscle groups using a combination of body weight, dumbbells, resistance bands, and exercise machines. Leslie will begin with three to four multijoint exercises performing 8–12 repetitions to fatigue and progressed by approximately 10% per week until she is able to perform 12 repetitions. One new exercise will be added approximately every week until a total of 8–10 exercises are performed two to three times per week. She will be instructed on flexibility exercises for each major muscle group to be performed after the completion of resistance training. Because her recreational goal involves spending more time with family, although feeling less fatigued, energy conservation education will be included to help her best direct her energy to the activities that are important to her.

Discussion: The etiology of this patient's disability is most likely sarcoidosis with end-organ damage involving the lungs, kidneys, and heart. Her prognosis is grim. Goals of her exercise program will be to maintain optimal functional status. Progress will likely be minimal and slow with multiple setbacks. The CEP should pay particular attention to factors limiting her exercise tolerance. Patients with this presentation are best served with a cardiopulmonary stress test to determine which system is the limiting function. Pulmonary hypertension, heart failure, and general deconditioning could all be the limiting factor. Cardiopulmonary exercise testing (CPET) will determine which system fails first and can guide the exercise prescription. However, as with all complex patients, the principles of specificity of training, overload, and progression will apply. The application of the prescription is, in all cases, symptom-limited regardless of the root cause of the symptoms. Severe pulmonary hypertension, critical aortic stenosis, intractable angina, and any other active symptomatology of hemodynamic instability should be carefully considered and evaluated prior to exercise testing.

Case Study 16.2 Questions

1. What four factors are considered in the BODE Index score? What information does the BODE Index score provide the CEP?

2. What important information would CPET provide for this patient? Why would that information be useful for a CEP?

Case Study 16.3

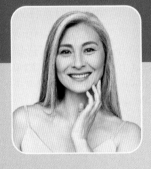

Situation: Victoria is a 57-year-old female who has severe asthma and a rare pulmonary condition tracheobronchomalacia. Other PMH: history of atrial fibrillation (A-fib), gastroesophageal reflux disease (GERD), anxiety, depression, widespread osteo-arthritis, and persistent back pain with cervical and lumbar fusions at C3–C5 and L4 S1. Victoria was referred to pulmonary rehabilitation for supervised exercise, with the goal of improving her strength and functional capacity.

Background: The patient has tracheobronchomalacia because of prolonged mechanical ventilation stemming from chlorine exposure. Her BMI is 21 $kg·m^{-2}$ and she has a history of lifelong exercise participation. Her providers have been concerned about the high recurrence of intubations because of frequent tracheal collapse. To address this concern, a surgical tracheal reconstruction was performed 3 years ago. The procedure improved the stability of the trachea. The patient is not currently exercising and would like to improve her functional capacity so she could return to her occupation in marketing and hike in the mountains again. The patient is concerned about exercising as shortness of breath and subsequent hypoxia evoke anxiety and feelings of panic. Providers documented additional concerns of post-traumatic stress disorder (PTSD) from the

(continued)

Case Study 16.3 (*continued*)

exceptionally high use of mechanical ventilation with 29 intubations. Victoria is currently using room air at rest and 2 L/m of O_2 during exercise. She does not use any assistive devices. She agreed to have a rescue inhaler available for each visit, prior to starting exercise.

Assessment: Victoria performed a 6MWT resulting in 1,500 feet (457.2 m) and 3.1 METs. Because of no history of falls in the past year, a TUG resulting in 6.6 seconds, and a 30-second sit-to-stand test result of 21, the patient was classified as a low fall risk. She demonstrated appropriate diaphragmatic breathing technique and will receive education on mindfulness, grounding, and relaxation techniques to reduce situational anxiety resulting from exercise. A combination of seated and standing exercise is initially recommended to accommodate back pain, with the goal of progressing to walking. Exercise will progress to incline treadmill walking to more closely mimic hiking.

Recommendation: The initial exercise prescription includes supervised cardiovascular exercise three times a week and strength training for all major muscle groups two times a week, gradually progressing exercise duration and intensity. An appropriate warm-up and cool-down will be implemented prior to starting and finishing exercise. The initial cardiovascular exercise prescription included a 10-minute bouts recumbent cycling followed by a 10-minute bought of treadmill walking as tolerated with max METs of 2.4 using 2 L/m of supplemental oxygen. Exercise goal is to elicit an RPE of 5–6/10 and RPD of less than 6. Oxygen flow rates will be titrated to maintain SpO_2 more than 90%.

Cycling and walking volume will be progressed at a maximum of 10% per week, attempted progression weekly. As cardiovascular endurance is her primary recreation goal, she will work up to 30 minutes of consistent well-tolerated incline walking. BP, $SpO_2\%$, HR, RPE, RPD scales, and patient feedback will be used to determine exercise tolerance. The initial strength training prescription will focus on challenging all major muscle groups using a combination of body weight, dumbbells, resistance bands, and exercise machines. Victoria will begin with three to four multijoint exercises performing 8–12 repetitions to fatigue and progressed by approximately 10% per week until she is able to perform 12 repetitions. One new exercise will be added approximately every week until a total of 8–10 exercises are performed two to three times per week.

Discussion: When rare conditions arise such as tracheobronchomalacia, it is helpful to use additional resources to supplement gaps in knowledge. Even experienced CEPs will run into conditions that they have never seen before. When this occurs, thoroughly review the clinical documentation to identify information needed to keep the patient safe during exercise. Identify clinicians who have experience working with the condition, such as an experienced respiratory therapist or pulmonologist. Use trusted search engines to locate peer-reviewed research to learn more about the condition and expected responses to exercise. The CEP should be aware of the status of the tracheostomy prior to the clinical interview. If the tracheostomy (commonly referred to as a trach) is fully closed, it would not be a concern. If the trach was open, additional precautions need to be observed, including a backup tube, a plan for hydration, and a communication plan in case speech is limited or difficult to understand. The history of A-fib is concerning in a pulmonary rehab setting as cardiac monitoring with an ECG is not a standard practice. Close monitoring through a HR monitor may help to provide Victoria with additional comfort and ensure that her HR response to exercise is safe and appropriate.

Case Study 16.3 Questions

1. What resources should the CEP consider using if the patient had a tracheostomy? If speech was difficult at rest or during exercise, what strategies could they consider using?

2. If Victoria were to experience acute respiratory distress (ARDS) during exercise, what steps should be taken to support her?

Case Study 16.4

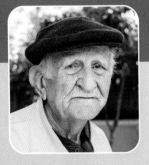

Situation: Noah is an 80-year-old male presented to the emergency department with a sudden onset of severe substernal chest pain/pressure and was diagnosed with ST-segment elevation MI (STEMI). Cardiac catheterization revealed 99% stenosis in the mid-left anterior descending coronary artery that was successfully stented with a drug-eluting stent. Residual 20% stenosis in distal RCA. ECHO showed some mild midseptal and anteroseptal as well as apical akinesis, and EF was 30%–35% with mild mitral regurgitation and mild tricuspid regurgitation. Repeat ECHO showed improved EF to 55%–60% with mild-to-moderate pulmonary hypertension. The patient developed bloody stools on the day of discharge with slight hematocrit drop from 39.3% to 37.5%, now stable at 38.6%. Benefits outweighed risks for aspirin (acetylsalicylic acid [ASA]) therapy and discharged on both ASA and Plavix. BP was too low for angiotensin-converting enzyme (ACE) inhibitor but was treated with Toprol ER 12.5 mg daily and Lipitor 80 mg daily.

Background: Noah is a retired farmer. He has hyperlipidemia with an LDL of 131. He is currently experiencing kidney stones, benign pulmonary nodules, and COPD (PFT = FEV_1/FVC 23%, FEV_1 20%) with baseline O_2 at 3 L/m and treated with Symbicort and Combivent with rare use of albuterol and theophylline. Patient also has history of gastroesophageal reflux disease (GERD), abdominal aortic aneurysm (AAA), history of tobacco abuse (quit after 94 pack-years), iodine allergy, chronic dermatitis on topical steroids, and known history of AAA repair. He states that he used to be very active when he was farming, but when he retired at 70 years, his health took a decline. Although very active 10 years ago, he has not done any formal exercise since his days in the air force.

Assessment: Noah performed a 6MWT for 459 feet (140 m), resulting in 1.7 METs. He desaturated to 83% during ambulation and needed O_2 titrated to 6 $L \cdot min^{-1}$ via nasal cannula to maintain saturation more than 90%. Patient had a history of two falls in the past year and completed the TUG in 12.7 seconds, placing him at a high risk for falls at time of initial intake. Patient surveys included the following: GAD-7 (Generalized Anxiety Disorder 7-item scale) total score: 2; PHQ-9 (Patient Health Questionnaire 9-item scale) total score: 3; COOP-Dartmouth Questionnaire (Dartmouth Cooperative Functional Assessment) score: 23; and CAT (COPD Assessment Test): 21. Noah is able to complete all the necessary ADLs, and he has no recreation or occupation goals, but stated that he wanted to breathe better, have less pain, feel stronger overall, and work around his shop.

Patient has significant limitations with advanced COPD. Patient is currently taking Combivent, Symbicort, and albuterol. According to the Global Initiative for Chronic Obstructive Lung Disease (GOLD) guidelines, patient could benefit from a long-acting muscarinic antagonist if deemed appropriate per medical provider. Patient also does not use rescue inhaler properly and has been scheduled to meet with respiratory therapy (RT). Patient will be educated on proper rescue inhaler use prior to exercise.

Recommendation: Noah will be started on a combination of an interval walking program and seated stepper at an initial MET level of 1.7. An appropriate warm-up and cool-down will be implemented prior to starting and finishing exercise. He will use two, 5-minute bouts on the seated stepper and two, 5-minute bouts on the treadmill, building exercise intensity and duration gradually. The initial strength training prescription will focus on challenging all major muscle groups using dumbbells, at his request because he has some available at home. Noah will begin with two multijoint exercises performing 6–12 repetitions to fatigue and progressed by approximately 10% per week until he is able to perform 12 repetitions. One new exercise will be added approximately every week until a total of 8–10 exercises are performed two to three times per week.

Discussion: This patient presents for a cardiac diagnosis, but after evaluation, it appears his underlying pulmonary disease is more functionally limiting. Primary goals will be to get his oxygen prescription and inhaled medications optimized and instruct the patient on pursed lip breathing techniques. This will have to be addressed prior to any significant increases in physical activity that can be tolerated. Of other concern would be his tendency toward anemia. There are a vast number of conditions that can cause and/or contribute to anemia and being on dual antiplatelet therapy will exacerbate this condition. Anemia will not show on routine pulse oximetry and will have to be monitored. Patients can be severely anemic but still have high pulse oxygen readings.

Case Study 16.4 Questions

1. Describe the results of the patient's initial and repeat ECHO. How would you classify his initial and repeat values in relation to normal values?

2. What might be a cause of the patient's anemia? Will routine pulse oximetry be useful in monitoring anemia?

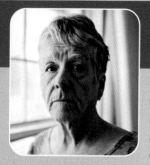

Case Study 16.5

Situation: Nancy is a 64-year-old woman referred for spontaneous coronary artery dissection and anterior wall MI was taken to emergent cardiac catheterization laboratory. No focal occlusion was found but there was narrowing of the mid-to-distal left anterior descending artery as well as anterior and apical akinesis. Medically managed only. Patient came back to emergency department a few weeks later with chest pain. Nuclear stress test revealed a prior infarction in the basal to mid-lateral wall. Apical akinesis has resolved and her EF had improved back to 60%–65%. She also had a recent diagnosis of costochondritis, which may be causing musculoskeletal pain, which in turn could be causing her recurring chest pain; patient is now on Voltaren topical gel. Patient is enrolled for chronic care management from insurance company and has home health caregivers daily.

Background: Nancy works at a grocery store, standing for the majority of her day. Her current HbA1c is 4.9, current tobacco use is one pack per day, COPD (chronically on 4 L·min^{-1} of oxygen), pulmonary cachexia, hypertension, major depressive disorder, severe anxiety, PTSD, pulmonary lung nodule to right mid-lung, genital herpes, leukocytosis, paroxysmal supraventricular tachycardia, hyperlipidemia, migraines, GERD, degenerative disc disease, history of lumbar compression fractures, chronic low back pain, and previous MI.

Assessment: Nancy is very concerned and has expressed that she needs to go back to work as soon as possible. She performed a 6MWT for 475 feet (145 m). Also of note, patient's prior 6MWT distance for pulmonary rehabilitation 3 months earlier was 258 m, showing significant decline in function. Patient reported no falls in the past year and completed TUG in 9.7 seconds, placing patient at moderate risk for falls at time of initial intake. However, the patient did request to use a four-wheel walker during cardiac rehabilitation sessions, which increased confidence and improved the ability to carry portable oxygen. She is struggling to perform some ADLs, she would like to return to work, and she would like to return to gardening.

Recommendation: Because Nancy would like to return to work that requires standing, exercise in a standing position will be prioritized to slowly rebuild endurance, using an initial MET level of 1.7. An appropriate warm-up and cool-down will be implemented prior to starting and finishing exercise. As she is still quite weak, she will alternate between a seated stepper and walking, using two 4-minute bouts for each modality, closely monitoring her cardiac rhythm, HR, BP, RPE, RDP, and SpO$_2$%. The goal is to build endurance by first adding duration to each modality, and then transitioning to walking as the dominant cardiovascular exercise. Nancy has expressed that she "hates" strength training but is open to try a more relaxing class like yoga. So, the initial compromise is to start strength training with a resistance band and three exercises for 6–12 repetitions, two to three times per week. The intension is to slowly add one additional exercise each week for 6 weeks. Additionally, she will attend a gentle yoga class once a week.

Discussion: The presentation of this patient is very common and generally very difficult to manage. Patients with multiple orthopedic concerns in conjunction with other major complicating conditions are difficult to motivate to exercise. Their exercise history is typically limited and their ability to progress is also limited. Increasing or even beginning exercise results in an exacerbation of their underlying orthopedic conditions. To further complicate this case, NSAIDs are contraindicated in patients with coronary disease because of the increased risk of major cardiac events with their usage. This eliminates one of the main tools to decrease orthopedic pain associated with a new physical activity program. The use of a four-wheel walker can provide some relief by off-loading partial body weight and aiding in balancing. The initial program will need to be very gentle and progressed very slowly until such time as her ability to tolerate the activity is evaluated and whether or not she will be able to have a good response. An initial exercise prescription that is too aggressive will, in all likelihood, result in poor compliance. Too many variables could be aggravated by activity that would result in the patient dropping from any activity at all. The light resistance training is intentional because of her expressed preference. Resistance training is frequently better tolerated than cardiovascular activity at the outset in these patients and will allow the connective tissues to adapt prior to more stressful activity.

Of particular concern is the decrease of approximately 100 m on the 6MWT in less than 6 months from a previous evaluation. This finding, in addition to the diagnosis of pulmonary cachexia, is significant prognostically. This large drop in functional capacity in such a short period indicates a rapid decline. The patient will have to be monitored closely for rhythm disturbances and SpO_2. Self-reported exertion levels will need to be used carefully. Particular attention should be paid to the patient's pain level and dyspnea. These patients frequently cannot distinguish between breathing hard because of the increased oxygen demand of exercise and dyspnea. High levels of pain also raise BP, anxiety, and myocardial oxygen demand, resulting in higher perception of work which may not accurately reflect musculoskeletal fatigue.

It is often helpful to have patients report their perception of effort, pain, and breathing separately.

The scripting may sound like: "How hard are you working on a scale of 1–10? This is an overall measure of your effort level." Then: "What is your pain level? What area is hurting you the most?" Then: "How hard are you breathing? If you stop exercise will your breathing get better soon? Are you short of breath or breathing hard?" This line of questioning often allows patients to begin to understand what is limiting their exercise.

Case Study 16.5 Questions

1. How would you describe apical akinesis to the patient?
2. What factors were considered in the initial exercise program for the patient? What are the benefits of this approach?

3. In addition to RPE and pain level, what other subjective factor was assessed during exercise and why?

Case Study 16.6

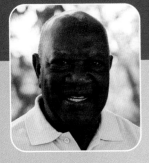

Situation: Jerry is a 74-year-old male status/post (S/P) transcatheter aortic valve replacement (TAVR). Post-op ECHO shows EF estimated at 80%. He was traveling when this event occurred, and he has decided to stay in the area to receive treatment. Because of the nature of his travels, some medical documentation was able to be obtained, but not complete records.

Background: Jerry is a snowbird who was on an RV (recreational vehicle) trip with his spouse when his TAVR occurred. He has Crohn disease with associated vasculitis resulting in bilateral below-the-knee amputations (BKAs) on both legs. He was released 12 weeks ago to ambulate as tolerated. PMH: macular degeneration and recent bilateral cataract surgery. Additionally, he experiences osteopenia, hypocalcemia, vitamin D and B_{12} deficiencies, vitamin K deficiency with history of coagulopathy, chronic pain syndrome, and stage 2 CKD/solitary kidney.

Assessment: Jerry performed a staged UBE test, resulting in 3.0 METs completed before test was stopped because of RPE of 6/10. Testing was well-tolerated with normal hemodynamic response and with no complaint of cardiac symptoms. Patient has bilateral lower extremity prostheses and reports that he is not able to walk much because rubbing on his legs has caused discomfort and wounds. Patient was unable to tolerate staged tests on recumbent stepper or recumbent cycle. TUG was not completed. Patient is placed at high risk for falls at time of initial intake. Patient is able to transfer from wheelchair to equipment with a stand-by assist. Patient is able to complete ADLs

(continued)

Case Study 16.6 (*continued*)

with minor assistance from his spouse. He is retired and has occupational goals at this time. His recreational goals are to gain body weight and return to his activities such as resistance training and bike riding on the recumbent bike/upright bike.

Recommendation: Jerry will need his residual limbs checked each pre- and post-exercise. The initial focus of his exercise will be on strength training, with a minor emphasis on cardiovascular exercise. He will be started on UBE and seated stepper at an initial MET level of 1.8 for 10 minutes each. When the patient is on the seated stepper, he will be using his arms only until his wounds are healed and he can tolerate the activity. Jerry will complete a resistance training program using 8–10 exercises targeting all major muscle groups, adapting around his lower limbs as he tolerates his prostheses. He will perform one to two sets of 6–12 repetitions for each exercise. Progression will be 10% per week of weight when patient can complete 12 repetitions to fatigue. The high use of his arms can result in muscular imbalances and tightness. Flexibility training will be incorporated 3 days a week, targeting all major muscle groups, with a focus on the upper body, after the completion of strength training.

Discussion: Several things will need to be evaluated and considered with this patient. The ECHO finding that his left ventricle is hyperdynamic is of moderate concern. Normal EF is 60%–65%, with 70% being the upper limit of what is considered normal. The fact that his aortic valve was just replaced, along with the ECHO finding, is suggestive of very tight aortic stenosis. A review of his preprocedure ECHO is indicated. Three things suggest aortic stenosis on ECHO: high aortic velocity (>4 m·s^{-1}), transaortic pressure gradient, and small aortic valve area. One or all three are present in patients with aortic stenosis. In order to maintain

homeostasis, the body's adaptation is to increase the force with which the heart contracts to maintain perfusion. If the valve was extremely tight as indicated by valve area, then an increase in force is required to maintain adequate cardiac output. With prolonged periods, the constant strain causes the myocardium to become thickened. Hypertrophic cardiomyopathy is the result. The ECHO should give some idea as to the severity of this hypertrophy. The concern here from an exercise standpoint is that the new valve does not require the same amount of force for circulation. However, the stroke volume will remain decreased from the hypertrophy for some time. Most often, with no other issues, EF and cardiac output will return to normal 6–12 months following valve replacement. In the interim, cardiac output will be limited by the decreased stroke volume and may limit exercise tolerance from inadequate perfusion. This patient has two BKAs and therefore has a decreased amount of possible working muscle mass demanding oxygenation, so the issue may be negligible; however, it should still be monitored. The BKA will need to be closely supervised to ensure that the healing is not slowed or worsened by the repetitive nature of aerobic conditioning. This patient would benefit from preferential emphasis on resistance training from a functional status standpoint. Increased strength would aid in his ability to transfer and potentially place less stress on his wound sites. Other issues with this particular patient are his abnormal electrolyte and clotting issues. Although this is more in the purview of his treating physician, the CEP should be aware of signs and symptoms that could present with physical activity. These include ECG rhythm abnormalities, unusual swelling, new-onset dyspnea, deep vein thrombosis (DVT), pulmonary emboli, and tachycardia. Should they arise, these issues would all need to be closely monitored.

Case Study 16.6 Questions

1. What three factors suggest aortic stenosis on the ECHO?
2. How does the body respond to aortic stenosis, and how does this lead to hypertrophic cardiomyopathy? How will this affect cardiac output during exercise?
3. Why would the patient benefit from an initial emphasis on resistance training?

REFERENCES

1. Boyd CM, Fortin M. Future of multimorbidity research: how should understanding of multimorbidity inform health system design? *Public Health Rev.* 2010;32:451–74.

2. Moffat K, Mercer SW. Challenges of managing people with multimorbidity in today's healthcare systems. *BMC Fam Pract.* 2015;16:129.

3. Feinstein AR. The pre-therapeutic classification of comorbidity in chronic disease. *J Chronic Dis.* 1970;23:455–68.

4. van den Akker M, Buntinx F, Knottnerus JA. Comorbidity or multimorbidity. *Eur J Gen Pract.* 1996;2:65–70.

5. Boyd CM, Fortin M. Future of multimorbidity research: how should understanding of multimorbidity inform health system design? *Public Health Rev.* 2010;32:451–74.

6. Prados-Torres A, Calderón-Larrañaga A, Hancco-Saavedra J, Poblador-Plou B, van den Akker M. Multimorbidity patterns: a systematic review. *J Clin Epidemiol.* 2014;67(3):254–66.

7. Zulman DM, Asch SM, Martins SB, Kerr EA, Hoffman BB, Goldstein MK. Quality of care for patients with multiple chronic conditions: the role of comorbidity interrelatedness. *J Gen Intern Med.* 2014;29(3):529–37.

8. Waits SA, Reames BN, Sheetz KH, Englesbe MJ, Campbell DA Jr. Anticipating the effects of Medicaid expansion on surgical care. *JAMA Surg.* 2014;149(7):745–7.

9. Astor BC, Hallan SI, Miller ER III, Yeung E, Coresh J. Glomerular filtration rate, albuminuria, and risk of cardiovascular and all-cause mortality in the US population. *Am J Epidemiol.* 2008;167(10):1226–34.

10. Booth FW, Roberts CK, Laye MJ. Lack of exercise is a major cause of chronic diseases. *Compr Physiol.* 2012;2(2):1143–211.

11. Cruz-Jentoft AJ, Landi F, Schneider SM, et al. Prevalence of and interventions for sarcopenia in ageing adults: a systematic review. Report of the International Sarcopenia Initiative (EWGSOP and IWGS). *Age Ageing.* 2014;43(6):748–59.

12. Erickson KI, Leckie RL, Weinstein AM. Physical activity, fitness, and gray matter volume. *Neurobiol Aging.* 2014;35 (Suppl 2):S20–8.

13. Erickson KI, Voss MW, Prakash RS, et al. Exercise training increases size of hippocampus and improves memory. *Proc Natl Acad Sci U S A.* 2011;108(7):3017–22.

14. Gregory SM, Parker B, Thompson PD. Physical activity, cognitive function, and brain health: what is the role of exercise training in the prevention of dementia? *Brain Sci.* 2012;2(4):684–708.

15. Murphy EA, Enos RT, Velazquez KT. Influence of exercise on inflammation in cancer: direct effect or innocent bystander? *Exerc Sport Sci Rev.* 2015;43(3):134–42.

16. Amoabeng Nti AA, Robins TG, Mensah JA, et al. Personal exposure to particulate matter and heart rate variability among informal electronic waste workers at Agbogbloshie: a longitudinal study. *BMC Public Health.* 2021;21(1):2161.

17. DeFronzo RA, Tripathy D. Skeletal muscle insulin resistance is the primary defect in type 2 diabetes. *Diabetes Care.* 2009;32(Suppl 2):S157–63.

18. Goodpaster BH, Thaete FL, Kelley DE. Thigh adipose tissue distribution is associated with insulin resistance in obesity and in type 2 diabetes mellitus. *Am J Clin Nutr.* 2000;71(4):885–92.

19. Kahn SE, Hull RL, Utzschneider KM. Mechanisms linking obesity to insulin resistance and type 2 diabetes. *Nature.* 2006;444(7121):840–6.

20. Kelley DE, He J, Menshikova EV, Ritov VB. Dysfunction of mitochondria in human skeletal muscle in type 2 diabetes. *Diabetes.* 2002;51(10):2944–50.

21. Anandacoomarasamy A, Caterson I, Sambrook P, Fransen M, March L. The impact of obesity on the musculoskeletal system. *Int J Obes.* 2008;32(2):211–22.

22. Hanefeld M, Pistrosch F, Bornstein SR, Birkenfeld AL. The metabolic vascular syndrome — guide to an individualized treatment. *Rev Endocr Metab Disord.* 2016;17(1):5–17.

23. Cree MG, Newcomer BR, Katsanos CS, et al. Intramuscular and liver triglycerides are increased in the elderly. *J Clin Endocrinol Metab.* 2004;89(8):3864–71.

24. Franceschi C. Inflammaging as a major characteristic of old people: can it be prevented or cured? *Nutr Rev.* 2007;65(12 Pt 2):S173–6.

25. Reaven GM. Relationships among insulin resistance, type 2 diabetes, essential hypertension, and cardiovascular disease: similarities and differences. *J Clin Hypertens.* 2011;13(4):238–43.

26. De Felice FG, Lourenco MV, Ferreira ST. How does brain insulin resistance develop in Alzheimer's disease? *Alzheimers Dement.* 2014;10(Suppl 1):S26–32.

27. Wood RJ, O'Neill EC. Resistance training in type II diabetes mellitus: impact on areas of metabolic dysfunction in skeletal muscle and potential impact on bone. *J Nutr Metab.* 2012;2012:268197.

28. Paneni F, Costantino S, Cosentino F. Molecular mechanisms of vascular dysfunction and cardiovascular biomarkers in type 2 diabetes. *Cardiovasc Diagn Ther.* 2014;4(4):324–32.

29. Austin V, Crack PJ, Bozinovski S, Miller AA, Vlahos R. COPD and stroke: are systemic inflammation and oxidative stress the missing links? *Clin Sci (Lond).* 2016;130(13):1039–50.

30. Egger G. In search of a germ theory equivalent for chronic disease. *Prev Chronic Dis.* 2012;9:E95.

31. Hossain IA, Akter S, Bhuiyan FR, Shah MR, Rahman MK, Ali L. Subclinical inflammation in relation to insulin resistance in prediabetic subjects with nonalcoholic fatty liver disease. *BMC Res Notes.* 2016;9:266.

32. Huang Z, Chen C, Li S, Kong F, Shan P, Huang W. Serum markers of endothelial dysfunction and inflammation increase in hypertension with prediabetes mellitus. *Genet Test Mol Biomarkers.* 2016;20(6):322–7.

33. Hwang SJ, Ballantyne CM, Sharrett AR, et al. Circulating adhesion molecules VCAM-1, ICAM-1, and E-selectin in carotid atherosclerosis and incident coronary heart disease cases: the Atherosclerosis Risk in Communities (ARIC) study. *Circulation.* 1997;96(12):4219–25.

34. Matsumoto K, Sera Y, Nakamura H, Ueki Y, Miyake S. Serum concentrations of soluble adhesion molecules are related to degree of hyperglycemia and insulin resistance in patients with type 2 diabetes mellitus. *Diabetes Res Clin Pract.* 2002;55(2):131–8.

35. Meigs JB, Hu FB, Rifai N, Manson JE. Biomarkers of endothelial dysfunction and risk of type 2 diabetes mellitus. *JAMA.* 2004;291(16):1978–86.

36. Pradhan AD, Manson JE, Rifai N, Buring JE, Ridker PM. C-reactive protein, interleukin 6, and risk of developing type 2 diabetes mellitus. *JAMA.* 2001;286(3):327–34.

37. Preston RA, Coffey JO, Materson BJ, Ledford M, Alonso AB. Elevated platelet P-selectin expression and platelet activation in high-risk patients with uncontrolled severe hypertension. *Atherosclerosis.* 2007;192(1):148–54.

38. Li L, Hu D, Zhang W, et al. Effect of short-term exposure to particulate air pollution on heart rate variability in normal-weight and obese adults. *Environ Health.* 2021;20(1):29.

39. Smitka K, Maresova D. Adipose tissue as an endocrine organ: an update on pro-inflammatory and anti-inflammatory microenvironment. *Prague Med Rep.* 2015;116(2):87–111.

40. Ntaios G, Gatselis NK, Makaritsis K, Dalekos GN. Adipokines as mediators of endothelial function and atherosclerosis. *Atherosclerosis.* 2013;227(2):216–21.

41. Zammit C, Liddicoat H, Moonsie I, Makker H. Obesity and respiratory diseases. *Int J Gen Med.* 2010;3:335–43.

42. Mankowski RT, Anton SD, Buford TW, Leeuwenburgh C. Dietary antioxidants as modifiers of physiologic adaptations to exercise. *Med Sci Sports Exerc.* 2015;47(9):1857–68.

43. Ozben T. Oxidative stress and apoptosis: impact on cancer therapy. *J Pharm Sci.* 2007;96(9):2181–96.

44. Rask-Madsen C, King GL. Vascular complications of diabetes: mechanisms of injury and protective factors. *Cell Metab.* 2013;17(1):20–33.

45. Seyfried TN, Shelton LM. Cancer as a metabolic disease. *Nutr Metab (Lond).* 2010;7:7.

46. Paneni F, Beckman JA, Creager MA, Cosentino F. Diabetes and vascular disease: pathophysiology, clinical consequences, and medical therapy: part I. *Eur Heart J.* 2013;34(31):2436–43.

47. Keske MA, Premilovac D, Bradley EA, Dwyer RM, Richards SM, Rattigan S. Muscle microvascular blood flow responses in insulin resistance and ageing. *J Physiol.* 2016;594(8):2223–31.

48. Wagenmakers AJ, Strauss JA, Shepherd SO, Keske MA, Cocks M. Increased muscle blood supply and transendothelial nutrient and insulin transport induced by food intake and exercise: effect of obesity and ageing. *J Physiol.* 2016;594(8):2207–22.

49. Biessels GJ, Deary IJ, Ryan CM. Cognition and diabetes: a lifespan perspective. *Lancet Neurol.* 2008;7(2):184–90.

50. Song J, Kim J. Degeneration of dopaminergic neurons due to metabolic alterations and Parkinson's disease. *Front Aging Neurosci.* 2016;8:65.

51. van Elderen SG, de Roos A, de Craen AJ, et al. Progression of brain atrophy and cognitive decline in diabetes mellitus: a 3-year follow-up. *Neurology.* 2010;75(11):997–1002.

52. Ellis T, Motl RW. Physical activity behavior change in persons with neurologic disorders: overview and examples from Parkinson disease and multiple sclerosis. *J Neurol Phys Ther.* 2013;37(2):85–90.

53. Madeddu C, Deidda M, Piras A, et al. Pathophysiology of cardiotoxicity induced by nonanthracycline chemotherapy. *J Cardiovasc Med.* 2016;17(Suppl 1):S12–8.

54. Maurea N, Coppola C, Piscopo G, et al. Pathophysiology of cardiotoxicity from target therapy and angiogenesis inhibitors. *J Cardiovasc Med.* 2016; 17(Suppl 1):S19–26.

55. Deidda M, Madonna R, Mango R, et al. Novel insights in pathophysiology of antiblastic drugs-induced cardiotoxicity and cardioprotection. *J Cardiovasc Med.* 2016; 17(Suppl 1):S76–83.

56. Kolewaski CD, Mullally MC, Parsons TL, Paterson ML, Toffelmire EB, King-VanVlack CE. Quality of life and exercise rehabilitation in end stage renal disease. *CANNT J.* 2005;15(4):22–9.

57. Longenecker CT, Sullivan C, Baker JV. Immune activation and cardiovascular disease in chronic HIV infection. *Curr Opin HIV AIDS.* 2016;11(2):216–25.

58. Carr A. Pathogenesis of cardiovascular disease in HIV infection. *Curr Opin HIV AIDS.* 2008;3(3):234–9.

59. Fox C, Walker-Bone K. Evolving spectrum of HIV-associated rheumatic syndromes. *Best Pract Res Clin Rheumatol.* 2015; 29(2):244–58.

60. Guerri-Fernandez R, Villar-Garcia J, Diez-Perez A, Prieto-Alhambra D. HIV infection, bone metabolism, and fractures. *Arq Bras Endocrinol Metabol.* 2014;58(5):478–83.

61. Centers for Disease Control and Prevention. Bridging the artificial gap between physical and mental illness. *Chronic Dis Notes Rep.* 2003;16(1):26–31.

62. Golbidi S, Frisbee JC, Laher I. Chronic stress impacts the cardiovascular system: animal models and clinical outcomes. *Am J Physiol Heart Circ Physiol.* 2015;308(12):H1476–98.

63. Marventano S, Grosso G, Mistretta A, et al. Evaluation of four comorbidity indices and Charlson Comorbidity Index adjustment for colorectal cancer patients. *Int J Colorectal Dis.* 2014;29(9):1159–69.

64. Centers for Disease Control and Prevention. National Center for Health Statistics. Early Release of Selected Estimates Based on Data From the 2018 National Health Interview Survey; May 30, 2019. Accessed July 15, 2022. https://www.cdc.gov/nchs/nhis/releases/released201905.htm#7A.

65. McKevitt S, Healey E, Jinks C, Rathod-Mistry T, Quicke J. The association between comorbidity and physical activity levels in people with osteoarthritis: secondary analysis from two randomised controlled trials. *Osteoarthr Cartil Open.* 2020;2:100057. doi:10.1016/j.ocarto.2020.100057.

66. Bull FC, Al-Ansari SS, Biddle S, et al. World Health Organization 2020 guidelines on physical activity and sedentary behaviour. *Br J Sports Med.* 2020;54(24):1451–62. doi:10.1136/bjsports-2020-102955.

67. Ghosh R, Hwang SM, Cui Z, Gilda JE, Gomes AV. Different effects of the nonsteroidal anti-inflammatory drugs meclofenamate sodium and naproxen sodium on proteasome activity in cardiac cells. *J Mol Cell Cardiol.* 2016;94:131–44.

68. American College of Sports Medicine. *ACSM's Guidelines for Exercise Testing and Prescription.* 11th ed. Philadelphia (PA): Wolters Kluwer/Lippincott Williams & Wilkins; 2021.

69. Ainsworth BE, Haskell WL, Whitt MC, et al. Compendium of physical activities: an update of activity codes and MET intensities. *Med Sci Sports Exerc.* 2000;32(Suppl 9):S498–504.

70. Bureau of Labor Statistics. *Occupational Requirements Survey.* Washington (DC): U.S. Department of Labor; 2016. Available from: https://www.bls.gov/ors/#data.

71. Stevens JA, Phelan EA. Development of STEADI: a fall prevention resource for health care providers. *Health Promot Pract.* 2013;14(5):706–14.

72. Antman EM, Cohen M, Bernink PJ, et al. The TIMI risk score for unstable angina/non-ST elevation MI: a method for prognostication and therapeutic decision making. *JAMA.* 2000;284(7):835–42.

73. Marzolini S, Sarin M, Reitav J, Mendelson M, Oh P. Utility of screening for obstructive sleep apnea in cardiac rehabilitation. *J Cardiopulm Rehabil Prev.* 2016;36(6):413–2

74. Celli BR, Cote CG, Marin JM, et al. The body-mass index, airflow obstruction, dyspnea and exercise capacity index in chronic obstructive pulmonary disease. *N Engl J Med.* 2004;350(10):1005–12.

Considerations for Exercise in Stressful Environments: Hot, Cold, Polluted, and High Altitude

INTRODUCTION

The human body responds to changes in the environment every day to maintain health and optimal performance. Hot, cold, air-polluted, and high-altitude environments present the most common and the most stressful situations for individuals engaged in fitness/recreational activities or sports. Even when exercise occurs in an air-conditioned facility, pollution and high-altitude stresses may alter normal physiologic responses or retard adaptations to exercise. Further, individuals who live with today's most prevalent diseases (*i.e.*, obesity, diabetes, chronic respiratory disease, and cardiovascular disease [CVD]) may find their exercise capacity limited by one or more of these environments or may be at increased risk of aggravated signs and symptoms.

The term "stressor" refers to an influence that perturbs a concentration, condition, or level that is either homeostatically regulated or maintained at a steady state. Stressors can be external (*e.g.*, noise, darkness, electric shock, viruses) or internal (*e.g.*, lack of sleep, malnutrition, intense negative memories). Table 17.1 summarizes the physiologic outcomes of stress encountered in hot, cold, air-polluted, and high-altitude environments. These

Table 17.1	Potential Negative Effects of Environmental Stress on Metabolism and Performance		
Environment	Physiologic Outcomes of Environmental Stress	Potential Negative Effects of Environmental Stressors	Conditions That May Increase the Risk of Morbidity and Mortality
Hot (*e.g.*, ≥85°F WBGT)	• Increased skin temperature • Increased internal body temperature • Increased cardiovascular strain • Increased sweating • Increased respiration	• Increased anaerobic metabolism and plasma lactate accumulation • Reduced maximal oxygen consumption • Reduced endurance, strength, and power performance • Increased perceived exertion • Fluid–electrolyte deficit (*e.g.*, dehydration, sodium depletion) • Exertional heat illnesses (*e.g.*, heat syncope, heat exhaustion, heatstroke, heat cramps)	• Cardiovascular disease (hypertension/cardiac failure) • Older age • Obesity • Diabetes • Multiple sclerosis • Paraplegia • Burns • Medications such as diuretics, β-blockers, vasodilators
Cold	• Reduced skin temperature • Reduced internal body temperature	• Increased heat production (one to four times resting metabolic rate) because of shivering • Increased water loss in urine (volume per 24 h)	• Peripheral vascular disease • Coronary artery disease • Hypertension • Chronic obstructive pulmonary disease, asthma

(continued)

Table 17.1	Potential Negative Effects of Environmental Stress on Metabolism and Performance *(continued)*		
Environment	**Physiologic Outcomes of Environmental Stress**	**Potential Negative Effects of Environmental Stressors**	**Conditions That May Increase the Risk of Morbidity and Mortality**
		• Reduced maximal oxygen consumption • Reduced endurance exercise performance • Strength and power decrease 4%–5% per 1°C drop of muscle temperature • Cold injuries (*e.g.*, hypothermia, frostnip, frostbite)	• Cold-induced bronchoconstriction • Low body fat • Serum hypoglycemia • Older age • Raynaud disease
Air pollution	• Reduced arterial oxygen saturation • Increased ventilation • Bronchoconstriction • Headache • Eye irritation	• Reduced maximal oxygen consumption • Increased heart rate during sub-maximal exercise • Reduced endurance exercise performance • Earlier onset of angina • Increased inflammation and oxidative stress (free radical formation) • Altered blood clotting	• Asthma • Chronic obstructive pulmonary disease • Bronchitis • Older age • Cardiovascular disease • Diabetes • Overweight/obesity
High altitude (*i.e.*, 1,500–3,500 m [4,921–11,483 feet])	• Reduced arterial oxygen saturation • Increased resting ventilation • Reduced sleep quality and duration • Sleep apnea	• Reduced oxygen delivery to skeletal muscle and other tissues • Increased perceived exertion and fatigue • Breathlessness during exercise • Reduced cardiac output during exercise and rest • Reduced maximal oxygen consumption • Reduced endurance performance • Increased water loss in urine and expired air (volume per 24 h) • Impaired mood and appetite • Increased oxidative stress (free radical formation) • Reduced cognitive performance (memory, decision-making, calculations) • High-altitude illnesses (see Table 17.3)	• Asthma • Congestive heart failure • Cardiac arrhythmias • Chronic obstructive pulmonary disease • Hypertension • Patent ductus arteriosus • Atrial septal defects • Upper respiratory tract infection • Bronchitis • Sickle cell anemia • Cystic fibrosis • Older age

WBGT, wet-bulb globe temperature.

Source: Armstrong LE. Nutritional strategies for football: counteracting heat, cold, high altitude, and jet lag. *J Sports Sci.* 2006;24(7):723–40; Pescatello LS, Arena R, Riebe D, Thompson PD. Exercise prescription for healthy populations with special considerations and environmental considerations. In: *American College of Sports Medicine's Guidelines for Exercise Testing and Prescription.* Baltimore (MD): Lippincott Williams & Wilkins; 2014. p. 194–226; Pescatello LS, Arena R, Riebe D, Thompson PD. Exercise prescription for populations with other chronic diseases and health conditions. In: *American College of Sports Medicine's Guidelines for Exercise Testing and Prescription.* Baltimore (MD): Lippincott Williams & Wilkins; 2014. p. 260–343.

stressors influence human health and exercise performance, as well as the acute responses and chronic adaptations within organ systems. Table 17.1 also describes diseases and conditions that increase the risk of environmental illness, reduced exercise performance, and diminished cognitive function.

The model presented by Riebe et al. (1) provides general guidance for the prescription of aerobic exercise. This logic model results from scientific and clinical evidence that shows exercise is safe for most people, it provides numerous health and fitness benefits, and cardiovascular events during exercise are often preceded by warning signs/symptoms and that these cardiovascular risks associated with exercise decrease with improved fitness. However, harsh environments (*i.e.*, heat, cold, air pollution, high altitude) present additional stressors that are not part of the logic model in Figure 3.1. This chapter describes the influences of these environmental stressors on specific populations.

EXERCISE IN HOT ENVIRONMENTS

With the global temperature rising and heat waves increasing in frequency, severity, and relative length (2), it is no surprise that heat stress has the potential to affect everyone. After identifying four forms of heat illness, this section explains how a healthy individual regulates their body temperature, with emphasis on how heat and humidity compound the stress of body temperature regulation (*i.e.*, thermoregulation). A wealth of information exists regarding heat stress effects on a healthy individual (3), but less is known about how heat stress affects individuals afflicted with chronic disease, including CVD and metabolic diseases (*i.e.*, clinical populations). Thus, the rest of this section focuses on individual factors such as disease and age, by introducing concepts that may be used as starting point to manage the physiologic stress of heat and humidity. The goals of the clinical exercise physiologist (CEP) are to understand the basic physiology of heat stress, factors to consider when managing heat stress (*i.e.*, wet-bulb globe temperature [WBGT]), and strategies to reduce the detrimental effects of increased heat stress and humidity.

Heat Illness and Acclimatization

In exercise and recreational settings, heat stress can decrease cognitive and physiologic performance and increase the risk for heat illness (3). Similar detriments occur when individuals are exposed to heat during work (*i.e.*, occupational heat stress), a setting that is unique because of the relatively larger number of individuals being exposed and the somewhat involuntary nature of the exposure (4). Regardless of whether exposure was occupational or recreational, direct heat-related fatalities were greater than any other weather-related death (*e.g.*, cold, flooding, tornados, hurricanes, lightning) over the last 30 years (5). These fatalities are because of heat illness.

Strenuous exercise in, or prolonged exposure to, a hot environment may result in one of four distinct heat illnesses (3). The first, heat syncope, involves a brief fainting spell and pale skin without increased internal temperature. Warning signals include weakness, vertigo, nausea, or tunnel vision. Heat cramps represent the second type of exertional heat illness. Although many types of muscular cramps exist, this variety specifically results from a whole-body sodium deficit that involves the large muscles of the extremities and the abdominal muscles. The third and most common heat illness is heat exhaustion, which involves great fatigue and inability to continue exercise in a hot environment. Sweating is profuse, mental function is mildly impaired, and body temperature rises moderately. Dehydration often is a predisposing factor. Finally, exertional heatstroke is a medical emergency requiring immediate action. Metabolic heat, produced during exercise, is stored in the internal organs, and body temperature rises above 39°C–40°C (102°F–104°F). Obvious changes occur in cognitive function and mental awareness of events/surroundings. Other signs and symptoms may include vomiting, diarrhea, coma, and convulsions. Cooling by immersion in cold or iced water should begin immediately (6).

Heat acclimatization reduces the risk and severity of all forms of exertional heat illness. A traditional heat acclimatization protocol involves approximately 16 repeated 90-minute exposures to heat where core temperature increases approximately 2.5°C. In the process, positive physiologic adaptations occur in multiple organ systems (Table 17.2). These adaptations are specific to the stressors encountered and allow the body to function more effectively with less risk of illness or injury. Adaptations to repeated days of exercise in the heat include reduced rise in internal body temperature, a lower heart rate (HR) and rating of perceived exertion, and a reduction in sodium losses in sweat and urine. Whole-body sweat rate increases, and an expansion of plasma volume occurs (7).

Table 17.2	Acclimatization in Specific Organ Systems During 8–14 Days of Exercise in Stressful Environments			
	Environment			
Organ System or Function	**Heat**	**Cold**	**Air Pollution**	**High Altitude**
Circulatory — cardiac	↑	↑	↔	↑
Renal (fluid–electrolyte balance)	↑			
Respiratory			↔	↑
Muscular	↑	↑		↑
Temperature regulation	↑	↑		
Exercise performance	↑		↔	↑

↑, enhanced function; ↔, adaptations to specific pollutants may occur.

Thermoregulation in Hot Environments

It is critical that the body's internal temperature remains below 41°C–42°C (106°F–108°F; 8). The body's primary way of responding to increased body temperature primarily involves increased sweating and skin blood flow. These controls are generally very effective; however, exercise and environmental factors such as heat and humidity add a thermoregulatory stress that exacerbates the increase in body temperature.

Any muscular action (*i.e.*, contraction of skeletal muscle) produces heat that must be dissipated. Convective heat losses involve the transport of this warmer blood from the core to the skin, where heat is then transferred to the environment. Concomitantly, heat is lost via evaporation of sweat from the skin surface. The cooled skin surface subsequently lowers the temperature of blood circulating through the skin. The increase in skin blood flow and evaporation of sweat are critical to controlling body temperature; without them an individual would succumb to a very high internal temperature within minutes of beginning exercise.

High ambient temperature (approximately >30°C) challenges the body's ability to thermoregulate secondary to increasing skin temperature. Increased skin temperature decreases the gradient in which heat is transferred from the skin to the environment by convection and radiation. When ambient temperature exceeds skin temperature (*i.e.*, >38°C), heat is gained from the environment (*i.e.*, termed "passive heating"). This gain of heat from the environment can also occur in situations in which protective clothing creates a microenvironment that does not allow for the dissipation of heat (9).

Increased relative humidity also stresses thermoregulation because of its effect on sweat evaporation. Humid air will inherently move from areas of high concentration to low concentration. Thus, when relative humidity increases, the gradient for sweat to evaporate is decreased, slowing the process of sweat evaporation. For example, in high-humidity environments, sweat often pools on the skin or drips off before evaporation can occur. The microenvironment that protective clothing creates not only increases temperature (discussed earlier) but also creates an environment in which evaporated sweat is trapped in the clothing. This leads to a high-humidity microenvironment that greatly hampers loss of heat by radiation and sweat evaporation (9).

Despite the stress that high heat and humidity place on the thermoregulatory system, the body has a remarkable capability to live, work, and play in extreme environments. However, it should be recognized that core body temperature will rise more quickly in these conditions, increasing the risk for excessive hyperthermia, which in turn impairs physical and cognitive function. There are certain populations that are at an increased risk for hyperthermia during heat stress. These populations, discussed next, should take special care when living, working, or exercising in conditions of high environmental heat and/or humidity (*e.g.*, ≥85°F WBGT). Likewise, practitioners should be aware of these risks when prescribing exercise and physical activity.

Thermoregulation and Obesity

Approximately 40% of U.S. adults are obese (10). This public health problem has brought increased attention to the physiologic consequences of increased adipose tissue. Epidemiologic data suggest that individuals who are obese have an increased risk of heat illnesses (11, 12). A proposed mechanism for this increased risk is that excess adipose tissue, especially subcutaneous adipose tissue, creates a layer of insulation that impairs the dissipation of body heat (13). When attempting to explain individual differences in core temperature during heat exposure, researchers have identified obesity as a contributing factor in some studies (14, 15), but not all (16–18).

However, direct thermoregulatory comparisons between individuals who are obese and nonobese exposed to heat, either actively (*i.e.*, exercise) or passively (*i.e.*, passive heat exposure), have mixed conclusions. Females who are obese and nonobese, at low-to-moderate exercise intensities, have a similar core temperature response to exercise in the heat (19, 20). This may (21, 22) or may not (21–25) be true for males who are obese. Part of the confusion in this area of study is because of findings that show impaired skin blood flow or sweating responses but no differences in core temperature (23). For example, using a passive heating model, females who are obese reach similar core temperatures as their counterparts who are nonobese, but they have signs of impaired sweating when examining sweat rate on specific areas of the chest and forearm (26). Also contributing to mixed findings is that some early studies did not control for different magnitudes of metabolic heat production between individuals of different body sizes, particularly during treadmill and cycling exercise (20, 25).

Regardless of these mixed findings, current evidence suggests that there is no compelling reason to dissuade individuals who are obese from exercising in conditions of high heat/humidity. However, when in competitive or group settings (*e.g.*, military, American football), individuals who are obese are more susceptible than individuals who are nonobese to heat illnesses, and most heat-related deaths occur during group activities (11). Therefore, there may not be a *physiologic* impairment in individuals who are obese per se, but behavioral factors may contribute to an increased risk of heat illness. Thus, practitioners and other individuals overseeing group/team activities should be aware of the potential for individuals who are obese to be more susceptible to heat illnesses. Lastly, further studies are needed because research in this area often avoids individuals with high levels of obesity (*i.e.*, morbid obesity), uses low exercise intensities (19), and/or fails to control for confounding factors such as hydration status (22).

Thermoregulation and Diabetes

Over the last 30 years, the global prevalence of diabetes has nearly tripled, with 35 million people in the U.S.

having either diagnosed or undiagnosed diabetes in 2016 (10). During heat waves, individuals with diabetes account for a disproportionate number of hospitalizations and deaths (27), suggesting that they are not able to tolerate heat stress in a similar manner as nondiabetics. The thermoregulatory investigation of individuals with diabetes is difficult because the extent of dysfunction depends on the progression of the disease. Although many studies explicitly examine individuals with either Type 1 diabetes mellitus (T1DM) or Type 2 diabetes mellitus (T2DM), no further insight is provided about the extent of dysfunction or progression of the disease and its impact on thermoregulation (28). In fact, most studies use individuals with diabetes that have good glucose control and minimal neuropathies.

When passively heated, individuals with T1DM and T2DM have a decreased ability to increase skin blood flow (29–31), with the magnitude of impairment likely affected by the degree of neuropathy (28). Sweating responses are impaired in passively heated individuals with T2DM (30), but similar findings are mixed among individuals with T1DM (32).

During exercise heat stress, the intensity of exercise influences whether an individual with diabetes experiences thermoregulatory dysfunction. For example, during mild-intensity exercise (40% of maximal oxygen update ($\dot{V}O_{2max}$) in a 35°C [95°F] environment), individuals with T1DM have similar thermoregulatory control (*i.e.*, increase in sweating and skin blood flow) and responses (*i.e.*, increase in skin and core body temperature) compared to individuals without diabetes (32). However, at high-intensity exercise (*i.e.*, 60% $\dot{V}O_{2max}$), individuals with T1DM and T2DM have a lower sweating response than individuals without diabetes; this can lead to a greater elevation of internal temperature (33, 34).

These findings suggest that individuals with diabetes have thermoregulatory impairments that become apparent when they become hyperthermic (either via prolonged physical activity or prolonged exposure to heat). Therefore, the CEP should consider modifying the exercise duration and/or intensity when patients (*i.e.*, individuals with diabetes who have poor glucose control and/or diagnosed neuropathies) are exposed to a hot environment, given that prior research has not investigated individuals with these complications (32, 33).

It should be emphasized that individuals who have T2DM often have confounding factors that exacerbate thermoregulatory impairment. For example, they are often older, have hypertension (HTN) and/or CVD, and are obese. There is little research examining various combinations and contributions of these conditions to thermoregulatory impairment in individuals with T2DM; however, the other sections within this chapter address these conditions independently.

Thermoregulation and Age

From 2008 to 2018, the proportion of U.S. adults more than 65 years increased by 35%; over the same time period, individuals less than 65 years increased by only 4% (35). Individuals are not only living longer but also working later in life (36). Aging leads to physiologic maladaptations of the cardiovascular and thermoregulatory systems that may explain why older adults are more susceptible to heat illness and death during heat waves (37). For example, during passive heat exposure at rest, older adults have a delayed sweating response and a reduced sweat rate response (38). The ability of skin blood vessels to increase blood flow (i.e., vasodilate) also decreases as we age (39); thus, the increased skin blood flow associated with passive heating is attenuated in older adults (40).

Similarly, during exercise in the heat, older adults have an impaired increase in skin blood flow (38). In contrast, age-related differences in sweating responses during exercise are not consistently observed. Several studies have observed reduced maximal sweating ability in older (i.e., 52–62 yr) versus younger (20–30 yr) adults, but these individual differences are quite varied and may be dependent on environmental conditions, heat acclimatization status (see below), and sex (38). For example, females, who often have a smaller body size, may be at a thermoregulatory disadvantage that is exacerbated when exercising at high intensities (41). Even if sweating does not differ in older individuals, decreased thirst in older individuals can lead to greater dehydration (42), which increases cardiovascular strain and reduced exercise capacity. Overall, despite some possible differences in skin blood flow and sweating between older and younger individuals, most studies observe similar increases in core temperature when exercising in the heat (38).

Most deaths during heat waves occur in older adults, and these deaths are attributed to cardiovascular causes secondary to thermal stress (37). This suggests that older adults experience a greater cardiovascular than thermoregulatory risk during heat stress. This greater cardiovascular stress in older adults reflects their smaller cardiac stroke volume, which cannot sufficiently increase to meet the cardiovascular demand of thermoregulation. This is compounded when dehydration in older adults reduces blood volume, a major predicator of stroke

volume. Given this cardiovascular stress, it may be of no surprise that older adults also have increased markers of myocardial damage in heat-related deaths relative to younger adults (43).

Clinicians and CEPs should be aware of these thermoregulatory differences in older adults. Perhaps more important is that older adults have an increased cardiovascular strain during exercise and/or passive heat exposure that puts them at greater risk for heat illnesses and death. Thus, countermeasures such as frequent rest periods, reduced exercise intensity, or a combination of these and other strategies should be employed. Exercise prescription also should include considerations of age, appetite, nutrition, sleep quality, aerobic fitness, and history of recent heat exposures.

Like older adults, children adapt to exercise in hot environments less effectively than young adults. This primarily involves three factors. First, children have a greater surface area-to-body mass ratio than adults, which causes a greater heat gain in hot air and a greater heat loss in cold air. Second, children are less efficient (vs. adults) during walking and running, and thus produce more metabolic heat per kilogram of body mass. Third, the maximal sweating capacity of children is considerably lower than adults; this results in reduced cooling via evaporation. Despite these qualities, exercising children can dissipate heat effectively in a neutral or mildly warm climate (44, 45). It is only when air temperature exceeds 35°C (95°F) that children have a lower exercise tolerance than do adults. Children seem to be especially affected by very humid environments (46).

Thermoregulation and CVD

Chronic HTN leads to vascular changes that may include modified vasoconstriction and vasodilation. In individuals who are normotensive, increased core temperature during exercise leads to vasodilation of the cutaneous blood vessels and subsequent increased blood flow to aid in thermoregulation (3). When exercising in the heat, mild hypertensives do not have the same increases in skin blood flow, even when core temperature is significantly elevated (47). Interestingly, local and whole-body sweat rate is similar in hypertensives and normotensives, and subsequent increases of core temperature are also the same. This suggests that, despite impaired skin blood flow responses, individuals with mild HTN have similar core temperature responses to exercise in the heat. Caution is warranted in other populations (i.e., stage-2 hypertensives) because some research indicates that HTN can manifest to thermoregulatory dysfunction that is central in origin.

The cardiovascular response to heat stress includes an increase of cardiac output secondary to increased HR to compensate for the increased distribution of blood to the skin. Individuals with impaired cardiac function may not have the appropriate cardiac response and/or have an increased risk of a cardiovascular event during exposure to heat. Indeed, patients with heart failure have inappropriate changes in HR and blood pressure during heat exposure (48). From a thermoregulatory standpoint, patients with heart failure, compared to healthy controls, exhibit a blunted increase of skin blood flow during passive heat exposure, but the sweating and core temperature responses are normal (48, 49). Given the importance of exercise as management of coronary artery disease (CAD) and heart failure, future research should investigate how exercising in the heat affects these patients.

Thermoregulation and Multiple Sclerosis

Multiple sclerosis (MS) is a disease that attacks the myelin sheaths of the nerves in the central nervous system. Many patients with MS experience multiple signs and symptoms that include fatigue, pain, dizziness, numbness, and cognitive dysfunction (50). With heat exposure, 60%–80% of patients with MS experience a worsening of symptoms (51). This can be in the form of passive (*e.g.*, sitting in the heat) or active (*e.g.*, exercise) exposure. Logically, this has led many clinicians to recommend avoiding heat and exercise. However, exercise is shown to be beneficial for patients with MS and the symptoms that occur because of exercise and/or heat exposure are easily reversible (51).

MS affects the thermoregulatory system in multiple ways. When heat stressed, patients with MS have reduced sweating responses that are not improved with exercise training. Interestingly, increases in skin blood flow remain intact and may be enhanced when patients with MS are heat stressed (51). Little is known about the core temperature response during exercise in the heat in patients with MS.

Clinicians working with patients with MS should be aware of these heat-related issues. Patients with MS have worsening of symptoms, particularly increased fatigue when core body temperature increases with physical activity (52). Decreased sweating can lead to increased core temperature, so management strategies should include avoiding excess heat exposure. However, many strategies (*e.g.*, cooling garments, swimming in cool water) act as countermeasures when heat exposure is unavoidable. Thus, patients with MS should work with their physician and CEP to develop strategies that allow them to exercise in a variety of conditions.

Thermoregulation and Skin Grafts

Severe burns that require split-thickness grafts involve excision of the epidermis and all (or part) of the dermis. The procedure disrupts the vascular bed and the associated neural connections in the grafted skin; moreover, the sweat gland ducts are either removed or disrupted (53). Therefore, when exposed to heat stress, grafted skin does not allow increased skin blood flow or sweating (54). This local impairment of thermoregulation can lead to whole-body hyperthermia during passive heating and exercise heat exposure (53). The amount of skin that is grafted influences the degree of impairment. Individuals with grafts covering as little as 20% of their skin surface area can have an exaggerated increase in core temperature relative to individuals with nongraft (53). However, the greatest predicator of thermoregulatory impairment is the surface area of *nongrafted* skin. That is, the magnitude of core temperature increase during exercise in the heat is best predicated by the magnitude of nongrafted skin, and individuals with less than 1.0 m^2 of nongrafted skin have the greatest impairment (53). This may seem counterintuitive, but the nongrafted skin is the tissue that is able to thermoregulate.

Regardless of these impairments, exercise should be encouraged for individuals with well-healed skin grafts, because, on average, they are less physically fit than individuals without skin grafts (55). Exercise in the heat should be monitored if individuals have a large proportion of their body covered with skin grafts. Such individuals may need to decrease exercise intensity, have more frequent rest periods, or explore cooling strategies (*e.g.*, swimming in cool water, wearing cooling garments) to mitigate the heat stress.

Thermoregulation and Spinal Cord Injury

As compared to adults who are healthy, individuals with spinal cord injuries (SCIs) have a greater increase in core temperature during exercise in the heat (56). The neural disruption with the injury impairs the sweating response and increases skin blood flow when the individual (*i.e.*, with low-level spinal cord lesion) is exposed to heat stress (56). The magnitude of thermoregulatory impairment varies according to the level of the SCI, such that individuals with a higher level of SCI will have a greater increase in core temperature. This same relationship can be observed when patients with SCI are exposed to passive heat exposure (56). In cooler temperatures (25°C or 77°F), when the thermoregulatory system is less stressed, impairments of thermoregulation are less apparent at rest and during exercise in patients with SCI (56).

Patients with SCI should take extra precautions when working/exercising in a hot environment. Impaired thermoregulation in regions below the injury impairs whole-body heat loss and will lead to increased heat storage in deep tissues. Thus, patients with SCI will be more susceptible to the negative side effects of heat stress.

Assessing and Mitigating the Risk of Heat Stress

Increased core body temperature leads to multiple cognitive and physiologic impairments that can greatly diminish an individual's ability to exercise and/or work in the heat and can threaten the individual's health and life. All other things being equal (*e.g.*, exercise intensity), individuals with impaired thermoregulation and/or low cardiorespiratory fitness will experience the detrimental effects of heat stress sooner than those who are healthy. As a result, they will decrease exercise intensity and perform less work. This is especially true in noncompetitive situations when an individual is not exercising alongside a competitor (57). Therefore, assessing and mitigating heat stress is essential.

One way of managing exercise intensity during heat exposures is by using target heart rate (THR). For example, a THR that is determined in a mild environment may be useful as a guide for exercise prescription in a hot environment, because increased heat stress causes the THR to be reached at a lower speed, distance, or resistance.

Figure 17.1 presents an important and simple way to determine heat stress in the environment using the dry bulb temperature (ambient air temperature not affected by moisture) and relative humidity, commonly provided as part of weather forecasts. The CEP can use this tool to determine the approximate risk of heat exhaustion and heatstroke before exercise begins. Doing so allows the CEP to modify the duration, intensity, and type of exercise to match the environmental heat stress on any given day.

The WBGT index is a more sophisticated heat index that is used in labor, sport, and military settings. Determining the WBGT requires specialized equipment that is

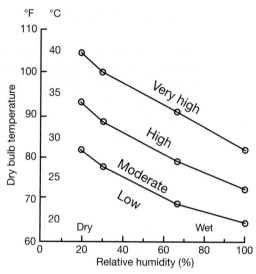

FIGURE 17.1 Approximate risk of heat exhaustion and heatstroke during strenuous exercise in a hot environment. Dry bulb temperature (air temperature) and relative humidity are commonly provided in weather forecasts. (Reprinted from Armstrong LE, Epstein Y, Greenleaf JE, et al. ACSM position stand: heat and cold illnesses during distance running. *Med Sci Sports Exerc.* 1996;28(10):139–48; using data from Armstrong LE. Nutritional strategies for football: counteracting heat, cold, high altitude, and jet lag. *J Sports Sci.* 2006;24(7):723–40; Pescatello LS, Arena R, Riebe D, Thompson PD. Exercise prescription for healthy populations with special considerations and environmental considerations. In: *American College of Sports Medicine's Guidelines for Exercise Testing and Prescription.* Baltimore (MD): Lippincott Williams & Wilkins; 2014. p. 194–226; Pescatello LS, Arena R, Riebe D, Thompson PD. *Exercise prescription for populations with other chronic diseases and health conditions. In: American College of Sports Medicine's Guidelines for Exercise Testing and Prescription.* Baltimore (MD): Lippincott Williams & Wilkins; 2014. p. 260–343.)

not available at weather stations. However, when air temperature, relative humidity, solar radiation, wind speed, and dew point temperature are available, WBGT can be calculated (58).

Multiple strategies can mitigate the risk and side effects of heat stress. This is important when high ambient temperature and/or high relative humidity cannot be avoided (*e.g.*, ≥85°F WBGT).

Acclimatization

Heat acclimatization (see Table 17.2) is one of the most effective preemptive measures that individuals can do to prepare their body for physical activity in the heat. This process involves 8–14 days of heat exposure, in which activity/exposure is progressively increased so that adaptations can occur. With full acclimatization, individuals will have a reduced core temperature response and an increased capacity to exercise in the heat relative to the period before acclimatization (3).

The acclimatization process can vary from person to person, but there is little evidence that the populations presented earlier are unable to acclimatize because of disease or personal idiosyncrasies. Specifically, it has been shown that heat acclimatization is effective in older adults, individuals who are obese, and individuals with well-healed skin grafts (38, 59). However, the process may take longer in certain clinical populations because of impaired thermoregulation relative to their healthy counterparts. Likewise, it is doubtful that the acclimatization process will "fix" impaired thermoregulation, although it may improve it (59).

Modifications for Exercise in a Hot Environment

Schedule exercise during a cooler time of the day, such as early morning, and select a location that is shaded from direct sunlight. Alternatively, exercise in an air-conditioned environment.

Patients who customarily use their THR to monitor exercise stress in a mild environment should use the same THR in a hot environment. Because HR increases in response to environmental heat stress, the THR will reduce the intensity and duration of the workout to an individualized, manageable level.

When possible, wear lightweight, loose-fitting clothing that encourages heat loss and sweat evaporation. Clothing that is worn for safety can create a microenvironment that greatly increases heat stress. Cooling garments may be worn in conjunction with other clothing throughout the activity or during rest periods (60). This area of research is still developing, but it is prudent to acknowledge that some garments may make individuals "feel better" without affecting their core temperature. This is important because a decrease in core temperature is required to reduce the risk of heat illnesses such as heatstroke (8).

Precooling (e.g., by cold water immersion, drinking ice-water mixtures, and packing ice on the neck, head, armpits, and groin areas) has been shown to enhance exercise performance in the heat because it lowers the internal body temperature, allowing a greater amount of heat to be stored before a critical body temperature is reached (61). Similar strategies may be effective for paraplegics and athletes with low spinal cord lesions (62).

Dehydration impairs exercise performance. A thorough review of the scientific literature indicated that endurance performance declines at approximately 3% body weight loss, and strength/power performance declines at about 5% body weight loss (63). Laboratory and field investigations also indicate that even mild dehydration of 1%–2% may reduce endurance exercise performance (64, 65). During training sessions, fluids should be readily available, chilled, and palatable.

Clinical Considerations for Exercise in Hot Environments

Clinical populations such as those who are obese and those who have diabetes, CVD, MS, skin grafts, or paraplegia have physiologic dysfunction that can lead to elevated body temperature during exercise heat exposure. Demographic factors such as age can also influence thermoregulation. Medications such as diuretics, β-blockers, and vasodilators may have a direct effect on thermoregulation and risk of heat illness. Individuals who take medications should consult with their physician.

The negative effects of elevated heat and humidity may be exacerbated in environments having significant air pollution. The effects of air pollution on health and exercise performance are discussed later in this chapter.

Heat acclimatization is the most effective method of reducing an individual's risk for heat illness, but it does not guarantee safety, especially if thermoregulation is inherently impaired. Other strategies to minimize heat stress include cooling modalities and optimizing rehydration.

Water and electrolyte losses usually are modest during brief exercise sessions (i.e., 20–40 min duration). A normal diet will replenish these deficits. Individuals who eat a low sodium diet (e.g., patients with HTN) should visit their physician to discuss the effects of exercise on whole-body sodium balance.

Although most individuals experience dehydration during exercise, it is possible to consume too much water or hypotonic fluid (e.g., sport drinks), to the point of illness or death, during exercise bouts lasting longer than 3–4 hours (66). Known as exertional hyponatremia (EHN) or water intoxication, this rare condition occurs when the volume of consumed fluid exceeds water losses in urine and sweat, causing dilution of body fluids, specifically a decrease of serum sodium concentration. Severe symptomatic EHN may involve signs and symptoms such as disorientation, depression, nausea, vomiting, seizure, coma, respiratory arrest, and lung or brain swelling (67). To avoid EHN, everyone should develop a personalized fluid intake plan that incorporates a measurement of sweat rate (easily accomplished by measuring nude body weight before after exercise, accounting for food/fluid intake and urine losses); this plan should be tested during field simulations involving anticipated environmental conditions, clothing, exercise duration, and exercise intensity.

EXERCISE IN COLD ENVIRONMENTS

In cold climates, several environmental stressors can affect health and exercise performance by disturbing homeostasis in the body's organ systems. These include very low air temperature that cools the skin, rain that moistens clothing and skin, high wind speed that accelerates heat loss via convection and evaporation, and minimal direct solar radiation. When even one of these conditions exists, anyone who exercises outdoors is at increased risk of hypothermia.

Hypothermia

Mild hypothermia is an internal body temperature of 34°C–35°C (94°F–95°F). Severe hypothermia is a temperature of 25°C–32°C (77°F–90°F). In terms of heat production and heat loss during exercise, hypothermia occurs when heat loss through the skin and lungs exceeds the metabolic heat produced by muscle contractions. The greatest risk of developing hypothermia during outdoor exercise exists on cloudy, cold, rainy, windy days. However, many factors interact to determine if outdoor exercise will result in hypothermia, including high wind speed, wet clothing, the percentage of skin surface covered, exercise intensity, health status, and age. As discussed shortly, air pollution can exacerbate the effects of cold exposure. Individual risk factors for hypothermia include low body fat, older age (*i.e.*, ≥60 yr), and serum hypoglycemia (68).

Cold acclimatization occurs during 8–14 days of exercise (see Table 17.2) but is subtle when compared to heat acclimatization. Whereas the initial (acute) responses to cold exposure include constriction of skin blood vessels, shivering, increased HR, and increased blood pressure, the process of cold acclimatization results in reduced shivering, blunted skin vasoconstriction, normal HR, and normal blood pressure (69).

Because a frigid, wet, windy environment can easily overwhelm thermoregulatory responses, individuals who exercise outdoors during winter months should optimize exercise performance by limiting the duration of cold exposure and insulating/covering skin surfaces with clothing. For optimal insulation and to be well prepared

for changing conditions during winter activity in a severe cold or cold-wet environment, clothing should be worn in three layers: a thin inner fabric (*i.e.*, polypropylene or polyester), an insulative middle layer (*i.e.*, wool or polyester fleece), and an outer layer that repels rain and wind, while allowing moisture to escape to the air. The latter must be worn when wind speed is high or when rain threatens to soak inner layers, because insulative layers are less effective when wet. Modern fabrics allow lightweight garments to be worn around the waist or carried in a small lumbar pack, then applied as needed. Advanced planning can reduce heat loss and the risk of hypothermia in three ways:

1. Select clothing layers to minimize sweating
2. Select the direction of walking, running, or cycling to avoid frontal wind exposure during the final stage of exercise, when clothing and skin are more likely to be wet
3. Remove wet clothing immediately after exercise ends (*i.e.*, as soon as metabolic heat production decreases) and after moving to a warm room

Cold Injuries

Frostbite (*i.e.*, cold-induced trauma in skin) occurs most commonly in the nose, fingers, toes, ears, and cheeks, when skin temperature falls below 0°C (32°F). Three clinical frostbite categories have been described (70):

- Frostnip involves freezing damage to the outer layer of skin. Frostnip often has the appearance of a first-degree burn and leads to frostbite if cold exposure continues. As it heals, it appears similar to sunburn.
- Superficial frostbite injures the outer layer of skin plus some of the underlying tissue. Blisters usually appear within 24 hours.
- Severe frostbite involves crystallization of fluid in the skin, formation of blood clots in arterioles, poor oxygen delivery to skin cells, and degeneration of the inner walls of blood vessels.

The Wind Chill Temperature Index provides one of the most effective means of preventing frostnip and frostbite (Figure 17.2). This index identifies the risk of freezing flesh on the face and incorporates both air temperature and wind speed, two critical determinants of cold injuries. It does not predict hypothermia.

Skin and underlying tissues can be damaged in the absence of freezing, when cold-wet conditions exist concurrently with air temperatures of 0°C–15°C (32°F–60°F) for prolonged periods of time. Known as nonfreezing cold injuries, they result from prolonged cold-wet exposure

Wind speed (mph)

Air temperature (°F)

	40	35	30	25	20	15	10	5	0	−5	−10	−15	−20	−25	−30	−35	−40	−45
5	36	31	25	19	13	7	1	−5	−11	−16	−22	−28	−34	−40	−46	−52	−57	−63
10	34	27	21	15	9	3	−4	−10	−16	−22	−28	−35	−41	−47	−53	−59	−66	−72
15	32	25	19	13	6	0	−7	−13	−19	−26	−32	−39	−45	−51	−58	−64	−71	−77
20	30	24	17	11	4	−2	−9	−15	−22	−29	−35	−42	−48	−55	−61	−68	−74	−81
25	29	23	16	9	3	−4	−11	−17	−24	−31	−37	−44	−51	−58	−64	−71	−78	−84
30	28	22	15	8	1	−5	−12	−19	−26	−33	−39	−46	−53	−60	−67	−73	−80	−87
35	28	21	14	7	0	−7	−14	−21	−27	−34	−41	−48	−55	−62	−69	−76	−82	−89
40	27	20	13	6	−1	−8	−15	−22	−29	−36	−43	−50	−57	−64	−71	−78	−84	−91
45	26	19	12	5	−2	−9	−16	−23	−30	−37	−44	−51	−58	−65	−72	−79	−86	−93
50	26	19	12	4	−3	−10	−17	−24	−31	−38	−45	−52	−60	−67	−74	−81	−88	−95
55	25	18	11	4	−3	−11	−18	−25	−32	−39	−46	−54	−61	−68	−75	−82	−89	−97
60	25	17	10	3	−4	−11	−19	−26	−33	−40	−48	−55	−62	−69	−76	−84	−91	−98

Frostbite times: ☐ Frostbite could occur in 30 min
▦ Frostbite could occur in 10 min
▩ Frostbite could occur in 5 min

FIGURE 17.2 The Wind Chill Temperature Index indicates frostbite exposure times for facial skin. (National Weather Service, United States. Available from: http://www.nws.noaa.gov/om/winter/resources/wind-chill-brochure.pdf.)

inside gloves or boots (70). In comparison to the minutes required to develop frostnip and frostbite (see Figure 17.2), nonfreezing cold injuries may develop across a span of half to 4 days. The most common are trench foot and chilblains. Trench foot occurs in tissues that are exposed to cold-wet conditions for prolonged periods of time, most commonly in the foot. Signs and symptoms include swelling, edema, numbness, aches, increased pain sensitivity, and infections. Chilblain (also known as pernio) is a superficial cold injury that occurs on fingers, ears, face, and exposed skin. Symptoms include swelling, tenderness, itching, and pain. Upon rewarming, the skin becomes inflamed, red and hot to the touch, and swollen, with an itching or burning sensation that may continue for several hours after exposure. There are no lasting effects from chilblain (70). Trench foot and chilblains are relatively uncommon in sports, but a higher incidence is observed during winter activities such as hiking. These injuries can be prevented by wearing dry socks, boots, and gloves and by reducing the length of periods of inactivity.

All the above cold injuries (*i.e.*, frostnip, frostbite, trench foot, and chilblains) require medical treatment. Patients should be evacuated immediately to a hospital.

Clinical Considerations for Exercise in Cold Environments

In a cold environment, individuals with asthma and CVD are more likely to experience exacerbated signs and symptoms (*e.g.*, angina) or cardiovascular-related mortality, because inhalation of cold-dry air stimulates the sympathetic nervous system, alters the temperature of blood, and reduces oxygen delivery to the heart muscle

via coronary arteries (71). Inhaling cold air (5°F–25°F, −15°C to −4°C) reduces upper airway temperature but not that of the lower respiratory tract and does not alter the pulmonary function of individuals who are healthy.

Strenuous exercise in cold air may trigger additional problems. First, bronchoconstriction may occur in individuals with allergies, because of facial cooling (72). Second, exercise-induced bronchospasm (EIB) describes the acute transient airway narrowing that occurs during or after exercise, in 10%–50% of elite athletes, depending upon the sport (73). Third, secretion and clearance of mucous may interfere with exercise that requires a high rate of ventilation (74).

Raynaud disease is a disorder of the cardiovascular system. Symptoms typically include intermittent, painful spasms of the blood vessels in the hands and feet. These spasms are induced by cold air or by contact with a cold object. Raynaud disease is five times more common in women than in men, but the physiologic mechanism is not clearly understood. It is believed that sympathetic nervous system activity and genetic predisposition underlie this annoying disorder (75). Both classical conditioning and biofeedback therapies have been used successfully to train patients with Raynaud disease to increase the temperature of their digits (76).

For individuals with CVD, the intensity, duration, and mode of exercise in a cold environment should be selected with care. Activities should be avoided if they involve the upper body (*e.g.*, chopping wood), require lifting the arms above the head, increase cardiovascular strain during usual activities (*e.g.*, walking on icy ground or in deep snow), or mask symptoms of angina (*e.g.*, swimming in cool water) (77). The best-known examples involve shoveling snow or chopping wood in cold air: arterial pressure, the force of contraction, and total cardiac work increase during exercise. These changes result in reduced exercise tolerance, angina pectoris symptoms, and increased risk of acute myocardial infarction (*i.e.*, heart attack) in patients with CAD, even during mild exercise (77, 78).

Considering the stresses that a cold environment presents to the body, individuals with HTN, CVD, or respiratory disease should consider their present level of fitness, how long they have been involved in a regular exercise program, and if signs or symptoms exist (see Figure 3.1). Depending on the interaction of these factors, approval by a health care professional may be necessary to engage in exercise (1). The prescription of duration, intensity, and frequency of exercise in a cold environment should be individualized to incorporate factors such as symptoms, age, recognized physical limitations, and present cardiorespiratory fitness. Some individuals may require a health-related fitness assessment, conducted by a certified exercise test technologist, before initiating exercise training in a cold environment.

Medications that improve oxygen demand, or oxygen delivery to the heart, should limit the stress effects of exercise in a cold environment. For example, calcium channel blockers, nitroglycerin, and nicorandil may reduce cold-induced coronary vasoconstriction in persons with CAD (78). Individuals with asthma or another breathing disorder should always have "rescue" medication available when exercising in cold air (79).

EFFECTS OF AIR POLLUTION ON HEALTH AND EXERCISE PERFORMANCE

Air pollution is a modern environmental stressor consisting of gases and particulates that are produced primarily by the combustion of fossil fuels. A growing body of scientific evidence shows that long-term exposure to air pollution is linked to increased risk of several chronic diseases, including CVD (80, 81), asthma (82–84), chronic obstructive pulmonary disease (COPD) (85, 86), T2DM (87, 88), incident atrial fibrillation (89, 90), and cancer (91, 92). From 1990 to 2019, ambient particulate matter pollution rose from 13th to 8th and 17th to 8th leading global risk factor for years of life lost because of premature mortality and years lived with disability or injury, respectively (10). Further, individuals with comorbidities, including HTN, diabetes, and COPD, are at an increased risk of adverse cardiovascular events in air pollution,

compared to those without these conditions (93). Overall, many studies suggest that individuals with comorbidities are more susceptible to the adverse health effects associated with air pollution (93–97).

Each airborne pollutant represents a unique stressor that exerts potentially detrimental effects on health and performance, primarily by affecting the respiratory and cardiovascular systems. Airborne pollutants are classified as primary or secondary (78, 98):

- Primary airborne pollutants (*e.g.*, carbon monoxide [CO], sulfur oxides, nitrogen oxides, fine particulates) are emitted directly from a source of pollution.
- Secondary pollutants (*e.g.*, ozone, peroxyacetyl nitrate [PAN]) are formed when primary pollutants interact with other compounds, ultraviolet light, or each other.

The following discussion summarizes the effects of each air pollutant on health and exercise performance in both healthy and clinical populations. Interactions between various air pollutants and other environmental factors are identified, as well as strategies to minimize the adverse health effects of air pollution.

Carbon Monoxide

CO is a colorless, odorless gas produced from the burning of fossil fuels and from cigarette smoke. Peak levels of CO are observed during the morning and afternoon automobile traffic rush hours and are higher in winter compared to summer months (see Figure 17.3) (99). CO

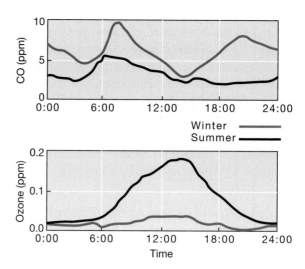

FIGURE 17.3 Daily and seasonal fluctuations of carbon monoxide (CO) and ozone concentrations in the Los Angeles area ("exercise and air pollution"; Adapted with permission from McCafferty W. *Air Pollution and Athletic Performance*. Springfield (IL): Charles C. Thomas Publisher Ltd; 1981.)

has a strong affinity for hemoglobin, which is the protein found in red blood cells responsible for approximately 99% of oxygen transport in blood. Hemoglobin combines with CO to form carboxyhemoglobin (HbCO), which blocks oxygen-binding sites on hemoglobin and decreases oxygen transport capacity. Also, HbCO inhibits the release of oxygen from hemoglobin in tissue capillaries. Environmental levels of CO sufficient to induce blood HbCO concentrations of 2.5%–20% result in a variety of cognitive and physiologic effects, including visual impairment, reduced maximal work capacity, headache, and decrements of cardiac function in individuals who are impaired (98).

In clinically healthy chronic smokers, smoking 15 cigarettes within 5 hours increased mean HbCO to 6.6% (compared to 1.8% on a nonsmoking day). These levels induce an adverse effect on cardiovascular responses to incremental exercise as evidenced by higher submaximal exercise HR and lower maximal oxygen consumption (100). These findings agree with Horvath et al. (101) who showed that the minimal HbCO threshold needed to decrease $\dot{V}O_{2max}$ was 4.3% in healthy men. In contrast, blood HbCO levels below 15% have little effect on physiologic responses to low- to moderate-intensity exercise of 35%–70% $\dot{V}O_{2max}$ (78, 102).

In patients with COPD who breathed CO (100 parts per million [ppm]) for 1 hour, blood HbCO levels increased to 4% and mean exercise time was reduced by 33% (103). In patients with ischemic heart disease exposed to CO levels sufficient to induce a blood HbCO concentration of 6%, an earlier onset of ventricular dysfunction, angina, and reduced exercise performance was observed (104). Further, the duration of exercise to the onset of angina symptoms was reduced by 22%–38% in patients with angina pectoris at blood HbCO levels of only 2% induced by passive smoke exposure (105), suggesting that exercise capacity is impaired in clinical patients at lower HbCO levels compared to individuals who are healthy. Overall, these findings support earlier evidence of a positive association between environmental levels of CO, the frequency of acute cardiorespiratory events (106, 107), and myocardial infarction mortality (108), suggesting that CO exposure may be a risk factor for cardiopulmonary disease.

Sulfur Dioxide

Sulfur dioxide (SO_2) is the primary sulfurous by-product of fossil fuel combustion. SO_2 is an upper respiratory tract irritant (80) that, when inhaled, can produce bronchoconstriction leading to increased airway resistance to breathing (109). At rest, exposure to SO_2 increases ventilation, augmenting the total volume of air inspired (and thus the total volume of SO_2), and decreases the effectiveness of nasal scrubbing (i.e., removal of gas when breathing through the nose) of SO_2 (110), thus increasing airway resistance to breathing as first described by Frank in 1962 (111). Exercise increases ventilation, suggesting that the large volume of inhaled SO_2 may exacerbate airway resistance and impair physical performance.

Studies have reported that exercise potentiates the effect of SO_2 on pulmonary function, compared to a control (untreated air) exposure, in adults who are healthy (112) and adults with asthma (113). Also, decrements of pulmonary function occur at lower levels of SO_2 exposure (i.e., 0.4–0.6 ppm) in asthmatics (113) compared to those without asthma (i.e., 1–3 ppm; 112), suggesting that individuals with asthma who are exercising are more sensitive to the bronchoconstrictive effects of SO_2. Additionally, air temperature and humidity alter the bronchoconstrictive effects of SO_2; bronchospasm occurs faster and is exacerbated in asthmatics who breathe SO_2 in cold-dry air, compared to breathing SO_2 in warm-moist air (114).

Nitrogen Dioxide

Nitrogen dioxide (NO_2) is one of six compounds in the nitrogen oxide family, which are air pollutants produced during automobile and aircraft engine combustion, firefighting, and cigarette smoking. NO_2 has been studied extensively because of its documented harmful effects on human health (102). Specifically, acute exposure to NO_2 increases airway resistance, impairs pulmonary diffusion capacity, induces hypoxemia, irritates the upper respiratory tract, and impairs pulmonary mucociliary activity in humans (115, 116).

Limited information exists that relate the effects of NO_2 with exercise performance. A review of this topic concluded that, in adults who are healthy, short-term low-level NO_2 exposure (0.5–2.0 ppm) does not induce adverse effects on pulmonary function or physical performance during submaximal exercise (80). Similar findings were observed in athletes exposed to 0.18 and 0.30 ppm NO_2 for 30 minutes while exercising on a treadmill (117).

Patients with existing respiratory disease, including chronic bronchitis, COPD, and asthma, are more susceptible to the adverse effects of NO_2 exposure (80, 118). Indeed, approximately 70% of individuals with asthma experienced an increase in airway responsiveness at rest following a 30- to 60-minute exposure to 0.1–0.3 ppm NO_2 (118). Minimal change of airway responsiveness occurred in asthmatics exposed to NO_2 during exercise (118), a finding consistent with others (119) and suggesting that exercise may reduce airway responsiveness to NO_2 in individuals with asthma. In contrast, others have shown that exposure to 0.30 ppm NO_2 for 30 minutes potentiates EIB in asthmatics (120). Exercise responses to NO_2 exposure have not been investigated at exercise intensities near or at $\dot{V}O_{2max}$.

Particulate Matter

Particulate matter includes a wide range of inhaled particles such as dust, soot, and smoke, which emanate primarily from automobile emissions, industrial combustion, pollens, molds, and wood burning. Particles are classified by aerodynamic diameter. Heightened levels of coarse (2.5–10 μm aerodynamic diameter) and fine (<2.5 μm) particles are associated with increased hospital admissions and CVD morbidity and mortality

(121–125). Fine and, especially, ultrafine (<0.1 μm) particles interact with environmental stressors (*e.g.*, wind, temperature, other air pollutants) and induce inflammatory and oxidative stress responses that impair pulmonary, cardiovascular, autonomic, hemostatic, and immune function; these may ultimately exert a chronic negative effect on health and exercise performance (Figure 17.4) (82, 83, 126).

A recent review highlights the mechanisms underlying particulate matter–associated CVD risk, including oxidative stress, inflammation, metabolic dysfunction, dyslipidemia, and autonomic dysfunction (127).

Sensitivity to increasing levels of particulate air pollution is demonstrated by increased emergency room visits, reduced pulmonary function, and increased reporting of respiratory symptoms when particulate levels are high (126–128). Moreover, recent prospective data from 114,537 middle-aged and older women enrolled in the

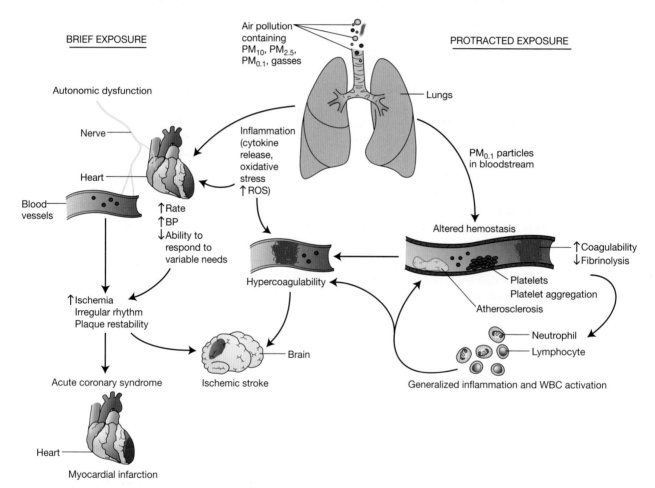

FIGURE 17.4 Pathophysiology of exposure to particulate matter in air. Potential outcomes are divided into brief (left) and long-term (right) consequences. Fine and ultrafine carbon particles carry toxic chemical products of combustion to the lungs, blood vessels, and the entire body. These microscopic particles may affect autonomic cardiovascular responses, induce inflammation, and alter blood clotting. These effects in turn may result in infarction. (Reprinted with permission from Strayer DS, Rubin E. *Rubin's Pathology*. 7th ed. Philadelphia (PA): Wolters Kluwer; 2014.)

Nurses' Health Study showed that increased long-term exposure to all sizes of particulate matter was associated with small, but not statistically significant, increased risks of incident CVD, coronary heart disease, and stroke (129). Compared to nondiabetic women, women with diabetes had significantly higher particulate matter–associated incident CVD risks, suggesting that patients with diabetes are more susceptible to the detrimental effects of particulate matter exposure on cardiovascular health (129). Data from a prospective community-based cohort study of more than 1,700 middle-aged adults showed that exposure to ambient fine particulate matter was associated with elevated blood glucose, impaired endothelial function, and increased incident CVD events and all-cause mortality (130). Ambient exposure to fine particulate matter was higher in Blacks compared to Whites, accounting, in part, for the higher risk of incident CVD events and all-cause mortality in Blacks (130). Further evidence supports a heightened cardiovascular risk to particulate matter exposure in the elderly, patients with diabetes, patients with preexisting cardiopulmonary disease, and individuals who are obese (80, 81). A large nationwide cohort study (>432,000 subjects) found a more profound effect of chronic particulate matter exposure on increased incidence of atrial fibrillation in males, older subjects ($\geq$60 yr), those characterized as obese, and those with a history of HTN or previous myocardial infarction (89). Two large prospective studies (n >132,000 women) found a stronger association between chronic particulate matter exposure and the occurrence of cardiovascular events with increasing obesity, as measured by body mass index (131, 132). These findings suggest that overweight/obesity may exacerbate the adverse health effects of air pollution. Future studies are warranted to explore this relationship, particularly because 71% and 41% of U.S. adults are considered overweight and obese, respectively (10).

The effects of particulate matter inhalation on exercise vary. In adults who are healthy, the fraction of inhaled ultrafine particles that remains in the lungs after inhalation increases by 4.5-fold (vs. rest) during moderate exercise (133). This finding suggests that exposure to particulate matter is greater during exercise, likely because of increased ventilation, and perhaps enhances the adverse effects of air pollution. Despite this, limited investigations to date have measured the effects of particulate matter on exercise performance. A recent review summarized evidence that acute exposure to particulate matter during exercise decreases pulmonary function and impairs submaximal and maximal exercise performance in adults who are healthy (126). Another study found that a 1-hour exposure to fine particulate matter prior to exercise increased exercise HR and attenuated exercise-induced bronchodilation in endurance-trained men (134).

In men with stable CAD, exposure to dilute diesel exhaust for 1 hour, at a concentration comparable to levels found in urban traffic, exacerbated exercise-induced myocardial ischemia compared to exercise performed in filtered air (135). These findings suggest that the adverse effects of air pollution persist for some time following exposure. In addition, longer time spent in traffic, thus increasing exposure to particulate matter, was directly associated with the onset of a myocardial infarction within 1-hour postexposure (122). The CEP should therefore consider the impact of travel (*i.e.*, to therapy and training) on health and exercise performance.

Ozone

Ozone (O_3), a major constituent of smog, is a secondary pollutant that is primarily produced by the atmospheric reaction between ultraviolet solar radiation (*i.e.*, sunlight) and exhaust from internal combustion engines. Peak levels of O_3 are observed year-round in the early afternoon and are markedly higher in the summer compared to winter months (see Figure 17.3) (99) when solar radiation is intense.

Armstrong (98) summarized numerous studies that investigated the effects of O_3 inhalation on exercise performance in adults who are healthy and concluded that short-term (*i.e.*, 15–120 min) O_3 exposure at concentrations that met or exceeded federal air quality standards (*i.e.*, 0.12 ppm) induced a variety of clinical symptoms (*e.g.*, cough, shortness of breath, nausea, headache), impaired pulmonary function during exercise, decreased endurance exercise performance, and increased subjective sensations of discomfort. Increased discomfort may result in earlier termination of exercise, an effect clinically important for novice exercisers or patients with limited exercise capacity. Also, compared to clean air, exposure to 0.3 ppm O_3 for 2 hours during intermittent exercise increased systemic and pulmonary markers of inflammation, impaired pulmonary function, and produced unfavorable changes of HR variability and cardiac repolarization in adults who are healthy (136).

In adults with asthma, O_3 exposure induced a greater pulmonary inflammatory response compared to nonasthmatics (137). Whether these changes increase the risk of a susceptible individual experiencing an adverse clinical event warrants future investigation. Nonetheless, these findings suggest potential pathophysiologic processes (*e.g.*, pulmonary inflammation) for the association between O_3 levels and increased cardiovascular morbidity (138, 139) and mortality (140, 141).

Peroxyacetyl Nitrate

Like O_3, PAN is a component of smog. Exposure causes eye irritation, blurred vision, and eye fatigue (142). The few studies investigating the effects of PAN exposure (0.24 ppm) during submaximal exercise showed no changes in a variety of cardiorespiratory, metabolic, and thermoregulatory responses in healthy men (78). Similarly, the limited research available during maximal exercise has shown no decrements of oxygen consumption, HR, exercise time, or ventilatory responses to PAN exposure (0.27 ppm) in healthy young and middle-aged men (143, 144). Historically, and even today, PAN concentrations over 0.50 ppm have been recorded in Los Angeles (102). Thus, further research is warranted using higher concentrations of this pollutant, especially in individuals with preexisting disease, before concluding that PAN exerts no detrimental effects on exercise performance (78).

Interactions Between Pollutants and Other Environmental Conditions

Air pollution consists of a mixture of pollutants that interact with each other and with other environmental conditions (*i.e.*, heat, cold, altitude), potentially posing a greater threat to human health and physical performance than single-pollutant exposure (81). Laboratory studies investigating the effects of air pollutant mixtures on physiologic responses during submaximal and maximal exercise in mostly individuals who are healthy suggest that most, if not all, pollutant mixtures exert a benign interaction; however, they either have no effect or have no effects beyond those induced by a single pollutant (98).

Because excessive heat and humidity increase cardiovascular mortality and emergency hospital admissions (145, 146), especially in elderly patients with chronic disease (146), and elevated air pollution levels often occur simultaneously with excessive heat and humidity (147), an assumption might be that the combined stresses of poor air quality and high heat and humidity further increase adverse events. Pandolf (78) summarized studies in individuals who are healthy performing exercise and found that heat stress and high relative humidity enhanced the adverse effects (*i.e.*, subjective complaints, pulmonary function decrements) of exposure to various air pollutants, including CO, PAN, O_3, and SO_2. However, only a few studies have specifically examined the interactive effects of high heat/humidity and elevated air pollution on adverse cardiovascular outcomes. In 694 older men, decreases in HR variability (indicative of an autonomic shift toward less parasympathetic and more

sympathetic activity) were greatest when both environmental temperature and O_3, but not fine particulate matter, levels were elevated (148). Further, findings from a large Chinese city characterized by high environmental temperatures and elevated air pollutant levels showed that increased concentrations of coarse particulate matter were associated with increased risk of CVD mortality and that the strongest particulate matter mortality effects occurred on extremely hot days (149). Future research is needed to better determine the adverse health effects of heat stress and/or humidity in combination with air pollution in clinical populations, particularly during exercise.

Few studies have evaluated the interactive effects of environmental cold and air pollution. Breathing cold and/or polluted air during exercise increases the risk for airway disorders, including asthma, in athletes (150). Epidemiologic findings from central Arkansas, a region characterized by high CVD morbidity and mortality rates, suggest stronger effects of short-term exposure to environmental fine particulate matter on CVD and respiratory disease hospital emergency visits during the colder months of October to March versus the warmer months of April to September (151). These findings were attributed to an increase in indoor wood burning during colder winter months. Interactive effects between airborne fine particulate matter and cardiovascular or respiratory hospitalizations during the winter months also have been reported in the Northeast U.S. (152). It remains to be determined if breathing cold, polluted air during exercise (compared to warm, polluted air) induces greater cardiorespiratory effects, impairs exercise performance, and/or increases the risk of adverse events in individuals who are susceptible.

Pandolf (78) reviewed the few studies that have examined the effects of CO inhalation during exercise at high altitude and found little to no impact of CO exposure on pulmonary function, oxygen consumption, and exercise performance compared to sea level. Additional research is necessary to determine if the adverse effects of CO or other air pollutants are enhanced at high altitude.

Clinical Considerations for Exercise in Polluted Environments

Multiple hours or repeated days of exposure to O_3 and SO_2 may result in minor, beneficial physiologic adaptations that represent a form of acclimatization (98). These adaptations (see Table 17.2) are not completely understood, but likely result from changes of bronchial inflammation and immune function and may last only a few days.

Individuals should engage in regular physical activity to reduce the likelihood of adverse effects attributed to air pollution (153–155). Strategies to minimize the adverse health effects of air pollution exposure during exercise are summarized below (80, 81, 98, 156).

Individuals should consider the environment prior to and during exercise. For example, they should check local air quality forecasts (157), schedule workouts accordingly, and reduce the amount of time spent performing vigorous activity or choose a less strenuous activity when air pollution levels are high. They should perform exercise away from heavy traffic and in the morning, especially in summer months, to minimize afternoon O_3 exposure. Further, individuals should minimize their exposure to air pollutants while traveling by closing windows and limiting air flow into their vehicle. Additionally, exposure to secondhand cigarette smoke should be avoided before, during, and after exercise.

Individuals more susceptible to the adverse effects of air pollution (*e.g.*, the elderly and those with cardiovascular or respiratory conditions) should consult with a physician before beginning an exercise program and should be educated about the potential health risks posed by air pollution. Pretreatment with antiasthmatic medications (*e.g.*, montelukast) before exercise may reduce exercise-induced bronchoconstriction (158). The CEP should know the ways that air pollution may affect exercise testing and prescription (*e.g.*, increased HR and myocardial ischemia), particularly in those with compromised cardiovascular function. Further, the CEP should advise patients to stop exercising immediately and seek medical advice if symptoms occur, such as tightness in the chest, coughing, wheezing, excess mucus, or shortness of breath.

EXERCISE AT ALTITUDE

The Earth's atmosphere changes with ascent to higher altitude. As air pressure decreases, the density of oxygen (*i.e.*, the number of oxygen molecules per liter) also decreases, causing a low partial pressure of oxygen, even though the percentage of oxygen in air remains constant (at ~20.9% of all gases). These differences — low air pressure and low partial pressure of oxygen — explain why the atmosphere at high altitude (*i.e.*, 1,500–3,500 m [4,921–11,483 feet]) is often described as "thin air."

In a healthy adult resting at sea level, 96%–98% of blood hemoglobin is saturated with oxygen. Upon initial resting exposure to hypobaric (low pressure) hypoxia (low oxygen content of inspired air) at an altitude of 4,300 m (14,107 feet), the blood oxygen saturation drops to approximately 80% (159). This decreased arterial saturation reduces delivery of oxygen to skeletal muscle during exercise. In response, the brain senses this lower level of oxygen in blood and increases the rate and depth of breathing (*i.e.*, hyperventilation) and increases HR to enhance the amount of blood pumped by the heart each minute (*i.e.*, cardiac output).

Altitude Illnesses

The three most common altitude illnesses are acute mountain sickness (AMS), high-altitude pulmonary edema (HAPE), and high-altitude cerebral edema (HACE). Table 17.3 compares their signs and symptoms, treatment, and prognosis. Notice that descent to lower altitude is the preferred treatment for all three types of altitude illness. Their common risk factors include rapid ascent, dehydration, and prolonged exercise.

The severity of AMS, the most common form, develops in direct proportion to the altitude and rate of ascent; thus, slow ascent across several days is advisable. The estimated incidence of AMS in individuals ascending to moderate altitude, high altitude, and very high altitude is 15% or less, 15%–70%, and 70%–85%, respectively. AMS symptoms usually maximize during the first day of exposure and recovery occurs across the next 24–48 hours (160). Prophylactic or therapeutic prescription of the medication acetazolamide (*i.e.*, Diamox) and dexamethasone (*i.e.*, Decadron, Hexadrol) may be helpful if other treatments are not available or effective. Headache is most effectively treated with ibuprofen.

Mitigating the Effects of High Altitude on Exercise

The exercise performance of most individuals decreases at altitudes of approximately 1,200 m (4,000 feet) or more. The most common effects involve an increased exercise time for a given task and more frequent rest periods (161). Exercise performance worsens as ascent progresses to high altitudes of 2,400–4,000 m (7,874–13,123 feet) and very high altitudes more than 4,000 m (>13,123 feet). This reduced performance is primarily because of reduced oxygen delivery to skeletal muscles. For example, declines by 8% at an altitude of 1,609 m (5,280 feet) and by 33% at 5,000 m (16,400 feet), which is the highest human habitation on Earth (162).

During the first few days at high altitudes, all adults should minimize their physical activity to reduce susceptibility to altitude illnesses. After several days of exposure,

Table 17.3	Recognition and Treatment of AMS, HAPE, and HACE	
	Signs and Symptoms	**Treatment**
Acute mountain sickness (AMS)	• Fatigue, dizziness • Headache • Irritability • Shortness of breath • Nausea, vomiting • Reduced appetite • Difficulty sleeping • Persistent, rapid pulse • Peripheral swelling • Cough and sore throat may also occur	• Descend to low altitude • Acetazolamide • Dexamethasone
High-altitude pulmonary edema (HAPE)[a]	• Symptoms resemble bronchitis • Persistent dry cough • Pink and frothy sputum • Fever with chills • Nasal congestion • Very rapid breathing • Breathless during exercise or at rest • Blue skin or mucous membranes	• Descend to low altitude • Furosemide • Nifedipine
High-altitude cerebral edema (HACE)[a]	• Headache does not respond to analgesics • Unsteady gait • Unilateral paralysis • Lethargy, weakness • Ashen-colored skin • Nausea • Mental impairment • Confusion, coma	• Descend to low altitude • Dexamethasone

For all the illnesses above, the prognosis and return to activity depend on clinical considerations of the following factors: complete alleviation of symptoms, highest altitude reached, severity of symptoms, duration of exposure, timing of descent to low altitude, and pharmacologic intervention.
[a]Life-threatening illness and medical emergency.

most adults can engage in the same number of weekly training sessions as performed at sea level, with a similar duration of each session. This phenomenon reflects adaptations in the cardiovascular, respiratory, and muscular systems (see Table 17.2). The THR utilized at sea level can be applied at high altitude, because the increased stress of hypobaric hypoxia causes the THR to be reached at a lower speed, distance, or resistance (163). Exercise prescription for adults who are healthy should also include considerations of appetite, nutrition, sleep quality, aerobic fitness, and history of recent altitude exposures.

Acclimatization

Acclimatization to high altitude (*i.e.*, repeated days of exercise, with gradually increasing duration and total work)

reduces symptoms of all altitude illnesses and optimizes cognitive and physical performance. As a result of 8–14 days of acclimatization, the following adaptations also occur:

- Improved physical performance
- Decreased HR at rest and during submaximal exercise
- Increased arterial oxygen saturation

Partial altitude acclimatization develops during living at a moderate elevation, known as staging, before ascending to a higher target elevation; in high and very high altitudes, ascent should be limited to 1,000 feet (305 m) per day.

Preparing for Competition at High Altitude

Athletes should plan their training and prepare carefully for competition at high altitude (164). Several

CHAPTER REVIEW QUESTIONS

1. The combination of cold air, high wind speed, rain, and/or sweat-soaked skin encourages the development of hypothermia. During exercise in such an environment, how would you use clothing to reduce the risk of hypothermia?

2. Explain how high environmental temperature and humidity decrease an individual's ability to maintain an internal temperature at 37°C (98.6°F).

3. List at least five clinical populations with an increased risk for a compromised ability to thermoregulate in a hot environment.

4. What strategies can be used to mitigate the thermoregulatory stress of exercising in a hot, humid environment? Identify at least five.

5. Explain (in terms of air oxygen content and red blood cells) why descent to a lower altitude is a valuable aspect of treatment for altitude illnesses.

6. Living at high altitude (2,500 m above sea level for 18 h a day) and training at a lower altitude (1,000–1,800 m for 24 h a day) increase blood hemoglobin mass and red cell volume in healthy, young athletes (179). What two environmental stressors stimulate these adaptations? Why are these adaptations important to athletic success?

7. Describe the physiologic processes by which particulate matter exposure may exert adverse effects on health and exercise performance.

8. Explain how CO can affect oxygen transport and endurance exercise performance.

9. As a health care professional working in an urban setting, what advice would you give to a patient with heart disease beginning a cardiac rehabilitation program to minimize the effects of air pollution on health and exercise performance?

10. Describe a simple method to self-assess hydration state, using body weight, urine color, and thirst. Explain how these three observations should be interpreted to determine the likelihood of whole-body dehydration.

Case Study 17.1

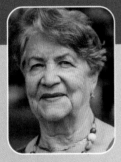

Natalie, a 67-year-old woman who is sedentary and obese, decided to begin a weight loss exercise program on the hottest day of the summer in Fort Lauderdale, Florida (USA). She walked 2.8 miles (4.5 km) briskly until she felt dizzy and nauseated, with a throbbing headache. At that point, she stood quietly for a few minutes, on the unshaded parking lot of an elementary school playground, hoping that she soon would feel better. Still not feeling better, she removed the jacket of her sweat suit. The next thing she recalled was waking, with a large swollen bruise on her forehead, in the emergency department of a nearby hospital. The attending nurse explained that she had fainted and struck her head on the asphalt surface of the playground.

Case Study 17.1 Questions

1. What environmental factors and personal characteristics resulted in Natalie's fainting (syncope) spell?

2. What role did her skin blood vessels, a hot environment, clothing, and exercise play in Natalie's syncopal episode?

3. What steps should Natalie take and who should she consult before resuming her exercise program?

Case Study 17.2

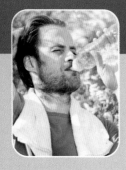

Miguel, a 40-year-old physically active man with asthma, decided to go for a bike ride on a 7°C (45°F) sunny afternoon in January. Ten miles from home, a fast-moving cold front suddenly dropped the outside temperature to 2°C (36°F), the wind speed increased to 15 mph, and it began sleeting. Miguel did not check the forecast before leaving his house and was not prepared for this sudden weather change. He was wearing only lightweight pants, a light jacket over a cotton short-sleeve shirt, a thin pair of gloves, and a helmet. He forgot his cell phone at home. Miguel decided to return home as quickly as possible. Five miles from home, Miguel was breathing heavily, sweating, shivering uncontrollably, and his face and fingers were numb. Miguel continued riding, finally arriving back home 30 minutes later. He quickly changed into dry clothes and turned up the thermostat to warm up.

Case Study 17.2 Questions

1. What factors increased the risk of Miguel developing hypothermia during his bike ride?

2. What specific steps should individuals who exercise outdoors during winter months take to reduce the risk of hypothermia?

Case Study 17.3

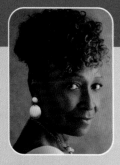

Elaine, a 58-year-old sedentary woman with Type 2 diabetes, lives in a large city. She wants to begin a walking program to improve her health. She decided to begin her walking program on a hot, hazy morning in the middle of summer. She walked 0.5 miles (0.8 km) briskly until she felt dizzy and nauseated, with moderate chest pain. She sat for a few minutes on a park bench, hoping that she would soon feel better. Still not feeling better, she caught the attention of a passing police officer. She was evaluated and quickly transported to the emergency department of a nearby hospital for treatment.

Case Study 17.3 Questions

1. What environmental factors and personal characteristics resulted in Elaine's symptoms?

2. What strategies should individuals who exercise outdoors in large cities take to reduce their exposure to air pollution?

REFERENCES

1. Riebe D, Franklin BA, Thompson PD, et al. Updating ACSM's recommendations for exercise preparticipation health screening. *Med Sci Sports Exerc.* 2015;47(11):2473–9.

2. Perkins SE, Alexander LV, Nairn JR. Increasing frequency, intensity and duration of observed global heat waves and warm spells. *Geophys Res Lett.* 2012;39:L20714.

3. Armstrong LE, Casa DJ, Millard-Stafford M, Moran DS, Pyne SW, Roberts WO. American college of sports medicine position stand. Exertional heat illness during training and competition. *Med Sci Sports Exerc.* 2007;39(3):556–72.

4. Kjellstrom T, Lemke B, Otto M. Mapping occupational heat exposure and effects in South-East Asia: ongoing time trends 1980–2011 and future estimates to 2050. *Ind Health.* 2013;51(1):56–67.

5. National Weather Service. *Weather Related Fatality and Injury Statistics.* Silver Spring (MD): National Weather Service; 2020. Available from: https://www.weather.gov/hazstat/.

6. Binkley HM, Beckett J, Casa DJ, Kleiner DM, Plummer PE. National Athletic Trainers' Association position statement: exertional heat illnesses. *J Athl Train.* 2002;37(3):329–43.

7. Armstrong LE, Maresh CM. The induction and decay of heat acclimatisation in trained athletes. *Sports Med.* 1991;12(5):302–12.

8. Casa DJ, DeMartini JK, Bergeron MF, et al. National Athletic Trainers' Association position statement: exertional heat illnesses. *J Athl Train.* 2015;50(9):986–1000.

9. Havenith G. Heat balance when wearing protective clothing. *Ann Occup Hyg.* 1999;43(5):289–96.

10. Virani SS, Alonso A, Aparicio HJ, et al; American Heart Association Council on Epidemiology and Prevention Statistics Committee and Stroke Statistics Subcommittee. Heart disease and stroke statistics — 2021 update: a report from the American Heart Association. *Circulation.* 2021;143(8):e2 54–e743.

11. Bedno SA, Li Y, Han W, et al. Exertional heat illness among overweight U.S. Army recruits in basic training. *Aviat Space Environ Med.* 2010;81(2):107–11.

12. Wallace RF, Kriebel D, Punnett L, et al. Risk factors for recruit exertional heat illness by gender and training period. *Aviat Space Environ Med.* 2006;77(4):415–21.

13. Anderson GS. Human morphology and temperature regulation. *Int J Biometeorol.* 1999;43(3):99–109.

14. Cramer MN, Jay O. Explained variance in the thermoregulatory responses to exercise: the independent roles of biophysical and fitness/fatness-related factors. *J Appl Physiol.* 2015;119(9):982–9.

15. Havenith G, Coenen JM, Kistemaker L, Kenney WL. Relevance of individual characteristics for human heat stress response is dependent on exercise intensity and climate type. *Eur J Appl Physiol Occup Physiol.* 1998;77(3):231–41.

16. Coso JD, Hamouti N, Ortega JF, Fernandez-Elias VE, Mora-Rodriguez R. Relevance of individual characteristics for thermoregulation during exercise in a hot-dry environment. *Eur J Appl Physiol.* 2011;111(9):2173–81.

17. Havenith G. Human surface to mass ratio and core temperature in exercise heat stress — a concept revisited. *J Therm Biol.* 2001;26(4–5):387–93.

18. Noakes TD, Myburgh KH, du Plessis J, et al. Metabolic rate, not percent dehydration, predicts rectal temperature in marathon runners. *Med Sci Sports Exerc.* 1991;23(4):443–9.

19. Adams JD, Ganio MS, Burchfield JM, et al. Effects of obesity on body temperature in otherwise-healthy females when controlling hydration and heat production during exercise in the heat. *Eur J Appl Physiol.* 2015;115(1):167–76.

20. Bar-Or O, Lundegren HM, Buskirk ER. Heat tolerance of exercising obese and lean women. *J Appl Physiol.* 1969;26(4):403–9.

21. Deren TM, Coris EE, Bain AR, Walz SM, Jay O. Sweating is greater in NCAA football linemen independently of heat production. *Med Sci Sports Exerc.* 2012;44(2):244–52.

22. Dervis SM, Coombs GB, Chaseling GK, Filingeri D, Smoljanic J, Jay O. A comparison of thermoregulatory responses to exercise between mass-matched groups with large differences in body fat. *J Appl Physiol.* 2016;120(6):615–23.

23. Cramer MN, Jay O. Selecting the correct exercise intensity for unbiased comparisons of thermoregulatory responses between groups of different mass and surface area. *J Appl Physiol.* 2014;116(9):1123–32.

24. Limbaugh JD, Wimer GS, Long LH, Baird WH. Body fatness, body core temperature, and heat loss during moderate-intensity exercise. *Aviat Space Environ Med.* 2013;84(11):1153–8.

25. Vroman NB, Buskirk ER, Hodgson JL. Cardiac output and skin blood flow in lean and obese individuals during exercise in the heat. *J Appl Physiol Respir Environ Exerc Physiol.* 1983;55(1 Pt 1):69–74.

26. Moyen NE, Burchfield JM, Butts CL, et al. Effects of obesity and mild hypohydration on local sweating and cutaneous vascular responses during passive heat stress in females. *Appl Physiol Nutr Metab.* 2016;41(8):879–87.

27. Schwartz J. Who is sensitive to extremes of temperature? A case-only analysis. *Epidemiology.* 2005;16(1):67–72.

28. Kenny GP, Sigal RJ, McGinn R. Body temperature regulation in diabetes. *Temperature.* 2016;3(1):119–45.

29. Khan F, Elhadd TA, Greene SA, Belch JJ. Impaired skin microvascular function in children, adolescents, and young adults with type 1 diabetes. *Diabetes Care.* 2000;23(2):215–20.

30. Petrofsky JS, Lee S, Patterson C, Cole M, Stewart B. Sweat production during global heating and during isometric exercise in people with diabetes. *Med Sci Monit.* 2005;11(11):CR515–21.

31. Wilson SB, Jennings PE, Belch JJ. Detection of microvascular impairment in type I diabetics by laser Doppler flowmetry. *Clin Physiol.* 1992;12(2):195–208.

32. Stapleton JM, Yardley JE, Boulay P, Sigal RJ, Kenny GP. Whole-body heat loss during exercise in the heat is not impaired in type 1 diabetes. *Med Sci Sports Exerc.* 2013;45(9):1656–64.

33. Carter MR, McGinn R, Barrera-Ramirez J, Sigal RJ, Kenny GP. Impairments in local heat loss in type 1 diabetes during exercise in the heat. *Med Sci Sports Exerc.* 2014;46(12):2224–33.

34. Kenny GP, Stapleton JM, Yardley JE, Boulay P, Sigal RJ. Older adults with type 2 diabetes store more heat during exercise. *Med Sci Sports Exerc.* 2013;45(10):1906–14.

35. Administration for Community Living. *Profile of Older Americans.* Washington (DC): U.S. Department of Health & Human Services; 2020. Available from: https://www.acl.gov/node/537.

36. Kenny GP, Groeller H, McGinn R, Flouris AD. Age, human performance, and physical employment standards. *Appl Physiol Nutr Metab.* 2016;41(6 Suppl 2):S92–107.

37. Kenney WL, Craighead DH, Alexander LM. Heat waves, aging and human cardiovascular health. *Med Sci Sports Exerc.* 2014;46(10):1891–9.

38. Kenney WL. Thermoregulation at rest and during exercise in healthy older adults. *Exerc Sport Sci Rev.* 1997;25:41–76.

39. Martin HL, Loomis JL, Kenney WL. Maximal skin vascular conductance in subjects aged 5–85 yr. *J Appl Physiol.* 1995;79(1):297–301.

40. Minson CT, Wladkowski SL, Cardell AF, Pawelczyk JA, Kenney WL. Age alters the cardiovascular response to direct passive heating. *J Appl Physiol.* 1998;84(4):1323–32.

41. Gagnon D, Kenny GP. Sex differences in thermoeffector responses during exercise at fixed requirements for heat loss. *J Appl Physiol.* 2012;113(5):746–57.

42. Phillips PA, Rolls BJ, Ledingham JG, et al. Reduced thirst after water deprivation in healthy elderly men. *N Engl J Med.* 1984;311(12):753–9.

43. Davido A, Patzak A, Dart T, et al. Risk factors for heat related death during the August 2003 heat wave in Paris, France, in patients evaluated at the emergency department of the Hospital European Georges Pompidou. *Emerg Med J.* 2006;23(7):515–8.

44. Drinkwater BL, Horvath SM. Heat tolerance and aging. *Med Sci Sports Exerc.* 1979;11(1):49–55.

45. Haymes EM, Buskirk ER, Hodgson JL, Lundegren HM, Nicholas WC. Heat tolerance of exercising lean and heavy prepubertal girls. *J Appl Physiol.* 1974;36(5):566–71.

46. Armstrong LE, Maresh CM. Exercise-heat tolerance of children and adolescents. *Pediatr Exerc Sci.* 1995;7(3):239–52.

47. Kenney WL, Kamon E, Buskirk ER. Effect of mild essential hypertension on control of forearm blood flow during exercise in the heat. *J Appl Physiol.* 1984;56(4):930–5.

48. Green DJ, Maiorana AJ, Siong JHJ, et al. Impaired skin blood flow response to environmental heating in chronic heart failure. *Eur Heart J.* 2006;27(3):338–43.

49. Cui J, Arbab-Zadeh A, Prasad A, Durand S, Levine BD, Crandall CG. Effects of heat stress on thermoregulatory responses in congestive heart failure patients. *Circulation.* 2005;112(15):2286–92.

50. National Multiple Sclerosis Society. *Multiple Sclerosis Symptoms* [Internet]. New York (NY): National Multiple Sclerosis Society. Available from: http://www.nationalmssociety.org/Symptoms-Diagnosis/MS-Symptoms.

51. Davis SL, Wilson TE, White AT, Frohman EM. Thermoregulation in multiple sclerosis. *J Appl Physiol.* 2010;109(5):1531–7.

52. Edlich RF, Buschbacher RM, Cox MJ, Long WB, Winters KL, Becker DG. Strategies to reduce hyperthermia in ambulatory multiple sclerosis patients. *J Long Term Eff Med Implants.* 2004;14(6):467–79.

53. Ganio MS, Schlader ZJ, Pearson J, et al. Nongrafted skin area best predicts exercise core temperature responses in burned humans. *Med Sci Sports Exerc.* 2015;47(10):2224–32.

54. Davis SL, Shibasaki M, Low DA, et al. Skin grafting impairs postsynaptic cutaneous vasodilator and sweating responses. *J Burn Care Res.* 2007;28(3):435–41.

55. Ganio MS, Pearson J, Schlader ZJ, et al. Aerobic fitness is disproportionately low in adult burn survivors years after injury. *J Burn Care Res.* 2015;36(4):513–9.

56. Yamasaki M, Kim KT, Choi SW, Muraki S, Shiokawa M, Kurokawa T. Characteristics of body heat balance of paraplegics during exercise in a hot environment. *J Physiol Anthropol Appl Human Sci.* 2001;20(4):227–32.

57. Noakes TD, St Clair Gibson A, Lambert EV. From catastrophe to complexity: a novel model of integrative central neural regulation of effort and fatigue during exercise in humans: summary and conclusions. *Br J Sports Med.* 2005;39(2):120–4.

58. Lemke B, Kjellstrom T. Calculating workplace WBGT from meteorological data: a tool for climate change assessment. *Ind Health.* 2012;50(4):267–78.

59. Schlader ZJ, Ganio MS, Pearson J, et al. Heat acclimation improves heat exercise tolerance and heat dissipation in individuals with extensive skin grafts. *J Appl Physiol.* 2015;119(1):69–76.

60. Adams JD, McDermott BP, Ridings CB, Mainer LL, Ganio MS, Kavouras SA. Effect of air-filled vest on exercise-heat strain when wearing ballistic protection. *Ann Occup Hyg.* 2014;58(8):1057–64.

61. Morris NB, Coombs G, Jay O. Ice slurry ingestion leads to a lower net heat loss during exercise in the heat. *Med Sci Sports Exerc.* 2016;48(1):114–22.

62. Goosey-Tolfrey V, Swainson M, Boyd C, Atkinson G, Tolfrey K. The effectiveness of hand cooling at reducing exercise-induced hyperthermia and improving distance-race performance in wheelchair and able-bodied athletes. *J Appl Physiol (1985).* 2008;105(1):37–43.

63. Judelson DA, Maresh CM, Anderson JM, et al. Hydration and muscular performance: does fluid balance affect strength, power and high-intensity endurance? *Sports Med.* 2007;37(10):907–21.

64. Armstrong LE, Costill DL, Fink WJ. Influence of diuretic-induced dehydration on competitive running performance. *Med Sci Sports Exerc.* 1985;17(4):456–61.

65. Bardis CN, Kavouras SA, Arnaoutis G, Panagiotakos DB, Sidossis LS. Mild dehydration and cycling performance during 5-kilometer hill climbing. *J Athl Train.* 2013;48(6):741–7.

66. Armstrong LE, McDermott BP, Hosokawa Y. Exertional hyponatremia. In: Casa DJ, Stearns RL, editors. *Preventing Sudden Death in Sport & Physical Activity.* Sudbury (MA): Jones & Bartlett Publishers; 2016. p. 219–38.

67. Hew-Butler T, Rosner MH, Fowkes-Godek S, et al. Statement of the 3rd international exercise-associated hyponatremia consensus development conference, Carlsbad, California, 2015. *Br J Sports Med.* 2015;49(22):1432–46.

68. Castellani JW, Young AJ, Ducharme MB, et al; American College of Sports Medicine. American College of Sports Medicine position stand: prevention of cold injuries during exercise. *Med Sci Sports Exerc.* 2006;38(11):2012–29.

69. Young AJ, Young PM. Human acclimatization to high terrestrial altitude. In: Pandolf KB, Sawka MN, Gonzalez RR, editors. *Human Performance Physiology and Environmental Medicine at Terrestrial Extremes.* Indianapolis (IN): Benchmark Press; 1988. p. 497–543.

70. U.S. Department of the Army. *Prevention and Management of Cold-Weather Injuries: Technical Bulletin Medical 508.* Washington (DC): Department of the Army; 2005. Available

from: https://www.usariem.army.mil/assets/doc s/publications/articles/2005/tbmed508.pdf.

71. Muller MD, Gao Z, Mast JL, et al. Aging attenuates the coronary blood flow response to cold air breathing and isometric handgrip in healthy humans. *Am J Physiol Heart Circ Physiol.* 2012;302(8):H1737–46.

72. Koskela H, Tukiainen H. Facial cooling, but not nasal breathing of cold air, induces bronchoconstriction: a study in asthmatic and healthy subjects. *Eur Respir J.* 1995;8(12):2088–93.

73. Rundell KW, Jenkinson DM. Exercise-induced bronchospasm in the elite athlete. *Sports Med.* 2002;32(9):583–600.

74. Giesbrecht GG. The respiratory system in a cold environment. *Aviat Space Environ Med.* 1995;66(9):890–902.

75. Surwit RS, Pilon RN, Fenton CH. Behavioral treatment of Raynaud's disease. *J Behav Med.* 1978;1(3):323–35.

76. Jobe JB, Sampson JB, Roberts DE, Kelly JA. Comparison of behavioral treatments for Raynaud's disease. *J Behav Med.* 1986;9(1):89–96

77. Manou-Stathopoulou V, Goodwin CD, Patterson T, Redwood SR, Marber MS, Williams RP. The effects of cold and exercise on the cardiovascular system. *Heart.* 2015;101(10):808–20.

78. Pandolf KB. Air quality and human performance. In: Pandolf KB, Sawka MN, Gonzalez RR, editors. *Human Performance Physiology and Environmental Medicine at Terrestrial Extremes.* Indianapolis (IN): Benchmark Press; 1988. p. 591–629.

79. Pescatello LS, Arena R, Riebe D, Thompson PD. Exercise prescription for populations with other chronic diseases and health conditions. In: *American College of Sports Medicine's Guidelines for Exercise Testing and Prescription.* Baltimore (MD): Lippincott Williams & Wilkins; 2014. p. 260–343.

80. Brook RD, Rajagopalan S, Pope CA III, et al. Particulate matter air pollution and cardiovascular disease: an update to the scientific statement from the American Heart Association. *Circulation.* 2010;121(21):2331–78.

81. Franklin BA, Brook R, Arden Pope C III. Air pollution and cardiovascular disease. *Curr Probl Cardiol.* 2015;40(5):207–38.

82. Bui DS, Burgess JA, Matheson MC, et al. Ambient wood smoke, traffic pollution and adult asthma prevalence and severity. *Respirology.* 2013;18(7):1101–7.

83. Jacquemin B, Schikowski T, Carsin AE, et al. The role of air pollution in adult-onset asthma: a review of the current evidence. *Semin Respir Crit Care Med.* 2012;33(6):606–19.

84. Kunzli N, Bridevaux PO, Liu LJ, et al; Swiss Cohort Study on Air Pollution and Lung Diseases in Adults. Traffic-related air pollution correlates with adult-onset asthma among never-smokers. *Thorax.* 2009;64(8):664–70.

85. Andersen ZJ, Hvidberg M, Jensen SS, et al. Chronic obstructive pulmonary disease and long-term exposure to traffic-related air pollution: a cohort study. *Am J Respir Crit Care Med.* 2011;183(4):455–61.

86. Schikowski T, Mills IC, Anderson HR, et al. Ambient air pollution: a cause of COPD? *Eur Respir J.* 2014;43(1):250–63.

87. Eze IC, Hemkens LG, Bucher HC, et al. Association between ambient air pollution and diabetes mellitus in Europe and North America: systematic review and meta-analysis. *Environ Health Perspect.* 2015;123(5):381–9.

88. Rao X, Montresor-Lopez J, Puett R, Rajagopalan S, Brook RD. Ambient air pollution: an emerging risk factor for diabetes mellitus. *Curr Diab Rep.* 2015;15(6):603.

89. Kim I, Yang P, Lee J, et al. Long-term exposure of fine particulate matter air pollution and incident atrial fibrillation in the general population: a nationwide cohort study. *Int J Cardiol.* 2019;283:178–83.

90. Shin S, Burnett RT, Kwong JC, et al. Ambient air pollution and the risk of atrial fibrillation and stroke: a population-based cohort study. *Environ Health Perspect.* 2019;127(8):87009.

91. Raaschou-Nielsen O, Andersen ZJ, Beelen R, et al. Air pollution and lung cancer incidence in 17 European cohorts: prospective analyses from the European Study of Cohorts for Air Pollution Effects (ESCAPE). *Lancet Oncol.* 2013;14(9):813–22.

92. Raaschou-Nielsen O, Andersen ZJ, Hvidberg M, et al. Air pollution from traffic and cancer incidence: a Danish cohort study. *Environ Health.* 2011;10:67.

93. Peel JL, Metzger KB, Klein M, Flanders WD, Mulholland JA, Tolbert PE. Ambient air pollution and cardiovascular emergency department visits in potentially sensitive groups. *Am J Epidemiol.* 2007;165(6):625–33.

94. Bateson TF, Schwartz J. Who is sensitive to the effects of particulate air pollution on mortality? A case-crossover analysis of effect modifiers. *Epidemiology.* 2004;15(2):143–9.

95. O'Neill MS, Veves A, Zanobetti A, et al. Diabetes enhances vulnerability to particulate air pollution-associated impairment in vascular reactivity and endothelial function. *Circulation.* 2005;111(22):2913–20.

96. Park SK, O'Neill MS, Vokonas PS, Sparrow D, Schwartz J. Effects of air pollution on heart rate variability: the VA normative aging study. *Environ Health Perspect.* 2005;113(3):304–9.

97. Sunyer J, Schwartz J, Tobias A, Macfarlane D, Garcia J, Anto JM. Patients with chronic obstructive pulmonary disease are at increased risk of death associated with urban particle air pollution: a case-crossover analysis. *Am J Epidemiol.* 2000;151(1):50–6.

98. Armstrong LE. Air pollution: exercise in the city. In: Armstrong LE, editor. *Performing in Extreme Environments.* Champaign (IL): Human Kinetics; 2000. p. 197–235.

99. McCafferty WB. *Air Pollution and Athletic Performance.* Springfield (IL): Charles C. Thomas; 1981.

100. Hirsch GL, Sue DY, Wasserman K, Robinson TE, Hansen JE. Immediate effects of cigarette smoking on cardiorespiratory responses to exercise. *J Appl Physiol (1985).* 1985;58(6):1975–81.

101. Horvath SM, Raven PB, Dahms TE, Gray DJ. Maximal aerobic capacity at different levels of carboxyhemoglobin. *J Appl Physiol.* 1975;38(2):300–3.

102. Horvath SM. Impact of air quality in exercise performance. *Exerc Sport Sci Rev.* 1981;9:265–96.

103. Aronow WS, Ferlinz J, Glauser F. Effect of carbon monoxide on exercise performance in chronic obstructive pulmonary disease. *Am J Med.* 1977;63(6):904–8.

104. Adams KF, Koch G, Chatterjee B, et al. Acute elevation of blood carboxyhemoglobin to 6% impairs exercise performance and aggravates symptoms in patients with ischemic heart disease. *J Am Coll Cardiol.* 1988;12(4):900–9.

105. Aronow WS. Effect of passive smoking on angina pectoris. *N Engl J Med.* 1978;299(1):21–4.

106. Kurt TL, Mogielnicki RP, Chandler JE. Association of the frequency of acute cardiorespiratory complaints with ambient levels of carbon monoxide. *Chest.* 1978;74(1):10–14.

107. Kurt TL, Mogielnicki RP, Chandler JE, Hirst K. Ambient carbon monoxide levels and acute cardiorespiratory complaints: an exploratory study. *Am J Public Health*. 1979;69(4):360–3.

108. Cohen SI, Deane M, Goldsmith JR. Carbon monoxide and survival from myocardial infarction. *Arch Environ Health*. 1969;19(4):510–7.

109. Nadel JA, Salem H, Tamplin B, Tokiwa Y. Mechanism of bronchoconstriction during inhalation of sulfur dioxide. *J Appl Physiol*. 1965;20:164–7.

110. Speizer FE, Frank NR. The uptake and release of SO$_2$ by the human nose. *Arch Environ Health*. 1966;12(6):725–8.

111. Frank NR, Amdur MO, Worcester J, Whittenberger JL. Effects of acute controlled exposure to SO2 on respiratory mechanics in healthy male adults. *J Appl Physiol*. 1962;17:252–8.

112. Kreisman H, Mitchell CA, Hosein HR, Bouhuys A. Effect of low concentrations of sulfur dioxide on respiratory function in man. *Lung*. 1976;154(1):25–34.

113. Linn WS, Venet TG, Shamoo DA, et al. Respiratory effects of sulfur dioxide in heavily exercising asthmatics. A dose-response study. *Am Rev Respir Dis*. 1983;127(3):278–83.

114. Gong H, Krishnareddy S. How pollution and airborne allergens affect exercise. *Phys Sportsmed*. 1995;23(7):35–43.

115. Helleday R, Huberman D, Blomberg A, Stjernberg N, Sandstrom T. Nitrogen dioxide exposure impairs the frequency of the mucociliary activity in healthy subjects. *Eur Respir J*. 1995;8(10):1664–8.

116. Horvath EP, doPico GA, Barbee RA, Dickie HA. Nitrogen dioxide-induced pulmonary disease: five new cases and a review of the literature. *J Occup Med*. 1978;20(2):103–10.

117. Kim SU, Koenig JQ, Pierson WE, Hanley QS. Acute pulmonary effects of nitrogen dioxide exposure during exercise in competitive athletes. *Chest*. 1991;99(4):815–9.

118. Brown JS. Nitrogen dioxide exposure and airway responsiveness in individuals with asthma. *Inhal Toxicol*. 2015;27(1):1–14.

119. Folinsbee LJ. Does nitrogen dioxide exposure increase airways responsiveness? *Toxicol Ind Health*. 1992;8(5):273–83.

120. Bauer MA, Utell MJ, Morrow PE, Speers DM, Gibb FR. Inhalation of 0.30 ppm nitrogen dioxide potentiates exercise-induced bronchospasm in asthmatics. *Am Rev Respir Dis*. 1986;134(6):1203–8.

121. Dockery DW, Pope CA III, Xu X, et al. An association between air pollution and mortality in six U.S. cities. *N Engl J Med*. 1993;329(24):1753–9.

122. Peters A, von Klot S, Heier M, et al; Cooperative Health Research in the Region of Augsburg Study Group. Exposure to traffic and the onset of myocardial infarction. *N Engl J Med*. 2004;351(17):1721–30.

123. Poloniecki JD, Atkinson RW, de Leon AP, Anderson HR. Daily time series for cardiovascular hospital admissions and previous day's air pollution in London, UK. *Occup Environ Med*. 1997;54(8):535–40.

124. Pope CA III, Thun MJ, Namboodiri MM, et al. Particulate air pollution as a predictor of mortality in a prospective study of U.S. adults. *Am J Respir Crit Care Med*. 1995;151(3 Pt 1):669–74.

125. Samet JM, Dominici F, Curriero FC, Coursac I, Zeger SL. Fine particulate air pollution and mortality in 20 U.S. cities, 1987–1994. *N Engl J Med*. 2000;343(24):1742–9.

126. Cutrufello PT, Smoliga JM, Rundell KW. Small things make a big difference: particulate matter and exercise. *Sports Med*. 2012;42(12):1041–58.

127. Aryal A, Harmon AC, Dugas TR. Particulate matter air pollutants and cardiovascular disease: strategies for intervention. *Pharmacol Ther*. 2021;223:107890.

128. Dockery DW, Pope CA III. Acute respiratory effects of particulate air pollution. *Annu Rev Public Health*. 1994;15:107–32.

129. Hart JE, Puett RC, Rexrode KM, Albert CM, Laden F. Effect modification of long-term air pollution exposures and the risk of incident cardiovascular disease in us women. *J Am Heart Assoc*. 2015;4(12):25.

130. Erqou S, Clougherty JE, Olafiranye O, et al. Particulate matter air pollution and racial differences in cardiovascular disease risk. *Arterioscler Thromb Vasc Biol*. 2018;38:935–42.

131. Miller KA, Siscovick DS, Sheppard L, et al. Long-term exposure to air pollution and incidence of cardiovascular events in women. *N Engl J Med*. 2007;356(5):447–58.

132. Puett RC, Schwartz J, Hart JE, et al. Chronic particulate exposure, mortality, and coronary heart disease in the nurses' health study. [Erratum appears in *Am J Epidemiol*. 2010;171(3):389]. *Am J Epidemiol*. 2008;168(10):1161–8.

133. Daigle CC, Chalupa DC, Gibb FR, et al. Ultrafine particle deposition in humans during rest and exercise. *Inhal Toxicol*. 2003;15(6):539–52.

134. Giles LV, Carlsten C, Koehle MS. The effect of pre-exercise diesel exhaust exposure on cycling performance and cardio-respiratory variables. *Inhal Toxicol*. 2012;24(12):783–9.

135. Mills NL, Tornqvist H, Gonzalez MC, et al. Ischemic and thrombotic effects of dilute diesel-exhaust inhalation in men with coronary heart disease. *N Engl J Med*. 2007;357(11):1075–82.

136. Devlin RB, Duncan KE, Jardim M, Schmitt MT, Rappold AG, Diaz-Sanchez D. Controlled exposure of healthy young volunteers to ozone causes cardiovascular effects. *Circulation*. 2012;126(1):104–11.

137. Scannell C, Chen L, Aris RM, et al. Greater ozone-induced inflammatory responses in subjects with asthma. *Am J Respir Crit Care Med*. 1996;154(1):24–9.

138. Chan CC, Chuang KJ, Chien LC, Chen WJ, Chang WT. Urban air pollution and emergency admissions for cerebrovascular diseases in Taipei, Taiwan. *Eur Heart J*. 2006;27(10):1238–44.

139. Yang CY. Air pollution and hospital admissions for congestive heart failure in a subtropical city: Taipei, Taiwan. *J Toxicol Environ Health A*. 2008;71(16):1085–90.

140. Bell ML, McDermott A, Zeger SL, Samet JM, Dominici F. Ozone and short-term mortality in 95 US urban communities, 1987–2000. *JAMA*. 2004;292(19):2372–8.

141. Ito K, De Leon SF, Lippmann M. Associations between ozone and daily mortality: analysis and meta-analysis. *Epidemiology*. 2005;16(4):446–57.

142. Gliner JA, Raven PB, Horvath SM, Drinkwater BL, Sutton JC. Man's physiologic response to long-term work during thermal and pollutant stress. *J Appl Physiol*. 1975;39(4):628–32.

143. Raven PB, Drinkwater BL, Horvath SM, et al. Age, smoking habits, heat stress, and their interactive effects with carbon monoxide and peroxyacetyl nitrate on man's aerobic power. *Int J Biometeorol*. 1974;18(3):222–32.

144. Raven PB, Drinkwater BL, Ruhling RO, et al. Effect of carbon monoxide and peroxyacetyl nitrate on man's maximal aerobic capacity. *J Appl Physiol.* 1974;36(3):288–93.

145. Ou CQ, Yang J, Ou QQ, et al. The impact of relative humidity and atmospheric pressure on mortality in Guangzhou, China. *Biomed Environ Sci.* 2014;27(12):917–25.

146. Wang XY, Barnett AG, Yu W, et al. The impact of heatwaves on mortality and emergency hospital admissions from non-external causes in Brisbane, Australia. *Occup Environ Med.* 2012;69(3):163–9.

147. Ellis FP. Mortality from heat illness and heat-aggravated illness in the United States. *Environ Res.* 1972;5(1):1–58.

148. Ren C, O'Neill MS, Park SK, Sparrow D, Vokonas P, Schwartz J. Ambient temperature, air pollution, and heart rate variability in an aging population. *Am J Epidemiol.* 2011;173(9):1013–21.

149. Qian Z, He Q, Lin HM, et al. Part 2. Association of daily mortality with ambient air pollution, and effect modification by extremely high temperature in Wuhan, China. *Res Rep Health Eff Inst.* 2010;(154):91–217.

150. Rundell KW, Sue-Chu M. Air quality and exercise-induced bronchoconstriction in elite athletes. *Immunol Allergy Clin North Am.* 2013;33(3):409–21, ix.

151. Rodopoulou S, Samoli E, Chalbot MC, Kavouras IG. Air pollution and cardiovascular and respiratory emergency visits in central Arkansas: a time-series analysis. *Sci Total Environ.* 2015;536:872–9.

152. Bell ML, Ebisu K, Peng RD, et al. Seasonal and regional short-term effects of fine particles on hospital admissions in 202 US counties, 1999–2005. *Am J Epidemiol.* 2008;168(11):1301–10.

153. Andersen ZJ, de Nazelle A, Mendez MA, et al. A study of the combined effects of physical activity and air pollution on mortality in elderly urban residents: the Danish diet, cancer, and health cohort. *Environ Health Perspect.* 2015;123(6):557–63.

154. Dong GH, Zhang P, Sun B, et al. Long-term exposure to ambient air pollution and respiratory disease mortality in Shenyang, China: a 12-year population-based retrospective cohort study. *Respiration.* 2012;84(5):360–8.

155. Wong CM, Ou CQ, Thach TQ, et al. Does regular exercise protect against air pollution-associated mortality? *Prev Med.* 2007;44(5):386–92.

156. Giles LV, Koehle MS. The health effects of exercising in air pollution. *Sports Med.* 2014;44(2):223–49.

157. Environmental Protection Agency. AirNow (Air Quality Index). Environmental Protection Agency; 2017. Available from: https://airnow.gov/.

158. Rundell KW, Spiering BA, Baumann JM, Evans TM. Bronchoconstriction provoked by exercise in a high-particulate-matter environment is attenuated by montelukast. *Inhal Toxicol.* 2005;17(2):99–105.

159. Young AJ, Reeves JT. Human adaptation to high terrestrial altitude. In: Lounsbury DE, Bellamy RF, Zajtchuk R, editors. *Medical Aspects of Harsh Environments.* Washington (DC): Office of the Surgeon General, Borden Institute; 2002. p. 647–91.

160. Beidleman BA, Tighiouart H, Schmid CH, Fulco CS, Muza SR. Predictive models of acute mountain sickness after rapid ascent to various altitudes. *Med Sci Sports Exerc.* 2013;45(4):792–800.

161. Muza SR, Fulco C, Beidleman BA, Cymerman A. *Altitude Acclimatization and Illness Management.* Washington (DC):

162. Fulco CS, Rock PB, Cymerman A. Maximal and submaximal exercise performance at altitude. *Aviat Space Environ Med.* 1998;69(8):793–801.

163. Pescatello LS, Arena R, Riebe D, Thompson PD. Exercise prescription for healthy populations with special considerations and environmental considerations. In: *American College of Sports Medicine's Guidelines for Exercise Testing and Prescription.* Baltimore (MD): Lippincott Williams & Wilkins; 2014. p. 194–226.

164. Chapman RF, Stickford JL, Levine BD. Altitude training considerations for the winter sport athlete. *Exp Physiol.* 2010;95(3):411–21.

165. LeMura LM, von Duvillard SP. *Clinical Exercise Physiology: Application and Physiological Principles.* Baltimore (MD): Lippincott Williams & Wilkins; 2014.

166. Armstrong LE. Assessing hydration status: the elusive gold standard. *J Am Coll Nutr.* 2007;26(Suppl 5):575S–84S.

167. Cheuvront SN, Sawka MN. Hydration assessment of athletes. *Gatorade Sports Sci Exchange.* 2005;18(2):1–5.

168. Cheuvront SN, Carter R III, Montain SJ, Sawka MN. Daily body mass variability and stability in active men undergoing exercise-heat stress. *Int J Sport Nutr Exerc Metab.* 2004;14(5):532–40.

169. Armstrong LE, Maresh CM, Castellani JW, et al. Urinary indices of hydration status. *Int J Sport Nutr.* 1994;4(3):265–79.

170. Human Hydration LLC. *HydrationCheck.* Hampton (VA): Human Hydration, LLC; 2017. Available from: http://www.hydrationcheck.com/.

171. Greenleaf JE. Problem: thirst, drinking behavior, and involuntary dehydration. *Med Sci Sports Exerc.* 1992;24(6):645–56.

172. Hoffman MD, Cotter JD, Goulet ED, Laursen PB. Rebuttal from "yes." *Wilderness Environ Med.* 2016;27(2):198–200.

173. Hoffman MD, Cotter JD, Goulet ED, Laursen PB. View: is drinking to thirst adequate to appropriately maintain hydration status during prolonged endurance exercise? Yes. *Wilderness Environ Med.* 2016;27(2):192–5.

174. Armstrong LE, Johnson EC, Bergeron MF. Counterview: is drinking to thirst adequate to appropriately maintain hydration status during prolonged endurance exercise? No. *Wilderness Environ Med.* 2016;27(2):195–8.

175. Armstrong LE, Johnson EC, Bergeron MF. Rebuttal from "no." *Wilderness Environ Med.* 2016;27(2):200–2.

176. Burchfield JM, Ganio MS, Kavouras SA, et al. 24-h void number as an indicator of hydration status. *Eur J Clin Nutr.* 2015;69(5):638–41.

177. Tucker MA, Caldwell AR, Ganio MS. Adequacy of daily fluid intake volume can be identified from urinary frequency and perceived thirst in healthy. *J Am Coll Nutr.* 2020;39(3):235–42

178. Tucker MA, Gonzalez MA, Adams JD, et al. Reliability of 24-h void frequency as an index of hydration status when euhydrated and hypohydrated. *Eur J Clin Nutr.* 2016;70(8):908–11.

179. Wehrlin JP, Zuest P, Hallen J, Marti B. Live high-train low for 24 days increases hemoglobin mass and red cell volume in elite endurance athletes. *J Appl Physiol.* 2006;100(6):1938–45.

Department of the Army Technical Bulletin: TB MED 505; 2010. Available from: https://www.usariem.army.mil/assets/doc s/partnering/TB-Med-505-Sept-2010.pdf.

Exercise System Genetics

INTRODUCTION

The study of genetics has impacted almost every academic discipline. Many research projects of genetics' effects on exercise and sport performance are getting a lot of attention. Terms and concepts such as genomics, clustered regularly interspaced short palindromic repeats (CRISPR), and the Human Genome Project have become part of the normal health care jargon, and the clinical exercise physiologist (CEP) may find it necessary to respond to client questions about these topics. However, the CEP may not have taken courses in genetics and thus may not be able to apply or even understand the advances in understanding and technology that are being reported and discussed — advances that may be coming to their clinic very soon.

Thus, this chapter provides a general overview of the fundamental concepts and potential applications of genetics that may augment the practice of a CEP. The technologies covered here are already in use and therefore promise to impact CEPs in a significant way. The CEP should not be afraid of, or worried about, these new ideas; indeed, once the basic concepts and terminology of genetics has been mastered (covered in Box 18.1), the discussion here may provide ideas about how to provide better services to the client.

THE PROMISE OF PRECISION MEDICINE

The Human Genome Project, an international effort to sequence the underlying genetic code of humans, was essentially completed in 2003. While it was ongoing, many researchers anticipated that having this genomic information would enable the development of health interventions based on an individual's genetic makeup, thereby allowing clinicians to deliver the most efficient

and optimal treatment for any condition or disease. This approach, called "personalized medicine," was listed as one of the future grand challenges of the Human Genome Project (Challenge II-3):

> Develop genome-based approaches to prediction of disease susceptibility and drug response, early detection of illness, and molecular taxonomy for disease states (1).

Although the term "precision medicine" is now more widely used than personalized medicine, the idea is still the same: to use an individual's genetic information to tailor health care interventions for that individual. Recent advances in gene technologies have further increased anticipation of the ready use of precision medicine.

Genetic Variability in Response to Exercise

The idea of precision medicine is not limited to the treatment of disease. The developers of the long-term goals of the Human Genome Project also saw precision medicine being applied to lifestyle interventions:

> The discovery of variants that affect risk for disease could potentially be used in individualized preventive medicine — including diet, exercise, lifestyle and pharmaceutical intervention — to maximize the likelihood of staying well (1).

Not surprisingly, then, discussions of the application of genomic information to exercise prescription in both healthy and clinical populations soon began. As early as 2008, Dr. Stephen Roth from the University of Maryland posed a simple question that was the basis for a series of commentary articles in the *Journal of Applied Physiology* (2):

> How can genomic factors be used to improve our ability to administer exercise interventions?

Like exercise physiology and other scientific specialties, genetics has its own vocabulary that allows users to communicate quickly and accurately; however, this functionality only works if everyone knows what the terms mean. Below are a few terms in the "genetic vocabulary" that will make understanding and using genetic information easier.

Gene — The term "gene" specifically refers to a distinct region of DNA that acts as a physical and functional unit of heredity. Genes are named according to an accepted convention in which the abbreviated gene name is italicized. For example, the actin beta gene is *ACTB*. Notice that abbreviated human gene names are written in all capitals. In contrast, abbreviated gene names from other mammals are written with just the first letter capitalized. Gene names can be confusing, but several good databases on the Internet can provide all the information needed about that gene. In most cases, type the gene name into an Internet browser and choose from a wide variety of sources (*e.g.*, Gene-cards — www.genecards.org).

Phenotype — The term "phenotype" refers to the set of measurable characteristics of an organism that are correlated with that organism's genome and its environment. Critically, the phenotype must be measurable and repeatable; this is the reason that often the first step in any genetic exploration is to link a particular characteristic with some genetic factor. Exercise endurance, voluntary activity, heart rate, and oxygen consumption are all aspects of an individual's phenotype that have been explored in the exercise genetics literature.

Polygenic risk score — It is a measurement that is calculated based on the contribution of various genetic factors such as genomic variation, gene expression, and/or other genetic factors to the phenotype of interest. The use of a polygenic risk score allows one number to represent the contributions of multiple genetic factors in determining a phenotype. This type of algorithm approach was first used to determine an individual's risk for particular diseases and, thus, the "risk" portion of the name. But the same concept can be used to determine the effect of many genetic variants on any physiological characteristic.

Polymorphism — The term "polymorphism" means "different forms." In genetics, it usually refers to a difference in one underlying nucleic acid at a specific location and is referred to as a "single-nucleotide polymorphism" or "SNP" (pronounced "snip"). For example, there may be an adenine nucleotide instead of a common guanine nucleotide at a specific genomic location. As described later in the chapter, SNPs are important markers and may cause functional differences in the proteins produced. The word "variant" may also be used to indicate a polymorphism.

Genotype — The broad term "genotype" refers to the unique genomic pattern of each individual. It encompasses everything, from the general overall genomic sequence to a specific SNP variant within a specific gene.

Exercise systems genetics — Because the genetic mechanisms that control any exercise phenotype involve multiple genetic factors, this term is a blanket term meaning "all heritable mechanisms, processes, and interactions that impact the capability and performance of sport and exercise" (6).

Dr. Roth's question reflected an understanding of the variability in response to exercise training that was identified by Dr. Claude Bouchard and Dr. Tuomo Rankinen in 2001 (3). When exposed to a standardized 20-week aerobic continuous exercise program, study participants showed a wide range of responses, from a more than 1,000 mL $O_2 \cdot min^{-1}$ increase in to a decrease of ≈ 100 mL $O_2 \cdot min^{-1}$ in oxygen consumption capacity (Figure 18.1). Thus, Dr. Roth proposed three training scenarios based on these responses to exercise. Training scenario 1 would be for responders to exercise. Scenario 2 would be for nonresponders (neutral) to exercise. Scenario 3 would be for negative responders to exercise. Roth estimated that up to 45% of individuals would fall into either scenario 2 or 3 (*i.e.*, nonresponders or negative responders). Roth's scenarios are described in more detail in Box 18.2.

As many exercise physiologists have noted, most notably Booth and Neufer (4), a challenge for the CEP is to determine how and when genetic information can be used to augment the traditional information used to prescribe exercise in both healthy and clinical populations. Given that variability in response to exercise training appears to be primarily genetically based, with estimates suggesting that genetics exerts about 50% of the influence on endurance training responses (3) and about 47% of the influence on resistance training responses (5), the challenge to

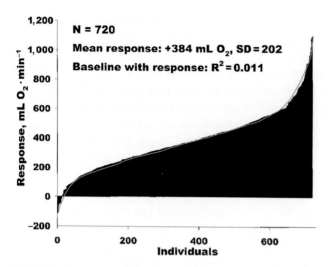

FIGURE 18.1 Heterogeneity of training response in the HERITAGE family study. The graph shows the individual variability in how much oxygen consumption changes when all the subjects underwent the same aerobic training protocol. The variability shown in this graph is one of the foundational observations, suggesting that genetics plays a large role in determining responses to an exercise training program and is the basis for Roth's scenarios, presented in Box 18.2. (From Bouchard C, Rankinen T. Individual differences in response to regular physical activity. *Med Sci Sports Exerc.* 2001;33:S446–51.)

CEPs is to determine if they should use genetic information in exercise prescriptions and, if so, what information should be used? The information in this chapter is meant to provide a background for CEPs so they can understand when the data in this area are trustworthy enough to be used in enhancing their exercise prescriptions.

Challenges of Precision Medicine in Exercise Prescription

Three facts significantly complicate the use of genetic information as part of exercise prescription:

- The rapid pace of change in our understanding of genetics, which causes our foundational understanding of how genetic mechanisms control any characteristic to continually change
- An evolving understanding of the complexity of genetic control and the many genetic factors that can play a role in controlling a physiological system
- The mostly exaggerated or false claims by commercial entities that genetic information (particularly genomic information) can be used to select and guide a wide range of health interventions, including exercise

---

Box 18.2   Roth's Scenarios

Although most CEPs assume that any client they put on an exercise program will benefit, exercise genetics studies suggest that in actuality, not all clients do. In this context, Dr. Stephen Roth from the University of Maryland postulated three different outcome scenarios based on the potential genetic control of responses to exercise training. These scenarios are useful to keep in mind as we consider how genetic information may be used in exercise prescriptions.

Scenario 1: Responder to exercise — This is the individual that most CEPs assume their clients to be, someone who when put on an exercise training program will increase their aerobic capacity or strength. Indeed, Dr. Roth estimated that approximately 55% of individuals would fall into this category. Given that these individuals respond to exercise as CEPs would expect, these individuals would be *least likely* to benefit from genetic factors being considered in the exercise prescription.

Scenario 2: Nonresponder to exercise — A nonresponder is an individual who shows little to no change with participation in an exercise training program. Depending on how "little to no change" is defined, between 30% and 40% of individuals may fall into this category. If genetic markers that characterize nonresponders can be found, it may be helpful to use this information to modify the exercise prescription.

Scenario 3: Negative responder to exercise — This category is one that is not familiar to most CEPs and a category that caused controversy for several years. This category includes individuals who actually show an adverse response to exercise training, including a decrease in aerobic capacity, as well as negative metabolic adaptations. Dr. Roth estimated that between 5% and 15% of all individuals fall into this category. For this population, genetic information could contribute significantly to the development of an exercise prescription that would provide health benefits despite decreases in aerobic capacity.

Regarding the first factor, concepts such as epigenetics, RNA interference, and exosomes (to name a few) have all entered the genetics literature since the year 2000. Thus, the basic understanding of how genetics regulates any physiological functioning is constantly undergoing revision and addition. For example, the Molecular Transducers of Physical Activity Consortium (MoTrPAC), funded by the National Institutes of Health (NIH) in 2016, promised to add literally thousands (if not more) of genetic factors that are integral to the physiological response to both endurance and resistance training to the body of knowledge that a CEP must understand. Results are still yet to be forthcoming from this effort, but should occur within the next several years.

Further, as we've learned more about different genetic factors, it is now understood that the actual control of most physiological phenotypes is very complicated. This genetic control may involve many genes, many transcriptional factors, translational controllers, epigenetic modifiers, to mention just a few. To date, there is no exercise phenotype that has been shown to have a few (less than five) genetic factors that control it. In fact, this is why the phrase "exercise systems genetics" (6) is now used to refer to the genetic controllers of exercise traits because of the large number of genetic-involved factors that are involved in controlling the simplest of exercise traits.

Coupled with the first two facts, the often aggressive and misleading marketing by entities that sell genomic testing directly to consumers — as opposed to those companies that work with health care providers/insurance carriers (see section on Influence of Genetics on the Efficiency and Efficacy of Pharmaceutical Regimens) — often lead to confusion in both clinicians and consumers interested in understanding how their genetics affect their health and exercise performance.

In short, the CEP working to apply genetic knowledge in developing exercise prescriptions must understand the basics of genetics so that they apply the newest genetic concepts to their practice and are not misled by the unfounded genetic claims so prevalent in today's aggressive advertising environment.

BASIC PRINCIPLES OF GENETICS

From the standpoint of a CEP, it is appealing to have another potential source of information available — genetic information — that may help determine whether a client will have positive changes with exercise training. However, the use of genetic information in developing

and implementing exercise prescriptions — whether for healthy or clinical populations — requires an up-to-date understanding of basic genetic principles. A wide variety of references are available for the CEP (*e.g.*, The "Lewin's Genes" series of textbooks, now up to the 12th edition) (7). However, even an abbreviated understanding of basic genetic principles will serve to help the CEP avoid many pitfalls in attempting to use genetic information.

The Central Dogma

The most fundamental genetic principles revolve around what is called the "central dogma," a foundational understanding of how genetic mechanisms work. The central dogma is readily applied to exercise questions. It has four primary steps (Figure 18.2).

Step 1: DNA and the Genetic Code

The first step of the central dogma is its foundation. That is, the central dogma cannot be understood without first understanding the genetic code — the genome. Scientists' appreciation of the need to understand the genome explains why there was, and still is, excitement over the completion of its sequencing in 2003.

A person's genome is encoded in the DNA packed into the nucleus of their body cells. DNA is made up of phosphates, sugars, and billions of nucleotides, of which there are only four types: adenine (A), cytosine (C), thymine (T), and guanine (G). The arrangement of these nucleotides gives rise to the specific amino acids assembled into proteins during the rest of the steps of the central dogma. Specifically, a sequence of three nucleotides, called a "codon," codes for a particular amino acid. CAG, for example, codes for glutamine.

Although approximately 99.9% of the human genome is the same among individuals, in some places, there are variations in the genomic code; for example, an A may occur where most individuals have a T. These variations are called "single-nucleotide polymorphisms," or SNPs, which literally means that there is a difference in one nucleotide at one spot in the genome. SNPs have been incredibly useful to scientists as guideposts/markers within the genome for mapping purposes and, in some cases, as indications of why the protein output is different between different people. However, a critical point to remember is that SNPs may or may not be functional. A *functional* SNP confers an alteration in the amino acid and possibly the protein produced, whereas a *nonfunctional* SNP does not alter the end amino acid or protein or change its function.

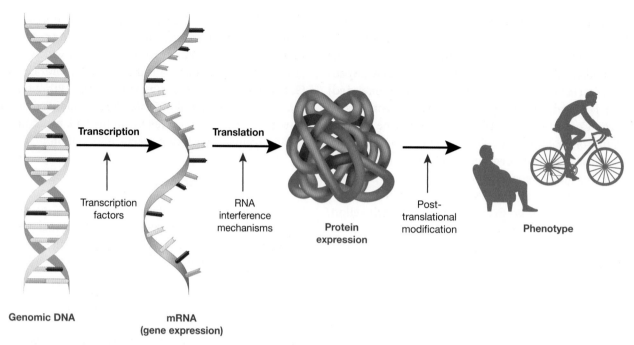

FIGURE 18.2 Central dogma. The central dogma begins with genomic DNA that is transcribed into mRNA that is then translated into proteins, which together with environmental factors determine the phenotype. Notice that the final protein expressed may be altered by the transcription factors present, inhibited by the RNA interference mechanisms, or altered by posttranslational modifications. Thus, although genomic DNA provides the blueprint, there are multiple steps that may alter the final protein.

Whether an SNP is functional or nonfunctional is hugely important in understanding whether a genomic marker (usually an SNP) that is associated with a specific characteristic actually means or does anything. Thus, anytime a CEP is told that an SNP is associated or correlated with a specific characteristic, the first question should be whether that SNP is actually functional and makes any difference in the physiology. The functionality of an SNP can often be easily determined by consulting the SNP database that is maintained by the National Center for Biotechnology Information (NCBI — www.ncbi.nlm.nih .gov/SNP). The CEP should also remember that our understanding of the functionality of an SNP can change. An SNP previously considered nonfunctional may be considered functional in the future if new studies or information suggest that it is involved in genetic processes. However, in general, if an SNP were nonfunctional, then using that SNP as potentially informative in an exercise prescription would be useless. Further, most exercise characteristics are not dependent on alterations in a single amino acid. Therefore, it is rare for an individual SNP to affect human exercise functioning.

Most commercial entities that do genomic testing (*e.g.*, www.23andme.com) merely check an individual's genome for SNPs. In most cases, any extrapolations about how the SNPs might affect exercise functioning is just speculation.

Think of the genome as a type of foundational cookbook with an assortment of recipes for proteins. Now consider how two people following the same recipe may produce very different outcomes. This variation is explained by the fact that the finished outcome (usually proteins) depends heavily on the rest of the steps of the central dogma.

Step 2: Transcription

The second step of the central dogma is the transcription of the genomic DNA into messenger RNA (or mRNA), which carries the genetic "message" from the nucleus into the cytosol. The process of transcription is thus the first step in the interpretation of the genetic "recipe." Many genetic factors either inhibit or augment transcription. Some of these "transcription factors" have gained a lot of attention in exercise science. One example is a molecule called "peroxisome proliferator-activated receptor delta" (*PPAR*d), which may play a role in exercise endurance (8). *PPAR*d actually turns on transcription of a number of genes and, as such, is thought to influence which genes are transcribed and which are not. Further, transcription factors can alter the interpretation of a gene's code. In a process known as "alternative splicing," regions of a gene can be joined or skipped during translation, producing an alternative protein. Many genes exhibit alternative splicing, so although in most cases expression of a particular gene will produce a particular protein, a single gene can sometimes code to produce multiple proteins.

Epigenetics, another mechanism that influences gene expression via transcription, has received a lot of research and media attention recently. Epigenetic mechanisms alter which genes are transcribed through a series of steps that are initiated by environmental exposures, including maternal attention, diet, exercise, and environmental toxins. Epigenetic factors do not alter the DNA itself. Rather, they alter the availability of a gene for transcription.

In summary, although two people's underlying genomic code may be very similar, differences in transcription factors, alternative splicing, and epigenetics can all markedly change the output of the transcription step. Bear in mind that all we have done to this point is move the "recipe" from the foundational "cookbook" in the nucleus to the cytosol. Step 3 is when the recipe gets made!

Step 3: Translation

During the third step of the central dogma, the mRNA from Step 2 travels to ribosomes, where it is "translated" into amino acids, which are then assembled into a protein. Continuing the previous analogy, translation is the act of making the recipe with the modifications that transcription has introduced. As with transcription, there are factors and mechanisms that can either inhibit or augment translation.

One such factor is micro-RNAs (or miRNA), which can inhibit or stop translation of specific strands of mRNA. The inhibition of translation by miRNA is a relatively new concept, first proposed in 1998 by Fire et al. (9), who were awarded the Nobel Prize in 2006. Thousands of miRNAs have been found, most of which can affect multiple genes. For example, miRNA-208a affects the synthesis of cardiac B-myosin heavy chains; in addition, it regulates the assembly of a protein complex called "MED13" (for "mediator component 13"), which is involved in energy homeostasis. MED13 has been shown to increase metabolism in adipose and liver cells in mice; thus, when MED13 is augmented (because miRNA-208 is turned down), body fat and weight in mice decrease (10).

Adding to the complexity that miRNA brings to the central dogma is the recent understanding that miRNA as well as RNA and other cellular products can be packaged in small vesicles called "exosomes" that are released from tissues and move to other cells throughout the body, where they release their contents for action (11). Thus, miRNA and other substances can act as a different type of cell-signaling mechanism that affects protein production all

over the body, greatly expanding the reach and impact of translational mechanisms. Thus, because of translational inhibitors, we cannot assume that a transcribed gene will always be translated into a protein. In fact, several studies have shown that gene transcription and translation are poorly correlated at best (12, 13), further supporting the saying common among geneticists, "Just because it transcribes, that doesn't mean it translates."

Step 4: Posttranslational Modification

After translation, proteins can undergo several modifications that alter their functioning. These posttranslational modifications include phosphorylation, acetylation, acylation, glycosylation, and/or myristoylation (4). Recalling our recipe analogy, this step is similar to adding seasoning to the finished recipe, thereby altering the taste of the dish. In the end, it is this modified protein that is the end product of the central dogma.

In summary, the central dogma starts with the genome and includes transcription, translation, and posttranslational modification. Within each step, several factors, conditions, and other mechanisms can influence the outcome — and subsequent downstream protein products. This variety of alterations during transcription, translation, and posttranslation is the primary reason why individuals with only slight genomic differences can be so diverse.

Step 5: Other Genetic Controllers

The central dogma primarily describes how the central genetic mechanisms turn genomic codes into protein. Although there are several controlling mechanisms that work within the central dogma — such as transcription, translation, and posttranslational modification — there are many other factors that control whether the overall dogma proceeds and directly regulates specific pieces of the process. These factors are also a form of genetic control that affects how a trait is expressed. Unfortunately, much of the exercise systems genetics has been undertaken without an appreciation of how these other genetic controllers increase the magnitude of complexity of understanding the underlying exercise systems genetics (14). For example, as has been emphasized in the case of exercise systems genetics, there are about 70,000 promoter regions, 400,000 enhancer regions, and many repressor sites encoded by DNA (14). Additionally, epistasis — where one gene's protein can affect how another gene functions — further complicates the genome to protein process. To get a true sense of how epistasis increases the complexity of genetic regulation, consider that there are as many as 250 protein-binding sites on a protein-coding gene; in other words, as many as 250 proteins can bind on each gene to alter its protein production. Our best computational models of epistasis only have enough power to describe one or two-gene epistasis! (15) As a result, all these steps from the genome to the end phenotype are complicated, involved, and often defy easy understanding.

In summary, the exercise systems genetics that control an exercise trait involves not only the components of the central dogma but also all the other genetic factors that influence and affect physiological phenotypes. Indeed, it is highly unlikely that any one factor contributes enough control of any exercise characteristic to definitively identify. As such, the CEP must recognize that any genetic information used for exercise prescription will have to be detailed and substantial!

Limitations of Association Studies for Exercise Prescription

The CEP must remember that because of the numerous steps between the genome and the finished, modified protein, in the large majority of cases, the client's genome does not solely determine the end protein that is made. This point has been largely lost in much of the exercise scientific literature; that is, many research studies have claimed that certain exercise traits are associated with a particular genomic SNP pattern. Although many studies reveal *associations* between SNPs and an exercise trait, all of these are large correlational studies using specialized statistical approaches. In particular, one type of genetic association study design that the CEP may hear of is a genome-wide association study, often shortened to GWAS (pronounced "G-Waz"). A GWAS can seem powerful because of the large number of subjects involved — often thousands. Unfortunately, GWAS studies tend to deliver quite a few false-positive results. Flint et al. (16) estimated that *less than 1% of the association studies* provided a true genetic mechanism for the characteristic studied. Put another way, Flint and colleagues' data suggested that about 99% of the time, the genetic association studies would not be able to identify the underlying mechanism responsible for controlling that characteristic. Although Fint's analysis was done on the existing animal studies at the time, there has been no other analysis like this so far in the genetics literature; so although dated, it is the best illustration of how difficult it is to use GWAS studies to understand the underlying control mechanisms for a phenotype.

Thus, "genomics-focused" association studies have three major weaknesses that generally prevent them from being used in exercise prescription:

1. They are associative/correlational and do not present causation.
2. They assume that the end protein product is directly represented by the variance in the genome (represented by SNPs) and thereby disregard three of the four steps in the central dogma, as well as other genetic factors that may influence an end characteristic.
3. These studies do not generally take into account other genetic factors that may be involved in regulating the characteristic of interest.

With a few exceptions (discussed later in the chapter), most of the existing research does provide an excellent starting point for further research; however, it is not a solid foundation to be used for exercise prescription. For example, there are many studies considering the angiotensin-converting enzyme (*ACE*) gene and its effect on a wide variety of exercise characteristics. Montgomery et al. (17) proposed that a particular genotype in the *ACE* gene would lead to a positive energy balance during rigorous training. This hypothesized effect was based on correlations found between the proposed genotype and body composition in 81 White male recruits in the British Army. To date, over 359 studies have investigated the relationship between *ACE* and exercise characteristics; however, careful examination of most of these studies shows a continued ambiguity over whether any specific *ACE* genotype confers any particular advantage during exercise. Thus, although most of the prominent direct-to-consumer (DTC) genetic services test the *ACE* genotype, it is unclear whether *ACE* actually has any role at all in determining exercise capacity, strength levels, and/or trainability (along with other characteristics to which *ACE* has been correlated). So, in the case of *ACE*, knowing a client's *ACE* genotype will not add to the information available for an exercise prescription. As noted by a recent review of the topic (18): "...this systematic review does not support the working hypothesis ... that adults with the *ACE I* allele exhibit superior endurance exercise performance than adults with the *D* allele."

The CEP may be tempted to make use of commercial products that promise "personalized exercise prescriptions based on an individual's genome," especially because doing so can add an air of sophistication and mystique that can help market a CEP's services. However, because of reasons pointed out above, current consensus among experts in the field hold that commercial genetic tests cannot predict exercise capacity, performance, capabilities, or many other exercise characteristics with any accuracy or should be used as an attempt to identify someone's talent or future performance in sport/exercise (19).

Although it is attractive to think that alterations in one or two genes may affect exercise responses, published data suggest that most exercise characteristics are regulated by a combination of many genes (*i.e.*, called "polygenic" or "multigenic" control). However, it is true that certain disorders are caused by a defective genomic code for a particular gene. These are often referred to as single-gene disorders. The following section discusses two single-gene disorders especially important for consideration by the CEP, as well as Down syndrome (DS), a chromosomal disorder.

SINGLE-GENE AND CHROMOSOMAL DISORDERS AFFECTING EXERCISE RESPONSE

Single-gene and chromosomal disorders can affect an individual's response to exercise and thus pose issues that the CEP needs to be aware of in developing an exercise prescription. The disorders discussed in this section include McArdle disease, sickle cell disease, and DS. Because these disorders severely compromise basic physiological functioning, affected individuals typically have compromised exercise capability or difficulty doing any exercise at all.

It is likely that individuals with these conditions have had extensive contact with health care providers, and thus additional genetic testing would not enhance the exercise prescription provided by the CEP. However, in general, the conditions discussed here are not covered under any specific currently published exercise prescription guidelines. Thus, the CEP should use ACSM's general exercise recommendations for individuals with chronic conditions referred to in *ACSM's Exercise Management for Persons with Chronic Disease and Disability* (20). Another helpful source is *ACSM's Guidelines for Exercise Testing and Prescription* (21). In conjunction with these established guidelines, the CEP should develop the appropriate exercise prescription in collaboration with the individual's existing health care team.

McArdle Disease

Most CEPs are familiar with McArdle disease because patients have been used in landmark studies of exercise metabolism (22). The disorder is caused by a defect in one gene, *myophosphorylase*, also known as glycogen phosphorylase muscle, or *PYGM*, which is located on chromosome 11 (23). This *PYGM* defect prevents the use of glycogen in glycolysis and generally prevents the development of lactate. McArdle disease is rare; the largest patient database available includes only 81 patients worldwide (24).

Patients suffering from McArdle disease exhibit extreme exercise intolerance that includes fatigue, myalgia, and muscle contractures. These consequences can lead to both myoglobinuria and rhabdomyolysis (a rapid breakdown of the muscle), thus leading to exercise contraindications in patients with McArdle disease. However, lack of exercise further exacerbates the exercise intolerance in these patients. In the largest cohort of patients with McArdle disease yet described ($n = 81$; age range 17–80 years; 42 males, 39 females; 21), patients exhibited significantly diminished exercise capacities with a $\dot{V}O_{2peak}$ ($mL \cdot kg^{-1} \cdot min^{-1}$) equaling 17.1 (range 15.9–18.3) with a peak power output equaling 74.7 W (range 68.3–81.1). However, patients with McArdle disease who engaged in higher levels of daily activity (using the International Physical Activity Questionnaire — IPAQ) generally showed higher $\dot{V}O_{2peak}$ (average = 20.0 $mL \cdot kg^{-1} \cdot min^{-1}$) and peak power output (average = 92.7 W) than patients who were inactive (24). These data suggest that greater physical activity improves cardiorespiratory functioning in patients with McArdle disease.

No adequate exercise guidelines are currently available for use in this population. It is possible that a recently developed mouse model of McArdle disease (25) will be useful in establishing initial exercise prescription parameters for human patients with McArdle disease. In the meantime, given the frank exercise intolerance demonstrated by patients with McArdle disease, the goal of any exercise program would be to encourage physical activity, even if it is light-intensity activity. Given the similarities in exercise discomfort and the need for energy budgeting in patients with chronic fatigue syndrome, another source of exercise programming information for patients with McArdle disease would be the exercise recommendations on chronic fatigue (26).

Sickle Cell Disease

Sickle cell disease is caused by an SNP (switch from A to T) in the seventh codon of the *beta-globulin* gene that is found on chromosome 11 (27). This SNP results in the production of abnormal hemoglobin that folds and deforms under low oxygen states (*e.g.*, at altitude or with extreme oxygen off-loading in the muscle). Sickle cell hemoglobin confers resistance to malaria, and the disease is more prevalent in individuals whose ancestors lived in sub-Saharan, Mediterranean, Central and South American, and other countries where malaria is widespread. Individuals with one affected gene have the sickle cell trait, whereas individuals who have inherited the affected gene from both parents have sickle cell disease.

In the U.S., the Centers for Disease Control and Prevention (CDC-P) estimates that approximately 1 in 13 Black or African American infants are born with sickle cell trait. Sickle cell disease occurs in approximately 1 in 365 Black or African American births, and 1 in 16,300 Hispanic-American births (28). In general, only individuals with sickle cell disease exhibit hemoglobin sickling, which causes pain, swelling, exercise intolerance, and other signs and symptoms, usually beginning within the first year of life. Individuals with sickle cell trait have one gene that still produces normal hemoglobin and, in general, they have few, if any, symptoms and can tolerate exercise.

In individuals with sickle cell disease, sickling of the hemoglobin is estimated to begin within 2–3 minutes of all-out exercise. Sickled cells block arteries, reducing blood flow and starving the muscle (and other tissues) of oxygen, thereby triggering rhabdomyolysis. The condition is life-threatening: the National Athletic Trainers' Association has attributed at least 15 deaths in football players to this type of exertional sickling (29). In 2010, the National Collegiate Athletic Association (NCAA) implemented a mandatory sickle cell screening program for all Division 1 athletes; although controversial, this program has been estimated to have resulted in the prevention of at least seven deaths per decade (30). Moreover, all 50 U.S. states and most U.S. territories (except Puerto Rico and the U.S. Virgin Islands) screen all newborns for sickle cell trait/disease (31).

Screening programs and the early onset of symptoms mean that each client the CEP works with should know whether they are positive for sickle cell trait or disease. With this knowledge, the CEP should modify the exercise prescription accordingly to decrease the risk of sickling and subsequent physiological issues. Given that higher-intensity exercise increases sickling, exercise in these patients should be confined to lower-intensity efforts using the general guidelines as proposed by Gordon et al. (32). In addition, some investigators have suggested that patients stay well hydrated during exercise, avoid extreme temperatures (especially cold) during exercise, and avoid contact sports that might lead to mechanical trauma (27).

Down Syndrome

DS, in most cases, is caused by an additional copy of chromosome 21 in the genome of an affected individual (see Chapter 12) (33). Although increased maternal age increases the risk of a newborn with DS (34), researchers have not determined why it occurs. Individuals with DS have a wide range of physiological and cognitive alterations, from minimal to severe.

In general, individuals with DS can exercise. However, approximately 45% of individuals with DS have congenital heart disease (35), and DS is associated with a reduced resting metabolic rate, which promotes obesity (36). Thus, as with the single-gene disorders just discussed, individuals with DS exhibit reduced exercise tolerance: it has been reported that the average $\dot{V}O_{2peak}$ of a male with DS is about 28 mL·kg^{-1}·min^{-1} and of a female with DS is about 22 mL·kg^{-1}·min^{-1} (37). These lower values are primarily because of a lower peak cardiac output in these individuals.

The application of an exercise training program can increase both quality of life and lifespan in the DS population. The CEP should consult the general exercise guidelines for individuals with chronic diseases (20) as well as the extensive discussion of exercise prescription for this population contained in *ACSM Guidelines for Exercise Testing and Prescription* (21) as a baseline for exercise programming. Additionally, for further information regarding DS and exercise programming, see Chapter 12. Although the underlying heart limitations will inhibit cardiac output, which will in turn reduce oxygen consumption, research has shown that there are a variety of health benefits with exercise programs in individuals with DS. These include the following:

- Increased reaction time after training (38)
- Increased work performance (39) and aerobic capacity (40)
- Increased strength (40)

THE USE OF GENETIC INFORMATION FOR THE EXERCISE PRESCRIPTION

As noted, most exercise characteristics are regulated not by a single gene, but by many genes along with many other genetic mechanisms (thus, exercise systems genetics). Thus, to prescribe exercise using genetic information, the CEP would require information regarding which genes, which central dogma mechanisms, and which other genetic interactions are involved with the exercise characteristic to truly understand the system genetics underpinning the characteristic. This type of extensive exercise systems genetics information is generally not available at this point in our understanding of how genetics regulates exercise characteristics. As more information on exercise genetics becomes available, the CEP may be able to apply that information in developing exercise prescriptions, but only if that information enhances the exercise prescription and provides a "more effective intervention strategy" (41). To this end, there are a few areas in which the amount of genetic information available is reaching critical mass and may indirectly and/or directly guide the CEP in developing the exercise prescription.

Exercise Genetics of β_2-Adrenergic Receptors

The β_2-adrenergic receptors, which respond primarily to epinephrine, play critical roles in exercise responses. β_2-Adrenergic receptors are thought to be involved in increases in bronchodilation, ventricular function, vasodilation, and lipolysis and may influence heart rate and ventricular contractility during exercise (42). They are the predominant type of β-receptor, estimated to make up 70%–80% of all β-receptors. Numerous studies (322

articles listed in PubMed as of this writing) have focused on the genomic variants present in β_2-adrenergic receptors and how these functional SNPs may alter responses to exercise (Table 18.1). Although most of these studies are of the genomic association design (*i.e.*, GWAS), the fact that the genetic variants in this receptor have been so well studied and that the results have been almost unanimous, in contrast to the research on the genotypes of *ACE* and *ACTN3* discussed earlier, lends strength to the use of the genomics of these receptors in developing exercise prescriptions.

The *ADRB2* gene encodes the β_2-adrenergic receptor. It is located on the long arm of chromosome 5, with primary functional polymorphisms located at the 16th (nucleotide 46) and 27th amino acid (nucleotide 79) positions. At the 16th amino acid, the polymorphism in the nucleotide leads to either a glycine or an arginine (designated as Gly16 or Arg16), and at the 27th amino acid, the polymorphism results in either a glutamine (Gln27) or glutamic acid (Glu27). Approximately 39% of individuals have the Gly16 variant on both chromosomes (*i.e.*, the individual is "homozygous" for the Gly16 variant), whereas the homozygous Arg16 occurs in approximately 15% of individuals. The heterozygous Gly/Arg (*i.e.*, the variant is on only one of the chromosomes) occurs in approximately

Table 18.1		Frequency and Cardiopulmonary Function According to Sequence Variation of the *ADRB2* at Amino Acids 16 and 27	
Codon	Substitutions	Frequency (%)	Function
46	Arg16Gly	AA = 15 AG = 47 GG = 39	GlyGly more prevalent in hypertensives
46	Arg16Gly	AA = 22 AG = 41 GG = 37	Patients with CHF with Gly allele have better pulmonary function compared with Arg
46	Arg16Gly		GlyGly more receptors, greater cardiac function, airway function, natriuretic function, and lung fluid clearance
46	Arg16Gly		GlyGly greater cardiac response to isometric handgrip
46	Arg16Gly		GlyGly sustained response to infused isoproterenol
79	Gln27Glu	GlnGln = 32 GlnGlu = 53 GluGlu = 16	GluGlu more prevalent in hypertensives

ADRB2, β_2-adrenergic receptors; CHF, congestive heart failure.

Source: Snyder EM, Johnson BD, Joyner MJ. Genetics of β_2-adrenergic receptors and the cardiopulmonary response to exercise. *Exerc Sport Sci Rev.* 2008;36(2):98–105.

47% of individuals (43, 44). Likewise, the glutamine (Gln) homozygosity at the 27th amino acid occurs in approximately 32% of individuals, with the glutamic acid (Glu) homozygosity occurring in approximately 16% and a glutamine/glutamic acid heterozygosity occurring in approximately 53% (43, 44).

The variants at both the 16th and 27th amino acids have been linked to multiple differential responses to exercise. An outstanding review delineating those altered responses is presented by Snyder et al. (42) (see Table 18.1). For example, an individual who is homozygous for Gly16 demonstrates greater stroke volume and cardiac output during absolute workload exercise (45) and has enhanced left ventricular function at rest (46), compared to those who are homozygous for the Arg16 variant. Further, individuals who are homozygous for Glu27 have a higher prevalence of hypertension (44) and may exhibit shifted metabolic use of carbohydrate during exercise, especially if they are obese (47). Additionally, although ventilation is not normally considered a limiting factor in exercise, individuals with the Gly16 genomic pattern have sustained bronchodilation and remove fluid from the lungs faster postexercise (48). Thus, Snyder et al. (42) suggested that individuals with the "Gly16Glu27" pattern have more "favorable responses to exercise" because individuals with this pattern generally show higher stroke volumes, cardiac outputs, and enhanced vasodilation during acute exercise. Thus, the CEP developing an exercise prescription for an individual who has the Gly16Glu27 genotype should understand that the current literature suggests that these clients will have an augmented cardiovascular response at any absolute workload during exercise, and predictably that these individuals' work capacity may be higher. However, in clinical patients with the Gly16Glu27 genotype, especially those in the early phases of recovery from cardiovascular procedures, the CEP should decrease the work rate to prevent elevated cardiovascular responses too soon postoperatively. Additionally, from a clinical perspective, it has been shown that patients with the Gly16 variant, primarily because of their increased vasodilation rates, require larger amounts of vasopressor drugs than do patients with the Arg16 variant (49).

In short, the type of *ADRB2* variant that a client has at the 16th and 27th positions can alter their responses to exercise, and the CEP should be aware of these potential alterations so the exercise prescription can reflect the different cardiovascular responses during exercise. This modification of the exercise prescription is especially important in clinical patients who have undergone recent cardiovascular procedures.

Given the potential dependency of exercise cardiovascular responses based on the *ADRB2* genotype, it would be tempting to suggest that an individual's exercise performance might be predicted from this genotype, especially because those individuals with the Gly16Glu27 seem to respond in an augmented manner during acute exercise. This hypothesis, although attractive, is still unproven, with at least one study (50) supporting it and one study not supporting it (51). Further, from the currently available literature, it is clear at this time that although the *ADRB2* genotype may lead to altered cardiovascular responses during exercise, the *ADRB2* genotype does not predict potential elite athletes (50).

Exercise Genetics and the *FTO* Gene

A gene that has received much scientific attention is the *alpha-ketoglutarate–dependent dioxygenase* gene, also known as the "*FTO*" gene. Although the exact function of *FTO* is not known, it has been extensively linked with obesity and predisposes to an increased risk of Type 2 diabetes. The SNP variant A/T *rs9939609* in the *FTO* gene (on chromosome 16) has drawn the most interest among obesity researchers. However, studies have not supported an association between *FTO* and energy intake, maximal oxygen consumption, or leisure-time activity levels (52, 53), general physical activity levels (54), or elite athletic status (55). Thus, the CEP should not use *FTO* genomic patterns to predict any of the mentioned exercise characteristics or behaviors.

However, studies (56) have shown that the activity status of an individual can affect the response of the *FTO* gene. Researchers have shown that if an individual is active, the obesity induction effect of *FTO* is reduced by approximately 30%. Thus, inclusion of an activity component within a weight loss program is thought to help reduce obesity by inhibiting *FTO*. Thus, although not useful for predicting exercise characteristics, knowing the *FTO* variant of the client, especially if they have the A/T *rs9939609* SNP, can help the CEP predict whether the client will be able to lose weight with exercise.

In summary, as noted before, the incorporation of genetic information into exercise prescription development should only be done when this information can enhance the exercise prescription. The CEP should continue to watch the literature: it is probable that other genetic variants like *FTO* will be found that, although not having a direct influence on exercise characteristics, will influence how their clients' physiology is altered with an exercise program.

Influence of Genetics on the Efficiency and Efficacy of Pharmaceutical Regimens

It is not normally in the CEP's scope of practice to determine appropriate pharmaceutical regimens for their patients. However, the CEP is often the frontline clinician, with regular interaction with patients. As such, the CEP is often the first to know if prescribed medication protocols are effective or not.

It has been estimated that 20%–95% of variations in pharmaceutical response can be attributed to genetic variation (57) that is individual or a result of a specific population having specific genetic variants. The wide range of responses to the same drug because of genetic variation can result in a variety of physiological differences in a patient's response to exercise. The Pharmacogenomics Knowledgebase (PharmGKB; www.pharmgkb.org) (58) is a concerted effort funded by the NIH and conducted by the national Clinical Pharmacogenetics Implementation Consortium housed at Stanford University to map and document the range of drug responses among different genotypes. One of the unique aspects of PharmGKB is that its noncorporate funding and managerial support reduce potential conflicts of interests regarding its conclusions. The patient genotype guidelines that PharmGKB publishes are based on the level of available evidence (ranked from the best evidence = 4 to the weakest evidence = 1). This ranking helps clinicians understand the strength of the evidence underlying any specific PharmGKB recommendation. PharmGKB also works in partnership with other entities around the world that are developing guidelines for pharmacogenetics, such as the Pharmacogenetics Working Group of the Royal Dutch Association for the Advancement of Pharmacy (59).

Where appropriate, the use of the PharmGKB database would entail the CEP cross-referencing a client's drug with their genotype and providing suggestions to the physician, as appropriate, on more efficacious options. As an example, up to 20% of commonly used pharmaceuticals, including many of the most popular β-blockers, are metabolized by an enzyme named cytochrome P450 2D6 (*CYP2D6*) in the liver (60). Different polymorphisms in the *CYP2D6* gene can alter the function of this enzyme and subsequently alter the metabolism of the pharmaceuticals that are disposed through this pathway. Starting in the early 1990s, there were extensive efforts to map the numerous genomic variants in *CYP2D6* that altered drug metabolism. The most common variant occurrences have been grouped into different "alleles" (*i.e.*, patterns of

variance). Currently, over 150 different alleles identified for *CYP2D6* change the functioning of the gene. Current information on *CYP2D6* variants is maintained at the Human Cytochrome P450 (CYP) Allele Nomenclature Database (61). Again, individuals with different allele patterns in the *CYP2D6* gene have different drug metabolism responses. Based on their *CYP2D6* genomic pattern, individuals are categorized as extensive metabolizers (EM), which is the most frequent pattern, poor metabolizers (PM), intermediate metabolizers (IM), or ultra-rapid metabolizers (UM) (60).

As an example especially relevant to CEPs, metoprolol, a popular β-blocking drug, was one of the first drugs that was observed to have adverse reactions in some individuals who were later shown to be PM because of their genome makeup (62, 63). In fact, current PharmGKB guidelines (www.pharmgkb.org) (58) indicate that for the three phenotypes (PM, IM, UM) of metoprolol metabolizers that do not occur as frequently, there is potential for heart failure. Therefore, recommended dosages for the patients with PM, IM, or UM are reduced by 50% (IM) or 75% (PM), or increased to a maximum of 250% normal with patients with UM. Alternatively, the clinician could switch the patient to a different drug that is not metabolized through the CYP2DG pathway. The evidence for pharmacogenetics interactions using metoprolol is generally considered the most rigorous available (level 4).

Several other β-blockers (atenolol, bisoprolol, propranolol) have level 3 dosing guidelines that consider the genotype of the client. Thus, although most CEPs will not be responsible for their clients' pharmaceutical regimens, it is helpful for the CEP to understand the potential genotype/pharmaceutical reactions that may complicate compliance or responses to a traditional exercise prescription.

Determining a client's genotypic pattern for a specific drug is a nontrivial task, especially given that for a well-known drug like metoprolol, over 150 different genetic variants can affect the drug's metabolism. Thus, if a pharmacological regimen is not having the expected effects, the CEP should consider consulting with the referring physician about pharmacogenomic testing. There are several companies available that specialize in pharmacogenomic testing and interpretation (*e.g.*, Admera Health — https://www.admerahealth.com), with these tests often covered by insurance. Although not directly related to exercise, the use of pharmacogenomic testing can help the CEP's client respond more appropriately to both their drug regimen and their exercise prescription.

Using Genomic Markers to Predict Responses to Aerobic Exercise Training

As noted, it is well established that genetic factors play a significant role in determining responses to both aerobic (3) and resistance exercise programs (5). However, the identity of the exercise systems genetic mechanisms that control these responses remains largely unknown. Thus, genetic biomarkers that could be used to predict who will respond, not respond, or have negative responses to training have generally been lacking. This is especially true for resistance training; that is, other than single-gene SNP speculations (*e.g.*, with *ACTN3* or *ACE*), there have been no efforts to develop predictor panels of genomic markers that could be used to inform an exercise prescription.

For aerobic exercise, there have been early efforts to develop and validate genomic markers that may predict training responses. In 2010, for example, a large international group of scientists, using muscle biopsies and mRNA from 24 young, sedentary European males, developed a potential predictor panel of 29 genes that were associated with the outcome of 6 weeks of high-intensity aerobic training (64). The use of mRNA (as opposed to genomic DNA) for prediction purposes is stronger from a theoretical perspective because mRNA is closer to the end of the genetic pathway (see Figure 18.2), and, as such, there is an increased probability that these results may more closely represent the end proteins that determine the training response. Importantly, this group then validated this mRNA-derived predictor panel against results from a different set of 17 young, sedentary European males and then validated the 29-gene predictor panel against previously collected results from approximately 500 subjects who were predominately of European ancestry. They found that 11 genes explained 23% of the aerobic adaptation to exercise, or about half of the known genetic role in endurance training. Although these results provided hope that genetic information could be used successfully in endurance training development, the fact that the predictor panel was primarily developed in European-descent males limited the possible application. Further, although the names of the genes used in the gene panel were published and the authors had applied for a patent on the gene panel, at this time, no commercial company offers screening using this predictor panel.

The use of muscle biopsy mRNA was one of the strengths of the previously discussed predictor panel,

but it represents a significant weakness when translating these findings to clinical use. As most CEPs appreciate, muscle biopsies are not typically performed to establish an exercise prescription and would represent unnecessary risk and pain for clients. Recognizing the limitations of the previous predictor panel, several researchers who were also involved in the earlier work presented a different predictor panel that was developed using genomic DNA from a large 20-week training study called the HERITAGE study that included 742 subjects of both European and African descent (65). This panel was developed based on genomic DNA, which are easier to collect saliva samples, making it more applicable to a larger population. The training paradigm used was also more representative of what CEPs normally prescribe. Additionally, this work was one of the first to calculate a "genetic predictor" score in which the actions of the genes in the predictor panel were mathematically summarized to give a single score. In the subjects of European descent who participated in this study, the published predictor panel revealed 21 genes that were related to 48% of the response to the 20-week training program, and the genetic predictor score was positively related to the change in oxygen consumption after training. However, only 5 of the 15 strongest genetic markers were significant in the subjects of African descent, suggesting that this predictor panel would not be appropriate to use with clients of African descent. This issue highlights one of the challenges in using genomic/genetic data of any kind to predict general characteristics; there are likely marked differences between ethnic groups in how genetic mechanisms adjust physiological adaptations, and, thus, separate predictor panels need to be developed for different ethnic groups. This ethnic genetic diversity is one reason why international efforts to map the human variability in genes, like the International HapMap Project (66), commonly recognize at least 11 different global populations in their genetic categorizations. Additionally, like the previous predictor panel, although the identities of genetic factors that make up the panel from Bouchard's group are freely available (65), no commercial entity at this point conducts prediction screening based on this predictor panel.

At about the same time as the previous prediction studies were published, Thomaes and coworkers (67) published a unique type of predictor study with almost 1,000 cardiac rehabilitation subjects in a study called the CAREGENE study (Cardiac Rehabilitation and GENetics of Exercise performance and training effect). What was unique about this study was that a seven-gene predictor score — now often called a "polygenic risk score" (PRS) — summarized the genetic results, instead of depending solely on associations with single genes. As with Bouchard's findings, Thomaes and coworkers found that the PRS correlated with the amount of change in $\dot{V}O_2$ after training. In other words, the higher the PRS, the greater the change in $\dot{V}O_2$. In summary, although it is not known why these genes are predictors, both Bouchard's group and Thomaes' group provide predictor panels/scores that positively correlate with the amount of change in aerobic capacity after training.

The use of PRS, instead of focusing on individual genes, takes advantages of and acknowledges what the literature on the genetic causes of most characteristics has shown: each physiological characteristic, like $\dot{V}O_2$ or the change in $\dot{V}O_2$ after training, is the result of many genes and genetic factors working together. As such, the use of a PRS can give a summary picture of the exercise systems genetics responsible for physiological characteristics.

Because you need to know a lot of genetic information to build a PRS that is reflective of the underlying characteristic, the development of these scores has been slow. One area that is starting to see some use of PRS to predict behavior is the area of physical activity prediction. There is a wide and deep pool of literature showing that an individual's daily physical activity is approximately 50% determined by their genetics (68). Recently, Kujala and colleagues (69) used the open-source data from the UK Biobank that has genetic data and physical activity data from approximately 321,000 individuals. The authors constructed an algorithm to predict the physical activity with a PRS and then applied that PRS to approximately 15,000 subjects from Finland. In short, the authors found that the PRS could predict daily activity, but the variation in that prediction was quite small, meaning it was not a very good fit. These results show that the use of a PRS may help apply genetic data to the prediction of physiological characteristics, but that additional work on the development of these PRS are needed before the CEP can use these in developing exercise prescriptions.

Although at a nascent stage, efforts to use genetic information to predict who can benefit the most and the least from exercise training will continue to advance, especially given the role of exercise in the management of chronic disease. The CEP should monitor the literature for further advances and make sure that any polygenetic prediction panels used are based on solid research supporting the PRS's effectiveness in enhancing exercise prescription.

GENE EDITING AND THE FUTURE

Altering exercise prescriptions to take genetic factors into account is one way to use genetic information to improve an individual's health, but altering the underlying genetic code to remove deleterious genomic factors is widely considered the end goal of much of precision medicine. Although scientists have had the capability to alter genetic coding since the 1970s, the methods used were often cumbersome and inefficient and could not be applied in a "real-world" setting. However, currently, several technologies being tested in humans may change medicine as we know it. In general, these technologies take two different approaches:

1. Blocking either transcription or translation to prevent protein production from certain genes
2. Editing out a piece of a gene or a whole gene to remove that gene or alter its function

Examples of each approach are currently being applied to some human models. Thus, it is incumbent upon the CEP to understand and be aware of these promising technologies.

Approaches That Block Protein Output

It has been known for several years that certain genetic structures, such as miRNAs, can interfere with transcription and/or translation. As understanding of miRNAs advanced, some researchers hypothesized that if short miRNA-like sequences (often called "oligos") based on a specific gene could be developed and delivered to the right place in the body, that gene's output could be turned on or off, at least for a short period of time. The trick was delivering the oligos in an efficient manner before they could be degraded by the body. One step forward in this technology occurred in early 2008 when Morcos et al. (70) developed a form of these oligos called "vivo-morpholinos" that resisted degradation for up to 7 days.

To date, vivo-morpholinos and the related morpholinos have been used in over 7,200 studies in many species. For example, they have been used in mice to block genes in both skeletal muscle and the brain that may control daily physical activity (71). This gene knockdown lasted about 7 days, and after this time, protein production from those genes resumed. Morpholinos also have been used in preliminary clinical trials in humans. For example, Kaye et al. treated boys 7–13 years old with Duchenne muscular dystrophy with a morpholino designed to produce functional dystrophin (72). These results (and others) were promising enough that the U.S. Food and Drug Administration (FDA) has recently given approval to three exon-skipping antisense oligonucleotides (similar to morpholinos) for treatment of Duchenne muscular dystrophy (73). Thus, the use of vivo-morpholinos (or similar substances) that inhibit transcription and/or translation may become a common therapy for controlling the deleterious effects of certain genes.

Direct Gene Editing

Whereas approaches that block transcription/translation can be beneficial both as physiological investigatory tools and as potential treatments, being able to cut out and replace either a deleterious gene or a defective piece of a gene would lead us closer to cures for many diseases, especially single-gene disorders such as McArdle disease and sickle cell disease. Approaches to gene editing have existed since 1985. The earliest technologies, called "zinc finger arrays," were joined in 2010 by transcription activator-like effectors (TALEN). These approaches were inefficient, often difficult, and expensive. In 2012, a team led by Drs. Jennifer Doudna and Emmanuelle Charpentier — who both were later awarded the 2020 Nobel Prize in Chemistry for this work — published the first use of a technology called CRISPR–Cas9 to enable quick, easy, and inexpensive gene editing (74). This technology was based on observations in bacteria of so-called CRISPR that were proposed to be a type of bacterial immune system against viruses. In short, CRISPR provided a genetic template for the viruses that the bacteria had overcome.

Researchers quickly found that most organisms have CRISPR. Further, an associated CRISPR protein, Cas9, provided the mechanism that actually edits the genome. With CRISPR as the template and Cas9 acting as the molecular scissors, the CRISPR–Cas9 system can effectively cut out any piece of the genome. Since 2012, CRISPR–Cas9 has been used effectively in literally thousands of studies for gene editing purposes (for more information, see the excellent review of CRISPR–Cas9 published in 2014 by Drs. Doudna and Charpentier in *Science*; 75). Because CRISPR–Cas9 is relatively inexpensive (some companies offer custom-designed CRISPR–Cas9 complexes for less than $200), is relatively easy to use, and has an approximately 80% editing efficiency, there has been both great excitement and trepidation concerning the potential uses of this technology.

The potential applications of CRISPR–Cas9 are almost infinite; for example, currently there is potential to use CRISPR–Cas9 to remove HIV in humans, make mosquitoes that cannot spread malaria, and even treat previously incurable human diseases like muscular dystrophy. Three studies (76–78) showed that the function of dystrophin was significantly (but not completely) restored using CRISPR–Cas9 in a mouse model of muscular dystrophy. Whether these results will apply to humans is still left to be determined. In addition, the first human trials of CRISPR–Cas9–based cancer treatments were approved in early 2016 with the first preliminary results recently published (79). Several ongoing trials are investigating the use of CRISPR–Cas9 in the treatment of multiple myelomas, melanoma, sarcoma, and several blood-related disorders, such as beta-thalassemia and sickle cell disorder. For example, it was recently reported that two patients — one with beta-thalassemia and one with sickle cell disease — were treated with CRISPR therapies, and after 1 year, both patients showed signs of alleviation of the symptoms of their underlying disease (80). In fact, the patient with sickle cell disease showed elimination of her vaso-occlusive episodes after 1 year of treatment. These early successful human trials will surely open the door to other therapeutic applications of CRISPR–Cas9, such as for heart disease, stroke, and hypertension. Therefore, the CEP should therefore stay informed about the development of these applications. In all, these types of results with CRISPR–Cas9 are paving the way toward a future in which the numbers of disorders that the CEP sees, and their treatment, may be very different from those in the current therapeutic environment.

As with any type of significant biomedical advance, there are concerns, controversies, and calls for caution in the use of CRISPR. These have been addressed, in part, by international collaboration. In response to the development of recombinant DNA technology in the early 1970s, the U.S. National Academy of Sciences convened the Asilomar Conference in 1975. There, conference attendees developed the guidelines that became the basis of federal and international policies regarding the use of recombinant DNA technologies. Similarly, in 2015, in conjunction with the Royal Society and the Chinese Academy of Sciences, the National Academy of Sciences, Engineering, and Medicine convened the International Summit on Human Gene Editing, with a follow-up summit in 2018, and a third summit scheduled in early 2023. These Summits addressed and discussed issues surrounding the use of CRISPR–Cas9 gene editing systems.

Whether by altering genetic output using transcription/translation blockers or by editing the genome, the treatment(s) that the CEP applies may be radically altered over a coming short span of years. As was noted at the beginning of the chapter, the exponential increase in genetic knowledge about many physiological conditions, as well as the almost unlimited therapeutic potential that technologies such as vivo-morpholinos and CRISPR–Cas9 represent, demand that the CEP not only be conversant regarding genetics but also be cautious and current with the newest advances. By applying these newest advances to help their patients and clients, the CEP will stand out as a truly innovative and effective health care practitioner.

SUMMARY

As CEPs, we are constantly looking for new information and techniques to help us develop an individualized exercise prescription that can provide maximal results for our clients, irrespective of their health status. However, despite our best efforts, CEPs understand that clients vary in how they respond physiologically to our prescriptions. It appears that approximately half of that physiological variation in response to the exercise prescription is determined by the client's genetic makeup. Whereas the advances in human genome sequencing and the explosion in understanding of how genetics regulates physiology over the past 20 years promised to provide us new information that could further refine our exercise prescriptions, unfortunately, that promise has not been met. The genetic information that can be used in exercise prescription, in general, is still at an embryonic stage. As such, the CEP should apply exercise systems genetic information to exercise prescriptions cautiously and with a full understanding of the strengths and weaknesses of the available data.

At this time, there are three areas in which the CEP may find it valuable to incorporate exercise systems genetics with extreme caution:

1. In considering the efficacy of the client's medication regimen
2. In relating the client's β_2-adrenergic receptor genotype to their exercise response
3. In predicting the client's aerobic responses to an endurance training program

The CEP is also encouraged to monitor the literature. As additional well-designed studies become available, especially those focusing on the variety of proteins involved with each characteristics (aka proteomics) and epigenetics, more exercise systems genetic indices applicable to exercise prescription will likely be developed. Moreover, with the advancement of technologies that can be used to alter the output of genes or to edit the underlying genome, the potential for breakthroughs in treatments that can be applied to patients with CEP and clients is high. Thus, the CEP should remain informed of advances in exercise systems genetic, as well as optimistic that whereas the uses available today appear meager, current applications are only the beginning of what will be possible in the near future.

CHAPTER REVIEW QUESTIONS

1. Precision medicine is often thought of in terms of clinical medicine. Why is it attractive to apply precision medicine techniques to exercise prescription, and should we necessarily do that?

2. Why is an "association" relationship between a phenotype and a genomic variant not necessarily indicative of a direct causal relationship?

3. Why have genomic targets been the most investigated associations with exercise characteristics as opposed to mRNA or protein targets?

4. Pharmacogenomics has been one of the early fields where precision medicine can be applied. As a CEP, why should you be concerned with pharmacogenomics?

5. Cardiovascular functioning during exercise is controlled by a variety of physiological mechanisms, including the β-receptors. Interestingly, the β_2-receptors, which make up less than 30% of the β-receptors, have been the target of quite a few genomic exercise studies. Individuals with a particular pattern (Gly16Glu27) appear to have an augmented cardiovascular response to exercise. How might this augmented response be incorporated into the exercise prescription?

6. A few early studies provide initial evidence that individuals with a certain genomic makeup may be either nonresponders or negative responders to an exercise program. Assuming that the testing becomes available, how could the CEP use this information to enhance an exercise prescription?

7. Certain chromosomal and single-gene disorders affect exercise responses. These include Down syndrome and sickle cell disease. In such cases, why does the CEP not necessarily have to be concerned with the genomic patterns of these patients?

8. What are the two approaches to regulating the output of a deleterious gene?

9. We now know that genetic regulation of any characteristic in most cases involves more than just genomic variation of protein-coding genes. Why does this discovery complicate the understanding of how a characteristic is regulated?

10. Why would a concept of polygenic risk scores be more applicable to predicting exercise performance than the existence of a particular genome variant?

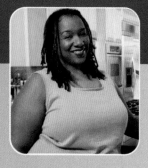

Case Study 18.1

"When I work, I get constriction and tightness in my chest that stops when I quit."

A 42-year-old woman of African descent named Janet presents to the emergency department. Her cardiovascular risk factors are hypertension, a sedentary lifestyle, and a diet high in fat. Her electrocardiogram (ECG) shows 2 mm of anterior ST-segment depression. She undergoes angioplasty with placement of a stent in her left anterior descending coronary artery. Twenty-four hours after stent placement, her cardiovascular variables appear normalized (ejection fraction normal and wall motion normal with echo). She is referred to cardiac rehabilitation as well as a new genomic screening/sequencing program in the Department of Genomic Medicine. Upon entry into cardiac rehabilitation, her symptoms have largely abated, but she does get symptoms if it has been more than 8 hours since taking medicines. Measurements taken upon admission into cardiac rehabilitation, 2 weeks poststent, include the following:

Height: 69 inches (1.75 m)
Weight: 253 lb (115 kg)
Body mass index (BMI): 37.4 kg·m^{-2}
Resting heart rate (HR): 68 contractions per minute
Resting blood pressure (BP): 135/82 mm Hg

PERTINENT EXAMINATION

No distress, heart rhythm normal, lung sounds normal.

Patient states that she continues to have slight discomfort even with adherence to medication schedule.

MEDICATIONS

Aspirin, metoprolol succinate (40 mg·d^{-1}; taken at 8 AM in the morning)

GRADED EXERCISE TEST

(Modified Balke protocol; conducted at 4 PM in the afternoon)

Completed 7.5 minutes (3 mph, 2.5%) ≈ 4 metabolic equivalents (METs) capacity, rate of perceived exertion (RPE) = 16 (complained of continued discomfort upon completion)

Peak HR: 182 contractions per minute (102% age-predicted max.)
Peak BP: 145/90 mm Hg
No ECG evidence of cardiac dysfunction

GENOMIC SCREENING RESULTS

ACE gene type: II (insertion/insertion) *Alu* repeat sequence — intron 16
ACTN3 gene type: *R577X*
β_2-Receptor functional polymorphisms: *Gly16Glu27*
CYPD26 classification: Ultra-metabolizer
Genetic prediction score based on Bouchard predictor panel: 12 (range of 0–42)

Assessment

Obesity

Coronary artery disease/postpercutaneous coronary intervention with stent placement

Genome results indicate that she may exhibit augmented cardiovascular response to exercise, a reduced efficacy of β-blocker medication, as well as a possible nonresponder type to aerobic exercise programs.

Exercise Plan and Special Considerations: Enhancement of Exercise Prescription With Genomic Information

Results with *ACTN3* and *ACE* still do not have universal support in the literature, especially among individuals of African descent. Thus, it is not certain that altering the exercise prescription based on Janet's genomic findings will translate into enhanced health outcomes. However, given the other genomic information available, there is a possibility that the exercise prescription would be enhanced by taking the following genomic-based issues into consideration.

1. Consult with Janet's supervising physician regarding her status as an ultra-metabolizer of CYP2DG drugs (*e.g.*, metoprolol being one of those). Her indication of long-term discomfort, even with strict adherence to medication schedule, and with the noted discomfort during the stress test that was conducted late in the day, may be a result of her ultra-metabolizer status because there are significant clinical data showing that ultra-metabolizers on metoprolol exhibit long-standing

discomfort. Her physician might consider increasing the metoprolol dose (up to 250% of normal dosing) or changing Janet to a β-blocker that is not metabolized through the CYP2DG pathway (*e.g.,* bisoprolol or carvedilol) (57).

2. Janet has the genomic variant Gly16Glu27 in the β₂-adrenergic receptor, suggesting that she may exhibit augmented cardiovascular responses to exercise. Her exhibited peak HR during the stress test, which was slightly above her age-predicted max. HR, coupled with her lower-than-expected RPE results, suggests that Janet showed augmented cardiovascular responses during the exercise test. This potential augmented response would be the basis of setting her intensity rates during exercise on the lower end of the suggested ranges during her cardiac rehabilitation exercise sessions.

3. Given that Janet has a low genetic predictor score on Bouchard's predictor panel, she might be a low responder to endurance training. Thus, it will be necessary to monitor her exercise tolerance closely to determine if she is making progress during her cardiac rehabilitation.

GOALS

Complete 12-week cardiac rehabilitation exercise program, four to five exercise sessions per week

Lose 20 lb with a monitored nutrition/exercise intervention

Increase flexibility, muscle mass, and decrease body fat percentage

Exercise Program (Modified from CAD/Stent case study/exercise prescription in Gordon BT, Durstine JL, Painter PL, Moore GE. Basic physical activity and exercise recommendations for persons with chronic conditions. In: Moore GE, Durstine JL, Painter PL, editors. *ACSM's Exercise Management for Persons With Chronic Diseases and Disabilities.* 4th ed. Champaign (IL): Human Kinetics. 2016. p. 15–32.):

Aerobic exercise program, four to five times per week

- Intensity: Exercise at RPE ≈ 13 (out of 20), and use talk test or target heart rate (THR; 60% of heart rate reserve [HRR])
- Modality: Cycle or walk on treadmill
- Duration: Starting at 20 minutes per session, with a break at 10 minutes, if needed

- Progression: Increase duration 5 minutes per week, with a goal of 45 minutes continuous exercise at the recommended intensity; increase intensity ≈ 5% per week to a goal of 75% HRR during exercise session.

Resistance training program, two times per week

- One cycle of 8–10 resistance exercises (*e.g.,* bench press, leg press, leg curls, leg extensions, shoulder press, lat pulls, abdominal curls, bicep curls, triceps curls, seated rows) at 10–12 reps (repetitions) each (monitor breathing pattern to ensure no Valsalva)
- Progress to two cycles of whole-body exercises at 8 reps each
  - Reduce aerobic program to 20 minutes on days with resistance training

Flexibility exercises, four to five times per week

- 20–30 seconds per stretch

Warm-up and cool-down phases, RPE = 7–9 for 10 minutes

Comment: This case study is a fairly standard cardiac rehabilitation case study for a client with a stent. However, what makes this study unique is the integration of genomic/genetic information that is normally not available. Although some of this information does not add to the prescription (*e.g., ACE* and *ACTN3* variants), other information can add to the prescription and explain the findings on the patient's intake into the cardiac rehabilitation program, from the initial stress test to the subsequent responses during the program. In particular, the ability to understand the patient's discomfort considering her pharmacogenetics is a powerful tool that helps get this patient on a more appropriate medication. Further, the β₂-receptor genomic information helps explain an obviously higher exercise response in the face of a moderate RPE value. This information makes planning the intensity tricky: Should the CEP prescribe as normal (60%–75% HRR), with the understanding that the patient's HR values may be augmented at each stage — which will lead to less work done at each stage? Or should the CEP reduce the work rate to a lower value to maintain THR in an acceptable range (and possibly prevent overtaxing the patient's cardiovascular system early in rehabilitation)? The literature pertaining to this question is still somewhat ambiguous, and it is not clear how the augmented cardiovascular responses because of

(*continued*)

Case Study 18.1 (*continued*)

the β₂-receptor variants should be handled. In the above case study, the CEP chose to implement a lower work rate at the beginning of the program — even if the total work completed is lower — with subsequent increases in THR as the program progresses. Additionally, although there is a possibility that the individual will be a low responder or nonresponder to the exercise program based on their prediction scores from the Bouchard prediction panel, the CEP will monitor weekly progression of duration and intensity responses to determine whether the patient is progressing as expected or will need other approaches to increase her fitness level.

Source: Adapted from CAD/Stent Case study/exercise prescription in Gordon BT, Durstine JL, Painter PL, Moore GE. Basic physical activity and exercise recommendations for persons with chronic conditions. In: Moore GE, Durstine JL, Painter PL, editors. *ACSM's Exercise Management for Persons With Chronic Diseases and Disabilities.* 4th ed. Champaign (IL): Human Kinetics. 2016. p. 15–32.

Case Study 18.1 Questions

1. From the verbiage above, it is clear that the CEP chose a lower work rate at the beginning of the program to offset the potential for augmented cardiovascular responses. How might this CEP alter the exercise prescription in the future if they find that Janet is a nonresponder to exercise?

2. Although the genomic/genetic data provided added another layer of information to determining the exercise prescription, what are the key factors that the CEP needs to monitor during Janet's exercise to support the genomic/genetic suggestions?

Case Study 18.2

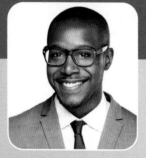

"I want to get bigger faster."

A 35-year-old man named Scott of African descent presents to the CEP for an evaluation of his current fitness status. After a complete physical work-up with his physician, his current health is good, with no cardiovascular risk indices and blood parameters all within the normal range. He had initiated this work-up because he has not observed the increases in his strength and size that he believes he should be achieving with his training program that is directed by a strength coach. He bases his expected changes on a genomic screening that was conducted by a large private company. Scott is not a competitive athlete, but rather works out because it "makes him feel good."

Measurements upon presentation to the CEP include the following:

Height: 72 inches (1.83 m)
Weight: 195 lb (88.6 kg)

Body mass index (BMI): 26.4 kg·m⁻²
Body fat %: 16%
Resting heart rate (HR): 62 contractions per minute
Resting blood pressure (BP): 120/76 mm Hg

MEDICATIONS
No prescribed medications
Over-the-counter (OTC) supplements including:

- Multivitamin one/day supplement (taken at 8 AM in the morning)
- Creatine: 7 g/day (taken at 8 AM in the morning)

GRADED EXERCISE TEST
(Modified Bruce treadmill protocol; conducted at 2 PM in the afternoon)

Completed 21.5 minutes (5 mph, 18% grade) ≈ 15.5 metabolic equivalents (METs) capacity, rate of perceived exertion (RPE) = 20

Peak HR: 194 contractions per minute (105% age-predicted max.)

Peak BP: 160/88 mm Hg

No ECG evidence of cardiac dysfunction

Bench press: 275 lb

Leg press: 450 lb

Push-ups per minute: 55

GENOMIC SCREENING RESULTS (FROM CLIENT SUPPLIED COMMERCIAL ANALYSIS)

ACE gene type (rs4340 SNP): II (insertion/insertion)

ACTN3 gene type (rs1815739 SNP): *R577RR*

Assessment

This client presents as healthy, with no signs/symptoms of underlying disease process. Subject has been using genome results to set his expectations regarding his gains with strength training. Genomic results for both *ACE* and *ACTN3* genes indicate that he has genome pattern that may be associated with increased results from training. However, CEP must stress to subject that *ACE* results association with strength gains have not been replicated and, thus, may not be indicative of his training results. The *ACTN3* result indicate that he has the genomic variants most often associated with elite power athletes, and, thus, may be indicative of an increased capacity for strength gain. However, results with *ACTN3* and *ACE* among individuals of African descent suggest that the *ACTN3* variant may not be associated with strength gain in this client. Additionally, the client already tests above the 90% level for his age and sex in both upper- and lower-body strength, as well as exhibiting a body fat percentage quite low for his age. Given these parameters, this subject would be considered a "highly trained" individual. Thus, the challenge with this client is to reset their expectations regarding their training gains, while working to put the client on a training program that will not increase the chance of injury.

GOALS

Continue current strength program with subject's current trainer.

Continue to increase flexibility, muscle mass, and decrease body fat percentage.

Educate client regarding recent findings related to strength training and *ACE* and *ACTN3* genomic variants.

Comment: This case study relates to the expectations that commercial entities can build in clients with the hyping of genomic results. The genomic results in *ACE* and *ACTN3* are common results that have been associated with higher strength gains reported in the literature. However, newer data with larger and more robust samples as well as more diverse sample populations have generally weakened the association of these genomic variants with strength gains, especially the *ACE* gene. The client's *ACTN3* variant is quite common for African-derived populations, and although this variant has been associated with strength gain after training, it only provides a predisposition for strength gain, not a predestination. Although the *ACTN3RR* variant (fully functioning gene) is highly prevalent in elite power athletes, there are also elite power athletes that have the *ACTN3XX* (or *ACTN3X*) variant (nonfunctioning gene). Thus, the gene results the client possesses are not a guarantee of higher-level strength gains. Thus, the challenge of this case is to reset the client's expectations through education and information.

Case Study 18.2 Questions

1. Why is it possible that Scott's initial suspicion that his strength gains are less than they could be, may be correct, despite the more recent literature suggesting that his genome may not give him a predisposition for larger gains in strength?

2. What type of education and information would you propose to share with Scott to reset his expectations regarding the certainty of genomic testing and strength gain?

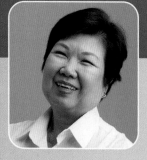

Case Study 18.3

"No one can figure out the right medication."

A 61-year-old woman named Elisa of Asian background was referred to the CEP for a standard exercise program after a diagnosis 2 months earlier of hypertension. She was put on a standard hypertension pharmaceutical regimen. Other than hypertension, Elisa presents as healthy with no other cardiovascular risk indices and all blood parameters within the normal ranges. Elisa stated that she has only exercised infrequently during her life and manages her weight primarily through her diet. Her diet of 20 years has been a plant-based, whole-food diet that has no eggs, dairy, oils, or meat (except seafood) in it. Elisa notes that since she has started taking the blood pressure (BP) medications (in the morning), she feels good until early afternoon.

Measurements upon presentation to the CEP include the following:

Height: 63 inches (1.6 m)
Weight: 130 lb (59.1 kg)
Body mass index (BMI): 23.0 kg·m^{-2}
Body fat %: 22%
Resting heart rate (HR): 74 contractions per minute
Resting BP: 166/84 mm Hg

MEDICATIONS

Metoprolol: 200 mg·day^{-1}
Irbesartan: 150 mg·day^{-1}
Amlodipine: 2.5 mg·day^{-1}
Over-the-counter (OTC) supplements: None

GRADED EXERCISE TEST

(Modified Bruce treadmill protocol; conducted at 4 PM in the afternoon)
Completed 9 minutes (1.7 mph, 10% grade) ≈ 5.0 metabolic equivalents (METs) capacity, rate of perceived exertion (RPE) = 18
Peak HR: 152 contractions per minute (96% age-predicted max.)
Peak BP: 196/98 mm Hg
Resting BP 30 minutes after exercise: 154/88 mm Hg
No ECG evidence of cardiac dysfunction

Assessment

This client presents as healthy, but with diagnosed hypertension and on a pharmaceutical protocol to reduce her BP. Her exercise testing revealed that while having a normal response to the exercise bout, she is in the Fair range for her fitness. Most importantly, the pharmaceutical regimen does not appear to reduce her BP to more appropriate levels. Upon questioning, Alisa states that she is timely with her prescription, taking them at the exact time daily, and in the exact dosages daily. Given the lack of BP control, the CEP sends Elisa back to her physician for further consultation, with a recommendation for pharmacogenomic testing.

GENOMIC SCREENING RESULTS (AS A RESULT OF PHARMACOGENOMIC TESTING)

Metoprolol — Gene assayed: *CYP2D6* — Genotype *1/*1; classified as ultra-rapid metabolizer, suggesting that this medication was being metabolized more quickly leaving her in a non-Beta controlled state.

Irbesartan — Gene assayed: *CYP2C9* (at rs1057910) — Genotype AC; associated with increased concentrations of irbesartan in East Asian individuals who are healthy. This finding suggested that irbesartan was not being cleared as normal, resulting in an accumulation of irbesartan.

Amlodipine — No negative genomic associations noted

FOLLOW-UP

Three months later, Elisa returned to the CEP for an exercise prescription and plan. Her BP was now considered stable by her general physician (resting: 124/78 mm Hg) using a pharmaceutical plan that was based on her genomic profile. Bisoprolol, an alternative beta-blocker that does not depend on *CYP2D6* metabolism was started at 5 mg·day^{-1}, but over the course of several weeks, was increased to 10 mg·day^{-1} to provide stable resting BPs. Given that there is no current literature suggesting how irbesartan should be modified given her genomic status, her physician had titrated her prescription to 75 mg·day^{-1}, which Elisa tolerated well. There was no change in the amlodipine dosage. Given that Elisa's BP was now stable, the CEP provided a full exercise plan based on Elisa's history.

Comment: This case study relates directly to patients that do not receive relief from traditional approaches to prescription (in this case, BP control). The key in this case (as it was in the earlier case study) was the tapering off of the pharmaceutical effect during the day in spite of the relatively high β-blocker dosage. As illustrated, genomic analysis illustrated that this client was an ultra-metabolizer, which was compensated for by employing a different β-blocker that used a different metabolism pathway. Additionally, the pharmacogenomic testing and analysis revealed that individuals of East Asian descent could show decreased metabolism of irbesartan. Although there is not literature suggesting how to compensate for this decreased irbesartan metabolism, Elisa's primary care physician decreased the irbesartan dosage. Elisa's case study shows how genomic variation because of both ethnic background and variation in the metabolism rate of specific drugs can ultimately affect the efficacy of the pharmaceutical intervention. Although out of the CEP's scope of practice, CEPs should be alert to potential genomic interference with expected pharmaceutical outcomes, especially if the client is compliant with their medication schedules. When the drug regimen is not effective, it increases the chances that the exercise prescription may also be ineffective. In this case study, the CEP was correct to consult with the physician before doing the exercise prescription when they saw that the drug regimen was not controlling the BP as intended. This point highlights that it is often as important to know when to do an exercise prescription as it is to know what to put in the exercise prescription.

Case Study 18.3 Questions

1. What would be a primary key for the CEP to suggest that a client be referred to the primary care physician for a pharmacogenomic work-up?

2. Although the above case study involved a simple case, what resources might the CEP use to check if there were further drug interactions between the three prescribed drugs from a genomic standpoint?

REFERENCES

1. Collins FS, Green ED, Guttmacher AE, Guyer MS; US National Human Genome Research Institute. A vision for the future of genomics research. *Nature.* 2003;422(6934):835–47. doi:10.1038/nature01626.

2. Roth SM. Perspective on the future use of genomics in exercise prescription. *J Appl Physiol (1985).* 2008;104(4):1243–5. doi:10.1152/japplphysiol.01000.2007.

3. Bouchard C, Rankinen T. Individual differences in response to regular physical activity. *Med Sci Sports Exerc.* 2001;33(Suppl 6):S446–51.

4. Booth FW, Neufer PD. Exercise genomics and proteomics. In: Farrell PA, Joyner MJ, Caiozzo VJ, editors. *ACSM's Advanced Exercise Physiology.* 2nd ed. Baltimore (MD): Wolters Kluwer; 2012. p. 669–97.

5. Thomis MA, Beunen GP, Van Leemputte M, et al. Inheritance of static and dynamic arm strength and some of its determinants. *Acta Physiol Scand.* 1998;163(1):59–71. doi:10.1046/j.1365-201x.1998.00344.x.

6. Lightfoot JT, Hubal MJ, Roth SM. Introduction. In: Lightfoot JT, Hubal MJ, Roth SM, editors. *Routledge Handbook of Sport and Exercise Systems Genetics.* London (UK): Routledge; 2019. p. 1–4.

7. Krebs JE, Goldstein ES, Kilpatrick ST. *Lewin's Genes XII.* Burlington (MA): Jones & Bartlett Learning; 2017.

8. Narkar VA, Downes M, Yu RT, et al. AMPK and PPARdelta agonists are exercise mimetics. *Cell.* 2008;134(3):405–15.

9. Fire A, Xu S, Montgomery MK, Kostas SA, Driver SE, Mello CC. Potent and specific genetic interference by double-stranded RNA in Caenorhabditis elegans. *Nature.* 1998;391(6669):806–11. doi:10.1038/35888.

10. Baskin KK, Grueter CE, Kusminski CM, et al. Med13-dependent signaling from the heart confers leanness by enhancing metabolism in adipose tissue and liver. *EMBO Mol Med.* 2014;6(12):1610–21. doi:10.15252/emmm.201404218.

11. Thery C. Exosomes: secreted vesicles and intercellular communications. *F1000 Biol Rep.* 2011;3:15.

12. Gygi SP, Rochon Y, Franza BR, Aebersold R. Correlation between protein and mRNA abundance in yeast. *Mol Cell Biol.* 1999;19(3):1720–30.

13. Perco P, Muhlberger I, Mayer G, Oberbauer R, Lukas A, Mayer B. Linking transcriptomic and proteomic data on the level of protein interaction networks. *Electrophoresis.* 2010;31(11):1780–9. doi:10.1002/elps.200900775.

14. Bouchard C. Exercise genomics, epigenomics, and transcriptomics: A reality check! In: Lightfooot JT, Hubal MJ, Roth SM, editors. *Routledge Handbook of Sport and Exercise Systems Genetics*. New York (NY): Routledge; 2019. p. 487–93.

15. Leamy LJ, Pomp D, Lightfoot JT. An epistatic genetic basis for physical activity traits in mice. *J Hered*. 2008;99(6):639–46. doi:10.1093/jhered/esn045.

16. Flint J, Valdar W, Shifman S, Mott R. Strategies for mapping and cloning quantitative trait genes in rodents. *Nat Rev Genet*. 2005;6:271–86.

17. Montgomery H, Clarkson P, Barnard M, et al. Angiotensin-converting-enzyme gene insertion/deletion polymorphism and response to physical training. *Lancet*. 1999;353(9152):541–5. doi:10.1016/S0140-6736(98)07131-1.

18. Pescatello LS, Corso LML, Santos LP, Livingston J, Taylor BA. Angiotensin-converting enzyme and the genomics of endurance performance. In: Lightfooot JT, Hubal MJ, Roth SM, editors. *Routledge Handbook of Sport and Exercise Systems Genetics*. New York (NY): Routledge; 2019. p. 216–49.

19. Mattsson CM, Wheeler MT, Waggott D, Caleshu C, Ashley EA. Sports genetics moving forward: lessons learned from medical research. *Physiol Genomics*. 2016;48(3):175–82. doi:10.1152/physiolgenomics.00109.2015.

20. Gordon BT, Durstine JL. Coronary artery disease and dyslipidemia, status/post-angioplasty with stent placement. In: Moore GE, Durstine JL, Painter PL, editors. *ACSM's Exercise Management for Persons With Chronic Diseases and Disabilities*. 4th ed. Champaign (IL): Human Kinetics; 2016. p. 322–4.

21. Liguori G, American College of Sports Medicine. Exercise testing and prescription for populations with other chronic diseases and health conditions. In: Liguori G, Feito Y, Fountaine C, Roy BA, editors. *ACSM's Guidelines for Exercise Testing and Prescription*. 11th ed. Baltimore (MD): Wolters Kluwer; 2021. p. 207–362.

22. Hagberg JM, Coyle EF, Carroll JE, Miller JM, Martin WH, Brooke MH. Exercise hyperventilation in patients with McArdle's disease. *J Appl Physiol Respir Environ Exerc Physiol*. 1982;52:991–4.

23. Gautron S, Daegelen D, Mennecier F, Dubocq D, Kahn A, Dreyfus JC. Molecular mechanisms of McArdle's disease (muscle glycogen phosphorylase deficiency). RNA and DNA analysis. *J Clin Invest*. 1987;79(1):275–81. doi:10.1172/JCI112794.

24. Munguía-Izquierdo D, Santalla A, Lucia A. Cardiorespiratory fitness, physical activity, and quality of life in patients with McArdle disease. *Med Sci Sports Exerc*. 2015;47(4):799–808. doi:10.1249/MSS.0000000000000458.

25. Fiuza-Luces C, Nogales-Gadea G, García-Consuegra I, et al. Muscle signaling in exercise intolerance: insights from the McArdle mouse model. *Med Sci Sports Exerc*. 2016;48(8):1448–58. doi:10.1249/MSS.0000000000000931.

26. Bailey SP, Nieman DC. Chronic fatigue syndrome. In: Moore GE, Durstine JL, Painter PL, editors. *ACSM's Exercise Management for Persons With Chronic Diseases and Disabilities*, 4th ed. Champaign (IL): Human Kinetics; 2016. p. 215–20.

27. Connes P, Machado R, Hue O, Reid H. Exercise limitation, exercise testing and exercise recommendations in sickle cell anemia. *Clin Hemorheol Microcirc*. 2011;49(1-4):151–63. doi:10.3233/CH-2011-1465.

28. Centers for Disease Control and Prevention. *Sickle Cell Disease: Data and Statistics*. 2016.

29. National Athletic Training Association. *Consensus Statement: Sickle Cell Trait and the Athlete*. 2007.

30. Tarini BA, Brooks MA, Bundy DG. A policy impact analysis of the mandatory NCAA sickle cell trait screening program. *Health Serv Res*. 2012;47(1 Pt 2):446–61. doi:10.1111/j.1475-6773.2011.01357.x.

31. South Carolina Newborn. *Baby's first test*. https://www.babysfirsttest.org/newbornscreening/states/south-carolina.

32. Gordon BT, Durstine JL, Painter PL, Moore GE. Basic physical activity and exercise precommendations for persons with chronic conditions. In: Moore GE, Durstine JL, Painter PL, editors. *ACSM's Exercise Management for Persons With Chronic Diseases and Disabilities*, 4th ed. Champaign (IL): Human Kinetics; 2016. p. 15–32.

33. Patterson D. Molecular genetic analysis of Down syndrome. *Hum Genet*. 2009; 126(1):195–214. doi:10.1007/s00439-009-0696-8.

34. Roizen NJ, Patterson D. Down's syndrome. *Lancet*. 2003; 361(9365):1281–9. doi:10.1016/S0140-6736(03)12987-X.

35. Freeman SB, Taft LF, Dooley KJ, et al. Population-based study of congenital heart defects in down syndrome. *Am J Med Genet*. 1998;80(3):213–7.

36. Rubin SS, Rimmer JH, Chicoine B, Braddock D, Mcguire DE. Overweight prevalence in persons with Down syndrome. *Ment Retard*. 1998;36(3):175–81. doi:10.1352/0047-6765(1998)0362.0.CO;2.

37. Fernhall B, Pitetti KH, Rimmer JH, et al. Cardiorespiratory capacity of individuals with mental retardation including down syndrome. *Med Sci Sports Exerc*. 1996;28(3):366–71.

38. Yildirim NU, Erbahçeci F, Ergun N, Pitetti KH, Beets MW. The effect of physical fitness training on reaction time in youth with intellectual disabilities. *Percept Mot Skills*. 2010;111(1):178–86. doi:10.2466/06.10.11.13.15.25.PMS.111.4.178-186.

39. Varela AM, Sardinha LB, Pitetti KH. Effects of an aerobic rowing training regimen in young adults with Down syndrome. *Am J Ment Retard*. 2001;106(2):135–44. doi:10.1352/0895-8017(2001)1062.0.CO;2.

40. Rimmer JH, Heller T, Wang E, Valerio I. Improvements in physical fitness in adults with down syndrome. *Am J Ment Retard*. 2004;109(2):165–74. doi:10.1352/0895-8017(2004)1092.0.CO;2.

41. Hawley JA. Commentary on viewpoint: perspective on the future use of genomics in exercise prescription. *J Appl Physiol (1985)*. 2008;104(4):1253. doi:10.1152/japplphysiol.00047.2008.

42. Snyder EM, Johnson BD, Joyner MJ. Genetics of beta$_2$-adrenergic receptors and the cardiopulmonary response to exercise. *Exerc Sport Sci Rev*. 2008;36(2):98–105. doi:10.1097/JES.0b013e318168f276.

43. Bray MS, Krushkal J, Li L, et al. Positional genomic analysis identifies the beta(2)-adrenergic receptor gene as a susceptibility locus for human hypertension. *Circulation*. 2000;101(25):2877–82.

44. Bray MS, Boerwinkle E. The role of beta(2)-adrenergic receptor variation in human hypertension. *Curr Hypertens Rep*. 2000;2(1):39–43.

45. Snyder EM, Beck KC, Dietz NM, et al. Arg16gly polymorphism of the beta2-adrenergic receptor is associated with differences in cardiovascular function at rest and during exercise in humans. *J Physiol.* 2006;571(Pt 1):121–30. doi:10.1113/jphysiol.2005.098558.

46. Tang W, Devereux RB, Kitzman DW, et al. The Arg16Gly polymorphism of the beta2-adrenergic receptor and left ventricular systolic function. *Am J Hypertens.* 2003; 16(11 Pt 1):945–51.

47. Macho-Azcárate T, Calabuig J, Martí A, Martínez JA. A maximal effort trial in obese women carrying the beta$_2$-adrenoceptor Gln27Glu polymorphism. *J Physiol Biochem.* 2002;58(2):103–8.

48. Snyder EM, Beck KC, Turner ST, Hoffman EA, Joyner MJ, Johnson BD. Genetic variation of the beta2-adrenergic receptor is associated with differences in lung fluid accumulation in humans. *J Appl Physiol (1985).* 2007;102(6):2172–8. doi:10.1152/japplphysiol.01300.2006.

49. Nielsen M, Staalsoe JM, Ullum H, Secher NH, Nielsen HB, Olsen NV. The Gly16 allele of the Gly16Arg single-nucleotide polymorphism in the β$_2$-adrenergic receptor gene augments perioperative use of vasopressors: a retrospective cohort study. *Anesth Analg.* 2016;122(5):1385–93. doi:10.1213/ANE.0000000000001167.

50. Sarpeshkar V, Bentley DJ. Adrenergic-beta(2) receptor polymorphism and athletic performance. *J Hum Genet.* 2010;55(8):479–85. doi:10.1038/jhg.2010.42.

51. Wolfarth B, Rankinen T, Mühlbauer S, et al. Association between a beta2-adrenergic receptor polymorphism and elite endurance performance. *Metabolism.* 2007;56(12):1649–51. doi:10.1016/j.metabol.2007.07.006.

52. Berentzen T, Kring SI, Holst C, et al. Lack of association of fatness-related FTO gene variants with energy expenditure or physical activity. *J Clin Endocrinol Metab.* 2008;93(7):2904–8. doi:10.1210/jc.2008-0007.

53. Hakanen M, Raitakari OT, Lehtimäki T, et al. FTO genotype is associated with body mass index after the age of seven years but not with energy intake or leisure-time physical activity. *J Clin Endocrinol Metab.* 2009;94(4):1281–7. doi:10.1210/jc.2008-1199.

54. Lee H, Ash GI, Angelopoulos TJ, et al. Obesity-related genetic variants and their associations with physical activity. *Sports Med Open.* 2015;1:34. doi:10.1186/s40798-015-0036-6.

55. Eynon N, Nasibulina ES, Banting LK, et al. The FTO A/T polymorphism and elite athletic performance: a study involving three groups of European athletes. *PLoS One.* 2013;8(4):e60570. doi:10.1371/journal.pone.0060570.

56. Leońska-Duniec A, Ahmetov II, Zmijewski P. Genetic variants influencing effectiveness of exercise training programmes in obesity: an overview of human studies. *Biol Sport.* 2016;33(3):207–14. doi:10.5604/20831862.1201052.

57. Kalow W, Tang BK, Endrenyi L. Hypothesis: comparisons of inter- and intra-individual variations can substitute for twin studies in drug research. *Pharmacogenetics.* 1998;8(4):283–9.

58. Whirl-Carrillo M, Huddart R, Gong L, et al. An evidence-based framework for evaluating pharmacogenomics knowledge for personalized medicine. *Clin Pharmacol Ther.* 2021; 110(3):563–72. doi:10.1002/cpt.2350.

59. Swen JJ, Nijenhuis M, De Boer A, et al. Pharmacogenetics: from bench to byte—an update of guidelines. *Clin Pharmacol Ther.* 2011;89(5):662–73. doi:10.1038/clpt.2011.34.

60. Zanger UM, Raimundo S and Eichelbaum M. Cytochrome P450 2D6: overview and update on pharmacology, genetics, biochemistry. *Naunyn Schmiedebergs Arch Pharmacol.* 2004;369(1):23–37. doi:10.1007/s00210-003-0832-2.

61. Gaedigk A, Ingelman-Sundbberg, M, Miller NA, Leeder JS, Whirl-Carrillo M, Klein TE, PharmVar Steering Committee. The Pharmacogene Variation (PharmVar) Consortium: Incorporation of the Human Cytochrome P450 (CYP) Allele Nomenclature Database. *Clin Pharmacol Ther.* 2018 Mar; 103(3):399–401. doi: 10.1002/cpt.910.

62. Lennard MS, Silas JH, Freestone S, Trevethick J. Defective metabolism of metoprolol in poor hydroxylators of debrisoquine. *Br J Clin Pharmacol.* 1982;14(2):301–3.

63. Lennard MS, Silas JH, Freestone S, Ramsay LE, Tucker GT, Woods HF. Oxidation phenotype: a major determinant of metoprolol metabolism and response. *N Engl J Med.* 1982;307(25):1558–60. doi:10.1056/NEJM198212163072505.

64. Timmons JA, Knudsen S, Rankinen T, et al. Using molecular classification to predict gains in maximal aerobic capacity following endurance exercise training in humans. *J Appl Physiol (1985).* 2010;108(6):1487–96. doi:10.1152/japplphysiol.01295.2009.

65. Bouchard C, Sarzynski MA, Rice TK, et al. Genomic predictors of the maximal O$_2$ uptake response to standardized exercise training programs. *J Appl Physiol (1985).* 2011;110(5):1160–70. doi:10.1152/japplphysiol.00973.2010.

66. Altshuler DM, Gibbs RA, Peltonen L, et al; International HapMap 3 Consortium. Integrating common and rare genetic variation in diverse human populations. *Nature.* 2010;467(7311):52–8. doi:10.1038/nature09298.

67. Thomaes T, Thomis M, Onkelinx S, et al. A genetic predisposition score for muscular endophenotypes predicts the increase in aerobic power after training: the CAREGENE study. *BMC Genet.* 2011;12:84. doi:10.1186/1471-2156-12-84.

68. Lightfoot JT, De Geus EJC, Booth FW, et al. Biological/genetic regulation of physical activity level: consensus from GenBioPac. *Med Sci Sports Exerc.* 2018;50(4):863–73. doi:10.1249/MSS.0000000000001499.

69. Kujala UM, Palviainen T, Pesonen P, et al. Polygenic risk scores and physical activity. *Med Sci Sports Exerc.* 2020;52(7):1518–24. doi:10.1249/MSS.0000000000002290.

70. Morcos PA, Li Y, Jiang S. Vivo-morpholinos: a non-peptide transporter delivers morpholinos into a wide array of mouse tissues. *Biotechniques.* 2008;45(6):613–23.

71. Ferguson DP, Schmitt EE, Lightfoot JT. Vivo-morpholinos induced transient knockdown of physical activity related proteins. *PLoS One.* 2013;8(4):e61472. doi:10.1371/journal.pone.0061472.

72. Kaye EM, Mendell JR, Rodino-Kapac L, et al. Eteplirsen, a phosphorodiamidate morpholino oligomer (PMO) for the treatment of Duchenne muscular dystrophy (DMD): 3.2 year update on six-minute walk test (6MWT), pulmonary function testing (PFT), and safety. *Eur J Paediatr Neurol.* 2015;19:S69.

73. Sheikh O, Yokota T. Developing DMD therapeutics: a review of the effectiveness of small molecules, stop-codon

readthrough, dystrophin gene replacement, and exon-skipping therapies. *Expert Opin Investig Drugs.* 2021;30(2):167–76. doi:10.1080/13543784.2021.1868434.

74. Jinek M, Chylinski K, Fonfara I, Hauer M, Doudna JA, Charpentier E. A programmable dual-RNA-guided DNA endonuclease in adaptive bacterial immunity. *Science.* 2012;337(6096):816–21. doi:10.1126/science.1225829.

75. Doudna JA, Charpentier E. Genome editing. The new frontier of genome engineering with CRISPR-Cas9. *Science.* 2014;346(6213):1258096. doi:10.1126/science.1258096.

76. Long C, Amoasii L, Mireault AA, et al. Postnatal genome editing partially restores dystrophin expression in a mouse model of muscular dystrophy. *Science.* 2016;351(6271):400–3. doi:10.1126/science.aad5725.

77. Nelson CE, Hakim CH, Ousterout DG, et al. In vivo genome editing improves muscle function in a mouse model of Duchenne muscular dystrophy. *Science.* 2016;351(6271):403–7. doi:10.1126/science.aad5143.

78. Tabebordbar M, Zhu K, Cheng JK, et al. In vivo gene editing in dystrophic mouse muscle and muscle stem cells. *Science.* 2016;351(6271):407–11. doi:10.1126/science.aad5177.

79. Stadtmauer EA, Fraietta JA, Davis MM, et al. CRISPR-engineered T cells in patients with refractory cancer. *Science.* 2020;367(6481):eaba7365. doi:10.1126/science.aba7365.

80. Frangoul H, Altshuler D, Cappellini MD, et al. CRISPR-Cas9 gene editing for sickle cell disease and β-thalassemia. *N Engl J Med.* 2021;384(3):252–60. doi:10.1056/NEJMoa2031054.

CHAPTER 19

Legal Considerations

INTRODUCTION

A clinical exercise physiologist (CEP) is sued when a client is thrown from a treadmill and fractures her ankle. The suit alleges that the CEP failed to provide the client with appropriate instruction and supervision for using the treadmill. Unfortunately, this example is not uncommon. Many CEPs are subjected to a lawsuit at some point in their career. Whether a lawsuit is legitimate or frivolous, it can be time consuming and costly for everyone involved. Accordingly, CEPs must learn to be proactive in identifying potential areas of legal liability and adopting preventative safety measures that will keep lawsuits to a minimum.

The purpose of this chapter is to provide CEPs with a rudimentary understanding of the legal issues that may arise as an employee or as a business owner. It therefore introduces CEPs to some basic legal terminology and concepts (Box 19.1) and explains how courts make decisions regarding the law. Ideally, this chapter provides the foundation to prevent or reduce the consequences of lawsuits. Should an injury occur, CEPs will be prepared to protect not only the legal interests of the injured person, but also their own legal interests and liability.

So, what is legal liability and how is it determined? Courts have consistently held that it is the responsibility of an individual to act in a specific way in certain circumstances. When an accident occurs that results in an injury, the legal questions include who was at fault and whether **damages** — monetary compensation for loss or injury caused by another — can be recovered by the injured party. Although the law can vary with every state and every case, this chapter presents an overview of legal liability in a manner that should apply to most regions and settings within the field. The information provided in this chapter does not constitute legal advice, however, and should not be used in lieu of seeking appropriate legal representation should an incident occur.

TORT LAW

A tort is a civil wrong or violation of a duty that causes an injury to another. Tort law, then, is the study of intentional or negligent injury to a person or their property. It is designed to render damages to the plaintiff for the tortfeasor's misconduct. A plaintiff is a person who files a lawsuit. A tortfeasor is an individual who causes an injury to another person. Because CEPs occasionally face charges of intentional or negligent injury, a thorough understanding of tort law is essential.

The standard of proof in a tort claim is by a preponderance of the evidence. In a voting process for a civic organization, this would be the equivalent of a vote by the majority. There are four general tort theories: negligence, intentional torts, strict liability, and product liability.

Negligence

Negligence is the most common theory in tort law. The question before the court is whether or not the defendant, the person charged with injuring the plaintiff, acted as a reasonable person would have acted in the same situation (*i.e.*, the reasonable CEP, nutritionist, team physician, athletic trainer, coach). Courts typically rely on certification or licensing entities or other experts in the field to identify what practices are considered reasonable. For cases of negligence, the plaintiff must demonstrate that the defendant failed to use the ordinary care of a reasonable person in that situation or circumstance. This standard of care is evaluated according to the general knowledge and skill of the profession and reflects how a practitioner in a specific field would act in a given situation or circumstance.

The standard of care required by a CEP is that they "must have and use the knowledge, skill, and care ordinarily possessed and employed by members of the

Box 19.1	Key Legal Terms

The following legal definitions will provide a basis for reading and understanding the terminology used within this chapter.

- Alternative dispute resolution — method of handling conflict that does not require the parties to go to court
- Answer — the defendant's response to the plaintiff's allegations or claims
- Appeal — request by a party to a lawsuit for a higher court to review a lower court's decision
- Arbitration — a neutral individual listens to the disputants and then makes a decision or award
- Civil law — area of the law that focuses on noncriminal acts/violations regarding the rights of people, corporations, or property
- Complaint/petition — document that summarizes the facts and identifies the plaintiff's claims against the defendant
- Contract — a valid and binding agreement between two or more parties
- Criminal law — area of the law that focuses on violations of criminal statutes
- Damages — monetary compensation for the loss or injury caused by another
- Defendant — the person who is believed to have injured another party
- Due process of the law — formal process that requires an individual to receive notice of an alleged violation and an opportunity to be heard or to defend the alleged violation
- Equal protection under the law — the right to receive equal treatment by the law
- Immune/immunity — exclusion or release from a duty or liability permitted by law or statute
- Informed consent — permission granted after receiving knowledge of potential harmful consequences
- Injunction — court order compelling an individual to act or not act in a particular situation
- Insurance — a guarantee of protection or compensation for a specified loss or damage
- Mediation — neutral individual assists the parties in reaching a settlement or agreement
- Meritorious claim — a valid legal claim that is likely to prevail on its merit or substance
- Motion to dismiss — granted when the plaintiff fails to sufficiently allege a set of facts that would support a claim against the defendant
- Motion for summary judgment — granted when there are no genuine issues regarding the facts of the case and the judge decides the case without conducting a full trial
- Plaintiff — the person who files a lawsuit
- Punitive damages — damages awarded to the plaintiff to punish the defendant
- Respondeat superior — employers are responsible for the negligent acts of their employees
- Settled/settlement — agreement between the plaintiff and the defendant to end a lawsuit
- Standard of care — acceptable conduct for an individual acting in the same or similar circumstance
- Statute of limitations — the legal time limit in which a plaintiff can file a lawsuit
- Tort — a civil wrong or violation of a duty that causes an injury to another
- Tortfeasor — an individual who causes an injury to another
- Waiver — intentionally relinquishing an individual's right or claim to legal recourse

profession in good standing" (1, p. 187). Courts will determine the appropriate professional standard of care through federal or state statutes and through published standards and guidelines by governing organizations/agencies, such as American College of Sports Medicine (ACSM), the National Athletic Trainers Association (NATA), and the National Strength and Conditioning Association (NSCA). If there are no published standards, courts will rely on the testimony of expert witnesses to identify the accepted practices within the field.

Characteristics of Negligence

Both the failure to act (omission) as well as improper action (commission) may result in legal action. For example, a personal fitness trainer's failure to supervise or spot a client who is lifting weights, or an athletic trainer advising a collegiate athlete that they should continue playing with a serious injury when playing could exacerbate the injury, could be deemed negligent conduct.

In all instances, CEPs are obligated to provide for the physical well-being of those in their care. Their duty is to act in a manner that is always in the best interest of the individual, patient, or athlete. Ignorance of the law as well as ignoring the law are no excuse for acting or failing to act in a circumstance involving an injured party.

Some courts have noted there are different levels of negligence, with the most severe being gross negligence. In cases of gross negligence, the defendant allegedly used so little care when dealing with the plaintiff that courts will hold that the defendant essentially intended to injure the plaintiff. For instance, if a personal fitness trainer fails to inquire about a client's prior cardiac risk factors, and during a training session, the client has a heart attack resulting in death, they may be liable for gross negligence.

Proof of Negligence

To prove a case of negligence, the plaintiff must demonstrate the following elements:

1. Defendant owed a duty to the plaintiff
2. Defendant breached that duty
3. Breach of the duty was the actual and proximate (or foreseeable) cause of the plaintiff's injury
4. Harm or injury

The third element, causation, can be examined under cause-in-fact or proximate cause. Cause-in-fact means that "but for" the defendant's breach, the injury would not have occurred. Proximate cause is segmented into direct causation and foreseeability. Under direct causation, the defendant is liable for all consequences of their negligent acts, provided no intervening acts occur. And foreseeability states the plaintiff must prove that the injury was foreseeable as a result of the defendant's negligent acts.

Defenses of Negligence

If faced with a negligence lawsuit, certain defenses or legal arguments could persuade a court that the defendant is not at fault for the plaintiff's injury. A few are discussed here.

All Elements of Ordinary Negligence Not Proven

As previously stated, specific elements are needed to prove a claim of negligence. If the plaintiff (or injured party) fails to prove that all elements of negligence exist, the lawsuit against the defendant will fail.

Assumption of Risk

At times, the plaintiff's injury can be attributed to the plaintiff voluntarily exposing themselves to an unreasonable risk of harm. Suppose a CEP advises a patient not to participate in a weekend 10K road race. The patient ignores the advice and suffers a heart attack. Courts will state the plaintiff assumed the risk of injury by ignoring the CEP's advice.

Contributory/Comparative Negligence

Courts will consider how much fault is attributable to the plaintiff and/or the defendant for the plaintiff's injuries based on a defense of contributory or comparative negligence. With contributory negligence, if the plaintiff is found to have caused their own injuries in any way, the plaintiff's lawsuit will fail. However, most states have done away with contributory negligence and have adopted comparative negligence to apportion damages based on fault. With comparative negligence, a plaintiff may be partially to blame for their own injuries; but as long as they are not more at fault than the defendant, they can recover damages minus their percentage of fault. In some states, even if the plaintiff is 90% at fault, they can still recover 10% of the damages. Other states limit the percentage of fault and recovery for damages at 50%–51%. In these states, where a patient ignores the advice of a CEP, courts are likely to rule that the patient was more than 50%–51% at fault and therefore will not be able to recover any damages.

Statutory Immunity

Some state statutes give a practitioner immunity — exclusion or release — from legal liability for malpractice claims in certain circumstances. Several states, for example, have enacted statutes protecting volunteers and Good Samaritans (professionals who provide emergency assistance gratuitously) from negligence arising from care in emergency situations. However, it is important for CEPs to realize that Good Samaritan statutes do not apply while on the job, where there is clearly a duty to aid an injured participant. A statute of limitations also can give a practitioner immunity from legal liability. In each state, a plaintiff has a certain amount of time to file a lawsuit against a defendant. Lawyers often will refer to this as a ticking clock for lawsuits. In tort law, after a plaintiff learns of an injury, they typically have 1–3 years to file a lawsuit for damages against a defendant.

Sovereign/Government Immunity

Practitioners employed by a (federal, state, or local) government agency may be immune from a lawsuit if they practiced discretionary acts of care within the scope and course of their employment. Traditionally, it was believed that a government entity could do no wrong. However, over time, the law has been modified or subjected to exceptions in most states allowing for government entities to be sued. This is based on the doctrine of *respondeat superior*, which means "let the principal answer." The idea is that if a party is injured, they may hold both the servant (employee) and the master (government entity) liable. Government employees are only immune from liability if they (a) act during the course of their employment and within the scope of their authority, (b) act in good faith, and (c) perform discretionary-decisional acts (2). Discretionary-decisional acts are those involving the use of personal deliberation or judgment as a function of a job. For example, a manager or supervisor makes a decision and expects the employee to execute the decision. Acts outside the scope of employment are not protected under an immunity defense.

Contractual Defenses

Informed consent and waivers are frequent contractual defenses. Prior to participating in any physical activity or receiving any medical treatment, the patient or client must give consent. The consent must be informed; that is, it must demonstrate the individual knew the risks prior to engaging in the activity or medical treatment. The consent can be either implied (based on the individual's behavior) or express (verbal or in writing). If the individual is a minor, consent must be received from a parent or legal guardian (3). For a medical emergency, consent may be implied. The law presumes that if the individual had been aware of their condition and was mentally competent, then they would have authorized appropriate treatment (4).

Waivers provide evidence, usually in writing, that an individual "knowingly and voluntarily [waives] his/her legal right to recover from future harm due to another's wrongful conduct" (1, p. 482–4). Conduct that is intentional, reckless, or involving gross negligence is generally not protected, even if the individual signs a waiver; that is, waivers only protect against ordinary negligence.

The informed consent and the waiver should be separate documents, each signed by the individual. Prior to signing the waiver and/or consent forms, participants should receive an explanation of the risks of the activity (being honest and clear), advise them of their own responsibility for their safety, provide opportunity for questions and clarification, and ensure the participant understands the documents. One should ensure participants understand and appreciate the risks of the activity prior to signing waivers and consents. If the waiver is included in the informed consent document, some courts have invalidated the informed consent. Both the informed consent and the waiver can strengthen the assumption of

risk defense, but they do not guarantee protection from a negligence lawsuit. In fact, waivers are not enforceable in all states. Therefore, it is imperative that CEPs seek the expertise of a licensed attorney regarding preparing and administering the informed consent and waiver agreements.

Cases Involving Claims of Negligence

Following an ankle injury, Alvin Howard, a football player at Greenville College in Greenville, Illinois, visited Missouri Bone and Joint Center (MBJC) seeking athletic training services to improve his football skills. Howard met with Kevin Templin, a certified athletic trainer at MBJC, for an initial evaluation. The initial evaluation included an interview, measurements, and some performance testing. Because of time constraints, Templin asked Howard to estimate the maximum amount of weight he could lift for a bench press and squat lift, rather than have Howard physically perform the exercises (a standard part of the MBJC evaluation). Templin did not ask Howard when he had last exercised, and Howard did not disclose that he had not performed any lower-body workouts for 12 weeks because of his ankle injury. A few months later, Howard started training under Templin's supervision. During his second workout with Templin, Howard felt a pop and a sharp pain in his lower back. When he informed Templin of the pain, Templin told him "no pain, no gain" and to "push through it" (5, p. 994). During the workout, Howard's pain escalated, and Templin instructed him to stretch and spend some time on a stationary bike. After several hospital visits, Howard was diagnosed with a herniated disc in his back. Howard filed a negligence claim against MBJC alleging the training service caused his back injury. At trial, Templin testified that during the initial evaluation he did not ask Howard when he last worked out and admitted this information is important to consider when designing a workout. Although MBJC's expert witness testified that Templin's evaluation was proper, the expert witness expressed that telling Howard to continue lifting after he complained of significant back pain was a violation of the standard of care. The District Court ruled in favor of Howard in the amount of $175,000, and MBJC filed a motion for a new trial. The motion was denied, and MBJC appealed the decision; that is, MBJC requested that a higher court review the decision. The appellate court agreed with the District Court's decision (5).

Jason Zimbauer, a major league pitcher for the Milwaukee Brewers, heard a pop in his shoulder while throwing a new pitch. He sought medical treatment from the team physician, who told him they had found no problems. Approximately 9 months later, Zimbauer again complained of pain because of the new pitch. The team physician diagnosed him with a recurrent subluxation of the shoulder. For almost 2 years, Zimbauer remained in the care of the team and its physician, and his pain continued. It was at this time Zimbauer consulted with another physician, who diagnosed him with a partial tear of the rotator cuff. No longer able to pitch, Zimbauer is now constantly in pain with limited movement of his arm, and he may need a shoulder replacement. Zimbauer filed a complaint — a summary of facts and claims — against the team and its physician alleging they misdiagnosed and mistreated his shoulder injury, and this negligence has caused him pain and permanent disability. At trial, Zimbauer failed to produce any evidence regarding the standard of care owed to the plaintiff by the defendants and that they had breached that standard of care. Zimbauer also failed to provide any evidence of causation. The court granted the defendant's motion for summary judgment requesting that the judge decide the case without conducting a trial, and the case was dismissed (6).

Joey Herren started working with a personal trainer a few weeks after he joined Nonstop Fitness Incorporated gym. Shortly after he began working with the personal trainer, Herren obtained a non–Food and Drug Administration (FDA)-approved dietary supplement from a co-worker. One day after working out with the personal trainer, Herren suffered a stroke. Herren filed a lawsuit against the gym, its owner, the personal trainer, a management company, and the original seller of the dietary supplement (defendants) alleging that he suffered a stroke as a result of taking the dietary supplement and overexercising with the personal trainer. His lawsuit included claims of negligence and gross negligence against the defendants. The defendants filed a motion for summary judgment stating that Herren had signed three separate agreements containing clauses waiving and releasing them from liability. They also argued that Herren had assumed the risk of his own injuries when he began working out at the gym. Herren claimed that the releases did not bar his gross negligence claims against the defendants. The trial court ruled in favor of the defendants. It found the waiver clauses enforceable, and Herren's gross negligence claims unwarranted. It upheld Herren's claims of ordinary negligence. Herren appealed the case, and the appellate court agreed with the trial court's decision (7).

Intentional Torts

Intentional torts are closely related to criminal law, which will be discussed later in this chapter. Any voluntary action intended to cause injury to another is considered an intentional tort.

Types of Intentional Torts

There are several different types of intentional torts; however, only a few that are relevant to the field of clinical exercise physiology are discussed here. These include assault, battery, invasion of privacy, and defamation.

Assault is defined as an intent to cause immediate harm through menacing or threatening behavior, apprehension of immediate harm, and lack of consent. For example, a defendant threatens to physically harm the plaintiff. No actual physical contact is needed for an assault to be committed. The victim only has to have an objectively reasonable belief that they may be harmed. In contrast, battery is the unauthorized or unwelcomed physical contact with another person (*e.g.*, providing medical treatment to an individual who has refused treatment). Here, the defendant intended to touch the plaintiff and an actual touching occurred. It is important to note the contact does not have to result in injury, nor is awareness required on the part of the person. If tort claims are filed for either an assault or battery, the tortfeasor may be liable to the plaintiff for monetary damages. The intentional torts of assault and battery may also be considered crimes.

Invasion of privacy is based on a generally recognized right to privacy. Although this right is not explicitly guaranteed in the U.S. Constitution, most states have recognized it either by statute or by judicial decisions. One tort associated with the invasion of privacy is known as the unreasonable disclosure of private facts. Here, the plaintiff must prove (a) whether the disclosed information was truly private or public and (b) if the disclosed information was highly offensive to an ordinary person. Even if the individual is a public person or official, there is still an expectation of privacy regarding some information. CEPs working in clinical settings should review the Health Insurance Portability and Accountability Act (HIPAA) of 1996 privacy rule prior to disclosing any health information about a client.

Defamation is similar to invasion of privacy. Defamation occurs when a false statement is published (libel) or spoken (slander) about the plaintiff who is a public official, a public figure, or a private figure. Public officials are individuals who have campaigned for, were elected to, or were appointed to a public office. A public figure is an individual who has generated public interest and attention based on behavior or status. Private figures are those who do not qualify as public officials or public figures and have the greatest expectation of privacy. A plaintiff in a defamation case is only likely to recover damages if they can prove the defendant made a statement that was knowingly false or had a reckless disregard of whether the statement was true or false. There are two defenses to a defamation claim. First, the defendant may be able to prove that the information disclosed was true. Even if the information is embarrassing, any statement having some element of truth will be protected speech. Second, the defendant may be able to prove that the individual consented to the information being published. If the individual authorized a verbal or written release of the information and is later embarrassed by the disclosure of this information, the defamation claim will fail.

A Case Involving a Claim of Intentional Tort

In *Chuy v. Philadelphia Eagles Football Club* (8), Don Chuy signed contracts to play in the National Football League (NFL) for the Philadelphia Eagles during the 1969–1971 seasons. During a game against the New York Giants in 1969, Chuy suffered a shoulder injury and was sidelined for the remainder of the season. In December 1969, Chuy was diagnosed with a pulmonary embolism, a blood clot in his lung, and was advised by his physician to end his professional football career. Chuy retired from the NFL, and requested the Eagles pay the salary remaining on his contracts. The Eagles responded with a request for Chuy to submit to a physical examination by a different doctor, Dr. Dick D. Harrell. Dr. Harrell conducted the examination in March 1970 and concluded Chuy suffered from an abnormal cell condition, most likely stress polycythemia vera, and suggested this condition predisposed Chuy to the formation of dangerous blood clots. Dr. Harrell recommended to the Eagles' General Manager Palmer Retzlaff that Chuy should end his career and no longer participate in contact sports.

Subsequently, General Manager Retzlaff informed Hugh Brown, a sports columnist for the *Philadelphia Bulletin*, of Chuy's condition and decision to end his football career. Chuy's story was picked up by multiple news outlets. The Eagles' team doctor, Dr. James Nixon, also commented on Chuy's status to the media by identifying the player's condition as *polycythemia vera* and stating that the disorder can lead to the formation of embolisms. After reading an article in the *Los Angeles Times* about his condition, Chuy became depressed and filed suit against the Eagles and the NFL for defamation and intentional infliction of emotional distress, along with other allegations.

The District Court awarded Chuy a sum of $115,590.96 but denied Chuy's defamation claim. Chuy filed a motion for a new trial, which was denied by the District Court. Both parties appealed. The appellate court affirmed the District Court's decision. Although Chuy was considered

a public figure and Dr. Nixon's statements injured Chuy's reputation, Pennsylvania law requires that the recipient of the communication must understand that the communication was defamatory. Because the news columnist did not understand the communication was defamatory, the court ruled in favor of the Philadelphia Eagles.

Strict Liability and Product Liability

Strict liability is a defendant's legal responsibility for an injury to a plaintiff without proof of intent or fault by the defendant. The plaintiff only has to prove that the tort occurred, and the defendant was responsible. Most commonly, strict liability applies to situations that are considered to be inherently dangerous or that involve a product. Product liability is an area of negligence involving equipment (*e.g.*, automated external defibrillator [AED], strength-training equipment). Plaintiffs bringing a product liability claim allege they suffered an injury after using a product that:

1. did not perform as it was expected to.
2. was defective in design.
3. was defective because of faulty manufacturing.

Plaintiffs also have brought claims when the manufacturer failed to properly warn the user of the potential dangers of using the product. In these types of cases, the seller as well as the manufacturer may be liable to the plaintiff. Liability applies even when the seller has exercised all possible care in the preparation and sale of the product. It also applies when the user has not bought the product from or entered into any contractual relationship with the seller.

In *Bloom v. ProMaxima Manufacturing Company v. M-F Athletic Company, Inc.* (9), Louis Bloom was an avid user of the Roman chair at the fitness facility, The Lodge at Woodcliff (Woodcliff). The Roman chair was a piece of exercise equipment Bloom had used three to four times per week over the course of 7 years. On May 16, 2004, Bloom was working out with the Roman chair and as he put his feet under the footrest restraint bar, the pin which was used to adjust the equipment to the user's personal preference dislodged and the plaintiff fell headfirst and sustained injuries. Bloom brought a personal injury action against the fitness facility, as well as the manufacturer and distributor of the exercise equipment.

Woodcliff procured the Roman chair through a distributor, M-F Athletic, in August 2000. The manufacturer, ProMaxima, assembled, packaged, and shipped the chair directly to Woodcliff, with no instruction manual or guide included on how to properly use the chair. However,

Woodcliff contends they had received no prior complaints about the Roman chair from other users and suggested Bloom may have improperly placed the restraining pin that holds the restraint bar in place. Woodcliff also had an independent company inspect all of their equipment on an annual basis, and no pins were found in need of repair during any of the inspections.

During the trial, Bloom obtained a settlement with M-F Athletic, which had previously agreed to protect Woodcliff from any financial loss because of their equipment. The jury reached a verdict of "no cause" against the manufacturing company, ProMaxima, stating Bloom failed to prove his injuries were caused by the lack of an instruction manual on how to correctly use the Roman chair.

CONTRACT LAW

A contract is a binding agreement between two or more parties. Although everyone enters into contracts in everyday life — for renting a car or apartment, taking out a student loan, or even charging a meal in a restaurant — contract law is especially important for CEPs.

Types of Contracts

Contracts may be express or implied. Express contracts are based on words that are oral or written, whereas implied contracts are based on the conduct/behavior of the parties. In some instances, contracts must be in writing; if not, the contract may be voided by one of the parties and will no longer be enforceable. All written contracts need to be reviewed by a competent lawyer prior to using them in the course of conducting business. Typical contracts used in clinical and fitness facilities may include, but are not limited to, informed consents, waivers, membership agreements, employment contracts (independent contractors and employees), personal training contracts, and lease agreements.

Parts of a Contract

There are five parts of a contract: offer, acceptance, consideration, legality, and capacity.

Offer

The person who makes the offer is responsible for determining the terms of the agreement. This individual will dictate *who* the contract will be with, *what* the contract will entail, and *how* the promises will be performed. Once an offer is made, an offeree can respond in four ways:

1. Accept the offer and a legally binding contract is created.
2. Reject the offer, and the offer is automatically terminated.
3. Counteroffer, in which case the original offeror is now the offeree.
4. Choose to do nothing and the offer will terminate after a reasonable amount of time has passed.

Acceptance

The acceptance of an offer must be by someone entitled to accept the offer and must also be in the manner permitted under the contract. If neither of these is present, the contract will be terminated. Furthermore, a contract can be terminated in one of the following manners: rejection or counteroffer, revocation, lapse of time, death or incapacity of the offeror and/or offeree, or destruction of an item essential to the performance of the contract.

Consideration

The next component of a contract is known as consideration, or the price of the promise. A contract is supported by consideration if the promisee acts or promises to act in exchange for the promisor's promise.

Legality and Capacity

Even if a contract meets the initial three components of a contract, it may still be deemed invalid or voidable because of the elements of legality and capacity.

A court will not enforce a contract that is illegal. A contract is illegal if it is entered into under duress by physical force; if one party signs the contract under fraudulent misrepresentation as to the very nature of the document itself; or if the contract calls for performance that is illegal or violates public policy.

A court will not enforce a contract involving a party who does not have the capacity to enter into a contract; for example, if the person lacks the mental capacity to understand that they are entering into an agreement. This includes the mentally ill and minors (typically people under 18 years of age). As a general rule, a minor may disaffirm, or opt out of, a contract they entered into prior to age 18. This option must be exercised before they turn 18 or the courts will regard the contract as ratified or agreeable to all parties.

Breach of Contract

Once the parties have a binding and valid agreement, it can be breached in either of two ways: an immaterial (or partial) breach or a material (total) breach.

These are instances in which a party to the contract excuses certain portions of the contract. For example, the contract stipulates that a weekly report is due on Mondays by 2 PM. The party for whom the report is due allows the report to be turned in at 2:15 PM. This would be considered an immaterial breach. An immaterial breach will not void the contract.

A breach can also be a material breach; that is, a party ceases performing under the contract. Once the contract is breached, the nonbreaching party may seek damages against the breaching party. The most common types of damages related to contracts are liquidated damages and specific performance. Liquidated damages are specified within the contract itself. For example, if a strength and conditioning coach leaves a university prior to the end of their contract, the contracts dictates that they must pay the university a specific amount of money. In contrast, specific performance requires a party who breached a contract to perform their obligations under the contract (*i.e.*, deliver the equipment that was the subject of the contract).

A Case Involving Contract Law

All parties to a contract should be careful to include all terms of the contract in writing. Westgate Hills Rehabilitation and Nursing Center, managed by Platinum Healthcare (Platinum), hired Helen Kane as a nutritionist. Kane's compensation package included a salary and eligibility for health care benefits. In 2009, Kane requested maternity leave, which Platinum approved. While Kane was on leave, Platinum hired a consulting company that recommended Kane's position be downgraded to part-time because the company determined the position's duties could be accomplished in less than 40 hours. When Kane returned to work following her 3-month leave, she discovered her position had been reduced to part-time and she was now ineligible for health care benefits. Kane agreed to the hourly wage and loss of benefit eligibility. Unable to complete her duties within the reduced number of hours, she continued to work additional hours at home. Platinum did not compensate her for these extra hours.

Platinum was later bought out by Global Healthcare Fiscal Services Group, LLC and Global Healthcare Services Group Corporation (Global Defendants). Kane notified the Global Defendants in 2010 that she had not been fully compensated by Platinum for the hours she worked at home. Global Defendants also did not pay Kane for the additional hours she worked at home. As a result, Kane filed a complaint against the Global Defendants alleging breach of express and implied contracts, failure to pay for hours worked, and unjust enrichment. The Global Defendants asserted that Kane did not have an employment contract and as a result could not claim breach of contract. The Court agreed with the Global Defendants, and the breach of contract claim was dismissed (10).

CONSTITUTIONAL LAW

Constitutional law is the body of law that details the fundamental principles for how a state is governed, including the nature and structure of the government, how it exercises and distributes its sovereign powers, and the relationship between the government entity and its citizens. More specifically, this area of law has evolved from both state and federal Supreme Court rulings, which interpret the U.S. Constitution as well as state constitutions. The primary aim of constitutional law is to ensure the application of the law does not violate the enumerated individual rights of citizens.

In all, 7 articles and 27 amendments comprise the U.S. Constitution; it is the foundation upon which all U.S. law is built. The first 10 amendments to the U.S. Constitution are known as the Bill of Rights. Each amendment to the U.S. Constitution identifies certain individual fundamental rights or privileges that must be protected against government infringement. These fundamental rights include (but are not limited to) freedom of religion, speech, press, and assembly; guarantee of a speedy trial in criminal cases; and protection against cruel and unusual punishment if you're convicted of a crime. In 1925, the U.S. Supreme Court ruled that the Bill of Rights applied to the states as well as the federal government (11). This decision provided the U.S. Supreme Court with the latitude and power to strike down state laws that it determined were in violation of the Bill of Rights.

Notable Constitutional Amendments

Two notable amendments to the U.S. Constitution are the First Amendment and the Fourteenth Amendment. The First Amendment states:

> Congress shall make no law respecting an establishment of religion, or prohibiting the free exercise thereof; or abridging the freedom of speech, or of

the press; or the right of the people peaceably to assemble, and to petition the Government for a redress of grievances.

The guarantee of freedom of speech allows citizens to express their thoughts and opinions without persecution or prosecution from the government. The prohibition against government establishment of religion, often referred to as the Establishment Clause, means not only that the government cannot establish a national church or religion, but also that it cannot be excessively involved in religion or religious activities. In contrast, the Free Exercise Clause states that the government cannot prohibit the free exercise of religious practices.

Sometimes the right to free speech and freedom of religion can be challenged simultaneously. In *Bishop v. Aronov* (12), Phillip Bishop was an assistant professor in the College of Education at the University of Alabama in the 1980s. Dr. Bishop taught exercise physiology, and occasionally referred to his personal biases and religious beliefs during class time. One afternoon, Dr. Bishop arranged a voluntary meeting with interested individuals for a lecture titled, "Evidences of God in Human Physiology." Five students from his class and one professor attended the lecture, which took place shortly before final examinations were set to begin. Under the belief that the timing of the class could have had a coercive effect on Bishop's students, in violation of the Establishment Clause, the University sent a memorandum to Bishop prohibiting him from discussing his religious preferences and/or beliefs that were not essential to class discussion or materials. Bishop filed a lawsuit against the University, seeking relief from the free speech encroachments the University had imposed. The Court agreed with Bishop citing the University had created a space for an interchange of ideas, and the after-class meeting was only an open exchange of ideas between individuals. The Court determined that Bishop did not violate the Establishment Clause and ordered the University to rescind its prohibition of Bishop's meetings and class (12).

Akin to the First Amendment, the Fourteenth Amendment protects the rights of citizens by ensuring that they are treated equally. Specifically, the Fourteenth Amendment prohibits discrimination and provides all citizens with equal protection under the law. The Amendment guarantees:

All persons born or naturalized in the United States, and subject to the jurisdiction thereof, are citizens of the United States and of the State where in they reside. No state shall make or enforce any law which shall abridge the privileges or immunities of citizens of the United States; nor shall any State deprive any person of life, liberty, or property, without due process of law; nor deny to any person within its jurisdiction the equal protection of the laws.

The most familiar clauses of the Fourteenth Amendment are the **Due Process** Clause and the **Equal Protection** Clause. The Due Process Clause prevents the government from depriving a citizen of life, liberty, or property without legislative permission. Citizens are granted the right to be notified, an opportunity to be heard, and opportunity to defend against any allegations. The Equal Protection Clause, explicitly, provides equal protection and treatment to all people regardless of nationality, race, gender, or religion, to name a few.

Notable Laws Based on the First and Fourteenth Amendments

These amendments are the foundation for several laws that have been enacted to work in conjunction with the U.S. Constitution to protect specific populations. These laws include the Civil Rights Act of 1964, which prohibits discrimination based on race, color, national origin, religion, sex, age, or disability. These characteristics are called protected classes. The 11 components of the Act are known as Titles. For instance, Title VII addresses employment discrimination. Under Title VII, it is prohibited to discriminate in any aspect of employment, including recruitment, hiring, terminations, and other decisions regarding employment. Claims related to employment discrimination are handled and enforced by the Equal Employment Opportunity Commission (EEOC). Although there is a Title IX of the Civil Rights Act of 1964, it should not be confused with Title IX of the Education Amendments Act of 1972. Title IX of the Civil Rights Act of 1964 allowed for the movement of civil cases from state courts to federal courts. This action was useful for cases in which either the plaintiff or defendant was concerned about receiving a fair and unbiased trial in state courts. Title IX of the Education Amendments Act of 1972 prohibits sex discrimination in federally funded education programs and activities. Title IX has been the law applied in cases related to gender equity and sexual harassment.

The Rehabilitation Act of 1973 (Act) (29 U.S.C. §§ 701–797(b)) (13) and the Americans with Disabilities Act (ADA) (42 U.S.C. §§ 12101–12213) (14) provide individuals with disabilities an equal opportunity for participation in athletics as well as in procuring and retaining employment. In both contexts, an individual with a disability is entitled to protection under the Act if they have a physical impairment that substantially limits a major life activity, and they are "otherwise qualified" to participate. Major life activities include, but are not limited to, seeing, hearing, speaking, eating, sleeping, walking, and breathing (42 U.S.C. § 12101) (14). Heart conditions, congenital back or spine abnormality, or loss of a paired organ are covered under the Act (29 U.S.C. § 705(9)(B)) (13).

If an individual or organization is found to have violated the Rehabilitation Act or the ADA, courts will generally require the individual or organization to allow the athlete to participate or the employee to work. In some instances, the individual or organization must provide a reasonable accommodation for the athlete or the employee. However, a reasonable accommodation will not be enforced if the change or modification will cause undue hardship for the individual or employer. An undue hardship is defined as significantly difficult, unduly extensive, or expensive (42 U.S.C. § 12112 (b)(5)(A)) (14).

In the area of sport, there have been occurrences where athletes have been medically disqualified by a team physician but possess the physical capabilities to participate. The litigation against the team and physician is usually based on the athlete obtaining medical clearance from another physician. Plaintiffs have successfully defended these lawsuits if the athlete's participation creates a significant increased risk of substantial harm to the athlete or other participants (15).

Cases Involving the ADA

Gavin Class transferred to Towson University (Towson) to play football in the fall of 2013. During practice drills, Class collapsed from exertional heat stroke and suffered multiorgan failure, which required a liver transplant and left him hospitalized for 2 months. After he recovered, Class expressed a desire to return to the football team and was referred by Towson to the Team Physician, Dr. Kindschi. Along with four other physicians, Dr. Kindschi concluded Class could not safely participate in Towson's football program, even though Dr. Kindschi recommended Class could participate in a cool environment that involved no contact conditioning. A few months after these results, Class took another heat tolerance test using an outside physician who recommended Class was at an acceptable risk to play football for the team, provided he had appropriate padding and protection. Towson again refused to clear Class to play football, stating the team physician has the final authority in deciding whether an injured student-athlete may return to competition or practice.

Class filed a suit against Towson, alleging the football program violated the ADA and Rehabilitation Act. He sought an injunction — a court order compelling Towson to allow him to participate. Class alleged his susceptibility to heat stroke was a disability that limited major life activities. But with reasonable accommodations such as abdominal padding and internal temperature monitoring, he would be able to fully return to football. Class also alleged a third heat tolerance test would conclude that he should be able to fully participate in football practices with recommended conditions. The District Court determined Class was an individual with a protected disability and determined Towson had discriminated against Class by refusing to provide reasonable accommodations. The court instructed Towson to allow Class to participate, and Towson filed an appeal. The Court of Appeals held that obtaining a physician's clearance for student-athletes to return from injury was an essential eligibility requirement, and the physician's refusal to clear the player did not constitute a failure to accommodate under the ADA and Rehabilitation Act. The judgment was reversed (16).

Nicholas Knapp was a promising high school basketball star who was verbally offered an athletic scholarship to Northwestern University (Northwestern) during his junior year in high school. Early into his senior year, Knapp suffered a sudden cardiac arrest during a pick-up game. Paramedics were able to restart his heart, and over the next few weeks doctors implanted an internal cardioverter defibrillator in Knapp's abdomen to detect arrhythmias and deliver shocks to the heart if the need arose. The day after his sudden cardiac arrest, Northwestern promised to honor Knapp's athletic scholarship, and Knapp signed a letter of intent to play for Northwestern. During his senior year, Knapp did not play basketball, although he remained on the team. During the fall semester, Knapp enrolled at Northwestern. In preparation for the upcoming basketball season at Northwestern, Dr. Howard Sweeney, the head team physician, reviewed Knapp's medical records and the recommendations of several treating physicians and declared Knapp was ineligible to participate on Northwestern's basketball team for the upcoming year. Following the season, Northwestern and the Big Ten declared Knapp permanently medically ineligible to play basketball. Knapp filed a complaint claiming Northwestern's actions violated the Rehabilitation Act and requested a permanent injunction. The District Court determined Knapp was medically eligible and prohibited Northwestern from excluding Knapp from playing on the basketball team because of reasons related to his cardiac condition. Northwestern appealed, and the appellate court decided that Northwestern must be allowed to determine its own conclusions of athlete substantial risk and severity of injury. As long as the conclusions are based on reliable evidence, the court would not replace its opinion with that of the school's team physicians. The appellate court returned the case to the District Court with instructions to decide the case in favor of Northwestern (17).

In March 2000, Kimberly Watson applied for a part-time PRN (as needed) nurse position at Hughston Sports Medicine Hospital (Hughston). Watson was conditionally offered the position, and one of the conditions was to complete a standard preemployment physical examination. Hughston screened for latex sensitivity with all potential employees, as it was a surgical hospital and used a multitude of products containing latex materials. Watson indicated she had suffered previous reactions to latex and voluntarily took the blood test. As a result of the blood test results, the Director of Human Services, Del Leftwich, and CEO of Hughston, Hugh Tappan, determined Watson had a high degree of sensitivity to latex and would be at risk of suffering allergic reactions as a nurse at Hughston. Thus, Watson was told she could not be offered the position. Afterward, Watson sought an opinion from an allergist, Dr. Robert Chrzanowski, who tested and diagnosed her with a latex allergy. His recommendations included avoiding latex at home and at work and advised Watson would be putting her health at risk if she continued to be exposed to latex. Watson then filed a lawsuit alleging Hughston violated the ADA by refusing to hire her because of her severe allergy to latex. Hughston moved for summary judgment, which was granted by the District Court. The court held that Watson was not actually disabled. Because of lack of evidence that the allergy substantially limited any major life activities, she was not viewed as disabled by the hospital (18).

CRIMINAL LAW

Criminal law is based on state or federal statutes defining specific actions that are unacceptable within a jurisdiction and are subject to punishment, which may include jail time and/or fines. In criminal law, the court must determine whether a perpetrator has formed the intent to commit a crime and then carried out that intent. The burden of proof in a criminal case is "beyond a reasonable doubt." Returning to the example of the voting process and a civic organization, the vote by a jury would need to be unanimous to convict an individual of a crime. For a CEP, it is important to understand criminal law, as certain

behaviors are considered crimes and may result in jail time, including stealing money from a place of employment, allowing an athlete to die from heat exhaustion, or providing incorrect treatment after an injury.

Types and Categories of Crimes

Certain acts/behaviors may be in violation of both federal and state law under what is called a "criminal (or penal) code." The federal and state criminal codes identify which offenses are prohibited by law within each jurisdiction. Based on the nature of the crime and the punishment associated with the crime, crimes are divided into three categories: infractions, misdemeanors, and felonies. Infractions, which are sometimes referred to as violations, are petty crimes typically punishable through fines, but no jail time. To illustrate, a speeding ticket is considered an infraction. Misdemeanors are minor crimes, which provide a punishment of incarceration for less than 1 year in county jail and/or a fine. The punishment may also include probation, community service, and restitution. An example of a misdemeanor is an assault that carries a maximum fine of $1,000 and maximum 6 months of jail time. Felonies, however, are the most serious in nature, involving serious physical harm or threat of harm to the victims. Felonies may also consist of financially motivated nonviolent crimes such as fraud, bribery, embezzlement, and forgery. Some states subdivide felonies into classes or degrees depending on severity. These crimes allow for penalty of more than 1 year in state or federal prison.

There are four major categories of crimes: crimes against the person, crimes related to property, crimes affecting the public health and welfare, and crimes against the government. For the purposes of this chapter, only crimes against the person and crimes against property will be discussed.

Crimes Against the Person

Crimes against the person typically include assault, battery, and homicide. As previously discussed under section Tort Law, an assault is an intent to cause immediate harm through menacing or threatening behavior, apprehension of immediate harm, and lack of consent. Conversely, battery is considered a successful assault. The difference between an assault or battery under criminal law and tort law is the penalty. Under tort law, a victim will seek damages; under criminal law, the perpetrator could be fined and/or incarcerated.

The most serious crime against a person is homicide. A homicide occurs when an individual's actions result in the death of another person. Depending on the mental state of the individual, there are several different categories of homicide depending on the jurisdiction. These can range from, but are not limited to, involuntary manslaughter, voluntary manslaughter, and varying degrees of murder.

Crimes Related to Property

Crimes related to property often include, but are not limited to, burglary, larceny, and vandalism. These distinct crimes do not involve the threat of force or actual force against a victim; the crimes are solely tied to property. Burglary is defined as entering into a building illegally with the intent to commit a crime. Larceny is the wrongful taking and carrying away of the personal property of another. Lastly, vandalism is deliberate destruction or damage to property.

As with tort law, statutes of limitations prohibit prosecutors from charging an individual with the commission of a crime against a person or property after a certain amount of time has passed. The statute of limitations countdown begins on the date the crime is committed and varies with each type of crime. However, not all crimes have a statute of limitation. For example, murder does not, and in some states sexual offenses with minors, kidnapping, forgery, and arson do not.

Defenses to Crimes

In criminal cases, determining guilt is often far from simple. Common defenses to crimes include consent, self-defense, and defense of a third party. These defenses must be raised when the defendant learns of the plaintiff's allegations.

Consent

In certain circumstances, the fact that a plaintiff consented to an act would absolve the defendant of a crime. The most conventional example is in the context of physical contact in sports. Courts will normally view sport participants as consenting to the physical contact and any potential harm that may occur. For instance, a boxer consents to being touched by another boxer during a boxing match. Outside of sport, this could be considered battery. To establish a consent defense, three requirements must be met:

1. An individual cannot consent to situations that may include serious bodily injury.

2. The injury or harm must be reasonably foreseeable.
3. The consent was justified, meaning the individual received a benefit from the conduct.

The application of the consent defense is extremely limited. Again, many cases have pertained to athletic or sport participation.

Self-Defense and Defense of a Third Party

Other defenses to a crime are self-defense — the act of protecting one's person or property — and defense of a third party being physically attacked. In order to assert a claim of defense, the defendant must show that the force used was reasonable. Reasonable force is the amount of force needed to halt the attack. Courts have been hesitant to apply this defense when the individual uses excessive force, such as force that results in the severe bodily harm or death of the assailant. Initially, some states limited the defense of a third party to include only close relatives, but most states acknowledge that a person may use reasonable force in defense of any other person, if that person had the right to use force themselves.

A Criminal Case

Tracy Brown was the owner and manager of the health care company Psalms 23 DME, LLC (Psalms) in New Orleans, Louisiana. During the course of her business, Brown negotiated with several parties regarding the amounts she would pay for patient referrals. Although Brown knew it was illegal to pay for patient names (a stipulation of her Medicare enrollment application), she actively engaged in paying patient recruiters for their referrals. In addition to the kickbacks, Brown submitted claims to Medicare for wheelchairs, orthotics, and other durable medical equipment that was not necessary or delivered. She also billed Medicare for more expensive versions of each type of equipment when she actually provided cheaper versions to patients (a practice referred to as "upcoding"). Over time, Psalms billed Medicare for $3.2 million in claims, and received almost $2 million from Medicare. Following complaints to Medicare from a considerable number of patients who were billed for equipment they did not need or receive, Brown was indicted by a grand jury on one count of conspiracy to pay illegal kickbacks, seven counts of paying illegal kickbacks, one count of conspiracy to commit health care fraud, and nine counts of health care fraud. Evidence at trial showed Brown was aware the kickbacks were illegal, and she ignored the Medicare rules for the billing of durable medical equipment. The federal jury convicted Brown on all 18 counts, and a motion for a new trial was denied (19).

EMPLOYMENT AND LABOR LAW

Employment law is rooted in contract law. Employment agreements identify the length of employment, duties and responsibilities, compensation, and how/when the employment agreement may be terminated. Some employment agreements also include restrictive covenants or covenants not to compete when the employment is ended. These provisions limit the ability of the employee to terminate the agreement early or to take a comparable job from an employer's competitor. If an employee does not have a contract for employment or there is no specified term of employment, the employment is known as "at will." This means the employer may terminate the employee at any time, with or without a reason.

Over many decades, the U.S. Congress has passed legislation to address labor conditions in the workplace related to standards of pay, time off from work because of medical circumstances, injuries sustained at work, and overall employee work environment. Many of these laws can impact work settings for CEPs, such as the conditions of their own employment as well as the employment of others. The next section will briefly discuss several labor laws that are essential for CEPs:

- Fair Labor Standards Act of 1938
- Equal Pay Act of 1963
- Age Discrimination in Employment Act
- Family Medical and Leave Act
- Title VII of the Civil Rights Act
- Occupational Safety and Health Administration Act of 1970
- Workers' Compensation Statutes

Fair Labor Standards Act

The Fair Labor Standards Act (FLSA) of 1938 was enacted to eradicate "labor conditions detrimental to the maintenance of the minimum standards of living necessary for health, efficiency, and well-being of workers" (29 U.S.C. § 202) (20). Based on this premise, the FLSA establishes guidelines for minimum wage, overtime pay, recordkeeping, and standards affecting the employment of minors. These guidelines cover employees in federal, state, and local government as well as the private sector. In general, they apply to any business that has at least two employees and at least $500,000 a year in sales or that has employees who regularly engage in activities or the production of goods involving interstate commerce (21).

Workers are classified as nonexempt (entitled to overtime pay) and exempt (not entitled to overtime pay). Nonexempt workers are entitled to a minimum wage of $7.25 per hour effective July 24, 2009. Nonexempt workers must also be paid overtime pay at a rate of not less than 1½ times their regular rates of pay after 40 hours of work in a week. To be classified as exempt, an employee must:

1. be paid not less than $684 per week.
2. be paid on a salary basis.
3. perform exempt job duties (22).

Four classes of job duties are considered exempt:

- Executive duties include supervision of two or more employees, or involvement in the hiring, promoting, and firing of employees.
- Professional duties require special education and the exercise of discretion or judgment. For example, lawyers, teachers, and registered nurses perform professional duties.
- Administrative duties involve office or nonmanual work directly related to the general business operations of the employer.
- Outside sales duties involve regular work distant from the employer's place of business (23).

Exempt jobs related to the field of clinical exercise physiology may include, but are not limited to, the manager of a fitness facility, college faculty, an athletic trainer, and a sales representative for a sports medicine supply company.

Any employer who violates an employee's rights under the FLSA will be liable to the employee in the amount of their unpaid minimum wages, their unpaid overtime compensation, liquidated damages, and any equitable relief that may be appropriate. Equitable relief may include, but is not limited to, employment, reinstatement, promotion, and lost wages (29 U.S.C. § 216(b)) (24).

The distinction between exempt and nonexempt employment status is not always clear. In 1999, a group of athletic trainers filed a suit against the San Antonio Independent School District (SAISD) pursuant to the FLSA over a disagreement regarding overtime benefits. SAISD claimed the athletic trainers were professionals and exempt from the FLSA's overtime benefits requirements. The athletic trainers argued that they were not considered professionals under

FLSA guidelines. Specifically, when responding to emergencies, they followed standard protocol but also called for emergency medical support that would qualify them as nonexempt. The District Court ruled in favor of the athletic trainers, and SAISD appealed the decision. The appellate court determined that athletic trainers have professional judgment and discretion to decide whether to treat the injury on-site or call for Emergency Medical Systems (EMS) help. Additionally, because the athletic trainers are mandated to take 15 hours of specific college-level courses, the position required custom learning or specialized instruction. In light of these facts, the athletic trainers were exempt professionals under the FLSA. The Court of Appeals rendered judgment in favor of SAISD, which meant the athletic trainers were not eligible for overtime benefits (25).

Equal Pay Act

The Equal Pay Act (EPA) of 1963 is a federal law subject to the FLSA mandating that individuals who perform substantially the same work must be paid equally. When suing under the EPA, an individual must prove the employer has paid them less than their counterpart for substantially equal work. There are exceptions for variances in pay based on an established seniority system, a merit system, or any other distinction based on a legitimate reason.

A 2005 case, *Dillow v. Wellmont Health System*, reveals that the concept of substantially equal work is not always easy to interpret. In 2001, Julie Cowan, the facility manager of the Wellness Wellmont Center (Center), requested a meeting to discuss a business proposition with Eric Deaton, the Vice President of Finance and Operations for Wellmont Bristol Regional Medical Center, the parent company of the Center. Cowan sought approval to develop a personal training fitness program at the Center. At that time, a limited amount of personal training was offered to new members of the Center during their orientation, and established members could pay an additional fee for private sessions with a personal trainer. Cowan believed these options were inadequate and envisioned a more extensive personal training program.

The plaintiffs, Dillow, McIlwain, and Stallard, were employees of the Center. Their responsibilities included management of various programs, working the front desk, and providing general orientation services to new members of the Center. Each was eager to help Cowan implement the changes to the program. However, Cowan stated that a new employee was needed with experience in managing a successful training program. Roger Altizer, an acquaintance of Cowan's, was known in the local health and fitness industry and was managing a personal training program at a fitness center in Tennessee. Altizer agreed to a starting salary of $35,000 a year in addition to health insurance and other benefits. Upon hiring Altizer, the Center established the "Wellfit Personal Training Program," which Altizer was charged with developing, managing, and overseeing. The plaintiffs learned of Altizer's salary, complained to Cowan that their own salaries were too low in comparison, and filed a formal grievance with the parent company. When their grievance was ignored and Cowan reprimanded them, they filed a lawsuit against the Center claiming violations of the EPA and Title VII of the Civil Rights Act. Cowan testified that Altizer's position was not equivalent to the plaintiffs', as Altizer's position was at risk and dependent on growing the Center's personal training clientele and generating revenue for the program, whereas the plaintiffs' personal training assignments were not tied to their normal duties. The Court found the plaintiffs were unable to establish that their positions were substantially equal to Altizer's. The Court also agreed that inconsiderate comments by Cowan and ignored requests from the plaintiffs had no adverse effect on their duties, salaries, or benefits. The Court concluded that the plaintiffs failed to prove a violation of the EPA or retaliation under Title VII of the Civil Rights Act (26).

Age Discrimination in Employment Act

In 1967, the Age Discrimination in Employment Act (ADEA) was passed to protect employees over the age of 40 years from being discriminated against in the workplace. The ADEA does not protect employees under the age minimum from discrimination — that is, from claims that they were not hired because they were too young for a position. In addition, the ADEA only applies to employers with 20 or more employees. Typical examples of age discrimination include, but are not limited to, age preferences in job announcements and forced retirement because of age (29 U.S.C. § 621) (27).

Family Medical and Leave Act

Enacted in 1993, the Family and Medical Leave Act (FMLA) entitles eligible employees to 12 weeks of unpaid, job-protected leave in a 12-month period for specified family and medical reasons or 26 weeks of leave to care for an active duty or service member of the Armed Forces who is covered by FMLA (29 U.S.C.A. § 2611(14–15)) (28). The specified reasons include the birth or adoption of a child; care for the employee's spouse, child, or parent who has a serious health condition; or a serious health condition that interferes with the employee's ability to perform their job. A serious health condition is defined as an "illness, injury, impairment, or physical or mental condition that involves [either] inpatient care in a hospital, hospice, or residential medical care facility or continuing treatment by a healthcare provider" (29 U.S.C.A. § 2611(14)) (28).

In order to qualify for leave under FMLA, four conditions must be met. First, the employee must work for a covered employer. The FMLA applies to public agencies, government agencies, public and private schools, and to businesses that employ 50 or more persons. Second, the employee must have worked for the employer for at least 12 months. This does not have to be a continuous 12 months; seasonal work is also considered in this time period. Third, the employee must have at least 1,250 hours of service with the employer during the previous 12 months, which is about 24 hours per week during the 12 weeks. Fourth, the employee must work in a location where the employer has at least 50 employees within 75 miles of the work site (29 U.S.C.A. § 2611(2)(A)) (28). If any of these conditions do not apply to the employee, they will not be eligible for FMLA leave.

When an employee is granted leave under the FMLA, they are entitled (a) to be restored by the employer to the position held by the employee when the leave began or (b) restored to an equivalent position with equivalent benefits, pay, and terms of employment (29 U.S.C.A. § 2614(a)(1)) (28). Any employer who violates an employee's rights under the FMLA may be liable to the employee for damages equal to the amount of wages, salary, and benefits. Additionally, the employer may be liable for any actual monetary losses the employee sustained as a result of the employer's violation, liquidated damages, and any additional relief that a court of law may determine as appropriate (29 U.S.C.A. § 2617(a)(1)) (28).

The right to be restored to the same or an equivalent position was upheld in *Carpo v. Wartburg Lutheran Home for the Aging* (29). Mediatrix Carpo was an employee at Wartburg Lutheran Home for the Aging (Wartburg) when she was injured in a car accident unrelated to her employment. Carpo sustained serious injuries that qualified her for leave under the FMLA. At the end of November 2003, Wartburg submitted a letter to Carpo requesting a doctor's note upon her return specifying that she could resume full duties. In January 2004, Carpo received another letter from Wartburg notifying her that her FMLA leave would expire on February 3, 2004. After 12 weeks of leave, Carpo returned to work on February 3 and presented a doctor's note handwritten on a prescription slip stating that Carpo could attempt to return to work. The Director of Human Services, Mary Ann Benton, notated

on the back of the doctor's prescription slip that the note was unacceptable, and the policy was for the employee to resume full duties, not to attempt to work. Carpo was then terminated from her position for failure to produce a doctor's certification that she was capable of resuming her full duties. As a result, Carpo filed a lawsuit against Wartburg. The suit claimed that Wartburg had no intention of rehiring her because her position had been filled in her absence. It also claimed Wartburg interfered with Carpo's right to return to work by refusing to accept her doctor's letter, and that Wartburg should have sought clarification from Carpo's doctor prior to termination. Both parties agreed that Carpo was an eligible employee, that she qualified for FMLA leave that had been approved, and that she returned to work in an appropriate amount of time. The disagreement was whether Carpo's doctor's note was an adequate certification for FMLA purposes, and if it was not, whether Wartburg had the right to terminate Carpo that day. The court determined the note was sufficient and approved of Carpo's ability to work. Although Wartburg demanded a definitive statement that an employee is able to return to full duties following approved leave, under the FMLA, a simple statement that an employee is able to return to work is sufficient. The Court supported Carpo's claim that Wartburg violated her FMLA rights by not seeking clarification from her doctor prior to termination and ruled in favor of Carpo.

Title VII of the Civil Rights Act

Title VII of the Civil Rights Act protects employees from workplace harassment, which is generally defined as unwelcome conduct. Sexual harassment is unwanted sexual behavior such as offensive comments about a person's sex, sexual advances, requests for sexual favors, and any verbal or physical conduct of a sexual nature (30). Harassment is an unlawful form of employment discrimination when the offensive conduct is a condition of continued employment or creates an uncomfortable work environment. The harasser could be the victim's co-worker or supervisor, a supervisor in another department, or the business client or customer. In cases of sexual harassment, the harasser may be of the opposite sex or the same sex as the victim. With harassment and sexual harassment, the victim also does not have to be the person being harassed. If another individual feels affected by the offensive conduct, they may file a claim.

The best method for eliminating harassment in the workplace is for employers to engage in practices that will prevent the behavior from occurring. All employees, managers, and executives should participate in anti-harassment training. Employers should also establish an effective grievance process, communicate this process to all employees, and take appropriate steps to investigate when an employee reports an incident.

Reznick v. Associated Orthopedics & Sports Medicine, P.A. (31) demonstrates that claims of harassment require adequate evidence. In July 1997, Associated Orthopedics & Sports Medicine, P.A. (AOSM) hired Lisa Reznick, an orthopedic surgeon with a specialty in hand, wrist, and elbow care. Reznick alleges that, shortly after she was hired, one of the partners of AOSM, Alex Glogau, made inappropriate and sexist comments to her in front of pharmaceutical representatives during lunch. When Reznick confronted Glogau afterward, he dismissed Reznick's concerns, told her that she was too sensitive, but apologized if he had seemingly offended her. That fall, according to Reznick, Glogau made more inappropriate comments about her sexuality and office attire and expressed a desire for her to wear skirts more often. In May 1998, Reznick overhead Glogau on the phone stating that she would not become a partner at the practice. Reznick believed this decision was based directly on her sex, not her job performance. Later that spring, AOSM hosted an open house for a new male physician who had recently joined the practice. Following a poor showing at the open house, AOSM resumed its previous policy of not hosting such events for new physicians. However, Reznick believed AOSM failed to host an open house to honor her employment based on her sex. In March 2000, Reznick submitted a resignation letter that included a 90-day notice. AOSM offered to pay her for the remaining 90 days if she wished to leave the practice earlier, but Reznick refused and continued to fulfill her 90 days of work. Following her resignation, Reznick filed suit alleging AOSM had violated the EPA and Title VII of the Civil Rights Act based on Glogau's sexist behavior toward her. Reznick also claimed her employer made her work environment unbearable, and she felt pressured to resign. AOSM submitted a motion for summary judgment, which was granted by the District court. Reznick appealed, and the Court of Appeals affirmed the District Court's ruling, citing that Reznick failed to provide adequate evidence that her work environment was unendurable and compelled her resignation.

Occupational Safety and Health Administration Act

The Occupational Safety and Health Administration Act (OSHA) of 1970 states that employers have a general duty to provide their employees with a safe and healthy work environment. The work environment must be free from any recognized hazards likely to cause serious physical harm or death to employees. Under OSHA, an employer is defined as any "person engaged in a business affecting commerce who has employees, but does not include the U.S. or any state or political subdivision of the state" (29 C.F.R. § 1910.2(c)) (32). Therefore, the law applies to most private industries, nonprofits, private educational institutions, and OSHA-approved state programs in such fields as agriculture, manufacturing, construction, retail, law, and medicine.

To further its purpose and scope, OSHA has two primary regulatory functions. The first is to set general industry safety standards (29 C.F.R. § 1903.1) (32). Several of the most common general industry standards deal with blood-borne pathogens, hazard communication, respiratory protection, occupational noise exposure, hazardous waste operations and emergency response, and personal protective equipment (33). For example, employers must establish an exposure control plan to eliminate or minimize employee exposures to blood-borne pathogens. This includes providing information and training to employees regarding preventative practices, imposing postexposure procedures, and the utilization of personal protective equipment such as gloves, gowns, and masks. For a CEP, knowledge of these OSHA standards is essential.

OSHA's second regulatory function is to conduct inspections to ensure that employers are providing safe and healthy workplaces (29 C.F.R. §1903.1) (32). If an employer is found to be in violation, OSHA provides for enforcement of the inspection, issuance of citations, and proposed penalties for the employer.

The OSHA also protects employees who report health or safety concerns and violations. Employers may not discriminate or retaliate against an employee who reports health or safety concerns within the workplace. If a complaint is filed with OSHA, employee remedies may include job reinstatement and payment of back wages (29 C.F.R. § 1977) (34).

Workers' Compensation Statutes

Over the past 100 years, every state in the U.S. has passed workers' compensation statutes to provide compensation for employees who have been injured, disabled, or become ill while performing their jobs. Before these statutes, injured employees or their dependents could not recover against their employers for job-related injuries. These statutes balanced the rights of both entities, thus creating an efficient, private no-fault system that was favorable for both workers and employers (35).

An employee is entitled to workers' compensation benefits for any work-related illness or injury. The illness or injury may be because of exposure to certain types of chemicals used in the work environment over a prolonged period of time or a single incident that resulted in physical harm. Because workers' compensation statutes are state-specific, the language of each statute may vary from state to state. However, most of the state statutes mirror the language provided in the Federal Employees' Compensation Act (FECA) (5 U.S.C. § 8101)) (36).

There are three essential elements for a workers' compensation claim:

1. The employer must have workers' compensation insurance.
2. The person must be an employee, not an independent contractor.
3. The employee's injury or illness must have arisen from or while performing employment duties (37).

If an employee files a claim seeking workers' compensation, the employee's only remedy will be under workers' compensation. This means the employee cannot be compensated under worker compensation laws, and then later decide to sue under tort law for additional monetary damages.

INTELLECTUAL PROPERTY

Intellectual property is defined as any creation of the mind that can be used in commerce (38). Creations of the mind may include literary and artistic works, inventions, symbols, names, and images. The primary goal of intellectual property law is to create and maintain an open and competitive marketplace, which allows creators of original work the right to control the use of their work (38).

Intellectual property is subdivided into three categories: copyright, trademark, and patent. Copyrights and patents are protected under Article 1, Section 8, Clause 8 of the U.S. Constitution, which states Congress has the power "to promote the progress of science and useful arts, by securing for limited times to authors and inventors the exclusive right to their respective writings and discoveries." Trademarks are protected based on Congress's ability to regulate interstate commerce under Article 1, Section 8, Clause 3. An understanding of intellectual property law can prevent CEPs from inadvertently infringing on copyright when writing academic papers or journal articles or when creating marketing materials for businesses, as well as from violating the intellectual property rights (*i.e.*, trademarks and patents) owned by others.

Copyright

In accordance with the powers granted under the U.S. Constitution, Congress enacted the U.S. Copyright Act of 1909 to protect original and artistic expressions. The law was revised in 1976 and modified multiple times over the years in response to changes in technology and the Internet.

Current copyright law specifies that its goal is to encourage creativity by extending protection to works of art, literature, music, and other works of authorship (17 U.S.C. § 102) (39).

Copyright law does not protect an individual's idea, but only the individual's fixed expression of the idea. Thus, there are two requirements to create a copyright. The work must be original, which means the material must be created by the author and possess some minimal amount of ingenuity. The work must be fixed or put into a tangible form, which may be written or an audio/visual recording. Notice that a copyright is created once an idea is put into an original and fixed form. This means that registration is not required for a copyright to exist. For example, the copyright to a CEP's written description of a case study belongs to the CEP from the moment it is written. Although registration of a copyright is not required, it does provide several benefits in the event there is unauthorized use of the author's work. These include receiving additional monetary damages, legal costs, and attorney's fees.

Copyrights are registered with the U.S. Copyright Office. The designation of a copyright includes the copyright symbol or word, the date, and the name of the author or copyright holder (*e.g.,* © 2022, Jane Doe or Copyright 2022, XYZ Publishing). Ownership of the copyright may belong to a sole author or joint authors. For collective works, such as a periodical, a book of essays, or a CD of conference proceedings, each single contribution has a separate copyright from the collective work as a whole. In contrast, the copyright to a work for hire — work prepared by an employee within the scope of their employment or work specifically ordered or commissioned for use by a third party — would be subject to the terms of an oral or written agreement (17 U.S.C. § 201) (39).

The duration of a copyright for works created prior to January 1, 1978, is 95 years from the date of creation. The copyright for works created after January 1, 1978, endures for the life of the author plus 70 years, or in the case of a work for hire, 95 years after the first publication or 120 years after creation, whichever is earlier (17 U.S.C. §§ 302–304) (39).

Types of Copyright Infringement

Copyright infringement is unauthorized use of a copyrighted work. There are three types: direct infringement, contributory infringement, and vicarious infringement.

Direct infringement occurs when a defendant violates one of the copyright owner's exclusive rights (17 U.S.C. § 501) (39). These rights may include, but are not limited to, the right to reproduce the copyrighted work, to prepare derivative works based on the copyrighted work, and to distribute copies of the copyrighted work to the public by sale or other transfer of ownership (17 U.S.C. § 106) (39). To prove direct copyright infringement, the copyright owner must prove the defendant had access to the copyrighted work and the allegedly infringing work is substantially similar to the copyrighted work. Even if the defendant accidentally or inadvertently copied the work, infringement may still exist.

Contributory infringement occurs when someone participates in or contributes to a direct infringement by another. The elements of contributory infringement are: (a) a direct infringement has occurred, (b) the defendant knew or should have known that the infringement was occurring, and (c) the defendant participated in the infringement by causing, inducing, or materially contributing to its occurrence.

Vicarious infringement arises from the relationship between a direct infringer and a defendant. Here, the defendant must have supervisory control over an infringing activity and some financial gain resulted from the infringing activity (40). For example, fitness facilities often play background music to enhance the environment as their clients work out. Because the businesses are benefiting financially from the music, they are required to obtain a license to play it. Music licensing organizations include the American Society of Composers, Authors, and Publishers (ASCAP), Broadcast Music, Inc. (BMI), the Society of European Stage Authors and Composers (SESAC), and commercial music services. Even if the facility has a business account with Pandora or SiriusXM, the facility may be in violation of federal law, as these accounts are only allowed "where people can be without paying a fee" (*e.g.*, a lobby or front desk area) (41). Some exemptions exist for small businesses, but businesses should take the proper steps to ensure that the necessary licenses are purchased. Without the correct license, facilities could be fined up to $150,000 for each copyrighted song played.

Defense of Copyright Infringement

The most common defense for copyright infringement is known as "fair use." Fair use is defined as use of a copyrighted work for purposes of criticism, comment, news reporting, teaching/classroom use, scholarship, or research. In determining whether a particular case involves fair use, courts will consider the purpose and character of the use (including whether the use is of a commercial nature or for nonprofit educational purposes), the nature of the copyrighted work, the amount and substantiality of the portion used in relation to the copyrighted work as a whole, and the effect of the use on the potential market for the copyrighted work (17 U.S.C. § 107) (39).

A Case Involving a Claim of Copyright Infringement

Lapine v. Seinfeld (42) demonstrates that copyright law protects only the individual's fixed expression of an idea. Missy Chase Lapine was a chef classically trained by the Institute of Culinary Education and the New School Culinary Arts in New York City. As faculty at the New School Culinary Arts, Lapine offered workshops and cooking classes instructing families on how to eat more health food. This experience led Lapine to decide to author a cookbook to help parents get their children to eat more vegetables. It took 2 years for her to write the book, and in February 2006, Lapine submitted her cookbook proposal as well as detailed chapters from the cookbook to HarperCollins, a book publisher. The submission was rejected, and the written work was not returned. Lapine then hired a literary agent, who resubmitted the proposal to HarperCollins in May 2006. It was rejected a second time, and again the written work was not returned. Later that year, Running Press, a subsidiary of Perseus Books Group, accepted her cookbook, titled *The Sneaky Chef: Simple Strategies for Hiding Healthy Food in Kids' Favorite Meals (Sneaky Chef)*. The cookbook was published in April 2007 and appeared on the *New York Times* bestseller list for the week of April 22, 2007.

In October 2007, HarperCollins published *Deceptively Delicious: Simple Secrets to Get Your Kids Eating Good Food (Deceptively Delicious)* by Jessica Seinfeld, the wife of comedian Jerry Seinfeld. Seinfeld indicated in her book that she was not a professional chef but was assisted by a chef in preparing and selecting her cookbook recipes. *Deceptively Delicious* achieved number-one on the *New York Times* bestseller list. Lapine sued Jessica Seinfeld and HarperCollins, alleging that *Deceptively Delicious* infringed upon the work published in *Sneaky Chef*. As was previously stated, to prove copyright infringement, a plaintiff must show that the "defendant has actually copied the plaintiff's work; and copying is illegal because a substantial similarity exists between the defendant's work and the protectable elements of plaintiff's" (43, p. 99).

In determining whether a "substantial similarity exits" between two works, the Court will examine the "total concept and feel of the contested works" (44, p. 268).

Lapine argued that the cookbooks were similarly themed, organized, structured, and sequenced. Although both cookbooks recommended camouflaging healthy food in a child's favorite meals, the Court ruled that similar themes are not enough to substantiate infringement nor was the arrangement of the book an actionable substantial similarity between the two books. Upon examining the "total concept and feel" of the two books, the court found that *Sneaky Chef* possessed an educational tone and consisted primarily of text with only a few photographs of the food items prepared. Conversely, *Deceptively Delicious* catered toward working or busy parents. The recipes were simple, and each was accompanied by color photographs of the final product and a brief commentary from the author. The Court concluded the two works were not substantially similar, and no reasonable observer would regard the aesthetic appeal of the two books as being the same. As a result, the copyright infringement claims were dismissed against Seinfeld and HarperCollins.

Trademark

Under the authority of Article 1, Section 8, Clause 3 of the U.S. Constitution, Congress enacted the Lanham Act in 1946 (amended in 1996). The Act provided federal protection for trademarks. Although many states afford common law protection of trademarks, the federal law serves as the predominant source of protection.

A trademark may be a word, name, symbol, device, slogan, or any combination thereof (15 U.S.C. § 1127) (45) that is used to identify the source or origin of a good or service and to distinguish it from others. This identification notifies the consumer about where a product or service comes from and protects consumers from confusion and deception about products that do not offer a consistent level of quality. A trademark is created when the mark is used in commerce; as with a copyright, it does not have to be registered before it may be used. Registration, however, provides certain benefits to the registrant at both the state and federal level. At the federal level, marks are registered with the U.S. Patent and Trademark Office (USPTO). If there is a conflict as to who owns a trademark, the first to use the mark has the superior rights to the mark (known as first use). Trademarks or service marks are identified by the following symbols: ᵗᵐ, ˢᵐ, or ® (46).

Trademark Infringement

A trademark infringement occurs when a person or entity uses in commerce a "reproduction, counterfeit, copy, or colorable imitation of a registered mark in connection with the sale, offering for sale, distribution, or advertising of any goods or services on or in connection with which such use is likely to cause confusion, or to cause mistake, or to deceive" without the consent or permission of the owner of the mark (15 U.S.C. § 1114) (45). The owner of the mark has the burden of proof to establish infringement. The key components of a trademark infringement claim are:

1. The plaintiff has a valid, protectable mark.
2. The plaintiff owns the trademark.
3. The defendant used the mark without the plaintiff's permission in a way that is likely to cause confusion among consumers regarding the source or origin of the good or service (15 U.S.C. § 1114(1)) (45).

Defense of Trademark Infringement

There are several defenses to a claim of trademark infringement. The first is fair use; this allows the use of another's trademark in connection with the sale of one's own goods or services as long as the use is not deceptive. The second defense is the word or symbol is generic and use of the word cannot be monopolized. The third defense is the owner of the mark abandoned or discontinued use of the mark and does not intend to resume using the mark within a reasonable amount of time. A fourth defense is there is no likelihood of confusion by consumers based on the services or products provided and/or the geographic location of the trademark owners. A fifth defense is known as functionality. Here, the defendant argues the mark being used by the plaintiff does not describe or distinguish the product or service but that it is necessary for the product to exist (15 U.S.C. § 1115(b)) (45). An example would be the wheels on a bicycle; a bicycle cannot properly function without wheels. Therefore, the wheels on a bicycle would not be eligible for trademark protection.

A Case Involving Trademark Infringement

In 1909, University of Arkansas coach Hugo Bezdeck described his football team as being as wild as Razorback hogs. Since that time, the University has identified itself with a trademark in the form of a RAZORBACK mark and a red hog design logo. In 1988, the University retained Collegiate Licensing Company (CLC) to oversee licensing and unauthorized usage of the RAZORBACK mark. The mark was officially registered in 1989. As of 1995, the mark had been registered by the University 25 times for purposes such as providing college courses and promoting sporting and musical events associated with the University. The RAZORBACK mark had been used for goods sold in the bookstore, the University credit card, and various other items. The University and the CLC also licensed the RAZORBACK mark to over 700 third-party vendors, for use in manufacturing, sale, and distribution of University of Arkansas memorabilia and souvenirs, which brought in over $400,000 from 1994 to 1995.

In 1989, Dean Weber, the former Director of Sports Medicine at the University of Arkansas, and Dave England, an athletic trainer at the University, became limited partners with a private business, the Physical Therapy Clinic, to help start a sports medicine clinic to provide specialized physical therapy for athletic injuries. In August 1991, the Clinic secured a fictitious name registration with the State of Arkansas to officially change their practice name to the Razorback Sports and Physical Therapy Clinic and chose a red hog for their logo. The Clinic used promotional materials to advertise their affiliation with the University, such as letters stating high school athletes deserved the same care as the Arkansas Razorbacks and promoting opportunities to attend Saturday Morning Sports Medicine clinics where a "Razorback Team Physician" would be available to speak to coaches, parents, and students. The University brought a suit against the Clinic, alleging trademark infringement and false designation under the Lanham Act. The University also claimed unfair competition, infringement, and trademark dilution. The Court found that the clinic's use of the logo and name infringed upon the University's rights under the Lanham Act and ruled in favor of the University (47).

Patent

Enacted in 1870 to promote science and invention, patent law establishes protection for those who invent or discover "any new and useful process, machine, manufacture, or composition of matter, or any new and useful improvement thereof" (35 U.S.C. § 101) (48). In order for a patent to be granted, the inventor must file an application with the USPTO. Registration provides the inventor with the exclusive rights to the invention for a specific period of time.

Requirements for Patents

As with copyrights and trademarks, a patent will not be granted for an idea. The patent must be a new machine, device, and so on, and the inventor must provide a complete description of the item to obtain registration.

The USPTO also requires the proposed patent be useful, novel, and nonobvious to a person having ordinary skill in the field related to the patent. *Useful* means the

invention has a useful purpose or that it was designed to operate for an intended purpose. *Novel* is defined as new. An invention normally cannot be patented if the invention was known to the public prior to the applicant filing the patent application or if the invention was described in a printed publication, in a published patent application, or in a patent issued prior to the applicant filing their patent application (35 U.S.C. § 102) (48). The *nonobvious* requirement is the most important; the invention must be suitably different from what has been previously used or described that it would not be obvious to a person possessing ordinary skill in the area or field related to the invention (35 U.S.C. § 103(a)) (48).

Types and Duration of Patents

There are three types of patents: utility, design, and plant. A utility patent is granted to anyone who invents any new and useful process, machine, or manufacture. A design patent covers inventions of any new and nonobvious ornate design for an object of manufacture. A plant patent is granted to anyone who invents or discovers and asexually reproduces any new and distinct variety of plant.

Once a patent is granted and depending on the type of patent, it will last for approximately 15–20 years from the date the application was filed with the USPTO (35 U.S.C. §§ 154, 161–163, 171–173) (48). The patent owner is also required to pay a maintenance fee to maintain the patent. Fees are due at 3.5, 7.5, and 11.5 years from the date the patent is granted. Failure to pay the maintenance fee may result in the expiration of the patent (49).

Patent Infringement

A patent infringement occurs when an individual or entity makes, uses, offers for sale, or sells any patented invention without the consent of the patent owner. There are several defenses to claims of patent infringement. The defendant can question the validity of the patent. If the court determines the patent owner does not have a valid patent, the case will be dismissed. The defendant accused of patent infringement can also argue their action do not constitute an infringement. Here, the courts will examine the language of the patent. If the defendant's actions are not within the language of the patent, there is no infringement.

A Case Involving Patent Law

An example of a patent dispute can be found in *IA Labs CA, LLC v. Nintendo Co., Ltd.* (50). On October 17, 2006, the USPTO issued the '982 patent to IA Labs CA, LLC.

The patent covered "an isometric exercise system that serves as a computer system peripheral and facilitates user interaction with a host computer system while the user performs isometric exercise" ('982 patent, col. 1 ll. 11-14). The patent explained that most isometric exercise devices only use isokinetic and/or isotonic exercise. Isometric exercise "involves the exertion of force by a user against an object that significantly resists movement as a result of the exerted force such that there is substantially minimal or no movement of the user's muscles during the force exertion" ('982 patent, col. 1 ll. 29-34). Isometric exercises can include "a person pushing against a stationary surface, attempting to pull apart tightly gripped hands, or attempting to bend or flex a rigid steel bar" ('982 patent, col. 1 ll. 34-37). Although these exercises are beneficial to fitness, training, and/or rehabilitation, they can be monotonous. Thus, isometric exercise devices are not as well-liked as isotonic and isokinetic exercise devices. Therefore, IA Labs CA, LLC created a device that could be used with a computer system. The device would allow users to perform the exercises in a virtual reality, thereby increasing the user's gratification in executing the exercises.

The device was based on two components. The first was a long, flexible, cylindrical bar with two sensors that are connected to the device's circuitry. Users could bend the bar in either direction. The force was measured by the device's circuitry. The second component was the cockpit, a supportive frame often used for computer games involving flying and driving simulations.

During the summer of 2007, Nintendo, the manufacturer of the Wii Console (a video game system designed to work with a user's movements and exercise), introduced the Wii Balance Board. The Balance Board resembled a household scale with four highly sensitive force sensors designed to measure the amount of force exerted by the user and any change in the user's center of gravity. This information was then sent wirelessly to the Wii Console, and the software inferred the user's motion by sensing changes in the user's center of gravity across the four load cells. The Balance Board was manufactured to be used with a collection of Nintendo games known as the Wii Fit and the Wii Fit Plus.

IA Labs CA challenged a Balance Board game called the Ski Jump. In this game, users simulated skiing down a ramp by crouching and, when reaching the edge of the virtual ramp, standing to execute a jump. The user was then awarded points for distance of the jump and the speed of the skier.

IA Labs CA claimed the Balance Board's peripheral, also known as the auxiliary device, directly infringed on their '982 patent and filed for a motion for summary judgment against Nintendo. IA Labs CA claimed the Balance Board was "an isometric exercise system according to the plain and ordinary meaning of the term because it does not significantly move in response to the application of force" (38, p. 454). They also claimed that the Balance Board required a user to engage in isometric exercise.

To determine infringement, the Court compares the accused device to the claims made by the patent holder. If the accused device encompasses every limitation of the patent holder's claim, either literally or substantially, the Court will find an infringement (51). The patentee must provide evidence that the accused device is an infringement.

In its decision, the Court ruled that IA Labs CA "failed to identify any allegedly isometric activity that can be performed in conjunction with the Balance Board that would satisfy the limitations of its '982 patent" (50, p. 455). Furthermore, each of the examples offered by IA Labs CA required the user to exert force against their own body and not against a Balance Board. As a result, the Court ruled in favor of Nintendo and dismissed the case.

Global Protection of Intellectual Property

For copyrights, trademarks, and patents, it is important to note that registration only protects against infringement within the U.S. or U.S. Territories. Protection against infringement by individuals or entities outside the U.S. may require additional registration procedures. For information regarding protecting intellectual property rights globally, rights holders should refer to the Berne Convention for the Protection of Literary Works, the Universal Copyright Convention, and the World Intellectual Property Organization. Additionally, for information on the requirements and protection provided by other countries, rights holders should seek advice from legal counsel familiar with foreign intellectual property laws.

MARKETING AND PROMOTIONS LAW

Individuals working in the field of clinical exercise physiology often will communicate to current or potential clients' information about their products and services or those provided by third parties. Many of these communications may be considered advertisements or marketing practices. As such, a CEP may encounter legal issues involving what information is communicated as well as how it is communicated.

All 50 states in the U.S. have adopted laws, either through common law or the enactment of a statute, to protect consumers from unfair, false, or deceptive practices. Under federal law, consumers and businesses are protected by the Federal Trade Commission (FTC). Founded in 1914, the FTC was established under the Federal Trade Commission Act (FTCA) to prevent false advertising and unfair competition (Act of Sept. 26, 1914, Ch. 111 § 5, 38 Stat. 719). Individual consumers cannot file lawsuits under the FTCA; instead, the consumer can file a complaint with the FTC, which then investigates allegations of unfair or deceptive practices.

Two sections of the FTCA are directly relevant to CEPs. One is a prohibition against false advertisements that are likely to influence consumer purchase behaviors. The second prohibits persons, companies, or organizations from engaging in unfair or deceptive acts in interstate commerce.

FTC Prohibitions Against False Advertising

According to the FTC, all advertising must be truthful, cannot be deceptive or unfair, and must be based on evidence (52). For an advertisement to be truthful, any claims made about the advantages, features, or benefits must be accurate. The FTC defines deceptive advertising as a representation, statement, or omission that is likely to mislead a reasonable consumer and is likely to influence the consumer's decision or conduct regarding the product or service (53).

For example, Soloflex, Inc. introduced its first exercise machine in 1978 (54). Since its inception, Soloflex has sold over 450,000 machines and earned revenues totaling over $426 million. A great deal of its profit is attributed to print, video, and television advertising. In 1991, a competitor to Soloflex called NordicTrack, Inc. launched an exercise machine called the NordicFlex Gold. NordicTrack implemented an advertising program that was similar to that of Soloflex. In its advertising, NordicTrack made untruthful comparisons with the Soloflex machine. One of the comparisons regarded pricing: NordicFlex stated that the price of the Soloflex machine without attachments was $1,500, whereas the price of a NordicFlex with attachments was only $999. Soloflex alleged that these assertions were false because the price of a Soloflex without attachments was $1,000. Soloflex, Inc. filed claims for false advertising alleging untrue statements of fact, which

deceived consumers and were likely to influence purchase decisions. NordicTrack acknowledged that the claims were false but argued that because the advertisements were no longer being aired, the claim was not an issue. Soloflex, however, presented evidence that at least one video and a brochure consistently used by NordicTrack were still being circulated. NordicTrack did not deny the allegations, and the Court issued an injunction prohibiting NordicTrack from using brochures, videos, and infomercials that falsely identified the price of a Soloflex without attachments as $1,500 (54).

The FTC also considers "puffery" when determining whether an advertisement is likely to mislead or deceive a consumer. Puffery is defined as "exaggerations reasonably to be expected of a seller as to the degree of quality of his product, the truth or falsity of which cannot be precisely determined" (55). Puffery is not considered deceptive under the FTC regulations. Embellishments such as "the best" and "the finest" are general statements that are not misleading claims or misrepresentations of fact. These types of claims are not actionable by the FTC (55). As a result, the FTC has acknowledged that not all advertisements are likely to deceive consumers who are acting reasonably (56).

In *Stokely-Van Camp, Inc. v. The Coca-Cola Company* (57), the Gatorade Thirst Quencher sports drink manufacturer Stokely-Van Camp, Inc. (Stokely) filed motion for a preliminary injunction against The Coca-Cola and Energy Brands Inc. (Coca-Cola) alleging that the company was making false and misleading claims in its advertising for Powerade ION4, a competing product introduced in March 2009. In its advertising campaign, Coca-Cola asserted that Powerade ION4 was more like human sweat than Stokely's Gatorade Thirst Quencher. These product claims were attributed to Powerade ION4's ingredients, which included small quantities of calcium and magnesium; both are lost in sweat during physical activity. Print advertisements depicted a half bottle of Gatorade with the caption "Don't settle for an incomplete sports drink" and "Introducing the Complete sports drink Powerade ION4" (57, p. 521). Coca-Cola also purchased a series of billboards using the same advertising messages and the tagline "Upgrade your formula. Upgrade your game" (57, p. 522). On March 24, 2009, Stokely sent a letter to Coca-Cola requesting they cease all false advertising for Powerade ION4, but received no response. On April 13, 2009, Stokely filed an action against Coca-Cola for false advertising, deceptive acts and practices, injury to business reputation, and unfair competition. The Court ruled in favor of Coca-Cola citing that the ads comparing

Powerade ION4 to Gatorade were discontinued in May 2009. It also ruled that the tagline "Upgrade your formula. Upgrade your game." was puffery, and no reasonable consumer reading the slogan would believe that drinking the sport beverage would provide them with increased athletic abilities (57, p. 529). Furthermore, during the lawsuit, evidence was presented that Stokely had also marketed the advantage of adding calcium and magnesium to its own Gatorade Endurance Formula. The Court stated that Stokely could not be granted a preliminary injunction for behavior the company had also practiced.

FTC Standards of Fairness

The FTC employs three standards to determine whether a specific business practice is unfair. The first is whether the practice injures a consumer. The injury must be substantial, could not have reasonably been avoided by the consumer, and is not outweighed by any countervailing benefits to the consumer or competition.

Second, the practice must violate a public policy that is clear and well established. However, the FTC recognizes some policies may support action by the FTC, whereas others may permit a practice the FTC may view as unfair. For example, the First Amendment of the U.S. Constitution protects consumers' rights to receive information, but the First Amendment also protects a company's commercial speech or speech proposing an economic transaction such as an advertisement. Therefore, when determining whether a practice is unfair, the FTC must consider the interests of the advertiser as well as the consumer.

Third, the practice must be unethical or unscrupulous. The FTC typically looks to the industry's recognized standards to determine if business's practices are unethical (58). Such practices may include withholding information that would be important to the consumer decision-making process, undue influence over a special class of consumer (*e.g.*, children, elderly), and unsubstantiated advertising claims. No company can make a claim about a product without having a reasonable basis for that claim. The FTC considers the following factors when assessing whether there is a reasonable basis for an advertiser's claims:

1. Type and specificity of the claim (*e.g.*, safety, efficacy, dietary, health, medical)
2. Type of product (*e.g.*, food, drug, potentially hazardous consumer product, other consumer product)
3. Possible consequences of a false claim (*e.g.*, personal injury, property damage)
4. Degree of reliance by consumers on the claims
5. Type and accessibility of evidence adequate to form a reasonable basis for making the particular claims (more specifically, there may be some types of claims for some types of products for which the only reasonable basis, in fairness and in the expectations of consumers, would be a valid scientific or medical basis) (59, p. 64)

Cautions on Endorsements

The same burdens are placed on endorsers for products or services. An endorsement is an advertising message a consumer is likely to believe reflects the opinions and experiences of an individual, group, or organization other than the advertiser (16 C.F.R. § 255(b)) (60). Before communicating information obtained from the advertiser, the endorser must substantiate the claims with at least one reliable independent source (61). Also, any endorsement of a product or service must be the honest opinions and beliefs of the endorser. Furthermore, if the endorser is engaged to promote a product or service and their opinion changes regarding the product or service, all advertisements using the endorser must no longer be used by the advertiser (16 C.F.R. § 255.1(b)) (60).

As a result, CEPs should be cautious about recommending products or services to clients. Before doing so, CEPs should research the product, service, business, and its principals and management. CEPs should also stay informed about food, drug, and medical device safety classifications, approvals, and recalls by the FDA, the federal agency responsible for regulating foods, drugs, and medical devices (21 C.F.R. § 3.1) (62). Failure to ascertain whether a product is approved (or recalled) by the FDA may have serious legal consequences for the CEP (21 C.F.R. § 7.12) (63).

Furthermore, if a benefit, either monetarily or through the receipt of free products or services, is received as a result of recommending a product or service to consumers, this arrangement must be disclosed to consumers. Failure to do so could result in potential FTCA violations. Even if a formal agreement does not exist, a CEP recommending a product or service could be held liable for any claims or representations they made about the product. For example, if a CEP promises a particular outcome from using a product or service, they may be legally considered as guaranteeing good results from treatment and may be subject to the rules and regulations of the FTC. Again, it is in the CEP's best interest to thoroughly evaluate any product, service, or business before recommending it to clients or consumers. For additional information about the FTC and the FDA, please visit http://www.ftc.gov or http://www.fda.gov.

PROTECTION VIA INSURANCE

As discussed, this chapter's overview of the types of legal issues associated with clinical exercise physiology was provided to train CEPs to be proactive rather than reactive to legal situations. Although improving legal knowledge will minimize the risks associated with practice, it will not eradicate all legal issues. Even the most careful CEP may be exposed to legal incidences. The goal, then, is to shift the burden of financial loss resulting from risks. This can be accomplished through the development and implementation of a comprehensive emergency action plan (EAP) and a risk management plan (RMP). ACSM publishes standards and guidelines (64) that address safety practices to aid CEPs with compliance. In addition, one of the most common strategies to shift the impact of financial loss is the procurement of insurance. Therefore, it is important to understand the types of insurance as well as the type of protection offered by each.

Types of Insurance

Several types of insurance can be obtained to meet personal or business needs. These include the following:

1. General liability insurance is for property losses or bodily injury to a third party.
2. Professional liability insurance (also known as errors and omissions insurance) covers the negligent acts, mistakes, or failures to do something by those who have professional knowledge or training.
3. Property insurance pertains to buildings, structures, or the contents thereof when certain natural disasters, theft, or vandalism occur. Typically, natural disasters such as floods or earthquakes are excluded from property insurance coverage.
4. Product liability insurance applies to injuries that result from the sale or use of products.
5. Employment practices liability insurance covers injury to employees caused by wrongful termination, sexual harassment, defamation, breach of the employment contract, and various types of employment discrimination.
6. Workers' compensation insurance is for injuries to employees while performing their duties at the workplace.
7. An umbrella policy is additional insurance designed to cover anything that exceeds the limits of any other previously mentioned policy.

When searching for liability insurance, it is important to understand what is covered under the policy as well as what is not covered. The title of the policy may state that all risks are covered, but the CEP will need to read all of the provisions as well as the exclusions section of the policy. The CEP should procure coverage that will cover damages as well as the cost of the legal defense. Depending on the type of legal claim and the amount of time the attorney will need to commit to the case, legal fees can range from thousands of dollars to even millions of dollars.

Some property insurance policies pay the actual cash value for the destroyed property, whereas others only cover replacement cost. If the policy says the insured will receive the actual cash value, this means the insured will receive the replacement value of the property minus 3 years of depreciation. Unfortunately, the proceeds from this insurance typically are not enough to buy new equipment. In contrast, a policy that pays replacement value will provide for the initial cost of the item or the current value of the exact item, if still available.

SUMMARY

This chapter has emphasized key legislation relevant to CEPs and examples of situations in which individuals and businesses have been involved in various types of litigation. Most lawsuits, however, are never deliberated and/or decided by a judge or jury. They are either settled out of court or resolved through alternative dispute resolution measures such as arbitration (a neutral individual listens to the disputants and then makes a decision or award) or mediation (a neutral individual assists the parties in reaching an agreement). Nevertheless, CEPs should take all available actions to protect themselves and their business. These include the following recommendations.

CEPs must abide by the procedures and guidelines in place at their place of employment. This encompasses possessing the requisite knowledge and skills to work with particular clients. CEPs should avoid practicing outside their scope of practice/training and be familiar with the appropriate standard of care for their field of expertise. They are also responsible for documenting any suggestions for treatment with a patient or client and informing the patient of any potential risks associated with a treatment or performing any physical activity. Prior to working with any patient or client, signatures for all paperwork (*e.g.,* informed consent and waivers) should be obtained and maintained electronically or securely stored in a file cabinet in a locked office. In addition, CEPs should be vigilant in maintaining the appropriate licenses and certifications as well as educating themselves about new developments or advances in the field. Courts have held practitioners liable for using outdated treatment methods that their field has established as no longer constituting acceptable or appropriate care.

Ultimately, CEPs should be cognizant of the wide range of legal issues that might arise during their career. Whether treating patients, cleaning and maintaining equipment, formalizing partnerships with a contract, accepting employment or hiring others, or advertising products and services, the safest course of action is to anticipate possible risks and take action to minimize those risks. CEPs can avoid a majority of legal issues by conducting themselves according to the best practices of the profession, and if faced with a lawsuit, seeking the advice of competent legal counsel.

Additional Legal Resources
- http://www.findlaw.com
- http://www.copyright.gov
- http://www.nolo.com
- http://www.uspto.gov
- http://www.wipo.int
- http://acsm.org/

CHAPTER REVIEW QUESTIONS

1. Explain the difference between the penalties for a civil battery and a criminal battery.
2. What are the five parts of a contract?
3. Explain the two ways a contract can be breached.
4. What standard of care is required of a CEP when practicing in the profession?
5. What is the difference between an exempt and non-exempt employee?
6. What constitutional rights are guaranteed under the First Amendment?
7. What is the difference between Title IX of the Civil Rights Act of 1964 and Title IX of the Education Amendments Act of 1972?
8. Define copyright infringement and the three types of copyright infringement. What is the most common defense against a copyright infringement claim?
9. According to the FTC, what are the three standards to determine whether a specific business practice is unfair?
10. Identify and explain at least three types of insurance that could shift or reduce financial loss resulting from a lawsuit.

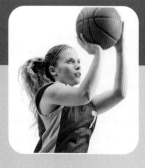

Case Study 19.1

The University of Hoffer (Wildcats) Women's basketball team (D-I) traveled to compete against the Tauern University (Eagles). The Wildcats normally travel with their Athletic Trainer (AT), Strength and Conditioning Coach (S&C), and their Sports Information Director (SID). However, for this trip, the S&C was unable to travel.

Unfortunately, the Wildcats were not playing well, and the Head Coach (HC) berated the athletes using derogatory terms throughout the game. The HC's comments to his players could be heard by the fans and the parents of the players. Ultimately, the Wildcats lost the game, and the HC was visibly upset.

After the game, instead of leading the players to the locker room for a post-game talk and shower, the HC led the players to the Eagles football field. The weather for that day indicated a heat index of 102°F, a temperature that was considered too extreme for outdoor sports. The HC then proceeded to make the players run the bleachers for losing (*i.e.*, conditioning) and added bear walks (which were not used in regular training) between the runs.

Throughout this session, many of the athletes complained and asked for water breaks. Grace, a freshman, fell while running and told the HC and AT she felt lightheaded and nauseous. The HC told Grace to keep running. The AT did nothing to stop the workout, cleared Grace to continue, and watched while the HC forced the players to complete the exercises. About 30 minutes later, the HC allowed the players to take a water break.

During the break, the HC called the S&C to ask for additional workouts to punish the players. The S&C informed the HC this coaching behavior was unacceptable and was not safe for the players. The HC threatened the S&C with obscene language and told the S&C if they were not comfortable with how the team was run, they should look for another job. Distraught after the phone conversation and fearful of losing their job, the S&C called the Associate AD

for Women's basketball to relay the situation. The Associate AD only listened to the S&C's account of what happened but did not report the situation to the AD or Compliance.

Meanwhile, the HC proceeded to direct the players to run the bleachers again. Upon reaching the top of the stairs, Sheila, who previously complained about being lightheaded, passed out. The paramedics were called, and she was rushed to the hospital. Sheila never regained consciousness and died later that evening. The medical examiner's report stated Sheila died from heat stroke.

Upon returning to campus, the other athletes started to experience pain in their hips and backs. They provided this information to the AT, who told them to deal with the pain. However, several weeks after the workout, the athletes still were experiencing pain. Some of the players could not go to class or function doing daily life activities. The athletes, again, expressed their concerns to the HC and AT. They were told to either ignore the pain or lose their financial support/scholarships.

Tracy, a senior, decided to seek medical advice outside of the AT. She was diagnosed with a stress fracture. The doctor recommended she seek physical therapy. When Tracy informed the AT of her diagnosis, the AT told her if she didn't think they could do their job, the athlete could leave the team. Because Tracy was predicted to be a first-round draft pick for the Women's National Basketball Association (WNBA) and needed the exposure, she followed the AT's advice and continued to play. At the end of the season, Tracy was diagnosed with an avascular necrosis. She now needs surgery, which will take her up to 12 months to recover and will have to forgo the WNBA draft.

Concerned about the welfare of the players, the S&C again contacted the Associate AD; during this conversation, the S&C indicated they wanted to file a complaint against the HC and AT. One week later, the S&C received a termination letter stating because the team had lost over 80% of their games in the past 2 years, the S&C's services were no longer needed. The Men's basketball team had an even worst record; however, their S&C was not terminated.

Case Study 19.1 Questions

1. Briefly evaluate the Sheila's parent's claims for negligence against the HC for their daughter's death.
2. Discuss the S&C's claim against the HC for assault under tort law and criminal law.
3. Assess the S&C's employment discrimination claims against the University and the Athletic Department for termination.
4. Discuss the recourse, if any, Tracy may have against the University and the AT for the injury preventing her from entering the draft.

Case Study 19.2

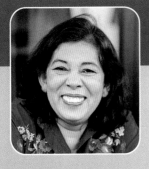

Gwen has owned the It Factor Total Body Center (TBC) for 8 years in Miami, Florida. The It Factor specializes in athletic training services for college athletes who would like additional training to further their athletics abilities. Gwen has one full-time and four part-time staff members.

It Factor TBC initially focused on athletic training services for softball, baseball, basketball, and soccer. Gwen then decided to expand the business to include tennis. Upon the recommendation of a friend, Gwen hired Theo, a former professional tennis player, to generate new business and train the tennis athletes who frequented It Factor TBC. After Theo had been at It Factor TBC for about 2 months, Gwen received a complaint from a staff member that Theo had made several unwelcome sexual comments regarding her work attire. Unsure of how to approach the subject with Theo, Gwen disregarded the complaint.

One evening Paul, an Olympic tennis hopeful, and his father Harry arrived at the facility for an appointment with Theo. Theo, however, had been called away for a family emergency, and had failed to reschedule the appointment. Harry was furious; he and Paul had traveled over 2 hours to train with Theo, and he demanded that someone at It Factor TBC compensate them for their time. While Gwen was discussing an agreeable solution with Harry, Paul decided to use the Center's Round Robin Elite Three Tennis Ball Machine to practice his backhand tennis stroke. The machine is capable of dispensing tennis balls at speeds of up to 80 miles an hour. Unknown to Gwen, Theo had earlier experienced problems with the machine randomly expelling balls in the off position. In his haste to leave the Center to address the family emergency, Theo asked Kate, a part-time staff member, to place a note on the machine

that it was not working. Kate forgot to place a note on the machine. As Paul was approaching the machine, a tennis ball exited the machine and hit him in his left eye. The paramedics were called, and it was later determined that Paul had an orbital blowout fracture, or a break in the facial bone around the eye. Paul and his father Harry are now suing Gwen and It Factor TBC for damages.

Because of Paul's status as an Olympic hopeful, the lawsuit received a great deal of publicity. After interviewing one of the responding paramedics, one news station reported that Paul had experienced a career-ending injury as a result of the negligence of It Factor TBC. Paul's doctor had determined, however, that with surgery and proper medical treatment Paul should be able to resume his career. It Factor TBC lost several clients as a result of the news report. Moreover, the report was picked up by a station in Topeka, Kansas, and was viewed by Ace, the owner of It Factor Athletic Training outside of Topeka. After watching the report, Ace filed a trademark infringement lawsuit claiming that he owned the right to the name "It Factor."

The stress of dealing with the lawsuits greatly affected Gwen, and she stayed away from work at It Factor TBC for over a month. Her full-time staff member, who had been with Gwen since she opened, began working extra hours to service Gwen's remaining athletic training clients. He contacted Gwen about receiving overtime pay but had no response. Gwen also missed last month's payment on her business loan, and the bank threatened to place a legal claim, or lien, on her business. While Gwen was running an errand, a reporter approached her for a comment about the incident. Gwen kindly asked the reporter to leave her alone, but the reporter jumped in front of her and shoved a microphone in Gwen's face. Furious, Gwen pushed the reporter, who dropped and damaged her recording device. The reporter yelled at Gwen that she intended to file a lawsuit.

Case Study 19.2 Questions

1. Identify at least three possible defenses that It Factor TBC could raise regarding Paul's injury.
2. Briefly discuss the steps Gwen should have taken to address the reported harassment issue with Theo and the staff member.
3. Discuss Gwen's options for arguing that the missed loan payment is an immaterial breach.
4. Evaluate the full-time staff member's employment claims for overtime pay.
5. Discuss the recourse, if any, Gwen may have against the news station that described Paul's injury as career-ending.
6. Assess Ace's claims for trademark infringement against It Factor TBC and Gwen.

Case Study 19.3

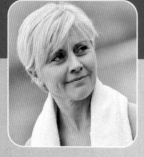

Stacey was a 49-year-old woman who joined Strong Fitness Gym (SFG) and signed up for three, 1-hour sessions with a personal trainer. SFG provides open floor space for working out with machines or free weights and also allows for classes and personal training sessions for clients. The day Stacey signed up for membership to the gym and for the sessions, the front desk attendant provided her with a contract for payment that Stacey saw had a liability waiver stapled to it. While the front desk attendant was assisting other customers, Stacey swiped her credit card for payment and quickly signed the waiver on the desk. The attendant then assigned her a personal trainer and told her to look around the facility to get comfortable with being inside of a gym.

According to Stacey, she had never visited a health facility or gym before in her life. She had also never used exercise equipment, including stationary machines such as a treadmill. Prior to her sessions, she and the personal trainer (Barry) sat down and went over her lifestyle and goals. Stacey told Barry she had led a pretty sedentary life and was unfamiliar with many exercises and machines because she had never been to a gym before. On her first day of personal training session with Barry, who had been with the gym for over 3 years as a personal trainer, she was told she would be doing a warm-up before moving onto weights and resistance exercises. Barry set her to walk on a treadmill at 3.5 miles per hours for 20 minutes, and then left Stacey alone to walk. Stacey claims Barry then proceeded to leave her alone during the warm-up without any instructions on how to adjust the treadmill's speed, how to stop the belt, or how to operate the control panel. She struggled to keep up with the speed of the treadmill and ended up drifting toward the back of the moving belt. Stacey attempted to speed up her walking pace but was thrown off the machine and injured her ankle in the process. Barry came back to check on her and ended up calling for help, as Stacey could not put any pressure on her right ankle. She was taken to the hospital where the doctor let her know her ankle was broken, and she would be unable to put weight on that leg for 6–10 weeks.

Following the injury, Stacey filed a lawsuit against SFG for negligence so that she could recover damages for the injury she sustained. Her claims included that (a) Barry did not properly instruct her on how to use a treadmill and the control panel, (b) he failed to supervise her while she was using the machine, and (c) she was never fully informed of the risks of the activity when signing her waiver. SFG claimed their responsibility to Stacey was to ensure that facility conditions were safe and that she signed a liability waiver and voluntarily participated in the training sessions. Thus, with her voluntary participation, she assumed the inherent risk of the sporting activity.

Case Study 19.3 Questions

1. Discuss what steps should have been taken throughout this case study to protect SFG and Barry from negligence claims?

2. According to SFG, Stacey signed a liability waiver that should protect them from her negligence claim. Why might this waiver not be effective in this case?

3. Describe the elements of negligence and what Stacey must prove to demonstrate SFG and Barry were negligent?

4. Why would an assumption of risk defense potentially fail in this instance?

REFERENCES

1. Dobbs DB, Keeton RE, Keeton WP, Owen DG. *Prosser and Keeton on the Law of Torts*. 5th ed. St. Paul (MN): West Publishing Company; 1984.
2. Ross v. Consumer Power Company, 420 Mich. 567 (1984).
3. Sullivan v. Montgomery, 279 N.Y.S. 575 (1935).
4. Gallup EM. *Law and the Team Physician*. Champaign (IL): Human Kinetics Publishers; 1995.
5. Howard v. Missouri Bone and Joint Center, 615 F.3d 991 (8th Cir. 2010).
6. Zimbauer v. Milwaukee Orthopaedic Group, Ltd., 920 F. Supp. 959 (E.D. Wis. 1996).
7. Herren v. Sucher, et al., 325 Ga. App. 219 (2013).
8. Chuy v. Philadelphia Eagles Football Club, 595 F.2d 1265 (3d Cir. 1979).
9. Bloom v. ProMaxima Manufacturing Company v. M-F Athletic Company, Inc. (2010).
10. Kane v. Platinum Healthcare, LLC, 2011 WL 248494 (E.D. Pa. Jan. 25, 2011).
11. Gitlow v. New York, 268 U.S. 652 (1925).
12. Bishop v. Aronov, 926 F.2d 1066 (11th Cir. 1991).
13. Rehabilitation Act of 1973, 29 U.S.C. §§ 701–797 (2015).
14. Americans with Disabilities Act, 42 U.S.C. §§ 12101–12213 (2009).
15. Mitten MJ. Enhanced risk of harm to one's self as a justification for exclusion from athletics. *Marq Sports Law J*. 1997;8:189.
16. Class v. Towson University, 806 F.3d 236 (4th Cir. 2015).
17. Knapp v. Northwestern University, 101 F.3d 473 (7th Cir. 1996).
18. Watson v. Hughston Sports Medicine Hospital, 231 F.Supp. 2d 1344 (M.D. Ga. 2002).
19. United States of America v. Tracy Richardson Brown, 2016 WL 3634127 (E.D. La. July 7, 2016).
20. Fair Labor Standards Act of 1938, 29 U.S.C. § 202–262 (2011).
21. U.S. Department of Labor [Internet]. *Handy Reference Guide to the Fair Labor Standards Act*. Washington (DC): DOL; 2014 [updated November 2014; cited 2016 July 25]. Available from: https://www.dol.gov/whd/regs/compliance/hrg.htm.
22. U.S. Department of Labor [Internet]. *Wage and Hour Division*. Washington (DC): DOL; 2019 [cited 2022 May 25]. Wage and Hour Division. Available from: https://www.dol.gov/agencies/whd/fact-sheets/17g-overtime-salary.
23. U.S. Department of Labor [Internet]. *FLSA Coverage*. Washington (DC): DOL; 2011 [cited 2016 August 2]. FLSA cover-age. Available from: https://www.dol.gov/whd/regs/statutes/FairLaborStandAct.pdf.
24. Fair Labor Standards Act of 1938, 29 U.S.C. § 216(b) (2011).
25. Owsley v. San Antonio Independent School Dist., 187 F.3d 521 (5th Cir. 1999).
26. Dillow v. Wellmont Health System, 2005 WL 3115424 (E.D. Tenn. Nov. 11, 2005).
27. Age Discrimination in Employment Act of 1967, 29 U.S.C. § 621–634 (2015).
28. Family Medical Leave Act of 1993, 29 U.S.C.A. § 2611 (14–15) (2015).
29. Carpo v. Wartburg Lutheran Home for the Aging, 2006 WL 2946315 (E.D.N.Y. 2006).
30. Equal Employment Opportunity Commission [Internet]. *About EEOC*. Washington (DC): EEOC; 2016 [cited 2016 July 17]. Available from: https://www.eeoc.gov/eeoc/.
31. Reznick v. Orthopedics & Sports Medicine, P.A., 104 Fed. Appx. 387 (5th Cir. 2004).
32. Occupational Safety and Health Administration Act of 1970, 29 C.F.R. § 1910.2(c) (2004).
33. U.S. Department of Labor [Internet]. *Occupational Safety and Health Administration*. Washington (DC): OSHA; 2016 [cited 2016 July 17]. Available from: https://www.osha.gov/laws-regs/regulations/standardnumber/1910.
34. Occupational Safety and Health Administration Act of 1970, 29 C.F.R. § 1977 (2004).
35. Midwest New Media, LLC. General Information about Workers' Compensation [Internet]. Workplace Fairness. 2016 [cited 2016 August 18]. Available from: https://www.workplacefairness.org/workers-compensation-general#1.
36. Federal Employees' Compensation Act, 5 U.S.C. § 8101 (1993).
37. DelPo A. Are You Eligible for Workers' Compensation Benefits? [Internet]. Nolo.com. 2016 [cited 2016 August 18]. Available from: http://www.nolo.com/legal-encyclopedia/are-you-eligible-workers-compensation-32963.html.
38. World Intellectual Property Organization [Internet]. *What Is Intellectual Property*. Geneva (Switzerland): WIPO; 2016 [cited 2016 July 17]. Available from: http://www.wipo.int/edocs/pubdocs/en/intproperty/450/wipo_pub_450.pdf.

39. U.S. Copyright Act of 1976, 17 U.S.C. §§ 102–1332 (2012).

40. Hollaar L [Internet]. Legal Protection of Digital Information; 2002. Available from: http://digital-law-online.info/lpdi1.0/treatise14.html.

41. SiriusXM Music for Business [Internet]. SiriusXM Music for Business; 2017 [cited 2017 July 9]. Available from: https://www.siriusxm.com/siriusxmforbusiness.

42. LaPine v. Seinfeld, 2009 WL 2902584 (S.D.N.Y. September 10, 2009).

43. Hamil America Inc. v. GIF, 193 F.3d 92 (2d Cir. 1999).

44. Boisson v. Banian, Ltd, 273 F.3d 262, 268 (2d Cir. 2001).

45. Lanham Act of 1946, 15 U.S.C. § 1127 (1996).

46. United States Patent and Trademark Office [Internet]. *Trademark Basics.* Virginia: USPTO; 2016 [cited 2016 July 29]. Available from: http://www.uspto.gov/patents-getting-started/general-information-concerning-patents#heading-25.

47. Board of Trustees of University of Arkansas v. Professional Therapy Services, 873 F.Supp. 1280 (W.D. Ark. 1995).

48. Patents, 35 U.S.C. §§ 101–390 (2017).

49. United States Patent and Trademark Office [Internet]. *Maintenance Fees.* Virginia: USPTO; 2014 October [cited 2016 July 29]. Available from: http://www.uspto.gov/trademarks-getting-started/trademark-basics

50. IA Labs CA, LLC v. Nintendo Co., Ltd., 863 F.Supp. 2d 430 (D.Md. 2012).

51. Nazomi Commc'ns, Inc. v. Arm Holdings, PLC, 403 F.3d 1364 (Fed. Cir. 2005).

52. Federal Trade Commission [Internet]. Advertising and Marketing Basics. Washington (DC): FTC; 2016 [cited 2016 July 15]. Available from: https://www.ftc.gov/tips-advice/business-center/advertising-and-marketing/advertising-and-marketing-basics.

53. Federal Trade Commission [Internet]. *FTC Policy Statement on Deception.* Washington (DC): FTC; 1983 October 14 [cited 2016 July 23]. Available from: http://www.ftc.gov/public-statements/1983/10/ftc-policy-statement-deception.

54. Soloflex, Inc. v. NordicTrack, Inc., 1994 WL 568401 (D. Or. Feb. 11, 1994).

55. Better Living, Inc. et al., 54 F.T.C. 648 (1957), aff'd, 259 F.2d 271 (3rd Cir. 1958).

56. Warner-Lambert, 86 F.T.C. 1398 (1975), aff'd, 562 F.2d 749 (D.C. Cir. 1977).

57. Stokely-Van Camp, Inc. v. The Coca-Cola Company, 646 F. Supp. 2d 510 (S.D.N.Y. 2009).

58. Federal Trade Commission [Internet]. *FTC Statement on Unfairness.* Washington (DC): FTC; 1980 December 17 [cited 2016 July 11]. Available from: https://www.ftc.gov/public-statements/1980/12/ftc-policy-statement-unfairness.

59. In re Pfizer, 81 F.T.C. 23 (1972).

60. FTC Guides Concerning the Use of Endorsements and Testimonials in Advertising, 16 C.F.R. § 255 (2009).

61. In re Leroy Gordon Cooper, Jr., 94 F.T.C 674 (1979).

62. Food and Drug Administration, Product Jurisdiction, 21 C.F.R. § 3.1 (2015).

63. Food and Drug Administration, Enforcement Policy, 21 C.F.R. § 7.12 (2015).

64. American College of Sports Medicine. *Guidelines for Exercise Testing and Prescription.* Baltimore (MD): Wolters Kluwer Health; 2017.

AAA	abdominal aortic aneurysm	APCs	antigen-presenting cells
AACVPR	American Association of Cardiovascular and Pulmonary Rehabilitation	APD	atrial premature depolarization
AAIDD	American Association on Intellectual and Developmental Disabilities	APOA1	apolipoprotein AI
		APOB	apolipoprotein B
ABGs	arterial blood gases	APPs	advanced practice professionals (physician assistants, nurse practitioners)
ABI	ankle/brachial systolic pressure index	APTA	American Physical Therapy Association
ACC	American College of Cardiology	APTT	activated partial thromboplastin time
ACE	angiotensin-converting enzyme	ARA	aldosterone receptor agonist
ACE-Is	angiotensin-converting enzyme inhibitors	ARB	angiotensin II receptor blocker
ACErg	arm cycling ergometer	ART	antiretroviral therapy
ACL	anterior cruciate ligament	AS	ankylosing spondylitis
ACLS	advanced cardiac life support	ASA	aspirin (acetylsalicylic acid)
ACP	American College of Physicians	AT	activity tracker
ACS	acute coronary syndrome	ATP	adenosine triphosphate
ACs	anticholinergics	ATS	American Thoracic Society
ACSM	American College of Sports Medicine	AV	atrioventricular
ACSM-CEP	American College of Sports Medicine certified Clinical Exercise Physiologist	AVNRT	atrioventricular nodal reentrant tachycardia
		BBB	bundle branch block
ACSM-EP	American College of Sports Medicine certified Exercise Physiologist	bid	twice daily
		BKA	below-the-knee amputation
ACSM-PS	ACSM Position Stand	BLS	basic life support
ACTH	adrenocorticotropic hormone	BMD	bone mineral density
ACTN3	actinin three	BMI	body mass index
ADA	American Diabetes Association	BMP	basic metabolic panel
ADHD	attention–deficit/hyperactivity disorder	BNP	brain natriuretic peptide
ADL	activities of daily living	BO	bronchiolitis obliterans
ADT	androgen deprivation therapy	BODE	body mass index, airflow obstruction, dyspnea, and exercise capacity index
AED	automated external defibrillator		
AGE	advanced glycosylated end products	BP	blood pressure
AGIs	α-glucosidase inhibitors	BPH	benign prostatic hyperplasia
AHA	American Heart Association	bpm	beats per minute
AIVR	accelerated idioventricular rhythm	BRM	biologic response modifier
ALS	amyotrophic lateral sclerosis	BTT	bridge-to-transplant
AMA	American Medical Association	Ca^{2+}	calcium
AMI	acute myocardial infarction	CAAHEP	Commission on Accreditation of Allied Health Education Programs
AML	acute myeloid leukemia		
AMP	adenosine monophosphate	CABG	coronary artery bypass graft
AMS	acute mountain sickness	CAD	coronary artery disease
APB	atrial premature beat	cAMP-PKA	cyclic adenosine monophosphate-protein kinase A
APC	atrial premature contraction		

CAMs	cell adhesion molecules	CRISPR	clustered regularly interspaced short palindromic repeats
CAV	cardiac allograft vasculopathy		
CBC	complete blood count	CRP	C-reactive protein
CBT	cognitive behavioral therapy	CRT	cardiac resynchronization therapy
CCB	calcium channel blocker	CSA	cross-sectional area
CCI	Charlson Comorbidity Index	CSEP	Canadian Society for Exercise Physiology
CCRP	AACVPR's Certified Cardiac Rehabilitation Professional	CSII	continuous subcutaneous insulin infusion
CD	clusters of differentiation	CT	computed tomography
CDC	U.S. Centers for Disease Control and Prevention	CVA	cerebrovascular accident
		CVD	cardiovascular disease
CDI	Children's Depression Inventory	Cx	circumflex artery
CEP	clinical exercise physiologist	CYP3A4	Cytochrome P450 Family 3 Subfamily A Member 4
CEPA	Clinical Exercise Physiology Association		
CES-D	Center for Epidemiological Studies Depression Scale	CysLT	cysteinyl leukotriene
		dB	decibel
CET	ACSM/ACS Certified Cancer Exercise Trainer	DCCT	Diabetes Control and Complication Trial
		DLCO	diffusing capacity or transfer factor of the lung for carbon monoxide
CFTR	cystic fibrosis transmembrane conductance regulator (gene)		
		DM	diabetes mellitus
CHD	coronary heart disease	DMARDs	disease-modifying antirheumatic drugs
CHF	congestive heart failure	DNA	deoxyribonucleic acid
CHOL	cholesterol	DPP	Diabetes Prevention Program
CIFT	ACSM/NCHPAD Certified Inclusive Fitness Trainer	DPP-4	dipeptidylpeptidase-4
		DRAs	dopamine receptor agonists
CIPN	chemotherapy-induced peripheral neuropathy	DRE	digital rectal examination
		DRI	direct renin inhibitor
CIS	clinically isolated syndrome	DS	Down syndrome
CK	creatine kinase	DSM-5	*Diagnostic and Statistical Manual of Mental Disorders–5th edition*
CKD	chronic kidney disease		
CKMB	creatine kinase myocardial isozyme	DT	destination therapy
CLAD	chronic lung allograft dysfunction	DTC	direct-to-consumer
CLL	chronic lymphocytic leukemia	DVT	deep venous thrombosis
CMS	Centers for Medicare and Medicaid Services	DXA	dual x-ray absorptiometry
		ECG	electrocardiogram
CMV	cytomegalovirus	ECHO	echocardiogram
CNS	central nervous system	ECT	electroconvulsive therapy
CO	carbon monoxide	EELV	end-expiratory lung volume
CoAES	Committee on Accreditation for the Exercise Sciences	EF	ejection fraction
		EHN	exertional hyponatremia
COMT	catechol-*O*-methyltransferase	EIA	exercise-induced asthma
COPD	chronic obstructive pulmonary disease	EIB	exercise-induced bronchoconstriction
COX	cyclooxygenase	EILV	end-inspiratory lung volume
CP	cerebral palsy	EIM	Exercise is Medicine
CPET	cardiopulmonary exercise test	EM	extensive metabolizers
CPR	cardiopulmonary resuscitation	EMD	electromechanical dissociation
CPX	cardiopulmonary exercise	EMG	electromyography
CR	cardiovascular rehabilitation	EMPA-REG	Empagliflozin, Cardiovascular Outcomes, and Mortality in Type 2 Diabetes Study
CREP	Coalition for the Registration for Exercise Professionals		
		ENRICHD	Enhancing Recovery in Coronary Heart Disease Trial
CRF	cardiorespiratory fitness	Epi	epinephrine

EPO	erythropoietin
EPOC	excess postexercise oxygen consumption
ER	external rotation
ERS	European Respiratory Society
ERV	expiratory reserve volume
ES	electrical stimulation
ESHF	end-stage heart failure
ESRD	end-stage renal disease
ESSA	Exercise and Sports Science Australia
ESWT	endurance shuttle-walk test
FAs	fatty acids
FDA	Food and Drug Administration
FDPS	Finnish Diabetes Prevention Study
FEF_{25-75}	forced expiratory flow between 25% and 75% of forced volume vital capacity
FENO	fractional concentration of exhaled nitric oxide
FES	functional electrostimulation
FEV_1	forced expiratory volume in 1 second
FEV_1/FVC	the proportion of vital capacity expired in the first second of forced expiration; also known as the Tiffeneau–Pinelli index
FHP	forward head posture
FIRSs	Forum of International Respiratory Societies
FITT	frequency, intensity, time, type
FITT-VP	frequency, intensity, time, type, volume, and progression
FMLA	Family and Medical Leave Act
FPG	fasting plasma glucose
FRC	functional residual capacity
FSH	follicle-stimulating hormone
FVC	forced vital capacity
GAD	generalized anxiety disorder
GAD-7	Generalized Anxiety Disorder 7-item scale
GCs	glucocorticoids
GDM	gestational diabetes mellitus
GERD	gastroesophageal reflux disease
GFR	glomerular filtration rate
GI	gastrointestinal
GINA	Global Initiative for Asthma
GIP	gastric inhibitory peptide
GLP-1	glucagon-like peptide-1
GLP-1RAs	glucagon-like peptide-1 receptor agonists
GLUT4	glucose transporter 4
GMP	guanylyl monophosphate
GOLD	Global Initiative for Chronic Obstructive Lung Disease
GVHD	graft-versus-host disease
GWAS	Genome-Wide Association Study

GXT	graded exercise test
H^+	positively charged ion of hydrogen
HACE	high-altitude cerebral edema
HAPE	high-altitude pulmonary edema
HbA1C	glycolated hemoglobin
HbCO	carboxyhemoglobin
HCTZ	hydrochlorothiazide
HDL	high-density lipoprotein cholesterol
HF	heart failure
HF ACTION	Heart Failure–A Controlled Trial to Investigate the Outcomes of Exercise Training
HFpEF	heart failure with a preserved left ventricular ejection fraction
HFrEF	heart failure with a reduced left ventricular ejection fraction
HGO	hepatic glucose output
HHS	U.S. Department of Health and Human Services
HII	Health Impact Index
HIIT	high-intensity interval training
HIPPA	Health Insurance Portability and Accountability Act
HIV	human immunodeficiency virus
HMG-CoA	3-hydroxy-3-methyl-glutaryl-CoA
HPV	human papillomavirus
HR	heart rate
HR_{max}	maximal heart rate
HR_{peak}	peak heart rate
HR_{rest}	resting heart rate
hs-CRP	high-sensitivity C-reactive protein
HSCT	hematopoietic stem cell transplantation
HT	heart transplantation
HTN	hypertension
IC	inspiratory capacity
ICAM-1	intercellular adhesion molecule-1
ICD	implantable cardioverter defibrillator
ICF	International Classification of Functioning, Disability and Health
iCREP	International Confederation of Registers for Exercise Professionals
ICU	intensive care unit
ID	intellectual disability
IDDM	insulin-dependent diabetes mellitus
IFG	impaired fasting glucose
IFN-γ	interferon-γ
Ig	immunoglobulin
IgE	immunoglobulin E
IGF-1	insulin-like growth factor 1
IGT	impaired glucose tolerance
IL-1	interleukin-1

IL-1β	interleukin-1β		LVEF	left ventricular ejection fraction
IL-2	interleukin-2		LVH	left ventricular hypertrophy
IL-6	interleukin-6		MACEP	Massachusetts Association of Clinical Exercise Physiology
IL-8	interleukin-8			
IMs	intermediate metabolizers		MADIT	Multicenter Automatic Defibrillator Implantation Trial
INR	International Normalized Ratio			
IPAQ	International Physical Activity Questionnaire		MAO	monoamine oxidase
			MAOIs	monoamine oxidase inhibitors
IQ	Intelligence Quotient		MAP	mean arterial pressure
IR	internal rotation		MCID	minimal clinically important difference
IRS-1	insulin receptor substrate-1		MCL	medial collateral ligament
IRT	immunoreactive trypsinogen		MCP-1	monocyte chemotactic protein-1
IRV	inspiratory reserve volume		MCS	mechanical circulatory support
ISWT	incremental shuttle-walk test		MD	Medical Doctor
ITB	iliotibial band		MDD	major depressive disorder
ITP	intrathoracic pressure		MDR1	multidrug resistance protein 1
IVCD	intraventricular conduction defect		MED13	mediator component 13
JPC	junctional premature complex		MET	metabolic equivalent
K-10	Kessler Psychological Distress 10-item scale		MFA	Medical Fitness Association
			MGF	mechano-growth factor
LA	lactic acidosis		MHC	major histocompatibility complex
LAA	left atrial abnormality		MI	myocardial infarction
LABA	long-acting β$_2$-agonists		MIP-1	macrophage inflammatory protein 1
LABS	Longitudinal Assessment of Bariatric Surgery		miRNA	micro-RNA
			mm	millimeter
LAD	left axis deviation		mmHg	millimeters of mercury
LADCA	left anterior descending coronary artery		MMP	matrix metalloproteinases
LAE	left atrial enlargement		MMP-9	matrix metalloproteinase-9
LAEP	Louisiana Association of Exercise Physiologists		MMRC	Modified Medical Research Council
			MoTrPAC	Molecular Transducers of Physical Activity Consortium
LAMAs	long-acting muscarinic antagonists			
LAS	Lung Allocation Scoring (system)		MRI	magnetic resonance imaging
LBBB	left bundle-branch block		mRNA	messenger RNA
LBP	low back pain		ms	millisecond
LCA	left coronary artery		MS	multiple sclerosis
LDCT	low-dose computed tomography		MSWS-12	12-item Multiple Sclerosis Walking Scale
LDL	low-density lipoprotein			
LEADER	Liraglutide Effect and Action in Diabetes: Evaluation of cardiovascular outcome Results		mV	millivolts
			MVC	maximal voluntary contraction
			MVPA	moderate-to-vigorous physical activity
L–G–L	Lown–Ganong–Levine		MVV	maximal voluntary ventilation
LH	luteinizing hormone		MyoD	myoblast determination protein
LHRH	luteinizing hormone–releasing hormone		NADP$^+$	nicotinamide adenine dinucleotide phosphate
LL	lower limb			
LM	lumbar multifidus		NATA	National Athletic Trainers Association
LMWH	low-molecular-weight heparin		NCAA	National Collegiate Athletic Association
Lp-PLA$_2$	lipoprotein-associated phospholipase A$_2$		NCBI	National Center for Biotechnology Information
LPS	lipopolysaccharide			
LTRAs	leukotriene-receptor antagonists		NCCA	National Commission for Certifying Agencies
LTRIs	leukotriene-receptor inhibitors			
LV	left ventricle		NCCN	National Comprehensive Cancer Network
LVAD	left ventricular assist device		NCEP	National Cholesterol Education Program

NCHPAD	National Center on Health, Physical Activity and Disability	PD	Parkinson disease
NEFAs	nonesterified fatty acids	PDA	patent ductus arteriosus
NEpi	norepinephrine	PE	pulmonary embolus
NHANES	National Health and Nutrition Examination Survey	PEA	pulseless electrical activity
		PEEP	positive end-expiratory pressure
NHLBI	National Heart, Lung, and Blood Institute	PEFR	peak expiratory flow rate
NIDDM	non-insulin-dependent diabetes mellitus	PET	positron emission tomography
		PFOS	Psychosocial Factors in Outcome Study
NIH	National Institutes of Health	PFPS	patellofemoral pain syndrome
NIVA	noninvasive vascular assessment	PFT	pulmonary function test
NK	natural killer cells	PG	prostaglandin
NO	nitric oxide	P-gp	P-glycoprotein
NO_2	nitrogen dioxide	PharmGKB	Pharmacogenomics Knowledgebase
NPAP	National Physical Activity Plan	PHQ-9	Patient Health Questionnaire 9-item scale
NPAS	National Physical Activity Society	PMs	poor metabolizers
NSAIDs	nonsteroidal anti-inflammatory drugs	PMH	pertinent medical history
NSCA	National Strength and Conditioning Association	PNS	parasympathetic nervous system
		POMC	proopiomelanocortin
NSTEMI	non–ST-segment elevation myocardial infarction	POTS	postural orthostatic tachycardia syndrome
		PPARδ	peroxisome proliferator-activated receptor delta
NTG	nitroglycerin		
NYFS	National Youth Fitness Survey	PPAR-γ	peroxisome proliferator-activated receptor-γ
NYHA	New York Heart Association	PPMS	primary progressive multiple sclerosis
O_3	ozone	PPT	prolonged prothrombin time
OA	osteoarthritis	PRN	*pro re nata*, as the occasion arise or as needed
OCD	obsessive-compulsive disorder		
OGTT	oral glucose tolerance test	PRS	polygenic risk score
OHG	oral hypoglycemic agent	PSA	prostate-specific antigen
1RM	one repetition maximum	PSVT	paroxysmal supraventricular tachycardia
OT	occupational therapist	PT	physical therapist
OTC	over-the-counter	PTSD	posttraumatic stress disorder
$P(A-a)O_2$	alveolar minus arterial oxygen and carbon dioxide difference	PVC	premature ventricular complex
		PYGM	glycogen phosphorylase muscle
$P(a-ET)CO_2$	arterial minus end-tidal carbon dioxide difference	qd	daily
		qid	four times daily
PA	physical activity	QOL	quality of life
PAC	premature atrial complex	RA	rheumatoid arthritis
$PaCO_2$	partial pressure of carbon dioxide in the arterial blood	RAA	right atrial abnormality
		RAAS	renin-angiotensin-aldosterone system
PAD	peripheral arterial disease	RAD	right axis deviation
PAG	Physical Activity Guidelines for Americans	RAE	right atrial enlargement
		RBBB	right bundle-branch block
PAL	Physical Activity and Lymphedema Trial	RCA	right coronary artery
PAN	peroxyacetyl nitrate	RCEP	ACSM Registered Clinical Exercise Physiologist
PaO_2	partial pressure of oxygen in the arterial blood		
		RD	registered dietitian
PAPHS	ACSM/NPAS Physical Activity in Public Health Specialist	REE	resting energy expenditure
		rhEPO	recombinant human erythropoietin
PAT	paroxysmal atrial tachycardia	RM	repetitions maximum
PCI	percutaneous coronary interventions	RMR	resting metabolic rate
PCP	primary care provider	ROM	range of motion

ROS	reactive oxygen species		TKA	total knee arthroplasty
RPD	rating of perceived dyspnea		TLC	total lung capacity
RPE	rating of perceived exertion		TNF-α	tumor necrosis factor-α
RPP	rate pressure product		tPA	tissue plasminogen activator
RRMS	relapsing–remitting multiple sclerosis		TPR	total peripheral resistance
RV	residual volume		TrA	transversus abdominis
RVH	right ventricular hypertrophy		TRIG	triglyceride
SA	sinoatrial		TSA	total shoulder arthroplasty
SABA	short-acting β_2-agonists		TSLP	thymic stromal lymphopoietin
SAISD	San Antonio Independent School District		TTM	transtheoretical model
SAM	sympatho-adrenomedullary system		TTP	thrombotic thrombocytopenic purpura
SAMA	short-acting muscarinic antagonist		TUG	Timed-Up & Go Test
SBAR	Situation, Background, Assessment, and Recommendation		TZDs	thiazolidinediones
			T1DM	Type 1 diabetes mellitus
SCAD	spontaneous coronary artery dissection		T2DM	Type 2 diabetes mellitus
SCD	sudden cardiac death		UA	unstable angina
SCD-HeFT	Sudden Cardiac Death in Heart Failure Trial		UL	upper limb
			UM	ultra-rapid metabolizers
SCI	spinal cord injury		UPDRS	Unified Parkinson Disease Rating Scale
SCM	sternocleidomastoid		US	ultrasound
SGLT2	sodium-glucose co-transporter 2		USD	United States Dollars
6MWT	6-minute walk test		USDA	United States Department of Agriculture
SLE	systemic lupus erythematosus		USREPS	United States Registry of Exercise Professionals
SNP	single-nucleotide polymorphism			
SNRIs	serotonin and norepinephrine reuptake inhibitors		VAD	ventricular assist device
			VAT	visceral adipose tissue
SNS	sympathetic nervous system		V_A/Q	alveolar ventilation perfusion
SO_2	sulfur dioxide		VC	vital capacity
SOB	shortness of breath		V_D	ventilatory dead space
SOLVD	Studies of Left Ventricular Dysfunction		V_D/V_T	dead space to tidal volume ratio
S/P	status/post		$\dot{V}_E$	minute ventilation
SPMS	secondary progressive multiple sclerosis		VEGF	vascular endothelial growth factor
SpO_2	oxygen saturation		VEGFR	vascular endothelial growth factor receptor
SS	Symptom Severity (Scale)			
SSRIs	selective serotonin reuptake inhibitors		VESs	ventricular extra-systoles
STEMI	ST-segment elevation myocardial infarction		V-Fib	ventricular fibrillation
sTNFR1	soluble TNF receptor 1		VI	visual impairment
SVT	supraventricular tachycardia		VLCD	very low-calorie diet
TALEN	transcription activator-like effectors		VLDL	very low-density lipoprotein
TAVR	transcatheter aortic valve replacement		$\dot{V}O_{2max}$	maximal oxygen consumption
TBI	traumatic brain injury		$\dot{V}O_{2peak}$	peak oxygen consumption
TCAs	tricyclic antidepressants		VPD	ventricular premature depolarization
T_H2	T-helper type 2 (specific cells)		VSMC	vascular smooth muscle cell
THA	total hip arthroplasty		V-Tach	ventricular tachycardia
THR	target heart rate		W	watts
TIA	transient ischemic attack		W_{peak}	peak work rate
tid	three times daily		WBC	white blood cell
TIMI	thrombolysis in myocardial infarction		WHO	World Health Organization
TJA	total joint arthroplasty		WPI	Widespread Pain Index
TJR	total joint replacement		WPW	Wolff–Parkinson–White

APPENDIX B

Editor and Contributors to ACSM's Clinical Exercise Physiology, First Edition*

FIRST EDITION

Senior Editor

Walter R. Thompson, PhD, FACSM, ACSM-CEP, RCEP, PD
Regents' Professor and Associate Dean
College of Education & Human Development
Georgia State University
Atlanta, Georgia

Contributors

Stamatis Agiovlasitis, PhD, FACSM, ACSM-CEP
Mississippi State University
Mississippi State, Mississippi

Lawrence E. Armstrong, PhD, FACSM
University of Connecticut
Storrs, Connecticut

Kevin D. Ballard, PhD, FACSM
Miami University
Oxford, Ohio

J. P. Barfield, DA
Emory & Henry College
Emory, Virginia

Melissa J. Benton, PhD, RN, FACSM
University of Colorado–Colorado Springs
Colorado Springs, Colorado

Marco Bernardi, MD
Sapienza University of Rome
Rome, Italy

C. Scott Bickel, PT, PhD, FACSM
Samford University
Birmingham, Alabama

Natasha T. Brison, JD, PhD
Texas A&M University
College Station, Texas

Katie M. Brown, PhD
Texas Tech University
Lubbock, Texas

Peter H. Brubaker, PhD, FACSM, PD
Wake Forest University
Winston-Salem, North Carolina

Kristin L. Campbell, BSc, PT, PhD, FACSM
University of British Columbia
Vancouver, British Columbia, Canada

Heather Chambliss, PhD, FACSM
St. Jude Children's Research Hospital
Memphis, Tennessee

Paul J. Chase, PhD, ACSM-CEP, EIM, RCEP
Ohio University
Athens, Ohio

Brian J. Coyne, MEd, ACSM-CEP, ACSM/NCHPAD-CIFT, RCEP
Duke University Health System
Durham, North Carolina

Sonja de Groot, PhD
Reade Centre for Rehabilitation and Rheumatology
Amsterdam, the Netherlands

---

*Degrees, certifications, and affiliations current at the time of publication of the edition listed.

Christopher C. Dunbar, PhD, MPH, FACSM, ACSM-CEP, RCEP
Brooklyn College
Brooklyn, New York

Gregory B. Dwyer, PhD, FACSM, ACSM-CEP, EIM, RCEP, ETT
East Stroudsburg University
East Stroudsburg, Pennsylvania

Ellen M. Evans, PhD, FACSM
University of Georgia
Athens, Georgia

Yuri Feito, PhD, MPH, FACSM, ACSM-CEP, EIM, RCEP
Kennesaw State University
Kennesaw, Georgia

Carl Foster, PhD, FACSM, MAACVPR
University of Wisconsin-La Crosse
La Crosse, Wisconsin

Judy Foxworth, PT, PhD, OCS
Winston-Salem State University
Winston-Salem, North Carolina

Matthew S. Ganio, PhD, FACSM
University of Arkansas
Fayetteville, Arkansas

Carol Ewing Garber, PhD, FACSM, ACSM-CEP, ACSM-EP, ETT, PD, RCEP
Teachers College, Columbia University
New York, New York

Sara Gregory, PhD, ACSM-CEP, RCEP
Cigna Healthcare
Bloomfield, Connecticut

Samuel A. E. Headley, PhD, FACSM, ACSM-CEP, EIM, ETT, RCEP
Springfield College
Springfield, Massachusetts

Maria Hipp, MS, ACSM-CPT
Wyoming Department of Health
Cheyenne, Wyoming

John M. Jakicic, PhD, FACSM, FTOS, ACSM-CEP, ETT
University of Pittsburgh
Pittsburgh, Pennsylvania

Carol Kennedy-Armbruster, PhD, FACSM, ACSM-EP, EIM
Indiana University
Bloomington, Indiana

G. Patrick Lara, MS, ACSM-CEP, RCEP
Saint Luke's Health System
Boise, Idaho

Shel Levine, MS, ACSM-CEP
Eastern Michigan University
Ypsilanti, Michigan

J. Timothy Lightfoot, PhD, FACSM, ACSM-CEP, RCEP
Texas A&M University
College Station, Texas

Laurie A. Malone, PhD, FACSM
University of Alabama at Birmingham
Birmingham, Alabama

A. Lynn Millar, PT, PhD, FACSM
Winston-Salem State University
Winston-Salem, North Carolina

Mark A. Patterson, MEd, ACSM-CEP, RCEP
Kaiser Permanente–Colorado Region
Denver, Colorado

Heather Phillips, MS, ACSM-CEP, RCEP
Clinical Exercise Physiologist
Kalamazoo, Michigan
Austin, Texas

John P. Porcari, PhD, FACSM, ACSM-CEP, PD, RCEP
University of Wisconsin-La Crosse
La Crosse, Wisconsin

Stacey A. Reading, PhD
University of Auckland
Auckland, New Zealand

Rachelle A. Reed, PhD
University of Georgia
Athens, Georgia

Deborah Riebe, PhD, FACSM, ACSM-EP
University of Rhode Island
Kingston, Rhode Island

Barry Saul, MD
New York Methodist Hospital
Brooklyn, New York

Kathryn H. Schmitz, PhD, MPH, FACSM
Pennsylvania State University
Hershey, Pennsylvania

Kevin R. Short, PhD, FACSM
The University of Oklahoma Health Sciences Center
Oklahoma City, Oklahoma

Andrew R. Smith, MS, ACSM-CEP, RCEP
North Colorado Medical Center—Banner Health
Greeley, Colorado

James W. Stinear, PhD
University of Auckland
Auckland, New Zealand

David E. Verrill, MS, ACSM-CEP, PD, RCEP
University of North Carolina at Charlotte
Charlotte, North Carolina

Christie L. Ward-Ritacco, PhD, ACSM-EP
University of Rhode Island
Kingston, Rhode Island

Tim Werner, PhD, ACSM-CEP, RCEP
Salisbury University
Salisbury, Maryland

Emma W. White, PT, DPT, OCS
Winston-Salem State University
Winston-Salem, North Carolina

Kenneth F. Whyte, MB, ChB, MD
University of Auckland
Auckland, New Zealand

Ciro Winckler, PhD
São Paulo Federal University
São Paulo, Brazil

Kerri Winters-Stone, PhD, FACSM
Oregon Health & Science University
Portland, Oregon

Index

X

Xadago. *See* Safinamide
Xanthine derivatives, 341*t*, 342
Xarelto. *See* Rivaroxaban
Xenical. *See* Orlistat
Xopenex. *See* Levalbuterol
Xylocaine. *See* Lidocaine
Xyzal. *See* Levocetirizine

Y

Yoga, 523, 525*f*
Young adults
  bone
    normal changes, 41
    physical activity and exercise, role of, 41
  cardiorespiratory
    normal changes, 41
    physical activity and exercise, role of, 41
  muscle
    normal changes, 39, 39*f*, 40*f*
    physical activity and exercise, role of,
      40–41
Youth, T2DM treatment, 498

Z

Zafirlukast (Accolate), 342*t*, 343
Zaroxolyn. *See* Metolazone

Zebeta. *See* Bisoprolol fumarate
Zestoretic. *See* Lisinopril + hydrochlorothiazide
Zestril. *See* Lisinopril
Zetia. *See* Ezetimibe
Zileuton (Zyflo), 342*t*
Zinbryta. *See* Daclizumab
Zipsor. *See* Diclofenac
Zocor. *See* Simvastatin
Zoledronic acid (Reclast), 365*t*, 366
Zontivity. *See* Vorapaxar
Zorvolex. *See* Diclofenac
Zyflo. *See* Zileuton
Zyrtec, Zyrtec-D. *See* Cetirizine